CONTEMPORARY ISSUES IN BIOETHICS

DICKENSON TITLES OF RELATED INTEREST

Problems of Moral Philosophy: An Introduction, Third Edition
  edited by Paul W. Taylor

Reason and Responsibility: Readings in Some Basic Problems of Philosophy, **Fourth Edition**
  edited by Joel Feinberg

The Logic of Grammar
  edited by Donald Davidson and Gilbert H. Harman

Individual Conduct and Social Norms
  by Rolf Sartorius

Principles of Ethics: An Introduction
  by Paul W. Taylor

Man in Conflict: Traditions in Social and Political Thought
  by Louis I. Katzner

Metaphysics: An Introduction
  by Keith Campbell

Understanding Moral Philosophy
  edited by James Rachels

Morality in the Modern World
  edited by Lawrence Habermehl

A Preface to Philosophy
  by Mark Woodhouse

A Guide Through the Theory of Knowledge
  by Adam Morton

Moral Philosophy: Classic Texts and Contemporary Problems
  edited by Joel Feinberg and Henry West

Philosophy of Religion
  by William L. Rowe

Philosophy of Law
  edited by Joel Feinberg and Hyman Gross

The following paperback volumes are adapted from *Philosophy of Law:*

Law in Philosophical Perspective: Selected Readings
  edited by Joel Feinberg and Hyman Gross

Liberty: Selected Readings
  edited by Joel Feinberg and Hyman Gross

Responsibility: Selected Readings
  edited by Joel Feinberg and Hyman Gross

Punishment: Selected Readings
  edited by Joel Feinberg and Hyman Gross

Justice: Selected Readings
  edited by Joel Feinberg and Hyman Gross

CONTEMPORARY ISSUES IN BIOETHICS

Edited, with Introductions, by

Tom L. Beauchamp
The Kennedy Institute, Georgetown University

and

LeRoy Walters
The Kennedy Institute, Georgetown University

With the advice and assistance of the Board of Editorial Advisors:

Alexander M. Capron
H. Tristram Engelhardt, Jr.
Joel Feinberg
William K. Frankena
James M. Gustafson
Judith Jarvis Thomson

WADSWORTH PUBLISHING COMPANY, INC.
BELMONT, CALIFORNIA

Printed in the United States of America
Printing (last digit) 9 8 7 6 5 4 3 2

Library of Congress Cataloging in Publication Data

Contemporary issues in bioethics.

  Bibliography
  1. Bioethics. I. Beauchamp, Tom L.
II. Walters, LeRoy.
QH332.C66   174'.2   77-9309
ISBN 0-8221-0200-5

Cover design by Preston J. Mitchell.

CONTENTS

PART II The Professional—Patient Relationship

PART III Life and Death

PART V Human Experimentation

PART VI Biomedical and Behavioral Technologies

Preface

Recent developments in the biomedical fields have led to considerable moral perplexity about the rights and duties of patients, health professionals, research subjects, and researchers. Since about 1970 members of numerous academic disciplines—including biology, medicine, philosophy, religious studies, and law—have become involved in an ongoing discussion of the complex ethical issues raised by these developments. This anthology provides a systematic overview of that discussion: it presents a brief introduction to ethical theory and a set of carefully selected readings on some of the most important contemporary issues in bioethics.

The eighty-seven essays in this book have been selected on the basis of their clarity of conceptual and ethical reflection, their teachability, and their significance for current controversies in bioethics. Throughout the book, wherever possible, the essays have been arranged in a debate-like format: divergent viewpoints have been juxtaposed, so that the reader may explore the strengths and weaknesses of alternative positions on the issues. In each chapter the readings are preceded by an editor's introduction, which sets the essays in context and surveys the major arguments on the chapter topic. At the end of each chapter we have listed approximately fifteen recommended readings. In addition, we have indicated bibliographical resources which contain numerous additional citations.

Many persons have contributed to the production of this book. Our greatest debt is to the members of the editorial advisory board—Alexander M. Capron, H. Tristram Engelhardt, Jr., Joel Feinberg, William K. Frankena, James M. Gustafson, and Judith Jarvis Thomson—who struggled through two different drafts of the entire work. Valuable advice on the book's outline and helpful comments on chapter introductions were provided by several of our colleagues at the Kennedy Institute, including Roy Branson, Kenneth Casebeer, James Childress, John Connery, André Hellegers, Leon Kass, Karen Lebacqz, Richard McCormick, Seymour Perlin, and Warren Reich. We also wish to thank Fred Carney, Norman Daniels, Gerald Dworkin, and Louis Katzner for exceptionally able criticisms of the manuscript. Finally, we owe special thanks to Arnold Davidson, for his constructive suggestions concerning the structure and content of the book, to James McCartney for his careful reading of the page proof, and to Lynn Taylor for her excellent editorial assistance.

T. L. B.
L. W.

Part I
M O R A L   A N D
C O N C E P T U A L
F O U N D A T I O N S

1.
Ethical Theory

This book is about ethics, and in particular about moral problems. It is also a book about science, medicine, and even the social sciences. But it concerns moral problems which arise in these disciplines, and hence cannot be said to be a scientific or medical work. In order to understand the nature of ethics and how it differs from scientific endeavors, it is important to understand the nature of moral problems, how ethical theory helps resolve moral problems, and the way in which ethical theory differs from scientific theory.

MORAL PROBLEMS AND MORAL REASONING

Ethical theory is the study of general ethical principles which may be applied to special areas where moral problems arise. While this book is a study of the most prominent issues in bioethics, there are many moral problems which are not connected with biology and medicine, e.g., moral problems in jurisprudence, business ethics, and the ethics of public trust. It will be useful to begin with a single practical problem which is both traditional and undeniably ethical in nature. We can then formulate some more general statements about the structure shared by all moral problems. The problem chosen here for illustrative purposes is the morality of civil disobedience.

In a now classic scene, Socrates was convicted both of corrupting the youth of Athens and of atheism. The aura of a witch hunt surrounded the trial, and Socrates was sentenced, quite unjustly, to death. While awaiting the end, he was visited in prison by his friend Crito, who informed him that an escape could be arranged and offered a number of *reasons to justify Socrates' escape:* He was innocent. He could continue his valuable work in philosophy. His friends would otherwise appear disloyal for not helping him escape. He would not have to abandon his sons. Socrates, however, regarded such reasons as emotionally tinged and as insufficient to warrant his escape. He countered with his own *reasons why he should stay:* Since he had always taught respect for the law, it would now be unprincipled and hypocritical of him to disobey the law. Moreover, if he disobeyed a law he did not like, such disobedience would seem to sanction general disobedience of the law. The law, he thought, could not survive such wanton disregard. Socrates further argued that one's tacit agreement to abide by the law was a binding obligation, even if the law could on occasion be turned by unscrupulous persons against those who had made the agreement. For these reasons Socrates contended that what we now call an act of civil disobedience against the law is itself an expression of ingratitude, as well as a violation of principles of justice.

On the other hand, Socrates also gave expression to a second and somewhat conflicting view about one's obligations to obey the laws of the state. He maintained at his trial that if the court were to find him guilty and were to stipulate as his punishment that he could no longer philosophize (which in his accusers' eyes meant practicing the corruption of youth), he would openly disobey such a sentence. Apparently Socrates thought that *some* legal decisions could not be supported because they are *too* unjust. They would therefore have to be disobeyed, though openly and without attempting to escape punishment for one's acts. In the end he left his followers with a nagging ethical puzzle: *How does one determine when obedience to the state is required and when it is not required?*

Several things about the structure of moral problems may be extracted from this example. First, *moral reasoning* is required. Socrates and Crito are presenting reasons in support of their moral positions. Each presents a moral argument, and their assertions are not merely emotional outbursts or statements of a personal creed. They are presenting reasons which they believe any reflective person would take seriously as a guide to action. Second, since they believe that these reasons are worthy of consideration by any person situated similarly to Socrates, they regard their reasons as *universally valid*. Socrates thinks, for example, that principles of justice which hold for everyone would be violated by his escape. Perhaps he is wrong about this, but right or wrong, he believes these are principles by which everyone should be guided. Third, the problem is an interesting and perplexing one because it faces us with a *moral dilemma*. The reasons on each side of the debate are weighty ones, and neither is in any obvious way the right set of reasons. If we act on either set of reasons, our actions will be desirable in some respects but undesirable in other respects. And yet we think that ideally we ought to act on all of these reasons, for each is, considered by itself, a good reason.

Practical reasoning, the use of presumably universally valid principles, and perplexing dilemmas are characteristic of moral problems. Yet none of the three notions is easily understandable. What are moral reasons and principles? Why must they be universally valid? What is the nature of a moral dilemma? These questions are taken up in the present chapter, especially in the first three readings by Lemmon, Taylor, and Frankena.

THE NATURE AND SCOPE OF ETHICS

Now that we have a clearer notion of a moral problem, it might still be asked, "What is morality?" While we cannot here explore what morality is as distinct from law, etiquette, custom, public policy, and religion, we can consider how inquiry into ethics is subdivided into different fields.

There are at least two *non-normative* fields of moral inquiry. First, there is the *scientific study of morality,* which is a factual investigation of moral behavior. Anthropologists, sociologists, and historians determine, for example, whether moral attitudes and codes differ from society to society. In doing so, they study different beliefs about sexual relations, about the treatment of the dying, etc. Second, there is a field referred to as *metaethics*. The task of this discipline, which has largely been pursued by philosophers, is to analyze the meanings of crucial ethical terms such as "right," "obligation," and "responsibility." Metaethicists also discuss the logic of moral reasoning, including the nature of moral justification. Metaethics and the scientific study of morality have in common (among other things) that they are not normative; that is, they do not attempt to provide prescriptive norms, rules, or proper guides to behavior. They attempt to establish what factually or conceptually *is* the case rather than to determine what ethically *ought* to be the case.[1]

There are also two *normative* fields of ethics. The first may be called *applied normative ethics*. Here ethicists attempt to explicate and defend positions on critical moral problems such as civil disobedience, abortion, and sexual discrimination. Most articles in this book are examples of applied ethics. The term "applied" is used because more general ethical principles are applied in an attempt to resolve these moral problems. For example, principles of justice, equality, welfare, and utility might be used to illuminate and resolve problems in the allocation of scarce medical resources. These general ethical principles, when systematically ordered into an ethical theory, constitute the second field of normative ethics, which may be called *general normative ethics*. Here ethicists attempt to formulate and defend a system of fundamental ethical principles which settle which actions are right and which are wrong. These principles are presumed to be valid for everyone. Ideally any such ethical theory will include the complete set of ethical principles and will defend the claim that they are universally valid. In order to obtain a clearer picture of this field of ethics, it will be useful to consider its most prominent schools of thought.

THEORIES OF GENERAL NORMATIVE ETHICS

Some ethicists have argued that there is one fundamental principle determining right action, which is roughly the following:

> An action is morally right if and only if it produces at least as great a balance of value over disvalue as any available alternative action.[2]

This principle is known as the principle of utility, and philosophers who subscribe to the view that this alone is the basic principle of morality are referred to as *utilitarians*. Though they frequently disagree concerning exactly what things are valuable and how value is to be determined, these ethicists are united by their appeal to the principle of utility both as the lone supreme principle and as underivable from other ethical principles. Paul Taylor provides a detailed analysis of the nature and limits of utilitarianism in this chapter.

Other ethicists have argued that there are one or more fundamental principles of ethics which differ from the principle of utility. For example, the following is offered as a non-utilitarian principle determining right action.

> An action is morally right if and only if it is the action required by a duty which is at least as strong as any other duty in the circumstances.

Philosophers who accept this non-utilitarian account of the principles of moral duty are referred to as *deontologists*. They are united by their conviction that the rightness of actions may be determined by features of the action other than the balance of value over disvalue which is produced by the action. W. K. Frankena provides a thorough account of deontological theories in his contribution to this chapter.

Many regard utilitarianism and deontologism as the *only* two major competing options in contemporary ethical theory, but others hold the view that a traditional theory known as *natural law ethics* is a living and viable option. Natural law is sometimes confused with the notion of scientific laws of nature, but the two have distinct meanings in the context of natural law ethics: "laws of nature" are empirical generalizations, while "natural laws" delimit the behavior which is morally appropriate for a human being. What is proper to a human differs from what is to be expected from other creatures insofar as their "natures" differ, and—according to this theory—their natures differ because they possess different essences with different potentialities. Moral rightness, then, is determined by reference to a theory of human nature. Until rather recent times writers in the area of medical ethics generally accepted some form of a natural law position. In the current literature, however, it is possible to find a wide variety of authors who subscribe to deontological, utilitarian, and natural law positions. (Some would say that natural law ethics is one type of deontological theory, and the above formulations do permit this interpretation.)

In the readings in this chapter the nature of utilitarianism, deontologism, and natural law, as well as the arguments used to defend and criticize them, are thoroughly explored—especially by Paul Taylor, W. K. Frankena, and Gerard Hughes. Also, two principles of justice which have had enormous influence on recent ethical theory are proposed by John Rawls. Whether or not Rawls's principles are correctly drawn, it is intriguing to consider whether they can be derived from the principle of utility, from some deontological system, or from some theory of human nature. (Rawls himself regards the principles as deontological.)

ETHICS AND PUBLIC AFFAIRS

Ethical theories often overlap with, and even provide theoretical foundations for, law and public policy. This occurs in two ways, corresponding roughly to the distinction between normative ethics and the non-normative study of ethics. First, there are (non-normative) conceptual problems which require careful explication in order that we communicate clearly and efficiently. What is meant when crucial terms are used such as "liberty," "justice," "equality," "rights," "responsibility," and "coercion by law"? At stake is not how justice and liberty should be ensured or what rights and responsibilities should be granted to what persons. The point of conceptual analysis of these fundamental terms is to be as clear and precise as possible without asserting any normative position or begging any substantive moral issue.

Second, however, normative problems require equally careful attention, in order that we determine what ought to be done in law and social policy. Here all issue-neutrality must be abandoned, for we are engaged in that controversial world of human affairs where there are conflicting interests, goals, and ideals. But even so, the objective is to formulate general principles which can be used to guide social policy without prejudicial regard to the interests and ideals of specific groups. For example, we would like a theory of human rights which determines which rights all persons have and a theory of justice which explains how goods should be distributed in society without regard to the special interest of any person or class of persons. (Chapter 8, on the allocation of scarce medical resources, deals with precisely these questions.)

The last few articles in this chapter are especially concerned with concepts and principles in ethical theory which may be directly related to public affairs. (The emphasis falls rather more heavily on the normative than on the non-normative contribution.) Joel Feinberg—one of the authors of these selections—has made a suggestive comment concerning how the problems raised in these essays might be viewed:

It is convenient to think of these problems as questions for some hypothetical and abstract political body. An answer to the question of when liberty should be limited or how wealth ideally should be distributed, for example, could be used to guide not only moralists, but also legislators and judges toward reasonable decisions in particular cases where interests, rules, or the liberties of different parties appear to conflict. . . . We must think of an ideal legislator as somewhat abstracted from the full legislative context, in that he is free to appeal directly to the public interest unencumbered by the need to please voters, to make "deals" with colleagues, or any other merely "political" considerations. . . . The principles of the ideal legislator . . . are still of the first practical importance, since they provide a target for our aspirations and a standard for judging our successes and failures.[3]

T. L. B.

NOTES

1. It is controversial for a variety of reasons whether such a sharp distinction can be drawn between metaethics and normative ethics.
2. Some utilitarians prefer a formulation in terms of *rules* rather than *actions*. Cf. Taylor's article below.
3. Joel Feinberg, *Social Philosophy* (Englewood Cliffs, New Jersey: Prentice-Hall, 1973), pp. 2-3.

JOHN LEMMON

Moral Dilemmas

In this paper, I attempt to characterize different varieties of moral dilemma. An assumption made throughout is that an affirmative answer can be given to the question: does a human being have free will? Without this assumption, in fact, there does not seem to be much for ethics to be about.

There are very many different kinds of moral situation in which a human agent can find himself or put himself. Without making any pretense of defining the distinction between moral and nonmoral situations, let us merely list some kinds of situation which it would be generally agreed can safely be called moral. I shall begin with the most straightforward and gradually move into areas which could be described as "dilemmatic."

1. The first, and it seems the simplest, class of moral situation is this: we know what we are to do, or have to do, or ought to do, and simply do it. Within this class, there are several subclasses, which it will be worth our while to distinguish, depending on the source of our knowledge of what we are to do. What sources are distinguished may well depend on the society to which the agent in question belongs. Thus, if I may stray, like so many philosophers, into the sociology of ethics for a while, our own society tends to distinguish such sources as duties, obligations, and moral principles (Classical Greek society, if we may go by its language, does not seem to have made a clear distinction between obligation and duty). For example, a soldier may receive a battle order, and act on it directly, because he knows that it is his *duty as a soldier* so to do. Or a man

Reprinted with permission of the publisher from *Philosophical Review,* Vol.71 (1962).

may know he is to attend a certain meeting, and do so, because, having given his word that he will be there, he is *under an obligation* to attend. Or a man may know that he ought to tell the truth, and do so, because he holds as a *moral principle* that one should always tell the truth—a slightly unrealistic example, since moral principles tend to be prohibitive rather than compelling: a better example would be that of a man who knows he is not to commit adultery with a certain woman, and does not do so, because he holds it to be a moral ruling that one should at no time commit adultery.

To summarize these three subcases: first, one may know what one is to do, and do it, because one knows it to be one's duty to do that thing, second, one may know what one is to do, and do it, because one knows oneself to be under an obligation to do that thing; third, one may know what one is to do, and do it, because one holds it to be the right thing to do in view of some moral rule.

It follows logically, I would wish to claim, that a man ought to do something, if it is his duty to do that thing, Equally, he ought to do it if he is under an obligation to do it, and he ought to do it if it is right, in view of some moral principle to which he subscribes, that he should do it. But the converse implications do not, I think, hold. It might be true that a man ought to do something, and yet it not be his duty to do it, because rather it is the case that he is under an obligation to do it; or, even though he ought to do it, he is under no obligation to do it, but rather it is his duty to do it; or, even though he ought to do it, it is not that it is right to do it in view of some moral principle which he holds, but rather a case of duty or obligation.

To see that these converse implications fail, it will be necessary to take a closer look at our (rather parochial) concepts of duty and obligation. A man's duties are closely related to his special status or position. It nearly always makes sense to ask of a duty "duty *as what?*" The most straightforward case is that of duties incurred in virtue of a job: thus one has duties as a policeman, duties as headmaster, duties as prime minister or garbage-collector. In many societies, family relationships are recognized as determining duties: thus there are duties as a father, mother, son, or daughter. Less clearly delineated duties, in our society at least, are those of a host, those of a friend, those of a citizen. . . .

If duties are related to a special position or status, which distinguishes the man holding the position or status from others, obligations on the other hand are typically incurred by previous committing actions. Of course, again what actions are regarded as committal will vary from society to society. To us, the most familiar committing actions are promising or giving one's word generally, and signing one's signature. If you swear to tell the truth, from the moment of swearing you are under an obligation to tell the truth.

.   .   .

Broadly speaking, then, duty-situations are status-situations while obligation-situations are contractual situations. Both duties and obligations may be sources of "ought's," but they are logically independent sources. And a third source, independent of the other two, is that it is right to do something in view of a moral principle. I have not discussed this here because it is well discussed in almost all contemporary ethical writing, while the concepts of duty and obligation tend to be neglected.

I shall not in fact be very disturbed to learn that there are aspects of the concept of duty or the concept of obligation which I have omitted, or even that I have missed either concept's most central aspect, as we have it. My main concern is rather that there are generically different ways in which it can come to be true that we ought to do something or ought not to do something. While "ought" is a very general word of ethical involvement, "duty" and "obligation" and "right," as I am using them at least, are highly specialized words. . . .

2. A second, slightly more complex, class of ethical situations in which agents find themselves may be described thus: we may know what we are to do, or ought to do, or have to do, and yet in various ways be tempted not to do it, and as a result either do or not do what we are or ought to do, either out of a conscious decision or not. This class includes as a subclass those cases commonly called cases of acrasia, where we know what we ought to do and for various reasons and in various ways fail to do it. There is a clear sense in which all examples in this second class of moral situation are dilemmatic. We are, as we often say, torn between duty and pleasure, or between our obligations and our interests, or between our principles and our desires. Nonetheless, I do not wish to call these cases *moral* dilemmas, because in all these cases our moral situation is perfectly clear. We know where our duties lie or what our obligations are or what our moral principles determine for us here, but for various *non*-moral reasons are tempted not to stick with morality. . . .

3. It is well past time to reach the main topic of this paper. My third class of moral situation constitutes what I take to be the simplest variety of moral dilemma in the full sense. The characterization of this class is as follows: a man both ought to do something and ought not to do that thing. Here is a simple example, borrowed from Plato. A friend leaves me with his gun, saying that he will be back for it in the evening, and I promise to return it when he calls. He arrives in a distraught condition, demands his gun, and announces that he is going to shoot his wife because she has been unfaithful. I ought to return the gun, since I promised to do so—a case of obligation. And yet I ought not to do so, since to do so would be to be indirectly responsible for a murder, and my moral principles are such that I regard this as wrong. I am in an extremely straightforward moral dilemma, evidently resolved by not returning the gun.

The description of this class of cases may perhaps cause alarm; for it may well be thought to be contradictory that a man both ought and ought not to do something. . . . It seems to me that "ought" and "ought not" may well both be true, and that this description in fact characterizes a certain class of moral dilemma. Indeed, the Platonic example cited would not be a dilemma at all unless it was true that the man both ought to return the gun and ought not to return it. It is a nasty fact about human life that we sometimes both ought and ought not to do things; but it is not a logical contradiction.

My motive for carefully distinguishing some of the sources for "ought's" earlier in this paper should now be apparent. For moral dilemmas of the sort we are at present considering will appear generally in the cases where these sources conflict. Our duty may conflict with our obligations, our duty may conflict with our moral principles, or our obligations may conflict with our moral principles. The Platonic case was an example of a conflict between principle and obligation. A simple variant illustrates a conflict between obligation and duty; the man with whom the gun is deposited may regard it as his duty as a friend not to return the gun, even though he is under an obligation to do so. And duty conflicts with principle every time that we are called on in our jobs to do things which we find morally repugnant.

A natural question to ask next is: how are moral dilemmas of this simple kind to be resolved? There are certain very simple resolutions, known from the philosophical literature, which we should discuss first; but I do not think they are in practice very common. First, we may hold to some very sweeping "higher-order principle" such as "Always prefer duty to obligation or "Always follow moral principles before duty to obligation." This last precept, for example, at once resolves the Platonic dilemma mentioned earlier, which, as I described it, was a simple clash between principle and obligation. Secondly, and rather less simply, we may have in advance a complex ordering of our various duties, obligations, and the like—putting, for example, our duties as a citi-

zen before our duties as a friend and our duties as a friend before any obligations we may have incurred—in virtue of which the moral dilemma is resolved. But dilemmas in which we are morally prepared, in which we, as it were, merely have to look up the solution in our private ethical code, are rare, I think, and in any case of little practical interest. Of greater importance are those dilemmas in this class where some decision of a moral character is required. And here it must be remembered that the failure to make a decision in one sense is itself to make a decision in another, broader, sense. For our predicament is here so described that, whatever we do, even if we do nothing at all (whatever that might mean), we are doing something which we ought not to do, and so can be called upon to justify either our activity or our inactivity. The only way we can avoid a decision is by ceasing to be any longer an agent (e.g., if we are arrested, or taken prisoner, or kidnapped, or die). This precise situation leads to [a] familiar pattern of bad faith, in which we pretend to ourselves either that no decision is called for or that in one way or another the decision has been taken out of our hands by others or that we are simply the victims of our own character in acting in this way or that, that we cannot help doing what we do do and so cannot be reproached for resolving the dilemma in this way or that. If, however, we are to act here in good faith, we shall recognize that the dilemma is what it is and make the best decision we can.

Now what kind of considerations may or should affect the decision? The situation is such that no moral, or at least purely moral, considerations are relevant, in the sense that no appeal to our own given morality can decide the issue. We may of course consult a friend, take moral advice, find out what others have done in similar situations, appeal as it were to precedent. But again none of these appeals will be decisive—we still have to decide to act in accordance with advice or precedent. Or again we may approach our decision by a consideration of ends—which course of action will, so far as we can see, lead to the best result. (I do not think it is an accident, by the way, that the word "good," or rather its superlative "best," makes its first appearance at this point in our discussion; for it is typically when we are torn between courses of conduct that the question of comparing different actions arises, and hence the word "good," a comparative adjective unlike "right," is at home here; the consequence, admittedly paradoxical, of this view of "good" is that it is not properly a word of moral appraisal at all, despite the vast attention it receives from ethical philosophers; and I think I accept this conclusion.) Thus a consideration of ends determines a solution to the Platonic dilemma discussed earlier. Although I ought to return the gun and also ought not to return the gun, in fact it is evidently best, when we weigh up the expected outcome, not to return the gun, and so to sacrifice one's obligation to utilitarian considerations. Of course, when I say that this solution is evidently the best, I do not mean that it cannot be questioned. What I do mean is that it can only be seriously questioned by someone whose whole attitude toward human life is basically different from that of a civilized western human being. Someone who thinks that it would really be better to return the gun must either hold the importance of a man's giving his word to be fantastically high or else hold human life to be extremely cheap, and I regard both these attitudes as morally primitive.

4. I shall pass on now to the next, more complex, class of moral situations which might be described as dilemmatic in the full sense. Roughly, the class I now have in mind may be described thus: there is some, but not conclusive, evidence that one ought to do something, and there is some, but not conclusive, evidence that one ought not to do that thing. All the difficulties that arose in the way of making a decision in the last class of cases arise typically here too, but there are now difficulties of a new kind as well. Moreover, in this class of cases there can be no preassigned moral solution to the dilemma in virtue of higher-order principles or a given ordering of one's duties and obligations and the like, because part of the very dilemma is just one's uncertainty as to one's actual moral situation, one's situation with respect to duties, obligations, and principles. . . .

A good illustration of the kind of complexity this type of situation may embrace is . . . from Sartre:

I will refer to the case of a pupil of mine who sought me out in the following circumstances. His father was quarrelling with his mother and was also inclined to be a "collaborator"; his elder brother had been killed in the German offensive of 1940 and this young man, with a sentiment somewhat primitive but generous, burned to avenge him. His mother was living alone with him, deeply afflicted by the semitreason of his father and by the death of her oldest son, and her one consolation was in this young man. But he, at this moment, had the choice between going to England to join the Free French Forces or of staying near his mother and helping her to live. He fully realized that this woman lived only for him and that his disappearance—or perhaps his death—would plunge her into despair. He also realized that, concretely and in fact, every action he performed on his mother's behalf would be sure of effect in the sense of aiding her to live, whereas anything he did in order to go and fight would be an ambiguous action which might vanish like water into sand and serve no purpose. For instance, to set out for England he would have to wait indefinitely in a Spanish camp on the way through Spain; or, on arriving in England or in Algiers he might be put into an office to fill up forms. Consequently, he found himself confronted by two very different modes of action; the one concrete, immediate, but directed towards only one individual; the other an action addressed to an end infinitely greater, a national collectivity, but for that reason ambiguous—and it might be frustrated on the way. At the same time, he was hesitating between two kinds of morality; on the one side, the morality of sympathy, of personal devotion and, on the other side, a morality of wider scope but of more debatable validity. He had to choose between these two.[1]

A crude oversimplification of this example might depict it thus: the boy is under some obligation to stay with his mother; or, perhaps better, his mother by her own position has put him under some obligation to stay with her, since she is now dependent on him for her own happiness. Consequently, he is conscious in some degree that he ought to stay with her. On

1. Sartre, *Existentialism and Humanism,* trans. by P. Mairet (London, 1948), pp. 35–36.

the other hand he feels some kind of duty to join the Free French in England—a duty perhaps to his country as a citizen. But this duty is far from being clearly given; as Sartre stresses, it is felt only ambiguously. It may be his duty to fight, but can it really be his duty, given his obligation to his mother, to sit in an office filling out forms? He is morally torn, but each limb of the moral dilemma is not itself here clearly delineated.

An interesting feature of this case, and of the class of cases in general which we are considering, is that, in attempting to reach a decision, the arguments which try to establish exactly what one's moral situation is are not distinguishable from those which attempt to resolve the dilemma itself. Thus the boy is unclear where his duty lies partly because he is unclear what exactly would be the outcome of his decision to leave his mother, and this outcome is also relevant to the decision itself, as a utilitarian consideration affecting his choice.

Sartre's example has an important further feature, which marks out a particular subclass of the class of moral dilemmas in general: the dilemma is so grave a one, personally speaking, that either decision in effect marks the adoption on the part of the agent of a changed moral outlook. It does not seem to have been much observed by ethical philosophers that, speaking psychologically, the adoption of a new morality by an agent is frequently associated with the confrontation of a moral dilemma. Indeed, it is hard to see what else would be likely to bring about a change of moral outlook other than the having to make a difficult moral decision. On the nature of such a change there is time here only to say a few things. First, the change frequently and always in serious cases is associated with a change in fundamental attitudes, such as the change from liberalism to conservatism in politics or the change from Christianity to atheism in the field of religion. And the reasons given for the moral change may well be identical with the reasons given for the change in fundamental attitudes. This last kind of change is neither fully rational nor fully irrational. To persuade someone to change his fundamental attitudes is like getting someone

to see an aesthetic point—to appreciate classical music or impressionist painting, for example. Arguments can be given, features of music or painting may be drawn to the person's attention, and so on and so forth, but none of these reasons is finally conclusive. Nonetheless, we should not rush to the opposite conclusion that matters of aesthetic taste are purely subjective. In a somewhat similar way we may persuade someone, or he may persuade himself, to change his fundamental attitudes, and so to change his moral outlook, at a time of moral crisis. Roughly speaking, Sartre's boy has to decide whether to be politically engaged or not, and this decision may well affect and be affected by his fundamental attitudes.

I am not at all saying that this kind of serious case is common; indeed, I think it is rare; but it is still of the greatest importance to ethics to investigate it, because it is of the greatest practical importance in a man's life. There may well be people who have never had to face a moral situation of these dimensions. But for Antigones and others who live faced with occasional major crises, the appropriate reasoning for this kind of moral dilemma is of vital importance. On the other hand, it is not at all clear what the role of the philosopher should be here. If we listen to much of contemporary ethical writing, his role is merely to analyze the discourse in which such reasoning is couched; the task of deciding what are good and what are bad ethical arguments belongs to someone else, though it is never quite made clear to whom. It is my own view that, even though it may be part and an important part of the philosopher's job to analyze the terminology of ethical arguments, his job does not stop there. Perhaps no one is properly equipped to give moral advice to anyone else, but if anyone is it is the philosopher, who at least may be supposed to be able to detect bad reasoning from good. It is a corollary of this view that a philosopher is not entitled to a private life—by which I mean that it is his duty to hold political and religious convictions in such a form as to be philosophically defensible or not to hold them at all. He is not entitled to hold such beliefs in the way in which many nonphilosophers hold them, as mere articles of faith.

5. After this brief digression, I must return to

my classification of moral dilemmas: for there is one more kind that, with some hesitation, I should like to introduce. This is an even more extreme kind of dilemma than the last and probably of even rarer occurrence. I mean the kind of situation in which an agent has to make a decision of a recognizably moral character though he is completely unprepared for the situation by his present moral outlook. This case differs from the last in that there the question was rather of the applicability of his moral outlook to his present situation, while here the question is rather how to create a new moral outlook to meet unprecedented moral need. This case is in some respects easier for the agent and in some respects harder to face than the last: easier, if he recognizes the situation for what it is, because he at least knows that for sure he had some basic moral rethinking to do, which is often not clear in the previous case; but harder, because basic moral rethinking is harder work in general than settling the applicability of given moral principles to a particular situation. A typical, but morally wrong, way of escape from this dilemma is again to act in bad faith, by pretending to oneself that the situation is one which one can handle with one's given moral apparatus.

A possible real instance of this kind of moral dilemma is that which faced Chamberlain in his negotiations with Hitler in 1938. He ought to have realized that he was dealing with a kind of person for which his own moral outlook had not prepared him, and that as Prime Minister he was called upon to rethink his moral and

political approach in a more realistic way. This he failed to do, either because he was genuinely deceived as to Hitler's real character or, as I suspect, because he deceived himself on this point: if the latter, then he was guilty of the type of bad faith to which I am alluding.

The main point of this variety of moral dilemma is that, at least if correctly resolved, it forces a man to develop a new morality; in the case of the last type of dilemma, this was a possible outcome but by no means a necessary one. So perhaps this is the place at which to say a little about what is involved in such a development. Here the analogy with aesthetics, which Sartre and others have cautiously drawn, may be useful. There may come a point in the development of a painter, say, or a composer, where he is no longer able to go on producing work that conforms to the canons of composition which he has hitherto accepted, where he is compelled by his authenticity as a creator to develop new procedures and new forms. It is difficult to describe what will guide him in the selection of new canons, but one consideration will often be the desire to be (whatever this means) *true to himself*. It may well be that an appropriate consideration in the development of a new moral outlook is the desire to be, in the relevant sense whatever that is, true to oneself and to one's own character. But I will not pursue this topic here, because I confess myself to be quite in the dark as to what the sense of these words is. . . .

PAUL TAYLOR

Utilitarianism

TWO KINDS OF ETHICAL SYSTEMS

A normative ethical system is an ordered set of moral standards and rules of conduct by reference to which, with the addition of factual knowledge, one can determine in any situation of choice what a person ought or ought not to do. . . . [There are] two normative ethical systems that are most widely discussed and defended in contemporary moral philosophy. The first system, utilitarianism, received its classical formulation in the writings of the British philosophers, Jeremy Bentham (1748–1832) and John Stuart Mill (1806–1873). The second system, which may be designated "ethical formalism," was originally propounded by the great German philosopher, Immanuel Kant (1724–1804). There is some disagreement among philosophers at present whether the two sets of doctrines are necessarily inconsistent with each other, although their earlier proponents thought that they were. . . . Whether there is a wider framework of moral principles within which both systems can be consistently integrated is a question to be left open here.

Utilitarianism and formalism are often contrasted with one another on the basis of the general type of ethical system each exemplifies. Utilitarianism is a *teleological* ethical system (from the Greek word *telos,* meaning end or purpose); formalism is a *deontological* ethical system (from the Greek word *deon,* meaning duty). The distinction between the two kinds of system may be conveniently summarized as follows. A teleological theory holds that an action is morally right either if a person's doing it brings about good consequences, or if the action is of a kind which, if everyone did it, would have good consequences. In either case, ultimately it is the goodness or badness of the consequences of actions that make them right or wrong. A deontological theory holds that an action is right if it accords with a moral rule, wrong if it violates such a rule. Moral rules are based on an ultimate principle of duty which, in contrast to teleological ethics, does not specify an end or purpose whose furtherance makes actions right. What the ultimate principle does specify is a set of conditions that are necessary and sufficient for any rule of moral obligation to apply to a kind of action. Let us take a closer look at this distinction.

In a teleological ethical system, the test of right and wrong actions consists in applying a standard of value to the consequences of the actions. If the consequences of someone's doing a particular action or of everyone's doing a type of action fulfill the standard of value, the consequences are good and the action or action-type is therefore right. If the consequences are bad (because they fail to meet the standard), the action or action-type is wrong. In this kind of ethical system the "consequences" of an action are understood to comprise *all* the effects which the action has in the future of the world. They include everything that happens *because* the action is done, that is, everything which would have been different in the future if the action had not occurred. Thus, suppose the assassination of Abraham Lincoln in 1865 by John Wilkes Booth caused a difference in United States history during the period of Reconstruction following the Civil War. Then that difference is to be considered one of the consequences of Booth's action. If what occurred as a result of Lincoln's murder is neither good nor bad (when judged by a certain standard of value), then even though it is a consequence of Booth's action, it has no bearing on the rightness or wrongness of that deed. If it is good or bad (to however slight a degree), it does have such a bearing.

On this point deontological ethics disagrees with teleological ethics. Deontologists hold that it is not the goodness or badness of the consequences of an action that make it right or wrong, but the *kind* of action it is. An action is right in their view if it is of a kind that all moral agents have an obligation to perform; it is wrong if it is one that all moral agents are obligated to avoid. The statement that all moral agents are obligated to do or to refrain from doing a certain kind of action is a *moral rule of conduct,* and deontologists believe that the ground of such obligation lies in the fact that the moral rule in question satisfies the requirements of an *ultimate norm* or *supreme principle* of duty, which is often designated as "the Moral Law.". . . For the present it is enough to point out that, in a deontological ethical system, the supreme principle of morality does not lay down, as either a necessary or a sufficient condition of a right action, that it bring about good consequences. It should be noted, however, that consequences may be relevant to *identifying the kind of action* required or prohibited by a deontological moral rule (and hence the kind of action we have a duty to perform or avoid). For example, the rule "Do not kill" tells us that we are obligated to refrain from intentionally taking the life of another. The rule forbids conduct of a certain type (killing). Now consider Booth's action of aiming and firing a loaded pistol at Lincoln. The fact that it caused Lincoln's death is relevant to its wrongness. For this consequence of the action —namely, Lincoln's dying—makes the action not merely one of aiming and firing a loaded pistol at a person, but one of intentionally *killing* someone. As such, the action is seen to fall under the rule of "Do not kill." Assuming that this rule is entailed by the ultimate principle of morality, the deontologist would conclude that Booth's conduct was morally wrong. Its wrongness, he would say, depends on its being of the type, killing. It is wrong, in other words, because it is a kind of act that includes someone's death among its consequences. It is not wrong because acts of killing have *further* consequences (occurring *after* someone's death) which, when judged by some standard of value, are bad.

Some moral philosophers hold that the grounds of right conduct are both teleological and deontological, and that there is no single supreme principle from which, ultimately, the moral rightness or wrongness of every action can be derived. According to this view, which is generally known as "ethical pluralism," the moral reasons for (or against) some actions lie in the consequences of those actions, while the moral reasons governing other actions arise from their being of a kind required (or prohibited) by a rule of duty or obligation. Ethical pluralists argue that both sorts of reasons, in fact, can apply to one and the same action. A person may therefore find himself in circumstances where he has moral reasons of the first sort *for* doing a particular action and moral reasons of the second sort *against* doing it, or vice versa. Consider the situation in which a policeman's carrying out his duty to apprehend a criminal might lead to a riot. If he does his duty, bad consequences are likely to result. If he avoids the consequences, he fails to do his duty. A contrasting case, where the reasons *for* an action are teleological and the reasons *against* deontological, occurs when a person can save someone's life only by stealing. An instance would be a poor man stealing medicine for his sick child.

In such situations, how is one to decide what the agent ought to do? The answer given by the ethical pluralist is that one must weigh the comparative importance of these various reasons to see which reasons outweigh or override any others applicable to the given action. Sometimes the consequences of an action will be so bad that it ought not to be done, despite a prima facie obligation to do it (that is, an obligation that would make the deed one's duty *if* there were no moral reasons against it). In other cases the prima facie obligation will be sufficiently heavy or stringent to outweigh the badness of the consequences. Only the development of a capacity for sensitive moral discrimination will enable one to decide how the weighing should go. Even among equally competent and sensitive moral thinkers, there will at times be disagreements about the relative importance of the various reasons for action. All that can fairly be demanded of anyone in such circumstances, say the ethical pluralists, is that the individual in question be thoroughly conscientious and impartial, weighing *all* the considerations morally relevant to *every* alternative course of action open to him. He must include in his deliberations, when applicable, both teleological and deontological factors, and he must not allow his self-interest, or the interests of his friends, relatives, class, nation, religion, or race to distort the importance he places on any given consideration (unless, of course, the furthering of one of these specified interests is itself a morally relevant factor that ought to be taken into account by *any* impartial and conscientious thinker in *any* situation of the given kind).

For [present] purposes . . . only "monistic" systems of ethics shall be examined—systems which have a single supreme principle, whether teleological or deontological, as the ultimate ground of morality. This will lead to a clear understanding of the fundamental differences between the two types of ethical systems. The reader will then have a firm grasp of the two sorts of moral reasons for (or against) an action: those based on the goodness or badness of the consequences of the action, and those based on the rules of obligation or duty under which the action falls. This will, in turn, enable the reader to consider on his own the possibility of constructing a form of ethical pluralism that would combine both sorts of reasons in one coherent system. . . .

UTILITY AS THE TEST OF RIGHT AND WRONG

The basic concept of utilitarian ethics is, as its name indicates, the idea of utility: an act is right if it is useful. As soon as this is said the question arises, Useful for what end? For unless we know the end to which something is to be judged as a means, we do not know how to decide whether it is useful or not.

The answer given by utilitarianism is that an act is right when it is useful in bringing about a *desirable* or *good* end, an end that has *intrinsic value.* . . . A preliminary account . . . must be given if we are to understand utilitarian ethics. By "intrinsic value" is meant the value something has as an end in itself, and not as a means to some further end. This may be explained as follows. There are certain things we value because of their consequences or effects, but we do not value them in themselves. Thus we think it is a good thing to go to the dentist because we want healthy teeth and we have reason to believe that the dentist is a person who can help bring about this end. But few people find visiting the dentist good in itself. In other words, the act of visiting the dentist is done not for its own sake but for the sake of something else. This something else may in turn be valued not as an end in itself but as a means to other ends. Eventually, however, we arrive at certain experiences or conditions of life that we want to have and enjoy just for their own sake. These are ends that we judge to be intrinsically good; they have for us intrinsic value. The experience of undergoing dental treatment, on the other hand, has only instrumental value for us. We consider it good only because we think it is a means to some further end. If we did not value the end, the means would lose its value. Thus suppose we did not mind losing our teeth or having toothaches. We would not then think going to the dentist was worthwhile. So the value of some things is entirely *derivative.* They derive all their value from the value of something else. Other things—things that are sought for their own sake—have *nonderivative* value. Their value is not derived from the value of something else and hence is intrinsic to them. Derivative value, in short, is instrumental value; nonderivative value is intrinsic value. Of course it is possible for one and the same thing to have both kinds of value. For example, if a person enjoys playing tennis and also does it for the exercise, the game of tennis has both intrinsic and instrumental value for him. In this case playing tennis is both intrinsically good and instrumentally good. In contrast to this, going to the dentist is intrinsically bad but instrumentally good. Two other combinations are also possible. Something can be intrinsically good but instrumentally bad (for example, eating too much of our favorite dessert), and something can be both intrinsically and instrumentally bad (for example, having a painful illness involving heavy medical expenses).

Now the basic principle of utilitarian ethics is that *the right depends on the good*. This means that we can know whether an act is morally right only by finding out what its consequences are and then determining the intrinsic goodness (or badness) of those consequences. The moral rightness of an act is not itself an intrinsic value. On the contrary, an act is right only when it is instrumentally good and its rightness consists in its instrumental goodness. Our next question is, What is the standard of intrinsic value by which utilitarians judge the goodness of the consequences of a right act? Classical utilitarians have proposed two different answers to this. Some, like Jeremy Bentham, have said "pleasure;" others, like John Stuart Mill, have said "happiness," and have added that happiness is not merely a sum total of pleasures. A third answer has been suggested by a twentieth century utilitarian, G. E. Moore (1873–1958), who has claimed that intrinsic goodness cannot be defined in terms of either pleasure or happiness, but is a unique and indefinable property of things. Thus we have three types of utilitarianism, categorized according to these three views of the end to which morally right conduct is a means. They are called "hedonistic utilitarianism" (from the Greek word *hedone,* meaning pleasure); "eudaimonistic utilitarianism" (from the Greek word *eudaimonia,* meaning happiness or well-being); and "ideal utilitarianism" or "agathistic utilitarianism" (from the Greek word *agathos,* meaning good). . . .

The fundamental norm of hedonistic utilitarianism may be stated thus: An act is right if it brings about pleasure (or prevents the bringing about of pain); an act is wrong if it brings about pain (or prevents the bringing about of pleasure). The fundamental norm of eudaimonistic utilitarianism may be stated in a corresponding way, merely by substituting "happiness" for "pleasure" and "unhappiness" for "pain." Similarly, ideal or agathistic utilitarianism may be formulated by substituting "intrinsic good" for "pleasure" and "intrinsic evil" for "pain." As soon as the norm of utilitarian ethics is stated in any of these ways, another question immediately arises: Pleasure or happiness or intrinsic good *for whom,* pain or unhappiness or intrinsic evil *for whom?*

Many alternative answers are possible. One can say, pleasure, happiness, or intrinsic good for the agent himself, that is, for the person doing the act. The resulting ethical system would then be a form of ethical egoism. . . . Another possible answer is, pleasure, happiness, or intrinsic good for the agent's family and friends, or for the members of his class or caste, his tribe or nation, his race, religion, or sex. This would yield an ethical system in which the interests of some people are understood to have a greater claim to fulfillment than the interests of others. Still another possibility is, pleasure, happiness, or intrinsic good for everyone *but* the agent. This answer would entail an ethics of pure altruism or brotherly love, in which the moral ideal for each agent is to devote himself to the welfare of others at whatever cost to his own interests. Finally, the answer to our question which utilitarians give is, *everyone's* pleasure, happiness, or intrinsic good.

According to utilitarianism, whether it be hedonistic, eudaimonistic, or agathistic, the standard of value for judging the consequences of actions must be completely impartial and universal in its application. In calculating the positive or negative value of consequences, one person's pleasure (or happiness or intrinsic good) is to count exactly as much as another's. The agent's own interests are to be considered along with everyone else's, but no greater (and no lesser) weight is to be given to his interests than to those of any other individual. Between his own pleasure (happiness, intrinsic good) and that of someone else, the agent must be strictly impartial, never allowing himself to be prejudiced in his own favor or in favor of those whom he happens to like. All human beings, for the utilitarian, have an equal right to the fulfillment of their interests.

Given this principle of impartiality, how does the utilitarian apply it in determining the rightness or wrongness of a particular action? For the sake of simplicity in answering this question, the differences among hedonistic, eudaimonistic, and agathistic forms of utilitarianism will be disregarded. . . . To find out what one morally ought to do in any situation of choice, utilitarianism prescribes the following decision-making procedure. First we specify all the alternatives that comprise the possible courses of action open to our choice. We then calculate to the best of our ability the probable consequences that would ensue if we were to choose each alternative. In this calculation we ask ourselves, How much pleasure (or happiness) and how much pain (or unhappiness) will result in my own life and in the lives of all people who will be affected by my doing this act? When we have done this for all the alternatives open to us, we then compare those consequences in order to find out which one leads to a greater amount of pleasure (or happiness) and a smaller amount of pain (or unhappiness) than any other alternative. The act that in this way is found to *maximize intrinsic value and minimize intrinsic disvalue* is the act we morally ought to do. To do any other act in the given situation would be morally wrong.

In the practical affairs of everyday life, of course, we cannot stop and make such detailed calculation every-time we have alternative courses of action open to us. Indeed, if we were to do this we might cause more unhappiness or less happiness to be brought about in the world than if we were to make choices on the basis of habits we had developed from our past experience. Thus it would be wrong for us, according to the principle of utility, to try to make an accurate calculation each time. What we must do is to use our common sense and choose on the basis of similar situations in the past. After all, it does not take much thought to predict that murdering someone is going to produce more unhappiness in the world than respecting the person's life. We need not have committed a murder in the past to know this. We need only to use our reason and imagination to be able to make a reasonable prediction about what would happen if we were to do such an act.

It is important to realize that for the utilitarian no act is morally wrong in itself. Its wrongness depends entirely on its consequences. Take the act of murder, for instance. If the consequences of murdering a particular man in a particular set of circumstances (say, assassinating Hitler in 1935) were to bring about less unhappiness in the world than would be caused by the man himself were he to remain alive, it is not wrong to murder him. Indeed, it is our duty to do so, since the circumstances are such that our refraining from doing the act will result in more unhappiness (intrinsic disvalue) and less happiness (intrinsic value) than our doing it. This might at first appear to be a shocking and outrageous teaching. But the utilitarian would argue, What, after all, is wrong with the act of murder? Is it not that it causes so much pain and unhappiness both to the victim and to his kin, and prevents the victim from having the chance to enjoy his right to the pursuit of happiness? Suppose the nature of man and the world were very different from what they in fact are, so that everyone at the age of thirty suddenly deteriorated physically and mentally and became incapable of having any pleasant experiences thereafter in life. Suppose, further, that there was a way of killing people at that age which gave them great pleasure up to the final moment of death. Finally, suppose that their death at this time in their lives was celebrated by others as a happy event, in the way births are often celebrated in our own culture. In such a world why should the murder of people at thirty be condemned? Since there would be more unhappiness in the world as a result of respecting their lives, what would be wrong in ending their lives? Indeed, it is just such considerations as these that have led some people in our actual world to advocate the painless killing of human beings under certain specified circumstances. Thus it has been suggested that a doctor be permitted to administer a drug that will painlessly cause the death of a person who has an incurable disease when, first, there is no likelihood that a cure will be discovered in the period the person will remain alive; second, when his suffering is intense and cannot be alleviated by medical means; and third, when both the person himself and his relatives have asked that such a drug be administered to him.

This example brings to light another aspect of utilitarian ethics. It shows that, from the utilitarian point of view, it is sometimes right to do an act which is known to bring about unhappiness. But this is true only when the act in question will bring about *less unhappiness than any possible alternative*. In that sort of situation to do anything else—even to "do nothing," that is, to let events take their course without trying to change them—would be deliberately to cause more unhappiness to people than is necessary. Situations of this unfortunate kind may occur in time of war or when there are natural disasters such as floods and earthquakes, as well as in cases of people suffering from incurable diseases.

ACT-UTILITARIANISM AND RULE-UTILITARIANISM

What is the function of moral rules of conduct, according to utilitarianism? Two different answers are given to this question by utilitarians, and this has been used as a basis for distinguishing two types of utilitarianism, one called "act" or "unrestricted" utilitarianism, the other called "rule" or "restricted" utilitarianism. The distinction may be put this way. For all utilitarians, the principle of utility is the *ultimate* test of the rightness or wrongness of human conduct. But in applying this test, do we apply it directly to particular acts, or do we restrict its application to rules of conduct, and let those rules determine whether a particular act is right or wrong? In the first case, which is unrestricted or act-utilitarianism, we must find out what are the consequences of a *particular act* in order to know whether it is right or wrong. It is this type of utilitarianism that has been presented in the foregoing paragraphs. The principle of utility is applied directly to each alternative act in a situation of choice. The right act is then defined as the one which has greater utility than any other alternative. It would be wrong for a person to do any of these other alternatives, be-

cause if he were to do any of them he would *not* thereby maximize intrinsic value and minimize intrinsic disvalue in the world, and a person's duty is always to do that act among all those open to his choice which has such consequences.

According to restricted or rule-utilitarianism, on the other hand, an act is right if it conforms to a valid rule of conduct and wrong if it violates such a rule. And it is the test of utility that determines the validity of rules of conduct. Thus the one true normative ethical system binding upon all mankind is a set of rules such that, if people regulated their conduct by these rules, greater intrinsic value and less intrinsic disvalue would result for everyone than if they followed a different code. To "regulate one's conduct by a rule" is explained by reference to the two kinds of rules, positive rules or requirements, and negative rules or prohibitions. A positive rule specifies the properties of an action-type which is required of everyone. It states that every person is to do a certain kind of action in circumstances where he can either do or refrain from doing such an act. Thus the rule "Keep your promises" tells us that when we have promised someone to do something and then have the choice to keep or to break our promise we must keep it. The right act is to do what the rule requires, the wrong conduct is not to do what it requires. A negative rule forbids everyone to do a certain kind of act. It requires that a person refrain from a certain kind of behavior when he has the choice of doing or not doing it. Thus the rule "Thou shalt not steal" tells us what we must not do rather than what we must do. Just as acting in accordance with a positive rule means doing what it requires, so acting in accordance with a negative rule means refraining from doing what it prohibits. And just as it is wrong to omit what is required by a positive rule, so it is wrong to perform an act contrary to a negative rule. In this way "right" and "wrong" can be defined as action that conforms to, or violates, a rule of conduct which is binding upon us. But how do we know, among all the possible rules that could regulate our conduct, which ones do really bind us? The rule-utilitarian's answer is, those rules which, when generally complied with, bring about more happiness or pleasure for everyone and less unhappiness or pain than would result from general compliance with any other set of rules.

Rule-utilitarianism has been proposed as a way out of certain difficulties that seem to be entailed by act-utilitarianism. Consider, for example, our ordinary moral judgments concerning the wrongness of acts perpetrated without the knowledge of others. Suppose a man were to commit the "perfect" crime by murdering someone without leaving any clues. As a result, the murderer is never caught and punished. Now compare this case with an exactly similar act of murder, except that the killer leaves some clues, is eventually caught, and is sentenced to life imprisonment. Ordinarily we would say that the two acts of murder were equally wrong, and that whether a murderer is caught has nothing to do with the wrongness of his act. Yet according to act-utilitarianism it would seem that the first act is not as bad as the second. For the consequences of the first act do not involve as much unhappiness as is involved in the consequences of the second, since the murderer gets away with his act and does not suffer imprisonment. The fact that his act is a "perfect" crime makes it better than the same crime done by someone who is careless about leaving evidence. This seems the very opposite of our ordinary moral judgments of the two cases. If there is any moral difference between them, we would say the first is worse than the second precisely because the criminal escapes punishment.

The act-utilitarian might reply that in fact the first case is worse than the second because, although the criminal does not suffer punishment by law, he will suffer the pangs of a bad conscience and will forever live in fear of the police. Furthermore, his not getting caught may encourage him and others to commit more crimes, and so bring about worse consequences than would have happened if he had been caught and imprisoned. Still, the argument against act-utilitarianism can be revised

to take at least some of these points into account. Suppose the man who commits the "perfect" crime is a hardened, amoral kind of man without a conscience, is fully confident that he will never be caught or even suspected by the police, and has no desire to commit another murder because the motive for his one crime was revenge directed at the particular person who was his victim. Again we would say that none of these facts makes the crime any the less wrong; indeed, we should say they are all completely *irrelevant* to the wrongness of his action. Yet by the theory of act-utilitarianism all of these factors *are* relevant, since they make a difference to the consequences of the action.

It should be observed that the foregoing type of argument cannot be used against the rule-utilitarian. According to his theory both acts of murder are equally wrong, since both are violations of the same rule of conduct—namely, that we ought to respect the lives of others. The consequences that follow the performance of each particular act do not determine the rightness or wrongness of the act, and therefore the crime can be judged to be wrong regardless of whether the criminal is caught, feels guilty, or will be encouraged to commit another crime. The rule that all murderers are to be punished by law is itself a valid rule for rule-utilitarians because the consequences of having such a rule regulating people's conduct are better than the consequences of not having it regulate their conduct. Hence, by the same reasoning that shows the act of murder to be wrong, the rule-utilitarian shows the act of apprehending and punishing a murderer to be right.

It is now possible to see how the two forms of utilitarianism differ with regard to the place of rules of conduct in an ethical system. For rule-utilitarianism, rules of conduct are the *criteria* of right and wrong action when those rules are utilitarian rules. By a "utilitarian rule" is meant a rule (like the one mentioned above: "All murderers are to be punished by law") the universal following of which would have greater utility than would universal compliance with any alternative rule applicable to the same action-type. To say that utilitarian rules are the criteria of right and wrong action is to say that conformity of a particular act (that is, an act which is performed at a particular time by a particular agent) to such a rule is what *makes* it right, while the fact that a particular act violates a utilitarian rule is what *makes* it wrong. In contrast, the function of rules of conduct in an act-utilitarian system is radically different. This can be made clear by the following considerations.

According to act-utilitarianism, the principle of utility itself (that is, productivity of maximum intrinsic value and minimum intrinsic disvalue) is applied directly to particular acts in order to determine their rightness or wrongness. What *makes* a particular act right is not its conformity with a valid rule (as is the case with rule-utilitarianism), but the actual consequences of its being performed at a specific time and place. If its performance results in more intrinsic value and less intrinsic disvalue than would result from any alternative in the given circumstances, it is the act that ought to be done. However, the act-utilitarian does say that there is a place for moral rules in practical life, even though they do not determine what acts are right or wrong.

. . .

UTILITY AND JUSTICE

Some contemporary philosophers claim that, whether or not act- and rule-utilitarianism are compatible with each other, *neither* theory is acceptable as a normative ethical system. In the present section the reasoning behind this rejection of both forms of utilitarianism is examined. . . .

The objection raised against both forms of utilitarian ethics is that *the principle of utility does not provide a sufficient ground for the obligations of justice*. Since the idea of justice is a fundamental moral concept, no normative ethical system can be considered adequate that does not show the basis for our duty to be just. The argument starts with a careful examination of the ultimate norm of utilitarian ethics, the principle of utility itself. Exactly what is utility? It has been described in the words, "the maximizing of intrinsic value and the minimizing of intrinsic disvalue." What, precisely, does this mean?

It will be helpful in answering this question to think of measurable units of intrinsic value and disvalue. We shall accordingly speak of units of happiness and unhappiness, respectively. This will enable us to see the difficulty more clearly, although no particular view of what is to be taken as the measurement of a unit of happiness or unhappiness will be presupposed. We all know in general what it means to be very happy, quite happy, not especially happy, rather unhappy, and extremely unhappy. Thus the idea of degrees of happiness corresponds to something in our experience. We also know what it means to be happy for a brief moment, or for a day, and we use such phrases as "It was a happy two-week vacation," "I was not very happy during my early teens," and "He has led an unhappy life." There is some basis, therefore, in our everyday concept of happiness (and also of pleasure) for giving meaning to the idea of quantities or amounts of happiness, even though we do not ordinarily measure these quantities in arithmetical terms.

What, then does the utilitarian mean by maximizing intrinsic value and minimizing intrinsic disvalue? There are three variables or factors that must be introduced in order to make this idea clear. First, it means to bring about, in the case of *one* person, the greatest balance of value over disvalue. Thus if one act or rule yields $+1000$ units of happiness and -500 units of unhappiness for a given person, while another act or rule yields $+700$ units and -100 units for that person, then, all other factors being equal, the second alternative is better than the first, since the balance of the second $(+600)$ is greater than the balance of the first $(+500)$. Similarly, to "minimize disvalue" would mean that an act or rule which yielded $+100$ and -300 for a given person would be better than one that yielded $+500$ and -1000 for the same person, other things being equal (even though more happiness is produced by the second than by the first).

The second factor is that the happiness and unhappiness of *all persons* affected must be considered. Thus if four persons, A, B, C, and D, each experiences some difference of happiness or unhappiness in his life as a consequence of the act or rule but no difference occurs in the lives of anyone else, then the calculation of maximum value and minimum disvalue must include the balance of pluses and minuses occurring in the experience of every one of the four persons. Suppose in one case the balance is $+300$ for A, $+200$ for B, -300 for C, and -400 for D. And suppose the alternative yields $+200$ for A, $+100$ for B, -400 for C, and $+500$ for D. Then if someone were to claim that the first is better than the second because D's happiness or unhappiness does not count (D, for example, might be a slave while A, B, and C are free men), this conclusion would not be acceptable to utilitarians. For them, the second alternative is better than the first because the second yields a higher total balance than the first when *all* persons are considered.

The third factor in the utilitarian calculus has been tacitly assumed in the foregoing discussion of the second factor. This is the principle that, in calculating the units of happiness or unhappiness for different persons, the same criteria for measuring quantity are used. If totals of $+500$ and -200 represent sums of happiness and unhappiness in the experience of A and $+300$ and -400 represent sums of happiness and unhappiness in the experience of B, then one unit of plus (or minus) for A must be equal to one unit of plus (or minus) for B. No differences between A and B are to be considered as grounds for assigning a different weight to one or the other's happiness or unhappiness. When utilitarians assert that everyone's happiness is to count *equally*, they mean that, in calculating consequences, it is irrelevant *whose* happiness or unhappiness is affected by the act or rule. This may be called the principle of the equality of worth of every person as a person. (It does not mean, of course, that everyone is just as morally good or bad as everyone else!)

Now when these three factors are used in calculating utility, it is still possible for some persons to be unfairly or unjustly treated. For the greatest total balance of pluses over minuses may be brought about in a given society by actions or rules which discriminate against certain persons on irrelevant grounds. Although a greater quantity of happiness and a lesser amount of unhappiness are produced, they are distributed unjustly among the persons affected. To illustrate this possibility, consider two societies, one of which distributes different amounts of happiness to people on the basis of their race or religion, the other dispensing them on the basis of people's different needs, abilities, and merits, where "merits" are determined by contributions to the common good or general happiness. In the first society, people belonging to one race or religion are favored in educational opportunities, comfortable housing, and high-paying jobs, while people of another race or religion are disfavored. Race and religion function in that society as grounds for discrimination. In the second society, on the other hand, race or religion do not matter as far as education, housing, and jobs are concerned. All that counts are such things as, Does the individual have a need for special treatment, a need which, if overlooked, would unfairly handicap him in matters of education, housing, or jobs? (For example, a blind person might be given special schooling and a special job, so that his blindness will not mean that he has less of a chance for happiness in life than others.) Or, has the individual, through fair and open competition, proven himself qualified for a high-paying job? Or, does he have exceptional abilities—such as musical genius or mathematical brilliance— which deserve the society's recognition, so that advanced education and scholarships are made available to him? Here race and religion do not function as grounds for discrimination, since they are not considered in determining the proper distribution of happiness and unhappiness throughout the population.

The problem of utility and justice arises when it is seen that, in the two societies described above, it is possible for the first to produce a greater total net balance of happiness over unhappiness than the second. Thus suppose the first society can force the members of the disfavored race or religion to work long hours for little or no pay, so that they produce much more and use up much less of what is produced than they would without such coercion. Then, even if the calculation of utility includes the unhappiness of the disadvantaged, the total balance of happiness over unhappiness could be greater than that resulting from the second society's system of production and consumption. A utilitarian, it seems, would have to say in that case that the first society was morally better than the second, since its policies and rules yielded a higher net utility. Yet the first society, if not simply and self-evidently unjust, would at least be considered (even by utilitarians) to be less just than the second. Hence, utility and justice are incompatible when applied to certain types of societies under certain conditions.

Such conflicts between utility and justice can occur because, as far as utility alone is concerned, it is always morally right to increase one person's happiness at the expense of another's, if the total net balance of pluses over minuses is greater than would be the case were the two persons treated equally. It would seem, in contrast to this, that justice requires that no individual serve as a mere instrument or means to someone else's happiness. (If a person freely consents to sacrifice his happiness for the sake of another, he is not, of course, being used merely as a means to someone else's ends.) On this point the opposition between justice and utility appears to be fundamental.

It should be noted in this connection that utility not only permits but actually requires one individual's being made unhappy if doing so adds to a group's happiness *however small an increase in happiness might be experienced by each of its members,* as long as the total amount of happiness to the group outweighs the unhappiness of the individual in question. Thus suppose an innocent man is made a scapegoat for the guilt of others and accordingly suffers punishment. If he experiences, say, -100 units of unhappiness and if there are 101 persons who, in victimizing him, gain $+1$ unit of happiness each (perhaps in relief at seeing another blamed for their own wrongdoing), then the principle of utility *requires* that the scapegoat be punished. This is not because the scapegoat's unhappiness is being ignored or is being assigned less intrinsic worth than the happiness of others. Each unit of unhappiness (-1) experienced by the scapegoat is equal in "weight" to a unit of happiness ($+1$) of someone in the group. It just happens that in the given situation the total quantity of the group's happiness is greater than that of the scapegoat's unhappiness. Consequently the principle of utility, when applied to this situation, entails that the scapegoat be made to suffer.

It is in this way that the idea of justice seems to present a major philosophical difficulty for all forms of utilitarianism. How might utilitarians reply to this criticism? They would begin by pointing out that, when we leave abstract speculations about theoretical possibilities behind and face the actual world around us, we find that any conflict between justice and utility is highly unlikely. The apparent plausibility of the cases given above, they would say, depends on their being abstracted from the real processes of historical and social development. They hold that when these processes are fully taken into account, it becomes clear that injustice inevitably yields great disutility.

In support of this claim, utilitarians ask us to consider how the principle of utility would apply to situations of social conflict, where one person's (or group's) interests can be furthered only if another person's (or group's) interests are frustrated. For this is where the concepts of justice and injustice are applicable. Now with regard to such situations, the principle of utility requires social rules which enable people to resolve their disagreements and live in harmony with one another. To live in harmony means, not that no social conflicts occur, but that whenever they do occur, there is a set of rules everyone can appeal to as a fair way to resolve them. Such rules will (a) take everyone's interests into account, (b) give equal consideration to the interests of each person, and (c) enable all parties to a dispute to decide issues on grounds freely acceptable by all. For it is only when everyone can appeal to such a system of conflict-resolving rules that the society as a whole can achieve its maximum happiness and minimum unhappiness.

This can be seen by referring to the condition of anyone who does *not* accept a set of conflict-resolving rules as fair. Such a person will simply consider himself to be under social coercion with respect to those rules. That is, he will conform to the rules only because he is forced to by society. If his interests are frustrated by their operation, he will believe he has legitimate moral complaints against the rest of society, and will then think any action necessary to right the wrongs carried out in the name of the rules to be justified. The greater the number of such disaffected persons, the deeper will be the state of social disharmony. It is obvious that very little happiness can be realized in such a society.

At this point the following objection might be raised. To make sure that social conflict will not get out of hand, let those who accept the rules establish a power structure which will ensure their domination over those who reject them. In this way, although some (the powerless) may suffer, those in power can maximize their happiness. To this the utilitarian replies, History has shown us that no such power structure can last for long; even while it does last, the effort spent by the "ins" on maintaining domination over the "outs" makes it impossible for the "ins" to obtain much happiness in life. A social system of this kind is constantly liable to break down. The need to preserve their position of power drives the "ins" to ever greater measures of surveillance and repression. The society as a whole becomes a closed system in which the freedom of all individuals is diminished. Accompanying this curtailment of human freedom is a dwindling in the very conception of man and his creative powers. Inevitably, there develops an intolerance of diversity in thought, in speech, in styles of life. A narrow conformity of taste, ideas, and outward behavior becomes the main concern of everyone. What kind of "happiness" is this? What amount of intrinsic value does such a narrow way of life really

make possible for people, even people who have the power to advance their interests at the expense of others?

The upshot of the argument is now apparent: Given a clearheaded view of the world as it is and a realistic understanding of man's nature, it becomes more and more evident that injustice will never have, in the long run, greater utility than justice. Even if the two principles of justice and utility can logically be separated in the abstract and even if they can be shown to yield contradictory results in hypothetical cases, it does not follow that the fundamental idea of utilitarianism must be given up. For it remains the case that, when we are dealing with the actual practices of people in their social and historical settings, to maximize happiness and minimize unhappiness requires an open, freely given commitment on the part of *everyone* to comply with the rules for settling conflicts among them. Anyone who is coerced into following the rules when he, in good conscience, cannot accept them as being fair to everyone (and consequently to himself) will not consider himself morally obligated to abide by them. Since he will either feel unjustly treated himself or see himself as a participant in the unfair treatment of others, society stands condemned in his judgment. From his point of view, he will have good reason to do what he can to change or abolish the rules. He will join with anyone else who rejects them as unfair, in an effort to overcome his powerlessness. Thus injustice becomes, in actual practice, a source of great social disutility. If society's reaction to the challenge of its dissidents is only a stronger attempt to impose its rules by force, this response will, sooner or later, bring about a situation in which no one really benefits. Not only is it profoundly true that "might does not make right," it is equally true that might cannot create the maximum balance of human happiness over human misery, when the lives of everyone are taken into account.

Whether this argument provides a successful rebuttal to the criticism of utilitarianism when viewed in the light of justice is a matter for the reader's own reflection.

· · ·

WILLIAM K. FRANKENA

Deontological Theories

. . . Moral philosophers have offered us a variety of alternative standards. In general their views have been of two sorts: (1) *deontological* theories and (2) *teleological* ones. A teleological theory says that the basic or ultimate criterion or standard of what is morally right, wrong, obligatory, etc., is the nonmoral value that is brought into being. The final appeal, directly or indirectly, must be to the comparative amount of good produced, or rather to the comparative balance of good over evil produced. Thus, an act is *right* if and only if it or the rule under which it falls produces, will probably produce, or is intended to produce *at least as great a balance of good over evil* as any available alternative; an act is *wrong* if and only if it does not do so. An act *ought to be done* if and only if it or the rule under which it falls produces, will probably produce, or is intended to produce *a greater balance of good over evil* than any available alternative.

It is important to notice here that, for a teleologist, the moral quality or value of actions, persons, or traits of character is dependent on the comparative nonmoral value of what they bring about or try to bring about. For the moral quality or value of something to depend on the moral value of whatever it promotes would be circular. Teleological theories, then, make the right, the obligatory, and the morally good dependent on the nonmorally good. Accordingly, they also make the theory of moral obligation and moral value dependent, in a sense, on the theory of nonmoral value.

. . .

Deontological theories deny what teleological theories affirm. They deny that the right, the obligatory, and the morally good are wholly, whether directly or indirectly, a function of what is nonmorally good or of what

William K. Frankena, *Ethics*, 2nd ed. © 1973, pp. 14,15,16,17, 23–30. Reprinted by permission of Prentice-Hall, Inc., Englewood Cliffs, New Jersey.

promotes the greatest balance of good over evil for self, one's society, or the world as a whole. They assert that there are other considerations that may make an action or rule right or obligatory besides the goodness or badness of its consequences—certain features of the act itself other than the *value* it brings into existence, for example, the fact that it keeps a promise, is just, or is commanded by God or by the state. Teleologists believe that there is one and only one basic or ultimate right-making characteristic, namely, the comparative value (nonmoral) of what is, probably will be, or is intended to be brought into being. Deontologists either deny that this characteristic is right-making at all or they insist that there are other basic or ultimate right-making characteristics as well. For them the principle of maximizing the balance of good over evil, no matter for whom, is either not a moral criterion or standard at all, or, at least, it is not the only basic or ultimate one.

To put the matter in yet another way: a deontologist contends that it is possible for an action or rule of action to be the morally right or obligatory one even if it does not promote the greatest possible balance of good over evil for self, society, or universe. It may be right or obligatory simply because of some other fact about it or because of its own nature. It follows that a deontologist may also adopt any kind of a view about what is good or bad in the nonmoral sense.

. . .

DEONTOLOGICAL THEORIES

Deontological theories are also of different kinds, depending on the role they give to general rules. *Act-deontological theories* maintain that the basic judgments of obligation are all purely particular ones like "In this situation I should do so and so," and that general ones like "We ought always to keep our promises" are unavailable, useless, or at best derivative from particular judgments. Extreme act-deontologists maintain that we can and must see or somehow decide separately in each particular situation what is the right or obligatory thing to do, without appealing to any rules and also without looking to see what will promote the greatest balance of good over evil for oneself or the world. Such a view was held by E. F. Carritt (in *Theory of Morals)* and possibly by H. A. Prichard; and was at least suggested by Aristotle when he said that in determining what the golden mean is "the decision rests with perception,"[1] and by Butler when he wrote that if:

. . . any plain honest man, before he engages in any course of action, ask himself, Is this I am going about right, or is it wrong? . . . I do not in the least doubt but that this question would be answered agreeably to truth and virtue, by almost any fair man in almost any circumstance [without any general rule].[2]

Today, with an emphasis on "decision" rather than "intuition" and with an admission of difficulty and anxiety, this is the view of most existentialists. In a less extreme form, act-deontologism allows that general rules can be built up on the basis of particular cases and may then be useful in determining what should be done on later occasions. But it cannot allow that a general rule may ever supersede a well-taken particular judgment as to what should be done. What is called "situation ethics" today includes both of these forms of act-deontologism.

Rule-deontologists hold that the standard of right and wrong consists of one or more rules—either fairly concrete ones like "We ought always to tell the truth" or very abstract ones like Henry Sidgwick's Principle of Justice: "It cannot be right for A to treat B in a manner in which it would be wrong for B to treat A, merely on the ground that they are two different individuals, and without there being any difference between the natures of circumstances of the two which can be stated as a reasonable ground for difference of treatment."[3] Against the teleologists, they insist, of course, that these rules are valid independently of whether or not they promote the good. Against act-deontologists, they contend that these rules are basic, and are not derived by induction from particular cases. In fact, they assert that judgments about what to do in particular cases are always to be determined in the light of these rules, as they were by Socrates in the *Apology* and *Crito*. The following writers are or were rule-deontologists: Samuel Clarke, Richard Price, Thomas Reid, W. D. Ross, Immanuel Kant, and perhaps Butler. People who take "conscience" to be our guide or standard in morality are usually either rule-deontologists or act-deontologists, depending on whether they think of conscience primarily as providing us with general rules or as making particular judgments in particular situations.

.   .   .

ACT-DEONTOLOGICAL THEORIES

[A] rather extreme reaction to the ethics of traditional rules, but one which remains on the deontological side as against egoists and other teleologists, is act-deontologism. The main point about it is that it offers us no standard whatsoever for determining what is right or wrong in particular cases; it tells us that particular judgments are basic and any general rules are to be derived from them, not the other way around. It presents a kind of method for determining what is right, namely, by becoming clear about the facts in the case and then forming a judgment about what is to be done, either by some kind of "intuition" as intuitionists would call it or by a "decision" of the kind that existentialists talk about. Act-deontologism, however, offers us no criterion or guiding principle, but at most only rules of thumb.

If we had a distinct intuitive faculty which perceives what is right or wrong, and speaks with a clear voice, matters might still be tolerable. But anthropological and psychological evidence seems to be against the existence of such a faculty, as does the everyday experience of disagreement about what is right in particular situations. . . . It seems imperative, therefore, to find a more satisfactory theory, if this is possible.

The other kind of act-deontological theory,

which makes "decision" rather than "intuition" central, is even less satisfactory. It leaves our particular moral judgments wholly up in the air, as existentialists think they are, subject to the "anxiety" of which they make so much. It does, indeed, tell one to take the "situation" one is in as his guide, and this must mean that one must look carefully to see just what his situation is, that is, one must be careful to get the facts about one's situation straight; but beyond that it has nothing to say, and it even insists that there is nothing else to guide one—one must simply "choose" or "decide" what to do, virtually making one's action right by choosing it. In effect, this gives us no guidance whatsoever, for merely looking at the facts does not tell one what to do if one does not also have some aim, ideal, or norm to go by. Just knowing that a car is coming tells me nothing about what to do unless I want to cross the street alive or have some notion of what I should be about. Certainly one can hardly call such unguided decisions morality. One wonders how one could even build up any rules of thumb on such a basis.

The main argument for act-deontologism, apart from the objections to prevailing rules that were listed earlier, is the claim that each situation is different and even unique, so that no general rules can possibly be of much help in dealing with it, except as mere rules of thumb. Now, it is true that each situation has something new or unique about it, but it does not follow that it is unique in all respects or that it cannot be like other situations in morally relevant respects. After all, events and situations are alike in some important respects, otherwise we could not make true general statements of a factual kind, as we do in ordinary life and in science. Therefore, there is no reason for thinking that we cannot similarly make general statements of a moral kind. For example, many situations are certainly alike in including the fact that a promise has been made, and this may be enough to warrant applying a rule to them.

On the other side, two lines of argument may be advanced against act-deontological theories. The first counts most against the more extreme ones, the other against them all. The first is that it is practically impossible for us to do without rules. For one thing, we cannot always put in the time and effort required to judge each situation anew. For another thing, rules are needed in the process of moral education. As R. M. Hare has said,

> . . . to learn to do anything is never to learn to do an individual act; it is always to learn to do acts of a certain kind in a certain kind of situation; and this is to learn a principle. . . . without principles we could not learn anything whatever from our elders. . . . every generation would have to start from scratch and teach itself. But . . . self-teaching like all other teaching, is the teaching of principles.[4]

An act-deontologist might reply that the only rules needed are rules of thumb arrived at on the basis of past experience. But this means rules arrived at on the basis of past intuitions or decisions, and we have already seen reason to question generalizations reached on such bases. In any case, it seems clear that the rules passed on in moral education must be perceived by the younger generation, at least for a time, as something stronger than rules of thumb that they may use or not use at their discretion—something more like the rules of prima facie duty that we shall come to in dealing with W. D. Ross.

The other line of argument is more technical. It holds that particular moral judgments are not purely particular, as the act-deontologist claims, but implicitly general. For the act-deontologist, "This is what X ought to do in situation Y" does not entail anything about what X or anyone else should do in similar situations. Suppose that I go to Jones for advice about what to do in situation Y, and he tells me that I morally ought to do Z. Suppose I also recall that the day before he had maintained that W was the right thing for Smith to do in a situation of the same kind. I shall then certainly point this out to Jones and ask him if he is not being inconsistent. Now suppose that Jones does not do anything to show that the two cases are different, but simply says, "No, there is no connection between the two cases. Sure, they are alike, but one was yesterday and involved Smith. Now it's today and you are involved." Surely, this would strike us as an odd response from anyone who purports to be taking the moral point of view or giving moral advice. The fact is that when one makes a moral judgment in a particular situation, one implicitly commits oneself to making the same judgment in any similar situation, even if the second situation occurs at a different time or place, or involves another agent. Moral and value predicates are such that if they belong to an action or object, they also belong to any other action or object which has the same properties. If I say I ought to serve my country, I imply that everyone ought to serve his country. The point involved here is called the Principle of Universalizability: if one judges that X is right or good, then one is committed to judging that anything exactly like X, or like X in relevant respects, is right and good. Otherwise he has no business using these words.

This point is connected with the fact, noted earlier, that particular ethical and value judgments can be supported by reasons. If Jones makes such a judgment, it is appropriate to ask him for his reason for believing that the act is right or the object good, and to expect an answer like, "Because you promised to do it" or "Because it gives pleasure." If he answers, "Oh, for no reason whatsoever," we are puzzled and feel that he has misled us by using ethical or value terms at all. Moral and value judgments imply reasons, and reasons cannot apply in a particular case only. If they apply in one case, they apply in all similar cases. Moreover, in order to give a reason in a particular case, one must presuppose a general proposition. If Jones answers your question "Why?" by saying "Because you promised to" or "Because it gives pleasure," he presupposes that it is right to keep promises or that what gives pleasure is good.

RULE-DEONTOLOGICAL THEORIES

It follows that act-deontological theories are untenable in principle. In choosing, judging, and reasoning morally, one is at least implicitly espousing rules or principles. This suggests rule-deontologism, which holds that there is a non-teleological standard consisting of one or more rules, though these need not be the prevailing ones. Usually rule-deontologists hold that the standard consists of a number of rather specific rules like those of telling the truth or keeping agreements, each one saying that we *always* ought to act in a certain way in a certain kind of situation. Here, the stock objection is that no rule can be framed which does not admit of exceptions (and excuses) and no set of rules can be framed which does not admit of conflicts between the rules. To this objection, one might say that an exception to a rule can only occur when it has to yield the right of way to another rule, and that the rules proposed may be ranked in a hierarchy so that they never can conflict or dispute the right of way. One might also say that the rules may have all the necessary exceptions built into them, so that, fully stated, they have no exceptions. Thus, for example, the case of the white lie, if we accept it, is an exception to the rule "We ought never to lie," but if we formulate the "exception" as part of the rule and say, "We ought not to lie, except for white lies," assuming that we have a way of telling when a lie is "white," then it is no longer an exception. It must be confessed, however, that no deontologist has presented us with a conflict-and-exception-free system of concrete rules about what we are actually to do. To this fact, the deontologist might retort, "That's the way things are. We can't be as satisfied with any other theory of obligation as with this one, but this one isn't perfect either. The moral life simply does present us with unsolvable dilemmas." But, of course, we need not agree without looking farther.

W. D. Ross, who is a rule-deontologist, deals with the difficulty pointed out in this stock objection partly by retorting in the way just indicated, but he also has another answer. He distinguishes between *actual* duty and *prima facie* duty, between what is *actually* right and what is *prima facie* right. What is actually right or obligatory is what we actually ought to do in a particular situation. About what we actually ought to do in the situations of life, which often involve the conflicts referred to, there are and can be, Ross admits, no rules that do not have exceptions. "Every rule has exceptions," that is, every rule of actual duty has exceptions. But there still may be and are, Ross contends, exceptionless rules of prima facie duty. Something is a prima facie duty if it is a duty other things being equal, that is, if it would be an actual duty if other moral considerations did not intervene. For example, if I have promised to give my secretary a day off, then I have a prima facie duty to give her the day off; and if there are no conflicting considerations that outweigh this prima facie duty, then I also have an actual duty to let her take the day off. Accordingly, Ross suggests that one can formulate a number of moral rules that hold without exception as rules of prima facie, though not of actual, duty. That one ought to keep one's promises is always valid as a rule of prima facie duty; it is always an obligation one must try to fulfill. But it may on occasion be outweighed by another obligation or rule of prima facie duty. Or, to use a different phrase, the fact that one has made a promise is always a right-making consideration, it must always be taken into account; but there are other such considerations, and these may sometimes outweigh it or take precedence over it when they conflict with it.

This view does much to meet the objection. It shows how we may have a set of rules that have no exceptions, namely, by conceiving of them as rules of prima facie, not actual, duty. But, of course, it does not help us in cases of conflict, since it allows that prima facie duties may come into conflict in actual situations. Ross could clear even this hurdle if he could provide us with a ranking of our prima facie duties that would always tell us when one takes precedence over the others, but he does not believe this to be possible. It is at this point that he says, "C'est la vie," and refers us to Aristotle's dictum, "The decision rests with perception." Nevertheless, as far as it goes, Ross's conception of a set of rules of prima facie duty is an important one which I shall accept and use. The main difficulty about it, besides the one just mentioned, is that a deontologist like Ross cannot give us any criterion by which to tell what our prima facie duties are, or in other words, what considerations are

always to be taken into account in determining what is morally right or wrong. We must at least try to look for such a criterion. Ross simply contends that his prima facie duties—fidelity, reparation, gratitude, justice, etc.—are self-evident, so that no criterion is needed; but to anyone who doubts the claim of self-evidence . . . this explanation will hardly suffice. Other rule-deontologists would say that their basic rules are not self-evident but arbitrarily decided on, divinely revealed, or deducible from metaphysics. Such claims also raise questions about the *justification* of moral judgments. . . .

Ross's standard consists of a fairly large number of relatively concrete rules of prima facie duty. A deontologist who is dissatisfied with such a scheme might, however, offer as a more satisfactory standard a small number of more abstract and highly general rules like the Golden Rule, or Sidgwick's Principle of Justice, previously quoted, or Rashdall's Axiom of Equity: "I ought to regard the good of one man as of equal intrinsic value with the like good of any one else."[5] He might then claim that more concrete rules and particular conclusions can be reached by applying these general principles. Such principles certainly capture some of the truth, for they entail a recognition of the Principle of Universalizability, but, as we shall see in discussing Kant, it may be doubted that they can actually suffice for the determination of our duties. In fact, Sidgwick and Rashdall argue that they must be supplemented by two teleological axioms—the Principle of Prudence or Rational Egoism . . . and the Principle of Beneficence or Utility. . . . Thus they come to a position much like the one I shall be advocating. Here we must notice that even if one has only a few basic axioms of this kind, one must allow that they may come into conflict (unless one postulates a divinely regulated universe in which this cannot happen, as Sidgwick does), and that one is not yet free from this difficulty in Ross's system. To be free from it we must find a view that has a single basic principle and is otherwise satisfactory. Can we find such a view?

THE DIVINE COMMAND THEORY

A rule-deontologist can avoid the problem of possible conflict between basic principles if he can show that there is a single basic non-teleological principle that is adequate as a moral standard. One such monistic kind of rule deontology with a long and important history is the Divine Command theory, also known as theological voluntarism, which holds that the standard of right and wrong is the will or law of God. Proponents of this view sometimes hold that "right" and "wrong" *mean,* respectively, commanded and forbidden by God, but even if they do not define "right" and "wrong" in this way, they all hold that an action or kind of action is right or wrong if and only if and *because* it is commanded or forbidden by God, or, in other words, that what ultimately *makes* an action right or wrong is its being commanded or forbidden by God and nothing else.

One who holds such a view may believe that we ought to do what is for the greatest general good, that one ought to do what is for his own good, or that we ought to keep promises, tell the truth, etc. Then his working ethics will be like that of the utilitarian, ethical egoist, or pluralistic deontologist. In any case, however, he will insist that such conduct is right because and only because it is commanded by God. If he believes that God's law consists of a number of rules, e.g., the Ten Commandments of the Old Testament, then, of course, like the pluralistic rule-deontologist, he may still be faced with the problem of conflicts between them, unless God somehow instructs us how to resolve them.

Sometimes, when asked why we should do what God wills, a theologian replies that we should do so because God will reward us if we do and punish us if we do not, if not in this life then in the hereafter. This reply may be meant only to motivate us to obey God, but if it is intended to justify the claim that we ought to obey God, then it presupposes a basic ethical egoism, for then the theologian is telling us that, basically, one ought to do what is to one's own interest, adding that God makes it to our interest to do what He commands, thus leading us to the conclusion that we ought to obey God. For him, then, the basic normative principle is not obedience to God but doing what is for one's own greatest good. In short, he is a teleologist of a kind we have already discussed, not a deontologist at all. Just now we are interested only in the theologian who really believes that what finally makes an action right or wrong is simply its being commanded or forbidden by God.

It should also be noticed that a religious person who believes that God only *reveals* the moral law to a mankind otherwise incapable of knowing adequately what is right or wrong is not a theological voluntarist. He will, of course, hold that the moral law coincides with what God tells us to do, but he does not assert that what it prescribes is right just because God commands it; he may even think that it would be right anyway.

It is not easy to discuss the Divine Command theory of right and wrong in a way that will satisfy both believers and nonbelievers. The latter find the theory hard to take seriously and the former find it hard to think that, if God commands something, it may still be wrong. We must remember, however, that many religious thinkers have rejected the Divine Command theory, at least in its voluntaristic form, e.g., St. Thomas Aquinas and Ralph Cudworth.

One question that arises at once is, "How can we know what God commands or forbids?" Socrates asked this in the *Euthyphro*. However, it raises problems that cannot be discussed here. More to the point is another question asked by Socrates. Euthyphro suggests in effect that what makes something right is the fact that God commands it, and Socrates then asks him, "Is something right because God commands it or does He command it because it is right?" Euthyphro answers that, of course, God commands it because it is right, and Socrates at once points out that, if this is true, then Euthyphro must give up his theory. Such an argument does not actually disprove theological voluntarism, but it does show that it is hard to hold consistently. Euthyphro's answer to Socrates' question seems to be the natural one, and it implies that what is right is so independently of whether God commands it or not, or, in other words, that God only reveals what is right and does not make it right or create its rightness merely by willing it.

Cudworth's kind of argument is more conclusive.[6] Like others, he points out that, if theological voluntarism is true, then, if God were to command cruelty, dishonesty, or injustice, these things would be right and obligatory. If God were to order the exact opposite of what we generally take him to have ordered or of what we take to be right, then, by the hypothesis in question, this would be what we ought to do. Now, a voluntarist could reply, "So be it!" But such a position is hard to accept, and voluntarists are themselves reluctant to accept it. They usually reply by saying that God would not or could not command cruelty, etc., because that would go against His nature, since He is good.

This answer may contain a circle. If, in saying that God is good, the voluntarist means that God does what is right or what He thinks is right, which is what we usually mean by being morally good, then he is in a kind of dilemma. He must either give up his voluntarism or say that God's goodness consists simply in the fact that He does what He himself commands or wills, which will be true no matter what He commands or wills, even if it is cruelty, etc.

To avoid this outcome a voluntarist may reply that, when we say God is good, we mean not that He does or tries to do what is right, but that He is benevolent or loving, and therefore would not order us to be cruel, etc. Such a line of thought would avoid the difficulty pointed to by Cudworth. But then we may ask how we know that God is benevolent or loving independently of knowing what He commands and whether He commands cruelty, etc., or not? To this objection a theologian may answer that God is by definition benevolent or loving, but then he is still faced with the problem of proving the existence of a Being that has the other attributes ascribed to God and is also benevolent or loving, and of doing so independently of knowing what this Being commands us to do. This problem, however, cannot be taken up here.

It may also be worth pointing out that what the theological voluntarist offers us as a guide to life is a kind of legal system, cosmic in scale and supernatural in origin, but still essentially a legal system. Since we ordinarily think that law and morality are rather different in character, we may then ask whether the action-guide of the voluntarist is a moral one at all. Theologians themselves sometimes even suggest that their religious system of life is "beyond morality" and should replace it, at least in the life of a believer. This raises the questions of what a morality is and what the moral point of view is, . . . and also the question of whether God takes the moral point of view in telling us what and what not to do, which we cannot try to deal with.

. . .

NOTES

1. *Nicomachean Ethics,* end of Book II.
2. Joseph Butler, *Five Sermons,* New York: Liberal Arts Press, 1949, p. 45.
3. *The Methods of Ethics,* 7th ed. (London: Macmillan and Co., Ltd., 1907), p. 380.
4. *The Language of Morals* (Oxford: Clarendon Press, 1952), pp. 60–61.
5. H. Rashdall, *The Theory of Good and Evil,* 2nd ed. (London: Oxford University Press, 1924), I, 185.
6. See D. D. Raphael, ed., *British Moralists 1650-1800* (Oxford: Clarendon Press, 1969), I, 105.

GERARD J. HUGHES

Natural Law

DEFINITIONS

The term "natural law" has been used in the history of philosophy to refer to a wide variety of different views. Some of these are concerned with particular approaches to legislation in human society; others are concerned with the connexion between moral philosophy and religious revelation. But those with which I shall deal here are particular views within moral philosophy itself about the values and duties which we have, and the methods by which we might set about discovering them.

NATURAL LAW THEORIES

Exactly which ethical theories can properly be described as natural law theories is perhaps a matter of terminology. I shall use the term to include all those theories which share two basic assumptions: first, that moral values and moral duties depend on the kind of being that man is; and secondly, that we can discover what man is by those processes of rational and scientific reflexion which we employ in other areas of human knowledge. Each of these assumptions can, of course, be challenged. To the first, it might be retorted that no scientific description of man, however well elaborated, can ever yield evaluative theories about what is *good* for him, or what he *ought* to do, or what an *ideal* man *should* be like. In short, one cannot derive an "ought" from an "is." But the natural law philosopher would simply reply to such an objection by saying that he *can* link morals to descriptions of man in a way which carries conviction. A full discussion of this problem (which afflicts other theories besides natural law theories) is beyond the scope of this article; suffice it to say that the issue is currently one over which there is considerable controversy.

To the second assumption, it might be replied that there is no *one* picture of man on

Reprinted with permission of the author and the publisher from *Journal of Medical Ethics*, Vol. 2, No. 1 (March 1976).

which a moral theory could (possibly) be based. And indeed in the history of moral philosophy there have been a bewildering variety of views each claiming to present *the* picture of man and his morality. I shall briefly mention two, and consider a third at somewhat greater length.

THREE PICTURES OF MAN

In an ambitious attempt to integrate biology, psychology and ethics, Thomas Hobbes regarded man as being, from one point of view, a pleasure-pain machine. He then argued that ethics must therefore consist in the rational study of how the individual might best go about maximizing his pleasures and minimizing his pain. From this picture of man, he thought that it followed that man had to be a moral egoist. But he was careful to point out that the enlightened egoist could not afford to be selfish, or unforgiving, or ungenerous or inconsiderate, and could not do without a state which enforced certain duties at law.

In sharp contrast, Kant regards man as above all a rational agent, whose principal concerns are with justice and freedom. Moreover, while Kant does not deny that the notion of happiness is required to make ultimate sense of morality, he resolutely refuses to interpret man's moral aims in terms simply of the satisfaction of physical or psychological needs, stressing instead man's freedom and his autonomy as moral values which must above all be respected. Kant's moral views differ from those of Hobbes precisely because they have quite different pictures of what it is to be a human being in the first place.

Yet a third picture of man is provided by Aristotle. On this view, man is comparable to other living organisms, which flourish when, and only when, each of their parts works properly and in harmony with one another. Man is, of course, much more complex than a flower or an animal such as a dog; nevertheless, man too will flourish only when his body, his emotions, and his intellect each is functioning as it should; and when man himself is functioning properly in a harmoniously organized society. This kind of functional approach to natural law is of particular importance, since, via Aquinas, it was taken over by many Roman Catholic theologians, and developed into one of the most influential of all natural law theories of ethics. I shall therefore examine it in somewhat more detail.

A FUNCTIONAL APPROACH TO NATURAL LAW: THE CONCEPT OF HEALTH

The analogy is perhaps seen at its best if we consider a concept such as "healthy." To say of a man that he is healthy is not just to describe his physical condition—it is to say that he is in a desirable physical condition. Moreover, it is desirable just because it is the kind of condition it is. He is healthy just because each of the organs of his body is functioning as it should, and in harmony with all the others. Each organ has a "purpose," and if it fails in this purpose the body as a whole will not succeed in functioning so well. It might further be suggested that we might in principle be able to approach the matter the other way round. We might be able to say—for example, in the case of the fossil remains of some extinct animal—what it would have been like for that animal to function at its best by a careful examination of its various organs and so on. In a similar way, some natural law philosophers have argued that we can discover what human happiness consists in either by looking at happy people or by an examination of the various features of human nature in order to see their role or purpose in the functioning of the whole man.

A functional analysis of health works reasonably well, I suggest, because it is comparatively easy to discover what the purpose of the various bodily organs is, and exactly how they interact with one another. Some organs have only one purpose, like the heart; others have more than one, such as the nose; and others again have purposes which are highly complex, like the brain or the endocrine glands. It is possible to give an uncontroversial account of what they are for. Moreover, to say that, other

things being equal, it is preferable to be healthy [rather] than unhealthy is to say something which there is no point in challenging.

THE EXTENSION INTO THE MORAL FIELD

Up to a point, it is not particularly difficult to extend this analogy into the moral field. Once it is admitted that the kind of being a man is can be taken as the basis of certain moral duties, it can be argued that it is immoral, other things being equal, to impede the natural functions of the various organs on which a man's health depends. People have a right to food, shelter and competent medical treatment precisely because they will not function so well if they are denied these things. One might even go further and argue that we have a duty to give people affection, support and a fairly clear role in society, since any great measure of deprivation in these areas produces neurosis or psychosis; and one could interpret these illnesses as failures to function properly on an emotional and social level. The boundaries here may be less sharply drawn, and the sense of "function" less clearly defined than in biology and physiology. Nevertheless, we are clear about many instances of mental illness and about the wrongness of treating people in such a way that they become mentally ill; and the functional analogy is by no means entirely unhelpful, at least as a model.

The difficulties arise when the analogy is extended still further. One might wish to say that it is wrong for a man to be an expert housebreaker; but there is surely a clear sense in which, when he is engaged upon his trade, he is functioning extremely well—his reflexes are sharp, he does not allow his feelings to cloud his judgment, his intelligence is working at a very high level. The general point is that man can use his body and his emotions and his mind for many *different* purposes, some of which are good and some bad. Man's body, mind and emotions cannot be said to be "for" a purpose in the clear and uncontroversial (even if at times complex) sense in which his heart, or his endocrine glands, are "for" a purpose in relation to his health. Hence, those natural law philosophers who have argued that sex is "for" the procreation of children and the expression of love, but not just "for" pleasure, have been criticized on the grounds that it is by no means as easy to say what sex is for in a human life as it might be to say what the heart is for in the human body; the functional analogy seems to break down at this point, just as it does if we try to argue that the sense of touch is not "for" the cracking of safes. Even if we admit that human fulfilment is analogous to bodily health, the contribution of the various elements in a human life is much more difficult to assess than the contribution to the human body of properly functioning organs.

NEW BASES FOR MORAL JUDGMENTS ACCORDING TO NATURAL LAW

Indeed, the very process of assessment itself seems to differ considerably from the way in which we might seek to discover the proper function of our bodily organs with respect to health, because "health" itself is a comparatively clear concept and "human fulfilment" is not. Hence, it is comparatively easy to determine when something has gone wrong with our health (even if we are not always in a position to say just what), and much more difficult to say when a person is, or is not, living a life of fulfilment. Critics of natural law theories would argue at this point that what is to count as fulfilment is simply not something which can be discovered by any kind of scientific method, nor is it something which can be ascertained independently of some moral commitment. At any rate it is clear that the three versions of natural law theory which we have given as illustrations here are each much too simple to be at all satisfactory. Most natural law philosophers now would insist that any picture of man which is going to be at all adequate as the basis for moral judgments will have to be elaborated by means of a whole range of enquiries, involving psychology, sociology, economics and political theory as well as biology and purely philosophical reflection. And they would admit that our knowledge of man in his society, and of the kinds of life in which men might find fulfilment, is in many respects very inadequate.

The natural law approach to moral philosophy, then, is best regarded not as a complete specification of the moral life, but as a spirit and a method of approach to be employed in discussing moral problems. It insists that the starting point for ethics is knowledge of human nature; and that this knowledge is to be gained as scientifically and critically as possible before any attempt is made to base moral conclusions upon it.

H. L. A. HART

Responsibility

1. [INTRODUCTION]

A wide range of different, though connected, ideas is covered by the expressions "responsibility," "responsible," and "responsible for," as these are standardly used in and out of the law. Though connexions exist between these different ideas, they are often very indirect, and it seems appropriate to speak of different *senses* of these expressions. The following simple story of a drunken sea captain who lost his ship at sea can be told in the terminology of responsibility to illustrate, with stylistically horrible clarity, these differences of sense.

As captain of the ship, X was responsible for the safety of his passengers and crew. But on his last voyage he got drunk every night and was responsible for the loss of the ship with all aboard. It was rumoured that he was insane, but the doctors considered that he was responsible for his actions. Throughout the voyage he behaved quite irresponsibly, and various incidents in his career showed that he was not a responsible person. He always maintained that the exceptional winter storms were responsible for the loss of the ship, but in the legal proceedings brought against him he was found criminally responsible for his negligent conduct, and in separate civil proceedings he was held legally responsible for the loss of life and property. He is still alive and he is morally responsible for the deaths of many women and children.

This welter of distinguishable senses of the word "responsibility" and its grammatical cognates can, I think, be profitably reduced by division and classification. I shall distinguish four heads of classification to which I shall assign the following names:

Reprinted by permission of the publisher from *Punishment and Responsibility* by H. L. A. Hart. © Oxford University Press 1968.

(a) Role-Responsibility
(b) Causal-Responsibility
(c) Liability-Responsibility
(d) Capacity-Responsibility.

I hope that in drawing these dividing lines, and in the exposition which follows, I have avoided the arbitrary pedantries of classificatory systematics, and that my divisions pick out and clarify the main, though not all, varieties of responsibility to which reference is constantly made, explicitly or implicitly, by moralists, lawyers, historians, and ordinary men. I relegate to the notes discussion of what unifies these varieties and explains the extension of the terminology of responsibility.

2. ROLE-RESPONSIBILITY

A sea captain is responsible for the safety of his ship, and that is his responsibility, or one of his responsibilities. A husband is responsible for the maintenance of his wife; parents for the upbringing of their children; a sentry for alerting the guard at the enemy's approach; a clerk for keeping the accounts of his firm. These examples of a person's responsibilities suggest the generalization that, whenever a person occupies a distinctive place or office in a social organization, to which specific duties are attached to provide for the welfare of others or to advance in some specific way the aims or purposes of the organization, he is properly said to be responsible for the performance of these duties, or for doing what is necessary to fulfil them. Such duties are a person's responsibilities. As a guide to this sense of responsibility this generalization is, I think, adequate, but the idea of a distinct role or place or office is, of course, a vague one, and I cannot undertake to make it very precise. Doubts about its extension to marginal cases will always arise. If two friends, out on a mountaineering expedition, agree that the one shall look after the food and the other the maps, then the one is correctly said to be responsible for the food, and the other for the maps, and I would classify this as a case of role-responsibility. Yet such fugitive or temporary assignments with specific duties would not usually be considered by sociologists, who mainly use the word, as an example of "role." So "role" in my classification is extended to include a task assigned to any person by agreement or otherwise. But it is also important to notice that not all the duties which a man has in virtue of occupying what in a quite strict sense of role is a distinct role, are thought or spoken of as "responsibilities." A private soldier has a duty to obey his superior officer and, if commanded by him to form fours or present arms on a given occasion, has a duty to do so. But to form fours or present arms would scarcely be said to be the private's responsibility; nor would he be said to be responsible for doing it. If on the other hand a soldier was ordered to deliver a message to H.Q. or to conduct prisoners to a base camp, he might well be said to be responsible for doing these things, and these things to be his responsibility. I think, though I confess to not being sure, that what distinguishes those duties of a role which are singled out as responsibilities is that they are duties of a relatively complex or extensive kind, defining a "sphere of responsibility" requiring care and attention over a protracted period of time, while short-lived duties of a very simple kind, to do or not do some specific act on a particular occasion, are not termed responsibilities. Thus a soldier detailed off to keep the camp clean and tidy for the general's visit of inspection has this as his sphere of responsibility and is responsible for it. But if merely told to remove a piece of paper from the approaching general's path, this would be at most his duty.

A "responsible person," "behaving responsibly" (not "irresponsibly"), require for their elucidation a reference to role-responsibility. A responsible person is one who is disposed to take his duties seriously; to think about them, and to make serious efforts to fulfil them. To behave responsibly is to behave as a man would who took his duties in this serious way. Responsibilities in this sense may be either legal or moral, or fall outside this dichotomy. Thus a man may be morally as well as legally responsible for the maintenance of his wife and children, but a host's responsibility for the comfort of his guests, and a referee's responsibility for the control of the players is neither legal nor moral, unless the word "moral" is unilluminatingly used simply to exclude legal responsibility.

3. CAUSAL RESPONSIBILITY

"The long drought was responsible for the famine in India." In many contexts, as in this one, it is possible to substitute for the expression "was responsible for" the words "caused" or "produced" or some other causal expression in referring to consequences, results, or outcomes. The converse, however, is not always true. Examples of this causal sense of responsibility are legion. "His neglect was responsible for her distress." "The Prime Minister's speech was responsible for the panic." "Disraeli was responsible for the defeat of the Government." "The icy condition of the road was responsible for the accident." The past tense of the verb used in this causal sense of the expression "responsible for" should be noticed. If it is said of a living person, who has in fact caused some disaster, that he *is* responsible for it, this is not, or not merely, an example of causal responsibility, but of what I term "liability-responsibility"; it asserts his liability on account of the disaster, even though it is also true that he is responsible in that sense *because* he caused the disaster, and that he caused the disaster may be expressed by saying that he was responsible for it. On the other hand, if it is said of a person no longer living that he was responsible for some disaster, this may be either a simple causal statement or a statement of liability-responsibility, or both.

From the above examples it is clear that in this causal sense not only human beings but also their actions or omissions, and things, conditions, and events, may be said to be responsible for outcomes. It is perhaps true that only where an outcome is thought unfortunate or felicitous is its cause commonly spoken of as responsible for it. But this may not reflect any aspect of the meaning of the expression "responsible for"; it may only reflect the fact that, except in such cases, it may be pointless and hence rare to pick out the causes of events. It is sometimes suggested that, though we may speak of a human being's action as responsible for some outcome in a purely causal sense, we do not speak of a person, as distinct from his actions, as responsible for an outcome, unless he is felt to deserve censure or praise. This is, I think, a mistake. History books are full of examples to the contrary. "Disraeli was responsible for the defeat of the Government" need not carry even an implication that he was deserving of censure or praise; it may be purely a statement concerned with the contribution made by one human being to an outcome of importance, and be entirely neutral as to its moral or other merits. The contrary view depends, I think, on the failure to appreciate sufficiently the ambiguity of statements of the form "X *was* responsible for Y" as distinct from "X *is* responsible for Y" to which I have drawn attention above. The former expression in the case of a person no longer living may be (though it *need* not be) a statement of liability-responsibility.

4. LEGAL LIABILITY-RESPONSIBILITY

Though it was noted that role-responsibility might take either legal or moral form, it was not found necessary to treat these separately. But in the case of the present topic of liability-responsibility, separate treatment seems advisable. For responsibility seems to have a wider extension in relation to the law than it does in relation to morals, and it is a question to be considered whether this is due merely to the general differences between law and morality, or to some differences in the sense of responsibility involved.

When legal rules require men to act or abstain from action, one who breaks the law is usually liable, according to other legal rules, to punishment for his misdeeds, or to make compensation to persons injured thereby, and very often he is liable to both punishment and enforced compensation. He is thus liable to be "made to pay" for what he has done in either or both of the senses which the expression "He'll pay for it" may bear in ordinary usage. But most legal systems go much further than this. A man may be legally punished on account of what his servant has done, even if he in no way caused or instigated or even knew of the servant's action, or knew of the likelihood of his servant so acting. Liability in such circumstances is rare in modern systems of criminal law; but it is common in all systems of civil law for men to be made to pay compensation for injuries caused by others, generally their servants or employees. The law of most countries goes further still. A man may be liable to pay compensation for harm suffered by others, though neither he nor his servants have caused it. This is so, for example, in Anglo-American law when the harm is caused by dangerous things which escape from a man's possession, even if their escape is not due to any act or omission of his or his servants, or if harm is caused to a man's employees by defective machinery whose defective condition he could not have discovered.

.   .   .

5. MORAL LIABILITY-RESPONSIBILITY

How far can the account given above of legal liability-responsibility be applied *mutatis mutandis* to moral responsibility? The *mutanda* seem to be the following: "deserving blame" or "blameworthy" will have to be substituted for "liable to punishment," and "morally bound to make amends or pay compensation" for "liable to be made to pay compensation." Then the moral counterpart to the account given of legal liability-responsibility would be the following: to say that a person is morally responsible for something he has done or for some harmful outcome of his own or others' conduct, is to say that he is morally blameworthy, or morally obliged to make amends for the harm, so far as this depends on certain conditions: these conditions relate to the character or extent of a man's control over his own conduct, or to the causal or other connexion between his action and harmful occurrences, or to his relationship with the person who actually did the harm.

In general, such an account of the meaning of "morally responsible" seems correct, and the striking differences between legal and moral responsibility are due to substantive differences between the content of legal and moral rules and principles rather than to any variation in meaning of responsibility when conjoined with the word "moral" rather than "legal." Thus, both in the legal and the moral case, the criteria of responsibility seem to be restricted to the psychological elements involved in the control of conduct, to causal or other connexions between acts and harm, and to the relationships with the actual doer of misdeeds. The interesting differences between legal and moral responsibility arise from the differences in the particular criteria falling under these general heads. Thus a system of criminal law may make responsibility strict, or even absolute, not even exempting very young children or the grossly insane from punishment; or it may vicariously punish one man for what another has done, even though the former had no control of the latter; or it may punish an individual or make him compensate another for harm which he neither intended nor could have foreseen as likely to arise from his conduct. We may condemn such a legal system which extends strict or vicarious responsibility in these ways as barbarous or unjust, but there are no conceptual barriers to be overcome in speaking of such a system as a legal system, though it is certainly arguable that we should not speak of "punishment" where liability is vicarious or strict. In the moral case, however, greater conceptual barriers exist: the hypothesis that we might hold individuals morally blameworthy for doing things which they could not have avoided doing, or for things done by others over whom they had no control, conflicts with too many of the central features of the idea of morality to be treated merely as speculation about a rare or inferior kind of moral system. It may be an exaggeration to say that there could not logically be such a morality or that blame administered according to principles of strict or vicarious responsibility, even in a minority of cases, could not logically be moral blame; none the less, admission of such a system as a morality would require a profound modification in our present concept of morality, and there is no similar requirement in the case of law.

Some of the most familiar contexts in which the expression "responsibility" appears confirm these general parallels between legal and moral liability-responsibility. Thus in the famous question "Is moral responsibility compatible with determinism?" the expression "moral responsibility" is apt just because the bogey raised by determinism specifically relates to the usual criteria of responsibility; for it opens the question whether, if "determinism" were true, the capacities of human beings to control their conduct would still exist or could be regarded as adequate to justify moral blame.

In less abstract or philosophical contexts, where there is a present question of blaming someone for some particular act, the assertion or denial that a person is morally responsible for his actions is common. But this expression is as ambiguous in the moral as in the legal case: it is most frequently used to refer to what I have termed "capacity-responsibility," which is the most important criterion of moral liability-responsibility; but in some contexts it may also refer to moral liability-responsibility itself. Perhaps the most frequent use in moral contexts of the expression "responsible for" is in cases where persons are said to be morally responsible for the outcomes or results of morally wrong conduct. . . .

6. CAPACITY-RESPONSIBILITY

In most contexts, as I have already stressed, the expression "he is responsible for his actions" is used to assert that a person has certain normal capacities. These constitute the most important criteria of moral liability-responsibility, though it is characteristic of most legal systems that they have given only a partial or tardy recognition to all these capacities as general criteria of legal responsibility. The capacities in question are those of understanding, reasoning, and control of conduct: the ability to understand what conduct legal rules or morality require, to deliberate and reach decisions concerning these requirements, and to conform to decisions when made. Because "responsible for his actions" in this sense refers not to a legal status but to certain complex psychological characteristics of persons, a person's responsibility for his actions may intelligibly be said to be "diminished" or "impaired" as well as altogether absent, and persons may be said to be "suffering from diminished responsibility" much as a wounded man may be said to be suffering from a diminished capacity to control the movements of his limbs.

No doubt the most frequent occasions for asserting or denying that a person is "responsible for his actions" are cases where questions of blame or punishment for particular actions are in issue. But, as with other expressions used to denote criteria of responsibility, this one also may be used where no particular question of blame or punishment is in issue, and it is then used simply to describe a person's psychological condition. Hence it may be said purely by way of description of some harmless inmate of a mental institution, even though there is no present question of his misconduct, that he is a person who is not responsible for his actions. No doubt if there were no social practice of blaming and punishing people for their misdeeds, and excusing them from punishment because they lack the normal capacities of understanding and control, we should lack this shorthand description for describing their condition which we now derive from these social practices. In that case we should have to describe the condition of the inmate directly, by saying that he could not understand what people told him to do, or could not reason about it, or come to, or adhere to any decisions about his conduct.

Legal systems left to themselves may be very niggardly in their admission of the relevance of liability to legal punishment of the several capacities, possession of which are necessary to render a man morally responsible for his actions. So much is evident from the history sketched in the preceding chapter of the painfully slow emancipation of English crim-

inal law from the narrow, cognitive criteria of responsibility formulated in the M'Naghten Rules. Though some continental legal systems have been willing to confront squarely the question whether the accused "lacked the ability to recognize the wrongness of his conduct and to act in accordance with that recognition,"[1] such an issue, if taken seriously, raises formidable difficulties of proof, especially before juries. For this reason I think that, instead of a close determination of such questions of capacity, the apparently coarser-grained technique of exempting persons from liability to punishment if they fall into certain recognized categories of mental disorder is likely to be increasingly used. Such exemption by general category is a technique long known to English law; for in the case of very young children it has made no attempt to determine, as a condition of liability, the question whether on account of their immaturity they could have understood what the law required and could have conformed to its requirements, or whether their responsibility on account of their immaturity was "substantially impaired," but exempts them from liability for punishment if under a specific age. It seems likely that exemption by medical category rather than by individualized findings of absent or diminished capacity will be found more likely to lead in practice to satisfactory results. . . .

Though a legal system may fail to incorporate in its rules any psychological criteria of responsibility, and so may apply its sanction to those who are not morally blameworthy, it is none the less dependent for its efficacy on the possession by a sufficient number of those whose conduct it seeks to control of the capacities of understanding and control of conduct which constitute capacity-responsibility. For if a large proportion of those concerned could not understand what the law required them to do or could not form and keep a decision to obey, no legal system could come into existence or continue to exist. The general possession of such capacities is therefore a condition of the

1. German Criminal Code, Art. 51.

efficacy of law, even though it is not made a condition of liability to legal sanctions. The same condition of efficacy attaches to all attempts to regulate or control human conduct by forms of *communication:* such as orders, commands, the invocation of moral or other rules or principles, argument, and advice.

"The notion of prevention through the medium of the mind assumes mental ability adequate to restraint." This was clearly seen by Bentham and by Austin, who perhaps influenced the seventh report of the Criminal Law Commissioners of 1833 containing this sentence. But they overstressed the point; for they wrongly assumed that this condition of efficacy must also be incorporated in legal rules as a condition of liability. This mistaken assumption is to be found not only in the ex-planation of the doctrine of *mens rea* given in Bentham's and Austin's works, but is explicit in the Commissioners' statement preceding the sentence quoted above that "the object of penal law being the prevention of wrong, the principle does not extend to mere involuntary acts or even to harmful consequences the result of inevitable accident." The case of morality is however different in precisely this respect: the possession by those to whom its injunctions are addressed of "mental ability adequate to restraint" (capacity-responsibility) has there a double status and importance. It is not only a condition of the efficacy of morality; but a system or practice which did not regard the possession of these capacities as a necessary condition of liability, and so treated blame as appropriate even in the case of those who lacked them, would not, as morality is at present understood, be a morality.

JOEL FEINBERG

Rights

Rights and liberties are bestowed by rules of many different kinds—rules of games such as chess and baseball, rules of nongovernmental institutions such as clubs and learned societies, even the rules of logic, which grant us, under certain conditions, the "right to infer." The concepts of a right and a liberty (as opposed to freedom generally) probably originated however, in systems of juridical law, and it is in legal systems that they have their most subtle and interesting applications and most thorough and detailed elaborations.

.   .   .

Joel Feinberg, *Social Philosophy,* © 1973, pp. 55–56, 67, 82–83, 84–88, 94–97. Reprinted by permission of Prentice-Hall, Inc., Englewood Cliffs, New Jersey.

I prefer to define rights as valid claims rather than justified ones, because I suspect that justification is too broad a qualification. "Validity," as I understand it, is justification of a peculiar and narrow kind, namely justification within a system of rules. A man has a legal right when the official recognition of his claim (as valid) is called for by the governing rules. This definition, of course, hardly applies to moral rights, but that is not because the genus of which moral rights are a species is something other than claims. A man has a moral right when he has a claim, the recognition of which is called for—not (necessarily) by legal rules— but by moral principles, or the principles of an enlightened conscience.

.   .   .

A guaranteed *right,* "absolute" within its established sphere, adds something of great importance to a liberty, or a "mere privilege," or a "right" that is vulnerable to overturning by interest-balancing procedures. When the government leaves me at liberty (merely) to do X, it tells me in effect that I may do X if I can, but it will not protect me by imposing a duty of noninterference upon others. A liberty is a permission without a protection. A "mere privilege" may or may not add protection to the permission. When it does, the privilege looks more like a right than like a mere liberty. Unlike rights, however, neither the permission nor the continued protection are assured; either can be withdrawn at any time at the state's pleasure, although the holder of a privilege will be warned in advance that withdrawal is coming. It would be otherwise with a so-called "nonabsolute right." When the government grants me a "right" that is vulnerable to interest-balancing tests even at its core, it tells me, in effect, that I may do X and others may not interfere, *but* that this permission cum protection does not apply whenever the state finds it useful to withdraw it, without prior warning, in a given case. "When you speak quietly at a private gathering," says the state, "you may say anything you please about the wisdom of a government policy *unless* a court later determines that interfering with your right at the time was more conducive to the public interest than protecting it." Such a right begins to resemble a so-called prima-facie right in that its exceptive clause is virtually unspecified and unlimited. It is only a small parody to interpret the prima-facie right as permission to do anything except what one shouldn't, and to interpret the nonabsolute "right" as permission to do anything for which permission is not subsequently withdrawn. These are hardly "rights" that one can stand upon, demand, fight for, or treasure. They are "rights" that make men humble, not claims that make men bold.

1. MORAL RIGHTS

Legal and institutional rights are typically conferred by specific rules recorded in handbooks of regulations that can be observed and studied by the citizens or members subject to the rules. But not all rights are derived from such clearly visible laws and institutional regulations. On many occasions we assert that someone has a right to something even though we know there are no regulations or laws conferring such a right. Such talk clearly makes sense, so any theory of the nature of rights that cannot account for it is radically defective.

The term "moral rights" can be applied to all rights that are held to exist prior to, or independently of, any legal or institutional rules. Moral rights so conceived form a genus divisible into various species of rights having little in common except that they are not (necessarily) legal or institutional. The following are the main specific senses of "moral right": (1) A *conventional right* is one derived from established customs and expectations, whether or not recognized by law (e.g., an old woman's right to a young man's seat on a subway train). (2) An *ideal right* is not necessarily an actual right of any kind, but is rather what *ought* to be a positive (institutional or conventional) right, and would be so in a better or ideal legal system or conventional code. (3) A *conscientious right* is a claim the recognition of which as valid is called for, not (necessarily) by actual or ideal rules or conventions, but rather by the principles of an enlightened individual conscience. (4) An *exercise right* is not, strictly speaking, a right at all, though it is so-called in popular usage; it is simply moral justification in the exercise of a right of some other kind, the latter right remaining in one's possession and unaffected by considerations bearing on the rightness or wrongness of its exercising. When a person speaks of a moral right, he may be referring to a generically moral right not further specified, or to a right in one of these four specific senses; sometimes the context does not reveal which sense of "moral" is employed, and the possibility of equivocation is always present.

2. HUMAN RIGHTS

Among the rights that are commonly said to be moral in the generic sense (that is, independent of legal or other institutional recognition) are some also called "human rights."

Human rights are sometimes understood to be ideal rights, sometimes conscientious rights, and sometimes both. In any case, they are held to be closely associated with actual claims. If a given human right is an ideal right, then human rightholders do or will have a claim against political legislators to convert (eventually) their "moral right" into a positive legal one. If the human right in question is a conscientious right, then it is an actual claim against private individuals for a certain kind of treatment—a claim that holds *now,* whatever the positive law may say about it.

I shall define "human rights" to be generically moral rights of a fundamentally important kind held equally by all human beings, unconditionally and unalterably. Whether these rights are "moral" in any of the more precise senses, I shall leave an open question to be settled by argument, not definition. Of course, it is also an open question whether there *are* any human rights and, if so, just what those rights are. All of the rights that have been characterized as "natural rights" in the leading manifestoes[1] can also be called human rights, but, as I shall be using the terms, not all human rights are also by definition natural rights. The theory of natural rights asserts not only that there are certain human rights, but also that these rights have certain further epistemic properties and a certain metaphysical status. In respect to questions of moral ontology and moral epistemology, the theory of human rights is neutral. Finally, it should be noticed that our definition includes the phrase *"all human beings"* but does not say *"only* human beings," so that a human right held by animals is not excluded by definition.

In addition to the characteristics mentioned in our definition, human rights have also been said to be "absolute." Sometimes this is simply a redundancy, another way of referring to the properties of universality and inalienability; but sometimes "absoluteness" is meant to refer to an additional characteristic, which in turn is subject to at least three interpretations. Human rights can be absolute, first, only in the sense that all rights are absolute, namely, unconditionally incumbent within the limits of their well-defined scope. Second, a human right might be held to be absolute in the sense that the rights to life, liberty, and the pursuit of happiness, as proclaimed in the Declaration of Independence, are most plausibly interpreted as absolute, namely, as "ideal directives" to relevant parties to "do their best" for the values involved. If the state has seriously considered Doe's right to his land, done its best to find alternative routes for a public road, and compensated Doe as generously as possible before expropriating him by eminent domain, it has faithfully discharged its duty of "due consideration" that is the correlative of his "right to property" conceived simply as an ideal directive. If a human right is absolute only in the sense in which an ideal directive is absolute, then it is satisfied whenever it is given the serious and respectful consideration it always deserves, even when that consideration is followed by a reluctant invasion of its corresponding interest.

The strongest and most interesting sense of "absolute" attributed to rights is that of being "absolutely exceptionless" not only within a limited scope but throughout a scope *itself* unlimited. The right to free speech would be absolute in this sense *if* it protected all speech without exception in all circumstances. In that case, the limits of the right would correspond with the limit of the form of conduct specified, and once these wide boundaries had been defined, no further boundary adjustments, incursions or encumbrances, legislative restrictions, or conditions for emergency suspensions would be permitted. For a human right to have this character it would have to be such that no conflicts with other human rights, either of the same or another type, would be possible.

Some formulations of human rights might be passed off as absolute in the strongest sense merely because they are so vaguely put. Some are formulated in conditional language ("a right to adequate nutrition *if* or *when* food is available") and then held to be absolute qua conditional. Other rights, put in glittering and general language ("a right to be treated like a human being," "a right to be treated like a person, not a thing") are safely held to be absolute because without detailed specification they yield few clear and uncontroversial injunctions. Others are formulated in language containing "standard-bearing terms" such as "reasonable," "proper," or "worthy," without any clue to the standards to be employed in applying these terms. Thus it is said that all men (like all animals) have a right not to be treated cruelly. So far, so good; there can be no exceptions to that right. But its "absoluteness" can be seen to be merely formal when one considers that cruel treatment is treatment that inflicts *unnecessary, unreasonable,* or *improper* suffering on its victim. The air of self-evidence and security beyond all controversy immediately disappears from this human right when men come to propose and debate precise standards of necessity, reasonableness, and propriety.

We should not despair, however, of finding explicit standards of (say) cruelty that will give human rights content and yet leave them plausible candidates for absoluteness in the strong sense. The right not to be *tortured,* for example, comes close to exhaustive definability in nonstandard-bearing terms, and may be such that it cannot conflict with other rights, including other human rights, and can therefore be treated as categorical and exceptionless. If torture is still too vague a term, we can give exact empirical descriptions of the Chinese Water Torture, the Bamboo Fingernail Torture, and so on, and then claim that everyone has an absolutely exceptionless right in every conceivable circumstance not to be treated in any of those precisely described ways. Does this right pass the test of nonconflict with other rights?

Suppose a foreign tyrant of Caligulan character demands of our government that it seize certain political critics, imprison them, and slowly torture them to death, and threatens that unless that is done, his police will seize the members of our diplomatic staff in his country and torture *them* to death. At first sight this appears to be an authentic case of conflict between human rights, in that it would be impossible to do anything that would have as its consequence the fulfillment of everyone's right not to be tortured. What we should say about

this blackmail situation if we wish to maintain that the right not to be tortured is nevertheless absolute (exceptionless and nonconflictable) is as follows. If the political critics in our grasp have a human right never to be tortured, then we have a categorical duty not to torture them. Thus, we ought not and will not torture them. We know, however, that this is likely to lead to the torture of the diplomatic hostages. We should therefore make every effort to dissuade Caligula, perhaps even through military pressure, not to carry out his threat. If Caligula nevertheless tortures his hostages, their rights have been infringed, but by Caligula, *not by us.*

All cases of apparent conflict of rights not to be tortured can be treated in this way. Whenever it is impossible to honor all of them, the situation causing that impossibility is itself the voluntary creation of human beings. Nothing in nature itself can ever bring such a conflict into existence. A tyrant's threat is in this respect unlike a plague that renders it impossible for everybody to get enough to eat. It would be idle to claim that the right to enough food is an absolute, categorical right, exceptionless in every conceivable circumstance, because we cannot legislate over nature. But we can legislate for man (the argument continues), and this is a plausible way to do it: *No acts of torture anywhere at any time are ever to be permitted.* All human beings can thus be possessed of a right that is absolutely exceptionless. That we have no guarantee that some people somewhere won't violate it or try to force us to violate it is no argument against the "legislation" itself.

There is therefore no objection in principle to the idea of human rights that are absolute in the sense of being categorically exceptionless. It is another question as to whether there are such rights, and what they might be. The most plausible candidates, like the right not to be tortured, will be passive negative rights, that is, rights not to be done to by others in certain ways. It is more difficult to think of active negative rights (rights not to be interfered with) or positive rights (rights to be done to in certain ways) as absolutely exceptionless. The positive rights to be given certain essentials—food, shelter, security, education—clearly depend upon the existence of an adequate supply, something that cannot be guaranteed categorically and universally.

If absoluteness in this strong sense is made part of the very meaning of the expression "human right," then it would seem that there is a lamentable paucity of human rights, if any at all. Clarity will best be served, I think, if we keep "absoluteness" out of the definition of "human right." Two questions can then be kept separate: (1) Are there any human rights, i.e., generically moral, unforfeitable, irrevocable rights held equally and universally by human beings (at least)? (2) If so, are any of these rights absolute? We turn now to a consideration of the grounds for thinking that there are human rights, so defined.

. . .

3. ABSOLUTE AND NONABSOLUTE HUMAN RIGHTS

In December 1948, the General Assembly of the United Nations adopted a Universal Declaration of Human Rights. Unlike the eighteenth-century manifestoes of natural rights, which were concerned almost exclusively with the individual's rights not to be interfered with by others, the U.N. Declaration endorses numerous basic positive rights to receive benefits and be provided with the means to satisfy basic human needs. Even the conception in the U.N. document of a basic need (in contrast to an unneeded but valuable commodity) reflected changes in the world's outlook and hopes since the eighteenth century. The U.N. Declaration contains the old-style negative rights, mostly pertaining to civic and political activities and criminal procedures, as well as the new "social and economic rights" that are correlated with the positive duties of others (usually of the state). Rights of the former kind impose duties upon private citizens and the state alike to keep hands off individuals in certain respects, to leave them alone.

Other articles, however, impose duties upon others that are so difficult that they may, under widely prevalent conditions of scarcity and conflict, be impossible for *anyone* to discharge. Articles 22–27, for example, state that "everyone, as a member of society . . . has the right to work, to free choice of employment . . . to protection against unemployment . . . to just and favorable remuneration . . . to rest and leisure . . . and periodic holidays with pay . . . to food, clothing, housing, and medical care . . . to education . . . to enjoy the arts and to share in scientific advancement and its benefits."[2] Now, as we have seen,[3] these positive (as opposed to negative) human rights are rights in an unusual new "manifesto sense," for, unlike all other claim-rights, they are not necessarily correlated with the duties of any assignable persons. The Declaration must therefore be interpreted to say that all men as such have a claim (that is, are in a position to make claim) to the goods therein mentioned, even if there should temporarily be no one in the corresponding position to be claimed against.

These social and economic human rights, therefore, are certainly not *absolute* rights, since easily imaginable and commonly actual circumstances can reduce them to mere claims. Moreover, these rights are clearly not non-conflictable. For example, where there are two persons for every job, there must be conflict between the claims of some workers to "free choice of employment," in the sense that if one worker's claim is recognized as valid, another's *must* be rejected.

Can any human rights plausibly be construed as absolutely exceptionless and therefore non-conflictable in principle, or must all rights in their very natures be vulnerable to legitimate invasion in some circumstances? The most plausible candidates for absoluteness are (some) *negative rights;* since they require no positive actions or contributions from others, they are less likely to be affected by conditions of scarcity. To say of a given negative right that it is nonconflictable is to say: (1) if conflicts occur with rights of other kinds, it must always win, and (2) no conflict is possible with other rights of its own kind. The right to speak freely is a plausible human right and is conferred by

Article 19 of the U.N. Declaration, but it is certainly not nonconflictable in the sense defined above, for it cannot plausibly be said always and necessarily to win out whenever it conflicts with another's right to reputation, privacy, or safety. In theory, of course, we could consistently hold that the free expression right always overrides rights of other kinds, but then that right would fail to satisfy the second condition for nonconflictability, no matter how stubbornly we back it. The requirement that the right in question be incapable in principle of conflicting with another person's right of the *same* kind is the real stumbling block in the path of absoluteness. Consider an audience of hecklers exercising *their* "free speech" to shout down a speaker, or some scoundrel using his "free speech" to persuade others to cut out the tongue of his hated rival. In these cases, free speech must be limited in its *own* interest. Similar examples can be provided, *mutatis mutandis,* for freedom of movement, free exercise of religion, the right to property, and to virtually all of the characteristically eighteenth-century rights of noninterference.

There remain at least three kinds of human rights that may very well be understood (without obvious absurdity) to be absolute and nonconflictable. Positive rights to "goods" that cannot ever, in the very nature of the case, be in scarce supply, are one possibility. Perhaps the right to a fair trial (really a package of positive and negative rights) or the right to equal protection of the law,[4] or "the right to equal consideration,"[5] fall into this category.

A second possibility is the negative right not to be treated inhumanely or cruelly, not to be tortured or treated barbarously.[6] Whether we as legislators (actual or ideal) should confer such an absolute right on everyone is entirely up to us. There may be good policy reasons against it, but if we are convinced by the powerful policy and moral reasons in favor of it, we needn't be deterred by the fear of conflictability. As I argued in the previous section, we can *decide* without absurdity to let this right override rights of all *other* kinds, and there is nothing in nature to bring this right into conflict with other persons' rights of the *same* kind. Article 5 of the U.N. Declaration, which forbids "torture or . . . cruel, inhuman . . . treatment," may be conceived as conferring a human right in a very strong sense, namely one which is not only universal and inalienable, but also absolute. It is still not a human right in the very strongest sense—one that applies absolutely and unalterably to all and *only* humans—for it is presumably the one right that the higher animals have, if they have any rights at all.

A third possibility is the right not to be subjected to exploitation or degradation even when such subjection is utterly painless and therefore not cruel. It is possible to treat human beings with drugs, hypnosis, or other brainwashing techniques so that they become compliant tools in the hands of their manipulators, useful as means to their manipulators' ends, but with all serious purposes of their own totally obliterated. Once human beings are in this condition, they may have no notion that they are being exploited or degraded, having come to accept and internalize their exploiters' image of themselves as their own. In this state, human beings might be raised, as Swift suggested, for food, fattened up for a few years, and then slaughtered (humanely, of course); or they might be harnessed, like donkeys, to wagons or millstones. It would be good business as well as good morals to treat them kindly (so long as they are obedient), for that way one can get more labor out of them in the long run. Clearly, kindness and "humanity," while sufficient to satisfy the rights of animals, are not sufficient for human beings, who must therefore have ascribed to them another kind of right that we deliberately withhold from animals. That is a right to a higher kind of respect, an inviolate dignity, which as a broad category includes the negative rights not to be brainwashed, not to be made into a docile instrument for the purposes of others, and not to be converted into a domesticated animal. Rights in this category are probably the only ones that are human rights in the strongest sense: unalterable, "absolute" (exceptionless and nonconflictable), and universally and *peculiarly* human.

NOTES

1. E.g., the American Declaration of Independence (1776), the Virginia Bill of Rights (1775), and the French Declaration of the Rights of Man and of Citizens (1789).

2. UNESCO, *Human Rights, a Symposium* (London and New York: Allan Wingate, 1949).

3. *Supra,* pp. 66 f. [Original source.]

4. As suggested by L. B. Frantz. Cf. *supra,* p. 81. [Original source.]

5. "Notice . . . that there is one ['natural'] right which . . . is to all intents and purposes an absolute right. That is the right to equal consideration—the right to be treated as the formula for justice provides. For this right is one which is the most basic of all, one which is under no conditions to be violated." Lucius Garvin, *A Modern Introduction to Ethics* (Boston: Houghton Mifflin Company, 1953), p. 491.

6. See *supra,* pp. 86–88. [Original source]

JOHN RAWLS

Justice as Fairness

I. THE ROLE OF JUSTICE

Justice is the first virtue of social institutions, as truth is of systems of thought. A theory however elegant and economical must be rejected or revised if it is untrue; likewise laws and institutions no matter how efficient and well-arranged must be reformed or abolished if they are unjust. Each person possesses an inviolability founded on justice that even the welfare of society as a whole cannot override. For this reason justice denies that the loss of freedom for some is made right by a greater good shared by others. It does not allow that the sacrifices imposed on a few are outweighed by the larger sum of advantages enjoyed by many. Therefore in a just society the liberties of equal citizenship are taken as settled; the rights secured by justice are not subject to political bargaining or to the calculus of social interests. The only thing that permits us to acquiesce in an erroneous theory is the lack of a better one; analogously, an injustice is tolerable only when it is necessary to avoid an even greater injustice. Being first virtues of human activities, truth and justice are uncompromising.

These propositions seem to express our intuitive conviction of the primacy of justice. No doubt they are expressed too strongly. In any event I wish to inquire whether these contentions or others similar to them are sound, and if so how they can be accounted for. To this end it is necessary to work out a theory of justice in the light of which these assertions can be interpreted and assessed. I shall begin by considering the role of the principles of justice. Let us assume, to fix ideas, that a society is a more or less self-sufficient association of persons who in their relations to one another recognize certain rules of conduct as binding and who for the most part act in accordance with them. Suppose further that these rules specify a system of cooperation designed to advance the good of those taking part in it. Then, although a society is a cooperative venture for mutual advantage, it is typically marked by a conflict as well as by an identity of interests. There is an identity of interests since social cooperation makes possible a better life for all than any would have if each were to live solely by his own efforts. There is a conflict of interests since persons are not indifferent as to how the greater benefits produced by their col-

Reprinted by permission of the publishers from *A Theory of Justice* by John Rawls, Cambridge, Mass.: The Belknap Press of Harvard University Press and Oxford University Press. Copyright © 1971 by the President and Fellows of Harvard College.

laboration are distributed, for in order to pursue their ends they each prefer a larger to a lesser share. A set of principles is required for choosing among the various social arrangements which determine this division of advantages and for underwriting an agreement on the proper distributive shares. These principles are the principles of social justice: they provide a way of assigning rights and duties in the basic institutions of society and they define the appropriate distribution of the benefits and burdens of social cooperation.

Now let us say that a society is well-ordered when it is not only designed to advance the good of its members but when it is also effectively regulated by a public conception of justice. That is, it is a society in which (1) everyone accepts and knows that the others accept the same principles of justice, and (2) the basic social institutions generally satisfy and are generally known to satisfy these principles. In this case while men may put forth excessive demands on one another, they nevertheless acknowledge a common point of view from which their claims may be adjudicated. If men's inclination to self-interest makes their vigilance against one another necessary, their public sense of justice makes their secure association together possible. Among individuals with disparate aims and purposes a shared conception of justice establishes the bonds of civic friendship; the general desire for justice limits the pursuit of other ends. One may think of a public conception of justice as constituting the fundamental charter of a well-ordered human association.

Existing societies are of course seldom well-ordered in this sense, for what is just and unjust is usually in dispute. Men disagree about which principles should define the basic terms of their association. Yet we may still say, despite this disagreement, that they each have a conception of justice. That is, they understand the need for, and they are prepared to affirm, a characteristic set of principles for assigning basic rights and duties and for determining what they take to be the proper distribution of the benefits and burdens of social cooperation. Thus it seems natural to think of the concept of justice as distinct from the various conceptions of justice and as being specified by the role

which these different sets of principles, these different conceptions, have in common.[1] Those who hold different conceptions of justice can, then, still agree that institutions are just when no arbitrary distinctions are made between persons in the assigning of basic rights and duties and when the rules determine a proper balance between competing claims to the advantages of social life. Men can agree to this description of just institutions since the notions of an arbitrary distinction and of a proper balance, which are included in the concept of justice, are left open for each to interpret according to the principles of justice that he accepts. These principles single out which similarities and differences among persons are relevant in determining rights and duties and they specify which division of advantages is appropriate. Clearly this distinction between the concept and the various conceptions of justice settles no important questions. It simply helps to identify the role of the principles of social justice.

Some measure of agreement in conceptions of justice is, however, not the only prerequisite for a viable human community. There are other fundamental social problems, in particular those of coordination, efficiency, and stability. Thus the plans of individuals need to be fitted together so that their activities are compatible with one another and they can all be carried through without anyone's legitimate expectations being severely disappointed. Moreover, the execution of these plans should lead to the achievement of social ends in ways that are efficient and consistent with justice. And finally, the scheme of social cooperation must be stable: it must be more or less regularly complied with and its basic rules willingly acted upon; and when infractions occur stabilizing forces should exist that prevent further violations and tend to restore the arrangement. Now it is evident that these three problems are connected with that of justice. In the absence of a certain measure of agreement on what is just and unjust, it is clearly more difficult for individuals to coordinate their plans efficiently

1. Here I follow H. L. A. Hart, *The Concept of Law* (Oxford, The Clarendon Press, 1961), pp. 155–159.

in order to insure that mutually beneficial arrangements are maintained. Distrust and resentment corrode the ties of civility, and suspicion and hostility tempt men to act in ways they would otherwise avoid. So while the distinctive role of conceptions of justice is to specify basic rights and duties and to determine the appropriate distributive shares, the way in which a conception does this is bound to affect the problems of efficiency, coordination, and stability. We cannot, in general, assess a conception of justice by its distributive role alone, however useful this role may be in identifying the concept of justice. We must take into account its wider connections; for even though justice has a certain priority, being the most important virtue of institutions, it is still true that, other things equal, one conception of justice is preferable to another when its broader consequences are more desirable.

II. TWO PRINCIPLES OF JUSTICE

I shall now state in a provisional form the two principles of justice that I believe would be chosen in the original position. . . .

First: each person is to have an equal right to the most extensive basic liberty compatible with a similar liberty for others.

Second: social and economic inequalities are to be arranged so that they are both (a) reasonably expected to be to everyone's advantage, and (b) attached to positions and offices open to all. . . .

By way of general comment, these principles primarily apply, as I have said, to the basic structure of society. They are to govern the assignment of rights and duties and to regulate the distribution of social and economic advantages. As their formulation suggests, these principles presuppose that the social structure can be divided into two more or less distinct parts, the first principle applying to the one, the second to the other. They distinguish between those aspects of the social system that define and secure the equal liberties of citizenship and those that specify and establish social and economic inequalitites. The basic liberties of citizens are, roughly speaking, political liberty (the right to vote and to be eligible for public office) together with freedom of speech and

assembly; liberty of conscience and freedom of thought; freedom of the person along with the right to hold (personal) property; and freedom from arbitrary arrest and seizure as defined by the concept of the rule of law. These liberties are all required to be equal by the first principle, since citizens of a just society are to have the same basic rights.

The second principle applies, in the first approximation, to the distribution of income and wealth and to the design of organizations that make use of differences in authority and responsibility, or chains of command. While the distribution of wealth and income need not be equal, it must be to everyone's advantage, and at the same time, positions of authority and offices of command must be accessible to all. One applies the second principle by holding positions open, and then, subject to this constraint, arranges social and economic inequalities so that everyone benefits.

These principles are to be arranged in a serial order with the first principle prior to the second. This ordering means that a departure from the institutions of equal liberty required by the first principle cannot be justified by, or compensated for, by greater social and economic advantages. The distribution of wealth and income, and the hierarchies of authority, must be consistent with both the liberties of equal citizenship and equality of opportunity.

It is clear that these principles are rather specific in their content, and their acceptance rests on certain assumptions that I must eventually try to explain and justify. A theory of justice depends upon a theory of society in ways that will become evident as we proceed. For the present, it should be observed that the two principles (and this holds for all formulations) are a special case of a more general conception of justice that can be expressed as follows.

All social values—liberty and opportunity, income and wealth, and the bases of self-respect—are to be distributed equally unless an unequal distribution of any, or all, of these values is to everyone's advantage.

Injustice, then, is simply inequalities that are not to the benefit of all. Of course, this conception is extremely vague and requires interpretation.

JOEL FEINBERG

Liberty-Limiting Principles

The distinction between self-regarding and other-regarding behavior, as Mill intended it to be understood, does seem at least roughly serviceable, and unlikely to invite massive social interference in private affairs. I think most critics of Mill would grant that, but reject the harm principle [below] on the opposite ground that it doesn't permit enough interference. These writers would allow at least one, and as many as five or more, additional valid grounds for coercion. Each of these proposed grounds is stated in a principle listed below. One might hold that restriction of one person's liberty can be justified:

1. To prevent harm to others, either a) injury to individual persons *(The Private Harm Principle)*, or b) impairment of institutional practices that are in the public interest *(The Public Harm Principle)*;

2. To prevent offense to others *(The Offense Principle)*;

3. To prevent harm to self *(Legal Paternalism)*;

4. To prevent or punish sin, i.e., to "enforce morality as such" *(Legal Moralism)*;

5. To benefit the self *(Extreme Paternalism)*;

6. To benefit others *(The Welfare Principle)*.

The liberty-limiting principles on this list are best understood as stating neither necessary nor sufficient conditions for justified coercion, but rather specifications of the *kinds* of reasons that are always relevant or acceptable in support of proposed coercion, even though in a given case they may not be conclusive.[1] Each principle states that interference might be permissible *if* (but not *only if*) a certain condition is satisfied. Hence the principles are not mutually exclusive; it is possible to hold two or more of them at once, even all of them to-

gether, and it is possible to deny all of them. Moreover, the principles cannot be construed as stating sufficient conditions for legitimate interference with liberty, for even though the principle is satisfied in a given case, the general presumption against coercion might not be outweighed. The harm principle, for example, does not justify state interference to prevent a tiny bit of inconsequential harm. Prevention of minor harm always counts in favor of proposals (as in a legislature) to restrict liberty, but in a given instance it might not count *enough* to outweigh the general presumption against interference, or it might be outweighed by the prospect of practical difficulties in enforcing the law, excessive costs, and forfeitures of privacy. A liberty-limiting principle states considerations that are always good reasons for coercion, though neither exclusively nor, in every case, decisively good reasons.

It will not be possible to examine each principle in detail here, and offer "proofs" and "refutations." The best way to defend one's selection of principles is to show to which positions they commit one on such issues as censorship of literature, "morals offenses," and compulsory social security programs. General principles arise in the course of deliberations over particular problems, especially in the efforts to defend one's judgments by showing that they are consistent with what has gone before. If a principle commits one to an antecedently unacceptable judgment, then one has to modify or supplement the principle in a way that does the least damage to the harmony of one's particular and general opinions taken as a group. On the other hand, when a solid, well-entrenched principle entails a change in a particular judgment, the overriding claims of consistency may require that the judgment be adjusted. This sort of dialectic is similar to the reasonings that are prevalent in law courts. When similar cases are decided in opposite ways, it is incumbent on the court to distinguish them in some respect that will recon-

Joel Feinberg, *Social Philosophy,* © 1973, pp. 33–35. Reprinted by permission of Prentice-Hall, Inc., Englewood Cliffs, New Jersey.

1. I owe this point to Professor Michael Bayles. See his contribution to *Issues in Law and Morality,* ed. Norman Care and Thomas Trelogan (Cleveland: The Press of Case Western Reserve University, 1973).

cile the separate decisions with each other and with the common rule applied to each. Every effort is made to render current decisions consistent with past ones unless the precedents seem so disruptive of the overall internal harmony of the law that they must, reluctantly, be revised or abandoned. In social and political philosophy every person is on his own, and the counterparts to "past decisions" are the most confident judgments one makes in ordinary normative discourse. The philosophical task is to extract from these "given" judgments the principles that render them consistent, adjusting and modifying where necessary in order to convert the whole body of opinions into an intelligible, coherent system. There is no a priori way of refuting another's political opinions, but if our opponents are rational men committed to the ideal of consistency, we can always hope to show them that a given judgment is inconsistent with one of their own acknowledged principles. Then something will have to give.

SUGGESTED READINGS FOR CHAPTER 1

Books and Articles

Beauchamp, Tom L., ed. *Ethics and Public Policy*. Englewood Cliffs, N.J.: Prentice-Hall, 1975.

Feinberg, Joel. *Social Philosophy*. Englewood Cliffs, N.J.: Prentice-Hall, 1973.

Feinberg, Joel, and Gross, Hyman, eds. *Philosophy of Law*. Encino, Calif.: Dickenson Publishing Co., 1976.

Frankena, William K. *Ethics*. 2nd edition. Englewood Cliffs, N.J.: Prentice-Hall, 1973.

Gert, Bernard. *The Moral Rules*. New York: Harper & Row, 1970.

Hare, R. M. *The Language of Morals*. New York: Oxford University Press, 1952.

Hudson, W. D. *Modern Moral Philosophy*. Garden City, N.Y.: Doubleday Anchor, 1970.

MacIntyre, Alasdair. *A Short History of Ethics*. New York: Macmillan, 1966.

Macklin, Ruth. "Moral Concerns and Appeals to Rights and Duties: Grounding Claims in a Theory of Justice." *Hastings Center Report* 6 (October, 1976), 31–38.

Nielsen, Kai. "Problems of Ethics." In Edwards, Paul, ed. *Encyclopedia of Philosophy*. New York: Macmillan and Free Press, 1967. Vol. 3, pp. 117–134.

O'Connor, Daniel J. *Aquinas and Natural Law*. New York: St. Martin's, 1968.

Outka, Gene, and Reeder, John, eds. *Religion and Morality*. Garden City, N.Y.: Anchor Books, 1973.

Rachels, James. *Understanding Moral Philosophy*. Encino, Calif.: Dickenson Publishing Co., 1976.

Rawls, John. *A Theory of Justice*. Cambridge, Mass.: Harvard University Press, 1971.

Reich, Warren T., ed. *Encyclopedia of Bioethics*. New York: Macmillan and Free Press, 1978.

Taylor, Paul. *Principles of Ethics: An Introduction*. Encino, Calif.: Dickenson Publishing Co., 1975.

Bibliographies

Hospers, John. *Human Conduct*. Shorter edition. New York: Harcourt Brace Jovanovich, 1972. Reading lists at the end of each section.

Philosopher's Index. Quarterly and annual volumes.

Taylor, Paul. *Principles of Ethics: An Introduction*. Suggested readings at the end of each section.

2.
Bioethics as a Field of Ethics

Bioethics is the branch of applied ethics which studies practices and developments in the biomedical fields. Although the term "bioethics" is a relatively modern invention, the subject matter of the field includes issues which have been debated for centuries. Viewing the field historically, one can identify distinct stages in the evolution of bioethics. From a more systematic perspective, it is possible to discover several major themes which have predominated in the literature of the field. These themes provide a basic continuity among the stages, linking the field of bioethics to traditional discussions in philosophical and religious ethics, political philosophy, and the philosophy of law.

STAGES IN THE DEVELOPMENT OF BIOETHICS

Medical Ethics. The oldest component of bioethics is "medical ethics," which since the time of Hippocrates has formulated ethical norms for the conduct of health professionals in the treatment of patients. The Hippocratic Oath, Percival's *Medical Ethics* (published in England in 1803), and the American Medical Association's *Code of Ethics* (1847) are landmark documents in this long tradition. During the past century these codes of ethics written by and for physicians have been supplemented by similar codes for several other groups of health professionals, for example, nurses. In addition, health professionals and members of numerous nonmedical professions alike have contributed to the rapidly expanding literature on ethical issues in clinical practice. (Chapter 4 discusses several general issues in the professional-patient relationship. In Chapters 5 through 7, three specific problems of contemporary clinical practice are analyzed. Chapter 8 explores the social dimension of clinical practice—the problem of health care allocation.)

Research Ethics. Ethical issues in the clinical relationship continue to constitute a very significant aspect of bioethics. However, especially since the seventeenth century a novel phenomenon has emerged within the biomedical fields—the effort to derive new knowledge through systematic human experimentation. In the nineteenth and twentieth centuries, as both the volume and the visible achievements of this research have increased, efforts have been made to discuss the ethical issues raised by biomedical research and its offspring, biomedical technology. One facet of this discussion has been the development of ethical codes concerning research involving human subjects. These codes propose guidelines for what might be called the microlevel of biomedical research; that is, they focus on the obligations of the individual researcher in his or her relationship to each individual subject. Although brief statements of researchers' obligations appeared during the nineteenth century, the first major code of research ethics was not developed until the late 1940s. The Nuremberg Code, as it came to be called, was drafted in response to the Nazi practice of performing high-risk and often lethal experiments on concentration camp inmates and other nonconsenting subjects. Since the formulation of the Nuremberg Code (1947), several additional international and national codes of research ethics have been drafted, and numerous books on ethical aspects of human experimentation have appeared. (Chapters 9 and 10 examine several major ethical issues in research involving human subjects.)

A rather different type of ethical analysis is applied to what might be called the macrolevel of biomedical research. Here one is not primarily concerned with the protection of individual research subjects, but rather seeks to assess the potential long-term social consequences—both positive and negative—of biomedical research and technology. The essay by Leon Kass in this chapter illustrates how the general principles of "technology assessment" can be applied to various biomedical technologies. (Chapters 11 and 12 provide more detailed discussion of sample biomedical and behavioral technologies.)

Public Policy. Since the early 1960s, a third stage in the development of bioethics has become apparent, the effort to formulate public policy guidelines for both clinical care and biomedical research. During this phase authors from various disciplines have advanced public policy recommendations on numerous issues, for example, the equitable allocation of scarce medical resources or the social control of human experimentation. In the case of several bioethical issues, discussion has been supplemented by the official enactment of policy—through legislation, regulation, or judicial decision. In turn, these official enactments have been subjected to ethical analysis and evaluation. Thus, bioethics, while distinct from law, has sought to test proposed or existing legal provisions by raising the question: What, if anything, *should* the law permit or require with respect to particular biomedical issues? Such questions of public policy arise in virtually all of the subsequent chapters of this book.

MAJOR THEMES IN THE LITERATURE OF BIOETHICS

A variety of principles, duties, rights, and values are analyzed or appealed to in the discussion of bioethical issues. The complex interplay of arguments cannot be reduced to a simple common denominator. However, three themes dominate much of the discussion: beneficence, justice, and self-determination.

1. *Principles of Beneficence*. Discussions of beneficence frequently include two distinct but related foci—the prevention of harm and the production of good. Traditionally, professional medical ethics has emphasized the first of these foci, adopting as its central norm the principle "Do no harm." Within the medical context the principle of not harming has meant that the health professional should take great care not to compound an ill patient's condition by causing further injury. Ethical codes governing biomedical research continue this tradition through their concern for the protection of human subjects. Similarly, bioethicists attempt to assess in advance the possible negative social consequences of new biomedical technologies in order to protect large groups of persons from potential harm. For example, critics of test tube fertilization argue that the use of the technique will constitute a major step toward the large-scale (and, in their view, dehumanizing) use of laboratory-based methods for human reproduction.

There are no sharp breaks on the continuum between "preventing harm" and "producing good." However, the positive principle of beneficence is generally thought to be more demanding since it requires the conferring of benefits rather than merely the avoidance of harm. At the same time, the positive principle may be less stringent than the negative in the sense that it allows at least the risk of some harm in the course of attempting to produce great benefits. The general justification of biomedical research is frequently based on the promise of advances in scientific knowledge or medical progress. Advocates of new biomedical and behavioral technologies—for example, gene therapy or new modes of behavior control—seek to demonstrate that the long-term benefits of the technologies outweigh their negative side-effects. (The reading on utilitarianism in Chapter 1 provides a helpful theoretical perspective on the assessment of harms and benefits.)

2. *Principles of Justice.* The principles of beneficence, by themselves, say nothing about the distribution of harms and benefits. The allocation issue is most frequently discussed under the general heading of justice, or equity. Principles of justice play a major role in several facets of bioethical discussion. Equal access to health care is identified as an important social goal. The overuse of the poor or the institutionalized in biomedical research is criticized as an inequitable distribution of research risks. Similarly, persons assessing the long-term consequences of technology seek to ensure that the benefits and harms of new biomedical technologies are allocated fairly among various social groups. (John Rawls' discussion of justice in the preceding chapter indicates one possible approach to the problem of equitable allocation.)

3. *The Right of Self-Determination.* Beneficence and justice are sometimes said to be adequate principles for the development of a normative theory. However, in the literature of bioethics there is a third theme which is not adequately represented by either beneficence or justice. This theme, self-determination, is grounded in the tradition of human rights which has had such a significant impact on Western social and political thought during the last four centuries.

The right of self-determination is perhaps the central element in the relatively recent emphasis on patients' rights. This right is also an important consideration in discussions of informed consent in both the clinical and the research setting. For example, there are debates concerning the capacity for self-determination of a prisoner who expresses a wish to take part in research or the right of an epileptic patient who desires psychosurgery. Self-determination is also a major theme in discussions of abortion (where the right to control one's body is often claimed) and euthanasia (where the right to die with dignity is often asserted). (The extent and limits of individual freedom are explored in the excerpts from Joel Feinberg's *Social Philosophy* reprinted in Chapter 1.)

In some of the readings which follow in this book one of these three themes is featured. In others, the authors attempt to strike a balance among beneficence, justice, and self-determination. The question of the proper relationship among the three themes constitutes one of the central problems in contemporary ethical discussions.

L. W.

SAMUEL GOROVITZ

Bioethics and Social Responsibility[1]

I

Bioethics is the critical examination of the moral dimensions of decision-making in health related contexts and in contexts involving the biological sciences. Many of the problems of bioethics are perennial, and those who have been involved in clinical medicine and in biological research have reflected on the moral limits on their activities as long as those activities have existed. In the past, however, medical capability fell so far short of commonly accepted medical aspirations that there was rarely any question about whether or not medical intervention ought to be employed. Now, the efficacy of medical intervention has increased so stunningly in many ways that the question is inescapable [as to] whether medical capability sometimes extends beyond reasonable aspirations. Bioethics has therefore begun to take on the trappings of a coherent discipline —traditions, a literature, an identifiable group of practitioners, a largely agreed upon subject matter, shared methodology, somewhat standardized conditions of professional admissibility, a sense of distinctiveness that arises out of these other components, and a market or constituency. There is even an encyclopedia in the works.[2]

Although concern with the moral aspects of the life sciences is ancient, such issues have historically been addressed primarily within the medical profession, especially as it has evolved explicit and implicit canons of professional conduct; among theologians, especially as they have sought to understand the natural processes of birth, human sexuality, and death; and by those who, through legislative action, have sought to protect or advance the public interest by the advocacy of legal constraints or entitlements pertaining to medical or scientific

matters. In these areas, and to a lesser extent in others, there has been published discussion of moral issues in medical and biological contexts. Thus, for source materials, a historian of medical ethics would look to writings in various fields in, or with an interest in, health care —but not to an independent literature in medical ethics. Now, the moral issues in medicine and biological science have aroused dramatically increased attention because of the dramatically increased efficacy of medical and scientific procedures, their greater visibility through mass media, and changing social expectations pertaining to health care. Philosophers have come lately to bioethical problems, as compared with theologians, lawyers, and some members of the medical and scientific communities, but . . . they have important contributions to make. Indeed, unable in this introductory survey to treat any particular problem in depth, I shall instead try to make the case that the contribution that philosophers can make to bioethics is unique and essential.

By "health related contexts" I refer to the full spectrum of activities pertaining to the maintenance and achievement of health. These include specific clinical interactions between a physician or other health care provider and patient, and also include social policy decisions about the allocation of national resources as between preventive and curative medicine, between therapeutic medicine and medical research, and between health related expenditures and other kinds of social programs. I would also include conceptual issues such as clarification of the concept of health and identification of what kinds of physiological, psychological, or sociological states carry entitlements to or justify medical intervention. By "the biological sciences" I refer to scientific inquiries into organic and biochemical processes—including both the results of such inquiries and the protocols by which such in-

Reprinted from *The Monist,* Vol. 60, No. 1 (January 1977) with the permission of the author and the publisher. This essay is adapted from the author's introduction to *Moral Problems in Medicine,* Prentice-Hall, 1976.

quiries are advanced. I take it that "social responsibility" refers ambiguously both to the responsibility borne by individuals toward the social community and also to the responsibilities that social organizations, including governments, have as agents of redistribution, protection, prevention, compensation, facilitation, and regulation, in the public interest.

I cannot here provide any exhaustive account of the issues that arise in bioethics, or even of the kinds of issues. A sense of the subject can be conveyed, however, by the brief citation of several fairly general issue areas, along with just one specific illustrative problem within each area. These citations are neither exhaustive nor mutually exclusive.[3]

The Allocation of Limited Resources. At every level, from the individual practitioner to the federal government, needs outstrip resources, and the resulting conflicts about priorities are laden with evaluative questions. Illustration: given limited governmental capacity to finance health related endeavors, how much of the available resources should be allocated to improving future health care through basic research, and how much to improving the quality of present health care through support for rural clinics, new medical schools, etc.?

The Regulation of Health Care. Medical practice has been largely self-regulatory, but there is a growing sense that it is too important for that. Yet the proper locus and limits of external regulation can only be determined in the light of a viewpoint about social and political organization, and the nature of the conflict between social needs and individual rights. Illustration: under what conditions and for what reasons should mass-screening for heritable diseases or severe birth defects via amniocentesis (examination of fetal cells drawn from the amniotic fluid) or other means be required or encouraged as a matter of public policy?

The Use of Human Subjects in Experimentation. Although this cluster of issues has received wide attention within the scientific community, with certain codes of conduct having gained acceptance, there are still questions that are vigorously disputed. Illustration: what, precisely, is the nature of informed consent to participation as a subject in an experiment on the part of persons who are disadvantaged with respect to making autonomous decisions—e.g., infants, the mentally retarded, or perhaps those who are involuntarily confined?

The Scope of Medical Prerogative. It has been largely conceded that medical decisions should be made by medical professionals, but it is a matter of some dispute what constitutes a medical decision. Illustration: are these strictly medical questions, and if not, what sort are they—whether a diabetic should be treated with insulin, whether a kidney patient should receive renal dialysis, whether a woman should have an abortion, whether a homosexual or drug user is sick, whether a new drug or surgical procedure is suitable for general use?

Constraint of Research Objectives. Here the issues go beyond the mores of using human subjects to the question of the fundamental purposes and possible effects of research. Illustration: should experimentation which may lead to the raising of experimental subjects in vitro, via nuclear implantation from human genetic material, be permitted or regulated?

Responsibility for Dependent Persons. Many people deviate from what may be considered normal in the functional capacity of a human being, the reasons for such diminished capacity including retardation, congenital deformity, blindness, severe illness, injury, advanced age, and the like. Medical practice is closely involved in the plight of such persons. But it is not clear what the nature and locus of responsibility are for those who, for whatever reason, are unable to function independently. Illustration: if social policy or law prohibits infanticide in cases of radical deformity or readily demonstrable severe retardation, is there also a communal responsibility to provide resources and facilities for the care of such individuals? Are the problems, principles, and responsibilities different in cases of severe senility or other geriatric infirmity?

Death and Dying. New criteria of death are being shaped, used as guidelines, and affirmed in the courts. But questions remain concerning policy toward the terminally ill. Illustration: what principles should govern decisions concerning euthanasia, withdrawal of costly or scarce life support systems, determination of narcotic dosages, aggressiveness of treatment of life-threatening infections, and the like, in the terminally ill patient, with what dependency, if any, on the patient's age?

Commitments of the Medical Profession. The physician's classical commitment to prolong life and relieve suffering places him in conflict situations where adherence to one value requires violation of the other. This is merely a special case of the conflicts inherent in the physician's multiple commitments to his patient, his profession, his own monetary or other career-related interests, the medical profession generally, and his own value structure. Illustration: the *Archives of Dermatology* recently included an FBI wanted poster in its "News and Notes" section, because the wanted woman was known to have recurrent dermatological problems, and the AMA, through its editorial processes, sanctioned this sort of cooperation with the FBI. If a dermatologist, already treating a patient, recognizes her in such a poster, has he an obligation to report her to authorities? Has he even the right to do so, as one who has a commitment to the patient's well-being and to confidentiality? Is the AMA's position credible that the inclusion of such notices in medical journals is unproblematic because "no issues of medical ethics are involved?"[4]

The Physician-Patient Relationship. Physicians have a uniquely privileged and powerful position with regard to their patients, and the nature of the actual and optimal relationship between physician and patient is thus a highly charged question for both. Illustration: when a physician discovers an infant to have a heritable disease, and upon testing the ostensible parents discovers that neither is the carrier, what should he tell to whom, and why?

Control of Behavior. The increasing prominence of psychopharmaceutical techniques of behavior control, psychosurgery, behavior modification by aversive conditioning, and the conjectured prospects for intervention via electrode implantation, have all received a good deal of public attention as issues raising moral dilemmas. Confronted by the power of such techniques, one can hardly help but ask what sorts of behavior may justifiably be controlled, by whom, in what ways, for what purposes, in accordance with what values. But less obvious issues also need to be brought to the surface. Illustration: the "medical model" has been debated at length with regard to its appropriateness for conceptualization in mental health or behavior problem areas. But in some ways, the medical model itself, with its fundamental dependence on classification of people by experts into categories of normal or deviant functioning, is an ominously powerful force in general. Given the influence that medical judgments have on attitudes and behavior—what Willard Gaylin has called the physician's special "rights to coercion"—should the concepts of normality that underlie medical practices and public health policy be subjected to greater critical scrutiny from outside the medical profession?[5] Just what are those concepts of normality—how do they limit or influence therapeutic intervention? Are there credible alternatives to them—and if so, how ought differing models of normality be evaluated?

II

In an earlier era, when considerations of medical ethics took place largely within the medical community, the phrase "medical ethics" would frequently be taken to refer to a variety of issues concerning the conventions of medical practice. This tradition is reflected even today in the views of the Judicial Council of the American Medical Association, which, in its statement on the Principles of Medical Ethics, addresses attention to such questions as whether physicians may advertise, collect referral commissions, lecture to groups of chiropractors, etc.[6] To distinguish these questions about the conventions of professional practice from questions of substantial philosophical interest, I refer to the former as questions of professional etiquette.

More recently, the taxonomy of problems in bioethics has come to be viewed differently. Instead of referring to the old issues of professional etiquette, medical ethics came to be taken as referring to a new variety of problems, of the sort exemplified above, characterizable largely in terms that are essentially medical or biological in origin. Thus, the focus shifted to problems of abortion, birth defects, confidentiality in the physician-patient relationship, dying, euthanasia, financing of health care, genetic counseling, human subjects in experimentation, involuntary confinement, etc. That taxonomy persists as the most prominent interpretation of the problems of bioethics. It is legitimate and useful; the problems thus described are real and important. However, I wish to argue for the concomitant importance, particularly for philosophers, of a different taxonomy.

Inquiry into many of the medical contexts that generate moral dilemmas reveals certain common threads of philosophical puzzlement. For example, questions about the right to suicide, about involuntary confinement, about the Jehovah's Witnesses' right to refuse blood transfusions, and about whether the adolescent patient should have access to medical treatment in confidence from parents (who perhaps directly or indirectly cover its costs), all involve issues of personal autonomy and the justifiability of paternalistic intervention. Similarly, questions about responsibility to sustain the lives of seriously deformed newborn infants, like questions about responsibility to sustain the lives of severely deteriorated, terminally ill victims of injury, illness, or advanced age, raise questions about the value of life and the relevance of considerations of quality of life to the assessment of value of life. Only a consistent point of view about personal autonomy, the justifiability of paternalistic intervention, and the considerations that are relevant to determining the value of life in general or a given life in particular, can allow one to develop a consistent perspective on the various different problems in bioethics that are reflected in a medically inspired taxonomy. There is thus a taxonomy of topics, fundamentally philosophical in conception, that must be addressed as a part of the process of dealing with the problems of bioethics and social responsibility. These philosophical topics are not new. What is perhaps new is the extent to which clarity about them is demanded for the resolution of pressing problems that arise elsewhere.

I will not attempt to enumerate such topics exhaustively; I will simply identify those that seem most obviously to arise, and illustrate in part their relation to bioethical problems.

Autonomy. To what extent is it morally required to allow individuals to act in pursuit of their own aspirations? Does an individual with self-destructive aspirations thereby lose the right to autonomy generally enjoyed by others? Should freedom to act include freedom to follow a foolish or tragic (e.g., suicidal) course of events, or is it justifiable to override another's autonomy paternalistically, as well as for reasons of social benefit? Does respect for a patient's autonomy require honesty on the part of the physician, even when deception seems medically prudent?

Coercion. When is an act voluntary? What conditions must be met for an experimental subject to have volunteered? Do federal programs related to public health or population planning become coercive if they are based on the provision of powerful incentives? Under what conditions is coercion justified in medical contexts?

Normalcy. Does it make any sense to try to characterize health or illness in terms of a notion of normalcy? What are the criteria for distinguishing between desirable and undesirable deviations from physiological or psychological normalcy for health related purposes, assuming that the notion of normalcy is useful?

Naturalness. Can the familiar case be sustained that it is sometimes right to prolong life using natural means but wrong to sustain it by artificial means? Is the distinction between artificial and natural means an intelligible one? Is "exotic" life-saving therapy any less natural than routine abdominal surgery or the use of antibiotics?

Rights. Much of the talk about ethical issues in medicine invokes the notion of rights. Is there a right of a fetus to be born, of a patient to have access to his medical record, of a sick person to receive medical treatment, or of a physician to practice where he pleases? Insofar as claims about rights and the resolution of conflicts of rights are obscure, so too are the arguments that involve such claims.

Dependency. Is there a sense in which some individuals can be identified as dependent persons in medically relevant ways? Is anyone genuinely independent? If the notion of dependency is a medically legitimate one, what consequence does a person's being dependent have for the justifiability of paternalistic intervention in his life?

Justice. Is it unjust to distribute health care as a free market commodity, or to consider the social utility of persons in distributing scarce medical resources?

Needs and Wants. Even granting that one's health-related needs should be met, how are needs to be distinguished from wants that would justify a lesser claim on the benefits of social organization? Insofar as it makes sense to speak of a right to health care, is there a distinction between the need for antibiotic intervention to combat a life-threatening infection on the one hand and the desire for cosmetic surgery to alleviate the evidence of aging on the other?

Responsibility. If there can be said to be a right to health care—in the sense that the body politic must make treatment available to individuals suffering from specific diseases the treatments for which are known—is this right to be limited in any way by considerations of personal responsibility? For example, under a system of federally financed free medical care, should the individual whose chronic smoking results in respiratory disease be entitled to treatment at public expense, when his imprudent behavior took place in the face of warnings in virtue of which his illness can be viewed to some extent as voluntary?

Personhood. Under what conditions is it appropriate to consider an organism to be a person? What is the relationship between this issue and questions of abortion, the use of fetal tissue in research, and the withdrawal of life support systems from an irreversibly comatose patient?

One could go on at length. My purpose here is merely to show that many familiar philosoph-ical topics are centrally important to the illumination of problems in bioethics—and, more importantly, that each such philosophical topic cuts across a variety of bioethical issues. Thus, a philosophical inquiry into bioethics might well focus, say, on the notion of paternalism, and investigate the variety of medical and scientific contexts in which that issue arises; likewise for each of the other entries in the philosophical taxonomy I have suggested. One of the virtues of such an approach is that it enables the philosopher to concentrate on new problems in a way that is familiar and in the use of which he has substantial expertise. An additional virtue of this approach is that it helps those outside philosophy to see connections among medical and scientific problems that are not so easily seen otherwise, and it thereby exhibits more plainly the importance of philosophical inquiry to the resolution of problems of broad social interest.

III

This [essay] is focused primarily on those problems in bioethics which arise out of new developments in biomedical research. Such problems, of course, do not exhaust the field of bioethics. The question of whether death is always and everywhere an evil, whether one has a right willingly to embrace it, and whether life has value independently of the experiences for which it is a precondition, are ancient questions. So too are a number of questions pertaining to the responsibilities of the physician in regard to his patient. Other problems, which seem to arise out of new developments in biomedical research, are largely old problems given new force by recent developments. But there are some genuinely new problems as well. I want now to focus some attention on what some of these problems are, and how they relate to the technical developments that have nurtured or spawned them.

Among the old problems given new force by recent developments, I would include many of those arising in clinical medicine. For example, it is not a new puzzlement to wonder about the appropriate societal constraints on parental reactions to newborn infants who are undesirable in virtue of having certain unanticipated and repugnant characteristics. What is new is the power of the medical profession to save malformed infants who would have died under earlier circumstances. Similarly, what gives deliberations about euthanasia a new urgency is our increased capacity to sustain life beyond reasonable hope of recovery. How one ought to die, and the extent to which one ought to be able to influence or determine the manner and mode of one's death, are old questions. What is new is the power of medical technology to intervene in what were previously dramas that played out largely in their own way.

Similarly, our new abilities to gain information intensify old conflicts. For example, that we can learn via amniocentesis that a fetus is defective sharpens the debate about abortion. We can now identify certain individuals as defective (sometimes grievously) prior to birth, and hence can circumvent the question of infanticide by advocating early abortion in such instances. Debate about the justifiability of abortion is not new; what is new is our power to perform safe abortions, and the quality of the information that we can bring to bear in some instances in stating the case for abortion.

The new problems arising from technical developments can be divided into those that arise from developments in health care technology and those that stem from developments of other sorts. Among the most important developments in health care technology that generate new moral problems are these: . . .

1. New techniques for obtaining and handling information, including both specific testing procedure such as amniocentesis, and an understanding of statistical phenomena such as are considered in epidemiology, as well as the powers of information-handling provided by computerization.

2. Increased understanding of both the physiological and psychological dimensions of a person each as a complex set of interrelated systems that can to some extent be separated and acted on independently—e.g., as respiration can be sustained despite renal failure.

3. The development of psycho-pharmaceuticals and other technological methods of influencing or controlling behavior.

4. The ability to conduct research or intervene therapeutically in a way that involves manipulation of human development.

Among the technical developments not directly related to health care, but with substantial impact on questions of health, are the developments in food technology, including the widespread use of chemical food additives, and industrialization, with its attendant pollution of the environment with substances directly related to the pathogenesis of a large variety of diseases.

Each of these areas of technical progress generates or intensifies a cluster of ethically troubling issues. Let me mention a few. . . . Our understanding of epidemiology raises some fundamental questions about the competing claims of curative and preventive medicine. Is it justifiable as social policy, for example, that we have allocated $600 million in quest of cures for malignant diseases, and only $30 million to exploration of the carcinogenic effects of environmental pollutants, when there seems to be increasing evidence that a large percentage of the malignant disease that we wish we knew how to cure arises from the presence in the environment of substances that we could regulate more easily than we can control the resulting diseases? To be sure, curing disease is more dramatic than preventing it, and hence has more appeal both politically and medically. Still, it is not implausible that reflection on the relationship between social responsibility and health would produce arguments in favor of shifting resources dramatically from curative to preventive medicine.

In older, simpler times, an individual was thought to be either alive or dead—the occasional problem being to determine which. Now that we realize that physiological systems deteriorate at different rates and in different ways, we are forced to recognize that, in some of the more difficult cases, whether we have an instance of death or not depends on decisions that we make about which systems have a fundamental importance to our conception of life. Thus, the respirating, digesting, irreversibly comatose quasi-person devoid of neocortical activity, challenges us, not to discover whether death or life is present, but to decide which physiological systems are to count in what ways in our deliberations about how to behave in regard to the person or corpse at issue. It is because we understand so much better than we used to what is happening physiologically, and have so much more ability to influence it, that the definition of death is now problematic.

There is no serious question that some use of chemotherapy for psychological purposes is laudable. For example, lithium compounds can transform the lives of certain manic-depressive patients, enabling even some who had required institutionalization to lead happy, productive, stable lives. There seems little basis for dispute about the justifiability of this sort of pharmacological intervention. But the use of drugs such as ritalin as a means of controlling the behavior of inattentive and disruptive school children who lack any identifiable organic deficiency seems a highly suspect use of chemicals to control behavior. Perhaps, after all, it is the school setting that is in need of therapy. But by what principles do we condemn the latter use of drugs while lauding the former?

The horror that some express at the prospects of genetic experimentation results in part from an unwarranted extrapolation from what is presently possible, or even plausible for the foreseeable future, to a fictionalized vision of malevolent geneticists manufacturing humans and quasi-humans in inhumane ways for inhumane purposes. But some genetic research, particularly that involving recombinatory use of genetic material, raises troubling questions now. Thus, the temporary self-imposed moratorium . . . on such research, and the stringent new guidelines suggested by the research community itself for conducting such experiments safely, reflect the fact that geneticists are now able to create new forms of life with characteristics that are not fully predictable and which, while they fall far short of the fictional mass production of human beings, nonetheless could have substantial impact on the well-being of human beings. And it is explicit in the programs of some of those engaged in such research that a possible future benefit of the work is direct intervention in the genetic development of individual human beings.

Scientific inquiry is a social enterprise supported and conducted at the pleasure of the public whom it ultimately serves. Yet, like medicine, it is practiced by a professional elite whose judgments are based on considerations that are essentially obscure in many ways to the public at large. Thus we find, in grappling with questions pertaining to public regulation and public accountability in regard to scientific research, that we must confront traditional questions concerning the proper scope of democratic processes, and the prudence of establishing and supporting social institutions that invest power in elite groups charged to act in the interest of a comparatively benighted public.

Two additional points bear mention. First, in the medical context issues of distributive justice and scarcity are particularly apposite. Medical science is in its infancy. Its successes, largely in the area of infectious diseases and surgical techniques, are impressive. Still, next to nothing is known about the pathogenesis of malignancies, circulatory or cardiac ailments, arthritis, degenerative neurological diseases, and most of the rest of what concerns medical science. The best and most advanced of medical care, as more and more is learned about the etiology and cure of disease, will for the foreseeable future be in scarce supply. Further, medicine in its entirety will be in competition with other socially valued enterprises for resources that are limited. It will be necessary to address these problems in terms of an unending need to allocate limited resources in the face of competing claims.

Finally, it is clear that there is an inherent conflict between epistemological and ethical aspects of experimentation. For certain kinds of experiments, to inform the subject of the nature of the experiment is to destroy the validity of the experiment at the same time. For example, if we wish to screen newborn infants for the notorious XYY syndrome, as the first step in a longitudinal study aimed at determining whether or not individuals born with that genetic anomaly are predisposed to antisocial behavior, we cannot inform the parents about the nature of our study without introducing a potentially distorting influence on the relationship between the parents and the children that might itself alter each child's propensity to engage in antisocial behavior. Yet it has been argued that no study of a child is morally permissible without the informed consent of the adults who have responsibility for the child's well-being. Other forms of experimentation that would likely contribute to the general welfare are simply morally repugnant because of their violation of individual rights. For example, we might learn a great deal about language acquisition, with a view toward improving the linguistic ability of underprivileged children, by raising a few children in total isolation from linguistic input for various periods of time— say, two or three years—prior to immersing them in verbal environments. There should be no question about the scientific utility of such an undertaking, nor should there be any question about its moral unacceptability.

IV

I have been able . . . only to highlight some of the areas and issues that seem to me most intriguing under the general heading of bioethics and social responsibility. These problems have a special urgency that distinguishes them from many of the issues that philosophers traditionally address. Decisions in clinical medicine do not await philosophical reflection. Nor do government agencies, in establishing regulations that can facilitate or cripple medical research, come to terms as a first step with conflicts between deontological and consequentalist ethical theories. Nor do the courts, in ordering life-sustaining treatment of a neonatal monster come first to some clear general view about the relationship between the value of an individual life and the characteristics of the person whose life it is. Yet these decisions do get made against a backdrop of assumptions and confusions about essentially philosophical topics. For philosophers to address themselves explicitly to those topics as they arise in bioethical contexts is in no way to abandon the essential character of their philosophical commitments. It is, on the contrary, to do philosophy in a particularly rewarding way, by bringing the strengths of philosophical analysis to bear on problems that

engage the immediate interest of physicians, lawyers, policy-makers, legislators, patients, and all the rest of the public in its grand diversity.

That science exists in the final analysis at the pleasure and for the benefit of society generally is a point to which philosophers generally accede readily. What is perhaps less often noted by them is that philosophy, too, is a social enterprise supported in the final analysis by the public to whose interest it ultimately accrues. It is entirely opportune that philosophers in increasing numbers are now addressing their attention to issues with which large portions of the non-philosophical public can readily identify. When rigorous philosophical work illuminates problems of interest to the public, it is far easier to make the case that the philosophical community, like the scientific, merits public support and respect because it, too, is prepared to respond constructively to pressing social concerns—both because of the essential philosophical interest of those concerns, and out of its own sense of social responsibility.

NOTES

1. Portions of this essay are adapted from my introduction to *Moral Problems in Medicine*, ed. S. Gorovitz, et al. (Englewood Cliffs, N.J.: Prentice Hall, 1976).

2. New journals include: the *Hastings Center Report*, now in its sixth year published by the Institute of Society, Ethics and the Life Sciences; the *Journal of Medicine and Philosophy*, published by the Society for Health and Human Values; and *Man and Medicine*, published by the College of Physicians and Surgeons of Columbia University. *The Encyclopedia of Bioethics* is an undertaking of the Center for Bioethics at the Kennedy Institute of Georgetown University, and will be published shortly by The Free Press.

3. Rather than provide illustrative bibliography for each of the topics described below, I refer the reader to several recent bibliographies in the area of medical ethics. These include The Hastings Center *Bibliography* (1974); *Ethical Issues in Health Services: A Report and Annotated Bibliography* (1971) prepared by James Carmody and published by the National Center for Health Services (Department of Health, Education and Welfare Publication HSM-73-3008), and Carmody's *Ethical Issues in Health Services,*

Supplement 1 (DHEW Publication HRA-74-3123, 1974); *Abortion and Euthanasia: An Annotated Bibliography* compiled by K. D. Clouser and A. Zucker (1974) and published by the Society for Health and Human Values; the *Bibliography of Bioethics*—the Kennedy Institute's comprehensive annual listing of English language print and nonprint media materials which discuss value problems in biology and medicine, edited by LeRoy Walters and pub-

lished by Gale Research (vol. 1, June 1975); and the many excellent specialized bibliographies in books on topics in bioethics.

4. See W. Gaylin, "What's an F.B.I. Poster Doing in a Nice Journal Like That?" *Hastings Center Report* 2 (April 1972), 1–3.

5. See Gaylin's foreword to Gorovitz, et al. *Moral Problems in Medicine.*

6. *Opinions and Reports of Judicial Council* (Chicago: American Medical Association, 1972).

LEON R. KASS

The New Biology: What Price Relieving Man's Estate?

Recent advances in biology and medicine suggest that we may be rapidly acquiring the power to modify and control the capacities and activities of men by direct intervention and manipulation of their bodies and minds. Certain means are already in use or at hand, others await the solution of relatively minor technical problems, while yet others, those offering perhaps the most precise kind of control, depend upon further basic research. Biologists who have considered these matters disagree on the question of how much how soon, but all agree that the power for "human engineering," to borrow from the jargon, is coming and that it will probably have profound social consequences.

These developments have been viewed both with enthusiasm and with alarm; they are only just beginning to receive serious attention. Several biologists have undertaken to inform the public about the technical possibilities, present and future. Practitioners of social science "futurology" are attempting to predict and describe the likely social consequences of and public responses to the new technologies. Lawyers and legislators are exploring institutional innovations for assessing new tech-

nologies. All of these activities are based upon the hope that we can harness the new technology of man for the betterment of mankind.

Yet this commendable aspiration points to another set of questions, which are, in my view, sorely neglected—questions that inquire into the meaning of phrases such as the "betterment of mankind." A *full* understanding of the new technology of man requires an exploration of ends, values, standards. What ends will or should the new techniques serve? What values should guide society's adjustments? By what standards should the assessment agencies assess? Behind these questions lie others: what is a good man, what is a good life for man, what is a good community? This article is an attempt to provoke discussion of these neglected and important questions.

While these questions about ends and ultimate ends are never unimportant or irrelevant, they have rarely been more important or more relevant. That this is so can be seen once we recognize that we are dealing here with a group of technologies that are in a decisive respect unique: the object upon which they operate is man himself. The technologies of energy or food production, of communication, of manufacture, and of motion greatly alter the implements available to man and the conditions in which he uses them. In contrast, the biomedical technology works to change the user

Reprinted with permission of the author and the publisher from *Science*, Vol. 174 (19 November 1971), pp. 779-788. Copyright 1971 by the American Association for the Advancement of Science.

himself. To be sure, the printing press, the automobile, the television, and the jet airplane have greatly altered the conditions under which and the way in which men live; but men as biological beings have remained largely unchanged. They have been, and remain, able to accept or reject, to use and abuse these technologies; they choose, whether wisely or foolishly, the ends to which these technologies are means. Biomedical technology may make it possible to change the inherent capacity for choice itself. Indeed, both those who welcome and those who fear the advent of "human engineering" ground their hopes and fears in the same prospect: *that man can for the first time recreate himself.*

Engineering the engineer seems to differ in kind from engineering his engine. Some have argued, however, that biomedical engineering does not differ qualitatively from toilet training, education, and moral teachings—all of which are forms of so-called "social engineering," which has man as its object, and is used by one generation to mold the next. In reply, it must at least be said that the techniques which have hitherto been employed are feeble and inefficient when compared to those on the horizon. This quantitative difference rests in part on a qualitative difference in the means of intervention. The traditional influences operate by speech or by symbolic deeds. They pay tribute to man as the animal who lives by speech and who understands the meanings of actions. Also, their effects are, in general, reversible, or at least subject to attempts at reversal. Each person has greater or lesser power to accept or reject or abandon them. In contrast, biomedical engineering circumvents the human context of speech and meaning, bypasses choice, and goes directly to work to modify the human material itself. Moreover, the changes wrought may be irreversible.

In addition, there is an important practical reason for considering the biomedical technology apart from other technologies. The advances we shall examine are fruits of a large, humane project dedicated to the conquest of disease and the relief of human suffering. The biologist and physician, regardless of their private motives, are seen, with justification, to be the well-wishers and benefactors of mankind.

Thus, in a time in which technological advance is more carefully scrutinized and increasingly criticized, biomedical developments are still viewed by most people as benefits largely without qualification. The price we pay for these developments is thus more likely to go unrecognized. For this reason, I shall consider only the dangers and costs of biomedical advance. As the benefits are well known, there is no need to dwell upon them here. My discussion is deliberately partial.

I begin with a survey of the pertinent technologies. Next, I will consider some of the basic ethical and social problems in the use of these technologies. Then, I will briefly raise some fundamental questions to which these problems point. Finally, I shall offer some very general reflections on what is to be done.

THE BIOMEDICAL TECHNOLOGIES

The biomedical technologies can be usefully organized into three groups, according to their major purpose: (i) control of death and life, (ii) control of human potentialities, and (iii) control of human achievement. The corresponding technologies are (i) medicine, especially the arts of prolonging life and of controlling reproduction, (ii) genetic engineering, and (iii) neurological and psychological manipulation. I shall briefly summarize each group of techniques.

CONTROL OF DEATH AND LIFE

Previous medical triumphs have greatly increased average life expectancy. Yet other developments, such as organ transplantation or replacement and research into aging, hold forth the promise of increasing not just the average, but also the maximum life expectancy. Indeed, medicine seems to be sharpening its tools to do battle with death itself, as if death were just one more disease.

More immediately and concretely, available techniques of prolonging life—respirators, cardiac pacemakers, artificial kidneys—are already in the lists against death. Ironically, the success of these devices in forestalling death has introduced confusion in determining that death has, in fact, occurred. The traditional signs of life—heartbeat and respiration—can now be maintained entirely by machines. Some physicians are now busily trying to devise so-called "new definitions of death," while others maintain that the technical advances show that death is not a concrete event at all, but rather a gradual process, like twilight, incapable of precise temporal localization.

The real challenge to death will come from research into aging and senescence, a field just entering puberty. Recent studies suggest that aging is a genetically controlled process, distinct from disease, but one that can be manipulated and altered by diet or drugs. Extrapolating from animal studies, some scientists have suggested that a decrease in the rate of aging might also be achieved simply by effecting a very small decrease in human body temperature. According to some estimates, by the year 2000 it may be technically possible to add from 20 to 40 useful years to the period of middle life.

Medicine's success in extending life is already a major cause of excessive population growth: death control points to birth control. Although we are already technically competent, new techniques for lowering fertility and chemical agents for inducing abortion will greatly enhance our powers over conception and gestation. Problems of definition have been raised here as well. The need to determine when individuals acquire enforceable legal rights gives society an interest in the definition of human life and of the time when it begins. These matters are too familiar to need elaboration.

Technologies to conquer infertility proceed alongside those to promote it. The first successful laboratory fertilization of human egg by human sperm was reported in 1969.[1] In 1970, British scientists learned how to grow human embryos in the laboratory up to at least the blastocyst stage [that is, to the age of 1 week].[2] We may soon hear about the next stage, the successful reimplantation of such an embryo into a woman previously infertile because of oviduct disease. The development of an artificial placenta, now under investigation, will make possible full laboratory control of fertilization and gestation. In addition, sophisticated biochemical and cytological techniques of monitoring the "quality" of the fetus have been and are being developed and used. These developments not only give us more power over the generation of human life, but make it possible to manipulate and to modify the quality of the human material.

CONTROL OF HUMAN POTENTIALITIES

Genetic engineering, when fully developed, will wield two powers not shared by ordinary medical practice. Medicine treats existing individuals and seeks to correct deviations from a norm of health. Genetic engineering, in contrast, will be able to make changes that can be transmitted to succeeding generations and will be able to create new capacities, and hence to establish new norms of health and fitness.

Nevertheless, one of the major interests in genetic manipulation is strictly medical: to develop treatments for individuals with inherited diseases. Genetic disease is prevalent and increasing, thanks partly to medical advances that enable those affected to survive and perpetuate their mutant genes. The hope is that normal copies of the appropriate gene, obtained biologically or synthesized chemically, can be introduced into defective individuals to correct their deficiencies. This *therapeutic* use of genetic technology appears to be far in the future. Moreover, there is some doubt that it will ever be practical, since the same end could be more easily achieved by transplanting cells or organs that could compensate for the missing or defective gene product.

Far less remote are technologies that could serve *eugenic* ends. Their development has been endorsed by those concerned about a general deterioration of the human gene pool and by others who believe that even an undeteriorated human gene pool needs upgrading. Artificial insemination with selected donors, the eugenic proposal of Herman Muller,[3] has been possible for several years because of the perfection of methods for long-term storage of human spermatozoa. The successful maturation of human oocytes in the laboratory and their subsequent fertilization now make it possible to select donors of ova as well. But a far more suitable technique for eugenic purposes will soon be upon us—namely, nuclear transplantation, or cloning. Bypassing the lottery of sexual recombination, nuclear transplantation permits the asexual reproduction or copying of an already developed individual. The nucleus of a mature but unfertilized egg is replaced by a nucleus obtained from a specialized cell of an adult organism or embryo (for example, a cell from the intestines or the skin). The egg with its transplanted nucleus develops as if it had been fertilized and, barring complications, will give rise to a normal adult organism. Since almost all the hereditary material (DNA) of a cell is contained within its nucleus, the renucleated egg and the individual into which it develops are genetically identical to the adult organism that was the source of the donor nucleus. Cloning could be used to produce sets of unlimited numbers of genetically identical individuals, each set derived from a single parent. Cloning has been successful in amphibians and is now being tried in mice; its extension to man merely requires the solution of certain technical problems.

Production of man-animal chimeras by the introduction of selected nonhuman material into developing human embryos is also expected. Fusion of human and nonhuman cells in tissue culture has already been achieved.

Other, less direct means for influencing the gene pool are already available, thanks to our increasing ability to identify and diagnose genetic diseases. Genetic counselors can now detect biochemically and cytologically a variety of severe genetic defects (for example, Mongolism, Tay-Sachs disease) while the fetus is still in utero. Since treatments are at present largely unavailable, diagnosis is often followed by abortion of the affected fetus. In the future, more sensitive tests will also permit the detection of heterozygote carriers, the unaffected individuals who carry but a single dose of a given deleterious gene. The eradication of a given genetic disease might then be attempted by aborting all such carriers. In fact, it was recently suggested that the fairly common disease cystic fibrosis could be completely eliminated over the next 40 years by screening all

pregnancies and aborting the 17,000,000 unaffected fetuses that will carry a single gene for this disease. Such zealots need to be reminded of the consequences should each geneticist be allowed an equal assault on his favorite genetic disorder, given that each human being is a carrier for some four to eight such recessive, lethal genetic diseases.

CONTROL OF HUMAN ACHIEVEMENT

Although human achievement depends at least in part upon genetic endowment, heredity determines only the material upon which experience and education impose the form. The limits of many capacities and powers of an individual are indeed genetically determined, but the nurturing and perfection of these capacities depend upon other influences. Neurological and psychological manipulation hold forth the promise of controlling the development of human capacities, particularly those long considered most distinctively human: speech, thought, choice, emotion, memory, and imagination.

These techniques are now in a rather primitive state because we understand so little about the brain and mind. Nevertheless, we have already seen the use of electrical stimulation of the human brain to produce sensations of intense pleasure and to control rage, the use of brain surgery (for example, frontal lobotomy) for the relief of severe anxiety, and the use of aversive conditioning with electric shock to treat sexual perversion. Operant-conditioning techniques are widely used, apparently with success, in schools and mental hospitals. The use of so-called consciousness-expanding and hallucinogenic drugs is widespread, to say nothing of tranquilizers and stimulants. We are promised drugs to modify memory, intelligence, libido, and aggressiveness.

The following passages from a recent book by Yale neurophysiologist José Delgado—a book instructively entitled *Physical Control of the Mind: Toward a Psychocivilized Society*— should serve to make this discussion more concrete. In the early 1950's, it was discovered that, with electrodes placed in certain discrete regions of their brains, animals would repeatedly and indefatigably press levers to stimulate their own brains, with obvious resultant enjoyment. Even starving animals preferred stimulating these so-called pleasure centers to eating. Delgado comments on the electrical stimulation of a similar center in a human subject[4] (p. 185).

[T]he patient reported a pleasant tingling sensation in the left side of her body 'from my face down to the bottom of my legs.' She started giggling and making funny comments, stating that she enjoyed the sensation 'very much.' Repetition of these stimulations made the patient more communicative and flirtatious, and she ended by openly expressing her desire to marry the therapist.

And one further quotation from Delgado[4] (p. 88).

Leaving wires inside of a thinking brain may appear unpleasant or dangerous, but actually the many patients who have undergone this experience have not been concerned about the fact of being wired, nor have they felt any discomfort due to the presence of conductors in their heads. Some women have shown their feminine adaptability to circumstances by wearing attractive hats or wigs to conceal their electrical headgear, and many people have been able to enjoy a normal life as out-patients, returning to the clinic periodically for examination and stimulation. In a few cases in which contacts were located in pleasurable areas, patients have had the opportunity to stimulate their own brains by pressing the button of a portable instrument, and this procedure is reported to have therapeutic benefits.

It bears repeating that the sciences of neurophysiology and psychopharmacology are in their infancy. The techniques that are now available are crude, imprecise, weak, and unpredictable, compared to those that may flow from a more mature neurobiology.

BASIC ETHICAL AND SOCIAL PROBLEMS IN THE USE OF BIOMEDICAL TECHNOLOGY

After this cursory review of the powers now and soon to be at our disposal, I turn to the questions concerning the use of these powers. First, we must recognize that questions of use

of science and technology are always moral and political questions, never simply technical ones. All private or public decisions to develop or to use biomedical technology—and decisions *not* to do so—inevitably contain judgments about value. This is true even if the values guiding those decisions are not articulated or made clear, as indeed they often are not. Secondly, the value judgments cannot be derived from biomedical science. This is true even if scientists themselves make the decisions.

These important points are often overlooked for at least three reasons.

1) They are obscured by those who like to speak of "the control of nature by science." It is men who control, not that abstraction "science." Science may provide the means, but men choose the ends; the choice of ends comes from beyond science.

2) Introduction of new technologies often appears to be the result of no decision whatsoever, or of the culmination of decisions too small or unconscious to be recognized as such. What can be done is done. However, someone is deciding on the basis of some notions of desirability, no matter how self-serving or altruistic.

3) Desires to gain or keep money and power no doubt influence much of what happens, but these desires can also be formulated as reasons and then discussed and debated.

Insofar as our society has tried to deliberate about questions of use, how has it done so? Pragmatists that we are, we prefer a utilitarian calculus: we weigh "benefits" against "risks," and we weigh them for both the individual and "society." We often ignore the fact that the very definitions of "a benefit" and "a risk" are themselves based upon judgments about value. In the biomedical areas just reviewed, the benefits are considered to be self-evident: prolongation of life, control of fertility and of population size, treatment and prevention of genetic disease, the reduction of anxiety and aggressiveness, and the enhancement of memory, intelligence, and pleasure. The assessment of risk is, in general, simply pragmatic— will the technique work effectively and reliably, how much will it cost, will it do detectable bodily harm, and who will complain if we proceed with development? As these questions are familiar and congenial, there is no need to belabor them.

The very pragmatism that makes us sensitive to considerations of economic cost often blinds us to the larger social costs exacted by biomedical advances. For one thing, we seem to be unaware that we may not be able to maximize all the benefits, that several of the goals we are promoting conflict with each other. On the one hand, we seek to control population growth by lowering fertility; on the other hand, we develop techniques to enable every infertile woman to bear a child. On the one hand, we try to extend the lives of individuals with genetic disease; on the other, we wish to eliminate deleterious genes from the human population. I am not urging that we resolve these conflicts in favor of one side or the other, but simply that we recognize that such conflicts exist. Once we do, we are more likely to appreciate that most "progress" is heavily paid for in terms not generally included in the simple utilitarian calculus.

To become sensitive to the larger costs of biomedical progress, we must attend to several serious ethical and social questions. I will briefly discuss three of them: (i) questions of distributive justice, (ii) questions of the use and abuse of power, and (iii) questions of self-degradation and dehumanization.

DISTRIBUTIVE JUSTICE

The introduction of any biomedical technology presents a new balance of an old problem—how to distribute scarce resources justly. We should assume that demand will usually exceed supply. Which people should receive a kidney transplant or an artificial heart? Who should get the benefits of genetic therapy or of brain stimulation? Is "first-come, first-served" the fairest principle? Or are certain people "more worthy," and if so, on what grounds?

It is unlikely that we will arrive at answers to these questions in the form of deliberate decisions. More likely, the problem of distribution will continue to be decided ad hoc and locally. If so, the consequence will probably be a sharp increase in the already far too great inequality of medical care. The extreme case will be longevity, which will probably be, at first, obtainable only at great expense. Who is likely to be able to buy it? Do conscience and prudence permit us to enlarge the gap between rich and poor, especially with respect to something as fundamental as life itself?

Questions of distributive justice also arise in the earlier decisions to acquire new knowledge and to develop new techniques. Personnel and facilities for medical research and treatment are scarce resources. Is the development of a new technology the best use of the limited resources, given current circumstances? How should we balance efforts aimed at prevention against those aimed at cure, or either of these against efforts to redesign the species? How should we balance the delivery of available levels of care against further basic research? More fundamentally, how should we balance efforts in biology and medicine against efforts to eliminate poverty, pollution, urban decay, discrimination, and poor education? This last question about distribution is perhaps the most profound. We should reflect upon the social consequences of seducing many of our brightest young people to spend their lives locating the biochemical defects in rare genetic diseases, while our more serious problems go begging. The current squeeze on money for research provides us with an opportunity to rethink and reorder our priorities.

Problems of distributive justice are frequently mentioned and discussed, but they are hard to resolve in a rational manner. We find them especially difficult because of the enormous range of conflicting values and interests that characterizes our pluralistic society. We cannot agree—unfortunately, we often do not even try to agree—on standards for just distribution. Rather, decisions tend to be made largely out of a clash of competing interests. Thus, regrettably, the question of how to distribute justly often gets reduced to who shall decide how to distribute. The question about justice has led us to the question about power.

USE AND ABUSE OF POWER

We have difficulty recognizing the problems of the exercise of power in the biomedical enterprise because of our delight with the wondrous fruits it has yielded. This is ironic because the notion of power is absolutely central to the modern conception of science. The ancients conceived of science as the *understanding* of nature, pursued for its own sake. We moderns view science as power, as *control* over nature; the conquest of nature "for the relief of man's estate" was the charge issued by Francis Bacon, one of the leading architects of the modern scientific project.[5]

Another source of difficulty is our fondness for speaking of the abstraction "Man." I suspect that we prefer to speak figuratively about "Man's power over Nature" because it obscures an unpleasant reality about human affairs. It is in fact particular men who wield power, not Man. What we really mean by "Man's power over Nature" is a power exercised by some men over other men, with a knowledge of nature as their instrument.

While applicable to technology in general, these reflections are especially pertinent to the technologies of human engineering, with which men deliberately exercise power over future generations. An excellent discussion of this question is found in *The Abolition of Man,* by C. S. Lewis.[6]

It is, of course, a commonplace to complain that men have hitherto used badly, and against their fellows, the powers that science has given them. But that is not the point I am trying to make. I am not speaking of particular corruptions and abuses which an increase of moral virtue would cure: I am considering what the thing called "Man's power over Nature" must always and essentially be. . . .

In reality, of course, if any one age really attains, by eugenics and scientific education, the power to make its descendants what it pleases, all men who live after it are the patients of that power. They are weaker, not stronger: for though we may have put wonderful machines in their hands, we have preordained how they are to use them. . . . The real picture is that of one dominant age . . . which resists all previous ages most successfully and dominates all subsequent ages most irresistibly, and thus is the real master of the human species. But even within this master generation (itself an infinitesimal minority of the species) the power will be exercised by a minority smaller still. Man's conquest of Nature, if the dreams of some scientific planners are realized,

means the rule of a few hundreds of men over billions upon billions of men. There neither is nor can be any simple increase of power on Man's side. Each new power won *by* man is a power *over* man as well. Each advance leaves him weaker as well as stronger. In every victory, besides being the general who triumphs, he is also the prisoner who follows the triumphal car.

Please note that I am not yet speaking about the problem of the misuse or abuse of power. The point is rather that the power which grows is unavoidably the power of only some men, and that the number of powerful men decreases as power increases.

Specific problems of abuse and misuse of specific powers must not, however, be overlooked. Some have voiced the fear that the technologies of genetic engineering and behavior control, though developed for good purposes, will be put to evil uses. These fears are perhaps somewhat exaggerated, if only because biomedical technologies would add very little to our highly developed arsenal for mischief, destruction, and stultification. Nevertheless, any proposal for large-scale human engineering should make us wary. Consider a program of positive eugenics based upon the widespread practice of asexual reproduction. Who shall decide what constitutes a superior individual worthy of replication? Who shall decide which individuals may or must reproduce, and by which method? These are questions easily answered only for a tyrannical regime.

Concern about the use of power is equally necessary in the selection of means for desirable or agreed-upon ends. Consider the desired end of limiting population growth. An effective program of fertility control is likely to be coercive. Who should decide the choice of means? Will the program penalize "conscientious objectors"?

Serious problems arise simply from obtaining and disseminating information, as in the mass screening programs now being proposed for detection of genetic disease. For what kinds of disorders is compulsory screening justified? Who shall have access to the data obtained, and for what purposes? To whom does information about a person's genotype belong? In ordinary medical practice, the patient's privacy is protected by the doctor's adherence to the principle of confidentiality. What will protect his privacy under conditions of mass screening?

. . .

There are many clinical situations which already permit, if not invite, the manipulative or arbitrary use of powers provided by biomedical technology: obtaining organs for transplantation, refusing to let a person die with dignity, giving genetic counseling to a frightened couple, recommending eugenic sterilization for a mental retardate, ordering electric shock for a homosexual. In each situation, there is an opportunity to violate the will of the patient or subject. Such opportunities have generally existed in medical practice, but the dangers are becoming increasingly serious. With the growing complexity of the technologies, the technician gains in authority, since he alone can understand what he is doing. The patient's lack of knowledge makes him deferential and often inhibits him from speaking up when he feels threatened. Physicians *are* sometimes troubled by their increasing power, yet they feel they cannot avoid its exercise. "Reluctantly," one commented to me, "we shall have to play God." With what guidance and to what ends I shall consider later. For the moment, I merely ask: "By whose authority?"

While these questions about power are pertinent and important, they are in one sense misleading. They imply an inherent conflict of purpose between physician and patient, between scientist and citizen. The discussion conjures up images of master and slave, of oppressor and oppressed. Yet it must be remembered that conflict of purpose is largely absent, especially with regard to general goals. To be sure, the purposes of medical scientists are not always the same as those of the subjects experimented on. Nevertheless, basic sponsors and partisans of biomedical technology are precisely those upon whom the technology will operate. The will of the scientist and physician is happily married to (rather, is the offspring of) the desire of all of us for better health, longer life, and peace of mind.

Most future biomedical technologies will probably be welcomed, as have those of the past. Their use will require little or no coercion. Some developments, such as pills to improve memory, control mood, or induce pleasure, are likely to need no promotion. Thus, even if we should escape from the dangers of coercive manipulation, we shall still face large problems posed by the voluntary use of biomedical technology, problems to which I now turn.

VOLUNTARY SELF-DEGRADATION AND DEHUMANIZATION

Modern opinion is sensitive to problems of restriction of freedom and abuse of power. Indeed, many hold that a man can be injured only by violating his will. But this view is much too narrow. It fails to recognize the great dangers we shall face in the use of biomedical technology, dangers that stem from an excess of freedom, from the uninhibited exercises of will. In my view, our greatest problem will increasingly be one of voluntary self-degradation, or willing dehumanization.

Certain desired and perfected medical technologies have already had some dehumanizing consequences. Improved methods of resuscitation have made possible heroic efforts to "save" the severely ill and injured. Yet these efforts are sometimes only partly successful; they may succeed in salvaging individuals with severe brain damage, capable of only a less-than-human, vegetating existence. Such patients, increasingly found in the intensive care units of university hospitals, have been denied a death with dignity. Families are forced to suffer seeing their loved ones so reduced, and are made to bear the burdens of a protracted death watch.

Even the ordinary methods of treating disease and prolonging life have impoverished the context in which men die. Fewer and fewer people die in the familiar surroundings of home or in the company of family and friends. At that time of life when there is perhaps the greatest need for human warmth and comfort, the dying patient is kept company by cardiac pacemakers and defibrillators, respirators, aspirators, oxygenators, catheters, and his intravenous drip.

But the loneliness is not confined to the dying patient in the hospital bed. Consider the increasing number of old people who are still alive, thanks to medical progress. As a group, the elderly are the most alienated members of our society. Not yet ready for the world of the dead, not deemed fit for the world of the living, they are shunted aside. More and more of them spend the extra years medicine has given them in "homes for senior citizens," in chronic hospitals, in nursing homes—waiting for the end. We have learned how to increase their years, but we have not learned how to help them enjoy their days. And yet, we bravely and relentlessly push back the frontiers against death.

. . .

Consider next the coming power over reproduction and genotype. We endorse the project that will enable us to control numbers and to treat individuals with genetic disease. But our desires outrun these defensible goals. Many would welcome the chance to become parents without the inconvenience of pregnancy; others would wish to know in advance the characteristics of their offspring (sex, height, eye color, intelligence); still others would wish to design these characteristics to suit their tastes. Some scientists have called for the use of the new technologies to assure the "quality" of all new babies.[7] As one obstetrician put it: "The business of obstetrics is to produce *optimum* babies." But the price to be paid for the "optimum baby" is the transfer of procreation from the home to the laboratory and its coincident transformation into manufacture. Increasing control over the product is purchased by the increasing depersonalization of the process. The complete depersonalization of procreation (possible with the development of an artificial placenta) shall be, in itself, seriously dehumanizing, no matter how optimum the product. It should not be forgotten that human procreation not only issues new human beings, but is itself a human activity.

Procreation is not simply an activity of the rational will. It is a more complete human activity precisely because it engages us bodily and spiritually, as well as rationally. Is there perhaps some wisdom in that mystery of nature which joins the pleasure of sex, the communication of love, and the desire for children in the very activity by which we continue the chain of human existence? Is not biological parenthood a built-in "mechanism," selected because it fosters and supports in parents an adequate concern for and commitment to their children? Would not the laboratory production of human beings no longer be *human* procreation? Could it keep human parenthood human?

The dehumanizing consequences of programmed reproduction extend beyond the mere acts and processes of life-giving. Transfer of procreation to the laboratory will no doubt weaken what is presently for many people the best remaining justification and support for the existence of marriage and the family. Sex is now comfortably at home outside of marriage; child-rearing is progressively being given over to the state, the schools, the mass media, and the child-care centers. Some have argued that the family, long the nursery of humanity, has outlived its usefulness. To be sure, laboratory and governmental alternatives might be designed for procreation and child-rearing, but at what cost?

This is not the place to conduct a full evaluation of the biological family. Nevertheless, some of its important virtues are, nowadays, too often overlooked. The family is rapidly becoming the only institution in an increasingly impersonal world where each person is loved not for what he does or makes, but simply because he is. The family is also the institution where most of us, both as children and as parents, acquire a sense of continuity with the past and a sense of commitment to the future. Without the family, we would have little incentive to take an interest in anything after our own deaths. These observations suggest that the elimination of the family would weaken ties to past and future, and would throw us, even more than we are now, to the mercy of an impersonal, lonely present.

Neurobiology and psychobiology probe most directly into the distinctively human. The technological fruit of these sciences is likely to be both more tempting than Eve's apple and more "catastrophic" in its result. One need only consider contemporary drug use to see what people are willing to risk or sacrifice for novel experiences, heightened perceptions, or just "kicks." The possibility of drug-induced, instant, and effortless gratification will be welcomed. Recall the possibilities of voluntary self-stimulation of the brain to reduce anxiety, to heighten pleasure, or to create visual and auditory sensations unavailable through the peripheral sense organs. Once these techniques are perfected and safe, is there much doubt that they will be desired, demanded, and used?

What ends will these techniques serve? Most likely, only the most elemental, those most tied to the bodily pleasures. What will happen to thought, to love, to friendship, to art, to judgment, to public-spiritedness in a society with a perfected technology of pleasure? What kinds of creatures will we become if we obtain our pleasure by drug or electrical stimulation without the usual kind of human efforts and frustrations? What kind of society will we have?

We need only consult Aldous Huxley's prophetic novel *Brave New World* for a likely answer to these questions. There we encounter a society dedicated to homogeneity and stability, administered by means of instant gratifications and peopled by creatures of human shape but of stunted humanity. They consume, fornicate, take "soma," and operate the machinery that makes it all possible. They do not read, write, think, love, or govern themselves. Creativity and curiosity, reason and passion, exist only in a rudimentary and multilated form. In short, they are not men at all.

True, our techniques, like theirs, may in fact enable us to treat schizophrenia, to alleviate anxiety, to curb agressiveness. We, like they, may indeed be able to save mankind from itself, but probably only at the cost of its humanness. In the end, the price of relieving man's estate might well be the abolition of man.

There are, of course, many other routes leading to the abolition of man. There are many other and better known causes of dehumanization. Disease, starvation, mental re-

tardation, slavery, and brutality—to name just a few—have long prevented many, if not most, people from living a fully human life. We should work to reduce and eventually to eliminate these evils. But the existence of these evils should not prevent us from appreciating that the use of the technology of man, uninformed by wisdom concerning proper human ends, and untempered by an appropriate humility and awe, can unwittingly render us all irreversibly less than human. For, unlike the man reduced by disease or slavery, the people dehumanized à la *Brave New World* are not miserable, do not know that they are dehumanized, and, what is worse, would not care if they knew. They are, indeed, happy slaves, with a slavish happiness.

SOME FUNDAMENTAL QUESTIONS

The practical problems of distributing scarce resources, of curbing the abuses of power, and of preventing voluntary dehumanization point beyond themselves to some large, enduring, and most difficult questions: the nature of justice and the good community, the nature of man and the good for man. My appreciation of the profundity of these questions and my own ignorance before them makes me hesitant to say any more about them. Nevertheless, previous failures to find a shortcut around them have led me to believe that these questions must be faced if we are to have any hope of understanding where biology is taking us. Therefore, I shall try to show in outline how I think some of the larger questions arise from my discussion of dehumanization and self-degradation.

My remarks on dehumanization can hardly fail to arouse argument. It might be said, correctly, that to speak about dehumanization presupposes a concept of "the distinctively human." It might also be said, correctly, that to speak about wisdom concerning proper human ends presupposes that such ends do in fact exist and that they may be more or less accessible to human understanding, or at least to rational inquiry. It is true that neither presupposition is at home in modern thought.

The notion of the "distinctively human" has been seriously challenged by modern scientists. Darwinists hold that man is, at least in origin, tied to the subhuman; his seeming distinctiveness is an illusion or, at most, not very important. Biochemists and molecular biologists extend the challenge by blurring the distinction between the living and the nonliving. The laws of physics and chemistry are found to be valid and are held to be sufficient for explaining biological systems. Man is a collection of molecules, an accident on the stage of evolution, endowed by chance with the power to change himself, but only along determined lines.

Psychoanalysts have also debunked the "distinctly human." The essence of man is seen to be located in those drives he shares with other animals—pursuit of pleasure and avoidance of pain. The so-called "higher functions" are understood to be servants of the more elementary, the more base. Any distinctiveness or "dignity" that man has consists of his superior capacity for gratifying his animal needs.

The idea of "human good" fares no better. In the social sciences, historicists and existentialists have helped drive this question underground. The former hold all notions of human good to be culturally and historically bound, and hence mutable. The latter hold that values are subjective: each man makes his own, and ethics becomes simply the cataloging of personal tastes.

Such appear to be the prevailing opinions. Yet there is nothing novel about reductionism, hedonism, and relativism; these are doctrines with which Socrates contended. What is new is that these doctrines seem to be vindicated by scientific advance. Not only do the scientific notions of nature and of man flower into verifiable predictions, but they yield marvelous fruit. The technological triumphs are held to validate their scientific foundations. Here, perhaps, is the most pernicious result of technological progress—more dehumanizing than any actual manipulation or technique, present or future. We are witnessing the erosion, perhaps the final erosion, of the idea of man as something splendid or divine, and its replacement with a view that sees man, no less than nature, as simply more raw material for manipulation and homogenization. Hence, our peculiar moral crisis. We are in turbulent seas without a landmark precisely because we adhere more and more to a view of nature and of man which both gives us enormous power and, at the same time, denies all possibility of standards to guide its use. Though well-equipped, we know not who we are nor where we are going. We are left to the accidents of our hasty, biased, and ephemeral judgments.

Let us not fail to note a painful irony: our conquest of nature has made us the slaves of blind chance. We triumph over nature's unpredictabilities only to subject ourselves to the still greater unpredictability of our capricious wills and our fickle opinions. That we have a method is no proof against our madness. Thus, engineering the engineer as well as the engine, we race our train we know not where.

While the disastrous consequences of ethical nihilism are insufficient to refute it, they invite and make urgent a reinvestigation of the ancient and enduring questions of what is a proper life for a human being, what is a good community, and how are they achieved. We must not be deterred from these questions simply because the best minds in human history have failed to settle them. Should we not rather be encouraged by the fact that they considered them to be the most important questions?

As I have hinted before, our ethical dilemma is caused by the victory of modern natural science with its nonteleological view of man. We ought therefore to reexamine with great care the modern notions of nature and of man, which undermine those earlier notions that provide a basis for ethics. If we consult our common experience, we are likely to discover some grounds for believing that the questions about man and human good are far from closed. Our common experience suggests many difficulties for the modern "scientific view of man." For example, this view fails to account for the concern for justice and freedom that appears to be characteristic of all human societies.[8] It also fails to account for or to explain the fact that men have speech and not merely voice, that men can choose and act and not merely move or react. It fails to explain why men engage in moral discourse, or, for that matter, why they speak at all. Finally, the "scientific view of man" cannot account for scientific inquiry itself, for why men seek to know. Might there not be something the matter with a knowledge of man that does not explain or take account of his most distinctive activities, aspirations, and concerns?

Having gone this far, let me offer one suggestion as to where the difficulty might lie: in the modern understanding of knowledge. Since Bacon, as I have mentioned earlier, technology has increasingly come to be the basic justification for scientific inquiry. The end is power, not knowledge for its own sake. But power is not only the end. It is also an important *validation* of knowledge. One definitely knows that one knows only if one can make. Synthesis is held to be the ultimate proof of understanding. A more radical formulation holds that one knows only what one makes: knowing *equals* making.

Yet therein lies a difficulty. If truth be the power to change or to make the object studied, then of what do we have knowledge? If there are no fixed realities, but only material upon which we may work our wills, will not "science" be merely the "knowledge" of the transient and the manipulatable? We might indeed have knowledge of the laws by which things change and the rules for their manipulation, but no knowledge of the things themselves. Can such a view of "science" yield any knowledge about the nature of man, or indeed, about the nature of anything? Our questions appear to lead back to the most basic of questions: What does it mean to know? What is it that is knowable?[9]

We have seen that the practical problems point toward and make urgent certain enduring, fundamental questions. Yet while pursuing these questions, we cannot afford to neglect the practical problems as such. Let us not forget Delgado and the "psychocivilized society." The philosophical inquiry could be rendered moot by our blind, confident efforts to dissect and redesign ourselves. While awaiting a reconstruction of theory, we must act as best we can.

WHAT IS TO BE DONE?

First, we sorely need to recover some humility in the face of our awesome powers. The arguments I have presented should make apparent the folly of arrogance, of the presumption that we are wise enough to remake ourselves. Because we lack wisdom, caution is our urgent need. Or to put it another way, in the absence of that "ultimate wisdom," we can be wise enough to know that we are not wise enough. When we lack sufficient wisdom to do, wisdom consists in not doing. Caution, restraint, delay, abstention are what this second-best (and, perhaps, only) wisdom dictates with respect to the technology for human engineering.

If we can recognize that biomedical advances carry significant social costs, we may be willing to adopt a less permissive, more critical stance toward new developments. We need to reexamine our prejudice not only that all biomedical innovation is progress, but also that it is inevitable. Precedent certainly favors the view that what can be done will be done, but is this necessarily so? Ought we not to be suspicious when technologists speak of coming developments as automatic, not subject to human control? Is there not something contradictory in the notion that we have the power to control all the untoward consequences of a technology, but lack the power to determine whether it should be developed in the first place?

What will be the likely consequences of the perpetuation of our permissive and fatalistic attitude toward human engineering? How will the large decisions be made? Technocratically and self-servingly, if our experience with previous technologies is any guide. Under conditions of laissez-faire, most technologists will pursue techniques, and most private industries will pursue profits. We are fortunate that, apart from the drug manufacturers, there are at present in the biomedical area few large industries that influence public policy. Once these appear, the voice of "the public interest" will have to shout very loudly to be heard above their whisperings in the halls of Congress. These reflections point to the need for institutional controls.

Scientists understandably balk at the notion of the regulation of science and technology. Censorship is ugly and often based upon ignorant fear; bureaucratic regulation is often stupid and inefficient. Yet there is something disingenuous about a scientist who professes concern about the social consequences of science, but who responds to every suggestion of regulation with one or both of the following: "No restrictions on scientific research," and "Technological progress should not be curtailed." Surely, to suggest that *certain* technologies ought to be regulated or forestalled is not to call for the halt of *all* technological progress (and says nothing at all about basic research). Each development should be considered on its own merits. Although the dangers of regulation cannot be dismissed, who, for example, would still object to efforts to obtain an effective, complete, global prohibition on the development, testing, and use of biological and nuclear weapons?

The proponents of laissez-faire ignore two fundamental points. They ignore the fact that not to regulate is as much a policy decision as the opposite, and that it merely postpones the time of regulation. Controls will eventually be called for—as they are now being demanded to end environmental pollution. If attempts are not made early to detect and diminish the social costs of biomedical advances by intelligent institutional regulation, the society is likely to react later with more sweeping, immoderate, and throttling controls.

The proponents of laissez-faire also ignore the fact that much of technology is already regulated. The federal government is already deep in research and development (for example, space, electronics, and weapons) and is the principal sponsor of biomedical research. One may well question the wisdom of the direction given, but one would be wrong in arguing that technology cannot survive social control.

Clearly, the question is not control versus no control, but rather what kind of control, when, by whom, and for what purpose. . . .

To repeat, the basic short-term need is caution. Practically, this means that we should shift the burden of proof to the *proponents* of a new biomedical technology. Concepts of "risk" and "cost" need to be broadened to include some of the social and ethical consequences discussed earlier. The probable or possible harmful effects of the wide-spread use of a new technique should be anticipated and introduced as "costs" to be weighed in deciding about the *first* use. The regulatory institutions should be encouraged to exercise restraint and to formulate the grounds for saying "no." We must all get used to the idea that biomedical technology makes possible many things we should never do.

But caution is not enough. Nor are clever institutional arrangements. Institutions can be little better than the people who make them work. However worthy our intentions, we are deficient in understanding. In the *long* run, our hope can only lie in education: in a public educated about the meanings and limits of science and enlightened in its use of technology; in scientists better educated to understand the relationships between science and technology on the one hand, and ethics and politics on the other; in human beings who are as wise in the latter as they are clever in the former.

NOTES

1. R. G. Edwards, B. D. Bavister, P. C. Steptoe, *Nature* 221, 632 (1969).

2. R. G. Edwards, P. C. Steptoe, J. M. Purdy, *ibid.*, 227, 1307 (1970).

3. H. J. Muller, *Science* 134, 643 (1961).

4. J. M. R. Delgado, *Physical Control of the Mind: Toward a Psychocivilized Society* (Harper & Row, New York, 1969).

5. F. Bacon, *The Advancement of Learning, Book I*, H. G. Dick, ed. (Random House, New York, 1955), p. 193.

6. C. S. Lewis, *The Abolition of Man* (Macmillan, New York, 1965), pp. 69–71.

7. B. Glass, *Science* 171, 23 (1971).

8. Consider, for example, the widespread acceptance, in the legal systems of very different societies and cultures,

of the principle and the practice of third-party adjudication of disputes. And consider why, although many societies have practiced slavery, no slaveholder has preferred his own enslavement to his own freedom. It would seem that some notions of justice and freedom, as well as right and truthfulness, are constitutive for any society, and that a concern for these values may be a fundamental characteristic of "human nature."

9. When an earlier version of this article was presented publicly, it was criticized by one questioner as being "antiscientific." He suggested that my remarks "were the kind that gave science a bad name." He went on to argue that, far from being the enemy of morality, the pursuit of truth was itself a highly moral activity, perhaps the highest. The relation of science and morals is a long and difficult question with an illustrious history, and it deserves a more extensive discussion than space permits. However, because some readers may share the questioner's response, I offer a brief reply. First, on the matter of reputation, we should recall that the pursuit of truth may be in tension with keeping a good name (witness Oedipus, Socrates, Galileo, Spinoza, Solzhenitsyn). For most of human history, the pursuit of truth (including "science") was not a reputable activity among the many, and was, in fact, highly suspect. Even today, it is doubtful whether more than a few appreci-

ate knowledge as an end in itself. Science has acquired a "good name" in recent times largely because of its technological fruit; it is therefore to be expected that a disenchantment with technology will reflect badly upon science. Second, my own attack has not been directed against science, but against the use of *some* technologies and, even more, against the unexamined belief—indeed, I would say, superstition—that all biomedical technology is an unmixed blessing. I share the questioner's belief that the pursuit of truth is a highly moral activity. In fact, I am inviting him and others to join in a pursuit of the truth about whether all these new technologies are really good for us. This is a question that merits and is susceptible of serious intellectual inquiry. Finally, we must ask whether what we call "science" has a monopoly on the pursuit of truth. What is "truth"? What is knowable, and what does it mean to know? Surely, these are also questions that can be examined. Unless we do so, we shall remain ignorant about what "science" is and about what it discovers. Yet "science"—that is, modern natural science—cannot begin to answer them; they are philosophical questions, the very ones I am trying to raise at this point in the text.

J A M E S   M.   G U S T A F S O N

Basic Ethical Issues in the Bio-Medical Fields

The "new biology" and developments in medical science and technology have aroused a great deal of public interest. Nothing less than the future of human development seems to be at stake. Although men have always affected the course of evolution through such things as wars, the exposure of infants, and the use of natural resources, we are now able to intervene purposively in ways that did not exist before in the developmental process to prolong, shorten, and direct human life. Commentary on this new set of circumstances has come from scientists, social critics, journalists, philosophers, theologians, lawyers, and many others. The public is sharply aware of the growth of

Reprinted with permission of the publisher from *Soundings,* Vol. 52, No. 2 (Summer 1970), pp. 151-159, 162-169, 172-180. This abridged version includes six of the original article's nine sections.

knowledge and understanding of the life processes, of the power that this provides for human intervention and control, and thus of the extent to which human destiny is in the hands of men themselves rather than being fated by natural evolution or immediately governed by Deity. Two Jesuit theologians have stated very well the human fact that bristles with potentialities for good and ill. Teilhard de Chardin, in *The Phenomenon of Man,* simply states, "We are evolution." He also makes the point more dramatically: "We have become aware that, in the great game that is being played, we are the players as well as being the cards and the stakes."[1] Karl Rahner, in an interesting and important essay, "Experiment: Man," asserts that "Human self-creation means quite simply that today man is changing himself. To be more precise: Man is consciously and deliberately changing himself." "Man today finds that he is manipulable. A radically new age is coming—new in every dimension."[2]

These writers, and others, are responding to many scientific developments. Both negative and positive eugenics lie within the scientific capacities of man. The technical capabilities exist for family planning and population control. Artificial environments can be constructed so that human beings can exist where the natural environment is hostile to them. Chemical and electrical interventions in the human brain make possible states of euphoria, but they also create new possibilities of controlling the responses of others.

.   .   .

I undertake in this paper to distinguish some of the basic human moral issues* that arise in the situation created by developments in biology and medicine, and to suggest some ways in which we can deal with them. The task is too extensive and complex to be managed fully and satisfactorily in one paper. There are several quite different matters involved in the differences of judgment that are being made. One is simply the matter of fact. What exactly are the present capabilities and what are their actual limits? Another is the matter of prediction or projection from present knowledge. Exactly what possibilities can be seriously entertained? What new knowledge is on the horizons, and to what might its uses lead? Another is the matter of the perspectives from which the human situation is understood and evaluated. Can we have confidence that men will use their new knowledge and powers wisely, and for the end of human welfare? Or are human propensities for evil so great that we must protect the human race against its own capabilities? Another matter is more distinctively and narrowly ethical. Are there certain human rights and prerogatives that cannot be infringed upon under

---

*I have not used "moral" and "ethical" in a restricted sense that meets the criteria set by some moral philosophers. The paper rather addresses what comes within the general range of "moral" in the vocabulary of most scientists with whom I have discussed these matters.

any possible circumstances? Or is a utilitarian ethic, calculating and weighing desired and undesired consequences, the proper one to adopt?

In the hope of clarifying this situation, and of suggesting some possible ways to move the discussion forward, I shall distinguish [six] pertinent issues, and state some conflicting propositions directed to each. I shall develop these issues and propositions in such a way that some of the reasons for contrasting judgments become clear. In some instances, the reasonable position appears to be a dialectical one between two *prima facie* opposing propositions. A fully developed constructive or systematic position cannot be elaborated here, but the direction which I believe a more complete development ought to take does become clear.

1. The same scientific situation generates opposing dispositions or outlooks toward the future. These dispositions can be characterized as confidence and hope on the one hand, and anxiety and fear on the other. The contrasts, and the reasons that can be given for each, can be developed in the following manner.

a. There are surely grounds for confidence and hope in the new bio-medical developments. (1) Scientists have uncovered new possibilities for human health and welfare: certain genetic defects might be eliminated, suffering can be decreased, human life can be prolonged, and even a genetically superior human race might be developed. (2) Many of the possibilities that frighten the masses are the products of irresponsible speculation and science fiction. (3) Members of the scientific community are humane moral persons who can be counted on to restrict the uses of knowledge to what enhances human health and welfare. (4) Men, in general (whether scientists, politicians, administrators, or philosophers), can be trusted to seek and to do what is beneficial for all mankind. (5) There is a providential process, or a providential Deity, that is ultimately working out its purposes, and these are beneficial to the development of man. For example, Teilhard de Chardin assures us that the developmental process is one of "hominization," "amorization," and "personalization," moving toward fulfillment in the Omega point. Or, Rahner assures us that God is "not only above us, as Lord and horizon of history, but also . . . he is ahead of us as our own future, that future which carries history forward."[3]

b. There is also a sharply contrasting outlook, for surely there are reasons for anxiety and fear. (1) Scientific developments now make it possible for human life as we know it to be altered radically, or perhaps even be destroyed. (2) Many of the most knowledgeable scientists are themselves alarmed by the growing destructive capabilities of science, and thus on their authority others ought to be deeply concerned. Gordon R. Taylor, for example, quotes Professor Salvador Luria of MIT as having said that his response has "not been a feeling of optimism but one of tremendous fear of the potential dangers that genetic surgery, once it becomes feasible, can create if misapplied."[4] (3) Members of the scientific community tend to become so engrossed in the pursuit of knowledge that they do not always think about the potential human consequences of their work. (4) Even those who are very morally sensitive do not always have it in their power to control the uses of knowledge. (5) History testifies to the fact that scientists in the past have not been able to control fully the uses of the power they create, and certainly some of them tend to use their knowledge for their own self-interest, or that of their particular group, rather than for the benefit of all mankind. Thus, on very general grounds, we need to be careful about expressing confidence in the moral wisdom of men. (6) Evolution is not governed by a purpose. Or, even if it is, many mistakes are made in the process, and there is no guarantee that its end is the fulfillment and benefit of the human species. (7) There is no providential Deity working out his purposes. Or, if there is, he has granted man such a degree of autonomy and power for self-creation that natural and historical developments are to be held to man's accountability, not God's.

It is important to note the different kinds of reasons that are given as warrants either for confidence or for anxiety. Some of them involve *factual judgments* and the *predictive ex-*trapolations made on the basis of them, such as whether both potential benefits and harms are likely, and which is most dominant. Thus some disputes could perhaps be settled by an objective assessment of the actual status of the biomedical sciences, though agreement of this will not necessarily lead to agreement on the most fitting outlook toward the future. Some reasons, however, are based on *evaluative assessments* of matters about which persons might have agreement with reference to the evidences. For example, does historical evidence support the judgment that men generally are to be trusted, or that we ought to be wary about excessive confidence in man's ability to know and to do what is good for all mankind? What one *believes about the human condition* makes a difference in his disposition toward the future, insofar as it is in human control. So also *theological* and *metaphysical* beliefs enter in, e.g., whether the evolutionary process is providential with regard to the human species, or whether there is a God whose purposes are to be trusted. Assessing the weight and functions of reasons like these is itself a logically complex task.

.   .   .

2. The issues of moral responsibility in biomedical developments are several, and they will concern us in a number of subsequent sections of this paper. At this point our concern is to ask what lies within the bounds of the moral or the ethical, and what lies outside of these bounds. Is bio-medical research ethically neutral? If it is, where does neutrality end? The answer given to these questions will begin to define where the researchers' moral responsibilities begin. Two contrasting positions may be taken.

a. Medical and biological research procedures, and the acquisition of knowledge, are morally neutral. Therefore the scientist, *qua* researcher, has no moral responsibility for his work.

b. Moral issues are so intertwined in research, in the gaining of knowledge from it, and the uses of this knowledge, that it is not possible to declare research procedures and the acquisition of knowledge to be morally neutral. Therefore the scientist, *qua* researcher, has moral responsibility for his work.

A little reflection on these alternatives makes it clear that the old term "value-free" is insufficiently precise to be of much use in dealing with the issue. It begs the question of what kinds of values, or of interests (and do "values" equal "interests"?) are involved in research. It is clear that research at least has a reference to the interests of the scientist. James D. Watson's widely read narrative of the discovery of the structure of DNA had a disenchanting, even demythologizing effect for many persons, for it demonstrated that scientists are motivated by a variety of interests in their pursuits even in the "purest" kind of research.[5] Research in that project did not have anything like the kind of disinterested rationality the scientist has in the widely popular stereotype. The motives of Professor Watson and others were not in any simple sense "value-free." They were in a highly competitive situation, seeking to gain the intellectual prize also being sought by others. But does the fact that the research had reference to the values and interests of the researcher in his pursuit of honor in any way involve a moral or ethical issue? Do we judge either the research or the scientists to be in any sense immoral because their motives are not as disinterested as common belief has assumed? It is by no means clear that we ought to. The fact that research is not "value-free," in the sense that it is motivated by the interests (including the self-interest) of the scientist, makes it neither moral nor immoral.

The fact that there is a morality of the pursuit and reporting of knowledge must be recognized. The biologist is at least obligated to conform to the rules of practice of his profession, whether or not he recognizes a wider sphere of moral responsibility. The rules include such things as being honest in reporting one's findings, acknowledging one's dependence upon the work of others, reporting procedures so that they can be critically examined by one's colleagues, and the like. The very possibility of a community of discourse among scientists is dependent upon a rigorous adherence to the established canons of practice in the field. While mistakes might be made and forgiven, deliberate deception leads to the immediate discreditation of the researcher. In the sense, then, that there is a code of rules of practice to which scientists have a moral obligation, no research is ethically neutral or "value-free." Thus when the question of the ethical neutrality of biological research is raised, it usually refers to some realm of values or principles other than the rules of practice of the profession.

When, then, do the moral questions arise with reference to bio-medical experimentation? Do they arise only with reference to the social *use* that is to be made of the findings? If they do, research and knowledge are in and of themselves ethically neutral; it is only in the employment of knowledge that questions of a moral nature arise. To make this claim is to take a position in favor of one major option involved in ethical theory. It is to choose a utilitarian view of ethics, and it opens the door to the intricate philosophical discussions of the viability and limitations of that view. Moral philosophers in the Anglo-Saxon world have for decades been arguing whether the morality of action is to be judged by its consequences, or whether other criteria need to be used. If one claims, for example, that because the transplantation of vital organs has led to the prolongation of life transplant surgery is "good," has one made a *moral* judgment, or some other kind of judgment? How is the "good" known? How is it measured? Are all "good" consequences to be assumed to have moral value?[6] Although this is not the place to develop these questions, the main point is important: to choose to judge the morality of scientists on the basis of the consequences of the use of their research is to take on the task of defending a point of view about ethics. Much can be said in its favor. Certainly one advantage of the utilitarian point of view for bio-medical researchers is that a clear line could be drawn between ethically neutral research and ethically laden uses of it. The scientist would not be held morally accountable for his research; others would be accountable for the uses made of it. Confronted with such a claim, however, many persons will quickly ask whether the scientist who makes certain uses possible by his research does not have some responsibility for their subsequent consequences. Certainly he has "causal" responsibility. But does causal responsibility imply moral responsibility?

Public clamor about the morality of science normally does not occur until after scientific knowledge has had some significant consequences for human welfare. Research in atomic and nuclear physics in the early decades of this century is a case in point; no one thought of making a public moral judgment about that work until it was used in military technology to develop weapons of mass destruction. Interestingly, theoretical physicists had different opinions about whether and, if so, where they were morally culpable for the development of those weapons. In the latter decades of the century, which reputedly "belong to the biologists" as the first did to the physicists, has it occurred to anyone to make a moral judgment about the Crick-Watson theory of the double helix structure of DNA? Surely not in and of itself. One can anticipate, however, that judgments will be made about the morality of genetic surgery and other forms of manipulation of the biological processes that the Crick-Watson theory and other information will have made possible.

The clearest difficulty in holding biologists culpable for their research lies in the fact that it can be used for both human good and human ill. Just as atomic physics made possible the destruction of Hiroshima and Nagasaki, it also opened a vast source of energy that is being used for socially useful purposes. Similarly, the same brain research that could lead to the control of human behavior by persons who gain control of certain resources can also make possible relief from mental anguish for deeply distressed persons. Is our only procedure one of *ex post facto* judgment? Do we calculate the benefits and the harms, and then decide whether research was morally justifiable? Even the entertainment of this possibility leads

to the conclusion that the uses of bio-medical research are morally ambiguous, and thus the research itself is at least morally ambiguous, if not neutral.

An alternative to the calculation of consequences in making moral judgments about scientists and their research would be to insist that certain things are morally right or wrong regardless of their effects. For example, Kant argued that it is morally wrong to tell a lie even from altruistic motives, with the intention of saving the life of a potential victim of assassination. But we will return to the consideration of this possibility in [the next section].

. . .

3. Moralists have puzzled for centuries over the proper answer to the questions, "Are there any intrinsically morally evil acts?" and "Are there any intrinsically morally good acts?" With reference to bio-medical research, some persons might argue that men have no moral right to conduct certain sorts of experiments, regardless of the potentially beneficial consequences, just as they would argue that it is morally wrong to torture a human being regardless of the value of the information that might be extricated from him through inflicting acute pain. This issue can be set in the following contrasts.

a. A scientist has *the right* to do anything he has the capacity to do in research, such as fertilize human eggs outside the uterus, "clone" a human being, alter the genotype of human beings, and manipulate brain responses. Various reasons might be given in support of this position, though most persons would not find all of them to be equally persuasive. (1) New knowledge is intrinsically valuable, and therefore worth getting regardless of the means required. (2) Men will do anything they have the capacity to do anyway, so it might as well be assumed that rights to do something arise from the capacity to do it. (Obviously this would lead to negative responses from almost everyone if it were generalized; for example, the capacity of the American military technologists to make poison gases does not give them the moral right to make them, and certainly not to use them.) (3) The "right to know" is one of the basic human liberties, and any restraint of this is an infringement on the freedom of the scientist. (4) Intellectual curiosity and growth are some of the most distinctive characteristics of human beings, and thus unrestricted fulfillment of their maximum possibilities is in accord with human nature. (5) If it had not been assumed that man has the right to do anything he has the capacity to do, many of the scientific and technical advances of the past would not have taken place. There have always been suspicions and superstitions that have led to restrictions of inquiry, and the effects of these have been to delay scientific advancement. Here one would be arguing that since the breaking of taboos in the past has had beneficial effects (both the intrinsic value of the knowledge secured and the beneficial uses to which it has been put), the same would also be true in the present.

b. A scientist has no right to intervene in the natural processes of human life because all life is sacred.

This position would not be advanced by any serious intelligent person in the modern world. Obviously men have intervened in the natural processes from the earliest time of human development in order to make human life more comfortable, healthier, and more rewarding. Thus, once the right to intervene has been granted, the lines of discussion can no longer be held to this fundamental proposition. . . .

c. A scientist has no right to intervene in the natural processes in such a way that he might alter what men believe to be most distinctively human.

This third proposition comes closest to the center of the anxieties of scientists and humanists alike. It assumes a distinction between the normal situation and the exceptional situation, and suggests that there might even be a different "logic" of rights on the borderline or unusual cases. Also it suggests that in our present scientific circumstances one of the oldest issues of thoughtful literature again takes on importance, namely the pursuit of a normative

understanding of humanity. A question discussed by Stoic, Platonic, Aristotelian, and ancient Christian thinkers takes on an acutely exacerbated quality in our situation.

Various reasons might be given in support of the third proposition as it is stated. (1) A qualitative difference in the meaning of human life would occur if the effects of research were radically to alter life as we know and value it. The risk is too great to give up the degree of certitude about life's meaning and values as we know them for the uncertainty of qualities and meanings that might emerge. (2) A qualitative difference in the powers to control human destiny would occur, and if these powers fell into the hands of those who do not share the same values most men share, they could lead to tyranny and worse. After all, it is not that "man" in general is in a new position to determine human destiny, an exaggeration made by theologians, philosophers, and popular commentators alike, but rather that *some* men will be in that position. (3) Man is made in the image of God, and to alter the fundamental image of man is to "play God," which is not only religious idolatry but also a movement beyond the healthy recognition of human finitude that keeps various forms of evil in check.

The important question raised by the third proposition is this: What constitutes the distinctively human? As we have noted, it is not a new question, but it takes on new importance now. On the surface this seems to be a factual question that could be answered through proper kinds of research. We might find that man has distinctive capacities for speech, for abstract reasoning, for intellectual exploration, for a qualitatively different kind of control over his destiny than other animals do, for certain kinds of aspirations, for a sense of moral responsibility, for love, etc., etc. But how would any such inquiries resolve the *normative* questions about what is to be most valued in human existence?

Some theologians are interested in arguing, for example, that what is distinctively human (and thus in the image of God) is the capacity for "self-creation," the capacity to control the development of life. If this is taken in isolation from other normative considerations, it might be inferred that it is morally right for man to do whatever enables him to further the control of human development. Yet it is precisely the haunting uncertainty of this that raises moral doubts of the most acute existential import, to which this paper is one exploratory response.

. . .

4. Can general moral principles or rules, or statements of normative humanity which might be developed, be applicable to the procedures and uses of scientific research? The question invites three sorts of more intensive inquiry. How would such principles, rules, or statements of human values be arrived at? What ought their content to be? And, if one had them, how would they be applied to particular circumstances? Thus the question invites a comprehensive treatise on ethics; here our concentration is on the third question, the issue of practical reasoning. Some attention will be paid to the other two sorts of inquiry subsequently.

a. The decisions about the procedures and uses of bio-medical research all depend upon the circumstances. It is useless to attempt to apply general moral principles and rules, or general statements about normative humanity.

b. General moral principles and rules, and statements of normative humanity, can determine or (weaker) give guidance to the morally licit interventions in the life processes and indicate norms and purposes of human life that should direct the intentions of those who use bio-medical research.

The first proposition suggests that each new development in research and technology raises significantly novel moral issues, and that any sort of ethical reasons used in previous circumstances is not readily applicable to the new ones. For example, it might be argued that the feasibility of transplantation of vital organs is not only a new stage in medical technology, but it consequently calls for an absolutely fresh rethinking of the problems of medical ethics. Or, in a different vein, it might be argued that reasoning from some traditional moral principles and human values when choices have to be made concerning which patient is to receive vital organs never settles the individual case in

hand. Thus one must rely upon the discerning intuitive judgment of the medical staff attending the case to choose what would be not only medically but also morally right in the particular circumstances. The medical, social, economic, and other circumstances of the particular case would be judged to be more decisive than any general principles or rules, or any statements of the priorities of values.

At least two important matters are at stake here. One is whether a high degree of novelty in the scientific and medical circumstances necessitates a high degree of novelty in the normative content of the ethical thinking that pertains to those circumstances. The other is how practical moral judgments ought to be made. This involves many problems of theoretical and practical importance, such as the place of reason, the place of emotions, sensibilities, and dispositions, the place of insight or intuition, the significance of technical data for the ethical determination of what ought to be done, and the authority and function of moral principles in a particular moral judgment.

The second proposition indicates the basic contrast between the stance that "everything depends upon the circumstances" and the stance that moral principles and statements of values ought to function in an important way in the determination of conduct. It does not settle two questions, as we have noted: how one derives such moral principles and statements of values, and what content they ought to have. Nor does it settle precisely how they ought to function in the process of making practical judgments.

Two important suppositions are present, however, if the second proposition is chosen. The first is that, regardless of the significant changes in scientific and medical developments, both certain *formal* and certain *contentual* ethics still pertain. Does transplant technology raise new ethical problems, or are persistent ones being raised in new circumstances. If it is the latter, one can define the ethical issues in more traditional terms. For example, the problem of to whom scarce resources (blood or organs) are to be given involves very seriously the issue of justice. The medical profession seeks to be just in the decisions it makes about the allocation of available resources. Two traditional concepts of formal justice might be recalled: "equals should be treated equally," and "to each his due." In the light of either of these, the determination of who will receive a vital organ raises the practical question of what constitutes a just claim to it. Should organs be available according to the principle "to each according to his need"? If they should, one must make precise what constitutes "need." Is it purely a medical need? Or should organs be available according to the principle "to each according to his worth to the community"? If this principle is used, a university president might be placed above an inveterate gambler on the preference list.[7] As the questions of transplants involve the choice of recipients, the questions of justice are indeed pertinent. New circumstances raise persistent ethical questions, and traditional concepts are applicable.

The second supposition is that rationality is of great importance in making practical moral decisions and in the determination of what possible course of events ought to be followed. The alternative to rationality might be the profundity and direction of one's immediate emotional response, or of one's steadier and more persistent sentiments. The possibility of intervening in the function of the brain to control responses through electrical stimulation might arouse anger, and this sense of indignation might be judged to be a sufficient basis for prohibiting such procedures. Or one's persistent sentiment of hopefulness might lead him to approve of anything that suggests promise for the benefit of mankind. Or the alternative might be more complex than either of these; it might be a kind of "perceptual intuitionism" that claims to discern what response is fitting in the light of the primacy and objectivity of the facts of the matter confronted.

. . .

5. . . . . Is the principal conflict that between the right of a single individual to bodily life and the benefits that might accrue to others from risking life? In the concrete moral issues of both procedures and uses of research are we forced to make a choice between an ethic whose content is determined by the *rights* of individuals and an ethic whose content is determined by the *benefits* for persons and society? This issue is not only in the center of controversies in ethical theory, but it is also at the heart of many practical matters in the bio-medical field. Before stating the contrasting propositions, this issue might be illustrated from the area of the ethics of population control. On the basis of predictions of the harm that uncontrolled population growth will bring, or of the benefits that population control will bring, there are those who would argue that the rights of individuals are of no significant moral importance, such as the right of husband and wife to determine how many children they will have, or the right of the fetus (if such is granted) to come to full term. The benefits anticipated are determinative. Others would obviously disagree with this. Our contrasting propositions follow.[8]

a. The rights of individuals are sacred and primary, and therefore under no circumstances are they to be violated in favor of benefits to others that might be gained from their violation.

b. Anticipated consequences judged in terms of the "good" that will be achieved, or the "evil" that will be avoided, ought to determine policy and action, regardless of the restrictions on individual rights that this might require.

c. Propositions *a* and *b* are both one-sided. Decisions require consideration both of individual rights and of benefits to others. Thus one of the two can be the base line, and the other can function as the principle which justifies the restrictions on, or the exceptions to, the base line.

With these propositions we return to an issue previously introduced. In a crude sense the issue is that of means and ends, but a statement made in terms of individual rights and benefits to others provides a sharper focus for the ethical issues. It is not difficult to find examples which would give persuasive evidence that either *a* or *b* taken by itself leads to consequences which make most persons morally uneasy. Dr. Henry K. Beecher of Harvard, for example, has vigilantly exposed instances in which individual rights have been violated in the pursuit of medical experimentation, and many of the instances are indeed disturbing.[9] Instances of experimentation on institutionalized children who have no possibility of giving informed consent readily arouse profound moral resentment, as do the many documented evidences of the infamous activities of physicians in Nazi Germany. Yet the insistence that every fetus has the right to be born, regardless of the consequences for itself (e.g., if it is known to be deformed), for its family, or for the society as a whole, evokes the indignation of many persons whose dedication is to proposition *b*.

It is interesting and important to note that many individuals would morally resent both examples. This suggests that while adherence to either proposition *a* or to proposition *b* would have the effect of providing consistency in action and policy, such consistency seems not to be in and of itself admirable. Most persons would question the admirable character of such consistency because of the consequences to which it leads. (The implications of this latter for ethical theory are matters of importance outside the bounds of our present concerns.) In the face of the *prima facie* unsatisfactory character of either *a* or *b*, proposition *c* suggests an alternative.

The alternative of *c* is deliberately general. It might well be that under certain circumstances it is morally responsible to make the thrust of individual rights the base line, and under other circumstances the accounting of benefits. Most of the literature with which I am acquainted that deals with experimentation on human beings seems to take the first. The concern to make certain that the subject gives free and informed consent to being used for experimental purposes suggests this. (Perhaps this is because much of this literature has legal questions in mind, or is prepared by lawyers, and it has been a primary function of the law to uphold human rights.) Also, the more specific kinds of questions that are raised in these discussions suggest the same thrust. For example, before experimentation takes place on human beings, has experimentation on animals that

might lead to the knowledge sought for been exhausted? The practice of sacrificing animals rather than human beings indicates the widespread acceptance of the intent of the question. Is the knowledge to be gained important enough to risk the violation of individual lives? This question leads to consideration of benefits. If, as in the case of Salk vaccine, the potential benefit is the virtual eradication of polio which reached epidemic proportions over and over again, there would be greater justification than if the benefits would accrue only to the acclaim of the experimenter by his colleagues, or if it would affect only a handful of persons. What are the chances of success in the experimentation? If they are meager, the situation is different from one in which they are great. What is the degree of risk to the human subject? Might it cost his life? Or impair his functions in such a way that he cannot live a "normal" life? Or only slightly impair his functions?

. . .

There might be other areas in which the counting of potential benefits, rather than individual rights, becomes the base line. As the possibilities of genetic surgery, of "cloning" human beings, and the like, emerge, the calculation of benefits appears to be the primary concern, and the secondary question is that of the cost to rights of individuals as we know them now.

The point of proposition *c* is by now clear. It offers a way to think with some ethical sophistication about complex questions that exist. It is possible that the concerns of *a* might be accounted for in a sophisticated statement of *b*, and thus that one might have a consistency of theory. But in the first order of discourse about the ethical problems confronting developments in the bio-medical field it is important to keep the polarity between them more clearly in mind for the practical benefit of forcing a sharp awareness of the seriousness and complexity of the issues that are involved. A refined and rigorous development of proposition *c* would have such an effect.

6. When men are confronted with develop-

ments that could lead to radical change, they are likely to respond in one or two extreme ways. On the one hand, there is an impulse to guard and preserve the good things that have been achieved, and not allow them to be subject to potential loss in the course of change. On the other hand, there is an impulse to enthusiasm for the novelty that the developments promise to bring, and with it a softening of rigorous concerns for the maintenance of values already achieved. This is evident, for example, in certain reactions to social revolutions that are moving toward a future that is not fully predictable. With these impulses come different basic styles or modes of ethical response. The first is concerned to conserve what exists against the threats that are posed against it; the second moves with freedom and openness toward the future. Something similar occurs when we ponder the issues that emerge from developments in the bio-medical field.

a. It is best to restrict the kinds of experimentation that will be permitted through civil legislation and regulation, and through clearly defined general moral rules, in order to preserve human rights and values as we know them.

b. It is best to ensure the maximum possible freedom for research and for the human capacities for self-development regardless of the risks that are involved.

c. It is best to maintain the maximum possible freedom for research, but at the same time to formulate principles and values that will provide guidelines both for procedures and for uses of research.

These propositions bring us around full circle to those introduced in the first issue, namely, whether there are primarily grounds for confidence and hope, or for anxiety and fear with reference to the future development of man. Those who would opt to support proposition *a* are likely to be those who respond with anxiety and fear, and their support of the use of restrictive regulation would appear to be the proper practical inference to be drawn from the reasons they would give for their anxiety. Those who would opt for proposition *b* are likely to be those who respond with confidence and hope, and this choice would appear to them to be the practical inference from their reasons given for confidence.

Proposition *c* is primarily a qualification of *b*. It shares some of the reasons that would be given in support of *b*, but not all of them. The proponent of *c* might reason in the following way. Man has always been developing new ways to control his own destiny, and that of the human race. His history is in part the story of his efforts to intervene in the "natural" course of events to give greater mastery and control over those powers to which he has appeared to be subject. He has not assumed that he is fated by the natural forces that have created pain and suffering, but he has constantly discovered new ways to fulfill many of his aspirations and ends. Indeed, in his development he has seen new dimensions of the meaning of being human; for example, he has found institutions like slavery and capital punishment to be inconsistent with what human fulfillment and life mean. His interventions into nature have led to the irrigation of wastelands, the manufacture of chemicals to increase his food production, and the development of means to control population growth. He has always assumed the right to intervene in nature to be consistent with his capacities for self-determination.

The priority here is on the capacities for exploration, or for intervention, or for what Karl Rahner has called "self-creativity." This is the kind of being man is. He will continue to attempt to do whatever he thinks he has the capacity to do, and his ability to do new things will expand with his knowledge of the fundamental processes of life. Thus far, perhaps the proponents of *b* and *c* share a common outlook.

But man, the active experimenter and intervener, discovers that many things he is capable of doing do not issue in the welfare of the human community. He does this not by reference to some fixed image of what man essentially is and ought to be, as an extrinsic and mechanical test of his deeds, but by responding in moral seriousness to the new possibilities that emerge under new circumstances. It is not that what is known from the past about the values and rights of man is not pertinent to the future, but rather that the ongoing biological development of human life needs a direction toward those values which preserve and enhance the qualities of life that give a sense of fulfillment. His ethical task involves the formulation of those ends and values which give direction to the ways in which he plays the card-game of life. It involves seeking out in particular circumstances the limits beyond which he will become destructive of humane qualities of life, and perhaps even enforcing those limits by civil law. But more importantly it involves an ongoing rigorous conversation between those who can best pose the questions of ethics and human values and those who are shaping the most significant developments in the bio-medical field.

What *c* envisages is not so much a restrictive morality that authoritatively addresses each new possibility with an exact determination of what is absolutely right and wrong, good and evil, but an ongoing moral discourse and activity that helps to shape the developments of even biological life toward the end of fulfillment of the valued qualities of human life.

If this approach has merit, the chief task is to develop with both sensitivity and clarity an understanding of the qualities or values of human life and a conception of the basic human rights that will provide the moral guidelines or touchstones for human development . . . . The task is obviously not a new one; it has occupied the attention of theologians and philosophers, poets, novelists, and dramatists, scientists, and many others for centuries. But it takes on a qualitatively new importance in the present time, and demands the most of all who can contribute to it. For at stake is the future of humanity.

NOTES

1. Teilhard de Chardin, *The Phenomenon of Man* (New York, 1961), p. 231, p. 229.
2. Karl Rahner, "Experiment: Man," *Theology Digest,* Sesquicentennial Issue (February 1968), p. 58.
3. Rahner, op. cit., p. 65.
4. Gordon R. Taylor, *The Biological Time Bomb* (New York, 1968), p. 183.

5. James D. Watson, *The Double Helix* (New York, 1968).
6. The vast literature was provoked most of all by G. E. Moore's *Principia Ethica* (Cambridge, 1903), and the statement of the "naturalistic fallacy."
7. The literature on justice is vast. A very influential recent analysis is that made by Chaim Perelman, *The Idea of Justice and the Problem of Argument* (London, 1963).
8. An older, but still useful discussion of this issue is W. D. Ross, *The Right and the Good* (London, 1930), especially Ch. II, "What Makes Right Acts Right?"
9. Among his many articles, the one in Daniel Labby, ed., *Life or Death: Ethics and Options* (Seattle, 1968), pp. 114–151, provides an excellent summary of both Beecher's evidences and his ethical position.

SUGGESTED READINGS FOR CHAPTER 2

Books and Articles

"Bioethics and Social Responsibility." *Monist* 60 (January, 1977). Special issue.

Branson, Roy. "Bioethics as Individual and Social: the Scope of a Consulting Profession and Academic Discipline." *Journal of Religious Ethics* 3 (Spring, 1975), 111–139.

Callahan, Daniel. "Bioethics as a Discipline." *Hastings Center Studies* 1 (No. 1, 1973), 66–73.

Campbell, Alastair V. *Moral Dilemmas in Medicine*. 2nd edition. Edinburgh: Churchill-Livingston, 1975.

Fletcher, Joseph. *Morals and Medicine*. Boston: Beacon Press, 1954.

Fox, Renée C. "Advanced Medical Technology—Social and Ethical Implications." In Inkeles, Alex, *et al.*, eds. *Annual Review of Sociology,* Volume 2. Palo Alto, Calif: Annual Reviews, 1976. Pp. 231–268.

Fox, Renée C. "Ethical and Existential Developments in Contemporaneous American Medicine: Their Implications for Culture and Society." *Milbank Memorial Fund Quarterly* 52 (Fall, 1974), 445–483.

Gorovitz, Samuel, *et al.*, eds. *Moral Problems in Medicine*. Englewood Cliffs, N.J.: Prentice-Hall, 1976.

Ramsey, Paul. *The Patient as Person*. New Haven: Yale University Press, 1970.

Reich, Warren T., ed. *Encyclopedia of Bioethics*. New York: Macmillan and Free Press, 1978.

Veatch, Robert M. "Medical Ethics in a Revolutionary Age." *Journal of Current Social Issues* (Fall, 1975), 4–19.

Journals

   Hastings Center Report

   Journal of Medical Ethics

   Journal of Medicine and Philosophy

Bibliographies

Sollitto, Sharmon, and Veatch, Robert M., comps. *Bibliography of Society, Ethics and the Life Sciences*. Hastings-on-Hudson, N.Y.: Institute of Society, Ethics and the Life Sciences. Updated periodically. See under "Introductory Readings in Ethics and the Life Sciences."

Walters, LeRoy, ed. *Bibliography of Bioethics*. Vols. 1- . Detroit: Gale Research Co. Issued annually. See under "Bioethical Issues," "Bioethics," and "Medical Ethics."

3.
Health and Disease

The controversies in every chapter of this book are either centrally or loosely connected with modern problems of disease treatment and prevention. Medical science, we often say, is dedicated to the restoration and maintenance of health. But what is disease? And what is health? To ask questions of this sort is to ask not only how disease and health are to be understood, but also how they are to be distinguished from other human conditions, such as misery and ecstasy or achievement and failure. The questions "What is health?" and "What is disease?" may be understood, then, as requests for comprehensive definitions or conceptual explications of health and disease.

An influential example examined in this chapter is the World Health Organization (WHO) definition of "health": "Health is a state of complete physical, mental, and social well-being and not merely the absence of disease or infirmity." This definition is not inconsequential, since it has important implications both for our understanding of the role of medical practitioners and for public policy. If the goal of medicine is the maintenance and restoration of health, and if this term is understood broadly as complete well-being, then the scope of medical practice will be assumed to be quite extensive. Its scope will include for example, problems of social deviancy and all personal difficulties in adapting to new environments. Private and public health policies, such as insurance coverage, would then be adjusted to this (WHO) understanding of health.

To some the analysis of health and disease is intrinsically interesting, for they would simply like to know for the sake of clarity and understanding what health and disease are. Others are interested in such knowledge as a means to the end of developing healthy persons. However, it is the implications such definitions have for both practical decisions and medical policies such as those mentioned above that give the issue its urgency and direct relevance to ethics.

THE DEFINITION OF HEALTH AND DISEASE

There have been three prominent and competing ways of approaching the definition of health. The major controversy concerns how much ground the term "health" covers. Does it encompass treatment of the body? The mind? Social adaptability? The WHO definition falls in the most inclusive class of definitions: "Health is a state of complete *physical, mental,* and *social* well-being. . . ." René Dubos also seems, in his selection in this chapter, to support the inclusion of all three measures of well-being. A second class of definitions, however, excludes the social dimension, while retaining the *physical and mental.* Daniel Callahan is tempted by this approach, but eventually accepts a third and even more restrictive definition of health as "a state of *physical* well-being . . . without significant impairment of function." The approach taken by Callahan has the weight of tradition behind it, since in both the history of medicine and the history of philosophy (especially in the works of Plato, Aristotle, and Descartes) health is primarily regarded as physical well-being. This traditional support is not in itself decisive, of course. Several authors have pointed out that only recently have plausible reasons emerged for extending the scope of the concept.

Controversies over the definition of disease have a rather different focus. Here one central issue is whether or not the term "disease" (and "illness," if different) refers to conditions objectively in nature, or whether diseases are social constructions which are determined (wholly or partially) by our positive or negative evaluations, or whether some third alternative is correct. In our readings H. Tristram Engelhardt gives a vivid example of the non-objectivity of some "diseases" by analyzing the history of medical views of masturbation; and Peter Sedgwick provides an account of the full thesis that disease is nothing but a human social construction created by our likes and dislikes. One of Sedgwick's chief examples and his most striking conclusion are linked in the following way:

> The blight that strikes at corn or at potatoes is a human invention, for if man wished to cultivate parasites (rather than potatoes or corn) there would be no blight, but simply the necessary foddering of the parasite-crop. . . . Outside the significances that man voluntarily attaches to certain conditions, *there are no illnesses or diseases in nature*.

Sedgwick is challenging views of health rooted in classical philosophy and medicine, in modern mechanistic views of the body, and in the germ theory of disease. Not surprisingly, there has been a reaction to this evaluative theory of disease. In this chapter Leon Kass represents what many would regard as a return to more traditional views, especially as found in classical philosophy and medicine. And Christopher Boorse offers a third position, which maintains the objectivity of "disease" and the normativeness of "illness."

It should not go unnoticed that questions concerning whether "disease" is an inherently normative or evaluative concept may also be asked about "health." These controversies directly relate to the problem of whether "mental health" and "mental disease" are inherently evaluative notions. One could, of course, decide that "health" and "disease" should be defined as Callahan suggests (as exclusively concerned with *physical* well-being) and are *non-evaluative* notions as applied to physical health, while also claiming that such notions are either inherently evaluative or stretched beyond the bounds of normal objectivity when used in expressions such as "mental health" and "social disease." This illustration of the interconnection between problems of defining health and problems of defining disease is only one indicator of the striking complexity and interrelatedness of the issues raised in this chapter.

TYPES OF DEFINITION

There are at least four different ways of defining terms, and it is important to distinguish them in attempting to define "health" and "disease." Since many other terms besides these two will be the subjects of definitional investigation in this book (prominent ones include "death," "euthanasia," "behavior control," and "insanity"), it will prove worthwhile to discuss here the general nature of these four different types of definition.

1. *Descriptive Definitions* attempt to report the usage of terms as we ordinarily employ them. All good dictionary definitions have this aim, since they inform us how the words of a particular language actually are used by those who speak the language. If there are different meanings or uses of the same term, they will be distinguished by such definitions. Sometimes these definitions are little more than the substitution of synonym for synonym. The better formulated definitions, however, explicate the common meaning of terms by specifying the conditions which

must hold for the word to apply correctly. For example, Plato occasionally defines "health" in terms of the unimpeded natural functioning of the body. He seems to be attempting to describe the most general meaning of the term. Such definitions are either true or false, since they are either correct or incorrect reports of common usage.

2. *Stipulative Definitions* are ones which, instead of reporting actual usage, stipulate the meanings of terms, usually for purposes of clarity where the ordinary meaning is vague. Often the stipulation is only temporary and for a special purpose. For example, if the term "health" were defined as "the state of successful adaptation to the pressures of city life," such a definition would be stipulative. There are reasons of convenience and clarity for using stipulative definitions such as this one (imagine a study of the pressures of city life being presented to a convention of social psychologists); and it is not wrong to use such definitions as long as they are explicitly said to be stipulative and do not masquerade as descriptive. Unlike descriptive definitions, stipulative ones are neither true nor false, since they are simply proposals or announcements of usage. They might appear useless and misleading, since ordinary uses are excluded, but they cannot be mistaken.

3. *Reforming Definitions* resemble both descriptive and stipulative definitions. They provide new meanings for old terms by suggesting new outlooks not incorporated in previous usage. But they are not simply stipulative, since they try to illuminate proper usage by giving a deeper insight into the meaning of a term. Also, they attempt to *reform* ordinary usage, whereas stipulative definitions often do not aim at reform (since they either introduce new meanings or are temporary and only for a special purpose). In the readings in this chapter, Daniel Callahan mentions an example of a reforming definition. He notes that the task of defining "health" is often not merely descriptive but (as in the case of the WHO definition) "is nothing less than a way of deciding what should be valued, how life should be understood, and what principles should guide individual and social conduct." If Callahan is correct, it is clear that reforming definitions may also be important and even programmatic attempts to change our actions and policies. Such definitions are usually offered as the result of a theory—perhaps a social theory or perhaps a scientific theory. To assess the adequacy of the definition will thus probably require an assessment of the adequacy of that part of the theory which generates it.

4. *Real Definitions* are attempts to state what the real properties of something are. Such definitions are of special importance when (as in the case of reforming definitions) it is believed that ordinary usage is mistaken and therefore descriptive definitions necessarily inadequate. It might be, for example, that ordinary usage reflects Aristotle's belief that the term "man" means "rational animal." But perhaps it is not truly necessary that man be rational, since human infants do not appear to be rational. (This topic will be discussed in Chapter 5, Abortion.) If so, we would like to know what "man" *really is,* not just what the term might mean. Similarly in the case of "mental illness," we want to know what such illness really is, (if it is illness at all) and not simply what is commonly meant by the term. Such definitions are usually reforming definitions (though not necessarily, since the language might not need reformulation); but not all reforming definitions are real definitions. Many persons are now skeptical that real definitions can be given at all, since they are doubtful that language and theory are capable of grasping the real properties of things without recourse to an evaluative or theoretical perspective; but whether or not this is so, attempts to provide real definitions recur frequently.

In the readings in this chapter, several authors provide definitions of "health," "disease," and "illness." It is important to analyze what type or mixture of types of definition is being offered, for only then can one be prepared to judge the definition's acceptability. This is especially important where an author claims to be providing a descriptive or a real definition but in fact is providing a stipulative or a reforming one.

T.L.B.

WORLD HEALTH ORGANIZATION

A Definition of Health

The States Parties to this Constitution declare, in conformity with the Charter of the United Nations, that the following principles are basic to the happiness, harmonious relations and security of all peoples:

Health is a state of complete physical, mental and social well-being and not merely the absence of disease or infirmity.

The enjoyment of the highest attainable standard of health is one of the fundamental rights of every human being without distinction of race, religion, political belief, economic or social condition.

The health of all peoples is fundamental to the attainment of peace and security and is dependent upon the fullest co-operation of individuals and States.

The achievement of any State in the promotion and protection of health is of value to all.

Unequal development in different countries in the promotion of health and control of disease, especially communicable disease, is a common danger.

Healthy development of the child is of basic importance; the ability to live harmoniously in a changing total environment is essential to such development.

The extension to all peoples of the benefits of medical, psychological and related knowledge is essential to the fullest attainment of health.

Informed opinion and active co-operation on the part of the public are of the utmost importance in the improvement of the health of the people.

Governments have a responsibility for the health of their peoples which can be fulfilled only by the provision of adequate health and social measures.

Accepting these principles, and for the purpose of co-operation among themselves and with others to promote and protect the health of all peoples, the Contracting Parties agree to the present Constitution and hereby establish the World Health Organization as a specialized agency within the terms of Article 57 of the Charter of the United Nations.

From the Preamble to the Constitution of the World Health Organization. Adopted by the International Health Conference held in New York from 19 June to 22 July 1946, and signed on 22 July 1946 by the representatives of sixty-one States (*Off. Rec. Wld Hlth Org.* 2, 100). Reprinted with permission of the publisher from *The First Ten Years of the World Health Organization, WHO*, 1958.

DANIEL CALLAHAN

The WHO Definition of "Health"

There is not much that can be called fun and games in medicine, perhaps because unlike other sports it is the only one in which everyone, participant and spectator, eventually gets killed playing. In the meantime, one of the grandest games is that version of king-of-the-hill where the aim of all players is to upset the World Health Organization (WHO) definition of "health." That definition, in case anyone could possibly forget it, is, "Health is a state of complete physical, mental, and social well-being and not merely the absence of disease or infirmity." Fair game, indeed. Yet somehow, defying all comers, the WHO definition endures, though literally every other aspirant to the crown has managed to knock it off the hill at least once. One possible reason for its presence is that it provides such an irresistible straw man; few there are who can resist attacking it in the opening paragraphs of papers designed to move on to more profound reflections.

But there is another possible reason which deserves some exploration, however unsettling the implications. It may just be that the WHO definition has more than a grain of truth in it, of a kind which is as profoundly frustrating as it is enticingly attractive. At the very least it is a definition which implies that there is some intrinsic relationship between the good of the body and the good of the self. The attractiveness of this relationship is obvious: it thwarts any movement toward a dualism of self and body, a dualism which in any event immediately breaks down when one drops a brick on one's toe; and it impels the analyst to work toward a conception of health which in the end is resistant to clear and distinct categories, closer to the felt experience. All that, naturally, is very frustrating. It seems simply impossible to devise a concept of health which is

Reprinted with permission of the author and the Institute of Society, Ethics and the Life Sciences from *The Hastings Center Studies*, Vol. 1, No. 3 (1973).

rich enough to be nutritious and yet not so rich as to be indigestible.

One common objection to the WHO definition is, in effect, an assault upon any and all attempts to specify the meaning of very general concepts. Who can possibly define words as vague as "health," a venture as foolish as trying to define "peace," "justice," "happiness," and other systematically ambiguous notions? To this objection the "pragmatic" clinicians (as they often call themselves) add that, anyway, it is utterly unnecessary to know what "health" means in order to treat a patient running a high temperature. Not only that, it is also a harmful distraction to clutter medical judgment with philosophical puzzles.

Unfortunately for this line of argument, it is impossible to talk or think at all without employing general concepts: without them, cognition and language are impossible. More damagingly, it is rarely difficult to discover, with a bit of probing, that even the most "pragmatic" judgment (whatever *that* is) presupposes some general values and orientations, all of which can be translated into definitions of terms as general as "health" and "happiness." A failure to discern the operative underlying values, the conceptions of reality upon which they are based, and the definitions they entail, sets the stage for unexamined conduct and, beyond that, positive harm both to patients and to medicine in general.

But if these objections to any and all attempts to specify the meaning of "health" are common enough, the most specific complaint about the WHO definition is that its very generality, and particularly its association of health and general well-being as a positive ideal, has given rise to a variety of evils. Among them are the cultural tendency to define all social problems, from war to crime in the streets, as "health" problems; the blurring of lines of responsibility between and among the professions, and between the medical profession and the political order; the implicit denial of human freedom which results when failures to achieve social well-being are defined as forms of "sickness," somehow to be treated by medical means; and the general debasement of language which ensues upon the casual habit of labeling everyone from Adolf Hitler to student radicals to the brat next door as "sick." In short, the problem with the WHO definition is not that it represents an attempt to propose a general definition, but it is simply a bad one.

That is a valid line of objection, provided one can spell out in some detail just how the definition can or does entail some harmful consequences. Two lines of attack are possible against putatively hazardous social definitions of significant general concepts. One is by pointing out that the definition does not encompass all that a concept has commonly been taken to mean, either historically or at present, that it is a partial definition only. The task then is to come up with a fuller definition, one less subject to misuse. But there is still another way of objecting to socially significant definitions, and that is by pointing out some baneful effects of definitions generally accepted as adequate. Many of the objections to the WHO definition fall in the latter category, building upon the important insight that definitions of crucially important terms with a wide public use have ethical, social, and political implications; defining general terms is not an abstract exercise but a way of shaping the world metaphysically and structuring the world politically.

Wittgenstein's aphorism, "don't look for the meaning, look for the use," is pertinent here. The ethical problem in defining the concept of "health" is to determine what the implications are of the various uses to which a concept of "health" can be put. We might well agree that there are some uses of "health" which will produce socially harmful results. To carry Wittgenstein a step further, "don't look for the uses, look for the abuses." We might, then, examine some of the real or possible abuses to which the WHO definition leads, recognizing all the while that what we may term an "abuse" will itself rest upon some perceived *positive* good or value.

HEALTH AND HAPPINESS

Let us examine some of the principal objections to the WHO definition in more detail. One of them is that, by including the notion of "social well-being" under its rubric, it turns the enduring probem of human happiness into one more medical problem, to be dealt with by scientific means. That is surely an objectionable feature, if only because there exists no evidence whatever that medicine has anything more than a partial grasp of the sources of human misery. Despite [the optimism of Dr. Brock Chisholm, the first Director of WHO], medicine has not even found ways of dealing with more than a fraction of the whole range of physical diseases; campaigns, after all, are still being mounted against cancer and heart disease. Nor is there any special reason to think that future forays against those and other common diseases will bear rapid fruits. People will continue to die of disease for a long time to come, probably forever.

But perhaps, then, in the psychological and psychiatric sciences some progress has been made against what Dr. Chisholm called the "psychological ills," which lead to wars, hostility, and agression? To be sure, there are many interesting psychological theories to be found about these "ills," and a few techniques which can, with some individuals, reduce or eliminate anti-social behavior. But so far as I can see, despite the mental health movement and the rise of the psychological sciences, war and human hostility are as much with us as ever. Quite apart from philosophical objections to the WHO definition, there was no empirical basis for the unbounded optimism which lay behind it at the time of its inception, and little has happened since to lend its limitless aspiration any firm support.

Common sense alone makes evident the fact that the absence of "disease or infirmity" by no means guarantees "social well-being." In one sense, those who drafted the WHO definition seem well aware of that. Isn't the whole point of their definition to show the inadequacy of negative definitions? But in another sense, it may be doubted that they really did grasp that point. For the third principle enunciated in the WHO Constitution says that, "the health of all peoples is fundamental to the attainment of peace and security. . . ." Why is it fundamental, at least to peace? The worst wars of the twentieth century have been waged by countries with very high standards of health, by nations with superior life expectancies for individuals and with comparatively low infant mortality rates. The greatest present threats to world peace come in great part (though not entirely) from developed countries, those which have combatted disease and illness most effectively. There seems to be no historical correlation whatever between health and peace, and that is true even if one includes "mental health."

How are human beings to achieve happiness? That is the final and fundamental question. Obviously illness, whether mental or physical, makes happiness less possible in most cases. But that is only because they are only one symptom of a more basic restriction, that of human finitude, which sees infinite human desires constantly thwarted by the limitations of reality. "Complete" well-being might, conceivably, be attainable, but under one condition only: that people ceased expecting much from life. That does not seem about to happen. On the contrary, medical and psychological progress have been more than outstripped by rising demands and expectations. What is so odd about that, if it is indeed true that human desires are infinite? Whatever the answer to the question of human happiness, there is no particular reason to believe that medicine can do anything more than make a modest, finite contribution.

Another objection to the WHO definition is that, by implication, it makes the medical profession the gate-keeper for happiness and social well-being. Or if not exactly the gate-keeper (since political and economic support will be needed from sources other than medical), then the final magic-healer of human misery. Pushed far enough, the whole idea is absurd, and it is not necessary to believe that the organizers of the WHO would, if pressed, have

been willing to go quite that far. But even if one pushes the pretension a little way, considerable fantasy results. The mental health movement is the best example, casting the psychological professional in the role of high priest.

At its humble best, that movement can do considerable good; people do suffer from psychological disabilities and there are some effective ways of helping them. But it would be sheer folly to believe that all, or even the most important, social evils stem from bad mental health: political injustice, economic scarcity, food shortages, unfavorable physical environments, have a far greater historical claim as sources of a failure to achieve "social well-being." To retort that all or most of these troubles can, nonetheless, be seen finally as symptoms of bad mental health is, at best, self-serving and, at worst, just plain foolish.

A significant part of the objection that the WHO definition places, at least by implication, too much power and authority in the hands of the medical profession, need not be based on a fear of that power as such. There is no reason to think that the world would be any worse off if health professionals made all decisions than if any other group did; and no reason to think it would be any better off. That is not a very important point. More significant is that cultural development which, in its skepticism about "traditional" ways of solving social problems, would seek a technological and specifically a medical solution for human ills of all kinds. There is at least a hint in early WHO discussions that, since politicians and diplomats have failed in maintaining world peace, a more expert group should take over, armed with the scientific skills necessary to set things right; it is science which is best able to vanquish that old Enlightenment bogey-man, "superstition." More concretely, such an ideology has the practical effect of blurring the lines of appropriate authority and responsibility. If all problems—political, economic, and social—reduce to matters of "health," then there ceases to be any ways to determine who should be responsible for what.

THE TYRANNY OF HEALTH

The problem of responsibility has at least two faces. One is that of a tendency to turn all problems of "social well-being" over to the medical professional, most pronounced in the instance of the incarceration of a large group of criminals in mental institutions rather than prisons. The abuses, both medical and legal, of that practice are, fortunately, now beginning to receive the attention they deserve, even if little corrective action has yet been taken. (Counterbalancing that development, however, are others, where some are seeking more "effective" ways of bringing science to bear on criminal behavior.)

The other face of the problem of responsibility is that of the way in which those who are sick, or purportedly sick, are to be evaluated in terms of their freedom and responsibility. Siegler and Osmond elsewhere in this issue discuss the "sick role," a leading feature of which is the ascription of blamelessness, of non-responsibility, to those who contract illness. There is no reason to object to this kind of ascription in many instances—one can hardly blame someone for contracting kidney disease —but, obviously enough, matters get out of hand when all physical, mental, and communal disorders are put under the heading of "sickness," and all sufferers (all of us, in the end) placed in the blameless "sick role." Not only are the concepts of "sickness" and "illness" drained of all content, it also becomes impossible to ascribe any freedom or responsibility to those caught up in the throes of sickness. The whole world is sick, and no one is responsible any longer for anything. That is determinism gone mad, a rather odd outcome of a development which began with attempts to bring unbenighted "reason" and free self-determination to bear for the release of the helpless captives of superstition and ignorance.

The final and most telling objection to the WHO definition has less to do with the definition itself than with one of its natural historical consequences. Thomas Szasz has been the most eloquent (and most single-minded) critic of that sleight-of-hand which has seen the concept of health moved from the medical to the moral arena. What can no longer be done in the name of "morality" can now be done in the name of "health": human beings labeled, incarcerated, and dismissed for their failure to toe the line of "normalcy" and "sanity."

At first glance, this analysis of the present situation might seem to be totally at odds with the tendency to put everyone in the blame-free "sick role." Actually, there is a fine, probably indistinguishable, line separating these two positions. For as soon as one treats all human disorders—war, crime, social unrest—as forms of illness, then one turns health into a normative concept, that which human beings must and ought to have if they are to live in peace with themselves and others. Health is no longer an optional matter, but the golden key to the relief of human misery. We *must* be well or we will all perish. "Health" can and must be imposed; there can be no room for the luxury of freedom when so much is at stake. Of course the matter is rarely put so bluntly, but it is to Szasz's great credit that he has discerned what actually happens when "health" is allowed to gain the cultural clout which morality once had. (That he carries the whole business too far in his embracing of the most extreme moral individualism is another story, which cannot be dealt with here.) Something is seriously amiss when the "right" to have healthy children is turned into a further right for children not to be born defective, and from there into an obligation not to bring unhealthy children into the world as a way of respecting the right of those children to health! Nor is everything altogether lucid when abortion decisions are made a matter of "medical judgment" (see *Roe vs. Wade*); when decisions to provide psychoactive drugs for the relief of the ordinary stress of living are defined as no less "medical judgment"; when patients are not allowed to die with dignity because of medical indications that they can, come what may, be kept alive; when prisoners, without their consent, are subjected to aversive conditioning to improve their mental health.

ABUSES OF LANGUAGE

In running through the litany of criticisms which have been directed at the WHO definition of "health," and what seem to have been some of its long-term implications and consequences, I might well be accused of beating a dead horse. My only defense is to assert, first, that the spirit of the WHO definition is by no means dead either in medicine or society. In fact, because of the usual cultural lag which requires many years for new ideas to gain wide social currency, it is only now coming into its own on a broad scale. (Everyone now talks about everybody and everything, from Watergate to Billy Graham to trash in the streets, as "sick.") Second, I believe that we are now in the midst of a nascent (if not actual) crisis about how "health" ought properly to be understood, with much dependent upon what conception of health emerges in the near future.

If the ideology which underlies the WHO definition has proved to contain many muddled and hazardous ingredients, it is not at all evident what should take its place. The virtue of the WHO definition is that it tried to place health in the broadest human context. Yet the assumption behind the main criticisms of the WHO definition seem perfectly valid. Those assumptions can be characterized as follows: 1) health is only a part of life, and the achievement of health only a part of the achievement of happiness; 2) medicine's role, however important, is limited; it can neither solve nor even cope with the great majority of social, political, and cultural problems; 3) human freedom and responsibility must be recognized, and any tendency to place all deviant, devilish, or displeasing human beings into the blameless sick-role must be resisted; 4) while it is good for human beings to be healthy, medicine is not morality; except in very limited contexts (plagues and epidemics) "medical judgment" should not be allowed to become moral judgment; to be healthy is not to be righteous; 5) it is important to keep clear and distinct the different roles of different professions, with a clearly circumscribed role for medicine, limited to those domains of life where the contribution of medicine is appropriate. Medicine can save some lives; it cannot save the life of society.

These assumptions, and the criticisms of the WHO definition which spring from them, have some important implications for the use of the words "health," "illness," "sick," and the like. It will be counted an abuse of language if the word "sick" is applied to all individual and communal problems, if all unacceptable conduct is spoken of in the language of medical pathologies, if moral issues and moral judgments are translated into the language of "health," if the lines of authority, responsibility, and expertise are so blurred that the health profession is allowed to pre-empt the rights and responsibilities of others by redefining them in its own professional language.

Abuses of that kind have no possibility of being curbed in the absence of a definition of health which does not contain some intrinsic elements of limitation—that is, unless there is a definition which, when abused, is self-evidently *seen* as abused by those who know what health means. Unfortunately, it is in the nature of general definitions that they do not circumscribe their own meaning (or even explain it) and contain no built-in safeguards against misuse, e.g., our "peace with honor" in Southeast Asia—"peace," "honor"? Moreover, for a certain class of concepts—peace, honor, happiness, for example—it is difficult to keep them free in ordinary usage from a normative content. In our own usage, it would make no sense to talk to them in a way which implied they are not desirable or are merely neutral: by well-ingrained social custom (resting no doubt on some basic features of human nature) health, peace, and happiness are both desired and desirable—good. For those and other reasons, it is perfectly plausible to say the cultural task of defining terms, and settling on appropriate and inappropriate usages, is far more than a matter of getting our dictionary entries right. It is nothing less than a way of deciding what should be valued, how life should be understood, and what principles should guide individual and social conduct.

Health is not just a term to be defined. Intuitively, if we have lived at all, it is something we seek and value. We may not set the highest value on health—other goods may be valued as well—but it would strike me as incomprehensible should someone say that health was a matter of utter indifference to him; we would well doubt either his sanity or his maturity. The cultural problem, then, may be put this way. The acceptable range of uses of the term "health" should, at the minimum, capture the normative element in the concept as traditionally understood while, at the maximum, incorporating the insight (stemming from criticisms of the WHO definition) that the term "health" is abused if it becomes synonymous with virtue, social tranquility, and ultimate happiness. Since there are no instruction manuals available on how one would go about reaching a goal of that sort, I will offer no advice on the subject. I have the horrible suspicion, as a matter of fact, that people either have a decent intuitive sense on such matters (reflected in the way they use language) or they do not; and if they do not, little can be done to instruct them. One is left with the pious hope that, somehow, over a long period of time, things will change.

.   .   .

MODEST CONCLUSIONS

Two conclusions may be drawn. The first is that some minimal level of health is necessary if there is to be any possibility of human happiness. Only in exceptional circumstances can the good of self be long maintained in the absence of the good of the body. The second conclusion, however, is that one can be healthy without being in a state of "complete physical, mental, and social well-being." That conclusion can be justified in two ways: (a) because some degree of disease and infirmity is perfectly compatible with mental and social well-being; and (b) because it is doubtful that there ever was, or ever could be, more than a transient state of "complete physical, mental, and social well-being," for individuals or societies;

that's just not the way life is or could be. Its attractiveness as an ideal is vitiated by its practical impossibility of realization. Worse than that, it positively misleads, for health becomes a goal of such all-consuming importance that it simply begs to be thwarted in its realization. The demands which the word "complete" entail set the stage for the worst false consciousness of all: the demand that life deliver perfection. Practically speaking, this demand has led, in the field of health, to a constant escalation of expectation and requirement, never ending, never satisfied.

What, then, would be a good definition of "health"? I was afraid someone was going to ask me that question. I suggest we settle on the following: "health is a state of physical well-being." That state need not be "complete," but it must be at least adequate, i.e., without significant impairment of function. It also need not encompass "mental" well-being; one can be healthy yet anxious, well yet depressed. And it surely ought not to encompass "social well-being," except insofar as that well-being will be impaired by the presence of large-scale, serious physical infirmities. Of course my definition is vague, but it would take some very fancy semantic footwork for it to be socially misused; that brat next door could not be called "sick" except when he is running a fever. This definition would not, though, preclude all social use of the language of "pathology" for other than physical disease. The image of a physically well body is a powerful one and, used carefully, it can be suggestive of the kind of wholeness and adequacy of function one might hope to see in other areas of life.

RENÉ DUBOS

Health as Ability to Function

THE MIRAGE OF HEALTH

Benjamin Franklin once expressed in a letter to the chemist Joseph Priestley his belief that a time would come when "all diseases may by sure means be prevented or cured, not excepting that of old age, and our lives lengthened at pleasure even beyond the antediluvian standard." Depending upon one's prejudices, this statement may appear as a prophetic view of modern medical achievements, or as a naive expression of wishful thinking. More probably, however, Franklin simply reflected the optimism that permeated life during the Age of Reason. Condorcet, for example, went even further than Franklin in his optimistic prediction of the future. In the *Sketch for a Natural History of the Progresses of the Human Mind* he wrote in 1794, "I will show . . . that Nature has set no limit to the perfecting of the human faculties, that the perfectability of man, henceforth independent of any power that might wish to arrest it, has no other limit than the duration of the globe on which Nature has placed us."

During the past two centuries, social reformers and natural scientists have gone far toward converting into reality the concept of the Golden Age, so vividly imagined by Franklin and Condorcet. Indeed, it is truly a prodigious feat that the era of plenty, which was but a vague utopian dream at the end of the eighteenth century, has come to pass within less than 200 years of that time in several countries of Western civilization. If the social philosophers of the Age of Reason had spelled out in detail what they considered to be the essential requirements of health and happiness, their imaginings would probably prove to have become part and parcel of everyday life in the United States. Yet it is plain that health and happiness have not necessarily followed in step

with social, economic, and medical advances. Political freedom, abundance of worldly goods, and the miracles of modern medicine obviously are not sufficient to deal with the problems of the body and the mind that continue to plague man even under conditions of peace and prosperity.

One of the paradoxical aspects of the health picture is that despite the improvements in sanitation and nutrition, despite effective protection against heat, cold, humidity, and physical fatigue, an increasingly large percentage of the population depends on medical help for its daily existence. Most of the great plagues of the past have been brought under control, and more people than ever enjoy safety and comfort; yet the need for medical care and for hospital facilities is increasing everywhere. This paradox is not peculiar to the United States; it is encountered in each and every prosperous country of the Western world.

. . .

A few examples contrasting the medical problems of recent history with those characteristic of the present times will suffice to show how the pattern of diseases rapidly changes with the conditions of life.

Whereas microbiological pollution of water used to be responsible for much disease among our ancestors, chemical air pollution is now taking the limelight. Chemical fumes from factories and exhausts from motor cars are causing a variety of pathological disorders that bid fair to continue increasing in frequency and gravity and may become serious health handicaps in the near future. . . . There is reason to fear also that various types of radiation will soon add their long-range and unpredictable effects to this pathology of the future.

During recent decades we have gone far toward controlling microbial spoilage of food,

Reprinted with permission of the publisher from *Man Adapting* by René Dubos. © 1965 by Yale University Press.

but some of the new synthetic products that have become part and parcel of modern life are responsible for an endless variety of allergic and other toxic effects.

Nutritional deficiencies have now become rare in wealthy countries; but a new kind of malnutrition is arising from the fact that the nutritional regimens formulated for physically active human beings are no longer suited to automobile-borne and air-conditioned life in the twentieth century.

In the past many human beings suffered from physical exhaustion; now labor-saving devices and especially automated operations threaten to generate a type of psychiatric disturbance that will greatly complicate the medicine of tomorrow; boredom is replacing fatigue.

Who could have dreamed a generation ago that hypervitaminoses would become a common form of nutritional disease in the Western world; that the cigarette industry, air pollutants, and ionizing radiations would be held responsible for the increase in certain types of cancer; that the introduction of detergents and various synthetics would increase the incidence of allergies; that advances in chemotherapy and other therapeutic procedures would create a new staphylococcus pathology; that patients with various forms of iatrogenic disease would occupy such a large number of beds in the modern hospital; that some maladies of our times could be referred to by an eminent British epidemiologist as "pathology of inactivity" and "occupational hazards of sedentary and light work"?

There is reason to believe that the changes in ways of life and in technology are responsible in part for the degenerative diseases characteristic of our civilization. . . . But while this state of affairs demands serious attention, it need not create panic. The increased prevalence of certain diseases is not a new phenomenon. Disease presents itself in different forms today simply because the world is changing and demands new adaptive responses from human beings.

HEALTH AS ABILITY TO FUNCTION

The complex nature of man's response to his environment accounts for many of the difficulties experienced in developing methods for the prevention of disease. It is also responsible for the fact that the precise meanings of the words health and disease differ from one social group to another or even from person to person. Furthermore, the meanings change with time as well as with the environment and ways of life.

The definitions of health and disease that are commonly given by encyclopedias and academies remind one of Diafoirus' statement in Molière's play *Le Médecin malgré lui* that "opium induces sleep by virtue of the fact that it possesses a sleep producing property." In words that bring to mind this empty definition by which Molière poured ridicule on the ignorant and pretentious physicians of his time, modern dictionaries define disease as any departure from the state of health and health as a state of normalcy free from disease or pain. In 1946 the medical experts of the World Health Organization tried to sharpen and to enlarge the meaning of the word health by affirming that it implies not merely the absence of disease but rather a *positive* attribute, like a kind of primeval euphoria that would enable men to take advantage of all their potentialities for vigor and happiness. The introductory paragraph of the Constitution of the World Health Organization states: "Health is a state of complete physical, mental, and social well-being and is not merely the absence of disease or infirmity."

Health will be considered in the following pages from a more prosaic point of view. Instead of assuming that an ideal state of positive health can be achieved by eradicating all diseases from a utopian world, I shall take the view that the man of flesh, bone, and illusions will always experience unexpected difficulties as he tries to adapt to the real world, which is often hostile to him. In this light, positive health is not even a concept of the ideal to be striven for hopefully. Rather it is only a mirage, because man in the real world must face the physical, biological, and social forces of his environment, which are forever changing, usually in an unpredictable manner, and frequently with dangerous consequences for him as a person and for the human species in general. In the picturesque words of an English public health officer, "Man and his species are in perpetual struggle—with microbes, with incompatible mothers-in-law, with drunken car-drivers, and with cosmic rays from Outer Space. . . . The 'positiveness' of health does not lie in the state, but in the struggle—the effort to reach a goal which in its perfection is unattainable" (Gordon, 1958).

The evaluation of health and disease varies from person to person because it is conditioned by highly individual requirements and subjective reactions. In consequence, the words health and disease cannot be defined universally or statically. A Wall Street executive, a lumberjack in the Canadian Rockies, a newspaper boy at a crowded street corner, a steeple chase jockey, a cloistered monk rising during the night to pray and chant, and the pilot of a supersonic combat plane have very different physical and mental needs. The various imperfections and limitations of the flesh and the mind do not have equal importance for them. As pointed out by Ruth Benedict in *Patterns of Culture,* social aggressiveness is socially unacceptable and regarded as a form of disease by the Pueblo Indians, whereas this attribute is desirable in the countries of Western civilization because it facilitates the achievement of power and the acquisition of wealth.

Health is an even more elusive concept in the case of women. A farmer's wife with several children and a New York fashion model of the same age have very different physical requirements and therefore have different concepts of health. Furthermore, it is apparent from the history of fashions and from contemporary tastes that ideals of the feminine figure and complexion have undergone a wide gamut of changes in the course of time, and still differ at present from one country to the other. The fleshiness of the Paleolithic Venuses or of Ruben's goddesses reflects an attitude toward womanhood oddly different from the tastes that generated the slenderness of the English pre-Raphaelite models or of the American flapper in the 1920s. Entertainingly enough, sexual selection of hyperthyroidism occurred in much of Southern Europe during the sixteenth and seventeenth centuries, because this disease was then considered to enhance the attractiveness of young women. Lest this should appear nonsensical to us, we should remember that the dictates of publicity certainly affect our own concepts of health and physical attractiveness.

It must be acknowledged that history records many situations in which human beings seem to have achieved a state of physical development that can be regarded as healthy according to any criterion. In the account of his travels, for example, Christopher Columbus expressed admiration for the beautiful physical state of the natives he had found in the West Indies. Captain Cook, Bougainville, and the other navigators who discovered the Pacific islands also marvelled at the vigor of the Polynesians at that time; and similar reports came from the European explorers who first saw the American Indians in the Great Plains and in the Rio Grande valley. Even in modern times, people like the Xavantes Indians or the Mebans of East Africa generally remain vigorous as long as they live in isolated communities and retain their ancestral ways of life. . . .

In practically all cases, however, primitive people have undergone physical decadence within one generation after having had extensive contacts with the white man. It would seem therefore that the health of primitive people, like that of animals in the wild state, depends upon their ability to reach and maintain some sort of equilibrium with their environment. . . . In contrast, all of them are likely to fall prey to disease when their ancestral conditions of existence suddenly break down. For them, and certainly for us also, health can be regarded as an expression of fitness to the environment, as a state of adaptedness.

The societies of Polynesians, American Indians, Eskimos and other people who appeared so vigorous when first seen by European explorers provide examples of what Arnold Toynbee has called "arrested civilizations." They represent societies that lived for long periods of time under fairly stable physical and social conditions and had little if any contact with the outside world. New diseases appeared among them as soon as their *status quo* was disturbed, because changed conditions made new adaptive demands for which they were not prepared.

The examples mentioned above, among countless others which could have been selected, illustrate that it is not possible to define health in the abstract. Its criteria differ with the environmental conditions and with the norms and history of the social group. The criteria of health are conditioned even more by the aspirations and the values that govern individual lives. For this reason, the words health and disease are meaningful only when defined in terms of a given person functioning in a given physical and social environment. The nearest approach to health is a physical and mental state fairly free of discomfort and pain, which permits the person concerned to function as effectively and as long as possible in the environment where chance or choice has placed him. "Work is more important than life," Katherine Mansfield confided to the last pages of her journal. Searching for a definition of health as she was dying of tuberculosis, she could only conclude: "By health I mean the power to live a full, adult, living, breathing life in close contact with what I love—the earth and the wonders thereof. . . . I want to be all that I am capable of becoming."

LEON R. KASS

Regarding the End of Medicine and the Pursuit of Health

American medicine is not well. Though it remains the most widely respected of professions, though it has never been more competent technically, it is in trouble, both from without and from within.

The alleged causes are many; I will mention a few. Medical care is very costly and not equitably available. The average doctor sees many more patients than he should, yet many fewer than would like to be seen. On the one hand, the physician's powers and prerogatives have grown, as a result of new technologies yielding new modes of diagnosis and treatment, and new ways to alter the workings of the body. His responsibilities have grown as well, partly due to rising patient and societal demands for medical help with behavioral and social problems. All kinds of problems now roll to the doctor's door, from sagging anatomies to suicides, from unwanted childlessness to unwanted pregnancy, from marital difficulties to learning difficulties, from genetic counseling to drug addiction, from laziness to crime. On the other hand, the physician's new powers have brought new dilemmas, concern over which has led to new attempts to regulate and control his practices, including statutes, codes, professional review bodies, ombudsmen, national commissions, and lawsuits brought by public interest law and consumer groups. More and more physicians are being dragged before the bar, and medical malpractice insurance has become both alarmingly scarce and exorbitantly expensive.

. . .

Medicine, as well as the community which supports it, appears to be perplexed regarding

Reprinted with permission of Leon Kass and National Affairs, Inc. from *The Public Interest*, No. 40, (Summer 1975). Copyright © 1975 by National Affairs, Inc.

its purpose. It is ironic, but not accidental, that medicine's great technical power should arrive in tandem with great confusion about the standards and goals for guiding its use. When its powers were fewer, its purpose was clearer. Indeed, since antiquity, medicine has been regarded as the very model of an art, of a rational activity whose powers were all bent towards a clear and identifiable end. Today, though fully armed and eager to serve, the doctor finds that his target is no longer clear to him or to us. Sometimes, it appears to be anything at which he can take aim; at other times, it appears nowhere to be found. In fact, the very existence of a target is implicitly questioned by those who have begun to change the name of the doctor from "physician" to "member of the helping professions."

At what should the medical art aim? What is the proper end—or the proper ends—of medicine? Continued confusion about this matter could bring about, more directly than any other cause, the demise of the profession, even if there were to remain people with M.D. degrees whom their clients called "Doctor." For without a clear view of its end, medicine is at risk of becoming merely a set of powerful means, and the doctor at risk of becoming merely a technician and engineer of the body, a scalpel for hire, selling his services upon demand. There is a connection between the two meanings of "end" suggested by the title of this article: Since an end-less profession is an ended profession, there will be an end *to* medicine unless there remains an end *for* medicine. It is in part for this reason that I have chosen to inquire regarding the end, or purpose, of medicine, with the hope that we might more seriously regard—that is, look back at, pay attention to, and finally, esteem—the end or purpose of the medical art. Moreover, only by again attaining clarity about the goal of medicine can we hope intelligently to evaluate efforts to reach that goal and wisely to plan for their improvement. Otherwise, for all our good intentions, our health policies will be mere tinkerings in the dark, at great risk of doing more harm than good.

THE END OF MEDICINE

I trust it will shock no one if I say that I am rather inclined to the old-fashioned view that health—or if you prefer, the healthy human being—is the end of the physician's art. That health is *a* goal of medicine few would deny. The trouble is, so I am told, that health is not the only possible and reasonable goal of medicine, since there are other prizes for which medical technique can be put in harness. Yet I regard these other goals—even where I accept their goodness as goals—as false goals for medicine, and their pursuit as perversions of the art.

Let us examine some of the false goals that tempt today's physicians. First, there is what is usually called "happiness" in its sadly shrunken meaning, but which might best be called pleasure—that is, gratifying or satisfying patient desires, producing contentment. This temptation arises largely because of the open-ended character of some contemporary notions of mental health, which consider frustration or anxiety or any unsatisfied desires, no matter how questionable, to be marks of ill health, requiring a remedy.

Some examples of gratification may be helpful. A woman gets a surgeon to remove a normal breast because it interfered with her golf swing. An obstetrician is asked to perform amniocentesis, and then abortion, if the former procedure shows the fetus to be of the undesired gender. "Dr. Feelgood" devotes his entire practice to administering amphetamine injections to people seeking elevations of mood. To these real but admittedly extreme examples, one could add, among others, the now generally accepted practices of performing artificial insemination or arranging adoptions, performing vasectomies and abortions[1] for non-medical reasons (i.e., for family planning), dispensing antibiotics or other medicines simply because the patient wants to take something as well as some activities of psychiatrists and many of cosmetic surgeons (e.g., where the surgery does not aim to correct inborn or acquired abnormality or deformity). I would also add the practice, now being advocated more and more, of directly and painlessly killing a patient who wants to die.

All these practices, the worthy and the unworthy alike, aim *not* at the patient's health but rather at satisfying his, albeit in some cases reasonable, wishes. They are acts not of medicine, but of indulgence or gratification, in that they aim at pleasure or convenience or at the satisfaction of some other desire, and not at health. Now, some indulgence may be necessary in the *service* of healing, as a useful means to the proper end: I see nothing wrong in sweetening bad tasting medicine. But to serve the desires of patients as *consumers* should be the task of agents other than doctors, if and when it should be the task of anyone.

Even in its fuller sense, happiness is a false goal for medicine. By gerrymandering the definition of health to comprise "a state of complete physical, mental, and social well-being," the World Health Organization has in effect maintained that happiness is the doctor's business (even if he needs outside partners in this enterprise). For complete mental well-being—not to speak of the more elusive and ambiguous "social well-being," which will certainly mean different things to Pope Paul, President Ford, and Chairman Mao—goes well beyond the medical province of sanity, depending as it does on the successful and satisfying exercise of intelligence, awareness, imagination, taste, prudence, good sense, and fellow feeling, for whose cultivation medicine can do little. (That *happiness,* even in its full sense, is different from *health* can be seen in considering whether it would ever make sense to say, "Call no man *healthy* until he is dead.")

BEHAVIOR MODIFICATION

A second false goal for medicine is social adjustment or obedience, or more ambitiously, civic or moral virtue. The prevention of crime, the taming of juvenile delinquents, the relief of poverty and racial discrimination, the reduction of laziness and philandering, the rearing of decent and moral men and women—all worthy goals in my opinion—are none of the doctor's business, except as the doctor is also a human being and a citizen. These are jobs for parents, policemen, legislators, clergymen, teachers, judges, and the community as a whole—not to speak of the individual citizens themselves. It is doubtful that the physician has the authority and competence, as physician, to serve these goals with his skills and techniques.

The difficulty is, of course, that only doctors are able and legally entitled to manipulate the body; hence the temptation to lend this licensed skill to any social cause. This temptation is bound to increase as we learn more about the biological contributions to behavior. . . . But even assuming that we should accept, for example, psychosurgery for some men committing frequent crimes of violence, or the dispensing of drugs in schools for some restless children, or genetic screening to detect genotypes that may in the future be shown to predispose to violent behavior, I doubt that it is the proper business of medicine to conduct these practices—even though, on balance, there may be overriding prudential reasons for not establishing a separate profession of bio-behavioral conditioners.

I reject, next, in passing, the claim that the alteration of human nature, or of some human natures, is a proper end for medicine, whether it be a proposal by a psychologist for pills to reduce human "aggressiveness," especially in our political leaders, or the suggestions of some geneticists for eugenic uses of artificial insemination, or the more futuristic and radical visions of man-machine "hybrids," laboratory-grown "optimum babies," and pharmacologically induced "peace of mind."

. . .

DEATH PREVENTION

Let me, with some misgivings, suggest one more false goal of medicine: the prolongation of life, or the prevention of death. It is not so clear that this is a false goal, especially as it is so intimately connected with the medical art, and so often acclaimed as the first goal of medicine, or, at least, its most beneficial product. Yet to be *alive* and to be *healthy* are not the same, though the first is both a condition of the second, and, up to a point, a consequence. One might well ask whether we desire to live in order to live healthily and well, or whether we desire to be healthy and virtuous merely in order to stay alive. But no matter how desirable life may be—and clearly to be alive *is* a good, and a condition of all the other human goods—for the moment let us notice that the prolongation of life is ultimately an impossible, or rather an unattainable, goal for medicine. For we are all born with those twin inherited and inescapable "diseases," aging and mortality. To be sure, we can still achieve further reductions in *premature* deaths; but it often seems doubtful from our words and deeds that we ever regard any particular death as other than premature, as a failure to today's medicine, hopefully avoidable by tomorrow's.

If medicine aims at death prevention, rather than at health, then the medical ideal, ever more closely to be approximated, must be bodily immortality. Strange as it may sound, this goal really *is* implied in the way we as a community evaluate medical progress and medical needs. We go after the diseases that are the leading causes of death, rather than the leading causes of ill health. We evaluate medical progress, and compare medicine in different nations, in terms of mortality statistics. We ignore the fact that for the most part we are merely changing one set of fatal illnesses or conditions for another, and not necessarily for milder or more tolerable ones. We rarely stop to consider of what and how we will die, and in what condition of body and mind we shall spend our last years, once we can cure cancer, heart disease, and stroke.

I am not suggesting that we cease investigating the causes of these diseases. On the contrary, medicine *should* be interested in preventing these diseases, or failing that, in restoring their victims to as healthy a condition as possible. But it is primarily because they are causes of *unhealth,* and only secondarily because they are killers, that we should be interested in preventing or combating them. That their prevention and treatment may enable the prospective or actual victims to live longer may be deemed, in many cases, an added good, though we should not expect too much on this score. The complete eradication of heart dis-

ease, cancer, and stroke—currently the major mortal diseases—would, according to some calculations, extend the average life expectancy at birth only by approximately six or seven years, and, at age 65, by no more than one-and-a-half to two years.[2] Medicine's contribution to longer life has nearly reached its natural limit.

By challenging prolongation of life as a true goal of medicine, I may be challenging less what is done by practicing clinicians and more how we think and speak about it. Consider a concrete case. An elderly woman, still active in community affairs and family life, has a serious heart attack and suffers congestive heart failure. The doctor orders, among other things, oxygen, morphine, and diuretics, and connects her to a cardiac monitor, with pacemaker and defibrillator handy. What is the doctor's goal in treatment? To be sure, his actions, if successful, will help to keep her alive. But his immediate intention is to restore her circulatory functions as near to their healthy condition as possible; his more distant goal is to return her to her pre-morbid activities. Should the natural compensating and healing processes succeed, with his assistance, and should the cardiac wound heal and the circulation recover, the patient will keep herself alive.

We all are familiar with those sad cases in which a patient's life has been prolonged well beyond the time at which there is reasonable hope of returning him to a reasonably healthy state. Yet even in such cases—say a long-comatose patient or a patient with end-stage respiratory failure—a sensible physician will acknowledge that there is no longer any realizable therapeutic or medical goal, and will not take the mere preservation of life as his objective. Sometimes he may justify further life-prolonging activities in terms of a hope for a new remedy or some dramatic turn of events. But when reasonable hope of recovery is gone, he acts rather to comfort the patient as a friend and not especially or uniquely as a physician.

I do not want to be misunderstood. Mine is not an argument to permit or to condone medical callousness, or euthanasia practiced by physicians. Rather it is a suggestion that doctors keep their eye on their main business, restoring and correcting what can be corrected and restored, always acknowledging that death will and must come, that health is a mortal good, and that as embodied beings we are fragile beings that must snap sooner or later, medicine or no medicine. To keep the strings in tune, not to stretch them out of shape attempting to make them last forever, is the doctor's primary and proper goal.

To sum up: Health is different from pleasure, happiness, civil peace and order, virtue, wisdom, and truth. Health is possible only for mortal beings, and we must seek it knowing and accepting, as much as we are able to know and accept, the transience of health and of the beings who are healthy. To serve health and only health is a worthy profession, no less worthy because it does not serve all other goods as well.

WHAT IS "HEALTH"?

There was a time when the argument might have ended here, and we could have proceeded immediately to ask how the goal of health may be attained, and what the character of public policy toward health should be. But since there is nowadays much confusion about the nature and meaning of "health," we may have made but little progress by our identification of health as the proper purpose of medicine.

If the previous section might be viewed as an argument against a creeping medical imperialism expanding under a view of health that is much too broad, there remains a need to confront the implications of a medical isolationism and agnosticism that reduces its province under a view of health that is much too narrow. Indeed, the tendency to expand the notion of health to include happiness and good citizenship is, ironically, a consequence of, or a reaction to, the opposite and more fundamental tendency—namely, to treat health as merely the absence of known disease entities, and more radically, to insist that health as such is, in reality, nothing more than a word.

We are thus obliged . . . to examine the question "What is health?"; for what was once self-evident, now requires an argument. I begin with some of the important difficulties that confound the search for the meaning of "health."

1. What is the domain of health? Is it body, or body and soul? Can only individuals be healthy, or can we speak univocally, and not analogically, about a healthy marriage, a healthy family, a healthy city, or a healthy society, meaning by these references something more than collections of healthy individuals? I think not. In its strict sense, "health" refers to individual organisms—plants and animals, no less than humans—and only analogically or metaphorically to larger groupings. I will set aside the question of whether only bodies or also souls are or can be "healthy," since it appears difficult enough to discover what health is even for the body. While there is disagreement about the existence of a standard of health for the soul—or, if you prefer, about whether there is "psychic health"—no one I think denies that if health exists at all, it exists as a condition at least of bodies. For the sake of simplicity, then, we shall confine our investigation in the present context to somatic or bodily health.[3]

2. Health appears to be a matter of more and less, a matter of degree, and standards of health seem to be relative to persons, and also relative to time of life for each person. Almost everyone's state of health could be better, and most of us—even those of us free of overt disease—can remember being healthier than we are now. Yet as Aristotle long ago pointed out, "health admits of degrees without being indeterminate." In this respect, health is like pleasure, strength, or justice, and unlike "being pregnant" or "being dead."

3. Is health a positive quality or condition, or merely the absence of some negative quality or condition? Is one necessarily "healthy" if one is not ill or diseased? One might infer from modern medical practice that health is simply the absence of all known diseases. Harrison's textbook, *Principles of Internal Medicine,* is a compendium of diseases, and apart from the remedies for specific diseases it contains no discussion of regimens for gaining and keeping health. Indeed, the term "health" does not even occur in the index.

Clinical medicine's emphasis on disease and its cure is understandable. It is the sick, and not the well, who seek out medical advice. The doctor has long been concerned with restoration and remedy, not with promotion and maintenance, which were originally the responsibilities of gymnastics and dietetics. This orientation has been encouraged by the analytic and reductive approach of modern medical science and by the proliferation of known diseases and treatments—both leading to a highly specialized but highly fragmented medicine. Doctors are too busy fighting disease to be bothered much about health, and, up to a point, this makes sense.

Yet among pediatricians, with their well-baby clinics and their concern for normal growth and development, we can in fact see medicine clearly pointing to an overall good rather than away from particular evils. The same goal also informs the practices of gymnastics (physical fitness programs) and of dietetics. Together, these examples provide a provisional ground for the claim that health is a good in its own right, not merely a privation of one or all evils. Though we may be led to *think* about health and to discover its existence only through discovering and reflecting on *departures* from health, health would seem to be the primary notion. Moreover, as I hope will become clear, disease, as the generic name for the cluster of symptoms and identifiable pathological conditions of the body, is not a notion symmetrical with, or opposite to, health. Health and *unhealth*—i.e., health and falling short of health—are true contraries, not health and disease.

DO DOCTORS KNOW BEST?

4. Who is the best judge of health, the doctor or the patient? On the surface, this looks like, and has increasingly been treated as, a question about the power and the locus of authority. . . . But the question has deeper roots and more important implications.

If medicine is an art which aims at health, and if an art implies knowledge of ends and means, then the physician is a knower. As unnatural as it may seem that someone else should know better than I whether or not I am healthy—after all, it is my body and my pain, and not the doctor's—still, the doctor as a knower *should* know what health and healthy functioning are, and how to restore and preserve them. In principle, at least, and to a great extent in practice, doctors *are* experts—i.e., men who know not only how we feel about, and what we wish for, our bodies, but how our bodies work and how they should work. . . .

Yet the case for health as an objective condition, in principle recognizable by an expert, and independent of patient wishes and opinions, needs to be qualified. Health and unhealth, as well as all diseases, occur only in particular living beings, each experiencing *inward* manifestations of health or its absence. The patient's feelings of illness or well-being must be reckoned with, not only because the patient insists, but because they are pertinent signs in the assessment of health. To be sure, there are people who feel fine but harbor unbeknownst to themselves a fatal illness (e.g., the vigorous athlete whose routine blood count shows early leukemia). Still, when a patient complains of headaches or backaches, funny noises in his ears, fatigue, weakness, palpitations on exertion, pains or cramps in the abdomen, or dizziness, *he is not healthy*—even if he looks and acts healthy and even if the doctor fails "to find anything wrong," i.e., fails to discover a cause for the symptoms. A *negative* report by the patient always, or almost always, counts.

There need be no discordance between the "objective" and "subjective" manifestations of health and unhealth. For the most part, they do correspond. The individual's state of health shows itself both to himself and to the outsider, including the expert.

THE RELATIVIST ARGUMENT

5. Health is said to be relative not only to the age of the person but also to external circumstances, both natural and societal. A person with hay fever can be well in the absence of ragweed pollen or cats, and incapacitated in their presence. The hereditary deficiency of a certain enzyme (glucose-6-phosphate-de-

hydrogenase) results in serious illness for the individual who eats fava beans or takes certain drugs, but is otherwise without known consequence. Eyeglasses, it is said, make myopia no longer a disability. Paraplegia may be only an inconvenience to a theoretical physicist or a President of the United States, whereas an ingrown toenail could cripple the career of a ballerina. If various functions and activities are the measure of health, and if functions are affected by and relative to circumstances, then health too, so the argument goes, is relative.

Yet all these points, however valid, do not prove the relativity of health and unhealth. They show, rather, the relativity of the *importance* of health and unhealth. The person without hay fever, enzyme deficiency, myopia, paraplegia, and ingrown toenails, is, other things being equal, *healthier* than those *with* these conditions. To be sure, various absences of health can be ignored, and others overcome by change of circumstance, while still others, even if severe, can be rendered less incapacitating. But none of this affects the fact that they *are* absences of health, or undermines the possibility that health is something in its own right.

The most radical version of the relativist argument challenges the claim that health is a *natural* norm. According to this view, what is healthy is dependent not only on time and circumstance, but even more on custom and convention, on human valuation. To apply the concept or construct "healthy" is to throw our judgment of value onto a factual, value-neutral condition of the body; without human judgment, there is no health and no illness. A recent commentator, Peter Sedgwick, argues that "all sickness is essentially deviancy" and that illness and disease, health and treatment are "social constructions":

All departments of nature below the level of mankind are exempt both from disease and from treatment. The blight that strikes at corn or at potatoes is a *human invention,* for if man wished to cultivate parasites rather than potatoes (or corn) there would be no "blight" but simply the necessary foddering of the parasite-crop. Animals do not have diseases either, prior to the presence of man in a meaningful relation with them. . . . Outside the significances

that man voluntarily attaches to certain conditions, *there are no illnesses or diseases in nature*. . . . Out of his anthropocentric self-interest, man has chosen to consider as "illnesses" or "diseases" those natural circumstances which precipitate the death (or failure to function according to certain values) of a limited number of biological species: man himself, his pets and other cherished livestock, and the plant-varieties he cultivates for gain or pleasure. . . . Children and cattle may fall ill, have diseases, and seem as sick; but who has ever imagined that spiders or lizards can be sick or diseased? . . . The medical enterprise is from its inception value-loaded; it is not simply an applied biology, but a biology applied in accordance with the dictates of social interest.[4]

Insofar as one considers only disease, there is something to be said for this position—but not much. Disease-entities may in some cases be constructs, but the departures from health and the symptoms they group together are not. Moreover, health, although certainly a good, is not therefore a good whose goodness exists merely by convention or by human decree. Health, illness, and unhealth all may exist even if not discovered or attributed. That human beings don't *worry* about the health of lizards and spiders implies nothing about whether or not lizards and spiders *are* healthy, and any experienced student of spiders and lizards can discover—and not merely invent—abnormal structures and functionings of these animals. Human indifference is merely that. Deer can be healthy or full of cancer, a partially eaten butterfly escaping from a blue jay is not healthy but defective, and even the corn used to nourish parasites becomes abnormal corn, to the parasite-grower's delight.

Sedgwick must be partly forgiven for his confusion, for he has no doubt been influenced by a medicine that focuses on disease-entities and not on health, by a biology that does not consider wholes except as mere aggregates, and by that conventional wisdom of today's social science which holds that *all* goods are good because they are valued, and *all* values are in turn mere conventions, wholly tied to the culture or the individual that invents them. To be sure, different cultures have different taxonomies of diseases, and differing notions of their cause. But the fact that *some* form of medicine is *everywhere* practiced—whether by medicine men and faith healers or by trained neurosurgeons—is far more significant than the differences in nosology and explanation: It strongly suggests that healers do not fabricate the difference between being healthy and being unhealthy; they only try to learn about it, each in his own way.

THE LANGUAGE OF HEALTH

I turn next away from these difficulties to the constructive part of the search for health. To begin with, I should say that I am not seeking a precise definition of health. I am rather inclined to believe that it is not possible to say definitively what health is, any more than it is possible to say wholly and precisely what "livingness" or "light" or "knowledge" or "human excellence" is. What I hope to show more clearly is what *sort* of a "thing" health is, so that we can be more secure in recognizing and promoting it, even if we are unable to capture it in speech.

. . .

Etymological investigations may provide some clues for what we recognize when we recognize health. The English word *health* literally means "wholeness," and *to heal* means "to make whole." (Both words go back to the Old English *hal* and the Old High German *heil,* as does the English word "whole.") To be whole is to be healthy, and to be healthy is to be whole. Ancient Greek has two etymologically distinct words translatable as "health," *hygeia* and *euexia. Hygeia,* the source of our word "hygiene," apparently stands for the Indo-European *sugwiges,* which means "living well," or more precisely, a "well way of living." *Euexia* means, literally, "well-habited-ness," and, in this context, "good habit of body."

Two observations are worth noting: 1) Both the Greek and the English words for health are totally unrelated to all the words for disease, illness, sickness. (This is also true in German, Latin, and Hebrew). The Greek words for health, unlike the English, are also completely unrelated to all the verbs of healing: Health is a state or condition unrelated to, and prior to, both illness and physicians. 2) The English emphasis on "wholeness" or "completeness" is comparatively static and structural, and the notion of a whole distinct from all else and complete in itself carries connotations of self-containedness, self-sufficiency, and independence. In contrast, both Greek terms stress the *functioning* and *activity* of the whole, and not only its working, but its working well.[5]

WHOLENESS

Aided by these etymological reflections, we turn now from words to things in search of instances of *wholeness* and of *working-well* in nature. We shall look, of course, only at part of what is today called nature. We are not tempted to seek health in mountains or rocks or hurricanes, for these are surely not organic wholes. We look only at *animate* nature, at plants, animals, and man—true wholes, if any there be.

But are plants and animals authentic wholes, or are they mere aggregates masquerading as wholes? I have tried elsewhere[6] to show at greater length why living things cannot even be looked at, much less understood, except as wholes—and in this sense at least, as teleological beings—regardless of whether or not the species originally came to be by non-teleological processes. I will here present only some of the evidence.

First, consider the generation of living things. Each organism comes to be not at random, but in an orderly manner, starting from some relatively undifferentiated but nevertheless specific seed or zygote produced by parents of the same species, and developing, unfolding itself from within, in successive stages that tend toward and reach a limit—itself, the fully formed organism. The adult which emerges from the process of self-development and growth is no mere outcome, but a completion, an end, a whole.

Second, a fully formed mature organism is an organic whole, an articulated whole, composed of parts. It is a structure and not a heap. The parts of an organism have specific functions which define their nature as parts: the bone marrow for making red blood cells; the lungs for exchange of oxygen and carbon dioxide; the heart for pumping the blood. Even at a biochemical level, every molecule can be characterized in terms of its function. The parts, both macroscopic and microscopic, contribute to the maintenance and functioning of the other parts, and make possible the maintenance and functioning of the whole.

But perhaps the best evidence that organisms are wholes, and that their wholeness and their healthiness correspond, is the remarkable power of self-healing. In hydra, planaria, and many plants, the power to restore wholeness shows itself in an amazing degree in the form of adult regeneration. A plant-cutting will regrow the missing roots, a hydra regrows amputated tentacles, and each half of a divided planarian will regenerate the missing half. In human beings, various organs and tissues—e.g., skin, the epithelia of the digestive tract, liver, bone marrow, and lymph nodes—have comparable regenerative powers. More generally, nearly all living things heal wounds or breaks and tend to restore wholeness. Foreign bodies are engulfed and extruded by amoebas and by man. This tendency to maintain wholeness by rejecting *additions* to the whole becomes marvelously elaborate in the immune system of higher animals, which sensitively recognizes and combats the entry of alien elements, whether in the form of infectious agents, tumors, or grafted tissue.

.   .   .

WELL-WORKING

.   .   .

What constitutes *well-working?* The answers will vary from species to species: among other things, web-spinning for a spider, flight for some birds, swimming for others. For a given species, there will be some variations among individuals, increasingly so as functions are dissected into smaller and smaller subfunctions. For certain functions, the norm will be a mean between excess and deficiency: for example, blood pressure can be too high or too low, as can blood sugar or blood calcium; blood can clot too quickly or too slowly; body temperature can be too high or too low. And while there is some arbitrariness in our deciding on the lower and upper limits of the so-called normal range in all these cases, this indistinctness of the margins does not indicate nature's arbitrariness or indifference about the norm. For we note that the body has elaborate mechanisms to keep these properties balanced, often very precisely, between excess and deficiency, to preserve homeostasis.

Yet it is at the whole animal that one should finally look for the measure of well-working, for the well-working of the whole. That there are mechanisms for restoring well-working at this level can be seen by considering the case of a dog missing one hind leg. Such a dog still runs —though certainly not as well as when he had four legs—by positioning his remaining hind leg as close as he can to the midline of his body, to become a more balanced tripod, and he does this without being taught or without previous experience in three-legged running. There appear to be "rules of rightness," as Polanyi calls them, unique to each level of bodily organization, whose rightness is not explicable in terms of the lower levels, even though failure at the lower levels can cause failure at the higher. For example, a broken wing can prevent flight, but two intact wings, good chest muscles, and hollow bones don't add up to flight. Think about trying to give a mechanical account of the rules of rightness for the well-functioning that is riding a bicycle or swimming or speaking.

Thus, it is ultimately to the workings of the whole animal that we must turn to discover its healthiness. What, for example, is a healthy squirrel? Not a picture of a squirrel, not really or fully the sleeping squirrel, not even the aggregate of his normal blood pressure, serum calcium, total body zinc, normal digestion, fertility, and the like. Rather, the healthy squirrel is a bushy-tailed fellow who looks and acts like a squirrel; who leaps through the trees with great daring; who gathers, buries, and covers but later uncovers and recovers his acorns; who perches out on a limb cracking his nuts, sniffing the air for smells of danger, alert, cautious, with his tail beating rhythmically; who chatters and plays and courts and mates, and rears his young in large improbable looking homes at the tops of trees; who fights with vigor and forages with cunning, who shows spirit-edness, even anger, and more prudence than many human beings.

To sum up: Health is a natural standard or norm—not a moral norm, not a "value" as opposed to a "fact," not an obligation, but a state of being that reveals itself in activity as a standard of bodily excellence or fitness, rela-tive to each species and to some extent to indi-viduals, recognizable if not definable, and to some extent attainable. If you prefer a more simple formulation, I would say that health is "the well-working of the organism as a whole," or again, "an activity of the living body in accordance with its specific ex-cellences."[7][The remainder of this essay is in-cluded in Chapter 8, pp. 347–398. Ed.]

NOTES

1. Abortion—nearly all of it non-therapeutic in this sense—is now the third most common surgical procedure in the United States, after circumcision and tonsillectomy.

2. During the period between 1900 and 1970, the average life expectancy among white males in the United States, calculated from birth, increased by about 22 years (the biggest contribution being a decline in infant mortality), but the average life expectancy for those who reached age 65 increased only 1.5 years.

3. In doing so, we are supported by a sensible tradition which held that health, like beauty or strength, was an excellence of the body, whereas moderation, wisdom, and courage were excellences of soul. While excluding these latter goods from the goal of medicine, I do not mean to deny to a more minimal state of psychic health—namely, sanity or "emotional equilibrium"—a possible place among the true ends of medicine.

4. Peter Sedgwick, "Illness—Mental and Otherwise," *Hastings Center Studies,* Vol. 1, No. 3 (1973), pp. 30–31 (italics in original). [Reprinted below, pp. 114–119.]

5. The Greek terms suggest that health is connected with the way we live and perhaps imply that health has largely an inner cause. Indeed, it seems reasonable to think of health understood as "living well" or "well-habited" as the cause of itself. Just as courage is the cause of cou-rageous action and hence also of courage—for we become brave by acting bravely—so "living well" *is* health, is the *cause* of health, and is *caused by* health. The activities which in English usage we might be inclined to see as *signs* or *effects* of health, might in the Greek usage appear as the *essence* of health.

Related to this, the Greek seems to imply that to stay healthy requires effort and care, that however much nature makes health possible, human attention and habit are re-quired to maintain and preserve it. Health is neither given nor usually taken away from the outside, nor is it the gratuitously expected state of affairs.

6. "Teleology and Darwin's *The Origin of Species:* Beyond Chance and Necessity?", a lecture given at St. John's College, Annapolis, Maryland (October 11, 1974).

7. Whatever progress we may have made in our search for health, large questions still remain, which I defer to another occasion. These questions include: What activities of the living body should be considered, and are all of them of equal rank? What are the specific excellences or fitnesses of various organisms, and can one hope to dis-cover these standards for a being as complex as man, whose activities are so highly diversified and differ-entiated? What is a living body, and what a specifically *human* living body? Finally, what is the relation of health of body to psychic health?

H. TRISTRAM ENGELHARDT, JR.

The Disease of Masturbation: Values and the Concept of Disease

Masturbation in the eighteenth and especially in the nineteenth century was widely believed to produce a spectrum of serious signs and symptoms, and was held to be a dangerous disease entity. Explanation of this phenomenon entails a basic reexamination of the concept of disease. It presupposes that one think of disease neither as an objective entity in the world nor as a concept that admits of a single universal definition: there is not, nor need there be, one concept of disease.[1] Rather, one chooses concepts for certain purposes, depending on values and hopes concerning the world.[2] The disease of masturbation is an eloquent example of the value-laden nature of science in general and of medicine in particular. In explaining the world, one judges what is to be significant or insignificant. For example, mathematical formulae are chosen in terms of elegance and simplicity, though elegance and simplicity are not attributes to be found in the world as such. The problem is even more involved in the case of medicine which judges what the human organism should be (i.e., what counts as "health") and is thus involved in the entire range of human values. This paper will sketch the nature of the model of the disease of masturbation in the nineteenth century, particularly in America, and indicate the scope of this "disease entity" and the therapies it evoked. The goal will be to outline some of the interrelations between evaluation and explanation.

The moral offense of masturbation was transformed into disease with somatic not just psychological dimensions. Though sexual overindulgence generally was considered debilitating since at least the time of Hippocrates,[3] masturbation was not widely accepted as a disease until a book by the title *Onania* appeared anonymously in Holland in 1700 and met with great success.[4] This success was reinforced by the appearance of S. A. Tissot's book on onanism.[5] Tissot held that all sexual activity was potentially debilitating and that the debilitation was merely more exaggerated in the case of masturbation. The primary basis for the debilitation was, according to Tissot, loss of seminal fluid, one ounce being equivalent to the loss of forty ounces of blood.[6] When this loss of fluid took place in an other than recumbent position (which Tissot held often to be the case with masturbation), this exaggerated the ill effects.[7] In attempting to document his contention, Tissot provided a comprehensive monograph on masturbation, synthesizing and appropriating the views of classical authors who had been suspicious of the effects of sexual overindulgence. He focused these suspicions clearly on masturbation. In this he was very successful, for Tissot's book appears to have widely established the medical opinion that masturbation was associated with serious physical and mental maladies.[8]

There appears to have been some disagreement whether the effect of frequent intercourse was in any respect different from that of masturbation. The presupposition that masturbation was not in accordance with the dictates of nature suggested that it would tend to be more subversive of the constitution than excessive sexual intercourse. Accounts of this difference in terms of the differential effect of the excitation involved are for the most part obscure. It was, though, advanced that "dur-

Reprinted with permission of the author and the publisher from *Bulletin of the History of Medicine*, Vol. 48, No. 2 (Summer 1974), pp. 234–248. © 1974 by The Johns Hopkins University Press.

ing sexual intercourse the expenditure of nerve force is compensated by the magnetism of the partner.''[9] Tissot suggested that a beautiful sexual partner was of particular benefit or was at least less exhausting.[10] In any event, masturbation was held to be potentially more deleterious since it was unnatural, and, therefore, less satisfying and more likely to lead to a disturbance or disordering of nerve tone.

At first, the wide range of illnesses attributed to masturbation is striking. Masturbation was held to be the cause of dyspepsia,[11] constrictions of the urethra,[12] epilepsy,[13] blindness,[14] vertigo, loss of hearing,[15] headache, impotency, loss of memory, "irregular action of the heart," general loss of health and strength,[16] rickets,[17] leucorrhea in women,[18] and chronic catarrhal conjunctivitis.[19] Nymphomania was found to arise from masturbation, occurring more commonly in blonds than in brunettes.[20] Further, changes in the external genitalia were attributed to masturbation: elongation of the clitoris, reddening and congestion of the labia majora, elongation of the labia minora,[21] and a thinning and decrease in size of the penis.[22] Chronic masturbation was held to lead to the development of a particular type, including enlargement of the superficial veins of the hands and feet, moist and clammy hands, stooped shoulders, pale sallow face with heavy dark circles around the eyes, a "draggy" gait, and acne.[23] Careful case studies were published establishing masturbation as a cause of insanity,[24] and evidence indicated that it was a cause of hereditary insanity as well.[25] Masturbation was held also to cause an hereditary predisposition to consumption.[26] Finally, masturbation was believed to lead to general debility. "From health and vigor, and intelligence and loveliness of character, they became thin and pale and cadaverous; their amiability and loveliness departed, and in their stead irritability, moroseness and anger were prominent characteristics. . . . The child loses its flesh and becomes pale and weak.''[27] The natural history was one of progressive loss of vigor, both physical and mental.

In short, a broad and heterogeneous class of signs and symptoms were recognized in the nineteenth century as a part of what was tantamount to a syndrome, if not a disease: masturbation. If one thinks of a syndrome as the concurrence or running together of signs and symptoms into a recognizable pattern, surely masturbation was such a pattern. It was more, though, in that a cause was attributed to the syndrome providing an etiological framework for a disease entity. That is, if one views the development of disease concepts as the progression from the mere collection of signs and symptoms to their interrelation in terms of a recognized causal mechanism, the disease of masturbation was fairly well evolved.

· · ·

As mentioned, the concept of the disease of masturbation developed on the basis of a general suspicion that sexual activity was debilitating.[28] This development is not really unexpected: if one examines the world with a tacit presupposition of a parallelism between what is good for one's soul and what is good for one's health, then one would expect to find disease correlates for immoral sexual behavior.[29] Also, this was influenced by a concurrent inclination to translate a moral issue into medical terms and relieve it of the associated moral opprobrium in a fashion similar to the translation of alcoholism from a moral into a medical problem.[30] Further, disease as a departure from a state of stability due to excess or under excitation offered the skeleton of a psychosomatic theory of the somatic alterations attributed to the excitation associated with masturbation.

· · ·

Those who held the disease of masturbation to be more than a culturally dependent phenomenon often employed somewhat drastic therapies. Restraining devices were devised,[31] infibulation or placing a ring in the prepuce was used to make masturbation painful,[32] and no one less than Jonathan Hutchinson held that circumcision acted as a preventive.[33] Acid burns or thermoelectrocautery[34] were utilized to make masturbation painful and, therefore, to discourage it. The alleged seriousness of this disease in females led, as Professor John Duffy has shown to the employment of the rather radical treatment of clitoridectomy.[35] The classic monograph recommending clitoridectomy, written by the British surgeon Baker Brown, advocated the procedure to terminate the "long continued peripheral excitement, causing frequent and increasing losses of nerve force. . . ."[36] Brown recommended that "the patient having been placed completely under the influence of chloroform, the clitoris [be] freely excised either by scissors or knife—I always prefer the scissors."[37] The supposed sequelae of female masturbation, such as sterility, paresis, hysteria, dysmenorrhea, idiocy, and insanity, were also held to be remedied by the operation.

Male masturbation was likewise treated by means of surgical procedures. Some recommended vasectomy[38] while others found this procedure ineffective and employed castration.[39] One illustrative case involved the castration of a physician who had been confined as insane for seven years and who subsequently was able to return to practice.[40]

. . .

There were, though, more tolerant approaches, ranging from hard work and simple diet[41] to suggestions that "If the masturbator is totally continent, sexual intercourse is advisable."[42] This latter approach to therapy led some physicians to recommend that masturbators cure their disease by frequenting houses of prostitution,[43] or acquiring a mistress.[44] Though these treatments would appear ad hoc, more theoretically sound proposals were made by many physicians in terms of the model of excitability. They suggested that the disease and its sequelae could be adequately controlled by treating the excitation and debility consequent upon masturbation. Towards this end, "active tonics" and the use of cold baths at night just before bedtime were suggested.[45] Much more in a "Brownian" mode was the proposal that treatment with opium would be effective. An initial treatment with $1/12$ of a grain of morphine sulfate daily by injection was followed after ten days by a dose of $1/16$ of a grain. This dose was continued for three weeks and gradually diminished to $1/30$ of a grain a day. At the end of the month the patient was

dismissed from treatment "the picture of health, having fattened very much, and lost every trace of anaemia and mental imbecility."[46] The author, after his researches with opium and masturbation, concluded, *"We may find in opium a new and important aid in the treatment of the victims of the habit of masturbation by means of which their moral and physical forces may be so increased that they may be enabled to enter the true physiological path."*[47] This last example eloquently collects the elements of the concept of the disease of masturbation as a pathophysiological entity: excitation leads to physical debilitation requiring a physical remedy. Masturbation as a pathophysiological entity was thus incorporated within an acceptable medical model of diagnosis and therapy.

In summary, in the nineteenth century, biomedical scientists attempted to correlate a vast number of signs and symptoms with a disapproved activity found in many patients afflicted with various maladies. Given an inviting theoretical framework, it was very conducive to think of this range of signs and symptoms as having one cause. The theoretical framework, though, as has been indicated, was not value free but structured by the values and expectations of the times. In the nineteenth century, one was pleased to think that not "one bride in a hundred, of delicate, educated, sensitive women, accepts matrimony from any desire of sexual gratification: when she thinks of this at all, it is with shrinking, or even with horror, rather than with desire."[48] In contrast, in the twentieth century, articles are published for the instruction of women in the use of masturbation to overcome the disease of frigidity or orgasmic dysfunction.[49] In both cases, expectations concerning what should be significant structure the appreciation of reality by medicine. The variations are not due to mere fallacies of scientific method,[50] but involve a basic dependence of the logic of scientific discovery and explanation upon prior evaluations of reality.[51] A sought-for coincidence of morality and nature gives goals to explanation and therapy.[52] Values influence the purpose and direction of investigations and treatment. Moreover, the disease of masturbation has other analogues. In the nineteenth century, there were such diseases in the South as "Drapetomania, the disease causing slaves to run away," and the disease "Dysaesthesia Aethiopis or hebetude of mind and obtuse sensibility of body—a disease peculiar to negroes—called by overseers 'rascality'."[53] In Europe, there was the disease of *morbus democritus*.[54] Some would hold that current analogues exist in diseases such as alcoholism and drug abuse.[55] In short, the disease of masturbation indicates that evaluations play a role in the development of explanatory models and that this may not be an isolated phenomenon.

This analysis, then, suggests the following conclusion: although vice and virtue are not equivalent to disease and health, they bear a direct relation to these concepts. Insofar as a vice is taken to be a deviation from an ideal of human perfection, or "well-being," it can be translated into disease language. In shifting to disease language, one no longer speaks in moralistic terms (e.g., "You are evil"), but one speaks in terms of a deviation from a norm which implies a degree of imperfection (e.g., "You are a deviant"). The shift is from an explicitly ethical language to a language of natural teleology. To be ill is to fail to realize the perfection of an ideal type; to be sick is to be defective rather than to be evil. The concern is no longer with what is naturally, morally good, but what is naturally beautiful. Medicine turns to what has been judged to be naturally ugly or deviant, and then develops etiological accounts in order to explain and treat in a coherent fashion a manifold of displeasing signs and symptoms. The notion of the "deviant" structures the concept of disease providing a purpose and direction for explanation and for action, that is, for diagnosis and prognosis, and for therapy. A "disease entity" operates as a conceptual form organizing phenomena in a fashion deemed useful for certain goals. The goals, though, involve choice by man and are not objective facts, data "given" by nature. They are ideals imputed to nature. The disease of masturbation is an eloquent example of the role of evaluation in explanation and the structure values give to our picture of reality.

NOTES

1. Alvan R. Feinstein, "Taxonomy and logic in clinical data," *Ann. N.Y. Acad. Sci.*, 1969, *161:* 450-459.

2. Horacio Fabrega, Jr., "Concepts of disease: logical features and social implications," *Perspect. Biol. Med.*, 1972, *15:* 583-616.

3. For example, Hippocrates correlated gout with sexual intercourse, *Aphorisms*, VI, 30. Numerous passages in the *Corpus* recommend the avoidance of overindulgence especially during certain illnesses.

4. René A. Spitz, "Authority and masturbation. Some remarks on a bibliographical investigation," *Yb. Psychoanal.*, 1953, *9:* 116. Also, Robert H. MacDonald, "The frightful consequences of onanism: notes on the history of a delusion." *J. Hist. Ideas*, 1967, *28:* 423-431.

5. Simon-André Tissot, *Tentamen de Morbis ex Manustrupatione* (Lausannae: M. M. Bousquet, 1758). An anonymous American translation appeared in the early 19th century: *Onanism* (New York: Collins & Hannay, 1832).

6. Simon-André Tissot, *Onanism* (New York: Collins & Hannay, 1832). p. 5.

7. *Ibid.,* p. 50.

8. E. H. Hare, "Masturbatory insanity: the history of an idea," *J. Mental Sco.*, 1962, *108:* 2-3.

9. Howe, *op. cit.* (n. 5 above), pp. 76-77.

10. Tissot, *op. cit.* (n. 6 above), p. 51.

11. J. A. Mayes, "Spermatorrhoea, treated by the lately invented rings," *Charleston Med. J. & Rev.*, 1854, *9:* 352.

12. Allen W. Hagenbach, "Masturbation as a cause of insanity," *J. Ner. Ment. Dis.*, 1879, *6:* 609.

13. Baker Brown, *On the Curability of Certain Forms of Insanity, Epilepsy, Catalepsy, and Hysteria in Females* (London: Hardwicke, 1866). Brown phrased the cause discreetly in terms of "peripheral irritation, arising originally in some branches of the pudic nerve, more particularly the incident nerve supplying the clitoris. . . ." (p. 7)

14. F. A. Burdem, "Self pollution in children," *Mass. Med. J.*, 1896, *16:* 340.

15. Weber Liel, "The influence of sexual irritation upon the diseases of the ear," *New Orleans Med. & Surg. J.*, 1884, *11:* 786-788.

16. Joseph Jones, "Diseases of the nervous system," *Trans. La. Med. Soc.* (New Orleans: L. Graham & Son, 1889), p. 170.

17. Howe, *op. cit.* (n. 5 above), p. 93.

18. J. Castellanos, "Influence of sewing machines upon the health and morality of the females using them," *South. J. Med. Sci.*, 1866-1867, *1:* 495-496.

19. Comment, "Masturbation and ophthalmia," *New Orleans Med. & Surg. J.*, 1881-1882, *9:* 67.

20. Howe, *op. cit.* (n. 5 above), pp. 108-111.

21. *Ibid.,* pp. 41,72.

22. *Ibid.,* p. 68.

23. *Ibid.,* p. 73.

24. Hagenbach, *op. cit.* (n. 12 above), pp. 603-612.

25. Jones, *op. cit.* (n. 16 above), p. 170.

26. Howe, *op. cit.* (n. 5 above), p. 95.

27. Burdem, *op. cit.* (n. 14 above), pp. 339,341.

28. Even Boerhaave remarked that "an excessive discharge of semen causes fatigue, weakness, decrease in activity, convulsions, emaciation, dehydration, heat and pains in the membranes of the brain, a loss in the acuity of the senses, particularly of vision, *tabes dorsalis,* simplemindedness, and various similar disorders." My translation of Hermanno Boerhaave's *Institutiones Medicae* (Viennae: J. T. Trattner, 1775), p. 315, paragraph 776.

29. "We have seen that masturbation is more pernicious than excessive intercourse with females. Those who believe in a special providence, account for it by a special ordinance of the Deity to punish this crime." Tissot, *op. cit.* (n. 6 above), p. 45.

30. ". . . the best remedy was not to tell the poor children that they were damning their souls, but to tell them that they might seriously hurt their bodies, and to explain to them the nature and purport of the functions they were abusing." Lawson Tait, "Masturbation. A clinical lecture," *Med. News,* 1888, *53:* 2.

31. C. D. W. Colby, "Mechanical restraint of masturbation in a young girl," *Med. Record in N.Y.,* 1897, *52:* 206.

32. Louis Bauer, "Infibulation as a remedy for epilepsy and seminal losses," *St. Louis Clin. Record,* 1879, *6:* 163-165. See also Gerhart S. Schwarz, "Infibulation, population control, and the medical profession," *Bull. N. Y. Acad. Med.,* 1970, *46:* 979, 990.

33. Jonathan Hutchinson, "On circumcision as preventive of masturbation," *Arch. Surg.,* 1890-1891, *2:* 267–269.

34. William J. Robinson, "Masturbation and its treatment," *Am. J. Clin. Med.,* 1907, *14:* 349.

35. John Duffy, "Masturbation and clitoridectomy. A nineteenth-century view," *J. A. M. A.,* 1963, *186:* 246-248.

36. Brown, *op. cit.* (n. 13 above), p. 11.

37. *Ibid.,* p. 17.

38. Timothy Haynes, "Surgical treatment of hopeless cases of masturbation and nocturnal emissions," *Boston Med. & Surg. J.,* 1883, *109:* 130.

39. J. H. Marshall, "Insanity cured by castration," *Med. & Surg. Reptr.,* 1865, *13:* 363-364.

40. "The patient soon evinced marked evidences of being a changed man, becoming quiet, kind, and docile." *Ibid.,* p. 363.

41. Editorial, "Review of European legislation for the control of prostitution," *New Orleans Med. & Surg. J.,* 1854-1855, *11:* 704.

42. Robinson, *op. cit.* (n. 34 above), p. 350.

43. Theophilus Parvin, "The hygiene of the sexual functions," *New Orleans Med. & Surg. J.,* 1884, *11:* 606.

44. Mayes, *op. cit.* (n. 11 above), p. 352.

45. Haynes, *op. cit.* (n. 38 above), p. 130.

46. B. A. Pope, "Opium as a tonic and alternative; with remarks upon the hypodermic use of the sulfate of morphia, and its use in the debility and amorosis consequent upon onanism," *New Orleans Med. & Surg. J.,* 1879, *6:* 725.

47. *Ibid.,* p. 727.

48. Parvin, *op. cit.* (n. 43 above), p. 607.

49. Joseph LoPiccolo and W. Charles Lobitz, "The role of masturbation in the treatment of orgasmic dysfunction," *Arch. Sexual Behavior,* 1972, *2:* 163-171.

50. E. Hare, *op. cit.* (n. 8 above), pp. 15-19.

51 Norwood Hanson, *Patterns of Discovery* (London: Cambridge University Press, 1965).

52. Tissot, *op. cit.* (n. 6 above), p. 45. As Immanuel Kant, a contemporary of S.-A. Tissot remarked, "Also, in all probability, it was through this moral interest [in the moral law governing the world] that attentiveness to beauty and the ends of nature was first aroused." (*Kants Werke,* Vol. 5, *Kritik der Urtheilskraft* [Berlin: Walter de Gruyter & Co., 1968], p. 459, A 439. My translation.) That is, moral values influence the search for goals in nature, and direct attention to what will be considered natural, normal, and non-deviant. This would also imply a relationship between the aesthetic, especially what was judged to be naturally beautiful, and what was held to be the goals of nature.

53. Samuel A. Cartwright, "Report on the diseases and physical peculiarities of the negro race," *New Orleans Med. & Surg. J.,* 1850-1851, *7:* 707-709. An interesting examination of these diseases is given by Thomas S. Szasz, "The sane slave," *Am. J. Psychoth.,* 1971, *25:* 228-239.

54. Heinz Hartmann, "Towards a concept of mental health," *Brit. J. Med. Psychol.,* 1960, *33:* 248.

55. Thomas S. Szasz, "Bad habits are not diseases: a refutation of the claim that alcoholism is a disease," *Lancet,* 1972, *2:* 83-84; and Szasz, "The ethics of addiction," *Am. J. Psychiatry,* 1971, *128:* 541-546.

PETER SEDGWICK

What Is "Illness"?

. . .

What, then, is "illness"? It will be recalled that critical theory in psychiatry has tended to postulate a fundamental separation between mental illnesses and the general run of human ailments: the former are the expression of social norms, the latter proceed from ascertainable bodily states which have an "objective" existence within the individual. One critic of psychopathological concepts, Barbara Wootton, has suggested that the expurgation of normative references from psychiatry is at least a theoretical ideal, though one immensely difficult of achievement:

. . . anti-social behavior is the precipitating factor that leads to mental treatment. But at the same time the fact of the illness is itself inferred from the behavior. . . . But any disease, the morbidity of which is established only by the social failure that it involves, must rank as fundamentally different from those of which the symptoms are independent of the social norms . . . long indeed is the road to be travelled before we can hope to reach a definition of mental-cum-physical health which is objective, scientific, and wholly free of social value judgments and before we shall be able, consistently and without qualification, to treat mental and physical disorders on exactly the same footing.[1]

. . .

If we examine the logical structure of our judgments of illness (whether "physical" or "mental") it may prove possible to reduce the distance between psychiatry and other streams of medicine by working in the reverse direction to Wootton: not by annexing psychopathology to the technical instrumentation of the natural sciences but by revealing the character of illness and disease, health and treatment, as social constructions. For social constructions

Reprinted with permission of the author, Harper & Row, Publishers, Inc., and Pluto Press Limited, from *Psycho Politics* by Peter Sedgwick. First published in *The Hastings Center Studies*, Vol. 1, No. 3 (1973).

they most certainly are. All departments of nature below the level of mankind are exempt both from disease and from treatment—until man intervenes with his own human classifications of disease and treatment. The blight that strikes at corn or at potatoes is a *human invention,* for if man wished to cultivate parasites (rather than potatoes or corn) there would be no "blight," but simply the necessary foddering of the parasite crop. Animals do not have diseases either, prior to the presence of man in a meaningful relation with them. A tiger may experience pain or feebleness from a variety of causes (we do not intend to build our case on the supposition that animals, especially higher animals, cannot have experiences or feelings). It may be infected by a germ, trodden by an elephant, scratched by another tiger, or subjected to the aging processes of its own cells. It does not present itself as being *ill* (though it may present itself as being highly distressed or uncomfortable) except in the eyes of a human observer who can discriminate illness from other sources of pain or enfeeblement. Outside the significances that man voluntarily attaches to certain conditions, *there are no illnesses or diseases in nature.* We are nowadays so heavily indoctrinated with deriving from the technical medical discoveries of the last century-and-a-half that we are tempted to think that nature does contain diseases. Just as the sophisticated New Yorker classes the excrement of dogs and cats as one more form of "pollution" ruining the pre-established harmony of pavements and gardens, so does modern technologized man perceive nature to be mined and infested with all kinds of specifically morbid entities and agencies. What, he will protest, are there no diseases in nature? Are there not infectious and contagious bacilli? Are there not definite and objective lesions in the cellular structures of the human body? Are there not fractures of bones, the fatal ruptures of tissues, the malignant multiplications of tumorous growths? Are not these, surely, events of nature? Yet these, as natural events, do not —prior to the human social meanings we attach to them—constitute illnesses, sicknesses, or diseases. The fracture of a septuagenarian's femur has, within the world of nature, no more significance than the snapping of an autumn leaf from its twig: and the invasion of a human organism by cholera germs carries with it no more the stamp of "illness" than does the souring of milk by other forms of bacteria.[2] Human beings, like all other naturally occurring structures are characterized by a variety of inbuilt limitations or liabilities, any of which may (given the presence of further stressful circumstances) lead to the weakening or the collapse of the organism. Mountains as well as moles, stars as well as shrubs, protozoa no less than persons have their dates of expiry set in advance, over a time-span which varies greatly over different classes of structure but which is usually at least roughly predictable. Out of his anthropocentric self-interest, man has chosen to consider as "illnesses" or "diseases" those natural circumstances which precipitate the death (or the failure to function according to certain values) of a limited number of biological species: man himself, his pets and other cherished livestock, and the plant-varieties he cultivates for gain or pleasure. Around these select areas of structural failure man creates, in proportion to the progress of his technology, specialized combat-institutions for the control and cure of "disease": the different branches of the medical and nursing profession, veterinary doctors, and the botanical specialists in plant-disease. Despite their common use of experimental natural science, these institutions operate according to very different criteria and codes; the use of euthanasia by vets, and of ruthless eugenic policies by plant-pathologists, departs from most current medical practice with human patients. All the same, the fact that these specialisms share the categories of disease and illness indicates the selective quality of our perceptions in this field. Children and cattle may fall ill, have diseases, and seem as sick; but who has ever imagined that spiders and lizards can be sick or diseased? Plant diseases may strike at tulips, turnips, or such prized features of the natural landscape as elm trees: but if some plant-species in which man had no interest (a desert grass, let us say) were to be attacked by a fungus or parasite, we should speak not of a disease, but merely of the competition between two species. The medical enterprise is from its inception value-loaded; it is not simply an applied biology, but a biology applied in accordance with the dictates of social interest.

It could be argued that the discussion of animal and plant pathology deals in cases that are too marginal to our central concepts of health and illness to form a satisfactory basis for analysis. Such marginal instances are of course frequently used by logicians in the analysis of concepts since their peripheral character often usefully tests the limits within which our ideas can be seen to be applicable or inapplicable. However, a careful examination of the concept of illness in man himself will reveal the same value-impregnation, the same dependency of apparently descriptive, natural-scientific notions upon our norms of what is desirable. To complain of illness, or to ascribe illness to another person, is not to make a descriptive statement about physiology or anatomy. Concepts of illness were in use among men for centuries before the advent of any reliable knowledge of the human body, and are still employed today within societies which favor a non-physiological (magical and religious) account of the nature of human maladies. Our own classification and explanation of specific illnesses or diseases is of course tremendously different from the categories that are current in earlier ages or in contemporary tribal societies, but it is implausible to suppose that the state of illness itself has no common logical features over different types of society. Homer's sick warriors were tended by magical incantations as well as by herbs and other primitive technical remedies, but the avowal and ascription of illness in Homer does not set up a distance between his characters and ourselves but rather (like his descriptions of bereavement or of sexual attraction) a powerful resonance across the ages.[3] Similarly, the meaning of illness among primitive peoples is usually sufficiently close to our own to enable them to take advantage of modern medical facilities when these are made accessible within their territories: tribesmen and peasants do not have to be indoctrinated into Western physiological concepts before they can accept help from physicians and nurses trained in advanced societies. Sickness and disease may be conceptualized, in different cultures, as originating within bodily states, or within perturbations of the spirit, or as a mixture of both. Yet there appear to be common features in the declaration or attribution of the sick state, regardless of the causal explanation that is invoked.

VALUATION AND EXPLANATION

All sickness is essentially deviancy. That is to say, no attribution of sickness to any being can be made without the expectation of some alternative state of affairs which is considered more desirable. In the absence of this normative alternative, the presence of a particular bodily or subjective state will not in itself lead to an attribution of illness. Thus, where an entire community is by Western standards "ill," because it has been infected for generations by parasites which diminish energy, illness will not be recognized in any individual except by outsiders.[4] The Rockefeller Sanitary Commission on Hookworm found in 1911 that this disease was regarded as part of normal health in some areas of North Africa.[5] And in one South American Indian tribe the disease of dyschromic spirochetosis, which is marked by the appearance of colored spots on the skin, was so "normal" that those who did not have them were regarded as pathological and excluded from marriage.[6] Even within modern urbanized nations we cannot assume that aches, pains and other discomforts are uniformly categorized as signs of illness among all sections of the community. Although little work has been done on social-class variations in the construction of what constitutes "health" and "sickness,"[7] the example of tooth-decay is suggestive: among millions of

British working-class families, it is taken for granted that children will lose their teeth and require artificial dentures. The process of tooth-loss is not seen as a disease but as something like an act of fate. Among dentists, on the other hand, and in those more-educated sections of the community who are socialized into dental ideology, the loss of teeth arises through a definite disease-process known as caries, whose aetiology is established.[8] Social and cultural norms also plainly govern the varying perception, either as essentially "normal," or as esentially "pathological," of such characteristics as baldness, obesity, infestation by lice, venereal infection, and the presence of tonsils and foreskins among children.

Once again it can be argued that these cultural variations apply only to marginal cases of sickness and health, that there are some physical or psychological conditions which are *ipso facto* symptomatic of illness, whether among Bushmen or Brobdignagians, duchesses or dockworkers. But there is no reason to believe that the "standardized" varieties of human pathology operate according to a different logic from the "culturally dependent" varieties. The existence of common or even universal illnesses testifies, not to the absence of a normative framework for judging pathology, but to the presence of very wide-spread norms. To be ill, after all, is not the same thing as to feel pain, or to experience weaknesses, or to fail to manifest this or that kind of behavior. Rather it is to experience discomfort (or to manifest behavioral failure) in a context of a particular kind. Consider the imaginary conversations between physician and client:

(a) *Client:* Doctor, I want you to examine me, I keep feeling terrible pains in my right shoulder.

Doctor: Really? What are they like?

Client: Stabbing and intense.

Doctor: How often do they happen?

Client: Every evening after I get home from work.

Doctor: Always in the same spot?

Client: Yes, just in the place where my wife hits me with the rolling-pin.

(b) *Client:* (Telephoning Doctor). Doctor, I haven't consulted you before but things are getting desperate. I'm feeling so weak, I can't lift anything heavy.

Doctor: Goodness, when does this come on you?

Client: Every time I try to lift something or make an effort. I have to walk quite slowly up the stairs and last night when I was packing the big suitcase I found I couldn't lift it off the bed.

Doctor: Well, let's have some details about you before you come in. Name?

Client: John Smith.

Doctor: Age?

Client: Ninety-two last February.

In the first example, the "patient's" pain is not an illness because we expect pain as a normal response to being hit in tender places; indeed, if he did *not* feel pain when he was hit or prodded he would be taken to be suffering from some disease involving nerve-degeneration. In the second example, the patients infirmity would usually be ascribed not to the category of "illness" but to that of "aging." (If he had given his age as "twenty-two" the case would be different). In our culture we expect old people to find difficulty in lifting heavy weights, although it is easy to conceive of a culture in which mass rejuvenation among the aged had been perfected (perhaps by the injection of hormones, vitamins or other pep-pills into the water-supply) and where, in consequence, a dialogue of the type recounted would lead to a perfectly ordinary referral for medical treatment. The attribution of illness always proceeds from the computation of a gap between presented behavior (or feeling) and some social norm. In practice of course we take the norm for granted, so that the broken arm or the elevated temperature is seen alone as the illness. But the broken arm would be no more of an illness than a broken fingernail unless it stopped us from achieving certain socially contructed goals; just as, if we could all function according to approved social requirements within any range of body-temperature, thermometers would disappear from the household medical kit.

This is not to say that illness amounts to any deviancy whatsoever from social expectations about how men should function. Some deviancies are regarded as instances not of sickness but of criminality, wickedness, poor upbringing or bad manners (though not all cultures do in fact draw a firm line between illness and these other deviations, e.g., primitive societies for whom illness is also a moral flaw and modern liberal circles for whom drug-addiction is categorized in medical as well as moral terms). Looking over the very wide range of folk-concepts and technical ideas about illness which exist in the history of human societies, one finds it difficult to discern a common structural element which distinguishes the notion of illness from other attributions of social failure. Provisionally, it is possible to suggest that illness is set apart from other deviancies insofar as the description (or, at a deeper level, the explanation) of the sick state is located within a relatively restricted set of causal factors operating within the boundaries of the individual human being. One may become ill as the result of being infected by germs, or through being entered by evil demons, or visited by a curse from the Almighty. Each culturally specific account of illness must involve a theory of the person, of the boundaries between the person and the world "outside" him, and of the ways in which adverse influences can trespass over these limits and besiege or grip him. If the current theory of the person is positivistic and physical, the agencies of illness will be seen as arising from factors within (or at the boundaries of) his body; in cultures with an animistic tradition, the invasion will be one of the spirit or soul. But, however variously the nature of illness is specified from culture to culture, the attribution of illness appears to include a *quest for explanation,* or at least the descriptive delimiting of certain types of causal factor, as well as the normative component outlined above. It is indeed likely that the concept of illness has arisen in close parallel with the social practice of therapy, i.e., with the development of techniques to control those human afflictions which can be controlled at the boundaries of the individual person. It is hard to see how the category of illness, as a distinct construction separate from other kinds of misfortune, could have arisen without the discovery that some varieties of pain and affliction could be succored through individual specialized attention to the afflicted person. In traditional societies, of course, the institution of medicine is not crystallized out as an applied branch of natural science: "Therapy" for the Greeks was simply the word used for looking after or tending somebody, and in Greece as well as elsewhere, a great deal of therapy goes on either in the patient's household or in conjunction with religious and magical specialisms. A specifically "medical" framework of treatment is not necessary to provide the link between illness and practical action.

Practice and concept continue their mutual modification over the ages. In a society where the treatment of the sick is still conducted through religious ritual, the notion of illness will not be entirely distinct from the notion of sinfulness or pollution. Correspondingly, with the growth of progressively more technical and more autonomous specialisms of therapy, the concepts of disease and illness themselves become more technical, and thereby more alienated from their implicit normative background. Thus we reach the position of the present day where any characterization of an "illness" which is not amenable to a diagnosis drawn from physiology or to a therapy based on chemical, electrical, or surgical technique becomes suspect as not constituting, perhaps, an illness at all. Such has been the fate of mental illness in our own epoch. It has been much easier for societies with an animistic theory of the person (and of his boundaries and susceptibilities to influence) to view mental disturbances on a par with bodily ailments. Ceremonies of ritual purgation and demon-expulsion, along with primitive "medical" methods of a herbal or surgical type, are used differently by traditional healers on patients with a mental or with a bodily dysfunction. Fever and madness, the broken limb or the broken spirit are situated within the same normative frame, within the same explanatory and therapeutic system. Even the development of a technical-physiological specialism of medicine, such as emerged with the Hippocratic

tradition which runs in fits and starts from antiquity to modern times, does not impair the possibility of a unitary perspective on physical and mental illness, *so long as a common structure of valuation and explanation applies over the whole range of disorders of the person*. The medicine of the seventeenth and eighteenth centuries in Western Europe, for instance, was able to interpret our present-day "mental" disorders as a group of illnesses inhabiting the embodied person on much the same plane as other sorts of malady: the insane or the emotionally disturbed patient was suffering from a fault of "the vapors," "the nerves," "the fluids," "the animal spirits," "the spleen," "the humors," "the head," or the forces and qualities of the body.[9] This unitary integration of human illnesses was of course only achieved at the cost of a stupendously inaccurate and speculative physiology. But an integrated theory of illness, whether achieved within a unitary-animistic or a unitary-physicalistic doctrine of the person, has one singular advantage over a more fragmentary perspective: it is not beset by the kind of crisis we now have in psychopathology and psychiatry, whose conceptual and moral foundation has been exploded now that "illness" has acquired a technical-physical definition excluding disorders of the whole person from its purview. Animistic and unitary-physicalistic accounts of illness both dealt in the whole embodied individual, but the medical technology of the nineteenth century and onwards has succeeded in classifying illness as particular states of the body only. Psychiatry is left with two seeming alternatives: either to say that personal, psychological, and emotional disorders are really states of the body, objective features of the brain tissue, the organism-under-stress, the genes or what have you; or else to deny that such disorders are illnesses at all. If the latter, then the way is open to treat mental illnesses as the expression of social value-judgments about the patient, and psychiatry's role will not belong to the disciplines of objective, body-state medicine. Instead, it will be analogous to the value-laden and non-medical disciplines of moral education, police interrogation, criminal punishment or religion (depending on how low or how loftly a view one takes of the values inherent in psychiatric practice).

This dilemma will perhaps seem somewhat to dissolve if we recapitulate what was previously said about the nature of illness as a social construction. *All* illness, whether conceived in localized bodily terms or within a larger view of human functioning, expresses both a social value-judgment (contrasting a person's condition with certain understood and accepted norms) and an attempt at explanation (with a view to controlling the disvalued condition). The physicalistic psychiatrists are wrong in their belief that they can find objective disease-entities representing the psychopathological analogues to diabetes, tuberculosis, and post-syphilitic paresis. Quite correctly, the anti-psychiatrists have pointed out that psychopathological categories refer to value-judgments and that mental illness is deviancy. On the other hand, the anti-psychiatric critics themselves are wrong when they imagine physical medicine to be essentially different in its logic from psychiatry. A diagnosis of diabetes, or paresis, includes the recognition of norms or values. Anti-psychiatry can only operate by positing a mechanical and inaccurate model of physical illness and its medical diagnosis.

In my own judgment, then, mental illnesses can be conceptualized just as easily within the disease framework as physical maladies such as lumbago or TB.

. . .

NOTES

1. Barbara Wootton, *Social Science and Social Pathology* (London, 1959), p. 225.

2. The above discussion is heavily indebted to René Dubos' masterly *The Mirage of Health* (New York: Harper & Row, 1971), especially pp. 30-128. [Partially reprinted above, pp. 96-99.]

3. See the excellent account of Homeric medicine in P. Lain Entralgo, *The Therapy of the Word in Classical Antiquity* (New Haven: Yale Univ. Press, 1970).

4. I have taken this observation from Dr. L. Robbins' discussion in Eron (ed.), *The Classification of Behavior Disorders*.

5. Cited by A. L. Knutson, *The Individual, Society and Health Behavior* (New York: Russell Sage, 1965), p. 49.

6. Cited by Mechanic, *Medical Sociology*, p. 16.

7. Knutson, *The Individual, Society and Health Behavior*, p. 48, quotes one New York study showing lower-class indifference to the need for medical attention for such conditions as ankle-swelling and backache. But these should still have been regarded as illnesses by the respondents, who could have had their own reasons (such as lack of cash) for refusing to consider medical treatment.

8. There is now some doubt among dental experts as to whether "caries" is a genuine disease-entity or an artifact of diagnostic labeling.

9. See Foucault, *Madness and Civilization*, pp. 119, 121, 123, 129, and 151ff. Entralgo, in *The Therapy of the Word in Classical Antiquity*, has similar explanations collected from ancient Hippocratic medicine.

CHRISTOPHER BOORSE*

On the Distinction between Disease and Illness

In this century a strong tendency has developed to debate social issues in psychiatric terms. Whether the topic is criminal responsibility, sexual deviance, feminism, or a host of others, claims about mental health are increasingly likely to be the focus of discussion. This growing preference for medicine over morals, which might be called the *psychiatric turn,* has an obvious appeal. In the paradigm health discipline, physiological medicine, judgments of health and disease are normally uncontroversial. The idea of reaching comparable certainty about difficult ethical problems is an inviting prospect. Unfortunately our grasp of the issues that surround the psychiatric turn continues to be impeded, as does psychiatric theory itself, by a fundamental misunderstanding of the concept of health. With few exceptions, clinicians and philosophers are agreed that health is an essentially evaluative notion. According to this consensus view, a value-free science of health is impossible. This thesis I believe to be entirely mistaken. I shall argue in this essay that it rests on a confusion between the theoretical and the practical senses of "health," or in other words, between disease and illness.

Two presuppositions of my whole discussion should be noted at the outset. The first is substantive: with Szasz and Flew, I shall assume that the idea of health ought to be analyzed by reference to physiological medicine alone.[1] It is a mistake to view physical and mental health as equally well-entrenched species of a single conceptual genus. In most respects, our institutions of mental health are recent offshoots from physiological medicine, and their nature and future are under continual

controversy. In advance of a clear analysis of health in physiological medicine, it seems an open question whether current applications of the health vocabulary to mental conditions have any justification at all. Such applications will therefore be put on probation in the first two sections below. The other presupposition of my discussion is terminological. For convenience in distinguishing theoretical from practical uses of "health," I shall adhere to the technical usage of "disease" found in textbooks of medical theory. In such textbooks "disease" is simply synonymous with "unhealthy condition." Readers who wish to preserve the much narrower ordinary usage of "disease" should therefore substitute "theoretically unhealthy condition" throughout.

NORMATIVISM ABOUT HEALTH

It is safe to begin any discussion of health by saying that health is normality, since the terms are interchangeable in clinical contexts. But this remark provides no analysis of health until one specifies the norms involved. The most obvious proposal, that they are pure statistical means, is widely recognized to be erroneous. On the one hand, many deviations from the average—e.g. unusual strength or vital capacity or eye color—are not unhealthy. On the other hand, practically everyone has some disease or other, and there are also particular diseases such as tooth decay and minor lung irritation that are nearly universal. Since statistical normality is therefore neither necessary nor sufficient for clinical normality, most writers take the following view about the norms of health: that they must be determined, in whole or in part, by acts of evaluation. More precisely, the orthodox view is that all judgments of health include value judgments as part of their meaning. To call a condition unhealthy is at least in part to condemn it; hence it is impossible to define health in nonevaluative

* I thank the Delaware Institute for Medical Education and Research and the National Institute of Mental Health (Grant RO₃ MH 24621) for support in writing this essay.

Normativism has many varieties, which are often not clearly distinguished from one another by the clinicians who espouse them. The common feature of healthy conditions may, for example, be held to be either their desirability for the individual or their desirability for society. The gap between these two values is a persistent source of controversy in the mental-health domain. One especially common variety of normativism combines the thesis that health judgments are value judgments with ethical relativism. The resulting view that society is the final authority on what counts as disease is typical of psychiatric texts, as illustrated by the following quotation:

While professionals have a major voice in influencing the judgment of society, it it the collective judgment of the larger social group that determines whether its members are to be viewed as sick or criminal, eccentric or immoral.[2]

For the most part my arguments against normativism will apply to all versions indiscriminately. It will, however, be useful to make a minimal division of normativist positions into strong and weak. Strong normativism will be the view that health judgments are pure evaluations without descriptive meaning; weak normativism allows such judgments a descriptive as well as a normative component.[3]

As an example of a virtually explicit statement of strong normativism by a clinician, consider Dr. Judd Marmor's remark in a recent psychiatric symposium on homosexuality:

. . . to call homosexuality the result of disturbed sexual development really says nothing other than that you disapprove of the outcome of the development.[4]

If we may substitute "unhealthy" for "disturbed," Marmor is claiming that to call a condition unhealthy is *only* to express disapproval of it. In other words—to collapse a few ethical distinctions—for a condition to be unhealthy it is necessary and sufficient that it be bad. Now at least half of this view, the sufficiency claim, is demonstrably false of physiological medicine. It is undesirable to be moderately ugly or, for that matter, to lack the manual dexterity of

Liszt, but neither of these conditions is a disease. In fact, there are undesirable conditions regularly corrected by physicians which are not diseases: Jewish nose, sagging breasts, adolescent fertility, and unwanted pregnancies are only a few of many examples. Thus strong normativism is an erroneous account of health judgments in their paradigm area of application, and its influence upon mental-health theorists is regrettable.

Unlike Marmor, however, many clinical writers take positions that can be construed as committing them merely to weak normativism. A good example is Dr. Marie Jahoda, who concludes her survey of current criteria of psychological health with these words:

Actually, the discussion of the psychological meaning of various criteria could proceed without concern for value premises. Only as one calls these psychological phenomena "mental health" does the problem of values arise in full force. By this label, one asserts that these psychological attributes are "good." And, inevitably, the question is raised: Good for what? Good in terms of middle class ethics? Good for democracy? For the continuation of the social *status quo?* For the individual's happiness? For mankind? . . . For the encouragement of genius or of mediocrity and conformity? The list could be continued.[5]

Jahoda may here mean to claim only that calling a condition healthy *involves* calling it good. Her remarks are at least consistent with the weak normativist thesis that healthy conditions are good conditions which satisfy some further descriptive property as well. On this view, "healthy" is a mixed normative-descriptive term of the same sort as "honest" and "courageous." The following passage by Dr. F. C. Redlich is likewise consistent with the weak view:

Most propositions about normal behavior refer implicitly or explicitly to ideal behavior. Deviations from the ideal obviously are fraught with value judgments; actually, all propositions on normality contain certain statements in various degrees.[6]

Redlich's term "contain" suggests that he too sees the goodness of something as merely one necessary condition of its healthiness, and similarly for badness and unhealthiness.

Yet even weak normativism runs into counterexamples within physiological medicine. It is obvious that a disease may be on balance desirable, as with the flat feet of a draftee or the mild infection produced by inoculation. It might be suggested in response that diseases must at any rate be prima facie undesirable. The trouble with this suggestion is that it is obscure. Consider the case of a disease that has infertility as its sole important effect. In what sense is infertility prima facie undesirable? Considered in abstraction from the actual effects of reproduction on human beings, it is hard to see how infertility is either desirable or undesirable. Possibly those who see it as "prima facie" undesirable assume that most people want to be able to have more children. But the corollary of this position will be that writers of medical texts must do an empirical survey of human preferences to be sure that a condition is a disease. No such considerations seem to enter into human physiological research, any more than they do into standard biological studies of the diseases of plants and animals. Here indeed is another difficulty for any normativist, weak or strong. It seems clear that one may speak of diseases in plants and animals without judging the conditions in question undesirable. Biologists who study the diseases of fruit flies or sharks need not assume that their health is a good thing for us. On the other hand, there is not much sense in talking about the best interests of, say, a begonia. So it seems that normativists must interpret health judgments about plants and lower animals as analogical, in the same way as would be statements about the courage or considerateness of wolves and rats.

If normativism about health is at once so influential and so objectionable, one must ask what persuasive arguments there are in its support. I know of only three arguments, of which one will be treated in the next section. A germ of an argument appears in the passage by Redlich just quoted. Health judgments involve a comparison to an ideal; hence, Redlich concludes, they are "fraught with value judgments." It seems evident, however, that Redlich is thinking of ideals such as beauty and holiness rather than the chemist's ideal gas or Weber's ideal bureaucrat. The fact that a gas or a bureaucrat deviates from the ideal type is nothing against the gas or the bureaucrat. There are normative and nonnormative ideals, as there are in fact normative and nonnormative norms. The question is which sort health is, and Redlich has here provided no grounds for an answer.

A second and equally incomplete argument for normativism is suggested by the first two chapters of Margolis' *Psychotherapy and Morality*.[7] Margolis argues in his first chapter that psychoanalysts have been mistaken in holding that their therapeutic activities can "escape moral scrutiny" (p. 13). From this he concludes that "it is reasonable to view therapeutic values as forming part of a larger system of moral values" (p. 37), and explicitly endorses normativism. But this inference is a non sequitur. From the fact that the promotion of health is open to moral review, it in no way follows that health judgments are value judgments. Wealth and power are also "values" in the sense that people pursue them in a morally criticizable fashion; neither is a normative concept. The pursuit of any descriptively definable condition, if it has effects on persons, will be open to moral review.

These two arguments, like the health literature generally, do next to nothing to rule out the alternative view that health is a descriptively definable property which is usually valuable. Why, after all, may not health be a concept of the same sort as intelligence, or deductive validity? Though the idea of intelligence is certainly vague, it does not seem to be normative. Intelligence is the ability to perform certain intellectual tasks, and one would expect that these intellectual tasks could be characterized without presupposing their value.[8] Similarly, a valid argument may, for theoretical purposes, be descriptively defined[9] roughly as one that has a form no instance of which could have true premises and a false conclusion. Intelligence in people and validity in arguments being generally valued, the statement that a person is intelligent or an argument valid does tend to have the force of a recommendation. But this fact is wholly irrelevant to the employment of the terms in theories of intelligence or validity. To insist that evaluation is still part of the very meaning of the terms would be to make an implausible claim to which there are obvious counterexamples. Exactly the same may be true of the concept of health. At any rate, we have already seen some of the counterexamples.

Since the distinction between force and meaning in philosophy of language is in a rather primitive state, it is doubtful that weak normativism about health can be either decisively refuted or decisively established. But I suggest that its current prevalence is largely the result of two quite tractable causes. One is the lack of a plausible descriptive analysis; the other is a confusion between theoretical and practical uses of the health vocabulary. The required descriptive analysis I shall try to sketch in the next section. As for the second cause, one should always remember that a dual commitment to theory and practice is one of the features that distinguish a clinical discipline. Unlike chemists or astronomers, physicians and psychotherapists are professionally engaged in practical judgments about how certain people ought to be treated. It would not be surprising if the terms in which such practical judgments are formulated have normative content. One might contend, for example, that calling a cancer "inoperable" involves the value judgment that the results of operating will be worse than leaving the disease alone. But behind this conceptual framework of medical practice stands an autonomous framework of medical theory, a body of doctrine that describes the functioning of a healthy body, classifies various deviations from such functioning as diseases, predicts their behavior under various forms of treatment, etc. This theoretical corpus looks in every way continuous with theory in biology and the other natural sciences, and I believe it to be value-free.

The difference between the two frameworks emerges most clearly in the distinction between disease and illness. It is disease, the theoretical concept, that applies indifferently to organisms of all species. That is because, as we shall see, it is to be analyzed in biological

rather than ethical terms. The point is that illnesses are merely a subclass of diseases, namely, those diseases that have certain normative features reflected in the institutions of medical practice. An illness must be, first, a reasonably *serious* disease with incapacitating effects that make it undesirable. A shaving cut or mild athlete's foot cannot be called an illness, nor could one call in sick on the basis of a single dental cavity, though all these conditions are diseases. Secondly, to call a disease an illness is to view its owner as deserving special treatment and diminished moral accountability. These requirements of "illness" will be discussed in some detail shortly, with particular attention to "mental illness." But they explain at once why the notion of illness does not apply to plants and animals. Where we do not make the appropriate normative judgments or activate the social institutions, no amount of disease will lead us to use the term "ill." Even if the laboratory fruit flies fly in listless circles and expire at our feet, we do not say they succumbed to an illness, and for roughly the same reasons as we decline to give them a proper funeral.

There are, then, two senses of "health." In one sense it is a theoretical notion, the opposite of "disease." In another sense it is a practical or mixed ethical notion, the opposite of "illness."[10] Let us now examine the relation between these two concepts more closely.

DISEASE AND ILLNESS

What is the theoretical notion of a disease? An admirable explanation of clinical normality was given thirty years ago by C. Daly King.

The normal . . . is objectively, and properly, to be defined as that which functions in accordance with its design.[11]

The root idea of this account is that the normal is the natural. The state of an organism is theoretically healthy, i.e. free of disease, insofar as its mode of functioning comforms to the natural design of that kind of organism. Philosophers have, of course, grown repugnant to the idea of natural design since its cooptation by natural-purpose ethics and the so-called argument from design. It is undeniable that the term "natural" is often given an evaluative force. Shakespeare as well as Roman Catholicism is full of such usages, and they survive as well in the strictures of state legislatures against "unnatural acts." But it is no part of biological theory to assume that what is natural is desirable, still less the product of divine artifice. Contemporary biology employs a version of the idea of natural design that seems ideal for the analysis of health.

The crucial element in the idea of a biological design is the notion of a natural function. I have argued elsewhere that a function in the biologist's sense is nothing but a standard causal contribution to a goal actually pursued by the organism.[12] Organisms are vast assemblages of systems and subsystems which, in most members of a species, work together harmoniously in such a way as to achieve a hierarchy of goals. Cells are goal-directed toward metabolism, elimination, and mitosis; the heart is goal-directed toward supplying the rest of the body with blood; and the whole organism is goal-directed both to particular activities like eating and moving around and to higher-level goals such as survival and reproduction. The specifically physiological functions of any component are, I think, its species-typical contributions to the apical goals of survival and reproduction. But whatever the correct analysis of function statements, there is no doubt that biological theory is deeply committed to attributing functions to processes in plants and animals. And the single unifying property of all recognized diseases of plants and animals appears to be this: that they interfere with one or more functions typically performed within members of the species.

The account of health thus suggested is in one sense thoroughly Platonic. The health of an organism consists in the performance by each part of its natural function. And as Plato also saw, one of the most interesting features of the analysis is that it applies without alteration to mental health as long as there are standard mental functions. In another way, however,

the classical heritage is misleading, for it seems clear that biological function statements are descriptive rather than normative claims.[13] Physiologists obtain their functional doctrines without at any stage having to answer such questions as, What is the function of a man? or to explicate "a good man" on the analogy of "a good knife." Functions are not attributed in this context to the whole organism at all, but only to its parts, and the functions of a part are its causal contributions to empirically given goals. What goals a type of organism in fact pursues, and by what functions it pursues them, can be decided without considering the value of pursuing them. Consequently health in the theoretical sense is an equally value-free concept. The notion required for an analysis of health is not that of a good man or a good shark, but that of a good specimen of a human being or shark.

All of this amounts to saying that the epistemology King suggested for health judgments is, at bottom, a statistical one. The question therefore arises how the functional account avoids our earlier objections to statistical normality. King did explain how to dissolve one version of the paradox of saying that everyone is unhealthy. Clearly all the members of a species can have some disease or other as long as they do not have the same disease. King somewhat grimly compares the job of extracting an empirical ideal of health from a set of defective specimens to the job of reconstructing the Norden bombsight from assorted aerial debris (p. 495). But this answer does not touch universal diseases such as tooth decay. Although King nowhere considers this objection, the natural-design idea nevertheless suggests an answer that I suspect is correct. If what makes a condition a disease is its deviation from the natural functional organization of the species, then in calling tooth decay a disease we are saying that it is not simply in the nature of the species—and we say this because we think of it as mainly due to environmental causes. In general, deficiencies in the functional efficiency of the body are diseases when they are unnatural, and they may be unnatural either by being atypical or by being attributable mainly to the action of a hostile environment. If this explanation is accepted,[14] then the functional account simultaneously avoids the pitfalls of statistical normality and also frees the idea of theoretical health of all normative content.

Theoretical health now turns out to be strictly analogous to the mechanical condition of an artifact. Despite appearances, "perfect mechanical condition" in, say, a 1965 Volkswagen is a descriptive notion. Such an artifact is in perfect mechanical condition when it conforms in all respects to the designer's detailed specifications. Normative interests play a crucial role, of course, in the initial choice of the design. But what the Volkswagen design actually *is* is an empirical matter by the time production begins. Thenceforward a car may be in perfect condition regardless of whether the design is good or bad. If one replaces its stock carburetor with a high-performance part, one may well produce a better car, but one does not produce a Volkswagen in better mechanical condition. Similarly, an automatic camera may function perfectly and take wretched pictures; guided missiles and instruments of torture in perfect mechanical condition may serve execrable ends. Perfect working order is a matter not of the worth of the product but of the conformity of the process to a fixed design. In the case of organisms, of course, the ideal of health must be determined by empirical analysis of the species rather than by the intentions of a designer. But otherwise the parallel seems exact. A person who by mutation acquires a sixth sense, or the ability to regenerate severed limbs, is not thereby healthier than we are. Sixth senses and limb regeneration are not part of the human design, which at any given time, for better or worse, just is what it is.

We have been arguing that health is descriptively definable within medical theory, as intelligence is in psychological theory or validity in logical theory. Nevertheless medical theory is the basis of medical practice, and medical practice unquestioningly presupposes the value of health. We must therefore ask how the functional view explains this presumption that health is desirable.

In the case of physiological health, there are at least two general reasons why the functional normality that defines it is usually worth having. In the first place, most people do want to pursue the goals with respect to which physiological functions are isolated. Not only do we want to survive and reproduce, but we also want to engage in those particular activities, such as eating and sex, by which these goals are typically achieved. In the second place—and this is surely the main reason the value of physical health seems indisputable—physiological functions tend to contribute to all manner of activities neutrally. Whether it is desirable for one's heart to pump, one's stomach to digest, or one's kidneys to eliminate hardly depends at all on what one wants to do. It follows that essentially all serious physiological diseases will satisfy the first requirement of an illness, namely, undesirability for its bearer.

This explanation of the fit between medical theory and medical practice has the virtue of reminding us that health, though an important value, is conceptually a very limited one. Health is not unconditionally worth promoting, nor is what is worth promoting necessarily health. Although mental-health writers are especially prone to ignore these points, even the constitution of the World Health Organization seems to embody a similar confusion:

Health is a state of complete physical, mental, and social well-being, and not merely the absence of disease or infirmity.[15]

Unless one is to abandon the physiological paradigm altogether, this definition is far too wide. Health is functional normality, and as such is desirable exactly insofar as it promotes goals one can justify on independent grounds. But there is presumably no intrinsic value in having the functional organization typical of a species if the same goals can be better achieved by other means. A sixth sense, for example, would increase our goal-efficiency without increasing our health; so might the amputation of our legs at the knee and their replacement by a nuclear-powered air-cushion vehicle. Conversely, as we have seen, there is no a priori reason why ordinary diseases cannot contribute to well-being under appropriate circumstances.

In such cases, however, we will be reluctant to describe the person involved as ill, and that is because the term "ill" *does* have a negative evaluation built into it. Here again a comparison between health and other properties will be helpful. Disease and illness are related somewhat as are low intelligence and stupidity, or failure to tell the truth and speaking dishonestly. Sometimes the presumption that intelligence is desirable will fail, as in a discussion of qualifications for a menial job such as washing dishes or assembling auto parts. In such a context a person of low intelligence is unlikely to be described as stupid. Sometimes the presumption that truth should be told will fail, as when the Gestapo inquires about the Jews in your attic. Here the untruthful householder will not be described as speaking dishonestly. And sometimes the presumption that diseases are undesirable will fail, as with alcoholic intoxication or mild rubella intentionally contracted. Here the term "illness" is unlikely to appear despite the presence of disease. One concept of each pair is descriptive; the other adds to the first evaluative content, and so may be withheld where the first applies.

If we supplement this condition of undesirability with two further normative conditions, I believe we have the beginning of a plausible analysis of "illness."

A disease is an *illness* only if it is serious enough to be incapacitating, and therefore is

    (i) undesirable for its bearer;
    (ii) a title to special treatment; and
    (iii) a valid excuse for normally criticizable behavior.

The motivation for condition (ii) needs no explanation. As for (iii), the connection between illness and diminished responsibility has often been argued,[16] and I shall mention here only one suggestive point. Our notion of illness belongs to the ordinary conceptual scheme of persons and their actions, and it was developed to apply to physiological diseases. Consequently the relation between persons and their illnesses is conceived on the model of their relation to their bodies. It has often been observed that physiological processes, e.g. digestion or peristalsis, do not usually count as actions of ours at all. By the same token, we are not usually held responsible for the results of such processes when they go wrong, though we may be blamed for failing to take steps to prevent malfunction at some earlier time. Now if this special relation between persons and their bodies is the reason for connecting disease with nonresponsibility, the connection may break down when diseases of the mind are at stake instead. I shall now argue, in fact, that conditions (i), (ii), and (iii) all present difficulties in the domain of mental health.

MENTAL ILLNESS

For the sake of discussion, let us simply assume that the mental conditions usually called pathological are in fact unhealthy by the theoretical standard sketched in the last section. That is, we shall assume both that there are natural mental functions and also that recognized types of psychopathology are unnatural interferences with these functions.[17] Is it reasonable to make a parallel extension of the vocabulary of medical practice by calling these mental diseases mental illnesses? Let us consider each condition on "illness."

Condition (i) was the undesirability of an illness for its bearer. Now there are obstacles to transferring our general arguments that physiological health is desirable to the psychological domain. Mental states are not nearly so neutral to the choice of actions as physiological states are. In particular, to evaluate the desirability of mental health we can hardly avoid consulting our desires; but in the mental-health context it could be those very desires that are judged unhealthy. From a theoretical standpoint desires must be assigned a motivational function in producing action. Thus our wants may or may not conform to the species design. But if our wants do not conform to the species design, it is not immediately obvious why we should want them to. If there is no good reason to want them to, then we have a disease which is not an illness. It is conceivable that this divergence between the two notions is illustrated by homosexuality. It can hardly be denied that one normal function of sexual desire is to promote reproduction. If one does not have a desire for heterosexual sex, however, the only good reason for wanting to have such a desire seems to be that one would be happier if one did. But this judgment needs to be supported by evidence. The desirability of having species-typical desires is not nearly so obvious on inspection as the desirability of having species-typical physiological functions.

One of the corollaries of this point is that recent debates over homosexuality and other disputable diagnoses usually ignore at least one important issue. Besides asking whether, say, homosexuality is a disease, one should also ask what difference it makes if it is. I have suggested that biological normality is an instrumental rather than an intrinsic good. We always have the right to ask, of normality, what is in it for us that we already desire. If it were possible, then, to maximize intrinsic goods such as happiness, for ourselves and others, with a psyche full of deviant desires and unnatural acts, it is hard to see what practical significance the theoretical judgment of unhealthiness would have. I do not actually have serious doubts that disorders such as neuroses and psychoses diminish human happiness. It is also true that what is desirable for a person need not coincide with what the person wants; though an anorectic may not wish to eat, it is desirable that he or she do so. But we must be clear that requests to justify the value of health in other terms are always in order, and there are reasons to expect that such justification will require more evidence in the psychological domain than in the physiological.

We have been discussing the value of psychological normality for the individual, as dictated by condition (i) on illness, rather than its desirability for society at large. Since clinicians often assume that mental health involves social adjustment, it may be well to point out that the functional account of health shows this too to be a debatable assumption requiring empirical support. Certainly nothing in the mere statement that a person has a mental disease entails that he or she is contributing less to the social order than an arbitrary normal individual. There is no contradiction in calling van Gogh or Blake or Dostoyevsky mentally disturbed while admiring their work, even if they would

have been less creative had they been healthier. Conversely, there is no a priori reason to assume that the healthy human personality will be morally worthy or socially acceptable. If Freud and Lorenz are right about the existence of an aggressive drive, there is a large component of the normal psyche that is less than admirable. Whether or not they are right, the suggestion clearly makes sense. Perhaps most psychiatrists would agree anyway that antisocial behavior is to be expected during certain developmental stages, e.g. the so-called anal-sadistic period or adolescence.

It must be conceded that *Homo sapiens* is a social species. Other organisms of this class, such as ants and bees, display elaborate fixed systems of social adaptations, and it would be remarkable if the human design included no standard functions at all promoting socialization. On the basis of the physiological paradigm, however, it is not at all clear that contributions to society can be viewed as requirements of health except when they also contribute to individual survival and reproduction. No matter how this issue is decided, the crucial point remains: the nature and extent of social functions in the human species can be discovered only empirically. Despite the contrary convictions of many clinicians, the concept of mental health itself provides no guarantee that healthy individuals will meet the standards or serve the interests of society at large. If it did, that would be one more reason to question the desirability of health for the individual.

Let us now go on to condition (ii) on a disease which is an illness: that it justify "special treatment" of its owner. It is this condition together with (iii) that gives some plausibility to the many recent attempts to explain mental illness as a "social status" or "role."[18] The idea that the "sick role" is a special one is consistent with the statistical normality of having some disease or other. Since illnesses are serious diseases that incapacitate at the level of gross behavior, everyone can be minimally diseased without being ill. In the realm of mental health, however, many psychiatrists suggest the stronger thesis that it is statistically normal to be significantly incapacitated by neurosis.[19] A similar problem may arise on Benedict's famous view that the characteristic personality type of some whole societies is clinically paranoid.[20] A statistically normal condition, according to our analysis, can be a disease only if it can be blamed on the environment. But one might plausibly claim that most or all existing *cultural* environments do injure children, filling their minds with excessive anxiety about sexual pleasure, grotesque role models, absurd prejudices about reality, etc. It is at least possible that some degree of neurosis or psychosis is a nearly universal environmental injury in our species. Only an empirical inquiry into the incidence and etiology of neurosis can show whether this possibility is a reality. If it is, however, one can maintain the idea that serious diseases are illnesses only by abandoning one of the presuppositions of the illness concept: that not everyone can be ill.[21]

The last and clearest difficulty with "mental illness" concerns condition (iii), the role of illness in excusing conduct. We said that the idea that serious diseases excuse conduct derives from the model of the relation of agents to their own physiology. Unfortunately the relation of agents to their own psychology is of a much more intimate kind. The puzzle about mental illness is that it seems to be an activity of the very seat of responsibility—the mind and character—and therefore to be beyond all hope of excuse.

This inference is hardly inescapable; there is room for considerable controversy to which I cannot do justice here. Strictly speaking, mental disorders are disturbances of the personality. It is persons, not personalities, who are held responsible for actions, and one central element in the idea of a person is certainly consciousness. This means that there may be some sense in contrasting responsible persons with their mental diseases insofar as these diseases lie outside their conscious personalities. Perhaps from a psychoanalytic standpoint this condition is often met in psychosis and neurosis. The unconscious processes that surface in these disorders seem at first sight more like things that happen within us, e.g. peristalsis, than like things we do. But several points make this classification look oversimplified. Unconscious ideas and wishes are still *our* ideas and wishes in a more compelling sense than movements of the gut are our movements. They may have been conscious at an earlier time or be made conscious in therapy, whereupon it becomes increasingly difficult to disclaim responsibility for them. It seems quite unclear that we are more responsible for many conscious desires and beliefs than for these unconscious ones. Finally, the hope for contrasting responsible people with their mental diseases grows vanishingly dim in the case of a character disorder, where the unhealthy condition seems to be integrated into the conscious personality.

In view of these points and the rest of the discussion, I think we must accept the following conclusion. While conditions (i), (ii), and (iii) apply fairly automatically to serious physical diseases, not one of them should be assumed to apply automatically to serious mental diseases. If the term "mental illness" is to be applied at all, it should probably be restricted to psychoses and disabling neuroses. But even this decision needs more analysis than I have provided in this essay. It seems doubtful that on any construal mental illness will ever be, in the mental-health movement's famous phrase, "just like any other illness."

What are the implications of our discussion for the social issues to which psychiatry is so frequently applied? As far as the criminal law is concerned, our results suggest that psychiatric theory alone should not be expected to define legal responsibility, e.g. in the insanity defense.[22] Although the notion of responsibility is a component of the notion of illness, it belongs not to medical theory but to ethics, and one can fix its boundaries only by rational ethical debate. It seems certain that such a simple responsibility test as that the act of the accused not be "the product of mental disease" is unsatisfactory. No doubt many of us have antisocial tendencies that derive from underlying psychopathology of an ordinary sort. When these tendencies erupt in a parking violation or negligent collision, it hardly seems inhumane or unjust to apply legal sanctions.[23] But this is not surprising, for no psychiatric concept is properly designed to answer moral questions. I am not saying that psychiatry is irrelevant to law and ethics. Anyone writing or applying a criminal code is certainly well advised to obtain the best available information about human nature, including the information about human nature that constitutes mental-health theory. The point is that one cannot expect to substitute psychiatry for moral debate, any more than moral evaluations can be substituted for psychiatric theory. Insofar as the psychiatric turn consists in such substitutions, it is fundamentally misconceived.

The other main implications of our discussion seem to me twofold. First, there is not the slightest warrant for the recurrent fantasy that what society or its professionals disapprove of is ipso facto unhealthy. This is not merely because society may disapprove of the wrong things. Even if ethical relativism were true, society still could not fix the functional organization of the members of a species. For this reason it could never be an infallible authority either on disease or on illness, which is a subclass of disease. Thus one main source of the tendency to call radical activists, Bohemians, feminists, and other unpopular deviants "sick" is nothing but a conceptual confusion.

The second moral suggested by our discussion is that it is always worth asking, in any particular case, how strong the presumption is that health is desirable. When the value of health is left both unquestioned and obscure, it has a tendency to undergo inflation. The diagnosis especially of a "mental illness" is then likely to become an amorphous and peculiarly repellent stigma to be removed at any cost. The use of muscle-paralyzing drugs to compel prisoners to participate in "group therapy" is a particularly gruesome example of this sort of thinking.[24] But there are many other situations in which everyone would profit by asking what exactly is wrong with being unhealthy. In a way liberal reformers tend to make the opposite mistake: in their zeal to remove the stigma of disease from conditions such as homosexuality, they wholly discount the possibility that these conditions, like most diseases,

are somewhat unideal. If the value of health, as I have argued in this essay, is nothing but the value of conformity to a generally excellent species design, then by recognizing that fact we may improve both the clarity and the humanity of our social discourse.

NOTES

1. Thomas S. Szasz, *The Myth of Mental Illness* (New York, 1961); Antony Flew, *Crime or Disease?* (New York, 1973), pp. 40,42.

2. Ian Gregory, *Fundamentals of Psychiatry* (Philadelphia, 1968), p. 32.

3. R. M. Hare, in *Freedom and Reason* (New York, 1963), chap. 2, argues that no terms have prescriptive meaning alone. If this view is accepted, the difference between strong and weak normativism concerns the question of whether "healthy" is "primarily" or "secondarily" evaluative.

4. Judd Marmor, "Homosexuality and Cultural Value Systems," *American Journal of Psychiatry* 130 (1973): 1208.

5. Marie Jahoda, *Current Concepts of Positive Mental Health* (New York, 1958), pp. 76-77. See also her remark in *Interrelations Between the Social Environment and Psychiatric Disorders* (New York, 1953), p. 142: ". . . inevitably at some place there is a value judgement involved. I think that mental health or mental sickness cannot be conceived of without reference to some basic value."

6. F. C. Redlich, "The Concept of Normality," *American Journal of Psychotherapy* 6 (1952): 553.

7. Joseph Margolis, *Psychotherapy and Morality* (New York, 1966).

8. Exactly what intellectual abilities are included in intelligence is, of course, unclear and may vary from culture to culture. (See N. J. Block and Gerald Dworkin, "IQ. Heritability and Inequality, Part I," *Philosophy and Public Affairs* 3, no. 4 [Summer 1974]: 333.) But this does not show that for any particular group of speakers "intelligent" is a normative term, i.e. has positive evaluation as part of its meaning.

9. The contrary view, which might be called normativism about validity, is defended by J. O. Urmson in "Some Questions Concerning Validity," *Revue Internationale de Philosophie* 25 (1953): 217-229.

10. Thomas Nagel has suggested that the adjective "ill" may have its own special opposite "well." Our thinking about health might be greatly clarified if "wellness" had some currency.

11. C. Daly King, "The Meaning of Normal," *Yale Journal of Biology and Medicine* 17 (1945): 493-494. Most definitions of health in medical dictionaries include some reference to functions. Almost exactly King's formulation also appears in Fredrick C. Redlich and Daniel X. Freedman. *The Theory and Practice of Psychiatry* (New York, 1966), p. 113.

12. "Wright on Functions," to appear in *The Philosophical Review.*

13. The view that function statements are normative generates the third argument for normativism. It is presented most fully by Margolis in "Illness and Medical Values," *The Philosophy Forum* 8 (1959): 55–76, section II. It is also suggested by Ronald B. de Sousa, "The Politics of Mental Illness," *Inquiry* 15 (1972): 187–201, p. 194, and possibly by Flew as well in *Crime or Disease?* pp. 39–40. I think philosophers of science have made too much progress in giving biological function statements a descriptive analysis for this argument to be very convincing.

14. For further discussion of environmental injuries and other details of the functional account of health sketched in this section, see my forthcoming essay "Health as a Theoretical Concept."

15. Quoted by Flew, *Crime or Disease?* p. 46.

16. A good discussion of this point and of the undesirability condition (i) is provided by Flew in the extremely illuminating second chapter of *Crime or Disease?* Flew takes these conditions as part of the meaning of "disease" rather than "illness"; but since he seems to be working from the ordinary usage of "disease," there may be no real disagreement here.

17. The plausibility of these two claims is discussed at length in my essay, "What a Theory of Mental Health Should Be," *Journal for the Theory of Social Behaviour,* 6 (1976): 61–84.

18. An example of this approach is Robert B. Edgerton, "On The 'Recognition' of Mental Illness," in Stanley C. Plog and Robert B. Edgerton, *Changing Perspectives in Mental Illness* (New York, 1969), pp. 49–72.

19. Only one example of this suggestion is Dr. Reuben Fine's statement that neurosis afflicts 99 percent of the population. See Fine's "The Goals of Psychoanalyis," in *The Goals of Psychotherapy,* ed. Alvin R. Mahrer (New York, 1967), p. 95. I consider the issue of whether all neurosis can be called unhealthy in the essay cited in note 17.

20. See the descriptions of the Kwakiutl and the Dobu in Ruth Benedict, *Patterns of Culture* (Boston: Houghton Mifflin, 1934).

21. A number of clinicians have seriously suggested that people who are ill can be distinguished from those who are well by their presence in your office. One such author goes as far as to calculate an upper limit on the incidence of mental illness from the number of members in the American Psychiatric Association. On a literal reading, this patient-in-the-office test implies that one could wipe out mental illness once and for all by dissolving the APA and outlawing psychotherapy. But the whole idea seems silly anyway in the face of various studies that indicate that the population at large is, by the ordinary descriptive criteria for mental disorder, no less disturbed than the population of clinical patients.

22. The same conclusion is defended by Herbert Fingarette in "Insanity and Responsibility," *Inquiry* 15 (1972): 6–29.

23. Thus I disagree with H.L.A. Hart, among others, who writes: ". . . the contention that it is fair or just to punish those who have broken the law must be absurd if the crime is merely a manifestation of a disease." The quotation is from "Murder and the Principles of Punishment: England and the United States," reprinted in *Moral Problems,* ed. James Rachels (New York, 1975), p. 274.

24. For this and other "therapeutic" abuses in our prison system, see Jessica Mitford, *Kind and Usual Punishment* (New York, 1973), chap. 8.

SUGGESTED READINGS FOR CHAPTER 3

Books and Articles

Boorse, Christopher. "What a Theory of Mental Health Should Be." *Journal for the Theory of Social Behaviour* 6 (April, 1976), 61–84.

"The Concept of Health." *Hastings Center Studies* 1 (No. 3, 1973). Special issue.

"Concepts of Health and Disease." *Journal of Medicine and Philosophy* 1 (September, 1976). Special issue.

Dubos, René. *Mirage of Health.* New York: Harper & Row, 1959.

Engelhardt, H. Tristram, Jr. "The Concepts of Health and Disease." In Engelhardt, H. Tristram, and Spicker, Stuart F., eds. *Philosophy and Medicine.* Vol. 1. Dordrecht: D. Reidel, 1974, pp. 125–141. Volume title: *Evaluation and Explanation in the Biomedical Sciences.*

Feinstein, Alvan R. *Clinical Judgment.* Baltimore: Williams & Wilkins, 1967.

Flew, Antony. *Crime or Disease?* New York: Barnes & Noble, 1973.

Kopelman, Loretta. "On Disease . . . ." In Engelhardt, H. Tristram, Jr., and Spicker, Stuart F., eds. *Philosophy and Medicine.* Vol. 1. Dordrecht: D. Reidel, 1974, pp. 143–150. Volume title: *Evaluation and Explanation in the Biomedical Sciences.*

Macklin, Ruth. "Mental Health and Mental Illness: Some Problems of Definition and Concept Formation." *Philosophy of Science* 39 (September, 1972), 341–365.

Macklin, Ruth. "The Medical Model in Psychoanalysis and Psychotherapy." *Comprehensive Psychiatry* 14 (January/February, 1973), 49–69.

Margolis, Joseph. *Negativities: The Limits of Life.* Columbus, Ohio: Charles Merrill Publishing Co., 1975. Chaps. 7 and 8.

Murphy, Edmond A., "The Normal and the Perils of the Sylleptic Argument." *Perspectives in Biology and Medicine* 15 (Summer, 1972), 566–582.

Osmond, Humphrey, and Siegler, Miriam. *Models of Madness, Models of Medicine.* New York: Macmillan, 1974.

Pellegrino, Edmund. "Medicine, History, and the Idea of Man." *Annals of the American Academy of Political and Social Science* 346 (March, 1963), 9–20.

Powles, John. "On the Limitations of Modern Medicine." *Science, Medicine and Man* 1 (April, 1973), 1–30.

Redlich, F. C. "The Concept of Health in Psychiatry." In Leighton, Alexander H., Claussen, John A., and Wilson, Robert N., eds. *Explorations in Social Psychiatry*. New York: Basic Books, 1957. Pp. 138–158.

Szasz, Thomas. *The Manufacture of Madness*. New York: Harper & Row, 1970.

Bibliographies

Journal of Medicine and Philosophy 1 (September, 1976). References at the ends of several articles.

Sollitto, Sharmon, and Veatch, Robert M., comps. *Bibliography of Society, Ethics and the Life Sciences*. Hastings-on-Hudson, N.Y.: Institute of Society, Ethics and the Life Sciences. Updated periodically. See under "Health Care Delivery."

Walters, LeRoy, ed. *Bibliography of Bioethics*. Vols. 1- . Detroit: Gale Research Co. Issued annually. See under "Genetic Defects," "Health," and "Mental Health."

Part II

THE PROFESSIONAL-PATIENT RELATIONSHIP

4.
Patients' Rights and Professional Responsibilities

That the practice of medicine is an applied science none would deny. But it also involves the common human transactions of contracts and services. Interesting professional responsibilities and patients' rights emerge from this human side of medical practice. Professional obligations have long been recognized in medical codes, but only recently has much systematic thought been given to the moral and legal rights of patients. In this chapter both the traditional conceptions of and the emerging problems in the professional-patient relationship are explored.

MEDICAL CODES OF ETHICS
The two codes of ethics included in this chapter are samples of the numerous codes which have been developed by health professionals in both ancient and modern times. The Hippocratic Oath took the form of a series of religious vows. More recent codes, including the International Code of Nursing Ethics, generally contain secular statements of ethical standards. The central affirmation of such codes is that, in treating the (frequently vulnerable) patient, the health professional will not exploit his or her position of relatively controlling power and influence.

Two questions arise concerning the status of these professional codes: (1) what is their relation to law? and (2) what is their relation to general ethical principles? The medical codes, though quasi-legal in form, are self-legislative documents developed by particular professions. As such, they have only the force which the profession chooses to attribute to them. In most professions, including medicine and nursing, professional self-discipline or self-policing has usually been less than vigorous.

Two possible relationships between codes of professional ethics and general ethical principles can be envisioned. Professional codes may constitute autonomous, self-contained systems of ethics which are unrelated to external validating principles. On the other hand, the codes may be viewed as specific applications of universal ethical principles.[1] According to this latter conception, the codes can and should be evaluated in the light of general ethical considerations such as the principles of beneficence and justice and the right of self-determination.

PATIENTS' RIGHTS
It is precisely the right of patient self-determination which has most frequently been deemphasized, or even ignored, in the codes of professional ethics. In part because of this lacuna, explicit declarations of patients' rights began to be formulated in the 1970s. Perhaps the best-known and most widely-distributed of these declarations is the American Hospital Association's "Statement on a Patient's Bill of Rights." This Bill was originally intended as a means of informing hospital

patients that they do not have to endure certain kinds of treatment. However, in his editorial comment in this chapter, Willard Gaylin argues that the AHA document merely restates the obvious and that its recommendations should be supplemented by more substantive demands of health care consumers.

Gaylin mentions, but does not elaborate upon, the complex interplay of rights and duties. In recent philosophical discussions of rights, a central question has been: What is the extent of the claim made when it is asserted that person X has a right to something? In its strongest form, the claim that person X has a right to something entails that someone else (Y) has a duty to provide the thing in question for X. A weaker conception of rights views the claim that X has a right to something as a warning that, other things being equal, no one should prevent X from pursuing the thing in question since X is entitled to it. A third and still weaker conception of rights considers declarations of rights to be catalogs of ideals, toward which the society as a whole should constantly work. A fourth, and somewhat radical, account holds that X has a right to something if and only if specifically granted that right by law.[2] It is not clear which of these conceptions, if any, is operative in the AHA "Statement on a Patient's Bill of Rights."

INFORMED CONSENT

Whatever the full complement of rights possessed by patients, it is widely believed that the physician has a moral obligation to make it possible for patients to decide important matters which affect their health. However, the ability to "make a decision" is largely dependent upon the information made available to the patient. A patient's consent to a medical procedure would be insignificant if important relevant information were withheld from him. For example, suppose it is believed but not confirmed that a patient has cancer. If this patient is asked to submit to dangerous exploratory surgery, it may be of fundamental importance to him that he understands *that he has cancer* before consenting to the surgery. If he is only informed that exploratory surgery is needed, a piece of true but incomplete information has been provided to him. Unless additional information is supplied the consent will probably be regarded as invalid. Moreover, even if the consent were genuinely informed, we would also insist that it be noncoercively obtained. Hence, it is often said that before a physician performs a medical procedure on a competent patient, he has an obligation to obtain the patient's voluntary informed consent. In recent years this principle has become virtually an axiom of medical ethics, though it has by no means always been put into practice in difficult cases.

There are two main problems of informed consent. The first problem is a conceptual issue. What is the proper meaning of informed consent? The *consent* element is relatively unproblematic, but what is it to give *informed* consent, as distinct from either partially informed or uninformed consent? Physicians are hardly in a position to give patients a course in medicine, as a way of explaining their problem. But how can patients make an informed decision if they incompletely comprehend their medical condition? Moreover, most medical decisions are made by doctors on what *they* know to be incomplete information, for the simple reason that not all the desired information can be obtained. Since neither the patient nor the doctor can in most situations have full information, the notion of informed consent might be regarded as an ideal which is not fully realizable but ought to be approximated. Still, even if "informed consent" functions as an ideal, the question remains how much information must be provided for informed consent, in any realistic sense, to be present. And a satisfactory analysis of the term "informed consent" appears again at this more basic level.

The second problem has to do with ascertaining that informed consent has been given. The requirement of informed consent is often regarded simply as a matter of obtaining the signature of a patient on a dotted line at the end of a so-called "consent form." But is the signature sufficient evidence of informed consent? One might argue that the proper standard of informed consent is the prevailing standard used in any given community. Yet this standard may be unacceptably low, and hence itself ethically unacceptable. In confronting this and other problems, some courts have adopted the standard of the "reasonable man": the physician must have informed the patient to the extent that *any reasonable man* (or woman) would have to be informed in order to make a decision about his (or her) case. Yet it is unclear precisely what this doctrine requires and even whether it is morally satisfactory.

REFUSAL OF TREATMENT

Problems of informed consent to therapies are closely related to problems of informed refusal of therapies. Notoriously, patients have refused such treatments as blood transfusions because their religious convictions do not permit them; but ethical problems of patient refusal involve broader issues than those of freedom of religious exercise. A patient might refuse these same treatments for nonreligious reasons, and the case might or might not involve emergency measures. Refusal of treatment also encompasses problems of proxy refusal in the case of children and certain classes of incompetent patients, though in this chapter the primary focus is on refusal by competent adult patients. (For special problems of children and proxy decisions, see Chapter 7.)

Some of the most interesting cases of refusal of treatment occur when the patient makes an informed decision to refuse treatment with the knowledge that his or her own death will ensue. A major moral and legal question here is whether in life and death situations a patient should be judicially compelled to accept such treatment. If, as was suggested above, the moral requirement of informed consent has become a basic moral principle governing medical procedure, it might seem that a patient's informed refusal would be decisive, whether the decision was reached on religious or nonreligious grounds. Many regard such a right to refuse as fundamental in a free society, both in medical and other contexts. Moreover, there is a long tradition in the law that invasion of a person's body without valid consent is an assault; and doctors are as subject to this legal sanction as anyone else. This general line of argument against compulsory lifesaving treatment is supported by Robert M. Byrn in this chapter.

On the other hand, many persons do not think that patients' rights at the end of life include a right to "allow themselves to die." According to those who share this view, there are at least some circumstances where competent, nonconsenting patients should be *required* to accept livesaving medical therapies. Different reasons have been cited in defense of this view. Some regard a refusal of lifesaving treatment as patently unreasonable, even if "competently" decided. Others think the state often has a "compelling interest" in preventing such deaths. Another reason for forcing therapy, closely connected to that of unreasonableness, is paternalistic:[3] one limits the competent adult person's liberty of choice for his or her own good in order to prevent harm from befalling the person. This kind of paternalistic intervention occurred in the interesting case of Dr. Symmers, who—with complete information on his own case—asked his colleagues to take no steps to prolong his life if he suffered another cardiovascular collapse, yet was re-suscitated against his wishes.[4] Still another reason for coercive treatment chal-lenges the *validity* of the patient's refusal on the grounds that patients in life and death situations do not possess the requisite mental or emotional stability to make an informed choice.

Many physicians feel strongly that in these cases they are morally required (perhaps by the Hippocratic Oath) to prevent harm to patients. On the other hand, they also believe that it is a moral obligation to grant a patient's request whenever it is a true exercise of liberty; and in the "Patient's Bill of Rights" in this chapter it is said that "The patient has the right to refuse treatment to the extent permitted by law and to be informed of the medical consequences of his action." It is the clash between these two convictions which creates the dilemma of whether to treat patients who may do the "ultimate harm" to themselves by refusing therapy, or to give priority instead to patient choice.

CONFIDENTIALITY

Unlike informed consent, which is a relatively recent topic in codes of profes-sional ethics, confidentiality was a significant theme in some of the earliest codes, including the Hippocratic Oath. There the physician vowed: "What I may see or hear in the course of treatment or even outside of the treatment in regard to the life of men, . . . I will keep to myself. . . . "

Two general types of justifications have been proposed for the confidentiality principle in health care relationships. The first type of justification is deontolog-ical in character and argues that the health professional does not show proper respect for the patient if he or she does not uphold the confidentiality of the professional-patient relationship. A variant of this deontological approach asserts that there is an implied promise of confidentiality inherent in the professional-patient relationship—a promise which ought to be honored, just because it is a promise. In contrast, rule-utilitarians justify the preservation of medical confidentiality by claiming that violations of confidentiality will make patients unwilling to reveal sensitive information to health professionals; this unwillingness, in turn, will render diagnosis and cure more difficult and will, in the long run, be highly detrimental to the health of patients.

Even if one accepts the principle of medical confidentiality as important, there remains the question whether it states an absolute duty, and if not, under what conditions it is permissible to reveal otherwise confidential information. Perhaps the most difficult test case comes in a situation like the one described in *Tarasoff v. Regents of the University of California*. In this case a patient confided to his psychologist that he intended to kill a third party. The psychologist then faced the choice of preserving the confidentiality of his relationship with the patient or of breaching the principle of confidentiality to warn a young woman that her life might be in danger. Of course, not all examples of the problem of confidentiality are so dramatic. More common problems concern how much of a patient's medical record can be fed into a relatively "public" data bank and how much information about a patient's genetic makeup may be revealed to a sexual partner where there is a substantial likelihood of the couple's producing genetically handicapped children.

The readings in this chapter provide only a few samples of the rich literature on the relationship between patients and health professionals. In the past, much of this literature was written by health professionals for health professionals. It therefore highlighted their own sense of their *obligations* to the patient. In the foreseeable future, it seems likely that most of the literature on this topic will have its origin outside the health professions and that it will emphasize the *rights* of patients.

T.L.B.
L.W.

NOTES

1. On this point, see Robert M. Veatch, "Medical Ethics: Professional or Universal?" *Harvard Theological Review* 65 (October, 1972), 531–559.

2. On the general problem of rights, see R. M. Hare, "Abortion and the Golden Rule," *Philosophy and Public Affairs* 4 (Spring, 1975), and the Feinberg selection on "Rights" in Chapter 1.

3. On problems of the role of paternalism in ethical theory, see the Feinberg selection on "Liberty-Limiting Principles" in Chapter 1, and the essays by Shapiro, Bedau, and Beauchamp in Chapter 11.

4. Jay Katz, with Alexander Morgan Capron and Eleanor Swift Glass, *Experimentation with Human Beings* (New York: Russell Sage Foundation, 1972), p. 709.

The Hippocratic Oath

I swear by Apollo Physician and Asclepius and Hygieia and Panaceia and all the gods and goddesses, making them my witnesses, that I will fulfil according to my ability and judgment this oath and this covenant:

To hold him who has taught me this art as equal to my parents and to live my life in partnership with him, and if he is in need of money to give him a share of mine, and to regard his offspring as equal to my brothers in male lineage and to teach them this art—if they desire to learn it—without fee and covenant; to give a share of precepts and oral instruction and all the other learning to my sons and to the sons of him who has instructed me and to pupils who have signed the covenant and have taken an oath according to the medical law, but to no one else.

I will apply dietetic measures for the benefit of the sick according to my ability and judgment; I will keep them from harm and injustice.

I will neither give a deadly drug to anybody if asked for it, nor will I make a suggestion to this effect. Similarly I will not give to a woman an abortive remedy. In purity and holiness I will guard my life and my art.

I will not use the knife, not even on sufferers from stone, but will withdraw in favor of such men as are engaged in this work.

Whatever houses I may visit, I will come for the benefit of the sick, remaining free of all intentional injustice, of all mischief and in particular of sexual relations with both female and male persons, be they free or slaves.

What I may see or hear in the course of the treatment or even outside of the treatment in regard to the life of men, which on no account one must spread abroad, I will keep to myself holding such things shameful to be spoken about.

If I fulfil this oath and do not violate it, may it be granted to me to enjoy life and art, being honored with fame among all men for all time to come; if I transgress it and swear falsely, may the opposite of all this be my lot.

Reprinted with permission of the publisher from "The Hippocratic Oath," in Ludwig Edelstein, *Ancient Medicine*, edited by Oswei Temkin and C. Lillian Temkin (Baltimore: Johns Hopkins University Press, 1967).

International Code of Nursing Ethics

Professional nurses minister to the sick, assume responsibility for creating a physical, social and spiritual environment which will be conducive to recovery, and stress the prevention of illness and promotion of health by teaching and example. They render health-service to the individual, the family, and the community and coordinate their services with members of other health professions.

Service to mankind is the primary function of nurses and the reason for the existence of the nursing profession. Need for nursing service is universal. Professional nursing service is therefore unrestricted by considerations of nationality, race, creed, colour, politics, or social status.

Inherent in the code is the fundamental concept that the nurse believes in the essential freedoms of mankind and in the preservation of human life.

The profession recognises that an international code cannot cover in detail all the activities and relationships of nurses, some of which are conditioned by personal philosophies and beliefs.

1. The fundamental responsibility of the nurse is threefold: to conserve life, to alleviate suffering, and to promote health.

2. The nurse must maintain at all times the highest standards of nursing care and of professional conduct.

3. The nurse must not only be well prepared to practise but must maintain her knowledge and skill at a consistently high level.

4. The religious beliefs of a patient must be respected.

From Etziony, M. B., *The Physician's Creed,* 1973. Courtesy of Charles C. Thomas, Publisher, Springfield, Illinois. The *Code* was adopted by the International Council of Nurses, July 1953.

5. Nurses hold in confidence all personal information entrusted to them.

6. A nurse recognises not only the responsibilities but the limitations of her or his professional functions; recommends or gives medical treatment without medical orders only in emergencies and reports such action to a physician at the earliest possible moment.

7. The nurse is under an obligation to carry out the physician's orders intelligently and loyally and to refuse to participate in unethical procedures.

8. The nurse sustains confidence in the physician and other members of the health team: incompetence or unethical conduct of associates should be exposed but only to the proper authority.

9. A nurse is entitled to just remuneration and accepts only such compensation as the contract, actual or implied, provides.

10. Nurses do not permit their names to be used in connection with the advertisement of products or with any other form of self advertisement.

11. The nurse cooperates with and maintains harmonious relationships with members of other professions and with her or his nursing colleagues.

12. The nurse in private life adheres to standards of personal ethics which reflect credit upon her profession.

13. In personal conduct nurses should not knowingly disregard the accepted patterns of behaviour of the community in which they live and work.

14. A nurse should participate and share responsibility with other citizens and other health professions in promoting efforts to meet the health needs of the public—local, state, national and international.

Statement on a Patient's Bill of Rights

The American Hospital Association presents a Patient's Bill of Rights with the expectation that observance of these rights will contribute to more effective patient care and greater satisfaction for the patient, his physician, and the hospital organization. Further, the Association presents these rights in the expectation that they will be supported by the hospital on behalf of its patients, as an integral part of the healing process. It is recognized that a personal relationship between the physician and the patient is essential for the provision of proper medical care. The traditional physician-patient relationship takes on a new dimension when care is rendered within an organizational structure. Legal precedent has established that the institution itself also has a responsibility to the patient. It is in recognition of these factors that these rights are affirmed.

1. The patient has the right to considerate and respectful care.

2. The patient has the right to obtain from his physician complete current information concerning his diagnosis, treatment, and prognosis in terms the patient can be reasonably expected to understand. When it is not medically advisable to give such information to the patient, the information should be made available to an appropriate person in his behalf. He has the right to know, by name, the physician responsible for coordinating his care.

3. The patient has the right to receive from his physician information necessary to give informed consent prior to the start of any procedure and/or treatment. Except in emergencies, such information for informed consent should include but not necessarily be limited to the specific procedure and/or treatment, the medically significant risks involved, and the probable duration of incapacitation. Where medically significant alternatives for care or treatment exist, or when the patient requests information concerning medical alternatives, the patient has the right to such information. The patient also has the right to know the name of the person responsible for the procedures and/or treatment.

4. The patient has the right to refuse treatment to the extent permitted by law and to be informed of the medical consequences of his action.

5. The patient has the right to every consideration of his privacy concerning his own medical care program. Case discussion, consultation, examination, and treatment are confidential and should be conducted discreetly. Those not directly involved in his care must have the permission of the patient to be present.

6. The patient has the right to expect that all communications and records pertaining to his care should be treated as confidential.

7. The patient has the right to expect that within its capacity a hospital must make reasonable response to the request of a patient for services. The hospital must provide evaluation, service, and/or referral as indicated by the urgency of the case. When medically permissible, a patient may be transferred to another facility only after he has received complete information and explanation concerning the needs for and alternatives to such a transfer. The institution to which the patient is to be

Reprinted with permission of the American Hospital Association from *Hospitals,* Vol. 4, No. 4 (February 16, 1973). The *Statement* was affirmed by the Board of Trustees, November 17, 1972.

8. The patient has the right to obtain information as to any relationship of his hospital to other health care and educational institutions insofar as his care is concerned. The patient has the right to obtain information as to the existence of any professional relationships among individuals, by name, who are treating him.

9. The patient has the right to be advised if the hospital proposes to engage in or perform human experimentation affecting his care or treatment. The patient has the right to refuse to participate in such research projects.

10. The patient has the right to expect reasonable continuity of care. He has the right to know in advance what appointment times and physicians are available and where. The patient has the right to expect that the hospital will provide a mechanism whereby he is informed by his physician or a delegate of the physician of the patient's continuing health care requirements following discharge.

11. The patient has the right to examine and receive an explanation of his bill regardless of source of payment.

12. The patient has the right to know what hospital rules and regulations apply to his conduct as a patient.

No catalog of rights can guarantee for the patient the kind of treatment he has a right to expect. A hospital has many functions to perform, including the prevention and treatment of disease, the education of both health professionals and patients, and the conduct of clinical research. All these activities must be conducted with an overriding concern for the patient, and, above all, the recognition of his dignity as a human being. Success in achieving this recognition assures success in the defense of the rights of the patient.

WILLARD GAYLIN

The Patient's Bill of Rights

A stay in a hospital exposes an individual to a condition of passivity and impotence unparalleled in adult life, this side of prison. You are dressed in an uncomfortable garment, leaving you exposed and ludicrous; told when you must sleep and when you must rise; informed of what you may eat and when you have to eat it; notified as to when you can have visitors, who they shall be, and how long they can stay. You are discussed in the third person in your presence as though you were some idiot child or inanimate object. If you are unfortunate enough to have an interesting case, you will be presented to a group of strangers who may take the invasion of your privacy as their privilege. Your chart, at the foot of the bed, will contain all the vital information that you would seem to be entitled to have; yet, should you attempt to examine it, you will be treated like a prepubescent caught with a copy of *Portnoy's Complaint*.

Some of this may be necessary for health and some for convenience, but most of it is simply the inevitable result of an authoritative person dealing with people who unquestionably accept his authority.

Hospital regulations are endured by a patient conditioned to seeing his physician as a benev-

Reprinted with permission of the publisher from *Saturday Review of the Sciences,* Vol. 1, No. 2 (February 24, 1973), p. 22.

olent father in whose reassuring presence he is prepared to play the role of the child. Beyond this, however, more serious rights are violated under the numbing atmosphere of the same paternalism.

Modern scientific medicine, as exemplified in complex teaching hospitals, has advanced technical skill at the cost of personal warmth. Often there is no one physician rendering care, rather a battery of specialists, and while "treatment" may be superior, "care" is absent. This depersonalization of medicine is having a predictable effect on the patient, causing him to abandon his tendency to romanticize the physician, and, by extension, the medical community. For this and other reasons the patient is now pressing for a reevaluation of the medical contract.

In response to this, the American Hospital Association recently presented, with considerable fanfare, a "Patient's Bill of Rights." It is a document worth examining, for nothing indicates the low estate of current hospital care (as distinguished from treatment) more graphically than the form of the proferred cure.

The substance of the document is amazingly innocent of controversy, It affirms that "the patient has the right to considerate and respectful care" and, beyond that, the right to "reasonable continuity of care." He is told that he may expect a modicum of personal privacy; that the usual medical concern for confidentiality should be respected; that he has a right to expect "a reasonable response" to his request for service; and, as in any other commercial transaction, that he has a right to receive an explanation of his bill.

In addition, he will be relieved to hear that, as a patient in a hospital, knowledge of the "rules and regulations" that apply to him is manifestly his due—just as it would be if he were a participant in a poker game. Similarly, the right to obtain information "concerning his diagnosis, treatment and prognosis" seems perfectly straightforward—no more than the minimum required of any standard commercial transaction. On the other hand, the patient's right to "obtain information as to any re-lationship of his hospital to other health care and educational institutions in so far as his care is concerned" is disquieting, for it anxiously suggests that while his exclusive reason for being in the hospital is his personal health, the hospital may have multiple, unstated other reasons influencing its treatment of him.

Finally, when the bill affirms the patient's right to "give informed consent prior to the start of any procedure," his "right to refuse treatment to the extent permitted by law," and his right to be advised "if the hospital proposes to engage in or perform human experimentation" on him, it seems to be merely belaboring the obvious. It says no more than that the hospital is subject to the same laws concerning assault and battery as any other institution or member of society.

The objection to this well-intended, though timid, document is that it perpetuates the very paternalism that precipitated the abuses. By presenting its considerations as a "Patient's Bill of Rights," it creates the impression that the hospital is "granting" these rights to the patient. The hospital has no power to grant these rights. They were vested in the patient to begin with. If the rights have been violated, they have been violated by the hospital and its hirelings. The title a "Patient's Bill of Rights" therefore seems not only pretentious but deceptive. In effect, all that the document does is return to the patient, with an air of largess, some of the rights hospitals have previously stolen from him. It is the thief lecturing his victim on self-protection—i.e., the hospital instructs the patient to make sure that the hospital treats him according to the rules of decency and law to which he is entitled. It would be more appropriate if the association addressed its 7,000 member hospitals, cautioning them that for years they have violated patient rights, some of which have the mandate of law, and warning them they must no longer presume on the innocence of their customers or the indifference of judicial authorities.

Since this is a patently decent document, the fact that the American Hospital Association takes the circuitous route of speaking to the patient of his rights, rather than to the hospital of its duties, reveals the essential weakness of such professional organizations. The AHA, like the American Medical Association and similar groups, is designed to be the servant of its constituent members—and not of the general public. A servant does not lay down the law to his master. In this regard the AHA can only state that it "presents these rights in the expectation that they will be supported" by the member hospitals. The fact that it feels the need to alert the patient indicates how insecure that "expectation" is.

A reevaluation of patient rights—one that goes beyond the old rights reaffirmed in this bill —is greatly needed. The public should not look to the professional association for leadership here. It is not for the hospital community to outline the rights it will offer, but rather for the patient consumer to delineate and then demand those rights to which he feels entitled, by utilizing all the instruments of society designed for that purpose—including the legislature and the courts.

Informed Consent and the Refusal of Treatment

UNITED STATES COURT OF APPEALS

Canterbury v. Spence

SPOTTSWOOD W. ROBINSON, III, Circuit Judge

. . .

Once the circumstances give rise to a duty on the physician's part to inform his patient, the next inquiry is the scope of the disclosure the physician is legally obliged to make. The courts have frequently confronted this problem but no uniform standard defining the adequacy of the divulgence emerges from the decisions. Some have said "full" disclosure,[1] a norm we are unwilling to adopt literally. It seems obviously prohibitive and unrealistic to expect physicians to discuss with their patients every risk of proposed treatment—no matter how small or remote—and generally unnecessary from the pa-

No. 22099, U. S. Court of Appeals, District of Columbia Circuit, May 19, 1972. 464 Federal Reporter, 2nd Series, 772. Reprinted by permission of West Publishing Company.

tient's viewpoint as well. Indeed, the cases speaking in terms of "full" disclosure appear to envision something less than total disclosure,[2] leaving unanswered the question of just how much.

The larger number of courts, as might be expected, have applied tests framed with reference to prevailing fashion within the medical profession.[3] Some have measured the disclosure by "good medical practice,"[4] others by what a reasonable practitioner would have bared under the circumstances,[5] and still others by what medical custom in the community would demand.[6] We have explored this rather considerable body of law but are unprepared to follow it. The duty to disclose, we have reasoned, arises from phenomena apart from medical custom and practice. The latter, we think, should no more establish the scope of the duty than its existence. Any definition of scope in terms purely of a professional standard is at odds with the patient's prerogative to decide on projected therapy himself. That prerogative, we have said, is at the very foundation of the duty to disclose, and both the patient's right to know and the physician's correlative obligation to tell him are diluted to the extent that its compass is dictated by the medical profession.[7]

In our view, the patient's right of self-decision shapes the boundaries of the duty to reveal. That right can be effectively exercised only if the patient possesses enough information to enable an intelligent choice. The scope of the physician's communications to the patient, then, must be measured by the patient's need, and that need is the information material to the decision. Thus the test for determining whether a particular peril must be divulged is its materiality to the patient's decision: all risks potentially affecting the decision must be unmasked. And to safeguard the patient's interest in achieving his own determination on treatment, the law must itself set the standard for adequate disclosure.

Optimally for the patient, exposure of a risk would be mandatory whenever the patient would deem it significant to his decision, either singly or in combination with other risks. Such a requirement, however, would summon the physician to second-guess the patient, whose ideas on materiality could hardly be known to the physician. That would make an undue demand upon medical practitioners, whose conduct, like that of others, is to be measured in terms of reasonableness. Consonantly with orthodox negligence doctrine, the physician's liability for nondisclosure is to be determined on the basis of foresight, not hindsight; no less than any other aspect of negligence, the issue on nondisclosure must be approached from the viewpoint of the reasonableness of the physician's divulgence in terms of what he knows or should know to be the patient's informational needs. If, but only if, the fact-finder can say that the physician's communication was unreasonably inadequate is an imposition of liability legally or morally justified.

Of necessity, the content of the disclosure rests in the first instance with the physician. Ordinarily it is only he who is in position to identify particular dangers; always he must make a judgment, in terms of materiality, as to whether and to what extent revelation to the patient is called for. He cannot know with complete exactitude what the patient would consider important to his decision, but on the basis of his medical training and experience he can sense how the average, reasonable patient expectably would react. Indeed, with knowledge of, or ability to learn, his patient's background and current condition, he is in a position superior to that of most others—attorneys, for example—who are called upon to make judgments on pain of liability in damages for unreasonable miscalculation.

From these considerations we derive the breadth of the disclosure of risks legally to be required. The scope of the standard is not subjective as to either the physician or the patient; it remains objective with due regard for the patient's informational needs and with suitable leeway for the physician's situation. In broad outline, we agree that "[a] risk is thus material when a reasonable person, in what the physician knows or should know to be the patient's position, would be likely to attach significance to the risk or cluster of risks in deciding whether or not to forego the proposed therapy."[8]

The topics importantly demanding a communication of information are the inherent and potential hazards of the proposed treatment, the alternatives to that treatment, if any, and the results likely if the patient remains untreated. The factors contributing significance to the dangerousness of a medical technique are, of course, the incidence of injury and the degree of the harm threatened. A very small chance of death or serious disablement may well be significant; a potential disability which dramatically outweighs the potential benefit of the therapy or the detriments of the existing malady may summon discussion with the patient.

There is no bright line separating the significant from the insignificant; the answer in any case must abide a rule of reason. Some dangers—infection, for example—are inherent in any operation; there is no obligation to communicate those of which persons of average sophistication are aware. Even more clearly, the physician bears no responsibility for discussion of hazards the patient has already discovered, or those having no apparent materiality to patients' decision on therapy. The disclosure doctrine, like others marking lines between permissible and impermissible behavior in medical practice, is in essence a requirement of conduct prudent under the circumstances. Whenever nondisclosure of particular risk information is open to debate by reasonable-minded men, the issue is for the finder of the facts.

Two exceptions to the general rule of disclosure have been noted by the courts. Each is in the nature of a physician's privilege not to disclose, and the reasoning underlying them is appealing. Each, indeed, is but a recognition that, as important as is the patient's right to know, it is greatly outweighted by the magnitudinous circumstances giving rise to the privilege. The first comes into play when the patient is unconscious or otherwise incapable of consenting, and harm from a failure to treat is imminent and outweighs any harm threatened by the proposed treatment. When a genuine emergency of that sort arises, it is settled that the impracticality of conferring with the patient dispenses with need for it.[9] Even in situations of that character the physician should, as current law requires, attempt to secure a relative's consent if possible.[10] But if time is too short to accommodate discussion obviously the physician should proceed with the treatment.

The second exception obtains when risk-disclosure poses such a threat of detriment to the patient as to become unfeasible or contraindicated from a medical point of view. It is recognized that patients occasionally become so ill or emotionally distraught on disclosure as to foreclose a rational decision, or complicate or hinder the treatment, or perhaps even pose psychological damage to the patient.[11] Where that is so, the cases have generally held that the physician is armed with a privilege to keep the information from the patient,[12] and we think it clear that portents of that type may justify the physician in action he deems medically warranted. The critical inquiry is whether the physician responded to a sound medical judgment that communication of the risk information would present a threat to the patient's well-being.

The physician's privilege to withhold information for therapeutic reasons must be carefully circumscribed, however, for otherwise it might devour the disclosure rule itself. The privilege does not accept the paternalistic notion that the physician may remain silent simply because divulgence might prompt the patient to forego therapy the physician feels the patient really needs. That attitude presumes instability or perversity for even the normal patient, and runs counter to the foundation principle that the patient should and ordinarily can make the choice for himself. Nor does the privilege contemplate operation save where the patient's reaction to risk information, as reasonable foreseen by the physician, is menacing. And even in a situation of that kind, disclosure to a close relative with a view to securing consent to the proposed treatment may be the only alternative open to the physician.

NOTES

1. *E. g.,* Salgo v. Leland Stanford Jr. Univ. Bd. of Trustees, 154 Cal.App.2d 560, 317 P.2d 170, 181 (1957); Woods v. Brumlop, *supra* note 13 [in original text], 377 P.2d at 524–525.

2. See, Comment, Informed Consent in Medical Malpractice, 55 Calif.L.Rv. 1396, 1402–03 (1967).

3. *E. g.,* Shetter v. Rochelle, 2 Ariz.App.358, 409 P.2d 74, 86 (1965), modified, 2 Ariz.App. 607, 411 P.2d 45 (1966): Ditlow v. Kaplan, 181 So.2d 226, 228 (Fla.App. 1965); Williams v. Menehan, 191 Kan. 6, 379 P.2d 292, 294 (1963); Kaplan v. Haines, 96 N.J.Super. 242, 232 A.2d 840, 845 (1967) aff'd, 51 N.J. 404, 241 A.2d 235 (1968): Govin v. Hunter, 374 P.2d 421, 424 (Wyo.1962). This is not surprising since, as indicated, the majority of American jurisdictions find the source, as well as the scope, of duty to disclose in medical custom. See text *supra* at note 38. [In original text.]

4. Shetter v. Rochelle, *supra* note 3, 409 P.2d at 86.

5. *E. g.,* Ditlow v. Kaplan, *supra* note 3, 181 So.2d at 228: Kaplan v. Haines, *supra* note 3, 232 A.2d at 845.

6. *E. g.,* Williams v. Menehan, *supra* note 3, 379 P.2d at 294; Govin v. Hunter, *supra* note 3, 374 P.2d at 424.

7. For similar reasons, we reject the suggestion that disclosure should be discretionary with the physician. See Note, 109 U.Pa.L.Rev. 768, 772–73 (1961).

8. Waltz and Scheuneman, Informed Consent to Therapy, 64, Nw.U.L. Rev. 628, 640(1970).

The category of risks which the physician should communicate is, of course, no broader than the complement he could communicate. See Block v. McVay, 80 S.D. 469, 126 N.W.2d 808, 812 (1964). The duty to divulge may extend to any risk he actually knows, but he obviously cannot divulge any of which he may be unaware. Nondisclosure of an unknown risk does not, strictly speaking, present a problem in terms of the duty to disclose although it very well might pose problems in terms of the physician's duties to have known of it and to have acted accordingly.

9. *E. g.,* Dunham v. Wright, *supra* note 13 [in original text], 423 F.2d at 941–942 (applying Pennsylvania law); Koury v. Follo, 272 N.C. 366, 158 S.E.2d 548, 555 (1968); Woods v. Brumlop, *supra* note 13 [in original text], 377 P.2d at 525; Gravis v. Physicians & Surgeons Hosp., 415 S.W.2d 674, 677, 678 (Tex.Civ.App.1967).

10. Where the complaint in suit is unauthorized treatment of a patient legally or factually incapable of giving consent, the established rule is that, absent an emergency, the physician must obtain the necessary authority from a relative.

11. See, *e.g.,* Salgo v. Leland Stanford Jr. Univ. Bd. of Trustees, *supra* note 1, 317 P.2d at 181 (1957): Waltz & Scheuneman, Informed Consent to Therapy, 64 Nw.U.L.Rev. 628, 641–43 (1970).

12. *E. g.,* Roberts v. Wood, 206 F.Supp. 579, 583 (S.D.Ala.1962); Nishi v. Hartwell, 52 Haw. 188, 473 P.2d 116, 119 (1970); Woods v. Brumlop, *supra* note 13 [in original text], 377 P.2d at 525; Ball v. Mallinkrodt Chem. Works, 53 Tenn.App. 218, 381 S.W.2d 563, 567–568 (1964).

RALPH J. ALFIDI

Controversy, Alternatives, and Decisions in Complying with the Legal Doctrine of Informed Consent

Recent decisions of the Supreme Courts of Rhode Island (1) and California (2) and the United States Court of Appeals, District of Columbia (3) have stated that the necessity of obtaining informed consent prior to diagnosis and treatment of disease "is not governed by the standard of practice in the community; rather it is the duty imposed by law"(2). In other words, a physician practicing in Rhode Island, California, or the District of Columbia is subject to court action solely on the basis of lack of informed consent, regardless of whether consent is routinely obtained in the community. These courts have also ruled that expert medical testimony is not required in the determination of whether consent was ob-

Reprinted with permission of the author and the publisher from *Radiology,* Vol. 114, No. 1 (January 1975), pp. 231-234.

tained. Whether these decisions will be adopted by other courts remains to be seen. It must be noted that to date, no case has been litigated solely on the basis of lack of informed consent, so that whether the individual physician prefers to rely on his attorney and malpractice insurance rather than obtaining informed consent is a matter of choice. Nevertheless, it is advisable to consider the alternatives available to the physician seeking advice about informed consent, in particular the methods by which informed consent should be obtained, which patients should be informed, and what constitutes a great enough risk to warrant obtaining consent. Whether it is truly possible to inform a patient of risks and whether it is good medical practice to obtain consent are also subjects of considerable debate.

Informed consent is presently obtained either in writing or verbally. Each method has its advantages and disadvantages. Written consent generally consists of mimeographed or printed forms which provide information concerning the benefits and risks of various procedures. Regrettably, none of these forms provide any guarantee that the physician who uses them will be protected from all legal risks from claims of lack of informed consent. Although written consent has evidentiary value, it is not required by law and does not by itself conclusively establish that informed consent was obtained. Moreover, it is frequently considered a cold and formal approach. However, written forms do provide a certain amount of information and may be useful in answering questions which patients may have. They are a simple means of collecting standardized information for studies of this nature, often in less time than it would take to obtain verbal consent, and they provide evidence that an *attempt* was made to obtain informed consent.

Verbal consent has the significant advantage of providing for direct physician-patient discussion. Apprehension can be allayed quickly and questions answered immediately. I consider a brief outline of the benefits, risks, and mortality to be adequate. An extensive mini-course in medical education is self-defeating, in my opinion, because it takes considerable time and frequently results in confusion and increased apprehension. If written evidence of verbal consent is desired, a simple notation in the patient's chart, describing the nature of the procedure and stating that the risks were explained to and accepted by the patient, is generally considered sufficient.

The lengths to which a physician must go to obtain informed consent, and in particular the amount of information concerning risks and benefits which should be included in the information given to the patient, are ill-defined at best. Court comments on this subject range from a "reasonable disclosure" (1,2), to "Thus the test for determining whether a particular peril must be divulged is its materiality to the patient's decision: all risks potentially affecting the decision must be unmasked" (3). Further, in broad outline, I agree that "[a] risk is thus material when a reasonable person, in what the physician knows or should know to be the patient's position, would be likely to attach significance to the risk or cluster of risks in deciding whether or not to forego the proposed therapy (3).

.   .   .

There are those who would argue that it is necessary to include virtually all known complications and risks in an explanation of informed consent. I personally believe that this is neither wise nor possible. If it is decided that a certain procedure warrants obtaining informed consent, the most common complications and mortality of the procedure should be explained as an absolute minimum. Lengthy discussions, forms, or booklets should be avoided. Either written or verbal informed consent should be aimed at establishing rapport with the patient, giving a reasonable explanation of risks if desired and outlining the benefits to be obtained, answering questions, and explaining alternatives if they exist.

WHICH PATIENTS SHOULD NOT BE INFORMED?

There is no rationale for informing the obtunded or comatose patient. The parent, legal guardian, or next of kin should be informed when the patient is under age or unable to understand. When there is a language barrier, it is often possible to contact a physician who speaks the patient's language. Verbal consent is naturally the only possibility with blind or illiterate patients, and there is no legal obligation to obtain informed consent in an emergency.

WHAT CONSTITUTES ENOUGH RISK TO WARRANT OBTAINING INFORMED CONSENT?

Legally, it is virtually impossible to define significant risk. Whether one death in 50,000 cases or one in 10 is significant remains to be determined. "There is no bright line separating the significant from the insignificant; the answer in any case must abide a rule of reason"(3). At present the individual physician must make this decision, and this might best be done with the aid of an attorney in most cases. As yet, there are no guidelines which legally define which procedures or treatment shall require consent, however, it does not seem reasonable to obtain informed consent for procedures which offer little risk, such as intravenous urography or cholangiography,* but only for those with the highest risks. For the most part, these fall into the realm of special procedures, and it is in this area that I have employed informed consent.

. . .

AN ALTERNATIVE

At present, once it has been decided that a procedure warrants obtaining informed consent, it has been standard practice to provide either a written or verbal explanation of the benefit-alternative-risk principle to *all* patients. Thus the patient has no choice but to read or listen to a barrage of complications and mortality statistics, which is both disagreeable and distressing for those who do not want to know about them. There is legal precedent for the belief that the patient has the right to choose what shall be done with his own body, as expressed in the landmark decision of Judge Benjamin N. Cardozo: "Every human being of

*Visualization of the bile ducts. ED.

adult years and sound mind has the right to determine what shall be done with his own body; and a surgeon who performs an operation without the patient's consent commits an assault for which he is liable in damages" (4). In my opinion, it therefore follows that he also has the right to know or not know the risks involved. If the physician chooses this seemingly reasonable path, it becomes obvious that the "all or nothing" approach can be replaced by a simple verbal or written statement that the proposed procedure has certain inherent risks which will be explained if desired. Patients not wishing to know the risks need not be told, while those desiring an explanation will be given one. The experimental form shown in Figure 1 does exactly this. An analysis of results obtained using this form indicates that most patients do not wish to be informed of risks, a response almost diametrically opposed to earlier studies in which risks, complications, and mortality were explained without giving the patient a choice (5–7).

Obviously, the manner in which this problem is brought to the patient's attention significantly affects his reaction to informed consent. In previous studies, approximately 75 percent of patients indicated that all patients should receive an explanantion of complications. In the present study (Table I), only about one-third of patients stated that they wished to be informed of the risks. It is interesting to note that patients undergoing arteriography requested information more frequently than those undergoing other procedures.

TABLE I   PATIENT RESPONSES TO QUESTIONNAIRE

Study	Total No. of Patients	No. Who Wished to Be Informed	No. Who Did Not Wish to Be Informed	Refused Study
Intravenous urography	149	45	103	1
Intravenous cholangiography	7	1	6	0
Bronchography	6	3	3	0
Renal cyst aspiration	1	0	1	0
Lymphangiography	11	3	8	0
Venography	26	8	18	0
Arteriography	75	38	37	0
TOTAL	275	98	176	1

HOSPITAL DEPARTMENT OF RADIOLOGY—CLEVELAND CLINIC

☐ Intravenous urogram	☐ Splenoportogram	☐ Renal cyst aspiration
☐ Intravenous cholangiogram	☐ Bronchogram	☐ Lymphangiogram
☐ Venogram	☐ Myelogram	☐ Transhepatic cholangiogram
☐ Arteriogram	☐ Aspiration biopsy	

Dear Patient,

The procedure which you are scheduled for is checked in one of the columns above. There are some significant hazards associated with it. Your doctor is aware of these risks and feels that the diagnostic information obtained outweighs the possible risks of the procedure. If you want information concerning risks and complications of the study, please check the box marked "YES" below. If you do not wish to be informed please check the box marked "NO" and sign your name.

☐ YES, please inform me of risks.   ☐ NO, I do not wish to be informed of risks.

The risks and complications of the study have been explained to my satisfaction. I accept these risks and authorize. you to proceed.   Please proceed with the study.

Signature _____

Signature _____   Date _____ Clinic No. _____

(Do not sign until you have been advised of risk.)

Date _____ Clinic No. _____

I do not wish to have this study performed because of the risks involved.

Date _____ Signature _____ Clinic No. _____

FIGURE 1. Questionnaire devised to facilitate compliance with the doctrine of informed consent.

Although this approach appears reasonable to me, it has been argued that the patient cannot make a truly informed decision unless he knows of the possible risks. The legal precedent for using the approach suggested here may be found in a decision of the Supreme Court of California (Cobbs *vs.* Grant) (2), in which the court stated, "Thus, a medical doctor need not make disclosure of risks when the patient requests that he not be so informed. . . ."

CONCLUSION

The doctrine of informed consent is law, and it is doubtful that it will or should be abandoned. However, its interpretation and implementation will require careful thought and action. Because of the numerous complexities involved in compliance, physicians must exert Solomon-like judgment so that reason will prevail. Otherwise it may someday become necessary to obtain informed consent for a venipuncture or chest film. The procedures which appear to warrant obtaining routine informed consent, in my estimation, are those which carry the highest risks. It is hoped that future court actions will permit more decisive action in this controversial area.

REFERENCES

1. Wilkinson *vs.* Vesey: No. 1479-1482, Supreme Court of Rhode Island, October 20, 1972. Atlantic Rep 295 (2d Series): 676-692, 20 Oct 1972.

2. Cobbs *vs.* Grant: S.F. 22887, Supreme Court of California in Bank, October 27, 1972. Pacific Rep 502 (2d Series): 1-12, 27 Oct 1972.

3. Canterbury *vs.* Spence: No. 22099, United States Court of Appeals, District of Columbia Circuit, May 19, 1972. Fed Rep 464 (2d Series): 772-796, 19 May 1972.

4. Schloendorff *vs.* New York Hospital: Court of Appeals of New York, April 18, 1940. North Eastern Rep 105:92-96, 18 Apr 1940.

5. Alfidi, R J: Informed consent. A study of patient reaction. JAMA 216:1325-1329, 24 May 1971.

6. Alfidi R J: Informed consent and special procedures. Cleve Clin Q 40:21-25, Spring 1973.

7. Meaney T F, Lalli A F, Alfidi R J: Complications and Legal Implications of Radiologic Special Procedures. St. Louis, Mo., Mosby, 1973, p. 184.

ROBERT M. BYRN

Compulsory Lifesaving Treatment for the Competent Adult

INTRODUCTION

A significant problem in any discussion of sensitive medical-legal issues is the marked, perhaps unconscious, tendency of many to distort what the law is in pursuit of an exposition of what they would like the law to be. Nowhere is this barrier to the intelligent resolution of legal controversies more obstructive than in the debate over patient rights at the end of life. Judicial refusals to order lifesaving treatment in the face of contrary claims of bodily self-determination or free religious exercise are too often cited in support of a preconceived "right to die," even though the patients, wanting to live, have claimed no such right. Conversely, the assertion of a religious or other objection to lifesaving treatment is at times condemned as attempted suicide, even though suicide means something quite different in the law.

The purpose of this article is to elucidate the present law and the current trends concerning the question of whether a competent, unwilling adult may be required to undergo lifesaving medical treatment. I begin with a consideration of five cases typical of the situations wherein courts, deferring to rights implicit in the American concept of personal liberty, have given priority to patient choice. In discussing these cases, I have not attempted in this first section

Reprinted with permission of the author and the publisher from *Fordham Law Review,* Vol. 44, No. 1 (October 1975), pp. 1-4, 10, 12-19, 22-26, 29-31, 33-36.

of the article to carry them beyond their facts and the exact language of the courts. Quite the contrary, my goal has been to provide a detailed, rigorous, and conservative critique for it is impossible to project the full sweep of the patient's right to forego lifesaving treatment without a close scrutiny of the situations in which courts have ordered the treatment.

The second section of the article examines five decisions in which various governmental and private interests have been found sufficiently compelling to overbalance patient choice. Obviously, to the extent that these limiting decisions are valid, they define the extent of patient rights.[1]

THE PARAMOUNTCY OF PATIENT CHOICE: FIVE MODELS

THE RIGHT OF BODILY CONTROL IN A NON-EMERGENCY—PROGNOSIS: POOR WITHOUT THE TREATMENT

In *Erickson v. Dilgard,*[2] a competent, conscious adult patient was admitted to a county hospital, suffering from intestinal bleeding. An operation was suggested, including a transfusion to replace lost blood. The transfusion was deemed necessary "to offer the best chance of recovery," in that "there was a very great chance that the patient would have little opportunity to recover without the blood."[3] The patient consented to the operation but refused the transfusion. The superintendent of the hospital, in seeking an order to compel the transfusion, stated that the refusal "represented the patient's calculated decision."[4] Although the patient's refusal was based on religious grounds,[5] the court chose another avenue for its decision:

The County argues that it is in violation of the Penal Law to take one's own life and that as a practical matter the patient's decision not to accept blood is just about the taking of his own life. The court [does not] agree . . . because it is always a question of judgment whether the medical decision is correct. . . . [I]t is the individual who is the subject of a medical decision who has the final say. . . . [T]his must necessarily be so in a system of government which gives the greatest possible protection to the individual in the furtherance of his own desires.[6]

· · ·

THE RIGHT TO PRIVACY IN A NON-EMERGENCY— PROGNOSIS: DEATH WITHOUT THE TREATMENT

In re Yetter[7] presents a case where death was perhaps inevitable, but not imminent. Mrs. Yetter, a sixty year old inmate of a state mental institution, was discovered to have a breast discharge, indicating the possible presence of a carcinoma. A biopsy with corrective surgery, if necessary, was recommended. Mrs. Yetter refused, because she felt that the death of her aunt had been caused by such surgery. "[I]t was her own body and she did not desire the operation."[8] Her brother petitioned for appointment as her guardian so as to consent to the surgery. At the hearing Mrs. Yetter stated that she was afraid of surgery, that it "might hasten the spread of the disease and do further harm" and that "she would die if surgery were performed."[9]

In fact, her aunt had died from unrelated causes fifteen years after breast surgery, and Mrs. Yetter, after her initial refusal, suffered from delusions concerning her problem. The court, however, found her competent, at the time of her original refusal, to understand and decide the question of the proposed surgery, and concluded that her subsequent delusions were not the primary reason for her rejection of the treatment.[10]

Citing the Supreme Court abortion case, *Roe v. Wade*,[11] the court held:

[T]he constitutional right of privacy includes the right of a mature competent adult to refuse to accept medical recommendations that may prolong one's life and which, to a third person at least, appear to be in his best interests; in short, that the right of privacy includes a right to die with which the State should not interfere where there are no minor unborn children and no clear and present danger to public health, welfare or morals. If the person was competent while being presented with the decision and in making the decision which she did, the court should not interfere even though her decision might be considered unwise, foolish or ridiculous. . . .

There is no indication that Mrs. Yetter's condition is critical or that she is in the waning hours of life. . . . Upon reflection, balancing the risk involved in our refusal to act in favor of compulsory treatment against giving the greatest possible protection to the individual in furtherance of his own desires, we are unwilling now to overrule Mrs. Yetter's original irrational but competent decision.[12]

· · ·

THE RIGHT OF FREE RELIGIOUS EXERCISE IN AN EMERGENCY—PROGNOSIS: DEATH WITHOUT THE TREATMENT

In *In re Estate of Brooks*,[13] the court formulated the following question:

When approaching death has so weakened the mental and physical faculties of a theretofore competent adult without minor children that she may properly be said to be incompetent, may she be judicially compelled to accept treatment of a nature which will probably preserve her life, but which is forbidden by her religious convictions, and which she has previously steadfastly refused to accept, knowing death would result from such refusal?[14]

The recommended treatment was a blood transfusion. For two years Mrs. Brooks had repeatedly informed the physician who was treating her for a peptic ulcer that her "religious and medical convictions" precluded her from receiving blood transfusions and she had gone as far as to release the doctor from liability for failing to give a transfusion. Although she was disoriented when she entered the hospital, the court obviously presumed that her prior competent refusal continued up to the point where the situation became urgent.[15]

Upon petition of her doctor, the state and the county public guardian, a lower court had appointed a conservator (guardian) of the person of Mrs. Brooks and the transfusion was performed before the appeal reached the Illinois Supreme Court. Finding a substantial public interest in a resolution of the controversy despite its mootness, the court held that there was no showing that Mrs. Brooks' exercise of her religious belief "endangers, clearly and presently, the public health, welfare or morals."[16] Lacking such endangerment, the right of free religious exercise predominated. Nor would the court inquire into the reasonableness of the belief underlying the conduct.

. . .

Brooks can be profitably compared to *Erickson* and *Yetter*. While *Brooks* was premised on free exercise of religion, *Erickson* and *Yetter* expounded rights of bodily self-determination (mislabeled personal privacy in *Yetter*) without regard to any underlying religious belief. As in *Erickson,* the objectionable procedure in *Brooks,* though not free from hazard, was relatively simple—unlike the radical surgery in *Yetter*. In neither *Erickson* nor *Yetter* was the situation urgent. Although in *Yetter* the court assumed that death was inevitable without treatment, nevertheless, the court hedged its opinion by noting that Mrs. Yetter's condition was not critical, nor was she in the waning hours of life.

The trend in the law favors *Brooks*. When there are no circumstances establishing a compelling interest in preserving the life of a competent adult patient for the welfare and safety of others, a court will not invade the religious conscience of the patient in compelling submission to medical treatment—even though the patient is in imminent danger of death and the lifesaving treatment is relatively simple and safe.[17]

The *Brooks* decision speaks of free religious exercise in the context of a medical emergency. In the next case, death was imminent, and the patient's objection to treatment was not based on any religious principle.

THE RIGHT TO ACQUIESCE IN IMMINENT AND INEVITABLE DEATH—PROGNOSIS: DEATH DESPITE THE TREATMENT

Mrs. Carmen Martinez, a 72-year-old Miami resident suffering from terminal hemolytic anemia, refused "cut down" transfusions and the removal of her spleen. Death was certain without treatment, but she "begged her family not to 'torture me any more' with further surgery."[18] The medical procedures might have prolonged her life, but there was no hope of a cure. In *Palm Springs General Hospital Inc. v. Martinez,*[19] her physician sought guidance as to his obligation to administer the treatment, lest he be accused of "in effect helping her to die."[20] The court ruled that Mrs. Martinez could not be forced to undergo the surgery. She died in less than a day.

Religious objections played no part in the patient's refusal of treatment. She apparently wanted to be left in peace, knowing full well that the disease from which she suffered would inevitably cause death. The court honored her decision, competently made. In so doing, the court confirmed accepted medical practice. As a matter of course, valuable hospital and medical resources are not expended upon a terminal patient who no longer desires arduous life-prolonging treatment which offers, at best, a brief reprieve from death.[21]

. . .

In *Erickson, Yetter,* and *Brooks,* the patients, although in varying degrees of danger and asserting different rights, all wanted to live and the recommended treatment promised a cure for their ills. Mrs. Martinez wanted to acquiesce in a death which no treatment could prevent. Next we consider a case in which the patient presumably wanted the treatment which would save his life but another objected.

PATIENT-IMPLIED CONSENT VS. NEXT OF KIN NONCONSENT IN AN EMERGENCY—PROGNOSIS: DEATH WITHOUT THE TREATMENT

Last November, newspapers in New York City reported the case of one Harry Murray, a critically wounded, unconscious adult, awaiting "a desperately needed operation" while two women argued over which was his wife. One woman consented to the operation and the other refused.[22] Unanimous consent was finally obtained after the hospital sought court permission for the procedure.[23] It is difficult to understand why the consent of the spouse is necessary in such situations.[24] The relationship of husband and wife, without more, does not confer authority to make a binding decision on the administration of emergency lifesaving treatment.[25]

A different question arises when the spouse's refusal to consent expresses the wishes of the unconscious patient. If there is a barrier to treatment, it is the patient's nonconsent, not the refusal of his spouse. Mr. Murray presumably wanted to live and desired the treatment that would heal the condition which threatened him. No third party had a right to interfere.

THE FIVE MODELS: IN SUM

The five models are not exhaustive of all situations where the validity of compulsory lifesaving medical treatment for a competent adult may come into issue. They do typify the five situations in which the issue has been raised and in which courts, in the absence of an overbalancing state interest, have given priority to patient choice. The relevant fundamental patient rights—all concomitants of the American concept of personal liberty—are: (1) the right to determine what shall be done with one's body in *Erickson, Yetter* and *Murray,* and its corollary, the right to acquiesce in imminent and inevitable death as in *Martinez;* and (2) the right of free exercise of religion, in *Brooks.* . . .

As a general rule the exercise of any right may be limited if it conflicts with compelling state interests, at least where there are no less drastic means available to accomplish the state purpose. A consideration of the cases in which a state interest has been held to overbalance the competent adult's decision to forego medical treatment will facilitate a projection, beyond the five models presented, of a more comprehensive set of situations wherein patient choice should be paramount.

THE SUBORDINATION OF PATIENT CHOICE: FIVE MODELS

THE STATE INTEREST IN PREVENTING SUICIDE

Since ignominious burial and forfeiture of goods have been abolished as forms of punishment in the United States, suicide, not being punishable, is not strictly speaking a crime. In some American jurisdictions attempted suicide remains criminal.[26] Even in those states that no longer punish attempted suicide, there is a recognized privilege to use reasonable force to prevent another from committing suicide or inflicting serious harm upon himself.[27] Is it possible to analogize the refusal of lifesaving treatment to an attempt at suicide or self-inflicted injury so that saving action by another is justified?

The answer requires some examination of ·the common law. From the earliest times, the law of suicide dealt with cases in which an individual *(felo de se)* purposefully set in motion a death-producing agent with the specific intent of effecting his own destruction or, at least, serious injury. Suicide was *malum in se,* the equivalent of murder.[28]

Thus, "in legal acceptation and in popular use, the word suicide is employed to characterize . . . . 'the act of designedly destroying one's own life, committed by a person of years of discretion and of sound mind.' "[29]

When an individual actively inflicts injuries upon himself in an attempt to take his own life, a justification for coerced medical treatment may be that the patient's refusal is an extension of the suicide attempt, and the medical procedures a privileged interference with the attempt.[30] Otherwise, given its elements of active causation and specific intent to end life, suicide would seem to have little application to a competent adult's refusal of lifesaving medical treatment. The confusion of the two probably had its genesis in Emile Durkheim's nineteenth century non-legal definition of suicide, which was predicated on the assumption that an "objective" analysis of ethical and social phenomena could take no account of so "intimate a thing" as specific intent.[31] Durkheim defined suicide as "all cases of death resulting directly or indirectly from a positive or negative act of the victim himself, which he knows will produce this result."[32] Obviously this is not the common law definition. Yet it was the one unwittingly adopted by the court in *John F. Kennedy Memorial Hospital v. Heston.*[33]

Delores Heston, aged 22 and unmarried, was severely injured in an automobile accident. She was taken to the plaintiff hospital where it was determined that surgery and a blood transfusion would be necessary to save her life. She was disoriented and incoherent, but her mother informed the hospital that the patient and the family, as Jehovah's Witnesses, were opposed to the transfusion, but not to the surgery. Upon petition of the hospital, a guardian was appointed to consent to the transfusion. Surgery was performed and the patient recovered.

As in *Brooks,*[34] the highest court of the state rendered its opinion after the transfusion had been administered. In affirming the denial of a motion to vacate the guardianship order, the court observed:

[T]here is no constitutional right to choose to die. Attempted suicide was a crime at common law . . . . It is now denounced [in New Jersey] as a disorderly person's offense.

Nor is constitutional right established by adding that one's religious faith ordains his death.[35]

The answer, of course, is that suicide at common law required a specific intent to die. Miss Heston did not want to die; she did not "claim a right to choose to die," nor did her religious faith "ordain" her death. Had the court resorted to the genuine common law test of specific intent, rather than unwittingly espousing Durkheim's theory, it would have perceived that an indispensable element of common law suicide was lacking.

Having set up the strawman of a "right to die," the court proceeded to knock it down: "Appellant suggests there is a difference between passively submitting to death and actively seeking it. The distinction may be merely verbal, as it would be if an adult sought death by starvation instead of a drug. If the

State may interrupt one mode of self-destruction, it may with equal authority interfere with the other.[36] Not only did the court impute a purpose to Miss Heston which she did not have ("an adult sought death"), it also failed to appreciate the second component of common law suicide—that the individual has purposefully set in motion the death-producing agent. Whether in other areas of law his conduct be called misfeasance or nonfeasance, the person who starts out to starve himself to death has no doubt deliberately set in motion the agency of his own destruction. Miss Heston had not. For this reason too her conduct cannot be called attempted suicide.[37]

. . .

Heston [is] *contra* to *Brooks,* but *Brooks* represents the trend in the law. In [both] cases, the patient undoubtedly wanted to live, and the distinction from suicide—especially considering the patient's religious motivation—is clear. Suicide was also not a problem in either *Erickson,* where the patient wanted to live and the prognosis, though poor, was not of death, or in *Yetter,* where the patient refused treatment because she believed it would cause her death. The active causation and specific intent components of suicide were absent in each case. In *Murray* the patient presumably wanted the treatment. And in *Martinez,* the patient, though willing to acquiesce in the inevitability of early death, did not set in motion the death-producing agency with the specific intent of causing her own death, nor could she have prevented her death by submitting to treatment.

More complex problems arise when one combines and permutes the facts of the five models. Consider the following hypothetical examples:

Patient *A,* an otherwise healthy athlete, requires a leg amputation. Without it he will die, perhaps immediately or at some later time, distinguishing the merely poor prognosis in *Erickson.* The amputation will cure completely the condition that threatens to cause his death, distinguishing *Martinez. A* does not fear the surgery itself, distinguishing *Yetter,* nor does he have religious objections, distinguishing

Brooks. Nevertheless, he refuses, distinguishing *Murray*, because "I came into life with two legs and I'm going out with two legs."

Patient *B* is paralyzed or otherwise seriously incapacitated by a disease or injury which threatens to cause B's death at some time unless he consents to medical treatment. The treatment will neutralize the condition but will not restore *B* to health. He refuses for no other reason than "I would rather die than live like this."

Patient *C* has a chronic and ultimately fatal disease. Medical treatment will enable him to live and function normally for an unpredictable period of time, but death from the existing condition is inevitable. Knowing that he is doomed by the disease, *C* refuses the treatment solely because, "I would rather go now than live in dread."

Patient *D* is elderly and in a debilitated condition. He suffers from a disease or injury which will cause death sooner or later unless cured or controlled by arduous medical treatment. Although he is a "good risk," *D* refuses treatment because, "I'm too old for all that trouble and it's too expensive for my family."

. . .

Neither the actual patients in the models [reviewed] above, nor the hypothetical patients *A*, *B*, *C* and *D* were attempting suicide as that term should be properly understood. Nor can interference in the competent adult's decision to forego lifesaving treatment be justified as a paternalistic exercise of the police power. Paternalism, in this respect, should be limited to preventing hazardous or fatal *acts*.[38]

Because the prevention of suicide and the paternalistic exercise of the police power do not, in general, appear to provide bases for compelling a competent adult to undergo lifesaving medical treatment, we are required to re-examine the breadth and application of the rights which underpin the models [cited] above. Various questions may be asked. Which right has the patient asserted? Does he want to live or would he rather accept death? Is the risk of death immediate? Is the proposed treatment simple or arduous, hazardous or non-hazardous? Will the treatment merely postpone inevitable death? Will the patient be, or remain incapacitated or mutilated after treatment? Despite the numerous possibilities, the principle is easily stated: Assuming no other external, compelling state interest, a patient's decision to reject treatment ought to prevail in every case, including : (a) where the prognosis is poor although life is not immediately threatened (*Erickson*); (b) where the patient wants to live, although his reasons for rejecting treatment are unreasonable (*Yetter* and *Brooks*); (c) where death is inevitable despite treatment (*Martinez* and patient *C*); and (d) where the treatment is particularly hazardous or arduous, or where the patient will remain seriously incapacitated or mutilated after treatment (patient *D*, patients *A* and *B*).

What then is left? The one situation not covered involves the patient who can be treated relatively easily and inexpensively, without discomfort or hazard, in such a way that the threat of death from his condition will be eliminated, and the patient will not be incapacitated or mutilated. This patient rejects treatment only because he wants to die. Given all the factors, one might argue that the individual has technically become the active cause of his own impending death—like the person who sets out to starve himself to death. It has been said, for example, that the diabetic who refuses to take insulin is attempting suicide.[39] The assertion may be technically correct, but there are substantial practical problems in so labelling the conduct. How do we determine the patient's real motives? Does he truly want to die or is his conduct traceable to some other, albeit unreasonable, motivation like that of Mrs. Yetter? Is he old, debilitated and resigned to an early death, or young, healthy and seeking death? Should we distinguish the two? At what point may the law properly intervene—early or when the situation becomes critical?

Perhaps it is the difficulty of resolving these questions, or the rarity of the case, or both, that have persuaded some judges to make sweeping statements like, "[a]s to an adult (except possibly in the case of a contagious disease which would affect the health of others) I think there is no power to prescribe what medical treatment he shall receive, and . . . he is entitled to follow his own election, whether that election be dictated by religious belief or other considerations.''[40]

It is impossible to predict how a court would deal with the last situation. It might never come to judicial attention. Because of the rarity of the case and the overwhelming difficulties of proof, it ought not give us further pause. We can therefore formulate a rule of general application, beyond the specifics of the five models [above]. I would state it as follows: aside from the individual with self-inflicted injuries resulting from a suicide attempt, a competent adult is free to reject lifesaving medical treatment unless some other compelling state interest overbalances his claim of right. It is as much an error to distort this freedom to include a right to commit suicide, as it is to condemn its exercise as an attempt at suicide. Rejection of lifesaving therapy and attempted suicide are, and should be, as different in law as the proverbial apples and oranges.

THE STATE INTEREST IN PROTECTING INCOMPETENTS

In *Long Island Jewish-Hillside Medical Center v. Levitt,*[41] an eighty-four year old man was admitted to plaintiff hospital with a gangrenous leg which, if not amputated, would cause his death. He was a good surgical risk, but vascular disease disabled him from making judgments and decisions concerning his own health. Emphasizing the value of the life of every human being and the necessity of maintaining society's concern for human life, the court ordered the amputation. The decision is reflective of judicial concern that the lives of the elderly, the ill, and the burdensome not be devalued. The state, as *parens patriae,* has a special duty to help the person who is mentally incompetent to make such vital decisions as whether to submit to necessary treatment.[42] This concern for life, along with recognition of the state's duty, has persuaded courts to order substantial surgery under circumstances where, as the court pointed out in *Levitt,* a competent adult's refusal of treatment would be binding.

By definition, an incompetent lacks the ability to choose, so that court-ordered lifesaving treatment is not the subordination of patient choice to a compelling state interest. Nevertheless, *Levitt* is appropriate for consideration of the efficacy of patient choice because it exemplifies the solicitude of the law for the right to live of the helpless. This commendable attitude sometimes unduly influences the position of the court and the medical community when an unconscious or disoriented patient is brought to a hospital in need of emergency lifesaving treatment, and the medical personnel are informed of a prior decision by the individual to forego treatment should an emergency occur. A conflict exists between the patient's right to reject treatment and the court's *parens patriae* concern for the lives of incompetents, given the usual implication of consent in an emergency,[43] and the fact that the patient's previously expressed objections were not voiced in the face of a real hazard of imminent death.

Since the choice belongs ultimately to the patient, the implication of consent is the key. It is a fiction based not on any conduct of the patient, but on an estimate of how a reasonable man would react under the circumstance.[44] Is the implication destroyed by a previously expressed objection to treatment?

Relevant to this question is the decision in *Application of President & Directors of Georgetown College, Inc.*[45] In *Georgetown College,* Mrs. Jesse Jones, a twenty-five year old woman, was brought to the hospital in imminent danger of death from the loss of two-thirds of her body blood due to a ruptured ulcer. After a district court judge refused to order a transfusion, a circuit judge visited Mrs. Jones in the hospital and told her that she would die without the blood, but that there was a better then fifty percent chance of survival with it. "The only audible reply I could hear was 'Against my will.' ''[46] The court concluded, "Mrs. Jones was *in extremis* and hardly *compos mentis* at the time in question; she was as little able competently to decide for herself as any child would be. Under the circumstances, it may well be the duty of a court ... to assume the responsibility of guardianship for her, as for a child, at least to the extent of authorizing treatment to save her life."[47] Incompetency became another basis for ordering the treatment. It is possible to challenge the court's finding of fact of incompetence since Mrs. Jones' reply to the court's question was entirely consistent with her long-held beliefs as a Jehovah's Witness.[48] But this aside, the court's decision is some authority for the proposition that the previously expressed sentiments of a patient are irrelevant when the patient has become disoriented or unconscious prior to being informed that rejection of treatment will bring imminent death.

Given the patient's fundamental right to reject treatment, the sole function of a court in this situation is to make a good faith finding with respect to what the desires of the patient would have been had he been conscious and competent.[49] Insofar as *Georgetown College* may be read to mean that previously articulated beliefs are irrelevant, it would be considered in error. Where: (a) the objections to a particular kind of treatment (for instance, blood transfusion in the case of Jehovah's Witnesses) or to any treatment at all (for example the faith-healing sects) are religiously motivated, (b) the evidence indicates a strong adherence to the tenets of the sect, and (c) there is no countervailing evidence of irresolution, I would urge that the usual implication of consent is destroyed, and the patient's right to reject lifesaving treatment should prevail. In other situations it would be more difficult for the court to determine the desires of the patient. Such variables as the basis, profundity and longevity of the patient's objections, his age and usual state of health, the nature and risks of the treatment, and the likelihood of medical success and return to health will all, no doubt, enter into the court's calculations. Because life hangs in the balance, it seems probable that a court, properly aware of the incalculable value of even the most burdened life, will more frequently decide in favor of the treatment. In any event, the decision must be ad hoc.

. . .

THE STATE INTEREST IN PROTECTING THE MEDICAL PROFESSION; THE MEDICAL PROFESSION'S INTEREST IN PROTECTING ITSELF

In *United States v. George*,[50] the court ordered transfusions for a thirty-nine year old Jehovah's Witness, the father of four, who had refused the transfusions for religious reasons while lucid but in a physically critical condition from a bleeding ulcer. The court adopted "where applicable"[51] the rationale of *Georgetown College*,[52] various aspects of which have already been discussed, and added a further reason:

In addition to the factors weighted by Judge Wright one consideration is added to the scale. In the difficult realm of religious liberty it is often assumed only the religious conscience is imperiled. Here, however, the doctor's conscience and professional oath must also be respected. In the present case the patient voluntarily submitted himself to and insisted upon medical care. Simultaneously he sought to dictate to treating physicians a course of treatment amounting to medical malpractice. To require these doctors to ignore the mandates of their own conscience, even in the name of free religious exercise, cannot be justified under these circumstances. The patient may knowingly decline treatment, but he may not demand mistreatment.[53]

Certainly there is nothing in professional ethics or plain logic which should require congruence between the doctor's conscience and the patient's choice. By this I do not mean that the doctor is bound by the patient's choice to do something contrary to the doctor's conscience. That is discussed below. I do mean that the patient is not bound by the doctor's conscience to do something contrary to the patient's choice, and consequently the doctor may have the right and choice to do nothing.

The law of informed consent[54] would be rendered meaningless if patient choice were subservient to conscientious medical judgment. Tort cases condemning unauthorized medical treatment as a battery,[55] or, in some instances, if there has been state action, as an invasion of constitutional rights,[56] would have to be overruled. The rule of the supremacy of the "doctor's conscience" finds no real support in law.[57]

Much more difficult is the problem raised by the court's reference to "a course of treatment amounting to medical malpractice.[58] A doctor is not bound to undertake treatment of a patient even in an emergency.[59] Once treatment is undertaken, the doctor owes his patient a duty of reasonable care,[60] which is breached by abandoning the patient.[61] In *Yetter*, it will be recalled that Mrs. Yetter was confined in a mental institution. The court mentioned as a factor in its decision that "the present case does not involve a patient who sought medical attention from a hospital and then attempted to restrict the institution and physicians from rendering proper medical care."[62] But the involuntarily confined are also owed a duty of reasonable medical care.[63] And they may, if competent adults, reject medical treatment unless the demands of institutional security require otherwise.[64] If the duty of care owed by the medical profession to a competent adult patient, in combination with the adult's subsequent rejection of treatment, creates a legal dilemma it is the same dilemma whether the patient is involuntarily confined, or voluntarily seeks medical aid, or is unconscious when brought to the hospital and thereafter becomes lucid.

The dilemma arises in the following way. If unauthorized treatment is administered, the patient has an action for battery or, perhaps, for invasion of his constitutional rights. On the other hand, if the doctor and the hospital fail to treat the patient, they may be civilly liable for abandoning him. Further, a person under a duty to provide medical treatment, whose unreasonable failure to do so causes death, may also be criminally liable.[65] Taking the middle course is also hazardous. The doctor and the hospital might subject themselves to a claim of negligence were they to defer to patient wishes and refrain from the forbidden treatment, for example, a blood transfusion, while performing another procedure, surgery, which is rendered more dangerous by the absence of the forbidden treatment, with consequent ill effects to the patient. A release given by the patient in this situation might be questioned on

the ground that the patient was not competent at the time,[66] or that the release does not protect against criminal prosecution,[67] or that the release is against public policy.[68]

The conclusions already reached can be of assistance in finding a way out of the dilemma. Since a competent adult has a comprehensive right to reject lifesaving treatment, the liability of the treating institution and the responsible medical personnel is narrowly circumscribed. If the patient rejects treatment entirely, the problem is simplified. His instructions prevail provided that he is competent, or if he is not, that the objections of others truly reflect his wishes and beliefs, so long as there are no compelling state interests which outbalance the patient's rights to the extent that coerced treatment is justified. If there be doubt on these questions, the doctor and the hospital must seek judicial direction on how to proceed in order to protect themselves against liability.[69] Full disclosure must be made, with notice to next of kin who have information on the patient's wishes, lest there be a question of fraud upon the court.[70] Treatment will be administered or omitted as the court directs, and the court's order protects the hospital and the doctor from liability.[71]

. . .

THE STATE INTEREST IN PROTECTING MINOR CHILDREN

In *Georgetown College,* the court gave as a further reason for ordering the transfusion: "[t]he patient, 25 years old, was the mother of a seven-month-old child. The state, as *parens patriae,* will not allow a parent to abandon a child, and so it should not allow this most ultimate of voluntary abandonments. The patient had a responsibility to the community to care for her infant. Thus, the people had an interest in preserving the life of this mother."[72]

One author found two separate alleged state interests in this statement: (a) prevention of psychic harm to the child by loss of the parent and (b) prevention of economic harm to the state by the child's becoming a public charge.[73] It has been held that a pregnant woman may be compelled to submit to a blood transfusion, contrary to her religious beliefs, when the transfusion is necessary to perserve the life of her unborn child.[74] In *Yetter* and *Brooks* the courts were careful to point out that no minor children were involved. In *George,* the court adopted *Georgetown College.*

Without disputing *Georgetown College,* a few courts have modified it. It has been argued: "[a]t best the State's interest in preserving two spouses to care for their children instead of one seems attenuated; one wonders if it would be a stronger interest if a sole surviving parent's life were at stake, so that public guardianship of the minors became an imminent reality."[75]

The state's interest is even more in doubt, it has been urged, when the surviving parent is in accord with the patient's decision and willing to provide for the child alone.[76] Perhaps this reasoning persuaded a court to decline to order lifesaving transfusions for a twenty-four year old mother of three whose husband conveyed to the court the family's religious objection to such treatment.[77]

At least within these limitations it would seem that the "minor child" interest of the state does limit the right of a competent adult to reject lifesaving treatment. Whether the rule will survive remains to be seen. It will, perhaps, be put to its ultimate test if the *parens patriae* interest is asserted in a situation wherein it is the disability, rather than the death of the parent that is threatened, or where the unwilling patient, asserting a religious objection to lifesaving treatment, does not share the Jehovah's Witnesses' abhorrence of physical resistance to the mandated procedure.

THE STATE INTEREST IN PROTECTING PUBLIC HEALTH

Jacobson v. Massachusetts[78] involved a challenge to the validity of a conviction under a state statute authorizing a fine for an adult who "refuses or neglects" to be vaccinated as required by the statute.[79] The court found defendant's claim of an "inherent right of every freeman to care for his own body"[80] to be overbalanced by the interest of the state in the protection of its inhabitants from a dangerous, contagious disease.[81]

The state interest in protecting the health of others in the community clearly justifies com-

pulsory medical procedures to neutralize the danger of contagion from potential carriers of disease. In an unusual case the treatment may also save the life of one already infected and in danger of death. The purpose, however, is not to save the patient's life but to prevent the spread of the disease. Very little controversy surrounds the power of the state to compel lifesaving treatment in such cases.

THE FIVE MODELS: IN SUM

It would seem that only the state interests in the welfare of the minor child,[82] and the protection of the public from communicable disease[83] may be said, with colorable legal basis, to impinge upon the competent adult's freedom to reject lifesaving medical treatment.

CONCLUSION

This article is not a morality play. By no means did I set out to judge whether, in the scenario of a particular case, the patient's choice to forego treatment was ethically defensible. I have attempted only to discover the law and its trends. From an examination of these I deduce the following:

First: Every competent adult is free to reject lifesaving medical treatment. This freedom is grounded, depending upon the patient's claim, either on the right to determine what shall be done with one's body or the right of free religious exercise—both fundamental rights in the American scheme of personal liberty. There is no "zone of privacy" involved.

Second: The patient's freedom of choice, like all fundamental freedoms, may be subordinated to a compelling state interest at least when there are no less drastic means available to effectuate the interest.

Third: Interference with the patient's right cannot be justified either by a claimed state interest in preventing suicide or by a paternalistic exercise of the police power. Rejection of lifesaving medical treatment, except for injuries self-inflicted in an active attempt by an individual to destroy his own life, is not an attempt at suicide. However, one cannot extrapolate a right to commit suicide from the patient's freedom to reject lifesaving medical treatment. For this reason alone it is misleading to characterize the patient's freedom as a "right to die."

Fourth: The state has a *parens patriae* interest in protecting incompetents. But the disorientation of a patient ought not be used as an excuse to thwart his objection to, and rejection of, medical treatment.

Fifth: The "medical dilemma" is neither a substantive state interest justifying coerced medical treatment nor a problem of balancing conflicting personal rights. It is merely a matter of judicial resolution of doubts on such issues as patient competency. Protection of the medical community against liability requires that doctors and hospitals have free access to the courts and expeditious direction on how to proceed whenever a patient in precarious condition rejects lifesaving treatment. But under no circumstances may medical personnel be required to engage in procedures which are contradicted by reasonable medical judgment.

Sixth: In the present state of the law, lifesaving medical treatment may be compelled to further governmental interests in preventing the spread of communicable disease and in protecting the spiritual and material welfare of minor children. As to the latter, it is possible that the interest becomes attenuated when one parent would survive and is willing to care for the child, or where the child's needs have otherwise been provided for.

Reported cases on compulsory treatment are relatively rare. Newspaper accounts of such cases are frequent enough to indicate that the problem, if not pressing, at least requires clarification. Such has been the end and aim of this article.

NOTES

1. Since the matter at hand always involves patients who are indisputably alive, the problem of defining death is irrelevant.

2. 44 Misc. 2d 27, 252 N.Y.S.2d 705 (Sup. Ct. 1962).

3. Id. at 28, 252 N.Y.S.2d at 706.

4. Id.

5. See 33 Fordham L. Rev. 513 (1965).

6. 44 Misc. 2d at 28, 252 N.Y.S.2d at 706.

7. 62 Pa. D & C.2d 619 (C.P., Northampton County Ct. 1973).

8. Id. at 621.

9. Id. at 622.

10. Id.

11. 410 U.S. 113 (1973).

12. 62 Pa. D. & C.2d at 623, 624 (footnote omitted).

13. 32 Ill. 2d 361, 205 N.F.,2d 435 (1965).

14. Id. at 365–66, 205 N.E.2d at 438.

15. Thus, the case is to be distinguished from situations where a present emergency justifies treatment of an unconscious adult under a theory of implied consent, absent evidence that the adult would have refused the treatment if conscious and aware of impending death. See note 24 infra.

16. 32 Ill. 2d at 372, 205 N.E.,2d at 441.

17. See Holmes V. Silver Cross Hosp., 340 F. Supp. 125 (N.D. Ill. 1972); In re Osborne, 294 A. 2d 272, 374 (D.C. Ct. App. 1972) Contra, United States v. George, 239 F. Supp. 752, 753 (D. Conn. 1965); John F. Kennedy Mem. Hosp. v. Heston, 58 N.J. 576, 584, 279 A.2d 670, 674 (1971).

18. Wash. Post, Jul. 5, 1971, at A10, col. 1.

19. Palm Springs Gen. Hosp., Inc. v. Martinez, Civil No. 71-12687 (Dade County Cir. Ct., filed July 2, 1971).

20. Wash. Post, Jul. 5, 1971, at A10, col. 2.

21. Sharpe & Hargest, Lifesaving Treatment for Unwilling Patients, 36 Fordham L. Rev. 695, 700 (1968). In accord with Martinez, see In re Raasch,. No. 455–996 (Milwaukee County Ct., filed Jan. 25, 1972), discussed Sullivan, The Dying Person—His Plight and His Right, 8 New England L. Rev. 197, 198, 205 (1973).

22. N.Y. Post, Nov. 19, 1974, at 13, col. 1.

23. Id.

24. There is a universally accepted principle that a present emergency justifies treatment of an unconscious, but previously competent adult, under a theory of implied consent, at least when there is no evidence that the adult would have refused the treatment if conscious and aware of impending death. See W. Prosser, Torts § 2504(3) (McKinney Supp. 1974).

25. Karp v. Cooley, 493 F.2d 408, 421 (5th Cir.), cert. denied, 419 U.S. 845 (1974), Application of Pres. & Dirs. of Georgetown College, Inc., 331 F.2d 1000, 1008 (D.C. Cir.), cert. denied, 377 U.S. 978 (1964).

26. See W. LaFave & A. Scott, Criminal Law 568–69 (1972). In New York and many states, aiding and abetting a suicide or an attempt is a crime. F. g., N. Y. Penal Law § § 120.30, 120.35, 125.15(3), 125.25(1)(b) (McKinney 1975)., see W. LaFave & A. Scott, supra, at 570–71.

27. See, e.g., Conn. Gen. Stat. Ann § 53a-18(4) (Ann. 1972); N.Y. Penal Law § 35.10(4) (McKinney 1975); Model Penal Code § 3.07(5) (1962); Comment, Unauthorized Rendition of Lifesaving Medical Treatment, 53 Calif. L. Rev. 860, 869 (1965).

28. Mikell, Is Suicide Murder?, 3 Colum. L. Rev. 379 (1903). "[A]s to the quality of the offence . . . it is in a degree of murder, and not of homicide or manslaughter, for homicide is the killing a man feloniously without malice prepense. . . . And here the killing of himself was prepensed and resolved in his mind before the act was done." Hales v. Petit, 75 Eng. Rep. 387, 399 (C.B. 1562).

29. Connecticut Mut. Life Ins. Co. v. Groom, 86 Pa. 92, 97 (1878). See also 83 C.J.S. Suicide § 1 (1953).

30. Cf. Myer v. Supreme Lodge, 178 N.Y. 63, 70 N.E. 111 (1904), aff'd. 198 U.S. 508 (1905).

31. E. Durkheim, Suicide 42–43 (1951).

32. Id. at 44 (emphasis omitted).

33. 58 N.J. 576, 279 A.2d 670 (1971).

34. See notes 42–47 supra and accompanying test. [In original text.]

35. 58 N.J. at 580, 279 A.2d at 672.

36. Id. at 581–82, 279 A.2d at 672–73.

37. See generally Ford, Refusal of Blood Transfusions by Jehovah's Witnesses, 10 Catholic Law. 212, 214–16 (1964).

38. See notes 13–56 supra and accompanying text. [In original text.]

39. Perr, Suicide Responsibility of Hospital and Psychiatrist, 9 Clev.-Mar. L. Rev. 427, 433 (1960).

40. People v. Pierson, 176 N.Y. 201, 212, 68 N.E. 243, 247 (1903) (Cullen, J., concurring); accord, In re Osborne, 294 A.2d 372, 376 (D.C. Ct. App. 1972) (Yeagley, J., concurring).

41. 73 Misc. 2d 395, 342 N.Y.S.2d 356 (Sup. Ct. 1973).

42. In re Weberlist, 79 M.c. 2d 753, 360 N.Y.S.2d 783 (Sup. Ct. 1974).

43. See note 24 supra.

44. W. Prosser, Torts § 18, at 103 (4th ed. 1971).

45. 331 F.2d 1000 (D.C. Cir.), cert. denied, 377 U.S. 978 (1964).

46. Id. at 1007.

47. Id. at 1008 (footnote omitted).

48. See 113 U. Pa. L. Rev. 290, 294 (1964).

49. See Cantor, A Patient's Decision to Decline Lifesaving Medical Treatment: Bodily Integrity Versus the Preservation of Life, 26 Rutgers L. Rev. 228, 231–32 n 15 (1973).

50. 239 F. Supp. 752 (D. Conn. 1965).

51. Id. at 754.

52. 331 F.2d 1000 (D.C. Cir.), cert. denied, 377 U.S. 978 (1964). See notes 45–50 supra and accompanying text. [In original text.]

53. 239 F. Supp. at 754.

54. See Plante, An Analysis of "Informed Consent," 36 Fordham L. Rev. 639 (1968).

55. See note 21 supra. [In original text.]

56. See Winters v. Miller, 446 F.2d 65 (2d Cir.), cert. denied, 404 U.S. 985 (1971); Holmes v. Silver Cross Hosp., 340 F. Supp. 125 (N.D. Ill. 1972).

57. One would hope, on the other hand, that the ethics of medical practice remain life-oriented, and that the day will not arrive when doctors are forced to destroy life.

58. 239 F. Supp. at 754. See Application of Pres. & Dirs. of Georgetown College, Inc., 331 F.2d 1000, 1009 (D.C. Cir.), cert. denied, 377 U.S. 978 (1964); Collins v. Davis, 44 Misc. 2d 622, 254 N.Y.S.2d 666 (Sup. Ct. 1964).

59. Hurley v. Eddingfield, 156 Ind. 416, 59 N.E. 1058 (1901). In the absence of statute or regulation, e.g., N.Y. Pub. Health Law § 2805-b (McKinney Supp. 1974), neither is a hospital, although it has been held that the opening of an emergency facility may be an undertaking to treat those for whose benefit it has been established and who rely on its existence. Annot., 35 A.L.R.3d 841, 846–47 (1971).

60. See 1 Louisell & Williams, supra note 121, ¶ 8.08. [In original text.] If there are no problems of charitable immunity, the hospital may also be liable. C. Kramer, Medical Malpractice 21–27 (rev. ed. 1965).

61. 1 Louisell & Williams, supra note 121, ¶ 8.08, at 217–20. [In original text.]

62. In re Yetter, 62 Pa. D. & C.2d 619, 623 (C.P. Northampton County Ct. 1973).

63. Fischer v. City of Elmira, 75 Misc. 2d 510, 347 N.Y.S.2d 770 (Sup. Ct. 1973); O'Neil v. State, 66 Misc. 2d 936, 323 N.Y.S.2d 56 (Ct. Cl. 1971).

64. Runnels v. Rosendale, 499 F.2d 733 (9th Cir. 1974).

65. Application of Pres. & Dirs. of Georgetown College, Inc., 331 F.2d 1000, 1009 n.18 (D.C. Cir.), cert. denied, 377 U.S. 978 (1964). See Annot., 100 A.L.R.2d 483 (1965).

66. United States v. George, 239 F. Supp. 752 (D. Conn. 1965).

67. Application of Pres. & Dirs. of Georgetown College, Inc., 331 F.2d 1000, 1009 n. 18 (D.C. Cir.), cert. denied, 377 U.S. 978 (1964).

68. Cf. 11 U.C.L.A. L. Rev. 639 (1964).

69. See Sharpe & Hargest, Lifesaving Treatment for Unwilling Patients, 36 Fordham L. Rev. 695, 696–97 (1968) (discussing the doubtfully competent patient).

70. Holmes v. Silver Cross Hosp., 340 F. Supp. 125, 131 (N.D. Ill. 1972).

71. W. Prosser, Torts § 18, at 102 (4th ed. 1971).

72. 331 F.2d at 1008.

73. Cantor, A Patient's Decision to Decline Life-Saving Medical Treatment: Bodily Integrity Versus the Preservation of Life, 26 Rutgers L. Rev. 228, 251–54 (1973).

74. See Byrn, An American Tragedy: The Supreme Court on Abortion, 41 Fordham L. Rev. 807, 844–49 (1973). ·

75. Sharpe & Hargest, Lifesaving Treatment for Unwilling Patients, 36 Fordham L. Rev. 695, 697 (1968).

76. 113 U. Pa. L. Rev. 290, 294 (1964).

77. See N.Y. Times, Nov. 14, 1968, at 23, col. 1.

78. 197 U.S. 11 (1905).

79. Id. at 12.

80. Id. at 26.

81. Id. at 24–31. "The right to practice religion freely does not include liberty to expose the community . . . to communicable disease . . . . " Prince v. Massachusetts, 321 U.S. 158, 166–67 (1944) (dictum). The state interest in preventing or arresting an epidemic must not, however, be confused with unauthorized human experimentation on the victim of the disease.

82. See notes 162–71 supra and accompanying text. [In original text.]

83. See notes 78–81 supra and accompanying text.

KENNEY F. HEGLAND

Unauthorized Rendition of Lifesaving Medical Treatment

Anglo-American law starts with the premise of thorough-going self determination. It follows that each man is considered to be master of his own body, and he may, if he be of sound mind, expressly prohibit the performance of lifesaving surgery. . . . [1]

Do our humane laws make it the duty of a physician to leave the bedside of a dying man, because he demands it, and, if he remains and relieves him by physical touch, hold him guilty of assault?[2]

An adult hospital patient refuses to consent to lifesaving medical treatment, such as a blood transfusion: The individual's right to determine what shall be done with his own body and the sanctity of life come into direct conflict. Should a court order that the treatment be given, or should it respect the individual's commands and let him die? The few courts which have faced this problem are divided as to the proper course.

In September 1963 the mother of a seven-month-old baby entered the Georgetown College Hospital.[3] Massive internal bleeding, caused by a ruptured ulcer, necessitated an immediate transfusion. Due to religious conviction,[4] both the patient and her husband refused to authorize the transfusion. Hospital officials sought a court order authorizing the transfusion. After a district judge had refused the order, Circuit Judge Wright was contacted and after conferring with the patient, her husband, and attending physicians, signed an order authorizing the administration of "such transfusions as are in the opinion of the physicians in attendance necessary to save . . . [her] life."[5] Transfusions were given and the patient recovered.[6]

Application of the President of Georgetown College, Inc.[7] is one of several cases in which a court has authorized lifesaving treatment on

Reprinted with permission of Fred B. Rothman and Co. from *California Law Review*, Vol. 53, No. 3 (August 1965), pp. 860–875, 877.

the adult patient who has refused to consent. The Illinois Supreme Court, however, has recently held that where the refusal of treatment was due to religious conviction, such action constituted an unconstitutional infringement of religious liberty.[8]

The thesis of this Comment is that the rendition of emergency lifesaving medical treatment on the person of the objecting adult patient is proper. It will be seen that neither the common law nor the "free exercise" clause of the first amendment of the United States Constitution give the individual a right to reject lifesaving treatment. The law's traditional view of the sanctity of human life and the importance of the individual's life to the welfare of society, deny the individual a right to, in effect, consent to his own death. It will be shown that denial of the right to reject lifesaving treatment will not result in wholesale substitution of medical opinion for that of the individual. It will also be argued that a prior court order is not necessary in such a situation and the physician should be allowed to save the patient's life without one.

RIGHT TO REFUSE MEDICAL TREATMENT

In most circumstances the individual is afforded the right to reject medical treatment. Both the common law and the first amendment afford protection of the individual's right to determine what shall be done with his own body. However, an examination of these two sources of protection indicates that they do not give the individual the right to reject lifesaving treatment in the emergency situation.

COMMON LAW PROTECTION: UNAUTHORIZED MEDICAL TREATMENT AS BATTERY

Common law recognizes the right to refuse medical treatment at least in the non-emergency situation. Tort liability is imposed on the physician who renders treatment without his patient's authorization,[9] or, having once obtained it, goes beyond it by rendering treatment different from,[10] or more extensive than that authorized.[11] The plaintiff suing for an intentional, as opposed to a negligent, tort need only show that the treatment was given without authorization, he need not rely on the expert witnesses generally required in a malpractice action.[12] Since the heart of the battery action is the absence of legal consent,[13] it is no defense that the unauthorized treatment was given with a high degree of skill[14] or that it actually benefitted the patient.[15]

The common law does not, however, afford an absolute right to reject medical treatment, at least under certain circumstances. An exception to the requirement of prior consent is recognized in the emergency situation where the patient is in a condition, such as unconsciousness, which renders him incapable of either giving or withholding his consent.[16] The physician is then privileged to give the emergency aid.[17] The privilege is supported on two grounds. First, it is assumed that the patient, if capable, would consent to the treatment and hence its rendition does not conflict with his right to determine what shall be done with his own body. Second, although the particular patient might reject the treatment were he able to do so, the lives of other patients in like circumstances would be lost if the physician were held to act at his peril, *i.e.,* if the physician were held liable for battery if it developed that the patient would have refused consent. Thus, without yet reaching the question of whether there is ever a right to reject lifesaving treatment, it appears proper in many emergencies to ignore the patient's refusal. Certainly the physician may ignore the refusal to consent of an insane or delirious patient.[18]

Where the patient is neither insane nor delirious, it would be proper in many cases to render the treatment over the patient's commands when failure to do so would mean the patient's death. Assuming that the individual has, in effect, a right to choose death, the law should require a high degree of certainty that he really desires to exercise this prerogative before giving it operative significance. In many emergency situations, such certainty is not possible.

Assume that an individual's leg has been crushed in an automobile accident. Without immediate amputation he will die of blood poisoning. Stating that he would rather die than live with one leg, the patient refuses to consent. Just as it is assumed that an unconscious patient, if capable, would consent to emergency treatment, it seems justified to assume that this refusal of lifesaving aid is due to weakness, confusion, and pain rather than deliberation.

Such an assumption could, of course, be overcome if the refusal had been confirmed by a course of conduct antedating the emergency. For example, refusal by a Jehovah's Witness to consent to a blood transfusion is probably an expression of true preference. Yet, in a case like *Georgetown,* where the patient is suddenly seized by a condition requiring a transfusion, his refusal may be due to his physically weakened condition.[19] Even here there may be insufficient certainty to allow the patient to die.

In many cases involving the refusal of lifesaving aid, the physician should, therefore, be allowed to proceed, either by prior judicial order or by holding him privileged in a subsequent battery action, because of the inherent difficulties in distinguishing the rash refusal from that representing true choice. Whether the refusal was in fact rash should not be determinative, for to require the physician to act at his peril would tend to deter all action, thus costing the lives of those whose refusal was due to confusion and weakened physical condition.

This rationale, however, cannot be applied where it is clear that the patient's true desire is to refuse consent. For example, physicians inform a pregnant woman that blood transfusions will be necessary to save her life after the delivery of her child. While in perfect health, before any loss of blood, she refuses to consent. Here the issue is clearly raised: Does the individual have a legally protected right to reject lifesaving treatment? The few cases which have faced the issue in the battery context have given no clear answer.[20] Does the Constitution afford such a right?

CONSTITUTIONAL PROTECTION: FREEDOM OF RELIGION

If the refusal of required treatment is due to religious belief, to ignore it might violate the free exercise of religion clause of the first amendment to the United States Constitution. Yet reliance on the first amendment raises rather than answers the question because that amendment has not been held to give absolute freedom to religious practice.

In the early case of *Reynolds v. United States*,[21] the private secretary of Brigham Young appealed his conviction for bigamy, arguing that the statute was unconstitutional as applied to him because his religion required its violation. The United States Supreme Court, affirming, held that whereas freedom of conscience was absolute, the right to free exercise of religion could not justify acts against the public well being.

In the cases since *Reynolds*, the question has been whether a religious practice is sufficently detrimental to the public good to justify its curtailment: Courts have held that the practice must present an immediate threat to a valid public interest.[22] Whether a religiously motivated refusal of lifesaving medical treatment is constitutionally protected turns on whether there is a valid public interest in the individual's life. In many analogous areas of the law, courts have recognized this interest.

PUBLIC INTEREST IN THE LIFE OF THE INDIVIDUAL

Refusal of lifesaving treatment does not constitute an immediate and direct threat to the well being of others; however, several areas of the law recognize the propriety of curtailing activities which do not directly endanger others.[23] Certain activities, because they adversely affect the participants and thus indirectly affect the welfare of society, have fallen under legal proscription. Polygamy, for example, does not present an immediate and direct threat to the welfare of other individuals but this practice may be made criminal even for those whose religion dictates it. It is likewise arguable that much of modern narcotics legislation is designed primarily to protect users. The use of narcotics presents primarily an indirect threat to society by harming the individual user.[24]

Similarly, this Comment argues that refusal of lifesaving treatment constitutes an activity which should be curtailed despite the fact that it does not endanger others. Such a refusal is tantamount to consenting to death. In the analogous areas of euthanasia, the "snake cases" and suicide, the law has uniformly denied operative significance to the individual's consent to his own death and consequently it should be expected that the same result will follow in the case of the refusal of lifesaving treatment.

EUTHANASIA

It is no defense to homicide prosecution that the decedent desired to die.[25] In effect, the individual cannot consent to his own death at the hands of a second party. The primary concern of the law in condemning "mercy killing" is apparently not with the difficult proof problems in the prosecution of homicide that the defense of consent would generate; hence, the case of taking life cannot be distinguished from that of saving it by unauthorized treatment. First, there is society's interest in the life of the individual.[26] If this is the reason why the individual has no right to consent to his own death in the euthanasia situation, then he would have no right to prohibit lifesaving medical treatment. Second, there is the fear that any exception to the sanctity of life cannot but cheapen it. The same fear would lead to hesitation before condemning any act which saves life, *e.g.,* the rendition of lifesaving aid. If the individual has the right to command his own death, the form of the command should not be determinative: that is, whether it commands another individual to do something, as in the case of euthanasia, or whether it commands him not to do something, as in the case of the refusal of required medical treatment.

POISONOUS SNAKE RITUALS

The "snake cases"[27] provide additonal precedent for the proposition that the state may act to prevent the individual from consenting to his own death. A small religious sect, known as the Holiness Church, believes that the true test of faith is the handling of poisonous snakes: The true believer will not be harmed. Several state legislatures made this practice criminal. Several state courts, upholding the constitutionality of the statutes, iterated the traditional language about the safety of onlookers, but a close reading of the cases indicates that the concern was with the individuals who handled the snakes.

It is difficult to find a meaningful distinction between an individual who handles a poisonous snake and one who refuses required medical treatment. A distinction between misfeasance and nonfeasance is nonsense; each individual is making basically the same decision. Walking into a burning house is tantamount to refusing to walk out. In terms of the danger to others presented by the two acts, there is little distinction. The ceremonies of the Holiness Church create a slight public danger in that the poisonous snake might escape. If minor considerations are determinative, then it could be argued that the hospital patient, in refusing lifesaving treatment, creates a danger to others by bringing otherwise unneeded physicians to his bedside and by generally interrupting the smooth operation of the hospital.

A stronger argument for curtailing religious practice can be made in the case of the hospital patient than in the case of the snake handler. First, the extent of social harm presented by the practice is greater because death from the refusal of lifesaving treatment is as certain as medical knowledge can be, whereas death from the handling of snakes is a mere possibility. Second, the extent that religious practice must be curtailed is less in the case of the hospital patient. Handling snakes is essential to the ritual of the Holiness Church; the proscription of a given form of medical treatment is generally just one of many proscriptions found in religious doctrines. In addition, while the members of the Holiness Church are forever barred from practicing the dictates of their religion, the members of a sect which prohibits a given form of treatment are free to follow their religious dictates in all but the most limited of situations: the life and death situation. As to the manner of curtailment, criminal sanctions

are imposed on the individual who handles snakes due to his religion, while in the case of the individual who refuses a form of medical treatment due to his religion, no such sanctions are imposed. When a patient refuses lifesaving treatment, the propriety of his decision is not at issue: The only question is whether a physician's act in violation of that decision is proper.

ANALOGY TO PREVENTION OF SUICIDE

It is obviously proper for a physician to save his patient's life by unauthorized treatment if the physician in doing so is in the same position as the individual who has prevented a suicide. It is not a legal wrong to prevent suicide. To hold the physician liable and the rescuer from suicide privileged, a distinction must be found either in their respective actions or in the actions of the person saved.

There are two possible ways to distinguish the acts of the suicide from that of the patient who refuses lifesaving treatment: first, by the misfeasance-nonfeasance analysis, and second, in terms of the motivation of the person saved. Neither, however, appear to justify intervention in one case but not in the other.

The misfeasance-nonfeasance analysis would be misapplied in this context because the concern is not with whether the individual is "guilty" of his own death but rather with the preservation of his life. The misfeasance-nonfeasance analysis is employed to determine an individual's culpability in relation to a given result which society has condemned, and not to reassess the social disutility of that result. For example, a defendant drowns another by pushing him in a lake. He is guilty of homicide. A second defendant refuses to take affirmative action which would effectuate an easy rescue. He is guilty of nothing.[28] In both cases, however, the man is dead, and the loss to society is equally great. Similarly, the result of the suicide's "misfeasance" and the patient's "nonfeasance" is the same.

The second ground for a possible distinction between the suicide and the hospital patient lies in their respective motivations. The suicide wishes to die, whereas the patient who declines treatment for religious reasons, wishes to live, but prefers death to a breach of religious commandment. The act of the patient does not "seem" like suicide. It may well be that society's condemnation of suicide is directed at the motivation behind the act and not at the act itself because, as one author explains:

Suicide shows contempt for society. It is rude. . . . This most individualistic of all actions disturbs society profoundly. Seeing a man who appears not to care for the things which it prizes, society is compelled to question all it has thought desirable. The things which make its own life worth living, the suicide boldly jettisons. Society is troubled, and its natural and nervous reaction is to condemn the suicide. Thus it bolsters up again its own values.[29]

This may be good psychology but to use motivation as a basis of legal distinction in this context would be absurd. Take, for example, two hospital patients both in dire need of blood transfusions. One rejects them because of a desire to die, the other because of religious conviction. Should the law allow the patient wishing to live but preferring death to breach of religious faith, to die, while forcing the one wishing to die, to live? To ask the question is to answer it.

In *Reynolds v. United States*,[30] the Court stated in a dictum that it is within the power of government to prevent a religious suicide.[31] The dictum makes sense. If the non-religious suicide may be prevented, so may the religious suicide. If judicial response were to vary in the two situations, it would be the sheerest of hypocrisies: Life may be saved, not because it is valuable, but rather because suicide is "rude."

Failure to find a meaningful distinction between the refusal of lifesaving treatment and suicide, either in their respective motivations or in the misfeasance-nonfeasance analysis, leads to the conclusion that, based on the quality of their respective conduct, neither the patient nor the suicide can demand legal protection from lifesaving touching. Consequently, if the physician who renders unauthorized treatment is to be held liable while the individual who prevents suicide is held privileged, a distinction must be found in the respective acts of the rescuers. It may be that the latter would be held privileged because he was justified in assuming that the would-be suicide was acting rashly.[32] However, it is apparent that not all suicide attempts are rash. If the rescuer knew that the would-be suicide was not acting rashly, would he commit a legal wrong if he prevented the suicide? If he would not be, then neither would the physician.

IS THERE A RIGHT TO CHOOSE DEATH?

To hold that a court order which allows the physician to proceed with lifesaving treatment over the religious objections of the patient is an unconstitutional infringement of religious liberty, or to hold that the physician who has rendered the treatment is liable for battery, is to hold that the individual has a legally enforceable right to choose death. Because of society's interest in the life of the individual, because of the law's traditional view of the sanctity of human life, and because life can be saved without too great a curtailment of the religious liberty of those patients who refuse treatment on religious grounds, the law should not give its protection to the individual's decision to choose death.

Society has an interest in the life of the individual. In the *Georgetown* case, the patient was the mother of a seven-month-old child and it is apparent that others than herself would have suffered had she died.[33] Once it is admitted that there is sufficient interest in the life of a particular patient to deny him a legal right to refuse lifesaving treatment,[34] then the decision must be the same for all patients. That is, the criterion of the "social worth" of the patient would lead the courts into insolvable problems. Any distinction based on "social worth" in this area is repugnant to the basic ideal of equality: If the mother of several children is to be saved, then so must the childless individual.

It would be out of line with the law's traditional affirmation of life were it to label the saving of life as either unconstitutional or as a civil wrong. To bring the issue into focus, take the case of a Buddhist monk's attempt to burn himself. Does the individual commit battery if he prevents the attempted suicide? Does a court unconstitutionally deny the free exercise of religion if it acts to prevent the suicide? There seems but one answer.

To deny the individual a legally enforceable right to reject lifesaving treatment for religious reasons does not greatly curtail his religious freedom, where objection to treatment is on this ground. First, no criminal sanctions are imposed on him. Second, he is allowed to practice the dictates of his religion in all but the most limited of circumstances: the life and death situation. Third, neither he nor his religion, at least in the case of the Jehovah's Witnesses, will deem him to have sinned. He did not voluntarily breach religious dictates.[35]

LIMITATIONS

If it is decided that the physician can properly ignore his patient's objections to lifesaving treatment, can application of this rule be limited to cases where medical treatment is immediately required to save life? Or will the result be a wholesale substitution of medical discretion for that of the individual?

Basically, two problems are found. The first concerns the type of medical treatment which would be justified, and the second concerns whether lifesaving treatment could be justified upon the individual who had not sought any medical treatment. As to the type of treatment, it would seem that only emergency medical treatment, with a high degree of probable success, would be justified. This limitation is inherent in a privilege to ignore a patient's refusal of consent in order to save his life. To justify his trespass, the physician would probably be required to sustain the burden of showing that the situation was clearly one of life and death. This clear choice is not present when the proposed treatment does not have a high degree of probable success.

If it is decided that the social interest in the patient's life is sufficient to deny him legal protection in his refusal to consent to lifesaving treatment, the question arises whether or not this decision would justify similar treatment on the individual who has refused to seek medical aid altogether. For example, would a physician be held privileged to enter the home of a Christian Scientist, uninvited, to render lifesaving

treatment? There appear to be three possible grounds to distinguish this case from the case where the patient has voluntarily consented to some medical treatment. First, to recognize a privilege in the case of an individual who has not sought medical treatment would be an additional curtailment of the rights of the individual. Like the case of the hospital patient, the individual's right to determine what shall be done with his own body is invaded, but here also the right of the individual to be "let alone" is curtailed. In the judicial balance, this additional burden on the individual could tip the scales in his favor. Second, the hospital patient, unlike the person who has not sought medical attention, has placed the physician in an extremely vulnerable position both legally and morally. Finally, the hospital patient, in entering the hospital, recognizes the propriety of medicine in general. Although it is arguable that the reasons supporting the denial of a legal right to reject lifesaving aid outweigh the above considerations, the judiciary may make the distinction between the patient who has sought aid and the one who has not.

. . .

CONCLUSION

The *Georgetown* case, in ordering that lifesaving treatment may be given to the objecting adult patient, seems to be in accord with the traditional legal view of the sanctity of human life and the interest society has in the life of the individual. To hold otherwise is to hold that the individual has a legally enforceable right, in effect, to choose death, and that the saving of human life, under these circumstances, is a legal wrong. . . .

NOTES

1. Natanson v. Kline, 186 Kan. 393, 406–07, 350 P.2d 1093, 1104 (1960) (dictum), cited with approval in Woods v. Brumlop, 71 N.M. 221, 227, 377 P.2d 520, 524 (1962) (dictum).

2. Meyer v. Knights of Pythias, 178 N.Y. 63, 67, 70 N.E. 111, 112 (1904) (dictum).

3. Application of President of Georgetown College, Inc., 331 F.2d 1000 (D.C. Cir.), *cert. denied,* 377 U.S. 978 (1964).

4. Mrs. Jones and her husband are members of the religious sect knows as the Jehovah's Witnesses. Objection to blood transfusions, which are equated with the drinking of blood, is based on the Biblical text. See Acts 15:28–29.

5. 331 F.2d at 1002 n.4.

6. Her petition for rehearing en banc was denied (apparently on the grounds of mootness). 331 F.2d at 1010.

7. 331 F.2d 1000 (D.C. Cir.), *cert. denied,* 377 U.S. 978 (1964).

8. *In re* Estate of Brooks, 32 Ill. 2d 361, 205 N.E.2d 435 (1965); *accord,* Erickson v. Dilgard, 44 Misc. 2d 27, 252 N.Y.S.2d 705 (Sup. Ct. 1962).

9. Gill v. Selling, 125 Ore. 587, 267 Pac. 812 (1928) (operation on wrong patient).

10. Mohr v. Williams, 95 Minn. 261, 104 N.W. 12 (1905) (operation on left ear instead of right as agreed to by the patient).

11. Tabor v. Scobee, 254 S.W.2d 474 (Ky. 1952) (during operation for appendicitis, diseased fallopian tubes removed).

12. See, *e.g.,* Beane v. Perley, 99 N.H. 309, 109 A.2d 848 (1954).

13. PROSSER, TORTS, § 9 at 33 (1955).

14. *E.g.,* Perry v. Hodgsen, 168 Ga. 678, 148 S.E. 659 (1929); Franklyn v. Peabody, 249 Mich. 363, 228 N.W. 681 (1930); Mohr v. Williams, 95 Minn. 261, 104 N.W. 12 (1905).

15. See, *e.g.,* Church v. Adler, 350 Ill. App. 471, 113 N.E.2d 327 (1953).

16. The classic case is Jackovach v. Yocum, 212 Iowa 914, 237 N.W. 444 (1931), where a boy of seventeen jumped from a freight train, sustaining severe head and arm injuries. Attending physicians, while the boy was anesthetized, amputated the arm due to their fear of gangrene. The efforts to reach the boy's parents had failed. The court held the physicians were privileged because of the emergency situation.

17. According to the *Restatement of Torts,* the physician must maintain an affirmative burden as to the following elements: (1) that an emergency existed involving a serious threat to the life or health of the patient; (2) that the patient could not give his consent (physical incapacity such as unconsciousness or delirium, or legal incapacity such as minority or insanity), and that pressures of time prevented conference with his legal representatives; (3) that a reasonable man would have consented to the treatment; and (4) that there was no reason to know that the patient would, in fact, object. RESTATEMENT, TORTS § 62 (1938).

18. See, *e.g.,* Pratt v. Davis, 224 Ill. 300, 79 N.E. 562 (1906) (dictum); Littlejohn v. Arbogast, 95 Ill. App. 605 (1900) (dictum); RESTATEMENT, TORTS § 62 (1938), note. 17 *supra.*

19. In the *Georgetown* case, Judge Wright found the patient *in extremis* and "hardly compos mentis" when he arrived at the hospital. 331 F.2d at 1008.

20. *Compare* Mulloy v. Hop, 1 West. Weekly R. (n.s.) 714 (1935), *with* Ollet v. Pittsburg & St. L. Ry., 201 Pa. 316, 50 Atl. 1011 (1902).

21. 98 U.S. 145 (1878). For the historical setting of this case, see Cawley, *Criminal Liability in Faith Healing,* 39 MINN. L. REV. 48, 49–53 (1954).

22. For example, in West Virginia State Bd. of Educ. v.

Barnette, 319 U.S. 624 (1943), the Supreme Court struck down a board of education requirement that school children salute the flag daily. Jehovah's Witness parents argued that their children were being forced to pay homage to a "graven image." See Exodus 20:4–5. The Court held that first amendment freedoms can be restricted "only to prevent grave and immediate danger to interests which the state may lawfully protect." 319 U.S. at 639.

23. Where the individual presents a direct threat to the well-being of others, his activities will be restricted. In the area of battery, compulsory vaccination against contagious disease has been upheld as a valid exercise of police power. Jacobson v. Massachusetts, 197 U.S. 11 (1905).

24. Numerous other examples could be cited. In State v. Congdon, 76 N.J. Super. 493, 185 A.2d 21 (Super. Ct. App. Div. 1963) the court held that the state, without violating the first amendment, could impose criminal sanctions on individuals refusing to take cover during an air raid drill. It stated that "the basis of the State's police power is the protection of its citizens. This protection must be granted irrespective of the fact that certain individuals may not wish to be saved or protected." *Id.* at 511–12, 185 A.2d at 31. Another example would be that of dueling, which is illegal though both parties consent. *E.g.,* CAL. PENAL CODE §§225–31.

25. Regarding the legal status of mercy killing in this country and elsewhere, see Silving, *Euthanasia: A Study in Comparative Criminal Law,* 103 U. PA. L. REV. 350 (1954).

26. SHARTEL, MEDICAL PRACTICE § 1–17 n.5 (1959).

27. Hill v. State, 38 Ala. App. 623, 88 So. 2d 880 (Ct. App. 1956), *cert. denied,* 38 Ala. 697, 88 So. 2d 887 (1956); Lawson v. Commonwealth, 291 Ky. 473, 164 S.W.2d 972 (Ct. App. 1942); State v. Massey, 229 N.C. 734, 51 S.E.2d 179 (1949), *appeal dismissed sub nom.* Dunn v. North Carolina, 336 U.S. 942 (1949); Harden v. State, 188 Tenn. 17, 216 S.W.2d 708 (1948).

28. Osterline v. Hill, 263 Mass. 73, 160 N.E. 301 (1928).

29. FEEDEN, SUICIDE 42 (1938) as quoted in WILLIAMS, THE SANCTITY OF LIFE AND THE CRIMINAL LAW 267 (1957).

30. 98 U.S. 145 (1878).

31. *Id.* at 166.

32. Studies indicate that most suicide attempts are, in fact, rash, or perhaps insincere. For example, of the 138 patients admitted to the suicide ward of a London hospital during a one-year period, only one had committed suicide five years later. ST. JOHN-STEVAS, THE RIGHT TO LIFE 74 (1963).

33. Judge Wright argued that the "state, as *parens patriae,* will not allow a parent to abandon a child, and so it should not allow this most ultimate of voluntary abandonments. The patient had a responsibility to the community to care for her infant. Thus the people had an interest in preserving the life of this mother." 331 F.2d at 1008.

34. *Cf.* Martin v. Industrial Acc. Comm'n, 147 Cal. App. 2d 137, 304 P.2d 828 (1956) (withholding death benefits under workman's compensation because of an "unreasonable" refusal by the decedent, a Jehovah's Witness, to consent to a blood transfusion).

35. The conscientious Jehovah's Witness is to do "everything possible within reason and right and without injury to another" to resist the court-ordered transfusion. However, he is not required to resist by physical violence. Letter From the Watchtower Bible and Tract Society of New York, Inc., to the Villanova Law Review, Oct. 6, 1964, as quoted in 10 VILL. L. REV. 140 n.3 (1964).

LEROY WALTERS

Ethical Aspects of Medical Confidentiality

I. THE PRINCIPLE OF MEDICAL CONFIDENTIALITY: HISTORICAL SKETCH

Within the ethical tradition, the most extensive and detailed references to the principle of medical confidentiality occur within codes of professional ethics. The ancient works of Hindu medicine mention the obligation of medical secrecy.[1] For the Western tradition of medical ethics, however, the fundamental statement concerning medical confidentiality occurs in the Hippocratic Oath. There we read:

What I may see or hear in the course of the treatment or even outside of the treatment in regard to the life of men, which on no account one must spread abroad, I will keep to myself, holding such things shameful to be spoken about.[2]

This affirmation of the principle of confidentiality in the Hippocratic Oath exerted a strong influence on the formulation of subsequent codes of medical ethics. The principle recurs in the first great modern textbook of professional ethics for physicians, Thomas Percival's *Medical Ethics,* published in 1803. Percival noted:

Secrecy and delicacy, when required by peculiar circumstances, should be strictly observed. And the familiar and confidential intercourse, to which the faculty are admitted in their professional visits, should be used with discretion and with the most scrupulous regard to fidelity and honour.[3]

Percival's statement was reproduced practically verbatim in the first major American code, *The Code of Medical Ethics,* adopted by the American Medical Association in 1847.[4]

In more recent times the principle of medical confidentiality has been reaffirmed in numerous codes of professional ethics. The International Code of Medical Ethics adopted by the World Medical Association contains a strong statement of the principle:

A doctor owes to his patient absolute secrecy on all which has been confided to him or which he knows because of the confidence entrusted in him.[5]

The most recent version of the AMA's "Principles of Medical Ethics" devotes a separate section to the topic of medical confidentiality.[6]

In addition to appearing in codes of professional ethics for physicians, the principle of confidentiality also plays a prominent role in the ethical codes of various other health professionals, including nurses, medical social workers, and medical record librarians.[7] Of particular interest is a statement in the Code of Ethics of the American Association of Medical Record Librarians:

As a member of one of the paramedical professions [the librarian] shall . . . (2) Preserve and protect the medical records in his custody and hold inviolate the privileged contents of the records and any other information of a confidential nature obtained in his official capacity, taking due account of applicable status and of regulations and policies of his employer.[8]

Professional codes of ethics have been the main locus of ethical discussion concerning the principle of medical confidentiality. However, there are two other non-legal sources which should at least be mentioned in passing. The first is the tradition of Western religious ethics. The literature of various religious groups, par-

This essay is a revised version of an article originally published in the *Journal of Clinical Computing,* Vol. 4 (1974), pp. 9–20. Copyright 1974 by LeRoy Walters.

ticularly Jews and Roman Catholics, has devoted substantial attention to questions of medical ethics.[9] On the specific issue of medical confidentiality Jewish religious ethics is totally silent.[10] In contrast, Catholic textbooks of moral theology frequently include detailed discussions of confidentiality in the physician-patient relationship, perhaps in part because of its obvious parallels with the confidential relationship of priest and penitent.[11] Within the moral-theology textbooks are extended analyses of the nature of a secret, mental reservation, and the circumstances under which professional secrets may or may or may not be revealed.[12]

The other major non-professional source of ethical discussion concerning medical confidentiality is the emergent patient's rights movement. Probably the most important document resulting from pressures generated by the movement is the "Patient's Bill of Rights," published by the American Hospital Association in 1973. In that document one reads:

The patient has the right to expect that all communications and records pertaining to his care should be treated as confidential.[13]

The legal tradition has also wrestled at length with the problem of medical confidentiality. In many cases, the law has simultaneously discussed the analogous questions of confidential communications between attorneys and clients and between ministers or rabbis and persons who solicit their advice. Two kinds of legal protection for medical confidentiality can be distinguished: positive protection and negative protection. Positive protection refers to legal sanctions which can be applied against physicians who reveal confidential information about their patients. In English and American law the patient injured by such a breach can seek a remedy at law by bringing suit. In contrast, on the European continent, the violation of medical secrecy by the physician is punishable or punished according to provisions of the criminal law.[14]

Negative protection of medical confidentiality is provided by laws which establish communications between physician and patient as privileged communications and which thereby exempt the physician from the normal obligation to testify before a court of law. The English Common Law did not consider as privileged the communications which pass between physicians and patients. Since the common law formed the basis for American jurisprudence, it was to be expected that early American law would also lack any provision protecting communication between physicians and patients. However, in 1828, New York State by statute made physician-patient communication privileged. The New York State statute, which became the model for similar statutes adopted in many other states of the Union, read as follows:

No person duly authorized to practice physic or surgery, shall be allowed to disclose any information which he may have acquired in attending any patient, in a professional character, and which information was necessary to enable him to prescribe for such patient as a physician, or to do any act for him as a surgeon.[15]

As of 1973, forty-three states and the District of Columbia, had enacted general physician-patient privilege statutes. In addition, at least seventeen states have recently adopted laws which protect psychiatrist-patient or psychologist-client communications.[16]

II. THE PRINCIPLE OF MEDICAL CONFIDENTIALITY: PHILOSOPHICAL JUSTIFICATION

We turn now from history to philosophy, from the question of when and how the principle of medical confidentiality was formulated to the question of why it is important. There are two primary philosophical arguments in favor of preserving medical confidentiality. The first argument is utilitarian and refers to possible long-term consequences. The second argument is non-utilitarian and speaks of respect for the rights of persons.

The utilitarian argument for the preservation of medical confidentiality is that without such confidentiality the physician-patient relationship would be seriously impaired. More specifically, the promise of confidentiality encourages the patient to make a full disclosure of his symptoms and their causes, without fearing that an embarrassing condition will become public knowledge.[17] Among medical professionals, psychotherapists have been particularly concerned to protect the confidentiality of their relationship with patients. In the words of one psychiatrist:

The patient in analysis must learn to free associate and to break down resistances to deal with unconscious threatening thoughts and feelings. To revoke secrecy after encouraging such risk-taking is to threaten all future interaction.[18]

A second argument for the principle of medical confidentiality is that the right to a sphere of privacy is a basic human right. In what is perhaps the classic essay concerning the right of privacy, Samuel Warren and Louis Brandeis wrote in 1890 that the common law secured "to each individual the right of determining, ordinarily, to what extent his thoughts, sentiments, and emotions shall be communicated to others."[19] Present-day advocates of the right of privacy frequently employ the imagery of concentric circles or spheres. In the center is the "core self," which shelters the individual's "ultimate secrets"—"those hopes, fears, and prayers that are beyond sharing with anyone unless the individual comes under such stress that he must pour out these ultimate secrets to secure emotional release."[20] According to this image, the next largest circle contains intimate secrets which can be shared with close relatives or confessors of various kinds. Successively larger circles are open to intimate friends, to casual acquaintances, and finally to all observers.

The principle of medical confidentiality can be based squarely on this general right of privacy. The patient, in distress, shares with the physician detailed information concerning problems of body or mind. To employ the imagery of concentric circles, the patient admits the physician to an inner circle. If the physician, in turn, were to make public the information imparted by the patient—that is, if he were to invite scores or thousands of other persons into the same inner circle—we would be justified in charging that he had violated the patient's right of privacy and that he had shown disrespect to the patient as a human being.

These two arguments for the principle of medical confidentiality—the argument based on probable consequences of violation and the argument based on the right of privacy—seem to constitute a rather strong case for the principle. However, we have not yet faced the question whether the principle of confidentiality is a moral absolute, or whether it can be overridden by other considerations.

III. THE PRINCIPLE OF CONFIDENTIALITY: POSSIBLE GROUNDS FOR VIOLATING THE PRINCIPLE.

There are, in my view, three general reasons which might conceivably justify violating the principle of confidentiality.[21] The first is that the principle may come into conflict with the rights of the patient himself. To illustrate, one can envision a situation in which a patient, in a temporary fit of depression, threatens to kill himself or herself or to perform an irrational act which will almost certainly destroy the patient's reputation. In the case of threatened suicide, one finds oneself weighing a secret vs. a life. Perhaps the physician should feel free, in such a case, to violate the principle of confidentiality and to involve a third party for the protection of the patient himself or herself.

A second possible ground for violating the principle of confidentiality is that it may conflict with the right of an innocent third party. In older textbooks of moral theology, one can discover hypothetical cases constructed to illustrate this dilemma. Often the case involves a physician and a young couple about to be married. Because of his professional relationship with the husband-to-be, the physician knows that the man is concealing a condition of infective syphilis or permanent impotence from his future wife. The question then arises whether the physician should violate the principle of confidentiality in order to warn the unsuspecting innocent party.[22]

In our own time the physician's dilemma is more likely to concern the case of a "battered child." If the abused child is brought to the physician by the battering parents, the physician faces an immediate conflict of loyalties. Does he or she owe it to his adult patients to keep confidential the fact that they have abused the child? Or, is the physician under the obligation to protect the child from further harm by disclosing the child's injuries to the proper public authorities? It should perhaps be noted in passing that most states in the United States require that the physician report child-abuse cases to the appropriate governmental agency.[23]

A third possible ground for violating the principle of confidentiality is a serious conflict between the principle and the rights or interests of society in general. The possibility of such a conflict was formally recognized in 1912, when the American Medical Association revised its code of ethics. A new clause was introduced into the confidentiality section of the code, specifically authorizing the physician to report communicable diseases, even if such reports were based on confidential information. The justification for this type of disclosure was, of course, the protection of society at large from the spread of infectious disease.[24]

At present, various states require reports of particular types of contagious disease. Almost universally, the physician is legally obligated to report cases of venereal disease to the proper government authorities. The reporting of tuberculosis is also frequently required. State provisions for protecting the confidentiality of such public health reports vary widely, with about half of the states taking measures to prevent public disclosure of the data.[25] Whenever states require physicians to report such data concerning communicable diseases, the general justification for the violation of physician-patient confidentiality is that society at large must be protected.

There is a second type of situation in which the principle of confidentiality and the public good seem to come into sharp conflict. In these cases the physician discovers a serious medical problem in a patient whose occupation makes him responsible for the lives of many other persons. Two standard examples are a railroad signalman who is discovered to be subject to attacks of epilepsy, or an airline pilot with failing eyesight. A case reported in a recent essay on medical secrecy reads as follows:

Last year, 30 people were killed when a bus driver had a heart attack and plunged his bus into the East River in New York City. The driver's physician had known about the bad heart, had cautioned him not to drive, but felt he could not report it to the company since the patient might lose his job.[26]

In cases involving such critical occupations, some would argue that the physician's duty to protect the lives of many persons overrides his obligation to observe the principle of medical confidentiality.

In the future we are likely to see vigorous battles waged over the question of medical confidentiality vs. the public good. Three examples can be briefly cited. Already one hears rhetoric which implies that genetic disorders are quasi-contagious diseases.[27] According to this viewpoint, members of future generations will be "infected" if decisive action is not taken now. Is it possible that such pressures will lead to the requirement that physicians routinely report genetic defects to public health authorities? To cite a second example, epidemiologists constantly pursue new correlations between chronic diseases and particular environmental factors or medical conditions. Their studies frequently require surveys of total populations or random samples of such populations.[28] Will the desire of patients to keep their medical records confidential and their refusal to take part in such epidemiological studies come to be seen as an anti-social act or as a failure to perform a civic duty? Third, it is at least conceivable that the concept of public health could be expanded to include "economic contamination." According to this view, any disease which prevents a person from being a fully-productive member of the labor force would be seen as a hazard to the society's overall economic health, particularly if public funds were being used to defray the expenses of the illness. Cost-benefit analysis would indicate that because of the illness, other persons in the society would need to work to subsidize the relatively-less-productive ill person. As one economist put it, well persons would become, at least partially, the "economic slaves" of the patient.[29] If the concept of public health is expanded in this economic direction, it seems likely that there will be tremendous pressure directed against maintaining the medical confidentiality of patients whose treatment is subsidized by public funds.

My own view is that the physician has a prima facie obligation to preserve the principle of medical confidentiality.[30] This obligation is based on the two considerations mentioned in Part II above, a concern for protecting the physician-patient relationship and a desire to respect the patient's right of privacy. Thus, the burden of proof must be assumed by anyone who wishes to argue that the principle of medical confidentiality should be violated. However, there are some cases in which this prima facie obligation can be overridden because of other very weighty considerations, for example, the desire to protect the patient's own life or the lives of other persons. According to this view, then, the physician's duty to observe the principle of medical confidentiality is a very important moral obligation, but not an absolute obligation or one's only obligation.

IV. THE PRINCIPLE OF MEDICAL CONFIDENTIALITY AND COMPUTERIZED HEALTH-DATA SYSTEMS

In a sense, computers introduce only a quantitative change into the traditional physician-patient relationship. Thus, it would seem at first glance that no fundamentally new challenges to the principle of medical confidentiality are raised by the development of computerized health data systems.

The increasing participation of sub-specialists and allied-health personnel in medical care has meant that an ever-widening circle of persons has access to the medical records of patients, particularly the records of hospital patients. We have noted that each new group with access has tended to develop a professional code which includes a pledge to preserve the confidentiality of the record. Automation does not fundamentally change this situation, provided that access is restricted to the same circle of persons. At most, the new situation would seem to require that the persons managing the computerized health data system adopt a similar code of confidentiality.

Similarly, the gathering of the patient's disparate medical records into a single comprehensive file does not seem to raise qualitatively new problems, any more than a manual operation of photocopying, cutting, and pasting scattered records into a single master record would. So long as the rules of access to particular parts of the file remain the same, the medical-confidentiality issue remains fundamentally the same.

However, the quantitative difference is perhaps significant. Because of the efficiency of automated systems, violations of medical confidentiality may appear to be easier. Because of the amount of data which may be included in a comprehensive patient file, the damage to the patient whose confidentiality is violated may be proportionately greater.

In addition, the transition from manual to automated health-data systems provides us with an occasion to think through ethical issues which we should perhaps have confronted before this point but which we have largely ignored. Three issues merit brief consideration.

The first is the issue of patient access to his or her own confidential medical record. This question has been the subject of considerable debate during the past two years.[31] In my view, the development of comprehensive health records in computerized health-data systems makes it more important than ever for the patient to have a way to correct misinformation in his or her file. If lifetime records are compiled, information more than several years old may be badly outdated and therefore convey a false impression of the patient's current medical condition. Moreover, since many sub-specialists do not know the patient personally, there is no built-in check against serious misinformation about the patient. The precise mechanism for patient access remains to be worked out. Majority opinion seems to favor access through an intermediary, perhaps a lawyer or an ombudsperson.[32]

A second issue which merits thorough discussion is the grading of confidential information according to different levels of sensitivity. The effort to determine degrees of sensitivity is reminiscent of our earlier discussion of concentric circles of privacy. It is perhaps Sweden which has gone furthest in attempting to deal with the question of assessing the relative sensitivity of medical data. In the Stockholm district, several hospitals are linked to a central data bank which stores all medical data on every patient. This information is graded for sensitivity into three categories; details are decided upon by a reference committee. The most sensitive grade of information includes data concerning psychiatric problems, venereal disease, and gynecological problems. Users of the system are assigned codes which provide access only to particular grades of confidential information.[33]

A final issue is the question of *guaranteeing* medical confidentiality. Until now, the primary positive protection for patients against unwarranted disclosure of medical data has been the development of various codes of professional ethics. In effect, various professional groups have solemnly promised not to violate the principle of medical confidentiality. Professional self-regulation has been the primary sanction against abuse; legal remedies have been, except in cases of gross abuse, relatively unavailable. Now that more complete data files are being stored in automated systems, it is perhaps time to go beyond codes of ethics and to seek more precise legal guarantees for medical confidentiality. One scholar has proposed, for example, that the patient should be expressly protected by law against injuries resulting from a "breach of [medical] confidence."[34]

In summary, the principle of medical confidentiality has a long history. The primary arguments in favor of the principle are that it preserves the physician-patient relationship and that it expresses respect for the patient's right of privacy. I have argued that the principle of medical confidentiality should be adhered to in most cases but that it may be violated when an important value—for example, human life—would be threatened by such adherence. Finally, we have noted that the development of computerized health-data systems throws into sharp relief a series of critical issues which urgently require further attention and discussion.

NOTES

1. See the English translation of the *"Charaka Samhita"* in M. B. Etziony, *The Physician's Creed* (Springfield, Ill.: Charles C. Thomas, 1973), pp. 15–17.

2. Translated in Ludwig Edelstein, "The Hippocratic Oath: Text, Translation and Interpretation," in Owsei Temkin and C. Lillian Temkin, eds., *Ancient Medicine: Selected Papers of Ludwig Edelstein* (Baltimore: Johns Hopkins University Press, 1967), p. 6.

3. Thomas Percival, *Medical Ethics,* edited by Chauncey D. Leake (Baltimore: Williams & Wilkins, 1927), p. 90.

4. American Medical Association, *Code of Medical Ethics* (New York: H. Ludwig & Co., 1848), p. 13.

5. Quoted by Etziony, *Physician's Creed,* p. 88.

6. American Medical Association, Judicial Council, *Opinions and Reports* (Chicago: American Medical Association, 1968), p. VII.

7. See Etziony, *Physician's Creed,* pp. 120–122, 127–128, 135–137.

8. *Ibid.,* p. 136.

9. For a survey of the professional and religious sources of medical ethics see LeRoy Walters, "Medical Ethics," in David Eggenberger, ed., *New Catholic Encyclopedia.* Vol. 16: Supplement 1967–1974. (New York: McGraw-Hill, 1974), pp. 290–291. Two standard textbooks of religious thought concerning medical ethics are Immanuel Jakobovits, *Jewish Medical Ethics* (New York: Bloch Publishing Company, 1959) and Charles J. McFadden, *Medical Ethics* (6th ed.; Philadelphia: F. A. Davis Co., 1967).

10. Jakobovits, *Jewish Medical Ethics,* p. 210.

11. On this point see Ralph Slovenko, *Psychiatry and Law* (Boston: Little, Brown and Company, 1973), p. 435. Within Catholic moral theology textbooks, discussion of medical confidentiality usually appears at one of three points: in the treatment of the Eighth Commandment (vs. lying) or of justice and right *(de justitia et jure),* or in the consideration of special duties which attach to particular professions or states in life (Robert E. Regan, *Professional Secrecy in the Light of Moral Principles: with an Application to Several Important Professions* (Washington, D.C.: Augustinian Press, 1943, p. 124).

12. See Regan's comprehensive survey in *Professional Secrecy,* pp. 114–48.

13. American Hospital Association, "Statement on a Patient's Bill of Rights," Hospitals 47(4): 41, 16 February 1973.

14. Regan, *Professional Secrecy*, p. 119.

15. New York Revised Statutes, 1828, II, 406, Part III, c. vii, art. 8, paragraph 3; quoted by Elyce Zenoff, "Confidential and Privileged Communications" *Journal of the American Medical Association* 182(6): 657, 10 November 1962. For a comprehensive discussion of the physician-patient privilege see Clinton DeWitt, *Privileged Communications Between Physician and Patient* (Springfield, Ill.: Charles C. Thomas, 1958).

16. Dennis Helfman, *et al.*, "Access to Medical Records" in the *Appendix* to U.S., Department of Health, Education and Welfare, *Report of the Secretary's Commission on Medical Malpractice* (Washington, D.C.: U.S. Government Printing Office, 1973), pp. 178–179. The authors of this report note that in the 1971 draft of the Proposed Federal Rules of Evidence, the physician-patient privilege is abolished but a psychotherapist-patient privilege is retained *(ibid., p. 182.)*.

17. A similar line or argument was advanced in favor of testimonial privilege for physicians in *Randa v. Bear*, 50 Wash. 2d 415, 312 P. 2d 640 (1957); cited by William J. Curran and E. Donald Shapiro, *Law, Medicine, and Forensic Science* (2nd ed.; Boston: Little, Brown and Company, 1970), p. 377.

18. Harvey L. Ruben and Diane D. Ruben, "Confidentiality and Privileged Communications: The Psychotherapeutic Relationship Revisited," *Medical Annals of the District of Columbia* 41(6): 365, June 1972.

19. The Warren-Brandeis article appeared in the *Harvard Law Review*, vol. 4, 1890, at p. 193. This quotation is taken from Susan Beggs-Baker, *et al.*, "Individual Privacy Considerations for Computerized Health Information Systems," *Medical Care* 12 (1): 79, January 1974. For a perceptive recent treatment of the right to privacy see Charles Fried, *An Anatomy of Values: Problems of Personal and Social Choice* (Cambridge, Mass.: Harvard University Press, 1970), chap. 9. The constitutional right of privacy has recently been affirmed by the U.S. Supreme Court in the cases *Griswold v. Connecticut* [381 U.S. 479, 85 S. Ct. 1678 (1965) and *Katz v. United States* (389 U.S. 347, 88 S. Ct. 507 (1967)].

20. Alan F. Westin, *Privacy and Freedom* (New York: Atheneum, 1967), p. 33.

21. The following analysis parallels, in part, Regan's discussion of "various conflicts between the duty of medical secrecy and other rights and duties" *(Professional Secrecy*, pp. 138–148).

22. This illustration is drawn from Regan, *Professional Secrecy*, pp. 143–147.

23. Helfman, *et al.*, "Access to Medical Records," pp. 180–181.

24. Regan, *Professional Secrecy*, p. 116. A similar, although more general, exception to the confidentiality obligation is included in the current AMA "Principles of Medical Ethics" (Judicial Council, *Opinions and Reports*, p. VII).

25. Helfman, *et al.*, "Access to Medical Records," p. 181. State laws requiring that cases of drug addiction be reported would be justified by means of analogous arguments *(ibid.)*.

26. Henry A. Davidson, "Professional Secrecy," in E. Fuller Torrey, ed., *Ethical Issues in Medicine: the Role of the Physician in Today's Society* (Boston: Little, Brown and Company, 1968), p. 194.

27. See for example, Amitai Etzioni, *Genetic Fix* (New York: Macmillan, 1973), especially chap. 4.

28. Great Britain, Medical Research Council, "Responsibility in the Use of Medical Information for Research," *British Medical Journal* 1 (5847): 213–216, 27 January 1973.

29. See the comments on the economist Lester Thurow on a related issue in Betty Cochran, "Conference Report: Conception, Coercion, and Control," *Hospital and Community Psychiatry* 25 (5), 287, May 1974.

30. William Frankena, *Ethics* (2nd ed.; Englewood Cliffs, N.J.: Prentice-Hall, 1973), p. 26–28.

31. See U.S. Department of Health, Education, and Welfare, *Medical Malpractice: Report of the Secretary's Commission on Medical Malpractice*, pp. 75–77; and Budd N. Shenkin and David C. Warner, "Giving the Patient His Medical Record: a Proposal to Improve the System," *New England Journal of Medicine* 289 (13): 688–692, 27 September 1973.

32. U.S., Department of Health, Education, and Welfare, *Medical Malpractice*, p. 77.

33. "Research and Confidentiality," *C.M.A. Journal* 108 (11): 1351, 2 June 1973.

34. Roedersheimer, "Action for Breach of Medical Secrecy Outside the Courtroom," *University of Cincinnati Law Review* 36 (1966), 103; cited by Helfman, *et al.*, "Access to Medical Records," p. 183.

CALIFORNIA SUPREME COURT

Tarasoff v. Regents of the University of California

Action was brought against university regents, psychotherapists employed by university hospital and campus police to recover for murder of plaintiffs' daughter by psychiatric patient. The Superior Court, Alameda County, Robert L. Bostick, J., sustained demurrers without leave to amend, and plaintiffs appealed. The Supreme Court, Tobriner, J., held that when a psychotherapist determines, or pursuant to the standards of his profession should determine, that his patient presents a serious danger of violence to another he incurs an obligation to use reasonable care to protect the intended victim against such danger, that discharge of such duty may require, the therapist to take one or more of various steps, depending on the nature of the case, that complaint could be amended to state cause of action against the therapists, to whom patient confided his intentions to kill plaintiffs' daughter, on theory of failure to warn, that therapists were entitled to statutory immunity from liability for failure to bring about patient's confinement but that plaintiffs pled no special relationship between the patient and the police defendants which would impose on them any duty to warn the daughter or other appropriate individuals and that the police were also entitled to statutory immunity for failure to confine the patient.

Affirmed in part and reversed and remanded in part for further proceedings.

Mosk, J., filed concurring and dissenting opinion.

Clark, J., filed dissenting opinion in which McComb, J., joined.

131 California Reporter 14. Decided July 1, 1976. Most footnotes and numerous references in the text of the decision and a dissent have been omitted. Reprinted by permission of West Publishing Co.

TOBRINER, Justice.

On October 27, 1969, Prosenjit Poddar killed Tatiana Tarasoff. Plaintiffs, Tatiana's parents, allege that two months earlier Poddar confided his intention to kill Tatiana to Dr. Lawrence Moore, a psychologist employed by the Cowell Memorial Hospital at the University of California at Berkeley. They allege that on Moore's request, the campus police briefly detained Poddar, but released him when he appeared rational. They further claim that Dr. Harvey Powelson, Moore's superior, then directed that no further action be taken to detain Poddar. No one warned plaintiffs of Tatiana's peril.

. . .

We shall explain that defendant therapists cannot escape liability merely because Tatiana herself was not their patient. When a therapist determines, or pursuant to the standards of his profession should determine, that his patient presents a serious danger of violence to another, he incurs an obligation to use reasonable care to protect the intended victim against such danger. The discharge of this duty may require the therapist to take one or more of various steps, depending upon the nature of the case. Thus it may call for him to warn the intended victim or others likely to apprise the victim of the danger, to notify the police, or to take whatever other steps are reasonably necessary under the circumstances.

. . .

1. PLAINTIFFS' COMPLAINTS

Plaintiffs, Tatiana's mother and father, filed separate but virtually identical second amended complaints. The issue before us on this appeal is whether those complaints now state, or can be amended to state, causes of action against defendants. We therefore begin by setting forth the pertinent allegations of the complaints.

Plaintiffs' first cause of action, entitled "Failure to Detain a Dangerous Patient," alleges that on August 20, 1969, Poddar was a voluntary outpatient receiving therapy at Cowell Memorial Hospital. Poddar informed Moore, his therapist, that he was going to kill an unnamed girl, readily identifiable as Tatiana, when she returned home from spending the summer in Brazil. Moore, with the concurrence of Dr. Gold, who had initially examined Poddar, and Dr. Yandell, assistant to the director of the department of psychiatry, decided that Poddar should be committed for observation in a mental hospital. Moore orally notified Officers Atkinson and Teel of the campus police that he would request commitment. He then sent a letter to Police Chief William Beall requesting the assistance of the police department in securing Poddar's confinement.

Officers Atkinson, Brownrigg, and Halleran took Poddar into custody, but, satisfied that Poddar was rational, released him on his promise to stay away from Tatiana. Powelson, director of the department of psychiatry at Cowell Memorial Hospital, then asked the police to return Moore's letter, directed that all copies of the letter and notes that Moore had taken as therapist be destroyed, and "ordered no action to place Prosenjit Poddar in 72-hour treatment and evaluation facility."

Plaintiffs' second cause of action, entitled "Failure to Warn On a Dangerous Patient," incorporates the allegations of the first cause of action, but adds the assertion that defendants negligently permitted Poddar to be released from police custody without "notifying the parents of Tatiana Tarasoff that their daughter was in grave danger from Prosenjit Poddar." Poddar persuaded Tatiana's brother to share an apartment with him near Tatiana's residence; shortly after her return from Brazil, Poddar went to her residence and killed her.

Plaintiffs' third cause of action, entitled "Abandonment of a Dangerous Patient," seeks $10,000 punitive damages against defendant Powelson. Incorporating the crucial allegations of the first cause of action, plaintiffs charge that Powelson "did the things herein

alleged with intent to abandon a dangerous patient, and said acts were done maliciously and oppressively."

Plaintiffs' fourth cause of action, for "Breach of Primary Duty to Patient and the Public," states essentially the same allegations as the first cause of action, but seeks to characterize defendants' conduct as a breach of duty to safeguard their patient and the public. Since such conclusory labels add nothing to the factual allegations of the complaint, the first and fourth causes of action are legally indistinguishable.

As we explain in part 4 of this opinion, plaintiffs' first and fourth causes of action, which seek to predicate liability upon the defendants' failure to bring about Poddar's confinement, are barred by governmental immunity. Plaintiffs' third cause of action succumbs to the decisions precluding exemplary damages in a wrongful death action.

.   .   .

(We direct our attention, therefore, to the issue of whether plaintiffs' second cause of action can be amended to state a basis for recovery.)

2. PLAINTIFFS CAN STATE A CAUSE OF ACTION AGAINST DEFENDANT THERAPISTS FOR NEGLIGENT FAILURE TO PROTECT TATIANA.

The second cause of action can be amended to allege that Tatiana's death proximately resulted from defendants' negligent failure to warn Tatiana or others likely to apprise her of her danger. Plaintiffs contend that as amended, such allegations of negligence and proximate causation, with resulting damages, establish a cause of action. Defendants, however, contend that in the circumstances of the present case they owed no duty of care to Tatiana or her parents and that, in the absence of such duty, they were free to act in careless disregard of Tatiana's life and safety.

In analyzing this issue, we bear in mind that legal duties are not discoverable facts of nature, but merely conclusory expressions that, in cases of a particular type, liability should be imposed for damage done. As stated in *Dillion v. Legg* (1968) 68 Cal.2d 728, 734, 69 Cal.Rptr. 72, 76, 441 P.2d 912, 916: "The assertion that liability must . . . be denied because defendant bears no 'duty' to plaintiff 'begs the essential question—whether the plaintiff's interests are entitled to legal protection against the defendant's conduct . . . [Duty] is not sacrosanct itself, but only an expression of the sum total of those considerations of polich which lead the law to say that the particular plaintiff is entitled to protection.' (Prosser, Law of Torts [3d ed. 1964] at pp. 332–333)"

In the landmark case of *Rowland v. Christian* (1968) 69 Cal.2d 108, 70 Cal.Rptr. 97, 443 P.2d 561, Justice Peters recognized that liability should be imposed "for an injury occasioned to another by his want of ordinary care or skill" as expressed in section 1714 of the Civil Code. Thus, Justice Peters, quoting from *Heaven v. Pender* (1883) 11 Q.B.D. 503, 509 stated: " ' whenever one person is by circumstances placed in such a position with regard to another . . . that if he did not use ordinary care and skill in his own conduct . . . he would cause danger of injury to the person or property of the other, a duty arises to use ordinary care and skill to avoid such danger.' "

We depart from "this fundamental principle" only upon the "balancing of a number of considerations"; major ones "are the foreseeability of harm to the plaintiff, the degree of certainty that the plaintiff suffered injury, the closeness of the connection between the defendant's conduct and the injury suffered, the moral blame attached to the defendant's conduct, the policy of preventing future harm, the extent of the burden to the defendant and consequences to the community of imposing a duty to exercise care with resulting liability for breach, and the availability, cost and prevalence of insurance for the risk involved."

The most important of these considerations in establishing duty is foreseeability. As a general principle, a "defendant owes a duty of care to all persons who are foreseeably endangered by his conduct, with respect to all risks which make the conduct unreasonably dangerous."

(Rodriguez v. Bethlehem Steel Corp. (1974) 12 Cal.3d 382, 399, 115 Cal.Rptr. 765, 776, 525 P.2d 669, 680; *Dillion v. Legg, supra,* 68 Cal.2d 728, 739, 69 Cal.Rptr. 72, 441 P.2d 912; *Weirum v. R.K.O. General, Inc.* (1975) 15 Cal.3d 40, 123 Cal.Rptr. 468, 539 P.2d 36; see Civ.Code, § 1714.) As we shall explain, however, when the avoidance of foreseeable harm requires a defendant to control the conduct of another person, or to warn of such conduct, the common law has traditionally imposed liability only if the defendant bears some special relationship to the dangerous person or to the potential victim. Since the relationship between a therapist and his patient satisfies this requirement, we need not here decide whether foreseeability alone is sufficient to create a duty to exercise reasonably care to protect a potential victim of another's conduct.

Although, as we have stated above, under the common law, as a general rule, one person owed no duty to control the conduct of another. . . . (Rest.2d Torts (1965) § 315), nor to warn those endangered by such conduct (Rest, 2d Torts, *supra,* § 314, com. c.; Prosser, Law of Torts (4th ed. 1971) § 56, p. 341), the courts have carved out an exception to this rule in cases in which the defendant stands in some special relationship to either the person whose conduct needs to be controlled or in a relationship to the foreseeable victim of that conduct (see Rest, 2d Torts, *supra,* §§ 315–320). Applying this exception to the present case, we note that a relationship of defendant therapists to either Tatiana or Poddar will suffice to establish a duty of care; as explained in section 315 of the Restatement Second of Torts, a duty of care may arise from either "(a) a special relation . . . between the actor and the third person which imposes a duty upon the actor to control the third person's conduct, or (b) a special relation . . . between the actor and the other which gives to the other a right of protection."

Although plaintiffs' pleadings assert no special relation between Tatiana and defendant therapists, they establish as between Poddar and defendant therapists the special relation that arises between a patient and his doctor or psychotherapist.[1] Such a relationship may support affirmative duties for the benefit of third persons. Thus, for example, a hospital must exercise reasonable care to control the behavior of a patient which may endanger other persons.[2] A doctor must also warn a patient if the patient's condition or medication renders certain conduct, such as driving a car, dangerous to others.[3]

Although the California decisions that recognize this duty have involved cases in which the defendant stood in a special relationship *both* to the victim and to the person whose conduct created the danger,[4] we do not think that the duty should logically be constricted to such situations. Decisions of other jurisdictions hold that the single relationship of a doctor to his patient is sufficient to support the duty to exercise reasonable care to protect others against dangers emanating from the patient's illness. The courts hold that a doctor is liable to persons infected by his patient if he negligently fails to diagnose a contagious disease (*Hofmann v. Blackmon* (Fla.App.1970) 241 So.2d 752), or, having diagnosed the illness, fails to warn members of the patient's family (*Wojcik v. Aluminum Co. of America* (1959) 18 Misc.2d 740, 183 N.Y.S.2d 351, 357–358; *Davis v. Rodman* (1921) 147 Ark. 385, 227 S.W. 612; *Skillings v. Allen* (1919) 143 Minn. 323, 173 N.W. 663; see also *Jones v. Stanko* (1928) 118 Ohio St. 147, 160 N.E. 456).

Since it involved a dangerous mental patient, the decision in *Merchants Nat. Bank & Trust Co. of Fargo v. United States* (D.N.D. 1967) 272 f.Supp.-409 comes closer to the issue. The Veterans Administration arranged for the patient to work on a local farm, but did not inform the farmer of the man's background. The farmer consequently permitted the patient to come and go freely during nonworking hours; the patient borrowed a car, drove to his wife's residence and killed her. Notwithstanding the lack of any "special relationship" between the Veterans Administration and the wife, the court found the Veterans Administration liable for the wrongful death of the wife.

In their summary of the relevant rulings Fleming and Maximov conclude that the "case law should dispel any notion that to impose on the therapists a duty to take precautions for the safety of persons threatened by a patient, where due care so requires, is in any way opposed to contemporary ground rules on the duty relationship. On the contrary, there now seems to be sufficient authority to support the conclusion that by entering into a doctor-patient relationship the therapist becomes sufficiently involved to assume some responsibility for the safety, not only of the patient himself, but also of any third person whom the doctor knows to be threatened by the patient." (Fleming & Maximov, *The Patient or His Victim: The Therapist's Dilemma* (1974) 62 Cal.L.Rev. 1025, 1030.)

Defendants contend, however, that imposition of a duty to exercise reasonable care to protect third persons is unworkable because therapists cannot accurately predict whether or not a patient will resort to violence. In support of this argument amicus representing the American Psychiatric Association and other professional societies cites numerous articles which indicate that therapists, in the present state of the art, are unable reliably to predict violent acts; their forecasts, amicus claims, tend consistently to overpredict violence, and indeed are more often wrong than right. Since predictions of violence are often erroneous, amicus concludes, the courts should not render rulings that predicate the liability of therapists upon the validity of such predictions.

The role of the psychiatrist, who is indeed a practitioner of medicine, and that of the psychologist who performs an allied function, are like that of the physician who must conform to the standards of the profession and who must often make diagnoses and predictions based upon such evaluations. Thus the judgment of the therapist in diagnosing emotional disorders and in predicting whether a patient presents a serious danger of violence is comparable to the judgment which doctors and professionals must regularly render under accepted rules of responsibility.

We recognize the difficulty that a therapist encounters in attempting to forecast whether a patient presents a serious danger of violence. Obviously we do not require that the therapist, in making that determination, render a perfect performance; the therapist need only exercise "that reasonable degree of skill, knowledge, and care ordinarily possessed and exercised by members of [that professional specialty] under similar circumstances." *(Bardessono v. Michels* (1970) 3 Cal.3d 780, 788, 91 Cal.Rptr. 760, 764, 478 P.2d 480, 484; *Quintal v. Laurel Grove Hospital* (1964) 62 Cal.2d 154, 159–160, 41 Cal.Rptr. 577, 397 P.2d 161; see 4 Witkin, Summary of Cal.Law (8th ed. 1974) Torts, § 514 and cases cited.) Within the broad range of reasonable practice and treatment in which professional opinion and judgment may differ, the therapist is free to exercise his or her own best judgment without liability; proof, aided by hindsight, that he or she judged wrongly is insufficient to establish negligence.

In the instant case, however, the pleadings do not raise any question as to failure of defendant therapists to predict that Poddar presented a serious danger of violence. On the contrary, the present complaints allege that defendant therapists did in fact predict that Poddar would kill, but were negligent in failing to warn.

Amicus contends, however, that even when a therapist does in fact predict that a patient poses a serious danger of violence to others, the therapist should be absolved of any responsibility for failing to act to protect the potential victim. In our view, however, once a therapist does in fact determine, or under applicable professional standards reasonably should have determined, that a patient poses a serious danger of violence to others, he bears a duty to exercise reasonable care to protect the foreseeable victim of that danger. While the discharge of this duty of due care will necessarily vary with the facts of each case, in each instance the adequacy of the therapist's conduct must be measured against the traditional negligence standard of the rendition of reasonable care under the circumstances. (Accord *Cobbs v. Grant* (1972) 8 Cal.3d 229, 243, 104 Cal.Rptr. 505, 502 P.2d 1.) As explained in Fleming and Maximov, *The Patient or His Victim: The Therapist's Dilemma* (1974) 62 Cal.L.Rev.

1025, 1067: " . . . the ultimate question of resolving the tension between the conflicting interests of patient and potential victim is one of social policy, not professional expertise. . . . In sum, the therapist owes a legal duty not only to his patient, but also to his patient's would-be victim and is subject in both respects to scrutiny by judge and jury."

Contrary to the assertion of amicus, this conclusion is not inconsistent with our recent decision in *People v. Burnick, supra,* 14 Cal.3d 306, 121 Cal.Rptr. 488, 535 P.2d 352. Taking note of the uncertain character of therapeutic prediction, we held in *Burnick* that a person cannot be committed as a mentally disordered sex offender unless found to be such by proof beyond a reasonable doubt. (14 Cal.3d at p. 328, 121 Cal.Rptr. 488, 535 P.2d 352.) The issue in the present context, however, is not whether the patient should be incarcerated, but whether the therapist should take any steps at all to protect the threatened victim; some of the alternatives open to the therapist, such as warning the victim, will not result in the drastic consequences of depriving the patient of his liberty. Weighing the uncertain and conjectural character of the alleged damage done the patient by such a warning against the peril to the victim's life, we conclude that professional inaccuracy in predicting violence cannot negate the therapist's duty to protect the threatened victim.

The risk that unnecessary warnings may be given is a reasonable price to pay for the lives of possible victims that may be saved. We would hesitate to hold that the therapist who is aware that his patient expects to attempt to assassinate the President of the United States would not be obligated to warn the authorities because the therapist cannot predict with accuracy that his patient will commit the crime.

Defendants further argue that free and open communication is essential to psychotherapy (see *In re Lifschutz* (1970) 2 Cal.3d 415, 431–434, 85 Cal.Rptr. 829, 467 P.2d 557); that "Unless a patient . . . is assured that . . . information [revealed by him] can and will be held in utmost confidence, he will be reluctant to make the full disclosure upon which diagnosis and treatment . . . depends." (Sen.Com. on Judiciary, comment on Evid. Code, § 1014.) The giving of a warning, defendants contend, constitutes a breach of trust which entails the revelation of confidential communications.

We recognize the public interest in supporting effective treatment of mental illness and in protecting the rights of patients to privacy (see *In re Lifschutz, supra,* 2 Cal.3d at p. 432, 85 Cal.Rptr. 829, 467 P.2d 557), and the consequent public importance of safeguarding the confidential character of psychotherapeutic communication. Against this interest, however, we must weigh the public interest in safety from violent assault. The Legislature has undertaken the difficult task of balancing the countervailing concerns. In Evidence Code section 1014, it established a broad rule of privilege to protect confidential communications between patient and psychotherapist. In Evidence Code section 1024, the Legislature created a specific and limited exception to the psychotherapist-patient privilege: "There is no privilege . . . if the psychotherapist has reasonable cause to believe that the patient is in such mental or emotional condition as to be dangerous to himself or to the person or property of another and that disclosure of the communication is necessary to prevent the threatened danger."

We realize that the open and confidential character of psychotherapeutic dialogue encourages patients to express threats of violence, few of which are ever executed. Certainly a therapist should not be encouraged routinely to reveal such threats; such disclosures could seriously disrupt the patient's relationship with his therapist and with the persons threatened. To the contrary, the therapist's obligations to his patient require that he not disclose a confidence unless such disclosure is necessary to avert danger to others, and even then that he do so discreetly, and in a fashion that would preserve the privacy of his patient to the fullest extent compatible with the prevention of the threatened danger. (See Fleming & Maximov, *The Patient or His Victim: The Therapist's Dilemma* (1974) 62 Cal.L.Rev. 1025, 1065–1066.)

The revelation of a communication under the above circumstances is not a breach of trust or

a violation of professional ethics; as stated in the Principles of Medical Ethics of the American Medical Association (1957), section 9: "A physician may not reveal the confidence entrusted to him in the course of medical attendance . . .*unless he is required to do so by law or unless it becomes necessary in order to protect the welfare of the individual or of the community.*" (Emphasis added.) We conclude that the public policy favoring protection of the confidential character of patient-psychotherapist communications must yield to the extent to which disclosure is essential to avert danger to others. The protective privilege ends where the public peril begins.

Our current crowded and computerized society compels the interdependence of its members. In this risk-infested society we can hardly tolerate the further exposure to danger that would result from a concealed knowledge of the therapist that his patient was lethal. If the exercise of reasonable care to protect the threatened victim requires the therapist to warn the endangered party or those who can reasonably be expected to notify him, we see no sufficient societal interest that would protect and justify concealment. The containment of such risks lies in the public interest. For the foregoing reasons, we find that plaintiffs' complaints can be amended to state a cause of action against defendants Moore, Powelson, Gold, and Yandell and against the Regents as their employer, for breach of a duty to exercise reasonable care to protect Tatiana.

.   .   .

CLARK, Justice (dissenting).

Until today's majority opinion, both legal and medical authorities have agreed that confidentiality is essential to effectively treat the mentally ill, and that imposing a duty on doctors to disclose patient threats to potential victims would greatly impair treatment. Further, recognizing that effective treatment and society's safety are necessarily intertwined, the Legislature has already decided effective and confidential treatment is preferred over imposition of a duty to warn.

The issue whether effective treatment for the mentally ill should be sacrificed to a system of warnings is, in my opinion, properly one for the Legislature, and we are bound by its judgment. Moreover, even in the absence of clear legislative direction, we must reach the same conclusion because imposing the majority's new duty is certain to result in a net increase in violence.

. . .

COMMON LAW ANALYSIS

Entirely apart from the statutory provisions, the same result must be reached upon considering both general tort principles and the public policies favoring effective treatment, reduction of violence, and justified commitment.

Generally, a person owes no duty to control the conduct of another. Exceptions are recognized only in limited situations where (1) a special relationship exists between the defendant and injured party, or (2) a special relationship exists between defendant and the active wrongdoer, imposing a duty on defendant to control the wrongdoer's conduct. The majority does not contend the first exception is appropriate to this case.

Policy generally determines duty. Principal policy considerations include foreseeability of harm, certainty of the plaintiff's injury, proximity of the defendant's conduct to the plaintiff's injury, moral blame attributable to defendant's conduct, prevention of future harm, burden on the defendant, and consequences to the community.

Overwhelming policy considerations weigh against imposing a duty on psychotherapists to warn a potential victim against harm. While offering virtually no benefit to society, such a duty will frustrate psychiatric treatment, invade fundamental patient rights and increase violence.

The importance of psychiatric treatment and its need for confidentiality have been recognized by this court. "It is clearly recognized that the very practice of psychiatry vitally depends upon the reputation in the community that the psychiatrist will not tell." (Slovenko,

Psychiatry and a Second Look at the Medical Privilege (1960) 6 Wayne L.Rev. 175, 188.)

Assurance of confidentiality is important for three reasons.

DETERRENCE FROM TREATMENT

First, without substantial assurance of confidentiality, those requiring treatment will be deterred from seeking assistance. It remains an unfortunate fact in our society that people seeking psychiatric guidance tend to become stigmatized. Apprehension of such stigma—apparently increased by the propensity of people considering treatment to see themselves in the worst possible light—creates a well-recognized reluctance to seek aid. This reluctance is alleviated by the psychiatrist's assurance of confidentiality.

FULL DISCLOSURE

Second, the guarantee of confidentiality is essential in eliciting the full disclosure necessary for effective treatment. The psychiatric patient approaches treatment with conscious and unconscious inhibitions against revealing his innermost thoughts. "Every person, however well-motivated, has to overcome resistances to therapeutic exploration. These resistances seek support from every possible source and the possibility of disclosure would easily be employed in the service of resistance." (Goldstein & Katz, 36 Conn.Bar J. 175, 179) Until a patient can trust his psychiatrist not to violate their confidential relationship, "the unconscious psychological control mechanism of repression will prevent the recall of past experiences." (Butler, *Psychotherapy and Griswold: Is Confidentiality a Privilege or a Right?* (1971) 3 Conn.L.Rev. 599, 604.)

SUCCESSFUL TREATMENT

Third, even if the patient fully discloses his thoughts, assurance that the confidential relationship will not be breached is necessary to maintain his trust in his psychiatrist—the very means by which treatment is effected. "[T]he essence of much psychotherapy is the contribution of trust in the external world and ultimately in the self, modelled upon the trusting relationship established during therapy.'' (Dawidoff, *The Malpractice of Psychiatrists,* 1966 Duke L.J. 696, 704.) Patients will be helped only if they can form a trusting relationship with the psychiatrist. All authorities appear to agree that if the trust relationship cannot be developed because of collusive communication between the psychiatrist and others, treatment will be frustrated. (See, e.g., Slovenko (1973) Psychiatry and Law, p. 61; Cross, *Privileged Communications Between Participants in Group Psychotherapy* (1970) Law and the Social Order, 191, 199; Hollender, *The Psychiatrist and the Release of Patient Information* (1960) 116 Am.J. Psychiatry 828, 829.)

Given the importance of confidentiality to the practice of psychiatry, it becomes clear the duty to warn imposed by the majority will cripple the use and effectiveness of psychiatry. Many people, potentially violent—yet susceptible to treatment—will be deterred from seeking it; those seeking it will be inhibited from making revelations necessary to effective treatment; and, forcing the psychiatrist to violate the patient's trust will destroy the interpersonal relationship by which treatment is effected.

VIOLENCE AND CIVIL COMMITMENT

By imposing a duty to warn, the majority contributes to the danger to society of violence by the mentally ill and greatly increases the risk of civil commitment—the total deprivation of liberty—of those who should not be confined. The impairment of treatment and risk of improper commitment resulting from the new duty to warn will not be limited to a few patients but will extend to a large number of the mentally ill. Although under existing psychiatric procedures only a relatively few receiving treatment will ever present a risk of violence, the number making threats is huge, and it is the latter group—not just the former—whose treatment will be impaired and whose risk of commitment will be increased.

Both the legal and psychiatric communities recognize that the process of determining potential violence in a patient is far from exact, being fraught with complexity and uncertainty. In fact precision has not even been attained in predicting who of those having already committed violent acts will again become violent, a task recognized to be of much simpler proportions.

This predictive uncertainty means that the number of disclosures will necessarily be large. As noted above, psychiatric patients are encouraged to discuss all thoughts of violence, and they often express such thoughts. However, unlike this court, the psychiatrist does not enjoy the benefit of overwhelming hindsight in seeing which few, if any, of his patients will ultimately become violent. Now, confronted by the majority's new duty, the psychiatrist must instantaneously calculate potential violence from each patient on each visit. The difficulties researchers have encountered in accurately predicting violence will be heightened for the practicing psychiatrist dealing for brief periods in his office with heretofore nonviolent patients. And, given the decision not to warn or commit must always be made at the psychiatrist's civil peril, one can expect most doubts will be resolved in favor of the psychiatrist protecting himself.

Neither alternative open to the psychiatrist seeking to protect himself is in the public interest. The warning itself is an impairment of the psychiatrist's ability to treat, depriving many patients of adequate treatment. It is to be expected that after disclosing their threats, a significant number of patients, who would not become violent if treated according to existing practices, will engage in violent conduct as a result of unsuccessful treatment. In short, the majority's duty to warn will not only impair treatment of many who would never become violent but worse, will result in a net increase in violence.

The second alternative open to the psychiatrist is to commit his patient rather than to warn. Even in the absence of threat of civil liability, the doubts of psychiatrists as to the seriousness of patient threats have led psychiatrists to overcommit to mental institutions. This overcommitment has been authoritatively documented in both legal and psychiatric studies. (Ennis & Litwack, *Psychiatry and the Presumption of Expertise: Flipping Coins in the Courtroom,* 62 Cal.L.Rev. 693, 711 et seq.; Fleming & Maximov, *The Patient or His Victim: The Therapist's Dilemma,* 62 Cal.L.Rev. 1025, 1044–1046; Am. Psychiatric Assn. Task Force Rep. 8 (July 1974) Clinical Aspects of the Violent Individual, pp. 23–24; see Livermore, Malmquist & Meehl, *On the Justifications for Civil Commitment,* 117 U.Pa.L.Rev. 75, 84.) This practice is so prevalent that it has been estimated that "as many as twenty harmless persons are incarcerated for every one who will commit a violent act." (Steadman & Cocozza, *Stimulus/Response: We Can't Predict Who Is Dangerous* (Jan. 1975) 8 Psych. Today 32, 35.)

Given the incentive to commit created by the majority's duty, this already serious situation will be worsened, contrary to Chief Justice Wright's admonition "that liberty is no less precious because forfeited in a civil proceeding than when taken as a consequence of a criminal conviction." *(In re W.* (1971) 5 Cal.3d 296, 307, 96 Cal.Rptr. 1, 9, 486 P.2d 1201, 1209.)

NOTES

1. The pleadings establish the requisite relationship between Poddar and both Dr. Moore, the therapist who treated Poddar, and Dr. Powelson, who supervised that treatment. Plaintiffs also allege that Dr. Gold personally examined Poddar, and that Dr. Yandell, as Powelson's assistant, approved the decision to arrange Poddar's commitment. These allegations are sufficient to raise the issue whether a doctor-patient or therapist-patient relationship, giving rise to a possible duty by the doctor or therapist to exercise reasonable care to protect a threatened person of danger arising from the patient's mental illness, existed between Gold or Yandell and Poddar. (See Harney, Medical Malpractice (1973) p. 7.)

2. When a "hospital has notice or knowledge of facts from which it might reasonably be concluded that a patient would be likely to harm himself *or others* unless preclusive measures were taken, then the hospital must use reasonable care in the circumstances to prevent such harm." *(Vistica v. Presbyterian Hospital* (1967) 67 Cal.2d 465, 469, 62 Cal.Rptr. 577, 580, 432 P.2d 193, 196.) (Emphasis added.) A mental hospital may be liable if it negligently permits the escape or release of a dangerous patient *(Semler v. Psychiatric Institute of Washington, D.C.* (4th Cir. 1976)

44 U.S.L.Week 2139; *Underwood v. United States* (5th Cir. 1966) 356 F.2d 92; *Fair v. United States* (5th Cir. 1956) 234 F. 2d 288). *Greenberg v. Barbour* (E.D.Pa. 1971) 322 F.Supp. 745, upheld a cause of action against a hospital staff doctor whose negligent failure to admit a mental patient resulted in that patient assaulting the plaintiff.

3. *Kaiser v. Suburban Transp. System* (1965) 65 Wash.2d 461, 398 P.2d 11: see *Freese v. Lemmon* (Iowa 1973) 210 N.W.2d 576 (concurring opn. of Uhlenhopp, J.).

4. *Ellis v. D'Angelo* (1953) 116 Cal.App.2d 310, 253 P.2d 675, upheld a cause of action against parents who failed to warn a babysitter of the violent proclivities of their child; *Johnson v. State of California* (1968) 69 Cal.2d 782, 73 Cal.Rptr. 240, 447 P.2d 352, upheld a suit against the state for failure to warn foster parents of the dangerous tendencies of their ward; *Morgan v. City of Yuba* (1964) 230 Cal.App.2d 938, 41 Cal.Rptr. 508, sustained a cause of action against a sheriff who had promised to warn decedent before releasing a dangerous prisoner, but failed to do so.

SUGGESTED READINGS FOR CHAPTER 4

Books and Articles

Alfidi, R. J. "Informed Consent: A Study of Patient Reaction." *Journal of the American Medical Association* 216 (May 24, 1971), 1325–1329.

Annas, George J. *The Rights of Hospital Patients.* New York: Avon Books, 1975.

Branson, Roy. "The Secularization of American Medicine." *Hastings Center Studies* 1 (No. 2, 1973), 17–28.

Brody, Howard. *Ethical Decisions in Medicine.* Boston: Little, Brown, 1976. Chaps. 4 and 5.

Cass, Leo J., and Curran, William J. "Rights of Privacy in Medical Practice." *Lancet* 2 (October 16, 1965), 783–785.

Etziony, M. B., comp. *The Physician's Creed: An Anthology of Medical Prayers, Oaths and Codes of Ethics Written and Recited by Medical Practitioners through the Ages.* Springfield, Ill.: Charles C. Thomas, 1973.

Fried, Charles. *Medical Experimentation: Personal Integrity and Social Policy.* New York: American Elsevier, 1974. Pp. 14–25.

Gorovitz, Samuel, *et al. Moral Problems in Medicine.* Englewood Cliffs, N.J.: Prentice-Hall, 1976. Chap. 2.

Gorovitz, Samuel, and MacIntyre, Alasdair. "Toward a Theory of Medical Fallibility." *Journal of Medicine and Philosophy* 1 (March, 1976), 51–71.

"Informed Consent—A Proposed Standard for Medical Disclosure." *New York University Law Review* 48 (June, 1973), 548–563.

Medical Research Council. "Responsibility in the Use of Medical Information for Research." *British Medical Journal* 1 (January 27, 1973), 213–216.

Meyer, Bernard C. "Truth and the Physician." In Torrey, E. Fuller, ed. *Ethical Issues in Medicine*. Boston: Little, Brown, 1968. Pp. 159–177.

Montange, Charles H. "Informed Consent and the Dying Patient." *Yale Law Journal* 83 (July, 1974), 1632–1664.

Morison, Robert S. "Rights and Responsibilities: Redressing the Uneasy Balance." *Hastings Center Report* 4 (April, 1974), 1–4.

Ramsey, Paul. *The Patient as Person*. New Haven: Yale University Press, 1970.

Toulmin, Stephen. "On the Nature of the Physician's Understanding." *Journal of Medicine and Philosophy* 1 (March, 1976), 32–50.

Veatch, Robert M., ed. *Case Studies in Medical Ethics*. Cambridge, Mass.: Harvard University Press, 1977.

Veatch, Robert M. "Models for Ethical Medicine in a Revolutionary Age." *Hastings Center Report* 2 (June, 1972), 5–7.

Bibliographies

Sollitto, Sharmon, and Veatch, Robert M., comps. *Bibliography of Society, Ethics and the Life Sciences*. Hastings-on-Hudson, N.Y.: Institute of Society, Ethics and the Life Sciences. Updated periodically. See under "Codes of Professional Ethics," "Confidentiality," "Health Care Delivery," and "Truth-Telling in Medicine."

Walters, LeRoy, ed. *Bibliography of Bioethics*. Vols. 1- . Detroit: Gale Research Co. Issued annually. See under "Codes of Ethics," "Confidentiality," "Disclosure," "Informed Consent," "Patient Care," "Patients' Rights," "Physician Patient Relationship," and "Treatment Refusal."

5.
Abortion

Recently laws which restrict abortion have either been sharply modified or struck down by courts in several Western nations, including the United States. While abortion is legally permitted in these nations, questions of its ethical acceptability continue to be widely debated. In addition, the adequacy of court decisions which have rendered highly restrictive abortion laws unconstitutional is also debated. In this chapter these contemporary ethical and legal issues will be examined.

THE PROBLEM OF JUSTIFICATION

Among the many reasons why abortions are commonly sought are cardiac complications, a suicidal condition of mind, psychological trauma, pregnancy caused by rape, the inadvertent use of fetus-deforming drugs, and many personal and family reasons such as the financial burden or intrusiveness of a child. Such reasons certainly *explain* why abortions are often viewed as an available way to extricate a woman or a family from difficult circumstances. But the primary ethical issue remains: Are any such reasons sufficient to *justify* the act of aborting a human fetus? An ethicist concerned to defend abortion seeks a principled justification where ethical reasons are advanced for one's conclusions. It might be decided, of course, that in only some of the above mentioned circumstances would an abortion be warranted, whereas in others it would not be justified. Even so, such a decision presupposes some set of general criteria that enable one to discriminate ethically justified abortions from ethically unjustified ones.

The central moral problem of abortion may be stated in the following general form: Under what conditions, if any, is abortion ethically permissible? Some ethicists contend that abortion is never acceptable, or at most is permissible only if abortion is required to save the pregnant woman's life. This view is commonly called the *conservative* theory of abortion. Roman Catholics have traditionally been among the leading exponents of the conservative approach, but they are by no means its only advocates. John Noonan defends such a conservative theory in the present chapter. Others hold that abortion is always permissible, whatever the state of fetal development. This view is commonly termed the *liberal* theory of abortion and has frequently been advocated by those adherents of women's rights who emphasize the right of a woman to make decisions which affect her own body; but again the position is advocated by others as well. Mary Anne Warren defends such a liberal theory in this chapter. Finally, many ethicists defend *intermediate* or *moderate* theories, according to which abortion is ethically permissible up to a certain stage of fetal development or for some limited set of moral reasons which is sufficient to warrant the taking of fetal life in this or that special circumstance. In the present chapter Baruch Brody defends an intermediate theory which leans toward conservatism, while Judith Thomson defends an intermediate theory which leans toward liberalism. (While the traditional terminology of "liberal" and "conservative" is here employed, this terminology can be both distracting and inaccurate. Whether or not one considers the fetus to be a person, for example, is an issue not at all clearly linked to political liberalism and conservatism.)

FACTS OF HUMAN BIOLOGICAL DEVELOPMENT

Since one immediate goal of some articles in this chapter is to establish the conditions under which human life begins, it is advisable first to explain the biological facts of human development, including the terminology used to designate different stages of human growth. Some important features of these biological facts, as related to abortion, are discussed in this chapter by a physician, André Hellegers.

Pregnancy does not begin with intercourse, since the earliest point at which it can be dated is during the fertilization of the female egg (the ovum) by the sperm of the male. Once fertilization has occurred, a new genetic entity results from the combination of the genetic contributions of the male and the female. This new unit is a single cell capable, under normal conditions, of a constant process of alteration and growth. This single cell has twenty-three pairs of chromosomes (each parent contributes one chromosome in each pair). It quickly divides into two cells, four cells, then eight cells—reaching sixteen at approximately the third day after fertilization. Organ systems gradually appear before the eighth week of growth, roughly the point at which brain waves can be detected. Between approximately the nineteenth and twenty-eighth week of growth, the fetus reaches the stage known as "viability," the point at which it is capable of survival outside the womb.

There exists a small but useful body of terminology frequently used by embryologists and others who discuss human biological development. *Conception* is said to occur when the male sperm and the female egg combine; during this process, the resultant entity is spoken of as a *conceptus* and is referred to in this way until its implantation, at the wall of the uterus. It is also referred to as a *zygote* until the completion of implantation, which occurs roughly two weeks after conception. Thereafter the term *embryo* is used to designate the developing entity, until about eight weeks, when it is referred to as a *fetus*. However, the term "fetus" is frequently used to designate the unborn entity in *any* state of development, and in the readings in this chapter the latter is the most common way of using the term.

THE ONTOLOGICAL STATUS OF THE FETUS

Recent controversies about abortion focus on ethical problems of how we ought and ought not to treat fetuses and on what rights, if any, are possessed by fetuses. But a more basic issue is that of *what kind of entities fetuses are*. Following current usage, we shall refer to this as the problem of *ontological status*. An account of what kind of entities fetuses are will, of course, have important implications for all issues of the permissible treatment of fetuses. But the two issues are distinct, and we must first attempt to resolve the preliminary question.

Although there is no single problem of ontological status, several layers of questions may be distinguished: (1) whether the fetus is *an individual organism,* (2) whether the fetus is *biologically a human being,* (3) whether the fetus is *psychologically a human being,* and (4) whether the fetus is a *person.* Some who write on problems of ontological status attempt to develop a theory which specifies the conditions under which the fetus can be said to be independent, individual, and alive, while others focus on the conditions, if any, under which the fetus is in some sense human, and still others are concerned to explain the conditions, if any, under which the fetus is a person. It would be generally agreed that one attributes a more significant status to the fetus by saying that it is a fully human being rather than by simply saying that it is an individual organism, and also that one enhances its status still further by claiming that it is a person.

Many would be willing to concede that an individual life begins at fertilization without conceding that there is a human being or a person at fertilization. Others would upgrade the fetus' status by claiming that the fetus is a human being at fertilization, but not a person. Still others would grant full personhood at fertilization. Those who espouse these views sometimes differ only because they define one or the other of these terms differently, but most of the differences come from serious theoretical disagreements about what constitutes either life or humanity or personhood, including disagreements over which category correctly applies to the fetus.

The Concept of Humanity. The concept of human life is an especially perplexing one, for it can mean at least two very different things. On the one hand, it can mean (a) *biological human life,* that set of biological classificatory characteristics (e.g., genetic ones) which set the human species apart from nonhuman species. (This sense *may* be coextensive with "individual organism.") On the other hand, "human life" can also be used to mean (b) *life which is distinctively human*—that is, a life which is characterized by those properties which define the essence of humanity. These are largely psychological, as contrasted with biological properties. It is often said, for example, that the ability to use symbols, to imagine, to love, and to perform various higher intellectual skills are the most distinctive human properties, those which define humans as human. To have these properties, we sometimes say, is to be a "human being."

A simple example will illustrate the differences between these two senses. Infants with various exotic diseases are often born and die after a short period of time. They are born of human parents and certainly are classifiable in all relevant biological ways as human. However, they never exhibit any distinctively human traits, and do not have the potential for doing so. For such individuals it is not possible to make human life in the "biological" sense human in the "distinctively human" or "psychological" sense. We do not differentiate these two levels of life in discourse about any other animal species. We do not, for example, speak of making feline life feline. But we do meaningfully speak of making human life human, and this usage makes sense precisely because there exists in the language the dual meaning just discussed. In discussions of abortion, it is imperative that one be specific about which meaning is being employed when using an expression like the "taking of human life." A great many proponents of abortion, and opponents as well, would agree that while biological human life is taken by abortions, human life in the second or psychological sense is not.

The Concept of Personhood. The concept of personhood may or may not be different from either the biological sense or the psychological sense of "human life" discussed above. That is, one might claim that what it means to be a person is simply to have some properties which make an organism human in one or both of these senses. But other writers have suggested a list of rather more demanding criteria for being a person. A list of conditions for being a person, similar to the following, is advanced by Mary Anne Warren in this chapter and has been put forward by several recent writers:

(a) consciousness
(b) self-consciousness
(c) freedom to act on one's own reasons
(d) capacity to communicate with other persons
(e) capacity to make moral judgments
(f) rationality

Sometimes it is said by those who propose such a list that in order to be a person an entity need only satisfy some one criterion on the list—e.g., it must be conscious (a) but need not also satisfy the other conditions (b–f). Others say that all of these conditions must be satisfied in order to be a person. We shall see that it makes a major difference which of these two views one accepts. But the dominant and prior question is whether one needs to accept anything like this list at all.

Two issues have emerged concerning the proper analysis of the concept of person. First, there is considerable dispute concerning the *range of factual characteristics* an entity must possess in order to be a person. One might analyze personhood in terms of a rather abbreviated list of factual, though not necessarily biological characteristics—e.g., in terms of physical characteristics such as genetic structure, characteristics of consciousness such as rationality and free choice, and perhaps characteristics which can at present be applied only to human developmental histories such as having learned a language. If personhood can by explicated in this way by listing only *elementary* properties such as genetic structure, then fetuses might well qualify as persons. But one might also analyze personhood in terms of a more demanding list of presumably factual properties, such as *b–f* above. Clearly one would be under a heavy burden of argument to show that a fetus is a person if criteria such as these must be satisfied. In any event, the first controversy is over precisely this issue of whether any of these more demanding properties must be present in order to be a person, and if so which such properties. In this chapter Noonan claims, against philosophers like Warren, that no such properties need be present. Jane English argues, against both, that the issue is not decidable by appeal to the concept of person.

A second dispute has emerged in connection with this first one. Several writers have suggested that the concept of personhood must be analyzed in terms of properties bestowed by human *evaluation* as well as in terms of factual properties possessed by persons. For example, it has been argued that in order to be a person one must be the bearer of legal rights and social responsibilities, and must be capable of being judged by others as morally praiseworthy or blameworthy. The central question in this controversy is whether fetuses are the sort of entity which it is appropriate to value in this way. (Brody specifically considers these theories and rejects them.)

It is certainly not self-evident that a fetus either is or is not a person in any of the above senses. If this issue can be resolved, and English seems to think it cannot be, careful argumentation is required. Anyone who claims to have resolved these controversies about persons must be prepared to defend a particular theory of personhood.

THE PROBLEM OF LINE-DRAWING

The problem of ontological status is complicated by a further factor related to the biological development of the fetus. It is important to state at what *point of development* an entity is to be distinguished as fully individual, or fully human, or fully a person. This involves specifying at what point *full ontological status* is gained. This issue turns directly on *when* fetuses achieve important ontological status and only indirectly concerns *what* status they have. But it is imperative that any theory be specific regarding whether it is status as an individual entity, a human being, or a person which is in question.

This problem is sometimes referred to as the problem of drawing the line between that which has full status and that which does not. One polar position (said to be the extreme liberal position) is that the fetus never achieves status in terms of any of the categories mentioned above, and therefore has *no ontological status* of any importance. Warren defends this view. The polar opposite position (often said to be the extreme conservative position) is that the fetus always has *full ontological status* in regard to all of the categories discussed above. Those who hold this view claim that the line must be drawn at conception, in which case the fetus is always an individual human person. Noonan defends such a position. Obviously there can be many intermediate positions. These are generally defended by drawing the line somewhere between the two extremes of conception and birth. For example, the line may be drawn at quickening or viability—or perhaps when brain waves are first present, as Brody argues in this chapter. Whichever point is chosen, it is essential that any theory be clear on two crucial matters: (1) It should be specified whether the ontological status of persons or human beings or some other category is under discussion; and (2) Whatever the point at which the line is drawn (viability, conception, birth, etc.), it should be argued that the line can be justifiably drawn at that point so that the theory is a nonarbitrary one.

As we saw previously, it remains controversial precisely what *ontological* status the fetus has. We shall now see that the fetus' *moral* status is equally controversial.

THE MORAL STATUS OF THE FETUS

The notion of moral status might be explicated in several ways, but probably is most easily understood in abortion contexts in terms of *rights*.[1] Accordingly, to say that a fetus possesses moral status is to say that it possesses rights. But which rights and how many, if any? Conservatives such as Noonan hold that unborn fetuses possess the same rights as those who are born and therefore have *full moral status*. At least some moderates contend that fetuses have only some rights and therefore have only a *partial moral status*. (Brody apparently defends this view, and Thomson's article might be so interpreted.) Liberals, on the other hand, maintain that fetuses possess no rights and therefore have *no moral status,* as Warren maintains. If this liberal account is accepted, then the unborn have no more right to life than a bodily cell or a tumor, and an abortion would seem to be no more morally objectionable than surgery to remove the tumor. On the other hand, if the conservative account is accepted, then the unborn possess all the rights possessed by other human beings; and an abortion would appear to be as objectionable as any common killing—except perhaps those killings committed in self-defense.

Theories of moral status are usually closely connected with theories of ontological status. The conservative holds that since the line between the human and the nonhuman must be drawn at conception, the fetus has full ontological status and therefore full moral status. The liberal may similarly tie his theory to an ontological account by contending that since the line between the human and the nonhuman must be drawn at birth, the fetus has no significant ontological status and therefore no moral status. However, recently a rather different approach has been more popular. Liberals have argued that even though the fetus is biologically human, and thus has full ontological status as biologically human, it nonetheless is not human in a morally significant sense and hence has no significant moral status. (Compare the second sense of human life previously mentioned.) This claim is usually accompanied by the thesis that only persons constitute the moral community, and since fetuses are not persons they do not have a moral status (cf. Warren). Moderates, on the other hand, use a wide mixture of arguments, which sometimes do and sometimes do not combine an ontological account with a moral one. Typical of moderate views is the claim that the line between the human and the nonhuman or the line between persons and nonpersons should be drawn at some point between conception and birth, and therefore that the fetus has no significant moral status during some stages of growth but does have significant moral status beginning at some later stage (cf. Brody). In many recent theories viability has been an especially popular point at which to draw the line, with the result that the fetus is given either full moral status or partial moral status at viability (cf. the Supreme Court opinion delivered by Justice Blackmun).

THE PROBLEM OF CONFLICTING RIGHTS

If either the liberal or the conservative view of the moral status of the fetus is adopted the problem of morally justifying abortion may appear to admit of rather easy resolution. If one endorses the liberal theory—that a fetus does not enjoy an ethically significant claim to treatment as a human being—the problem may seem to quickly disappear, for it is then arguable that abortions are not morally reprehensible and are prudentially justified much as other surgical procedures are. On the other hand, if one endorses the conservative theory—that a fetus at any stage of development is a human life with full moral status, and possibly a person—the equation "abortion is murder" might be accepted. By this reasoning abortion is never justified under any conditions, or at least could be permitted only if it were an instance of "justified homicide." Many conservative theories would not accept the claim that homicide in such circumstances is ever justified. Killing of the innocent, they would argue, is never permitted. Since intended abortion is a case of the deliberate destruction of innocent human life, it must under no circumstances be permitted and cannot be correctly classified as justifiable homicide.

A conservative theory, however, is not committed by its account of the fetus (as a human being with full moral status) to take precisely this latter ethical position. Instead, it may be argued that there are cases of justified homicide involving the unborn. For example, it might be argued that a pregnant woman may legitimately "kill" the fetus in "self-defense" if only one of the two may survive or if both will die unless the life of the fetus is terminated. In order to claim that abortion is always wrong, conservatives must justify maintaining the position that the fetus's "right to life" *always* overrides (or at least is equal to) all the pregnant woman's rights, including *her* "right to life."

Even if the conservative theory is construed so that it entails that human fetuses have equal rights because of their moral status, nothing in the theory requires that these moral rights always override all other moral rights. Here a defender of the conservative theory confronts the problem of the morality of abortion on the level of conflicting rights: the unborn possess some rights (including a right to life) and pregnant women also possess rights (including a right to life). Those who possess the rights have a (prima facie) moral claim to be treated in accordance with their rights. But what is to be done when these rights conflict?

This problem is in some respects even greater for those who hold a moderate theory of the moral status of the fetus. These theories provide moral grounds against arbitrary termination of fetal life (the fetus has some claim to protection against the actions of others) yet do not grant to the unborn (at least in some stages) the same right to life possessed by those already born. Accordingly, advocates of these theories are faced with the problem of specifying which rights or claims are sufficiently weighty to take precedence over other rights or claims. More precisely, one must decide which rights or claims justify or fail to justify abortions. Is the woman's right to decide what happens to her body sufficient to justify abortion? Is pregnancy as a result of rape sufficient? Is the likely death of the mother sufficient? Is psychological damage (sometimes used to justify "therapeutic abortion") sufficient? Is knowledge of a grossly deformed fetus, which produces severe mental suffering to the pregnant woman, sufficient? These issues of conflicting rights are raised in a striking manner by Thomson, who in turn is criticized by both Noonan and Warren.

Finally, it could be argued that neither the moral status of the fetus nor the problem of conflicting rights is the central issue in the abortion dispute. One could take the utilitarian position that abortion is a practice whose justification is a *social* issue. From this perspective the permissibility of abortion must be judged in terms of the consequences it has for society as a whole: if the consequences are generally better than the consequences of not allowing abortion then it should be permitted, either as a rule or in particular cases, depending on the kind of utilitarian argument being advanced.

T. L. B.

NOTES

1. The notion of moral status could be explicated in ways other than by reference to rights. To say that a fetus possesses some form of moral status might be simply to say that it is *wrong* to do certain things to it. This is important since some who deny that fetuses have rights still believe that certain ways of treating fetuses are wrong, just as some who believe that animals do not have rights nonetheless believe that it is wrong to do certain things to them.

ANDRÉ E. HELLEGERS

Fetal Development

No [treatment of] abortion would be complete without a chapter on the fetus. He or she (in the absence of knowledge of the sex, we shall use the neutral "it") is, after all, one of the subjects in the debate. Frequently in the discussions on abortion, the physician is asked when life begins. Some seem to imply that there would be no problem of abortion if only a definitive statement could be made about the beginning of human life. This, however, is far from so, for the presence of human life has never precluded our taking it if we felt justified in doing so. In this [treatment of] abortion the question (when life begins) is therefore asked not to endorse or prohibit abortion, but rather because the layman is baffled by the fetus, since he cannot see it.

Since society has imagery and definitions of its own, which it has inherited from the past, it may be well in the description which follows to highlight those stages of development to which, for one reason or another, men have attached importance in the past.[1]

I

First, let us ask in what way the ovum, or female egg, and the sperm, or male eggs, differ from the fertilized ovum. The essential difference is that an ovum or a sperm will inevitably die unless they are combined together in the process of fertilization, while the fertilized egg will automatically develop unless untoward events occur. The first definition of life, then, could be the ability to reproduce oneself, and this the fertilized egg has while the individual ovum and sperm do not.

Reprinted with permission of the author and the publisher from *Theological Studies*, Vol. 31, No. 1 (March 1970), pp.3–9.

How is this process of fertilization brought about? At intercourse, about 300,000,000 sperm are deposited in the vagina and will begin their journey upwards through the uterus, or womb, and up into the tube leading from the uterus towards the ovary. If an ovum has been released from the woman's ovary, it in turn will pass from the ovary down the same tube towards the uterus. The survival time of this ovum will be about twenty-four hours. If fertilization has not occurred in that time, both the ovum and the sperm will die. From a variety of mammalian species it has been learned that the sperm, as ejaculated, are not capable of immediately fertilizing an ovum. They must undergo a chemical change called "capacitation," without which they cannot fertilize the ovum.[2] The process is as yet little understood, but it is thought that a substance in the female uterus or tube changes the sperm in such a way that they gain the ability to fertilize. In most species this process occurs in a matter of hours, say six or eight. Although the process has not yet been proven in the human, it is commonly assumed to exist, since it occurs in other mammalian species studied. Following intercourse, there would therefore be a period of several hours in which interference with reproduction would fall under the generally recognized heading of contraception rather than abortion, since no ovum would yet have been fertilized. Several hours after intercourse, then, fertilization may occur. The significance of this event lies in the fact that a totally new genetic package is now produced. The fertilized ovum contains genetic information brought from the father through the sperm, and from the mother through the ovum, so that a new combination of genetic information is created. This newly fertilized egg, sometimes called a zygote, has within it the hereditary characteristics of both the father and the mother, one half from each. The characteristics are derived from the genetic thread of life called DNA, contained in each.

This single fertilized cell will then proceed to divide into two cells, then four, then eight, etc., and this it will do at a rate of almost one division per day.[3]

It is well known that in this early stage of development the sphere of cells may split into identical parts to form identical twins. Twinning in the human may occur until the fourteenth day, when conjoined twins can still be produced. Less well known is the fact that it is also in these first few days that twins or triplets may be recombined into one single individual.

Experiments carried out in mice by Mintz showed that it was possible to recombine the early dividing cell stages from black parents and from white parents into a single black—and —white—striped mouse.[4] The significance of this phenomenon would seem to be that up until this stage the new individual mammal is not as yet irreversibly an individual, since it still may be recombined with others into one new, final being.

In the last few years this phenomenon has also been found in man. From the genetic make-up of these human individuals and from the make-up of their red blood cells it is clear that these human so-called chimeras, whose genetic type is XX-XY, are in fact recombinations into one human being of the products of more than one fertilization. The subject has recently been extensively reviewed by Benirschke,[5] and a prototype case can be found in the report of Myhre et al.[6] It is not as yet clear up to precisely what stage of development this can occur in the human, but in mice the recombination can still be performed at the 32-cell stage. The diagnostic criteria for such cases are that their genetic karyotype is XX-XY, that they are gonadally disturbed consisting as they do of a genetic mixture of male and female, that they can contain two different populations of red blood cells, and that they may have heterochromia of the eyes. Six human cases meeting these requirements have been reported up to the present time.

The initial stages of cell division of the fertilized egg do not seem to be dependent on any paternal genetic material brought to the fertilized egg by the sperm. It would seem as if genetic material brought to the fertilized egg in the mother's ovum suffices to take the fertilized egg through the earliest stages of cell division.

All these matters are brought forth to point out that, although at fertilization a new genetic package is brought into being within the confines of one cell, this anatomical fact does not necessarily mean that all of the genetic material in it becomes crucially activated at that point, or that final irreversible individuality has been achieved.

Modern genetic studies therefore suggest that, in old standard Catholic language, one could say: "If by means of two fertilizations two souls are infused, and if a single body only contains one soul, then we are beginning to see cases in which one of the two souls must have disappeared without any fertilized egg having died."

It is also important to realize that in these first few days of life it is quite impossible for the woman to know that she is pregnant, or for the doctor to diagnose the condition by a pregnancy test.

The fact that the first seven days of the reproductive process take place entirely in the tube, and not in the uterus itself, has several major implications for the subject of abortion. These should be fully understood. If within seven days of intercourse, as for instance following rape, the lining of the uterus is removed by curettage, abortion, in its legal sense, has not taken place. It would be impossible to prove that an abortion had been performed when all pregnancy tests were shown to be negative and the lining of the uterus was shown, under the microscope, to have contained no pregnancy. Indeed the operation of curettage is a common gynecological one, which is frequently carried out in the second half of the menstrual cycle, when a fertilized ovum may well be present in the tube. There has never been a medical tradition to perform the curettage only immediately following menstruation, in order to assure that no fertilized egg could be present in the tube (since ovulation would not as yet have occurred). By the same token, women scheduled to undergo a curettage are not instructed to forgo intercourse lest there be present in the tube a fertilized ovum which would be unable to implant into the uterus due to the removal of its lining. Moreover, there is some evidence that modern "contraceptive" techniques such as the intrauterine loop, and even some of the steroid pills, may well exert their effect in pregnancy prevention by acting after fertilization of the ovum has occurred, but before implantation in the uterus.[7] Although the action of these agents is not yet fully understood, there has never been a suggestion that they would be considered abortifacient under the civil law, since no evidence of pregnancy could possibly be obtained.

II

After approximately six or seven days of this cell-division process (all of which occurs in the tube), the next critical stage of development starts. The sphere of cells will now enter the uterus and implant itself into the uterine lining. This process of implantation is highly critical, for it is during these days that one pole of the sphere of cells, the trophoblast (later to become the placenta), burrows its way into the lining of the uterus. The opposite pole of this sphere will become the fetus. The part which becomes the placenta produces hormones. These enter the maternal blood stream and serve a critical function in preventing the mother from menstruating. Since the time interval between ovulation and menstruation is approximately fourteen days, and since the first seven days of the new life have been passed in the tube, it is obvious that the implanting trophoblast only has about seven days to produce enough hormone to stop the mother from menstruating and thus sloughing off the fetal life. These same hormones, circulating in the mother, form the basis for the chemical tests which enable us to diagnose pregnancy. After this second week of pregnancy the zygote rapidly becomes more complex and is now called the embryo. Somewhere between the third and fourth week the differentiation of the embryo will have been sufficient for heart pumping to occur,[8] although the heart will by no means yet have reached its final configuration. At the end of six weeks all of the internal organs of the fetus will be present, but as yet in a rudimentary stage. The blood vessels leading from the heart will have been fully deployed, although they too will continue to grow in size with growth of the fetus. By the end of seven weeks tickling of the mouth and nose of the developing embryo with a hair will cause it to flex its neck, while at the end of eight weeks there will be readable electrical activity coming from the brain.[9] The meaning of the activity cannot be interpreted. By now also the fingers and toes will be fully recognizable. Sometime between the ninth and the tenth week local reflexes appear such as swallowing, squinting, and tongue retraction. By the tenth week spontaneous movement is seen, independant of stimulation. By the eleventh week thumb-sucking has been observed and X rays of the fetus at this time show clear details of the skeleton. After twelve weeks the fetus, now 3½ inches in size, will have completed its brain structure, although growth of course will continue. By this time also it has become possible to pick up the fetal heart by modern electrocardiographic techniques, via the mother.

The twelve-week stage is also important for an entirely different reason. It is after this stage that the performance of an abortion by the relatively simple D&C (scraping of the womb) becomes dangerous. Thereafter abortion must be performed either by abdominal operation or by the more recently developed technique of the injection of a concentrated fluid into the amniotic cavity.

Sometime between the twelfth and sixteenth week "quickening" will occur. This event, long considered important in law, denotes the fact that fetal movements are first felt by the mother. Quickening, therefore, is a phenomenon of maternal perception rather than a fetal achievement. It is subjective and varies with the degree of experience and obesity of the mother.

Sometime between the sixteenth and twentieth week it will also become possible to hear the fetal heart, not just by the refined EKG, but also by the simple stethoscope.

The twentieth-week stage again has definite importance. Before this date delivery of the product of conception is called an abortion in medical terminology. After this date we no longer speak of abortion but of premature delivery. The fetus at this stage will weigh about one pound. Between the twentieth and twenty-eighth week fetuses born have an approximately 10% chance of survival. At twenty-eight weeks the fetus will weigh slightly over two pounds. In former days the medical profession defined fetuses of less than twenty-eight weeks of age as abortions, but this was impossible to maintain when 10% of such infants

TABLE 1   SOME MAJOR NORMAL STAGES IN FETAL DEVELOPMENT

Time	Cardiovascular system	Nervous system	Other criterion
Some Hours	—	—	Intercourse followed by "capacitation"
0 Hours	—	—	Fertilization; 1 cell, often called zygote
About 22 hours	—	—	2 cell ⎞ Possible recombination
About 44 hours	—	—	4 cell ⎟ until day ?
About 66 hours	—	—	8 cell ⎟ Possible twinning
About 4 days	—	—	16 cell ⎠ until day 14 "Morula" stage
About 6–7 days	—	—	Implantation—often called "blastocyst" stage
2 weeks	—	—	Name changed from zygote to embryo
3–4 weeks	Heart pumping	—	—
6 weeks	—	—	All organs present
7–8 weeks	—	Mouth or nose tickling-neck flexing	—
8 weeks	—	Readable brain electric activity	Name change from embryo to fetus. Length 3 cm.
9–10 weeks	—	Swallowing, squinting, local reflexes	
10 weeks	—	Spontaneous movement	
11 weeks	—	—	Thumb sucking
12 weeks	Fetal EKG via mother	—	Brain structure complete Length 10 cm.
13 weeks*	—	—	D & C contraindicated hereafter
12–16 weeks*	—	—	"Quickening." Length 18 cm. at 16 weeks
16–20 weeks*	Fetal heart heard	—	Length 25 cm. at 20 weeks
20 weeks*	—	—	Name change from abortus to premature infant
20–28 weeks*	—	—	10% survive
28 weeks*	—	—	Fetus said to be "viable" in some definitions
40 weeks*	—	—	Birth

*Calculated from the first day of the last menstrual period.

might survive. As a consequence, a discrepancy may now exist between possible definitions of viability in legal and in medical circles; at least the ability to ensure survival of fetuses has progressively occurred at earlier stages.

After the twenty-eighth week little change in outward appearance of the fetus occurs, although growth obviously continues, and with this growth the chances of survival also increase.

These, then, are the major stages of fetal development in the order of their occurrence. Grouped systematically, and therefore rather arbitrarily, by genetic factors, by cardiovascular or nervous system development, and by chances of survival, they can be summarized as in the accompanying Table.

Throughout the analysis of the beginning of life it is important to bear several factors in mind. First, the understanding of the processes described is the understanding of today. The eliciting of fetal responses depends on the methods available today. Second, it is not a function of science to prove, or disprove, where in this process *human* life begins, in the sense that those discussing the abortion issue so frequently use the word "life," i.e., human dignity, human personhood, or human inviolability. Such entities do not pertain to the science or art of medicine, but are rather a societal judgment. Science cannot prove them; it can only describe the biological development and predict what will occur to it with an accuracy that depends on the stage of development of the particular science. In the ultimate analysis the question is not just to forecast when life begins, but rather: How should one behave when one does not know whether dignity is or is not present in the fetus?

NOTES

1. I shall stress heavily the new biology on the developmental processes in the first seven days, while the "fetus" is in the tube. This is crucial, I believe, (1) by reason of its own biological interest; (2) because of the action of the pill and intrauterine devices, which may act during these seven days; (3) because this stage precedes the period when a diagnosis of pregnancy can be made, i.e., it is the stage commonly described as "the normal second half of the normal menstrual cycle"; (4) because it is the stage when the "morning-after pill" may act; (5) because it is not presently covered under abortion laws, inasmuch as it precedes the stage when the woman knows she is pregnant (for she has not yet missed a period) and precedes the stage when a diagnosis can be made; (6) because it is a stage upon which the Catholic Hospital Association has not yet reflected, since we frequently do operations after ovulation but before a period is missed, i.e., during these seven days.

2. Cf. C. E. Adams, "The Influence of Maternal Environment on Preimplantation Stages of Pregnancy in the Rabbit," in *Preimplantation Stages of Pregnancy,* ed. G. E. W. Wolstenholme and M. O'Connor (Boston, 1965) p. 345; K. A. Rafferty, "The Beginning of Development," in *Intrauterine Development,* ed. A. C. Barnes (Philadelphia, 1968).

3. Cf. Rafferty, *op. cit.*

4. Cf. B. Mintz, "Experimental Genetic Mosaicism in the Mouse," in *Preimplantation Stages of Pregnancy* (n. 1 above) p. 194.

5. Cf. K. Benirschke, *Current Topics in Pathology* 1 (1969) 1.

6. Cf. A. Myhre, T. Meyer, J. N. Opitz, R. R. Race, R. Sanger, and T. J. Greenwalt, "Two Populations of Erythrocytes Associated with XX-XY Mosaicism," *Transfusion* 5 (1965) 501.

7. Cf. P. A. Corfman and S. J. Segal, "Biologic Effects of Intrauterine Devices," *American Journal of Obstetrics and Gynecology* 100 (1968) 448; also "Hormonal Steroids in Contraception," *WHO Technical Report Series, 1968* (Geneva, 1968) p. 386.

8. Cf. J. W. C. Johnson, "Cardio-Respiratory Systems," in *Intrauterine Development* (n. 2 above).

9. Cf. D. Goldblatt, "Nervous System and Sensory Organs," in *Intrauterine Development* (n. 2 above).

JUDITH JARVIS THOMSON

A Defense of Abortion[1]

Most opposition to abortion relies on the premise that the fetus is a human being, a person, from the moment of conception. The premise is argued for, but, as I think, not well. Take, for example, the most common argument. We are asked to notice that the development of a human being from conception through birth into childhood is continuous; then it is said that to draw a line, to choose a point in this development and say "before this point the thing is not a person, after this point it is a person" is to make an arbitrary choice, a choice for which in the nature of things no good reason can be given. It is concluded that the fetus is, or anyway that we had better say it is, a person from the moment of conception. But this conclusion does not follow. Similar things might be said about the development of an acorn into an oak tree, and it does not follow that acorns are oak trees, or that we had better say they are. Arguments of this form are sometimes called "slippery slope arguments"—the phrase is perhaps self-explanatory—and it is dismaying that opponents of abortion rely on them so heavily and uncritically.

I am inclined to agree, however, that the prospects for "drawing a line" in the development of the fetus look dim. I am inclined to think also that we shall probably have to agree that the fetus has already become a human person well before birth. Indeed, it comes as a surprise when one first learns how early in its life it begins to acquire human characteristics. By the tenth week, for example, it already has a face, arms and legs, fingers and toes; it has

internal organs, and brain activity is detectable.[2] On the other hand, I think that the premise is false, that the fetus is not a person from the moment of conception. A newly fertilized ovum, a newly implanted clump of cells, is no more a person than an acorn is an oak tree. But I shall not discuss any of this. For it seems to me to be of great interest to ask what happens if, for the sake or argument, we allow the premise. How, precisely, are we supposed to get from there to the conclusion that abortion is morally impermissible? Opponents of abortion commonly spend most of their time establishing that the fetus is a person, and hardly any time explaining the step from there to the impermissibility of abortion. Perhaps they think the step too simple and obvious to require much comment. Or perhaps instead they are simply being economical in argument. Many of those who defend abortion rely on the premise that the fetus is not a person, but only a bit of tissue that will become a person at birth; and why pay out more arguments than you have to? Whatever the explanation, I suggest that the step they take is neither easy nor obvious, that it calls for closer examination than it is commonly given, and that when we do give it this closer examination we shall feel inclined to reject it.

I propose, then, that we grant that the fetus is a person from the moment of conception. How does the argument go from here? Something like this, I take it. Every person has a right to life. So the fetus has a right to life. No doubt the mother has a right to decide what shall happen in and to her body; everyone would grant that. But surely a person's right to life is stronger and more stringent than the mother's right to

Reprinted with permission of the publisher from *Philosophy and Public Affairs*, Vol. 1, No. 1 (1971), pp. 47–66. Copyright © 1971 by Princeton University Press.

decide what happens in and to her body, and so outweighs it. So the fetus may not be killed; an abortion may not be performed.

It sounds plausible. But now let me ask you to imagine this. You wake up in the morning and find yourself back to back in bed with an unconscious violinist. A famous unconscious violinist. He has been found to have a fatal kidney ailment, and the Society of Music Lovers has canvassed all the available medical records and found that you alone have the right blood type to help. They have therefore kidnapped you, and last night the violinist's circulatory system was plugged into yours, so that your kidneys can be used to extract poisons from his blood as well as your own. The director of the hospital now tells you, "Look, we're sorry the Society of Music Lovers did this to you—we would never have permitted it if we had known. But still, they did it, and the violinist now is plugged into you. To unplug you would be to kill him. But never mind, it's only for nine months. By then he will have recovered from his ailment, and can safely be unplugged from you." Is it morally incumbent on you to accede to this situation? No doubt it would be very nice of you if you did, a great kindness. But do you *have* to accede to it? What if it were not nine months, but nine years? Or longer still? What if the director of the hospital says, "Tough luck, I agree, but you've now got to stay in bed, with the violinist plugged into you, for the rest of your life. Because remember this. All persons have a right to life, and violinists are persons. Granted you have a right to decide what happens in and to your body, but a person's right to life outweighs your right to decide what happens in and to your body. So you cannot ever be unplugged from him." I imagine you would regard this as outrageous, which suggests that something really is wrong with that plausible-sounding argument I mentioned a moment ago.

In this case, of course, you were kidnapped; you didn't volunteer for the operation that plugged the violinist into your kidneys. Can those who oppose abortion on the ground I mentioned make an exception for a pregnancy

due to rape? Certainly. They can say that persons have a right to life only if they didn't come into existence because of rape; or they can say that all persons have a right to life, but that some have less of a right to life than others, in particular, that those who came into existence because of rape have less. But these statements have a rather unpleasant sound. Surely the question of whether you have a right to life at all, or how much of it you have, shouldn't turn on the question of whether or not you are the product of a rape. And in fact the people who oppose abortion on the ground I mentioned do not make this distinction, and hence do not make an exception in case of rape.

Nor do they make an exception for a case in which the mother has to spend the nine months of her pregnancy in bed. They would agree that would be a great pity, and hard on the mother; but all the same, all persons have a right to life, the fetus is a person, and so on. I suspect, in fact, that they would not make an exception for a case in which, miraculously enough, the pregnancy went on for nine years, or even the rest of the mother's life.

Some won't even make an exception for a case in which continuation of the pregnancy is likely to shorten the mother's life; they regard abortion as impermissible even to save the mother's life. Such cases are nowadays very rare, and many opponents of abortion do not accept this extreme view. All the same, it is a good place to begin: a number of points of interest come out in respect to it.

1. Let us call the view that abortion is impermissible even to save the mother's life "the extreme view." I want to suggest first that it does not issue from the argument I mentioned earlier without the addition of some fairly powerful premises. Suppose a woman has become pregnant, and now learns that she has a cardiac condition such that she will die if she carries the baby to term. What may be done for her? The fetus, being a person, has a right to life, but as the mother is a person too, so has she a right to life. Presumably they have an equal right to life. How is it supposed to come out that an abortion may not be performed? If mother and child have an equal right to life, shouldn't we perhaps flip a coin? Or should we add to the

mother's right to life her right to decide what happens in and to her body, which everybody seems to be ready to grant—the sum of her rights now outweighing the fetus' right to life?

The most familiar argument here is the following. We are told that performing the abortion would be directly killing[3] the child, whereas doing nothing would not be killing the mother, but only letting her die. Moreover, in killing the child, one would be killing an innocent person, for the child has committed no crime, and is not aiming at his mother's death. And then there are a variety of ways in which this might be continued. (1) But as directly killing an innocent person is always and absolutely impermissible, an abortion may not be performed. Or, (2) as directly killing an innocent person is murder, and murder is always and absolutely impermissible, an abortion may not be performed.[4] Or, (3) as one's duty to refrain from directly killing an innocent person is more stringent than one's duty to keep a person from dying, an abortion may not be performed. Or, (4) if one's only options are directly killing an innocent person or letting a person die, one must prefer letting the person die, and thus an abortion may not be performed.[5]

Some people seem to have thought that these are not further premises which must be added if the conclusion is to be reached, but that they follow from the very fact that an innocent person has a right to life.[6] But this seems to me to be a mistake, and perhaps the simplest way to show this is to bring out that while we must certainly grant that innocent persons have a right to life, the theses in (1) through (4) are all false. Take (2), for example. If directly killing an innocent person is murder, and thus is impermissible, then the mother's directly killing the innocent person inside her is murder, and thus is impermissible. But it cannot seriously be thought to be murder if the mother performs an abortion on herself to save her life. It cannot seriously be said that she *must* refrain, that she *must* sit passively by and wait for her death. Let us look again at the case of you and the violinist. There you are, in bed with the violinist, and the director of the hospital says to you, "It's all most distressing, and I deeply sympathize, but you see this is putting an additional strain on your kidneys, and you'll be dead within the month. But you *have* to stay where you are all the same. Because unplugging you would be directly killing an innocent violinist, and that's murder, and that's impermissible." If anything in the world is true, it is that you do not commit murder, you do not do what is impermissible, if you reach around to your back and unplug yourself from that violinist to save your life.

The main focus of attention in writings on abortion has been on what a third party may or may not do in answer to a request from a woman for an abortion. This is in a way understandable. Things being as they are, there isn't much a woman can safely do to abort herself. So the question asked is what a third party may do, and what the mother may do, if it is mentioned at all, is deduced, almost as an afterthought, from what it is concluded that third parties may do. But it seems to me that to treat the matter in this way is to refuse to grant to the mother that very status of person which is so firmly insisted on for the fetus. For we cannot simply read off what a person may do from what a third party may do. Suppose you find yourself trapped in a tiny house with a growing child. I mean a very tiny house, and a rapidly growing child—you are already up against the wall of the house and in a few minutes you'll be crushed to death. The child on the other hand won't be crushed to death; if nothing is done to stop him from growing he'll be hurt, but in the end he'll simply burst open the house and walk out a free man. Now I could well understand it if a bystander were to say, "There's nothing we can do for you. We cannot choose between your life and his, we cannot be the ones to decide who is to live, we cannot intervene." But it cannot be concluded that you too can do nothing, that you cannot attack it to save your life. However innocent the child may be, you do not have to wait passively while it crushes you to death. Perhaps a pregnant woman is vaguely felt to have the status of house, to which we don't allow the right of self-defense. But if the woman houses the child, it should be remembered that she is a person who houses it.

I should perhaps stop to say explicitly that I am not claiming that people have a right to do anything whatever to save their lives. I think, rather, that there are drastic limits to the right of self-defense. If someone threatens you with death unless you torture someone else to death, I think you have not the right, even to save your life, to do so. But the case under consideration here is very different. In our case there are only two people involved, one whose life is threatened, and one who threatens it. Both are innocent: the one who is threatened is not threatened because of any fault, the one who threatens does not threaten because of any fault. For this reason we may feel that we by-standers cannot intervene. But the person threatened can.

In sum, a woman surely can defend her life against the threat to it posed by the unborn child, even if doing so involves its death. And this shows not merely that the theses in (1) through (4) are false; it shows also that the extreme view of abortion is false, and so we need not canvass any other possible ways of arriving at it from the argument I mentioned at the outset.

2. The extreme view could of course be weakened to say that while abortion is permissible to save the mother's life, it may not be performed by a third party, but only by the mother herself. But this cannot be right either. For what we have to keep in mind is that the mother and the unborn child are not like two tenants in a small house which has, by an unfortunate mistake, been rented to both: the mother *owns* the house. The fact that she does adds to the offensiveness of deducing that the mother can do nothing from the supposition that third parties can do nothing. But it does more than this: it casts a bright light on the supposition that third parties can do nothing. Certainly it lets us see that a third party who says "I cannot choose between you" is fooling himself if he thinks this is impartiality. If Jones has found and fastened on a certain coat, which he needs to keep him from freezing, but which Smith also needs to keep him from freezing, then it is not impartiality that says "I cannot

choose between you" when Smith owns the coat. Women have said again and again "This body is *my* body!" and they have reason to feel angry, reason to feel that it has been like shouting into the wind. Smith, after all, is hardly likely to bless us if we say to him, "Of course it's your coat, anybody would grant that it is. But no one may choose between you and Jones who is to have it."

We should really ask what it is that says "no one may choose" in the face of the fact that the body that houses the child is the mother's body. It may be simply a failure to appreciate this fact. But it may be something more interesting, namely the sense that one has a right to refuse to lay hands on people, even where it would be just and fair to do so, even where justice seems to require that somebody do so. Thus justice might call for somebody to get Smith's coat back from Jones, and yet you have a right to refuse to be the one to lay hands on Jones, a right to refuse to do physical violence to him. This, I think, must be granted. But then what should be said is not "no one may choose," but only "*I* cannot choose," and indeed not even this, but "*I* will not *act*," leaving it open that somebody else can or should, and in particular that anyone in a position of authority, with the job of securing people's rights, both can and should. So this is no difficulty. I have not been arguing that any given third party must accede to the mother's request that he perform an abortion to save her life, but only that he may.

I suppose that in some views of human life the mother's body is only on loan to her, the loan not being one which gives her any prior claim to it. One who held this view might well think it impartiality to say "I cannot choose." But I shall simply ignore this possibility. My own view is that if a human being has any just, prior claim to anything at all, he has a just, prior claim to his own body. And perhaps this needn't be argued for here anyway, since, as I mentioned, the arguments against abortion we are looking at do grant that the woman has a right to decide what happens in and to her body.

But although they do grant it, I have tried to show that they do not take seriously what is done in granting it. I suggest the same thing will reappear even more clearly when we turn away from cases in which the mother's life is at stake, and attend, as I propose we now do, to the vastly more common cases in which a woman wants an abortion for some less weighty reason than preserving her own life.

3. Where the mother's life is not at stake, the argument I mentioned at the outset seems to have a much stronger pull. "Everyone has a right to life, so the unborn person has a right to life." And isn't the child's right to life weightier than anything other than the mother's own right to life, which she might put forward as ground for an abortion?

This argument treats the right to life as if it were unproblematic. It is not, and this seems to me to be precisely the source of the mistake.

For we should now, at long last, ask what it comes to, to have a right to life. In some views having a right to life includes having a right to be given at least the bare minimum one needs for continued life. But suppose that what in fact *is* the bare minimum a man needs for continued life is something he has no right at all to be given? If I am sick unto death, and the only thing that will save my life is the touch of Henry Fonda's cool hand on my fevered brow, then all the same, I have no right to be given the touch of Henry Fonda's cool hand on my fevered brow. It would be frightfully nice of him to fly in from the West Coast to provide it. It would be less nice, though no doubt well meant, if my friends flew out to the West Coast and carried Henry Fonda back with them. But I have no right at all against anybody that he should do this for me. Or again, to return to the story I told earlier, the fact that for continued life that violinist needs the continued use of your kidneys does not establish that he has a right to be given the continued use of your kidneys. He certainly has no right against you that *you* should give him continued use of your kidneys. For nobody has any right to use your kidneys unless you give him such a right; and nobody has the right against you that you shall give him this right—if you do allow him to go on using your kidneys, this is a kindness on your part, and not something he can claim from you as his due. Nor has he any right against any-

body else that *they* should give him continued use of your kidneys. Certainly he had no right against the Society of Music Lovers that they should plug him into you in the first place. And if you now start to unplug yourself, having learned that you will otherwise have to spend nine years in bed with him, there is nobody in the world who must try to prevent you, in order to see to it that he is given something he has a right to be given.

Some people are rather stricter about the right to life. In their view, it does not include the right to be given anything, but amounts to, and only to, the right not to be killed by anybody. But here a related difficulty arises. If everybody is to refrain from killing that violinist, then everybody must refrain from doing a great many different sorts of things. Everybody must refrain from slitting his throat, everybody must refrain from shooting him—and everybody must refrain from unplugging you from him. But does he have a right against everybody that they shall refrain from unplugging you from him? To refrain from doing this is to allow him to continue to use your kidneys. It could be argued that he has a right against us that *we* should allow him to continue to use your kidneys. That is, while he had no right against us that we should give him the use of your kidneys, it might be argued that he anyway has a right against us that we shall not now intervene and deprive him of the use of your kidneys. I shall come back to third-party interventions later. But certainly the violinist has no right against you that *you* shall allow him to continue to use your kidneys. As I said, if you do allow him to use them, it is a kindness on your part, and not something you owe him.

The difficulty I point to here is not peculiar to the right to life. It reappears in connection with all the other natural rights; and it is something which an adequate account of rights must deal with. For present purposes it is enough just to draw attention to it. But I would stress that I am not arguing that people do not have a right to life—quite to the contrary, it seems to me that the primary control we must place on the acceptability of an account of rights is that it should turn out in that account to be a truth that all persons have a right to life. I am arguing only that having a right to life does not guarantee having either a right to be given the use of or a right to be allowed continued use of another person's body—even if one needs it for life itself. So the right to life will not serve the opponents of abortion in the very simple and clear way in which they seem to have thought it would.

4. There is another way to bring out the difficulty. In the most ordinary sort of case, to deprive someone of what he has a right to is to treat him unjustly. Suppose a boy and his small brother are jointly given a box of chocolates for Christmas. If the older boy takes the box and refuses to give his brother any of the chocolates, he is unjust to him, for the brother has been given a right to half of them. But suppose that, having learned that otherwise it means nine years in bed with that violinist, you unplug yourself from him. You surely are not being unjust to him for you gave him no right to use your kidneys, and no one else can have given him any such right. But we have to notice that in unplugging yourself, you are killing him; and violinists, like everybody else, have a right to life, and thus in the view we were considering just now, the right not to be killed. So here you do what he supposedly has a right you shall not do, but you do not act unjustly to him in doing it.

The emendation which may be made at this point is this: the right to life consists not in the right not to be killed, but rather in the right not to be killed unjustly. This runs a risk of circularity, but never mind: it would enable us to square the fact that the violinist has a right to life with the fact that you do not act unjustly toward him in unplugging yourself, thereby killing him. For if you do not kill him unjustly, you do not violate his right to life, and so it is no wonder you do him no injustice.

But if this emendation is accepted, the gap in the argument against abortion stares us plainly in the face: it is by no means enough to show that the fetus is a person, and to remind us that all persons have a right to life—we need to be shown also that killing the fetus violates its right to life, i.e., that abortion is unjust killing. And is it?

I suppose we may take it as a datum that in a case of pregnancy due to rape the mother has not given the unborn person a right to the use of her body for food and shelter. Indeed, in what pregnancy could it be supposed that the mother has given the unborn person such a right? It is not as if there were unborn persons drifting about the world, to whom a woman who wants a child says "I invite you in."

But it might be argued that there are other ways one can have acquired a right to the use of another person's body than by having been invited to use it by that person. Suppose a woman voluntarily indulges in intercourse, knowing of the chance it will issue in pregnancy, and then she does become pregnant; is she not in part responsible for the presence, in fact the very existence, of the unborn person inside her? No doubt she did not invite it in. But doesn't her partial responsibility for its being there itself give it a right to the use of her body?[7] If so, then her aborting it would be more like the boy's taking away the chocolates, and less like your unplugging yourself from the violinist—doing so would be depriving it of what it does have a right to, and thus would be doing it an injustice.

And then, too, it might be asked whether or not she can kill it even to save her own life: If she voluntarily called it into existence, how can she now kill it, even in self-defense?

The first thing to be said about this is that it is something new. Opponents of abortion have been so concerned to make out the independence of the fetus, in order to establish that it has a right to life, just as its mother does, that they have tended to overlook the possible support they might gain from making out that the fetus is *dependent* on the mother, in order to establish that she has a special kind of responsibility for it, a responsibility that gives it rights against her which are not possessed by any independent person—such as an ailing violinist who is a stranger to her.

On the other hand, this argument would give the unborn person a right to its mother's body only if her pregnancy resulted from a voluntary act, undertaken in full knowledge of the chance a pregnancy might result from it. It would leave out entirely the unborn person whose existence is due to rape. Pending the availability of some further argument, then, we would be left with the conclusion that unborn persons whose existence is due to rape have no right to the use of their mothers' bodies, and thus that aborting them is not depriving them of anything they have a right to and hence is not unjust killing.

And we should also notice that it is not at all plain that this argument really does go even as far as it purports to. For there are cases and cases, and the details make a difference. If the room is stuffy, and I therefore open a window to air it, and a burglar climbs in, it would be absurd to say, "Ah, now he can stay, she's given him a right to the use of her house—for she is partially responsible for his presence there, having voluntarily done what enabled him to get in, in full knowledge that there are such things as burglars, and that burglars burgle." It would be still more absurd to say this if I had had bars installed outside my windows, precisely to prevent burglars from getting in, and a burglar got in only because of a defect in the bars. It remains equally absurd if we imagine it is not a burglar who climbs in, but an innocent person who blunders or falls in. Again, suppose it were like this: people-seeds drift about in the air like pollen, and if you open your windows, one may drift in and take root in your carpets or upholstery. You don't want children, so you fix up your windows with fine mesh screens, the very best you can buy. As can happen, however, and on very, very rare occasions does happen, one of the screens is defective; and a seed drifts in and takes root. Does the person-plant who now develops have a right to the use of your house? Surely not—despite the fact that you voluntarily opened your windows, you knowingly kept carpets and upholstered furniture, and you knew that screens were sometimes defective. Someone may argue that you are responsible for its rooting, that it does have a right to your house, because after all you *could* have lived out your life with bare floors and furniture, or with sealed windows and doors. But this won't do—for by the same token anyone can avoid a pregnancy due to rape by having a hysterectomy, or anyway by never leaving home without a (reliable!) army.

It seems to me that the argument we are looking at can establish at most that there are *some* cases in which the unborn person has a right to the use of its mother's body, and therefore *some* cases in which abortion is unjust killing. There is room for much discussion and argument as to precisely which, if any. But I think we should sidestep this issue and leave it open, for at any rate the argument certainly does not establish that all abortion is unjust killing.

5. There is room for yet another argument here, however. We surely must all grant that there may be cases in which it would be morally indecent to detach a person from your body at the cost of his life. Suppose you learn that what the violinist needs is not nine years of your life, but only one hour: all you need do to save his life is to spend one hour in that bed with him. Suppose also that letting him use your kidneys for that one hour would not affect your health in the slightest. Admittedly you were kidnapped. Admittedly you did not give anyone permission to plug him into you. Nevertheless it seems to me plain you *ought* to allow him to use your kidneys for that hour—it would be indecent to refuse.

Again, suppose pregnancy lasted only an hour, and constituted no threat to life or health. And suppose that a woman becomes pregnant as a result of rape. Admittedly she did not voluntarily do anything to bring about the existence of a child. Admittedly she did nothing at all which would give the unborn person a right to the use of her body. All the same it might well be said, as in the newly emended violinist story, that she *ought* to allow it to remain for that hour—that it would be indecent in her to refuse.

Now some people are inclined to use the term "right" in such a way that it follows from the fact that you ought to allow a person to use your body for the hour he needs, that he has a right to use your body for the hour he needs, even though he has not been given that right by any person or act. They may say that it follows also that if you refuse, you act unjustly toward him. This use of the term is perhaps so common that it cannot be called wrong; nevertheless it seems to me to be an unfortunate loosening of what we would do better to keep a tight rein on. Suppose that box of chocolates I mentioned earlier had not been given to both boys jointly, but was given only to the older boy. There he sits, stolidly eating his way through the box, his small brother watching enviously. Here we are likely to say "You ought not to be so mean. You ought to give your brother some of those chocolates." My own view is that it just does not follow from the truth of this that the brother has any right to any of the chocolates. If the boy refuses to give his brother any, he is greedy, stingy, callous—but not unjust. I suppose that the people I have in mind will say it does follow that the brother has a right to some of the chocolates, and thus that the boy does act unjustly if he refuses to give his brother any. But the effect of saying this is to obscure what we should keep distinct, namely the difference between the boy's refusal in this case and the boy's refusal in the earlier case, in which the box was given to both boys jointly, and in which the small brother thus had what was from any point of view clear title to half.

A further objection to so using the term "right" that from the fact that A ought to do a thing for B, it follows that B has a right against A that A do it for him, is that it is going to make the question of whether or not a man has a right to a thing turn on how easy it is to provide him with it; and this seems not merely unfortunate, but morally unacceptable. Take the case of Henry Fonda again. I said earlier that I had no right to the touch of his cool hand on my fevered brow, even though I needed it to save my life. I said it would be frightfully nice of him to fly in from the West Coast to provide me with it, but that I had no right against him that he should do so. But suppose he isn't on the West Coast. Suppose he has only to walk across the room, place a hand briefly on my brow—and lo, my life is saved. Then surely he ought to do it, it would be indecent to refuse. Is it to be said

"Ah, well, it follows that in this case she has a right to the touch of his hand on her brow, and so it would be an injustice in him to refuse"? So that I have a right to it when it is easy for him to provide it, though no right when it's hard? It's rather a shocking idea that anyone's rights should fade away and disappear as it gets harder and harder to accord them to him.

So my own view is that even though you ought to let the violinist use your kidneys for the one hour he needs, we should not conclude that he has a right to do so—we would say that if you refuse, you are, like the boy who owns all the chocolates and will give none away, self-centered and callous, indecent in fact, but not unjust. And similarly, that even supposing a case in which a woman pregnant due to rape ought to allow the unborn person to use her body for the hour he needs, we should not conclude that he has a right to do so; we should conclude that she is self-centered, callous, indecent, but not unjust, if she refuses. The complaints are no less grave; they are just different. However, there is no need to insist on this point. If anyone does wish to deduce "he has a right" from "you ought," then all the same he must surely grant that there are cases in which it is not morally required of you that you allow that violinist to use your kidneys, and in which he does not have a right to use them, and in which you do not do him an injustice if you refuse. And so also for mother and unborn child. Except in such cases as the unborn person has a right to demand it—and we were leaving open the possibility that there may be such cases—nobody is morally *required* to make large sacrifices, of health, of all other interests and concerns, of all other duties and commitments, for nine years, or even for nine months, in order to keep another person alive.

6. We have in fact to distinguish between two kinds of Samaritan: the Good Samaritan and what we might call the Minimally Decent Samaritan. The story of the Good Samaritan, you will remember, goes like this:

A certain man went down from Jerusalem to Jericho, and fell among thieves, which stripped him of his raiment, and wounded him, and departed, leaving him half dead.

And by chance there came down a certain priest

that way; and when he saw him, he passed by on the other side.

And likewise a Levite, when he was at the place, came and looked on him, and passed by on the other side.

But a certain Samaritan, as he journeyed, came where he was; and when he saw him he had compassion on him.

And went to him, and bound up his wounds, pouring in oil and wine, and set him on his own beast, and brought him to an inn, and took care of him.

And on the morrow, when he departed, he took out two pence, and gave them to the host, and said unto him, "Take care of him; and whatsoever thou spendest more, when I come again, I will repay thee."

(Luke 10:30–35).

The Good Samaritan went out of his way, at some cost to himself, to help one in need of it. We are not told what the options were, that is, whether or not the priest and the Levite could have helped by doing less than the Good Samaritan did, but assuming they could have, then the fact they did nothing at all shows they were not even Minimally Decent Samaritans, not because they were not Samaritans, but because they were not even minimally decent.

These things are a matter of degree, of course, but there is a difference, and it comes out perhaps most clearly in the story of Kitty Genovese, who, as you will remember, was murdered while thirty-eight people watched or listened, and did nothing at all to help her. A Good Samaritan would have rushed out to give direct assistance against the murderer. Or perhaps we had better allow that it would have been a Splendid Samaritan who did this, on the ground that it would have involved a risk of death for himself. But the thirty-eight not only did not do this, they did not even trouble to pick up a phone to call the police. Minimally Decent Samaritanism would call for doing at least that, and their not having done it was monstrous.

After telling the story of the Good Samaritan, Jesus said "Go, and do thou likewise." Perhaps he meant that we are morally required to act as the Good Samaritan did. Perhaps he was urging people to do more than is morally required of them. At all events it seems plain that it was not morally required of any of the thirty-eight that he rush out to give direct assis-

tance at the risk of his own life, and that it is not morally required of anyone that he give long stretches of his life—nine years or nine months—to sustaining the life of a person who has no special right (we were leaving open the possibility of this) to demand it.

Indeed, with one rather striking class of exceptions, no one in any country in the world is *legally* required to do anywhere near as much as this for anyone else. The class of exceptions is obvious. My main concern here is not the state of the law in respect to abortion, but it is worth drawing attention to the fact that in no state in this country is any man compelled by law to be even a Minimally Decent Samaritan to any person; there is no law under which charges could be brought against the thirty-eight who stood by while Kitty Genovese died. By contrast, in most states in this country women are compelled by law to be not merely Minimally Decent Samaritans, but Good Samaritans to unborn persons inside them. This doesn't by itself settle anything one way or the other, because it may well be argued that there should be laws in this country—as there are in many European countries—compelling at least Minimally Decent Samaritanism.[8] But it does show that there is a gross injustice in the existing state of the law. And it shows also that the groups currently working against liberalization of abortion laws, in fact working toward having it declared unconstitutional for a state to permit abortion, had better start working for the adoption of Good Samaritan laws generally, or earn the charge that they are acting in bad faith.

I should think, myself, that Minimally Decent Samaritan laws would be one thing, Good Samaritan laws quite another, and in fact highly improper. But we are not here concerned with the law. What we should ask is not whether anybody should be compelled by law to be a Good Samaritan, but whether we must accede to a situation in which somebody is being compelled—by nature, perhaps—to be a Good Samaritan. We have, in other words, to look now at third-party interventions. I have been arguing that no person is morally required to make large sacrifices to sustain the life of another who has no right to demand them, and this even where the sacrifices do not include life itself; we are not morally required to be Good Samaritans or anyway Very Good Samaritans to one another. But what if a man cannot extricate himself from such a situation? What if he appeals to us to extricate him? It seems to me plain that there are cases in which we can, cases in which a Good Samaritan would extricate him. There you are, you were kidnapped, and nine years in bed with that violinist lie ahead of you. You have your own life to lead. You are sorry, but you simply cannot see giving up so much of your life to the sustaining of his. You cannot extricate yourself, and ask us to do so. I should have thought that—in light of his having no right to the use of your body—it was obvious that we do not have to accede to your being forced to give up so much. We can do what you ask. There is no injustice to the violinist in our doing so.

7. Following the lead of the opponents of abortion, I have throughout been speaking of the fetus merely as a person, and what I have been asking is whether or not the argument we began with, which proceeds only from the fetus' being a person, really does establish its conclusion. I have argued that it does not.

But of course there are arguments and arguments, and it may be said that I have simply fastened on the wrong one. It may be said that what is important is not merely the fact that the fetus is a person, but that it is a person for whom the woman has a special kind of responsibility issuing from the fact that she is its mother. And it might be argued that all my analogies are therefore irrelevant—for you do not have that special kind of responsibility for that violinist, Henry Fonda does not have that special kind of responsibility for me. And our attention might be drawn to the fact that men and women both *are* compelled by law to provide support for their children.

I have in effect dealt (briefly) with this argument in section 4 above; but a (still briefer) recapitulation now may be in order. Surely we do not have any such ''special responsibility'' for a person unless we have assumed it, explicitly or implicitly. If a set of parents do not try to prevent pregnancy, do not obtain an abortion, and then at the time of birth of the child do not put it out for adoption, but rather take it home with them, then they have assumed responsibility for it, they have given it rights, and they cannot *now* withdraw support from it at the cost of its life because they now find it difficult to go on providing for it. But if they have taken all reasonable precautions against having a child, they do not simply by virtue of their biological relationship to the child who comes into existence have a special responsibility for it. They may wish to assume responsibility for it, or they may not wish to. And I am suggesting that if assuming responsibility for it would require large sacrifices, then they may refuse. A Good Samaritan would not refuse—or anyway, a Splendid Samaritan, if the sacrifices that had to be made were enormous. But then so would a Good Samaritan assume responsibility for that violinist; so would Henry Fonda, if he is a Good Samaritan, fly in from the West Coast and assume responsibility for me.

8. My argument will be found unsatisfactory on two counts by many of those who want to regard abortion as morally permissible. First, while I do argue that abortion is not impermissible, I do not argue that it is always permissible. There may well be cases in which carrying the child to term requires only Minimally Decent Samaritanism of the mother, and this is a standard we must not fall below. I am inclined to think it a merit of my account precisely that it does *not* give a general yes or a general no. It allows for and supports our sense that, for example, a sick and desperately frightened fourteen-year-old schoolgirl, pregnant due to rape, may *of course* choose abortion, and that any law which rules this out is an insane law. And it also allows for and supports our sense that in other cases resort to abortion is even positively indecent. It would be indecent in the woman to request an abortion, and indecent in a doctor to perform it, if she is in her seventh month, and wants the abortion just to avoid the nuisance of postponing a trip abroad.

The very fact that the arguments I have been drawing attention to treat all cases of abortion, or even all cases of abortion in which the mother's life is not at stake, as morally on a par ought to have made them suspect at the outset.

Secondly, while I am arguing for the permissibility of abortion in some cases, I am not arguing for the right to secure the death of the unborn child. It is easy to confuse these two things in that up to a certain point in the life of the fetus it is not able to survive outside the mother's body; hence removing it from her body guarantees its death. But they are importantly different. I have argued that you are not morally required to spend nine months in bed, sustaining the life of that violinist; but to say this is by no means to say that if, when you unplug yourself, there is a miracle and he survives, you then have a right to turn round and slit his throat. You may detach yourself even if this costs him his life; you have no right to be guaranteed his death, by some other means, if unplugging yourself does not kill him. There are some people who will feel dissatisfied by this feature of my argument. A woman may be utterly devastated by the thought of a child, a bit of herself, put out for adoption and never seen or heard of again. She may therefore want not merely that the child be detached from her, but more, that it die. Some opponents of abortion are inclined to regard this as beneath contempt—thereby showing insensitivity to what is surely a powerful source of despair. All the same, I agree that the desire for the child's death is not one which anybody may gratify, should it turn out to be possible to detach the child alive.

At this place, however, it should be remembered that we have only been pretending throughout that the fetus is a human being from the moment of conception. A very early abortion is surely not the killing of a person, and so is not dealt with by anything I have said here.

NOTES

1. I am very much indebted to James Thomson for discussion, criticism, and many helpful suggestions.

2. Daniel Callahan, *Abortion: Law, Choice and Morality* (New York, 1970), p. 373. This book gives a fascinating survey of the available information on abortion. The Jewish tradition is surveyed in David M. Feldman, *Birth Control in Jewish Law* (New York, 1968), Part 5, the Catholic tradition in John T. Noonan, Jr., "An Almost Absolute Value in History," in *The Morality of Abortion,* ed. John T. Noonan, Jr. (Cambridge, Mass., 1970).

3. The term "direct" in the arguments I refer to is a technical one. Roughly, what is meant by "direct killing" is either killing as an end in itself, or killing as a means to some end, for example, the end of saving someone else's life. See note 6, below, for an example of its use.

4. Cf. *Encyclical Letter of Pope Pius XI on Christian Marriage,* St. Paul Editions (Boston, n.d.), p. 32: "however much we may pity the mother whose health and even life is gravely imperiled in the performance of the duty allotted to her by nature, nevertheless what could ever be a sufficient reason for excusing in any way the direct murder of the innocent? This is precisely what we are dealing with here." Noonan *(The Morality of Abortion,* p. 43) reads this as follows: "What cause can ever avail to excuse in any way the direct killing of the innocent? For it is a question of that."

5. The thesis in (4) is in an interesting way weaker than those in (1), (2), and they rule out abortion even in cases in which both mother *and* child will die if the abortion is not performed. By contrast, one who held the view expressed in (4) could consistently say that one needn't prefer letting two persons die to killing one.

6. Cf. the following passage from Pius XII, *Address to the Italian Catholic Society of Midwives:* "The baby in the maternal breast has the right to life immediately from God. —Hence there is no man, no human authority, no science, no medical, eugenic, social, economic or moral 'indication' which can establish or grant a valid juridical ground for a direct deliberate disposition of an innocent human life, that is a disposition which looks to its destruction either as an end or as a means to another end perhaps in itself not illicit. —The baby, still not born, is a man in the same degree and for the same reason as the mother" (quoted in Noonan, *The Morality of Abortion,* p. 45).

7. The need for a discussion of this argument was brought home to me by members of the Society for Ethical and Legal Philosophy, to whom this paper was originally presented.

8. For a discussion of the difficulties involved, and a survey of the European experience with such laws, see *The Good Samaritan and the Law,* ed. James M. Ratcliffe (New York, 1966).

JOHN T. NOONAN

How To Argue About Abortion

At the heart of the debate about abortion is the relation of person to person in social contexts. Analogies, metaphors, and methods of debate which do not focus on persons and which do not attend to the central contexts are mischievous. Their use arises from a failure to appreciate the distinctive character of moral argument—its requirement that values be organically related and balanced, its dependence on personal vision, and its rootedness in social experience. I propose here to examine various models and methods used in the debate on abortion. . . . I write as a critic of abortion, with no doubt a sharper eye for the weaknesses of its friends than of its foes, but my chief aim is to suggest what arguments count.

ARTIFICIAL CASES

One way of reaching the nub of a moral issue is to construct a hypothetical situation endowed with precisely the characteristics you believe are crucial in the real issue you are seeking to resolve. Isolated from the clutter of detail in the real situation, these characteristics point to the proper solution. The risk is that the features you believe crucial you will enlarge to the point of creating a caricature. The pedagogy of your illustration will be blunted by the uneasiness caused by the lack of correspondence between the fantasized situation and the real situation to be judged. Such is the case with two recent efforts by philosophers, Judith Jarvis Thomson and Michael Tooley, to construct arguments justifying abortion.

Suppose, says Thomson, a violinist whose continued existence depends on acquiring new kidneys. Without the violinist's knowledge—he remains innocent—a healthy person is kidnapped and connected to him so that the violinist now shares the use of healthy kidneys. May the victim of the kidnapping break the

Published by the Ad Hoc Committee in Defense of Life, Inc. and reprinted with permission of the author. © 1974 by John T. Noonan, Jr.

connection and thereby kill the violinist? Thomson intuits that the normal judgment will be Yes. The healthy person should not be imposed upon by a lifelong physical connection with the violinist. This construct, Thomson contends, bears upon abortion by establishing that being human does not carry with it a right to life which must be respected by another at the cost of serious inconvenience.[1]

This ingenious attempt to make up a parallel to pregnancy imagines a kidnapping; a serious operation performed on the victim of the kidnapping; and a continuing interference with many of the activities of the victim. It supposes that violinist and victim were unrelated. It supposes nothing by which the victim's initial aversion to his yoke-mate might be mitigated or compensated. It supposes no degree of voluntariness. The similitude to pregnancy is grotesque. It is difficult to think of another age or society in which a caricature of this sort could be seriously put forward as a paradigm illustrating the moral choice to be made by a mother.

While Thomson focuses on this fantasy, she ignores a real case from which American tort law has generalized. On a January night in Minnesota, a cattle buyer, Orlando Depue, asked a family of farmers, the Flateaus, with whom he had dined, if he could remain overnight at their house. The Flateaus refused and, although Depue was sick and had fainted, put him out of the house into the cold night. Imposing liability of the Flateaus for Depue's loss of his frostbitten fingers the court said, "In the case at bar defendants were under no contract obligation to minister to plaintiff in his distress; but humanity demanded they do so, if they understood and appreciated his condition . . . The law as well as humanity required that he not be exposed in his helpless condition to the merciless elements."[2] Depue was a guest for supper although not a guest after supper. The American Law Institute, generalizing, has said that it makes no difference whether the helpless person is a guest or a trespasser. He has the privilege of staying. His host has the duty not to injure him or put him into an environment where he becomes nonviable. The obligation arises when one person "understands and appreciates" the condition of the other.[3] Although the analogy is not exact, the case seems closer to the mother's situation than the case imagined by Thomson; and the emotional response of the Minnesota judges seems to be a truer reflection of what humanity requires.

Michael Tooley's artificial case in defense of abortion is put forward in the course of an even broader defense by him of infanticide, horror of which he likens to other unreasoned cultural taboos. He attacks "the potentiality principle," the principle that the fetus or baby is entitled to respect because the fetus or baby will develop into an adult human being with an admitted right to life. He does so in this way. Suppose, he says, a chemical which could be injected into a kitten which would enable it to develop into a cat possessed of the brain and psychological capabilities of adult human beings. It would not be wrong, he intuits, to refrain from giving a kitten the chemical and to kill the kitten instead. Would it be wrong, he asks, to kill a kitten who had been injected? To do so would be to prevent the development of a rational adult cat. Yet, Tooley intuits, the answer must be that it would not be wrong to kill the injected kitten. Potentiality for rational adulthood, he concludes, does not enhance a kitten's claim to life, or a fetus'.[4]

Leaving the world of humans altogether, Tooley, like Thomson, has fashioned a hypothetical to give light on a very abstract question, "Who has a right to life?" The hypothetical is framed as though the subject of this question were indifferent. To get an answer we are asked to test our reactions to a fantasy. We do not have the experience to tell us what we would decide if we were confronted by his hypothetical cat or hypothetical kitten. Cat-lovers would probably respond very differently from dog-lovers. We are asked to respond to a construct, and to respond we need to see or feel the flesh and blood of a humanoid.

Cats may be treated on their own merits, apart from chemical injections, as humans. But

then the work of personification is consciously done by attention to the human analogues. . . .

HARD CASES AND EXCEPTIONS

In the presentation of permissive abortion to the American public, major emphasis has been put on situations of great pathos—the child deformed by thalidomide, the child affected by rubella, the child known to suffer from Tay-Sachs disease or Downs syndrome, the raped adolescent, the exhausted mother of small children. These situations are not imagined, and the cases described are not analogies to those where abortion might be sought; they are themselves cases to which abortion is a solution. Who could deny the poignancy of their appeal?

Hard cases make bad law, runs the venerable legal adage, but it seems to be worse law if the distress experienced in situations such as these is not taken into account. If persons are to be given preeminence over abstract principle, should not exceptions for these cases be made in the most rigid rule against abortion? Does not the human experience of such exceptions point to a more sweeping conclusion—the necessity of abandoning any uniform prohibition of abortion, so that all the elements of a particular situation may be weighted by the woman in question and her doctor?

So far, fault can scarcely be found with this method of argumentation, this appeal to common experience. But the cases are oversimplified if focus is directed solely on the parents of a physically defective child or on the mother in the cases of rape or psychic exhaustion. The situations are very hard for the parents or the mother; they are still harder for the fetus who is threatened with death. If the fetus is a person as the opponents of abortion contend, its destruction is not the sparing of suffering by the sacrifice of a principle but by the sacrifice of a life. Emotion is a proper element in moral response, but to the extent that the emotion generated by these cases obscures the claims of the fetus, this kind of argumentation fosters erroneous judgment.

In three of the cases—the child deformed by drugs, disease, or genetic defect—the neglect of the child's point of view seems stained by hypocrisy. Abortion is here justified as putting the child out of the misery of living a less than normal life. The child is not consulted as to the choice. Experience, which teaches that even the most seriously incapacitated prefer living to dying, is ignored. The feelings of the parents are the actual consideration, and these feelings are treated with greater tenderness than the fetal desire to live. The common unwillingness to say frankly that the abortion is sought for the parents' benefit is testimony, unwillingly given, to the intuition that such self-preference by the parents is difficult for society or for the parents themselves to accept.

The other kind of hard case does not mask preference for the parent by a pretense of concern for the fetus. The simplest situation is that of a pregnancy due to rape—in presentations to some legislatures it was usual to add a racist fillip by supposing a white woman and a black rapist—but this gratuitous pandering to bias is not essential. The fetus, unwanted in the most unequivocal way, is analogized to an invader of the mother's body—is it even appropriate to call her a mother when she did nothing to assume the special fiduciary cares of motherhood? If she is prevented from having an abortion, she is being compelled for nine months to be reminded of a traumatic assault. Do not her feelings override the right to life of her unwanted tenant?

Rape arouses fear and a desire for revenge, and reference to rape evokes emotion. The emotion has been enough for the state to take the life of the rapist.[5] Horror of the crime is easily extended to horror of the product, so that the fetal life becomes forfeit too. If horror is overcome, adoption appears to be a more humane solution than abortion. If the rape case is not being used as a stalking horse by proponents of abortion—if there is a desire to deal with it in itself—the solution is to assure the destruction of the sperm in the one to three days elapsing between insemination and impregnation.

Generally, however, the rape case is presented as a way of suggesting a general principle, a principle which could be formulated as follows: Every unintended pregnancy may be interrupted if its continuation will cause emotional distress to the mother. Pregnancies due to bad planning or bad luck are analogized to pregnancies due to rape; they are all involuntary.[6] Indeed many pregnancies can without great difficulty be assimilated to the hard case, for how often do persons undertake an act of sexual intercourse consciously intending that a child be the fruit of that act? Many pregnancies are unspecified by a particular intent, are unplanned, are in this sense involuntary. Many pregnancies become open to termination if only the baby consciously sought has immunity.

This result is unacceptable to those who believe that the fetus is human. It is acceptable to those who do not believe the fetus is human, but to reach it they do not need the argument based on the hard case. The result would follow immediately from the mother's dominion over a portion of her body. Opponents of abortion who out of consideration for the emotional distress caused by rape will grant the rape exception must see that the exception can be generalized to destroy the rule. If, on other grounds they believe the rule good, they must deny the exception which eats it up.

DIRECT AND INDIRECT

From paradigmatic arguments, I turn to metaphors and especially those which, based on some spatial image, are misleading. I shall begin with "direct" and "indirect" and their cousins, "affirmative" and "negative." In the abortion argument "direct" and "indirect," "affirmative" and "negative" occur more frequently in these kinds of questions: If one denies that a fetus may be killed directly, but admits that indirect abortion is permissible, is he guilty of inconsistency? If one maintains that there is a negative duty not to kill fetuses, does he thereby commit himself to an affirmative obligation of assuring the safe delivery of every fetus? If one agrees that there is no affirmative duty to actualize as many spermatic, ovoid, embryonic, or fetal potentialities as possible, does one thereby concede that it is generally permissible to take steps to destroy fertilized ova? The argumentative implications of these questions can be best unravelled by looking at the force of the metaphors invoked.

"Direct" and "indirect" appeal to our experience of linedrawing and of travel. You reach a place on a piece of paper by drawing a straight or crooked line—the line is direct or indirect. You go to a place without detours or you go in a roundabout fashion—your route is direct or indirect. In each instance, whether your path is direct or indirect your destination is the same. The root experience is that you can reach the same spot in ways distinguished by their immediacy and the amount of ground covered. "Indirectly" says you proceed more circuitously and cover more ground. It does not, however, say anything of the reason why you go circuitously. You may go indirectly because you want to disguise your destination.

The ambiguity in the reason for indirectness —an ambiguity present in the primary usage of the term—carries over when "indirect" is applied metaphorically to human intentions. There may be a reason for doing something indirectly—you want to achieve another objective besides the indirect action. You may also act indirectly to conceal from another or from yourself what is your true destination. Because of this ambiguity in the reason for indirection, "indirect" is apt to cause confusion when applied in moral analysis.

Defenders of an absolute prohibition of abortion have excepted the removal of a fertilized ovum in an ecotopic pregnancy and the removal of a cancerous uterus containing an embryo. They have characterized the abortion involved as "indirect." They have meant that the surgeon's attention is focused on correcting a pathological condition dangerous to the mother and he only performs the operation because there is no alternative way of correcting it.[7] But the physician has to intend to achieve not only the improvement of the mother but the performance of action by which the fertilized ovum becomes nonviable. He necessarily intends to perform an abortion, he necessarily intends to kill. To say that he acts indirectly is to conceal what is being done. It is a confusing and improper use of the metaphor.[8]

A clearer presentation of the cases of the cancerous uterus and the ectopic pregnancy would acknowledge them to be true exceptions to the absolute inviolability of the fetus. Why are they not exceptions which would eat up the rule? It depends on what the rule is considered to be. The principle that can be discerned in them is, whenever the embryo is a danger to the life of the mother, an abortion is permissible. At the level of reason nothing more can be asked of the mother. The exceptions do eat up any rule of preferring the fetus to the mother— any rule of fetus first. They do not destroy the rule that the life of the fetus has precedence over other interests of the mother. The exceptions of the ectopic pregnancy and the cancerous uterus are special cases of the general exception to the rule against killing, which permits one to kill in self-defense. Characterization of this kind of killing as "indirect" does not aid analysis.[9]

It is a basic intuition that one is not responsible for all the consequences of one's acts. By living at all one excludes others from the air one breathes, the food one eats. One cannot foresee all the results which will flow from any given action. It is imperative for moral discourse to be able to distinguish between injury foreseeably inflicted on another, and the harm which one may unknowingly bring about.

· · ·

LINEDRAWING

The prime linear metaphor is, of course, linedrawing. It is late in the history of moral thought for anyone to suppose that an effective moral retort is, "Yes, but where do you draw the line?" or to make the inference that, because any drawing of a line requires a decision, all linedrawing is arbitrary. One variant or another of these old ploys is, however, frequently used in the present controversy. From living cell to dying corpse a continuum exists. Proponents of abortion are said to be committed to murder, to euthanasia, or, at a minimum, to infanticide. Opponents are alleged to be bound to condemn contraception—after all, spermatazoa are living human cells. Even if contraception is admitted and infanticide rejected, the range of choice is still large enough for the line drawn to be challenged—is it to be at nidation, at formation of the embryo, at quickening, at viability, at birth? Whoever adopts one point is asked why he does not move forward or backward by one stage of development. The difficulty of presenting apodictic reasons for preferring one position is made to serve as proof that the choice may be made as best suits the convenience of an individual or the state.[10]

The metaphor of linedrawing distracts attention from the nature of the moral decision. The metaphor suggests an empty room composed of indistinguishable grey blocks. In whatever way the room is divided, there are grey blocks on either side of the line. Or if the metaphor is taken more mathematically, it suggests a series of points, which, wherever bisected, are fungible with each other. What is obscured in the spatial or mathematical model is the variety of values whose comparison enters into any moral decision. The model appeals chiefly to those novices in moral reasoning who believe that moral judgment is a matter of pursuing a principle to its logical limit. Single-mindedly looking at a single value, they ask, if this is good, why not more of it? In practice, however, no one can be so single-hearted. Insistence of this kind of logical consistency becomes the preserve of fanatics or of controversialists eager to convict their adversaries of inconsistency. If more than one good is sought by a human being, he must bring the goods he seeks into relationship with each other; he must limit one to maintain another; he must mix them.

. . .

Is, however, the choice of the stage of development which should not be destroyed by abortion a choice requiring the mixing of multiple goods? Is not the linear model appropriate when picking a point on the continuum of life? Are not the moral choices which require commitment and mixing made only after the selection of the stage at which a being becomes a person? To these related questions the answers must all be negative. To recognize a person is a moral decision; it depends on objective data but it also depends on the perceptions and inclinations and ends of the decision makers; it cannot be made without commitment and without consideration of alternative values. Who is a person? This is not a question asked abstractly, in the air, with no purpose in mind. To disguise the personal involvement in the response to personhood is to misconceive the issue of abortion from the start.

. . .

In the case of abortion, it is the contention of its opponents that in such a process the right response to the data is that the fetus is a human being.[11]

BALANCING

The process of decisionmaking just described is better caught by the term "balancing." In contrast to linedrawing, balancing is a metaphor helpful in understanding moral judgment. Biologically understood, balancing is the fundamental metaphor for moral reasoning. A biological system is in balance when its parts are in the equilibrium necessary for it to live. To achieve such equilibrium, some parts—the heart, for example—must be preserved at all costs; others may be sacrificed to maintain the whole. Balance in the biological sense does not demand an egalitarian concern for every part, but an ordering and subordination which permit the whole to function. So in moral reasoning the reasoner balances values.

The mistaken common reading of this metaphor is to treat it as equivalent to weighing, so that balancing is understood as an act of quantitative comparison analogous to that performed by an assayer or a butcher. This view tacitly supposes that values are weights which are tangible and commensurate. One puts so many units on one pan of the scales and matches them with so many units on the other to reach a "balanced" judgment. To give a personal example, Daniel Callahan has questioned my position that the value of innocent life cannot be sacrificed to achieve the other values which abortion might secure. The "force of the rule," he writes, "is absolutist, displaying no 'balance' at all.''[12] He takes balancing in the sense of weighing and wonders how one value can be so heavy.

. . .

But some values are more vital than others, as the heart is more vital to the body than the hand. A balanced moral judgment requires a sense of the limits, interrelations, and priority of values. It is the position of those generally opposed to abortion that a judgment preferring interests less than human life to human life is unbalanced, that a judgment denying a mother's fiduciary responsibility to her child is unbalanced, that a judgment making killing a principal part of the profession of a physician is unbalanced, that a judgment permitting agencies of the state to procure and pay for the destruction of the offspring of the poor or underprivileged is unbalanced. They contend that such judgments expand the right limits of a mother's responsibility for herself, destroy the fiduciary relation which is a central paradigm for the social bond, fail to relate to the physician's service to life and the state's care for its citizens. At stake in the acceptance of abortion is not a single value, life, against which the suffering of the mother or parents may be balanced. The values to be considered are the child's life, the mother's faithfulness to her dependent, the physician's commitment to preserving life; and in the United States today abortion cannot be discussed without awareness that if law does not prohibit it, the state will fund it, so that the value of the state's abstention from the taking of life is also at issue. The judgment which accepts abortion, it is contended, is unbalanced in subordinating these values to the personal autonomy of the mother and the social interest in population control.

SEEING

The metaphor of balancing points to the process of combining values. But we do not combine values like watercolors. We respond to values situated in subjects. ''Balancing'' is an inadequate metaphor for moral thinking in leaving out of account the central moral transaction—the response of human beings to other

human beings.[13] In making moral judgments we respond to those human beings whom we see.

The metaphor of sight is a way of emphasizing the need for perception, whether by eyes or ears or touch, of those we take as subjects to whom we respond. Seeing in any case is more than the registration of a surface. It is a penetration yielding some sense of the other's structure, so that the experiencing of another is never merely visual or auditory or tactile. We see the features and comprehend the humanity at the same time. Look at the fetus, say the anti-abortionists, and you will see humanity. How long, they ask, can a man turn his head and pretend that he just doesn't see?

. . .

Is there a contradiction in the opponents of abortion appealing to perception when fetuses are normally invisible? Should one not hold that until beings are seen they have not entered the ranks of society? Falling below the threshold of sight, do not fetuses fall below the threshold of humanity? If the central moral transaction is response to the other person, are not fetuses peculiarly weak subjects to elicit our response? These questions pinpoint the principal task of the defenders of the fetus—to make the fetus visible. The task is different only in degree from that assumed by defenders of other persons who have been or are ''overlooked.'' For centuries, color acted as a psychological block to perception, and the blindness induced by color provided a sturdy basis for discrimination. Minorities of various kinds exist today who are ''invisible'' and therefore unlikely to be ''heard'' in the democratic process. Persons literally out of sight of society in prisons and mental institutions are often not ''recognized'' as fellow humans by the world with which they have ''lost touch.'' In each of these instances those who seek to vindicate the rights of the unseen must begin by calling attention to their existence. ''Look'' is the exhortation they address to the callous and the negligent.[14]

Perception of fetuses is possible with not substantially greater effort than that required to pierce the physical or psychological barriers to recognizing other human beings. The main difficulty is everyone's reluctance to accept the extra burdens of care imposed by an expansion of the numbers in whom humanity is recognized. It is generally more convenient to have to consider only one's kin, one's peers, one's country, one's race. Seeing requires personal attention and personal response. The emotion generated by identification with a human form is necessary to overcome the inertia which is protected by a vision restricted to a convenient group. If one is willing to undertake the risk that more will be required in one's action, fetuses may be seen in multiple ways—circumstantially, by the observation of a pregnant woman; photographically, by pictures of life in the womb; scientifically, in accounts written by investigators of prenatal life and child psychologists; visually, by observing a blood transfusion or an abortion while the fetus is alive or by examination of a fetal corpse after death.[15] The proponent of abortion is invited to consider the organism kicking the mother, swimming peacefully in amniotic fluid, responding to the prick of an instrument, being extracted from the womb, sleeping in death. Is the kicker or swimmer similar to him or to her? Is the response to pain like his or hers? Will his or her own face look much different in death?

RESPONSE

Response to the fetus begins with grasp of the data which yield the fetus' structure. That structure is not merely anatomical form; it is dynamic—we apprehend the fetus' origin and end. It is this apprehension which makes response to the nameless fetus different from the conscious analogizing that goes on when we name a cat. Seeing, we are linked to the being in the womb by more than an inventory of shared physical characteristics and by more than a number of made-up psychological characteristics. The weakness of the being as potential recalls our own potential state, the helplessness of the being evokes the human

condition of contingency. We meet another human subject.

Seeing is impossible apart from experience, but experience is the most imprecise of terms. What kind of experience counts, and whose?

. . .

Vicarious experience appears strained to the outer limit when one is asked to consider the experience of the fetus. No one remembers being born, no one knows what it is like to die. Empathy may, however, supply for memory, as it does in other instances when we refer to the experience of infants who cannot speak or to the experience of death by those who cannot speak again. The experience of the fetus is no more beyond our knowledge than the experience of the baby and the experience of dying.

. . .

Another kind of experience is that embedded in law. In Roman law where children generally had little status independent of their parents, the fetus was "a portion of the mother or her viscera." This view persisted in nineteenth century American tort law, Justice Holmes in a leading case describing the fetus as "a part of the body of the mother." In recent years, however, the tort cases have asked, in Justice Bok's phrase, if the fetus is a person; and many courts have replied affirmatively. The change, a striking revolution in torts law, came from the courts incorporating into their thought new biological data on the fetus as a living organism.[16] Evidence on how the fetus is now perceived is also provided by another kind of case where abortion itself is not involved—the interpretation in wills and trusts of gifts to "children" or "issue." In these cases a basic question is, "What is the common understanding of people when they speak of children?" The answer, given repeatedly by American courts, is that "the average testator" speaking of children means to include a being who has been conceived but not born.[17] Free from the distorting pressures of the conflict over abortion, this evidence of the common understanding suggests that social experience has found the fetus to be within the family of man.

. . .

NOTES

1. Judith Thomson, "A Defense of Abortion," *Philosophy & Public Affairs* I (Princeton, N.J.: Princeton University Press, 1971) 48–49, 55–56. [Reprinted above, pp. 199–209]

2. *Depue v. Flateau* 100 Minn. 299, 111 W.W. 1 (1907).

3. American Law Institute, *Restatement of Torts, Second* (1965) sec. 197.

4. Michael Tooley, "Abortion and Infanticide," *Philosophy & Public Affairs* II (Princeton, N.J.: Princeton University Press, 1972) 60–62.

5. See Note, "Constitutional Law: Capital Punishment for Rape Constitutes Cruel and Unusual Punishment When No Life is Taken or Endangered," *Minnesota Law Review* 95 (1971) 56.

6. See Thomson, *op. cit:* "A Defense of Abortion." 59.

7. See my "An Almost Absolute Value in History," Noonan, ed., *The Morality of Abortion* (Cambridge, Mass.: Harvard University Press, 1970) 46–50.

8. To say that the act is in itself good seems to me to be an impossible supposition—there is no human act "in itself" apart from intent. See, for a contrary analysis, Germain Grisez, *Abortion: The Myths, The Realities, and the Arguments* (Washington: Corpus Books, 1970) 329.

9. For a comparable analysis of the use of direct and indirect in constitutional law, see D. J. Farage, "That Which 'Directly' Affects Interstate Commerce," *Dickinson Law Review* XLII (Carlisle, Pa.: Dickinson Law School, 1937) 71.

10. Even Roger Wertheimer, who has made a good explication of the anti-abortion argument from the point of view of one who does not accept it, ends his article by a question-begging device—the burden of proof of fetal humanity, he says, is on the state. Wertheimer, "Understanding the Abortion Argument," *Philosophy & Public Affairs* I (*op. cit.* 1971) 94–95. From the viewpoint of opponents of abortion, his argument may be reshaped: the state has the burden of proving that its actions are legitimate; laws which permit the killing of the fetus seriously threaten human life; they may be sustained only if the state can show that the fetus is not human; and this cannot be done.

11. E.g., my article, "Deciding Who is Human," *Natural Law Forum* XII (South Bend, Ind.: Notre Dame School of Law, 1968) 134–140.

12. Daniel Callahan, *Abortion: Law, Choice, and Morality* (New York: Macmillan, 1970) 430–431.

13. See Enda McDonagh, "The Structure and the Basis of the Moral Experience," *Irish Theological Quarterly* XXXVIII, No. 1 (Maynooth, Ireland: St. Patrick's College, 1971) 3–20.

14. On our complaisance if we cannot see mutilations or the mutilated, David Daube, *Legal Problems in Medical Advance* (Jerusalem, 1971) 19–22. See also the extensive treatment of the meaning of touch in Ashley Montagu, *Touching* (New York: Columbia, 1972).

15. See, e.g., Beth Day and H. M. I. Liley, *Modern Motherhood: Pregnancy, Childbirth, and the Newborn Baby* (1967 ed.) 23–24, 30–31. In the brief [for] the state in *Roe v. Wade,* Supreme Court of the United States, October Term, 1970, number 980, possibly the most effective argument was the photograph of an outstretched fetal hand; it was recognizably a human hand.

16. On this development, see Noonan, ed., *The Morality of Abortion (op. cit.)* 6–7, 226–230; William Prosser, *Handbook of the Law of Torts* (St. Paul: West Publ. Co., 3d ed., 1964) sec. 56; Edwin W. Patterson, *Law in a Scientific Age* (New York: Columbia, 1963) 65.

17. A. James Casner, ed., *American Law of Property* (Boston: Little, Brown, 1952) vol. VII, sec. 22.3; 249; sec. 22, 42, 358.

MARY ANNE WARREN

On the Moral and Legal Status of Abortion

We will be concerned with both the moral status of abortion, which for our purposes we may define as the act which a woman performs in voluntarily terminating, or allowing another person to terminate, her pregnancy, and the legal status which is appropriate for this act. I will argue that, while it is not possible to produce a satisfactory defense of a woman's right to obtain an abortion without showing that a fetus is not a human being, in the morally relevant sense of that term, we ought not to conclude that the difficulties involved in determining whether or not a fetus is human make it

Reprinted from *The Monist,* Vol. 57, No. 1 (January 1973) with the permission of the author and the publisher.

impossible to produce any satisfactory solution to the problem of the moral status of abortion. For it is possible to show that, on the basis of intuitions which we may expect even the opponents of abortion to share, a fetus is not a person, and hence not the sort of entity to which it is proper to ascribe full moral rights.

Of course, while some philosophers would deny the possibility of any such proof,[1] others will deny that there is any need for it, since the moral permissibility of abortion appears to them to be too obvious to require proof. But the inadequacy of this attitude should be evident from the fact that both the friends and the foes of abortion consider their position to be morally self-evident. Because pro-abortionists have never adequately come to grips with the conceptual issues surrounding abortion, most if not all, of the arguments which they advance in opposition to laws restricting access to abortion fail to refute or even weaken the traditional antiabortion argument, i.e., that a fetus is a human being, and therefore abortion is murder.

These arguments are typically of one of two sorts. Either they point to the terrible side effects of the restrictive laws, e.g., the deaths due to illegal abortions, and the fact that it is poor women who suffer the most as a result of these laws, or else they state that to deny a woman access to abortion is to deprive her of her right to control her own body. Unfortunately, however, the fact that restricting access to abortion has tragic side effects does not, in itself, show that the restrictions are unjustified, since murder is wrong regardless of the consequences of prohibiting it; and the appeal to the right to control one's body, which is generally construed as a property right, is at best a rather feeble argument for the permissibility of abortion. Mere ownership does not give me the right to kill innocent people whom I find on my property, and indeed I am apt to be held responsible if such people injure themselves while on my property. It is equally unclear that I have any moral right to expel an innocent person from my property when I know that doing so will result in his death.

Furthermore, it is probably inappropriate to describe a woman's body as her property, since it seems natural to hold that a person is something distinct from her property, but not from her body. Even those who would object to the identification of a person with his body, or with the conjunction of his body and his mind, must admit that it would be very odd to describe, say, breaking a leg, as damaging one's property, and much more appropriate to describe it as injuring one*self*. Thus it is probably a mistake to argue that the right to obtain an abortion is in any way derived from the right to own and regulate property.

But however we wish to construe the right to abortion, we cannot hope to convince those who consider abortion a form of murder of the existence of any such right unless we are able to produce a clear and convincing refutation of the traditional antiabortion argument, and this has not, to my knowledge, been done. With respect to the two most vital issues which that argument involves, i.e., the humanity of the fetus and its implication for the moral status of abortion, confusion has prevailed on both sides of the dispute.

Thus, both proabortionists and antiabortionists have tended to abstract the question of whether abortion is wrong to that of whether it is wrong to destroy a fetus, just as though the rights of another person were not necessarily involved. This mistaken abstraction has led to the almost universal assumption that if a fetus is a human being, with a right to life, then it follows immediately that abortion is wrong (except perhaps when necessary to save the woman's life), and that it ought to be prohibited. It has also been generally assumed that unless the question about the status of the fetus is answered, the moral status of abortion cannot possibly be determined.

Two recent papers, one by B. A. Brody,[2] and one by Judith Thomson,[3] have attempted to settle the question of whether abortion ought to be prohibited apart from the question of whether or not the fetus is human. Brody examines the possibility that the following two statements are compatible: (1) that abortion is the taking of innocent human life, and therefore wrong; and (2) that nevertheless it ought not to be prohibited by law, at least under the present circumstances.[4] Not surprisingly, Brody finds it impossible to reconcile these two statements, since, as he rightly argues, none of the unfortunate side effects of the prohibition of abortion is bad enough to justify legalizing the *wrongful* taking of human life. He is mistaken, however, in concluding that the incompatibility of (1) and (2), in itself, shows that "the legal problem about abortion cannot be resolved independently of the status of the fetus problem" (p. 369).

What Brody fails to realize is that (1) embodies the questionable assumption that if a fetus is a human being, then of course abortion is morally wrong, and that an attack on *this* assumption is more promising, as a way of reconciling the humanity of the fetus with the claim that laws prohibiting abortion are unjustified, than is an attack on the assumption that if abortion is the wrongful killing of innocent human beings then it ought to be prohibited. He thus overlooks the possibility that a fetus may have a right to life and abortion still be morally permissible, in that the right of a woman to terminate an unwanted pregnancy might override the right of the fetus to be kept alive. The immorality of abortion is no more demonstrated by the humanity of the fetus, in itself, than the immorality of killing in self-defense is demonstrated by the fact that the assailant is a human being. Neither is it demonstrated by the *innocence* of the fetus, since there may be situations in which the killing of innocent human beings is justified.

It is perhaps not surprising that Brody fails to spot this assumption, since it has been accepted with little or no argument by nearly everyone who has written on the morality of abortion. John Noonan is correct in saying that "the fundamental question in the long history of abortion is, How do you determine the humanity of a being?"[5] He summarizes his own antiabortion argument, which is a version of the official position of the Catholic Church, as follows:

. . . it is wrong to kill humans, however poor, weak, defenseless, and lacking in opportunity to develop their potential they may be. It is therefore morally wrong to kill Biafrans. Similarly, it is morally wrong to kill embryos.[6]

Noonan bases his claim that fetuses are human upon what he calls the theologians' criterion of humanity: that whoever is conceived of human beings is human. But although he argues at length for the appropriateness of this criterion, he never questions the assumption that if a fetus is human then abortion is wrong for exactly the same reason that murder is wrong.

Judith Thomson is, in fact, the only writer I am aware of who has seriously questioned this assumption; she has argued that, even if we grant the antiabortionist his claim that a fetus is a human being, with the same right to life as any other human being, we can still demonstrate that, in at least some and perhaps most cases, a woman is under no moral obligation to complete an unwanted pregnancy.[7] Her argument is worth examining, since if it holds up it may enable us to establish the moral permissibility of abortion without becoming involved in problems about what entitles an entity to be considered human, and accorded full moral rights. To be able to do this would be a great gain in the power and simplicity of the pro-abortion position, since, although I will argue that these problems can be solved at least as decisively as can any other moral problem, we should certainly be pleased to be able to avoid having to solve them as part of the justification of abortion.

On the other hand, even if Thomson's argument does not hold up, her insight, i.e., that it requires *argument* to show that if fetuses are human then abortion is properly classified as murder, is an extremely valuable one. The assumption she attacks is particularly invidious, for it amounts to the decision that it is appropriate, in deciding the moral status of abortion, to leave the rights of the pregnant woman out of consideration entirely, except possibly when her life is threatened. Obviously, this will not do; determining what moral rights, if any, a fetus possesses is only the first step in determining the moral status of abortion. Step two, which is at least equally essential, is finding a just solution to the conflict between whatever rights the fetus may have, and the rights of the woman who is unwillingly pregnant. While the historical error has been to pay far too little attention to the second step, Ms. Thomson's suggestion is that if we look at the second step first we may find that a woman has a right to obtain an abortion *regardless* of what rights the fetus has.

Our own inquiry will also have two stages. In Section I, we will consider whether or not it is possible to establish that abortion is morally permissible even on the assumption that a fetus is an entity with a full-fledged right to life. I will argue that in fact this cannot be established, at least not with the conclusiveness which is essential to our hopes of convincing those who are skeptical about the morality of abortion, and that we therefore cannot avoid dealing with the question of whether or not a fetus really does have the same right to life as a (more fully developed) human beng.

In Section II, I will propose an answer to this question, namely, that a fetus cannot be considered a member of the moral community, the set of beings with full and equal moral rights, for the simple reason that it is not a person, and that it is personhood, and not genetic humanity, i.e., humanity as defined by Noonan, which is the basis for membership in this community. I will argue that a fetus, whatever its stage of development, satisfies none of the basic criteria of personhood, and is not even enough *like* a person to be accorded even some of the same rights on the basis of this resemblance. Nor, as we will see, is a fetus's *potential* personhood a threat to the morality of abortion, since, whatever the rights of potential people may be, they are invariably overridden in any conflict with the moral rights of actual people.

I

We turn now to Professor Thomson's case for the claim that even if a fetus has full moral rights, abortion is still morally permissible, at least sometimes, and for some reasons other than to save the woman's life. Her argument is based upon a clever, but I think faulty, analogy. She asks us to picture ourselves waking up one day, in bed with a famous violinist. Imagine that you have been kidnapped, and your bloodstream hooked up to that of the violinist, who happens to have an ailment which will certainly kill him unless he is permitted to share your kidneys for a period of nine months. No one else can save him, since you alone have the right type of blood. He will be unconscious all that time, and you will have to stay in bed with him, but after the nine months are over he may be unplugged, completely cured, that is provided that you have cooperated.

Now then, she continues, what are your obligations in this situation? The antiabortionist, if he is consistent, will have to say that you are obligated to stay in bed with the violinist: for all people have a right to life, and violinists are people, and therefore it would be murder for you to disconnect yourself from him and let him die (p. 49). But this is outrageous, and so there must be something wrong with the same argument when it is applied to abortion. It would certainly be commendable of you to agree to save the violinist, but it is absurd to suggest that your refusal to do so would be murder. His right to life does not obligate you to do whatever is required to keep him alive; nor does it justify anyone else in forcing you to do so. A law which required you to stay in bed with the violinist would clearly be an unjust law, since it is no proper function of the law to force unwilling people to make huge sacrifices for the sake of other people toward whom they have no such prior obligation.

Thomson concludes that, if this analogy is an apt one, then we can grant the antiabortionist his claim that a fetus is a human being, and still hold that it is at least sometimes the case that a pregnant woman has the right to refuse to be a Good Samaritan towards the fetus, i.e., to obtain an abortion. For there is a great gap between the claim that x has a right to life, and the claim that y is obligated to do whatever is necessary to keep x alive, let alone that he ought to be forced to do so. It is y's duty to keep x alive only if he has somehow contracted a *special* obligation to do so; and a woman who is unwillingly pregnant, e.g., who was raped, has done nothing which obligates her to make the enormous sacrifice which is necessary to preserve the conceptus.

This argument is initially quite plausible, and in the extreme case of pregnancy due to rape it is probably conclusive. Difficulties arise, however, when we try to specify more exactly the range of cases in which abortion is clearly justifiable even on the assumption that the fetus is human. Professor Thomson considers it a virtue of her argument that it does not enable us to conclude that abortion is *always* permissible. It would, she says, be "indecent" for a woman in her seventh month to obtain an abortion just to avoid having to postpone a trip to Europe. On the other hand, her argument enables us to see that "a sick and desperately frightened schoolgirl pregnant due to rape may *of course* choose abortion, and that any law which rules this out is an insane law" (p. 65). So far, so good; but what are we to say about the woman who becomes pregnant not through rape but as a result of her own carelessness, or because of contraceptive failure, or who gets pregnant intentionally and then changes her mind about wanting a child? With respect to such cases, the violinist analogy is of much less use to the defender of the woman's right to obtain an abortion.

Indeed, the choice of a pregnancy due to rape, as an example of a case in which abortion is permissible even if a fetus is considered a human being, is extremely significant; for it is only in the case of pregnancy due to rape that the woman's situation is adequately analogous to the violinist case for our intuitions about the latter to transfer convincingly. The crucial difference between a pregnancy due to rape and the *normal* case of an unwanted pregnancy is that in the normal case we cannot claim that the woman is in no way responsible for her predicament; she could have remained chaste, or taken her pills more faithfully, or abstained on dangerous days, and so on. If on the other hand, you are kidnapped by strangers, and hooked up to a strange violinist, then you are free of any shred of responsibility for the sit-

uation, on the basis of which it would be argued that you are obligated to keep the violinist alive. Only when her pregnancy is due to rape is a woman clearly just as nonresponsible.[8]

Consequently, there is room for the anti-abortionist to argue that in the normal case of unwanted pregnancy a woman has, by her own actions, assumed responsibility for the fetus. For if *x* behaves in a way which he could have avoided, and which he knows involves, let us say, a 1 percent chance of bringing into existence a human being, with a right to life, and does so knowing that if this should happen then that human being will perish unless *x* does certain things to keep him alive, then it is by no means clear that when it does happen *x* is free of any obligation to what he knew in advance would be required to keep that human being alive.

The plausibility of such an argument is enough to show that the Thomson analogy can provide a clear and persuasive defense of a woman's right to obtain an abortion only with respect to those cases in which the woman is in no way responsible for her pregnancy, e.g., where it is due to rape. In all other cases, we would almost certainly conclude that it was necessary to look carefully at the particular circumstances in order to determine the extent of the woman's responsibility, and hence the extent of her obligation. This is an extremely unsatisfactory outcome, from the viewpoint of the opponents of restrictive abortion laws, most of whom are convinced that a woman has a right to obtain an abortion regardless of how and why she got pregnant.

Of course a supporter of the violinist analogy might point out that it is absurd to suggest that forgetting her pill one day might be sufficient to obligate a woman to complete an unwanted pregnancy. And indeed it *is* absurd to suggest this. As we will see, the moral right to obtain an abortion is not in the least dependent upon the extent to which the woman is responsible for her pregnancy. But unfortunately, once we allow the assumption that a fetus has full moral rights, we cannot avoid taking this absurd suggestion seriously. Perhaps we can make this point more clear by altering the violinist story just enough to make it more analogous to a normal unwanted pregnancy and less to a pregnancy due to rape, and then seeing whether it is still obvious that you are not obligated to stay in bed with the fellow.

Suppose, then, that violinists are peculiarly prone to the sort of illness the only cure for which is the use of someone else's bloodstream for nine months, and that because of this there has been formed a society of music lovers who agree that whenever a violinist is stricken they will draw lots and the loser will, by some means, be made the one and only person capable of saving him. Now then, would you be obligated to cooperate in curing the violinist if you had voluntarily joined this society, knowing the possible consequences, and then your name had been drawn and you had been kidnapped? Admittedly, you did not promise ahead of time that you would, but you did deliberately place yourself in a position in which it might happen that a human life would be lost if you did not. Surely this is at least a prima facie reason for supposing that you have an obligation to stay in bed with the violinist. Suppose that you had gotten your name drawn deliberately; surely *that* would be quite a strong reason for thinking that you had such an obligation.

It might be suggested that there is one important disanalogy between the modified violinist case and the case of an unwanted pregnancy, which makes the woman's responsibility significantly less, namely, the fact that the fetus *comes into existence* as the result of the result of the woman's actions. This fact might give her a right to refuse to keep it alive, whereas she would not have had this right had it existed previously, independently, and then as a result of her actions become dependent upon her for its survival.

My own intuition, however, is that x has no more right to bring into existence, either deliberately or as a foreseeable result of actions he could have avoided, a being with full moral rights (y), and then refuse to do what he knew

beforehand would be required to keep that being alive, than he has to enter into an agreement with an existing person, whereby he may be called upon to save that person's life, and then refuse to do so when so called upon. Thus, x's responsibility for y's existence does not seem to lessen his obligation to keep y alive, if he is also responsible for y's being in a situation in which only he can save him.

Whether or not this intuition is entirely correct, it brings us back once again to the conclusion that once we allow the assumption that a fetus has full moral rights it becomes an extremely complex and difficult question whether and when abortion is justifiable. Thus the Thomson analogy cannot help us produce a clear and persuasive proof of the moral permissibility of abortion. Nor will the opponents of the restrictive laws thank us for anything less; for their conviction (for the most part) is that abortion is obviously *not* a morally serious and extremely unfortunate, even though sometimes justified act, comparable to killing in self-defense or to letting the violinist die, but rather is closer to being a morally neutral act, like cutting one's hair.

The basis of this conviction, I believe, is the realization that a fetus is not a person, and thus does not have a full-fledged right to life. Perhaps the reason why this claim has been so inadequately defended is that it seems self-evident to those who accept it. And so it is, insofar as it follows from what I take to be perfectly obvious claims about the nature of personhood, and about the proper grounds for ascribing moral rights, claims which ought, indeed, to be obvious to both the friends and foes of abortion. Nevertheless, it is worth examining these claims, and showing how they demonstrate the moral innocuousness of abortion, since this apparently has not been adequately done before.

II

The question which we must answer in order to produce a satisfactory solution to the problem of the moral status of abortion is this: How are we to define the moral community, the set of beings with full and equal moral rights, such that we can decide whether a human fetus is a member of this community or not? What sort of entity, exactly, has the inalienable rights to life, liberty, and the pursuit of happiness? Jefferson attributed these rights to all *men,* and it may or may not be fair to suggest that he intended to attribute them *only* to men. Perhaps he ought have attributed them to all human beings. If so, then we arrive, first, at Noonan's problem of defining what makes a being human, and, second, at the equally vital question which Noonan does not consider, namely, What reason is there for identifying the moral community with the set of all human beings, in whatever way we have chosen to define that term?

1. ON THE DEFINITION OF 'HUMAN'

One reason why this vital second question is so frequently overlooked in the debate over the moral status of abortion is that the term 'human' has two distinct, but not often distinguished, senses. This fact results in a slide of meaning, which serves to conceal the fallaciousness of the traditional argument that since (1) it is wrong to kill innocent human beings, and (2) fetuses are innocent human beings, then (3) it is wrong to kill fetuses. For if 'human' is used in the same sense in both (1) and (2) then, whichever of the two senses is meant, one of these premises is question-begging. And if it is used in two different senses then of course the conclusion doesn't follow.

Thus, (1) is a self-evident moral truth,[9] and avoids begging the question about abortion, only if 'human being' is used to mean something like 'a full-fledged member of the moral community.' (It may or may not also be meant to refer exclusively to members of the species *Homo sapiens*.) We may call this the *moral* sense of 'human.' It is not to be confused with what we will call the *genetic* sense, i.e., the sense in which *any* member of the species is a human being, and no member of any other species could be. If (1) is acceptable only if the moral sense is intended, (2) is non-question-begging only if what is intended is the genetic sense.

In "Deciding Who is Human," Noonan argues for the classification of fetuses with human beings by pointing to the presence of the full genetic code, and the potential capacity for

rational thought (p. 135). It is clear that what he needs to show, for his version of the traditional argument to be valid, is that fetuses are human in the moral sense, the sense in which it is analytically true that all human beings have full moral rights. But, in the absence of any argument showing that whatever is genetically human is also morally human, and he gives none, nothing more than genetic humanity can be demonstrated by the presence of the human genetic code. And, as we will see, the *potential* capacity for rational thought can at most show that an entity has the potential for *becoming* human in the moral sense.

2. DEFINING THE MORAL COMMUNITY

Can it be established that genetic humanity is sufficient for moral humanity? I think that there are very good reasons for not defining the moral community in this way. I would like to suggest an alternative way of defining the moral community, which I will argue for only to the extent of explaining why it is, or should be, self-evident. The suggestion is simply that the moral community consists of all and only *people,* rather than all and only human beings;[10] and probably the best way of demonstrating its self-evidence is by considering the concept of personhood, to see what sorts of entity are and are not persons, and what the decision that a being is or is not a person implies about its moral rights.

What characteristics entitle an entity to be considered a person? This is obviously not the place to attempt a complete analysis of the concept of personhood, but we do not need such a fully adequate analysis just to determine whether and why a fetus is or isn't a person. All we need is a rough and approximate list of the most basic criteria of personhood, and some idea of which, or how many, of these an entity must satisfy in order to properly be considered a person.

In searching for such criteria, it is useful to look beyond the set of people with whom we are acquainted, and ask how we would decide whether a totally alien being was a person or not. (For we have no right to assume that genetic humanity is necessary for personhood.) Imagine a space traveler who lands on an unknown planet and encounters a race of beings utterly unlike any he has ever seen or heard of. If he wants to be sure of behaving morally toward these beings, he has to somehow decide whether they are people, and hence have full moral rights, or whether they are the sort of thing which he need not feel guilty about treating as, for example, a source of food.

How should he go about making this decision? If he has some anthropological background, he might look for such things as religion, art, and the manufacturing of tools, weapons, or shelters, since these factors have been used to distinguish our human from our prehuman acestors, in what seems to be closer to the moral than the genetic sense of 'human.' And no doubt he would be right to consider the presence of such factors as good evidence that the alien beings were people, and morally human. It would, however, be overly anthropocentric of him to take the absence of these things as adequate evidence that they were not, since we can imagine people who have progressed beyond, or evolved without ever developing, these cultural characteristics.

I suggest that the traits which are most central to the concept of personhood, or humanity in the moral sense, are, very roughly, the following:

1. consciousness (of objects and events external and/or internal to the being), and in particular the capacity to feel pain;

2. reasoning (the *developed* capacity to solve new and relatively complex problems);

3. self-motivated activity (activity which is relatively independent of either genetic or direct external control);

4. the capacity to communicate, by whatever means, messages of an indefinite variety of types, that is, not just with an indefinite number of possible contents, but on indefinitely many possible topics;

5. the presence of self-concepts, and self-awareness, either individual or racial, or both.

Admittedly, there are apt to be a great many problems involved in formulating precise definitions of these criteria, let alone in developing universally valid behavioral criteria for deciding when they apply. But I will assume that both we and our explorer know approximately what (1)–(5) mean, and that he is also able to determine whether or not they apply. How, then, should he use his findings to decide whether or not the alien beings are people? We needn't suppose that an entity must have *all* of these attributes to be properly considered a person; (1) and (2) alone may well be sufficient for personhood, and quite probably (1)–(3) are sufficient. Neither do we need to insist that any one of these criteria is *necessary* for personhood, although once again (1) and (2) look like fairly good candidates for necessary conditions, as does (3), if 'activity' is construed so as to include the activity of reasoning.

All we need to claim, to demonstrate that a fetus is not a person, is that any being which satisfies *none* of (1)–(5) is certainly not a person. I consider this claim to be so obvious that I think anyone who denied it, and claimed that a being which satisfied none of (1)–(5) was a person all the same, would thereby demonstrate that he had no notion at all of what a person is—perhaps because he had confused the concept of a person with that of genetic humanity. If the opponents of abortion were to deny the appropriateness of these five criteria, I do not know what further arguments would convince them. We would probably have to admit that our conceptual schemes were indeed irreconcilably different, and that our dispute could not be settled objectively.

I do not expect this to happen, however, since I think that the concept of a person is one which is very nearly universal (to people), and that it is common to both proabortionists and antiabortionists, even though neither group has fully realized the relevance of this concept to the resolution of their dispute. Furthermore, I think that on reflection even the antiabortionists ought to agree not only that (1)–(5) are central to the concept of personhood, but also that it is a part of this concept that all and only people have full moral rights. The concept of a person is in part a moral concept; once we have admitted that x is a person we have recognized, even if we have not agreed to respect, *x*'s right to be treated as a member of the moral community. It is true that the claim that *x* is a *human being* is more commonly voiced as part of an appeal to treat *x* decently than is the claim that *x* is a person, but this is either because 'human being' is here used in the sense which implies personhood, or because the genetic and moral senses of 'human' have been confused.

Now if (1)–(5) are indeed the primary criteria of personhood, then it is clear that genetic humanity is neither necessary nor sufficient for establishing that an entity is a person. Some human beings are not people, and there may well be people who are not human beings. A man or woman whose consciousness has been permanently obliterated but who remains alive is a human being which is no longer a person; defective human beings, with no appreciable mental capacity, are not and presumably never will be people; and a fetus is a human being which is not yet a person, and which therefore cannot coherently be said to have full moral rights. Citizens of the next century should be prepared to recognize highly advanced, self-aware robots or computers, should such be developed, and intelligent inhabitants of other worlds, should such be found, as people in the fullest sense, and to respect their moral rights. But to ascribe full moral rights to an entity which is not a person is as absurd as to ascribe moral obligations and responsibilities to such an entity.

3. FETAL DEVELOPMENT AND THE RIGHT TO LIFE

Two problems arise in the application of these suggestions for the definition of the moral community to the determination of the precise moral status of a human fetus. Given that the paradigm example of a person is a normal adult being, then (1) How like this paradigm, in particular how far advanced since conception, does a human being need to be before it begins to have a right to life by virtue, not of being fully a person as of yet, but of being *like* a person? and (2) To what extent, if any, does the fact that a fetus has the *potential* for becoming a person endow it with some of the same rights? Each of these questions requires some comment.

In answering the first question, we need not attempt a detailed consideration of the moral rights of organisms which are not developed enough, aware enough, intelligent enough, etc., to be considered people, but which resemble people in some respects. It does seem reasonable to suggest that the more like a person, in the relevant respects, a being is, the stronger is the case for regarding it as having a right to life, and indeed the stronger its right to life is. Thus we ought to take seriously the suggestion that, insofar as "the human individual develops biologically in a continuous fashion . . . the rights of a human person might develop in the same way."[11] But we must keep in mind that the attributes which are relevant in determining whether or not an entity is enough like a person to be regarded as having some of the same moral rights are no different from those which are relevant to determining whether or not it is fully a person—i.e., are no different from (1)–(5)—and that being genetically human, or having recognizably human facial and other physical features, or detectable brain activity, or the capacity to survive outside the uterus, are simply not among these relevant attributes.

Thus it is clear that even though a seven- or eight-month fetus has features which make it apt to arouse in us almost the same powerful protective instinct as is commonly aroused by a small infant, nevertheless it is not significantly more personlike than is a very small embryo. It is *somewhat* more personlike; it can apparently feel and respond to pain, and it may even have a rudimentary form of consciousness, insofar as its brain is quite active. Nevertheless, it seems safe to say that it is not fully conscious, in the way that an infant of a few months is, and that it cannot reason, or communicate messages of indefinitely many sorts, does not engage in self-motivated activity, and has no self-awareness. Thus, in the *relevant* respects, a fetus, even a fully developed one, is considerably less personlike than is the average mature mammal, indeed the average fish. And I think that a rational person must conclude that if the right to life of a fetus is to be based upon its resemblance to a person, then it cannot be said to have any more right to life than, let us say, a newborn guppy (which also seems to be capable of feeling pain), and that a right of that magnitude could never override a woman's right to obtain an abortion, at any stage of her pregnancy.

There may, of course, be other arguments in favor of placing legal limits upon the stage of pregnancy in which an abortion may be performed. Given the relative safety of the new techniques of artificially inducing labor during the third trimester, the danger to the woman's life or health is no longer such an argument. Neither is the fact that people tend to respond to the thought of abortion in the later stages of pregnancy with emotional repulsion, since mere emotional responses cannot take the place of moral reasoning in determining what ought to be permitted. Nor, finally, is the frequently heard argument that legalizing abortion, especially late in the pregnancy, may erode the level of respect for human life, leading, perhaps, to an increase in unjustified euthanasia and other crimes. For this threat, if it is a threat, can be better met by educating people to the kinds of moral distinctions which we are making here than by limiting access to abortion (which limitation may, in its disregard for the rights of women, be just as damaging to the level of respect for human rights).

Thus, since the fact that even a fully developed fetus is not personlike enough to have any significant right to life on the basis of its personlikeness shows that no legal restrictions upon the stage of pregnancy in which an abortion may be performed can be justified on the grounds that we should protect the rights of the older fetus; and since there is no other apparent justification for such restrictions, we may conclude that they are entirely unjustified. Whether or not it would be *indecent* (whatever that means) for a woman in her seventh month to obtain an abortion just to avoid having to postpone a trip to Europe, it would not, in itself, be *immoral,* and therefore it ought to be permitted.

We have seen that a fetus does not resemble a person in any way which can support the claim that it has even some of the same rights. But what about its *potential,* the fact that if nurtured and allowed to develop naturally it will very probably become a person? Doesn't that alone give it at least some right to life? It is hard to deny that the fact that an entity is a potential person is a strong prima facie reason for not destroying it; but we need not conclude from this that a potential person has a right to life, by virtue of that potential. It may be that our feeling that it is better, other things being equal, not to destroy a potential person is better explained by the fact that potential people are still (felt to be) an invaluable resource, not to be lightly squandered. Surely, if every speck of dust were a potential person, we would be much less apt to conclude that every potential person has a right to become actual.

Still, we do not need to insist that a potential person has no right to life whatever. There may well be something immoral, and not just imprudent, about wantonly destroying potential people, when doing so isn't necessary to protect anyone's rights. But even if a potential person does have some prima facie right to life, such a right could not possibly outweigh the right of a woman to obtain an abortion, since the rights of any actual person invariably outweigh those of any potential person, whenever the two conflict. Since this may not be immediately obvious in the case of a human fetus, let us look at another case.

Suppose that our space explorer falls into the hands of an alien culture, whose scientists decide to create a few hundred thousand or more human beings, by breaking his body into its component cells, and using these to create fully developed human beings, with, of course, his genetic code. We may imagine that each of these newly created men will have all of the original man's abilities, skills, knowledge, and so on, and also have an individual self-concept, in short that each of them will be a bona fide (though hardly unique) person. Imagine that the whole project will take only seconds, and that its chances of success are extremely high, and that our explorer knows all of this, and also knows that these people will be treated fairly. I maintain that in such a situation he would have every right to escape if he could, and thus to deprive all of these potential people of their potential lives; for his right to life outweighs all of theirs together, in spite of the fact that they are all genetically human, all innocent, and all have a very high probability of becoming people very soon, if only he refrains from acting.

Indeed, I think he would have a right to escape even if it were not his life which the alien scientists planned to take, but only a year of his freedom, or, indeed, only a day. Nor would he be obligated to stay if he had gotten captured (thus bringing all these people-potentials into existence) because of his own carelessness, or even if he had done so deliberately, knowing the consequences. Regardless of how he got captured, he is not morally obligated to remain in captivity for *any* period of time for the sake of permitting any number of potential people to come into actuality, so great is the margin by which one actual person's right to liberty outweighs whatever right to life even a hundred thousand potential people have. And it seems reasonable to conclude that the rights of a woman will outweigh by a similar margin whatever right to life a fetus may have by virtue of its potential personhood.

Thus, neither a fetus's resemblance to a person, nor its potential for becoming a person provides any basis whatever for the claim that it has any significant right to life. Consequently, a woman's right to protect her health, happiness, freedom, and even her life,[12] by terminating an unwanted pregnancy, will always override whatever right to life it may be appropriate to ascribe to a fetus, even a fully developed one. And thus, in the absence of any overwhelming social need for every possible child, the laws which restrict the right to obtain an abortion, or limit the period of pregnancy during which an abortion may be performed, are a wholly unjustified violation of a woman's most basic moral and constitutional rights.[13]

Postscript on Infanticide

Since the publication of this article, many people have written to point out that my argument appears to justify not only abortion, but infanticide as well. For a new-born infant is not significantly more person-like than an advanced fetus, and consequently it would seem that if the destruction of the latter is permissible so too must be that of the former. Inasmuch as most people, regardless of how they feel about the morality of abortion, consider infanticide a form of murder, this might appear to represent a serious flaw in my argument.

Now, if I am right in holding that it is only people who have a full-fledged right to life, and who can be murdered, and if the criteria of personhood are as I have described them, then it obviously follows that killing a new-born infant isn't murder. It does *not* follow, however, that infanticide is permissible, for two reasons. In the first place, it would be wrong, at least in this country and in this period of history, and other things being equal, to kill a new-born infant, because even if its parents do not want it and would not suffer from its destruction, there are other people who would like to have it, and would, in all probability, be deprived of a great deal of pleasure by its destruction. Thus, infanticide is wrong for reasons analogous to those which make it wrong to wantonly destroy natural resources, or great works of art.

Secondly, most people, at least in this country, value infants and would much prefer that they be preserved, even if foster parents are not immediately available. Most of us would rather be taxed to support orphanages than allow unwanted infants to be destroyed. So long as there are people who want an infant preserved, and who are willing and able to provide the means of caring for it, under reasonably humane conditions, it is, *ceteris paribus,* wrong to destroy it.

But, it might be replied, if this argument shows that infanticide is wrong, at least at this time and in this country, doesn't it also show that abortion is wrong? After all, many people value fetuses, are disturbed by their destruction, and would much prefer that they be preserved, even at some cost to themselves. Furthermore, as a potential source of pleasure to some foster family, a fetus is just as valuable as an infant. There is, however, a crucial difference between the two cases: so long as the fetus is unborn, its preservation, contrary to the wishes of the pregnant woman, violates her rights to freedom, happiness, and self-determination. Her rights override the rights of those who would like the fetus preserved, just as if someone's life or limb is threatened by a wild animal, his right to protect himself by destroying the animal overrides the rights of those who would prefer that the animal not be harmed.

The minute the infant is born, however, its preservation no longer violates any of its mother's rights, even if she wants it destroyed, because she is free to put it up for adoption. Consequently, while the moment of birth does not mark any sharp discontinuity in the degree to which an infant possesses the right to life, it does mark the end of its mother's right to determine its fate. Indeed, if abortion could be performed without killing the fetus, she would never possess the right to have the fetus destroyed, for the same reasons that she has no right to have an infant destroyed.

On the other hand, it follows from my argument that when an unwanted or defective infant is born into a society which cannot afford and/or is not willing to care for it, then its destruction is permissible. This conclusion will, no doubt, strike many people as heartless and immoral; but remember that the very existence of people who feel this way, and who are willing and able to provide care for unwanted infants, is reason enough to conclude that they should be preserved.

NOTES

1. For example, Roger Wertheimer, who in "Understanding the Abortion Argument" *(Philosophy and Public Affairs,* 1, No. 1 [Fall, 1971], 67–95), argues that the problem of the moral status of abortion is insoluble, in that the dispute over the status of the fetus is not a question of fact at all, but only a question of how one responds to the facts.

2. B. A. Brody, "Abortion and the Law," *The Journal of Philosophy,* 68, No. 12 (June 17, 1971), 357–69.

3. Judith Thomson, "A Defense of Abortion," *Philosophy and Public Affairs,* 1, No. 1 (Fall, 1971), 47–66.

4. I have abbreviated these statements somewhat, but not in a way which affects the argument.

5. John Noonan, "Abortion and the Catholic Church: A Summary History," *Natural Law Forum,* 12 (1967), 125.

6. John Noonan, "Deciding Who is Human," *Natural Law Forum,* 13 (1968), 134.

7. "A Defense of Abortion."

8. We may safely ignore the fact that she might have avoided getting raped, e.g., by carrying a gun, since by similar means you might likewise have avoided getting kidnapped, and in neither case does the victim's failure to take all possible precautions against a highly unlikely event (as opposed to reasonable precautions against a rather likely event) mean that he is morally responsible for what happens.

9. Of course, the principle that it is (always) wrong to kill innocent human beings is in need of many other modifications, e.g., that it may be permissible to do so to save a greater number of other innocent human beings, but we may safely ignore these complications here.

10. From here on, we will use 'human' to mean genetically human, since the moral sense seems closely connected to, and perhaps derived from, the assumption that genetic humanity is sufficient for membership in the moral community.

11. Thomas L. Hayes, "A Biological View," *Commonweal,* 85 (March 17, 1967), 677–78; quoted by Daniel Callahan, in *Abortion, Law, Choice, and Morality* (London: Macmillan & Co., 1970).

12. That is, insofar as the death rate, for the woman, is higher for childbirth than for early abortion.

13. My thanks to the following people, who were kind enough to read and criticize an earlier version of this paper: Herbert Gold, Gene Glass, Anne Lauterbach, Judith Thomson, Mary Mothersill, and Timothy Binkley.

BARUCH BRODY

On the Humanity of the Foetus

In earlier essays,[1] I have argued that if there is some point in the development of the foetus from which time on it is a living human being with all the rights of such an entity, then it would be wrong (except in one special case) to abort the foetus even to save the life of the mother, and then there should be strong laws prohibiting such abortions. In neither of those essays did I consider the question as to whether there is such a point, so I should like, in this essay, to outline an approach to finding the answer to that question.

I

Moral philosophers are in definite disagreement about this issue. Among positions as to when the foetus becomes a living human being with all the rights of such an entity are the claims that it does so at the moment of conception, at the time (around the seventh or eighth day) at which segmentation, if it is to take place, takes place, at the time (around the end of the sixth week) at which foetal brain activity commences, at the moment (sometime between the thirteenth and twentieth week) of quickening when the mother begins to feel the movements of the foetus, at the time (around the twenty-fourth week) at which the foetus becomes viable, i.e., has reasonable chance of survival if born, and at the moment of birth.

It is difficult to see how one is to decide between these conflicting claims. The trouble is not merely that there are conflicting claims; the trouble is that the proponents of each of these claims seem to have somewhat persuasive arguments for their claims. Let us begin, therefore, by trying to understand each of these positions by looking at the arguments offered for them by their adherents.

The following seem to be the major reasons for supposing that the foetus becomes a living

Reprinted with permission of the publisher from *Abortion: Pro and Con,* edited by Robert L. Perkins (Cambridge, Mass.: Schenkman Publishing Co., Inc., 1974).

human being with all the rights that such an entity normally has at the moment of conception:

(1) At the moment of conception, the foetus is biologically determined by its genetic code. It is, from that point on, an individual unique creature, and everything that happens to it after that point is merely an unfolding of its unique selfhood. As Paul Ramsey[2] put it:

Thus it might be said that in all essential respects the individual is whoever he is going to become from the moment of impregnation. He already is this while not knowing this or anything else. Therefore, his subsequent development cannot be described as becoming something he is not now. It can only be described as a process of achieving, a process of becoming the one he already is. Genetics teaches us that we were from the beginning what we essentially still are in every cell and in every generally human attribute and in every individual attribute.

(2) Until the moment of conception, the likelihood of whatever is present (the spermatozoa, the ova) developing into a clear-cut living human being is very small. But once conception has taken place, the resulting fertilized cell has a very high probability of developing into a clear-cut living human being. Indeed, four out of five of these entities do survive to birth. So these new entities, as opposed to the spermatozoa and ova, do have human right to life. John Noonan, the leading advocate of this argument, put it[3] as follows:

. . . part of the business of a moralist is drawing lines. One evidence of the nonarbitrary character of the line drawn is the difference of probabilities on either side of it. If a spermatozoon is destroyed, one destroys a being which had a chance of far less than 1 in 200 million of developing into a reasoned being, possessed of the genetic code, a heart and other organs, and capable of pain. If a fetus is destroyed, one destroys a being already possessed of the genetic code, organs, and sensitivity to pain, and one which had an 80 percent chance of developing further into a baby outside the womb, who, in time, would reason.

(3) There is a continuity of development from the moment of conception on. There are constant changes in the foetal condition; the foetus is constantly acquiring new structures and characteristics, but there is no one stage which is radically different from any other. Since that is so, there is no one stage in the process of foetal development, after the moment of conception, which could plausibly be picked out as the moment at which the foetus becomes a living human being. The moment of conception is, however, different in this respect. It marks the beginning of this continuous process of development and introduces something new which is radically discontinuous with what has come before it. Therefore, the moment of conception, and only it, is a plausible candidate for being that moment at which the foetus becomes a living human being. Roger Wertheimer (who is not, himself, an advocate of this position) summarized this argument[4] very well as follows:

. . . going back stage by stage from the infant to the zygote, one will not find any differences between successive stages significant enough to bear the enormous moral burden of allowing wholesale slaughter at the earlier stage while categorically denying that permission at the next stage.

In order to understand the second position, the position that the foetus becomes a living human being at that moment at which, if it is to take place, segmentation takes place, it is necessary to remind ourselves of one or two key points about early foetal development. In a case in which there are identical twins, a primitive streak across the blastocyst signals the separation of the two twins. This occurs about the seventh day after fertilization. Although it occurs around the same time as implantation, it is an entirely separate process. And, of course, it is only a process that occurs when there are identical twins.

Now the argument for treating the foetus as a living human being only from this point on is really very simple. The individual in question only comes into existence, as a unique individual, at this point. Until then, for all we know, there may be two entities in the blastocyst.

Paul Ramsey, the first one to raise this argument (which we shall label argument[4]), put it as follows.[5]

It might be asserted that it is at the time of segmentation, not earlier, that life comes to be the individual human being it is thereafter to be . . . If there is a moment in the development of these nascent lives of ours subsequent to fertilization and prior to birth (or graduation from college) at which it would be reasonable to believe that a human life begins and therefore begins to be inviolate, that moment is arguably at the stage when segmentation may or may not take place.

The next three positions to be considered (the moment at which foetal brain activity begins, the moment of quickening, and the moment of viability), all share in common two basic ideas, the idea that the foetus does not become human until some point at which it has far more of the abilities and structures of a developed human being than it has at the moment of conception, and the idea that there is some point between conception and birth at which the foetus has acquired enough of these significant characteristics so that it becomes plausible to think of the foetus as a living human being. These three positions differ only over the question as to when this point is.

The proponents of the claim that the foetus becomes a living human being at about six weeks are primarily impressed with the fact that it is about that time that electroencephalographic waves have been noted,[6] and that, therefore, the foetal brain must clearly be functioning after this date. There are two main reasons for taking this development to be the one that marks the time at which the foetus becomes a living human being:

(5) It is just this indicator which is used in determining the moment of death, the moment at which the entity in question is no longer a living human being. So, on grounds of symmetry, it would seem appropriate to treat it as the moment at which the entity in question becomes a living human being.[7] Callahan (who is not entirely convinced by this argument) puts it as follows:[8]

. . . it is very rare, for instance, to find a discussion of when life begins (pertinent to abortion) related to a discussion of when life ends (pertinent to euthanasia and the artificial prolongation of life). Yet both problems turn on what is meant by human life, and the illumination we gain in dealing with one of the problems will be useful when we deal with the other. Similarly, there is much to be said for trying to work out some consistent standards regarding the use of empirical data.

(6) One of the characteristics that are certainly essential to being a living human being is that the entity in question is capable of conscious experience, at least of a primitive level. Before the sixth week, it is not. Thereafter, it is. Consequently, that is the time at which the foetus becomes a living human being.

Those who claim that the foetus becomes a living human being at the moment of quickening seem to be impressed with its significance for the following two reasons:

(7) Quickening is an indication of foetal movement. We would certainly want to think of the ability to move as one of those characteristics that are essential to living human beings (not, of course, only to living human beings). So it is only at quickening, when there is a definite indication of foetal movement, that we are justified in thinking of the foetus as a living human being.

(8) There is an important sense in which it is true that quickening is that occasion from which the foetus can be perceived by other human beings. From that point on, the foetus can at least be felt by the mother. And anything which is not perceivable by other human beings cannot be thought of as a living human being. So the foetus becomes a living human being only at the moment of quickening, only at the moment at which it enters into the realm of the perceivable.

The following seems to be the main argument for supposing that the foetus becomes a living human being at the moment of viability:

(9) There is no doubt that the foetus is human from the moment of conception; it is certainly a human foetus. The question that we have to consider, however, is about when it becomes a living human being, and that is an entirely different matter. How can anything be a living human being if it is incapable of existing on its own? The foetus cannot do so until it becomes viable, so it cannot be a living human being until then. But when it does become vi-

able, then it has that degree of independence that is required for its being a living human being.

We come finally to the position that the foetus becomes a living human being only at its birth. It is clear that there is no special structure or capacity that it develops at that point. Indeed, this is so, in the last few months of pregnancy. So those who argue for birth as the moment at which the foetus becomes a living human being cannot be doing so on the grounds that it is then that they develop that which makes them a living human being. It is this that sets this position off from the last three that we have considered. What then are the main arguments for supposing that the foetus becomes a living human being at the moment of birth? These seem to be the main points:

(10) As long as the foetus is in the mother, it is more appropriate to think of it as a part of the mother, rather than as an individual separate living human being. That status can accrue to the foetus, therefore, only when it emerges from the mother at the moment of birth.

(11) While it is true that the foetus has the capacity for independent existence from the time of viability, it does not actually have that independent existence until birth. Until then, its intake of oxygen and food, and its expelling of wastes (among other things) is parasitic on that of the mother's. So it is only at the moment of birth at which the foetus acquires that independence that is essential for its being a living human being.

(12) It is only after that birth that the foetus can interact with other humans, and vice versa. But certainly it is this interaction, and not the mere abstract possibility of it, that is essential for being a living human being. So the foetus can be considered as a living human being only after its birth.

II

In light of the existence of these arguments, one can easily understand how many would conclude that something has gone wrong and that a fundamentally different approach is required. There is one such fundamental alternative that we should consider. It claims that there is a common but questionable presupposition of all the positions and arguments that we have been considering, viz., that there is an answer to the question as to when the foetus becomes a living human being with all the associated rights, an answer whose truth is independent of what we think or feel. It is just this presupposition that is rejected by the adherents of this fundamental alternative. According to them, the humanity of the foetus depends upon certain decisions involving it made by, and/or certain reactions to it of, other human beings.

One such version of this thesis is held by Professor John O'Connor.[9] While agreeing that once the criterion for humanity (for having the rights of a living human being) is settled, the question of the humanity of a foetus is a purely scientific one, O'Connor claims that it is we who have to decide upon the criterion of humanity, and, therefore, in an indirect way, it is we who ultimately have to make the decisions that will determine whether the foetus has the rights that a living human being has:[10]

I suggest that the fundamental defect in Noonan's account is his assumption that the criterion of humanity needs to be discovered. Rather I suggest that we must decide what the criterion is to be.

In another passage, O'Connor puts his point as follows:[11]

It is possible to agree with Noonan that, in a sense, it is certainly an objective matter whether or not a being is human, but point out that it becomes objective only when human beings have decided what the criterion of humanity is.

There are a variety of objections that might be raised against this view. But the most important one is that this seems to place the matter of human rights open to too many objectionable decisions. After all, there are all types of people with all types of prejudices about what is or is not required for being a living human being. And would we want to say that members of some minority group are really not living human beings just because they fail to meet the criterion of humanity established by some prejudiced majority, where the criterion in question reflects the prejudices of that majority group? If there were a vast majority prejudiced against redheads, and if that prejudice were reflected in some decision to include non-redheadedness as one of the necessary conditions for being a living human being, should we feel, as O'Connor's position seems to entail, that redheads then have no rights as living human beings? I think not. So O'Connor's position seems wrong.

O'Connor is, of course, aware of this possible objection, and he attempts to state the basis for his rejection of it in the following passage:[12]

This is not, of course, to say that it is a subjective matter. Rather, there are good and bad reasons for deciding in the way we do.

There are two questions that naturally arise in response to such a remark: (1) what is the basis for distinguishing between good and bad reasons for such a decision; (2) is that basis such that it does not also serve as a basis for distinguishing between correct and incorrect answers to the question as to what is the criterion for being a living human being? It is extremely important that O'Connor should be able to say 'no' in response to this second question, for if he cannot, then he will have avoided the subjectivism he recognizes as dangerous only at the cost of giving up his idea that the criteria of humanity are a matter to be decided upon and at the cost of adopting our position that there is an objectively true answer to the moral question 'when is something a living human being?' It can, of course, be done. One way would be to provide a basis that picked out the reasons for several conflicting, but not all, proposed decisions as good reasons.

Let us now look at exactly what O'Connor does set out as his theory of good reasons and bad reasons. He puts it as follows:[13]

The reason that humanity is of interest to a person concerned with the moral status of abortion is that he wants a way to decide the scope of the moral principle to the effect that the taking of human life is wrong. Hence humanity should be characterized in terms of those features which are in fact related to the moral sensibility of human beings. . . It will do little good to couch the criterion of humanity in such a way that the moral judgments we now make concerning human beings would be felt to have no moral force when applied to the "newly qualified" humans, whose humanity was first recognized only by the new criterion of humanity.

There is something obscure about this passage in this context, because it looks like a statement of a basis for distinguishing good decisions from bad ones (although not, of course, correct answers from incorrect ones) rather than good reasons for adopting one decision from bad reasons for adopting one. So there seems to be a shift here in O'Connor's strategy. But it is close enough to what we want anyway, since having a criterion for good decisions is, for O'Connor's purpose, as satisfactory as having a criterion for good reasons for decisions.

But there is a great deal of trouble with O'Connor's answer. After all, it fails to meet the original objection. In a highly prejudiced society that has incorporated its prejudices into its criterion of humanity, it will be the case, according to O'Connor, that the only good criteria of humanity will be those that retain these prejudicial features. If we try to drop them out, so as to extend human rights to the minority in question, our new criterion of humanity will be a bad one, according to O'Connor's criterion, since it is not related to the moral sensibility of the human beings in that society. Going back once more to the case of redheads who, in their society, are not viewed as living human beings entitled to human rights, one would have to say that, according to O'Connor, it would be a bad decision to leave non-redheadedness out of the criterion for humanity.

Moreover, the reasons that O'Connor gives for adopting his criterion for good and bad decisions are not very convincing. To be sure, if one's decision extends the rules about human rights to entities not generally recognized as living human beings by most people, there is a very good chance that those rules will be broken in connection with these entities. In that sense, then, such a decision "would do little good." It might, however, do a great deal of good in other ways; it might serve an educational role (by making people think again about whether this minority is human), it might serve as an important protest of principle, etc. So it is not at all clear that such a decision would be a

bad one. Moreover, the mere fact that a correct decision will not have the desired consequences should not, by itself, take away from its correctness.

In short, then, O'Connor's way of distinguishing good from bad decisions will not do, partially because it does not solve the problem raised by prejudiced societies and partially because the reasons for it are unconvincing. So we are left with our original objection to his whole approach, viz., that it seems to allow for the loss of human rights by some minority merely because some society has adopted a criterion of humanity that excludes that minority.

A very similar difficulty is faced by Professor Wertheimer, who offers another version of the thesis we are considering now. Professor Wertheimer is sympathetic to the suggestion[14] that

. . . what our natural response is to a thing, how we naturally react, cognitively, affectively, and behaviorally, is partly definitive of how we ought to respond to that thing. Often only an actual confrontation will tell us what we need to know, and sometimes we may each respond differently, and thus have different understandings.

It is just this suggestion that we want to consider now.

Wertheimer himself is pessimistic of using his approach in the near future to resolve the problem of the status of the foetus. He feels that there would have to be serious modifications in the foetal condition before we could have enough interactions with, and responses to, the foetus so that we could see what we feel about it. Moreover, what we would feel about this new type of creature is not clearly relevant to the status of foetuses as they now exist.

It is not clear that Wertheimer's pessimism here is justified. Paul Ramsey[15] has called our attention to one possibility of studying human reactions to foetuses, even given their current condition, by letting people see pictures of foetuses and of foetal behavior and studying the response to viewing these pictures. Such an experiment has never been carried out, but there is at least some data that suggests that its results might be quite significant. When Lennart Nilsson's photographs of foetuses were published in *Life* in 1965, many readers wrote in reporting their reactions, which generally tended to be that they could no longer view the foetus, at least in the later stages, as a disposable thing. Naturally, no conclusions should be drawn from this small sample, but it does at least suggest that, were we to adopt Wertheimer's approach to the question of when something is a living human being, some progress could be made on the question of foetal humanity.

Of course the question that we must consider first is whether we want to adopt Wertheimer's approach. The question is, once more, whether his approach can meet the problem raised by the responses of a prejudiced society. He puts the problem as follows:[16]

We surely want to say that Negroes are and always have been full-fledged human beings, no matter what certain segments of mankind may have thought, and no matter how numerous or unanimous those segments were.

His problem is how to reconcile this with the view that humanity is determined by how people respond to the entity in question.

It is obvious that Wertheimer can meet this problem only by ruling out certain responses, only by showing that certain responses are not relevant to the determination of the status of the creature in question. He offers us no full account of how he would do this, but we get some idea of what he has in mind when we see how he rules out as irrelevant to the status of the Negro slave the response to him of the slaveholders:[17]

We argue that his form of life is, so to speak, an accident of history, explicable by reference to special sociopsychological circumstances, that are inessential to the nature of blacks and whites. The fact that Negroes can, and, special circumstances aside, naturally would be regarded and treated no differently than a Caucasian is at once a necessary and a sufficient condition for its being right to so regard and treat them.

Looking at this remark from our perspective, we see the following theory suggested here. A decision to count an entity as a human being is a good one only if it is in accord with the natural responses of clearcut human beings to the entity in question. This criterion is thought reasonable because it reflects our privileged natural response and it solves the problem of the responses of the prejudiced society on the grounds that their responses are conditioned rather than natural.

Does this suggestion work? I think not. To begin with, can the distinction between the natural response and the socio-psychologically determined response do the work that Wertheimer needs it to do? I do not now want to raise the standard challenges to this distinction; rather, I would like to point out just how unclear the notion of the natural response is in this context. In one important sense, the slaveholder's response to the Negro is perfectly natural. Wertheimer himself points this out (without, I think, recognizing its full significance) in a footnote to his discussion of the slaveholder's response:[18]

We develop our concept of a human through our relations with those near us and like us, and thus, at least initially, an isolated culture will generally perceive and describe foreigners as alien, strange, and not foursquare human.

On the other hand, there is an important sense in which the response of the integrationist is the natural one. As Huck Finn learnt, it is very natural, when put into situations in which one lives with Negroes, to respond to them as living human beings. So, the viability of Wertheimer's solution to the problem raised by the reactions of the prejudiced society is very unclear, because, in this context, appeals to what is a natural response seem to lead to hopelessly conflicting results.

Secondly, it is not clear that this criterion is reasonable. Why should we ascribe to the natural response the special status implicit in Wertheimer's proposal? Why should we suppose that the natural response gives us any deeper insight into the status of the entity in question than some historically and/or socio-psychologically determined response? I think that we have lurking here a new, and far more dangerous, naturalistic fallacy, the fallacy of supposing that what is natural is necessarily insightful.

Given, then, that neither Wertheimer nor O'Connor have been able to meet the problem of the prejudiced society, we cannot help but feel that this problem is going to destroy any version of this fundamental alternative approach that we are considering. This leads us then to the conclusion that we should return to the positions and arguments discussed in section I, that we should return to attempting to answer the question as to when the foetus really does become a living human being with all the rights that such an entity normally has.

III

As one looks over the various arguments, one is struck by the fact that they divide into two groups. The arguments in one group (consisting of arguments (3),(5),(6),(7),(8),(9),(11), and (12)) are based upon the consideration of the nature of foetal development, and whether there are some essential properties of being human that the foetus acquires at some point in its development that makes that point sharply discontinuous from what has come before it and which is therefore the time at which the foetus becomes a living human being. All of the arguments except (3) assert that there are such properties. We will be concerned with these arguments, and the theoretical issues that they raise, in the final sections of this article. But before doing so, we must first see why the remaining group of arguments ((1),(2),(4) and (10)), each of which is based upon some special feature, can be disregarded.

Argument (1), the genetic argument, begins from the biological fact that, at the moment of conception, the fertilized cell has the unique chromosomal structure that will be found in all of the cells of the living human being that will develop from this cell. But it goes on to conclude from that that the entity in question is, from the moment of conception, whatever it is going to become, and that therefore it is a living human being. But how are these conclusions supposed to follow from the premise in question?

As we reflect upon the argument, it seems to come to the following: For any living human being there is a set of properties which can properly be considered the basic attributes of that human being. Some of these are shared with others, while others of these attributes are unique to the particular living human being in question. Now, that human being has these characteristics because of the chromosomal makeup of his cells; it is that that gives him these characteristics. But the foetus has already got that chromosomal makeup from the moment of conception; so it is also a living human being identical with the adult living human being.

The first thing that one should note about this argument is its somewhat dubious assumption that all of the basic characteristics of a human being (including those which he alone possesses) are genetically determined. That is to say, this argument presupposes that none of them is environmentally determined. It is, of course, difficult to decide whether or not this is so without an account of which characteristics are basic to that individual living human being, but the justification for assuming that they are all genetically determined is very unclear.

There is, moreover, a fallacy in the logic of this argument. Even if it is true that anything that possesses the basic properties of some living human being a is identical with a and is like a, a living human being, and even if it is true that these characteristics are determined by the chromosomal structure that the foetus already has, it doesn't follow, and it is clearly not true, that the foetus already has all of these characteristics; therefore, it certainly does not follow that the foetus out of which a will develop is identical with a and is like a, a living human being.

We turn now to argument (2), the argument from probabilities. This argument certainly does call attention to an important difference between foetuses (even from the moment of conception) on the one hand, and spermatazoa and ova, on the other hand. But it is not immediately clear why this difference is supposed to show that the foetus (from the moment of conception) is a living human being.

There is one passage in which Noonan[19] explains the rationale for his argument:

I had supposed that the appeal to probabilities was the most common-sensical of arguments, that to a greater or smaller degree all of us based our actions on probabilities, and that in morals, as in law, prudence and negligence were often measured by the account one had taken of the probabilities. If the chance were 300,000,000 to 1 that the movement in the bushes into which you shot was a man's, I doubt if many persons would hold you careless in shooting; but if the chances were four out of five that the movement was a human being's few would acquit you of blame in shooting.

It is difficult to know what to make of this argument. To begin with, Noonan switches, at the key point where he provides us with his example, from the question of the morality of the action to the very different question of whether you are to blame for something you did, and the considerations that are relevant to one type of question are not necessarily relevant to the other type. But more importantly, the analogy is very unapt. In the case of the movement in the bushes, the probability of 4/5 is the probability of the entity in question already being a living human being. In the case of the foetus, the probability of 4/5 is the probability of the entity in question developing into a clear-cut living human being. And I cannot see how it follows from the fact that one ought to suppose that the entity in question is a living human being when the probability of its already being one is 4/5 that one therefore ought to suppose that the entity in question is a living human being when the probability of its developing into a clearcut living human being is 4/5.

There is however, a different suggestion that might be advanced as to the relevance of this probability data. The following argument is often advanced for the claim that the foetus, from the moment of conception, is a living human being: from the moment of conception, the foetus has the potentiality for engaging in all of those activities that are typically human. Now,

it is the potentiality for doing that that makes one a living human being. So the foetus is a living human being from the moment of conception. In connection with this argument, the question naturally arises as to whether the foetus does indeed already have these potentialities at the moment of conception. It might be felt that he does so just because of this difference in probabilities. An entity, like the foetus even from the moment of conception, who has a 4/5 probability of developing into a being that actually engages in these activities is an entity that has the potentiality of engaging in them.

Two additional points should be noted about this argument: (a) the claim that the foetus has these potentialities can be reinforced by an appeal to the facts about the genetic code. After all, there is, because of the presence of the genetic code in the foetal cells, a biological basis for these potentialities; (b) the argument we are considering now is not claiming that the foetus is a living human being because it is a potential human being. Such a claim is, of course, incoherent, for to be at a given time a potential P is precisely not to be, at that time, a P. Rather, it is arguing that the foetus is a living human being from the moment of conception because it has, from that moment, the potentiality of engaging in typically human activities, and it has that potentiality because of the probability consideration raised by Noonan (together, perhaps, with the facts about the genetic code).

There are several very difficult issues raised by this argument. The first has to do with what it is to possess the potentiality of engaging in human activities. It might be argued that, contra the argument we are considering, something more is required if the foetus is to be said to possess those potentialities. After all, consider as an example of a typical human activity, the activity of thinking. We have good reason to suppose that thinking can only take place in a living human being when certain physiological structures (in this case, neural structures) are present and operating. Would it not then be reasonable to say that an entity has the potentiality of engaging in these activities only when these structures are present? And if so, we certainly cannot say of the foetus, at the moment of conception, that it has the potentiality of engaging in thought. And, of course, a similar argument could be raised in connection with other typically human activities.

There is, moreover, a second objection to the whole argument that the foetus is a living human being because of its potentialities. Perhaps some actual human activity, in addition to the potentiality (in any sense) of human activity, is required if the entity in question is to be a living human being? There is, after all, a certain intuitive plausibility to this claim. If we suppose that a sufficient condition for being a living human being is the engagement in typically human activities, then isn't it plausible to suppose (admittedly, it does not follow) that the potentiality of engaging in these activities is sufficient only for being a potential human being? So even if we grant the foetus's potentialities on the basis of Noonan's statistical considerations, it hardly seems to follow that the foetus is a living human being.

We come now to argument (4), the argument for the time of segmentation as the time at which the foetus becomes a living human being. If we were to formalize this argument, it would run as follows:

(a) Until the time of segmentation, but not thereafter, it is physically possible that more than one living human being develop out of that which resulted from the fertilization of the ovum by the sperm.

(b) Therefore, that which results from the fertilization of the ovum by the sperm (i) cannot be a living human being until the time of segmentation and (ii) is a living human being after that time.

The trouble here is, of course, that it is totally unclear as to how either part of (b) follows from (a). Why should (i) be true just because (a) is true? The following suggests itself: if the foetus were a living human being at some time before segmentation, and then it were to split into two living human beings, then we would have one living human being becoming two, and that is not possible. Unfortunately, although initially persuasive, this argument must be rejected. One amoeba can become two,[20] so why can't one living human being become two?

It is equally unclear as to why it should be thought that (ii) should follow from (a). Even if we suppose that (i) follows, this only means that the foetus, by the time of segmentation, has passed one hurdle in its path towards becoming a living human being. It is now a unique individual that will not split into two others. But it certainly does not follow that it has passed all the hurdles; it certainly does not follow that it is now a living human being.

We come finally to the very weak argument (10), the argument that claims that the foetus is not a living human being until the moment of birth because, until then, it is only a part of the mother since it is in the mother. The inference here seems to be from the foetus's (a) being in the mother (b) to its being a part of the mother and not an independent entity. But one certainly cannot infer merely from the fact that *a* is in *b* that *a* is a part of *b* (and certainly not that *a* is not an independent entity). I am in this room, but I am certainly not a part of this room. Jonah in the whale was not a part of the whale. To be sure, the foetus is in the mother in the stronger sense that it is dependent upon the mother, etc. That is, of course, a very different matter, and argument (11) which raises it is a serious argument which cannot be dismissed so easily and which we will consider below. For the moment, we need only note that the mere fact that the foetus is in the mother says nothing about its status as a living human being.

IV

We turn finally to a consideration of the remaining arguments. With the exception of (3), the argument from the continuity of foetal development, they all seem to be of the following form:

(a) there is a property P which is such that every living human being must have it; it is essential for its being a living human being.

(b) when the foetus acquires P, it becomes a living human being. And even argument (3) is best viewed as denying that, at any point after conception, the foetus acquires any property that satisfies premise (a).

In this final section, I would like to consider some of the difficulties that might be involved in trying to defend an argument of this type and briefly sketch a possible way of dealing with them. The first point to be noted is that none of the arguments, as currently formulated, is valid. After all, if there are two such properties P and Q, the mere possession of one cannot make the foetus a living human being so long as it does not possess the other. So (b) cannot follow from (a). In order to meet this point, one would have to modify our arguments so that they would be of the following structure:

(c) there is a property P which is such that every living human being must have it; it is essential for its being a living human being.

(d) by the time an entity acquires P, it has every other property Q which is essential for its being a living human being.

(e) when the foetus acquires P, it becomes a living human being.

Even with this reformulation, however, none of these arguments would be valid. As they stand, all that the premises guarantee is that, by the time the foetus has acquired P, it will have also acquired all those other properties that living human beings must have, i.e., it will have satisfied all of the necessary conditions for being a living human being. But they do not guarantee that the foetus will have satisfied any condition that is sufficient for its being a living human being, i.e., they do not guarantee that (e) is true.

So the first major problem that any proponents of our arguments will have to consider is the following: is it possible to develop a theory of what properties are essential for being a human being according to which it will be true that

(d) when an entity acquires every property which is essential for its being a living human being, it becomes a living human being? It is only if such a premise is true that any of the arguments that we are considering will be valid.

There is, of course, a second problem that the proponents of any of our arguments will have to face: how are we to determine whether or not the possession of a given property is or is not essential for being a living human being? It should be kept in mind that this is an extremely difficult problem given our reformulation of the arguments. It is not enough that we know whether or not the given property P is essential for being a living human being. It would seem that we have to have a complete list of all of the properties that are essential for being a living human being. Otherwise, how would we know that the premise of type (d) is true? And how are we going to ascertain what is the full list of these properties essential to being human?

So much for the problems. Now for a brief sketch of a possible way of dealing with them.[21] Let us begin with the following account[22] of when it is that an object has a property essentially. An object a has a property P essentially just in the case that a cannot lose it without going out of existence, while a has P accidentally just in the case that a can change and lose the property without going out of existence. Thus, it is an accidental property of my tree that it has 832 leaves on it since it could grow an additional leaf and still continue to exist. But it is an essential property of it that it is a tree, for if it were chopped down and cut into lumber (so that it were no longer a tree), it would no longer exist. Now, we shall say that any property had essentially by some object and accidentally by none (whether actual or potential) determines a natural kind, and that the set of objects having that property is a natural kind. In short, a natural kind is a set of objects each of which has a certain property essentially, and nothing else has that property. Now, the set of white objects is not a natural kind, since the only property that all white objects, but nothing else, has is the property of being white, and not all white objects have that property essentially. After all, my desk, which is white, could be painted blue and still exist. On the other hand, the set of living human beings seems to be a natural kind, since there seems to be a property which only its members have (the property of being a living human being) and they all seem to have it essentially. After all, when we die, when we stop being a living human being, we (but not our body and perhaps not our soul) cease to exist. Surely that is why we treat death so differently than anything else that might happen to us. As Wittgenstein[23] put it, ''Death is not an event in life: we do not live to experience death.''

With these preliminaries out of the way, I should now like to introduce several claims about what properties are essential for membership in a natural kind:

(1) only the possession of properties had essentially by every member of a natural kind is essential for membership in that natural kind.

(2) only the possession of all properties had essentially by every member of a natural kind is sufficient for membership in that natural kind. Claim (1) tells us what properties are such that their possession is essential (necessary) for membership in natural kinds while claim (2) tells us what properties are such that their joint possession is sufficient for membership in the class in question.

Both of these claims are false if we are dealing with classes in general, and not just with natural kinds. Consider once more the class of white objects which is, as we have seen, not a natural kind. Certainly, being white is essential for membership in that class but being white is not, as we have seen, an essential property of every member of that class. So claim (1) would be false for this non-natural kind. Similarly, the only properties had essentially by every member of this class are those had essentially by all colored objects (i.e., those had essentially by all objects and the property of being colored), but the possession of those properties is not sufficient for membership in the class of white objects (a blue object would, after all, also have them). What is sufficient is being white. So claim (2) would also be false for this non-natural kind.

Intuitively, what is happening here is the following: assume that, for every class, there are some properties[24] which are such that the possession of each of them is necessary and their joint possession is sufficient for membership in the class in question. Now (1) claims that the only necessary properties are those had essentially by all members of that class and (2) claims that their joint possession is the only sufficient condition. This must be false in the case of non-natural kinds for precisely what

they lack are some properties that their members, and only their members, have essentially and the possession of which could therefore be the necessary and sufficient conditions for membership in the class in question. But in the case of natural kinds, where all members have some properties essentially, and nothing else has them at all, it is plausible to conjecture that it is the possession of these properties, and only them, which is necessary and sufficient for membership in the natural kind. This is, of course, precisely what is claimed in (1) and (2).

I have no proof that (1) and (2) are true. But they are intuitively plausible and no counterexamples seem to be immediately forthcoming. So I will tentatively adopt them in this sketch. Given, then, (1) and (2), and our previous claim that humanity is a natural kind, we are now in a position to properly evaluate our remaining arguments. Their common structure was the following:

(c) there is a property P which is such that its possession is essential for being a living human being.

(d) by the time an entity acquires P, it has every other property Q which is essential for being a living human being.

(e) when the foetus acquires P, it becomes a living human being.

And there were two major problems with each of these arguments, viz., how to tell whether their essentialist claims are true and how to fix up their logic so that (e) will follow from the appropriate (c) and (d). We can now see how to solve these problems. Since humanity is a natural kind, given assumption (1), the only properties essential for being a human being are those had essentially by every human being, i.e., those which are such that their loss would mean that the entity in question has gone out of existence. We can therefore use the going-out-of-existence test to determine the truth of claims (c) and (d) in any given argument. And given assumption (2), (e) does follow straightforwardly from (c) and (d).

In short, then, our technical excursus has put us into a position for dealing with the problem of the essence of humanity. And it suggests to us that the soundest argument is (5), the brain-function argument. After all, it and only it seems to rest upon the claim that the foetus becomes a living human being when it acquires that characteristic which is such that its loss entails that a living human being no longer exists. But this, like all other points in this sketch, needs further investigation.

V

Where, then, do we stand on this vexing issue of foetal humanity? We have seen pretty clearly that it is not a matter to be resolved upon the basis of human decisions and reactions; it is, in that sense, a more objective matter. We have seen, moreover, that the crucial objective factors are ones having to do with the essence of humanity and not ones having to do with genetic codes and with probabilities of development. Finally, we have sketched (although certainly not proved the truth of) an approach to the essence of humanity according to which the foetus would be a living human being from about six weeks, the time at which we begin to note foetal brain activity.

NOTES

1. "Abortion and the Law," *Journal of Philosophy* (1971) and "Abortion and the Sanctity of Human Life," *American Philosophical Quarterly* (1973).

2. In "Points in Deciding about Abortion" in Noonan's *The Morality of Abortion* (Harvard, 1970), pp. 66–67. In that essay, Ramsey seems to alternate between that position and the time-of-segmentation position.

3. In "An Almost Absolute Value In History" in his *The Morality of Abortion* (Harvard, 1970), pp. 56–57.

4. In his "Understanding the Abortion Argument," *Philosophy and Public Affairs* (1971), p. 83.

5. *Op. cit.,* p. 66

6. It is interesting to note that Glanville Williams, in his *The Sanctity of Life and the Criminal Law* (Stevens, 1961) thinks of the presence of foetal brain activity as a good compromise date for the beginning of foetal humanity, but

only because he mistakenly thought that foetal brain activity is first detectable in the seventh month.

7. This argument is sometimes turned around in very strange ways. Thus, writing in a letter to the *New York Times* (dated March 6, 1972), Cyril C. Means, Professor of Constitutional Law at New York Law School, argued as follows:

An adult heart donor, suffering from irreversible brain damage, is also a living human "being," but he is no longer a human "person." That is why his life may be ended by the excision of his heart for the benefit of another, the donee, who is still a human person. If there can be human "beings" who are non persons at one end of the life span, why not also at the other end?

Professor Means seems to be missing the point. If we took the analogy he, and the argument we are considering both suggest, then, in his terminology, the foetus will be a person, as well as a human being, from the sixth week on and will, from that point on, be entitled to the full rights of such an entity.

8. In his *Abortion: Law, Choice, and Morality* (Macmillan, 1970), p. 334.

9. In his "On Humanity and Abortion," *Natural Law Forum* (1968).

10. *Ibid.,* p. 131.

11. *Ibid.*

12. *Ibid.*

13. *Ibid.*

14. *Op. cit.,* p. 92.

15. *Op. cit.,* p. 74. It should be noted that Ramsey himself is dubious about the value and importance of these results: "Medical science knows the babies to be present in all essential respects earlier in foetal development than the women who wrote into *Life* magazine perceived them in the pictures. It is the rational account of the nature of foetal development that matters most."

16. *Op. cit.,* p. 86.

17. *Ibid.,* p. 87.

18. *Ibid.*

19. "Deciding Who Is Human," *Natural Law Forum* (1968), p. 136.

20. A whole literature has arisen about this so-called splitting problem and the difficulties that arise for the theory of personal identity. See, for example, D. Parfit's "Personal Identity," *Philosophical Review* (1971). But the example of the amoeba shows that, one way or another, we can live with it.

21. I hope to be able to present in the not-too-far future a fuller version of this sketched approach.

22. For a full defense of this account, see my "De Re and De Dicto Interpretations of Modal Logic," *Philosophia* (1972) and "Why Settle for Anything Less than Good Old-Fashioned Aristotilean Essentialism?" *Nous* (1973).

23. *Tractatus Logico-Philosophicus* (Routledge and Kegan Paul, 1961), 6.4311.

24. To make this assumption plausible, we have to keep in mind disjunctive and degree-of-resemblance properties. Even with that complication, there may be further difficulties, but we shall ignore them for now.

JANE ENGLISH

Abortion and the Concept of a Person*

The abortion debate rages on. Yet the two most popular positions seem to be clearly mistaken. Conservatives maintain that a human life begins at conception and that therefore abortion must be wrong because it is murder. But not all killings of humans are murders. Most notably, self defense may justify even the killing of an innocent person.

Liberals, on the other hand, are just as mistaken in their argument that since a fetus does not become a person until birth, a woman may do whatever she pleases in and to her own body. First, you cannot do as you please with your own body if it affects other people adversely.[1] Second, if a fetus is not a person, that does not imply that you can do to it anything you wish. Animals, for example, are not persons, yet to kill or torture them for no reason at all is wrong.

At the center of the storm has been the issue of just when it is between ovulation and adulthood that a person appears on the scene. Conservatives draw the line at conception, liberals at birth. In this paper I first examine our concept of a person and conclude that no single criterion can capture the concept of a person and no sharp line can be drawn. . . .

The several factions in the abortion argument have drawn battle lines around various proposed criteria for determining what is and what is not a person. For example, Mary Anne Warren[2] lists five features (capacities for reasoning, self-awareness, complex communication, etc.) as her criteria for personhood and argues for the permissibility of abortion because a fetus falls outside this concept. Baruch Brody[3] uses brain waves. Michael Tooley[4] picks having-a-concept-of-self as his criterion and concludes that infanticide and abortion are justifiable, while the killing of adult animals is not. On the other side, Paul Ramsey[5] claims a certain gene structure is the defining characteristic. John Noonan[6] prefers conceived-of-humans and presents counterexamples to various other candidate criteria. For instance, he argues against viability as the criterion because the newborn and infirm would then be non-persons, since they cannot live without the aid of others. He rejects any criterion that calls upon the sorts of sentiments a being can evoke in adults on the grounds that this would allow us to exclude other races as non-persons if we could just view them sufficiently unsentimentally.

These approaches are typical: foes of abortion propose sufficient conditions for personhood which fetuses satisfy, while friends of abortion counter with necessary conditions for personhood which fetuses lack. But these both presuppose that the concept of a person can be captured in a strait jacket of necessary and/or sufficient conditions.[7] Rather, 'person' is a cluster of features, of which rationality, having a self concept and being conceived of humans are only part.

What is typical of persons? Within our concept of a person we include, first, certain biological factors: descended from humans, having a certain genetic make-up, having a head, hands, arms, eyes, capable of locomotion, breathing, eating, sleeping. There are psychological factors: sentience, perception, having a concept of self and of one's own interests and desires, the ability to use tools, the ability to use language or symbol systems, the ability to joke, to be angry, to doubt. There are rationality factors: the ability to reason and draw conclusions, the ability to generalize and

* I am deeply indebted to Larry Crocker and Arthur Kuflik for their constructive comments.

Reprinted from Vol. 5, No. 2 (October 1975) of the *Canadian Journal of Philosophy*, by permission of the Canadian Association for Publishing in Philosophy.

to learn from past experience, the ability to sacrifice present interests for greater gains in the future. There are social factors: the ability to work in groups and respond to peer pressures, the ability to recognize and consider as valuable the interests of others, seeing oneself as one among "other minds," the ability to sympathize, encourage, love, the ability to evoke from others the responses of sympathy, encouragement, love, the ability to work with others for mutual advantage. Then there are legal factors: being subject to the law and protected by it, having the ability to sue and enter contracts, being counted in the census, having a name and citizenship, the ability to own property, inherit, and so forth.

Now the point is not that this list is incomplete, or that you can find counterinstances to each of its points. People typically exhibit rationality, for instance, but someone who was irrational would not thereby fail to qualify as a person. On the other hand, something could exhibit the majority of these features and still fail to be a person, as an advanced robot might. There is no single core of necessary and sufficient features which we can draw upon with the assurance that they constitute what really makes a person; there are only features that are more or less typical.

This is not to say that no necessary or sufficient conditions can be given. Being alive is a necessary condition for being a person, and being a U.S. Senator is sufficient. But rather than falling inside a sufficient condition or outside a necessary one, a fetus lies in the penumbra region where our concept of a person is not so simple. For this reason I think a conclusive answer to the question whether a fetus is a person is unattainable.

Here we might note a family of simple fallacies that proceed by stating a necessary condition for personhood and showing that a fetus has that characteristic. This is a form of the fallacy of affirming the consequent. For example, some have mistakenly reasoned from the premise that a fetus is human (after all, it is a human fetus rather than, say, a canine fetus), to

the conclusion that it is a human. Adding an equivocation on 'being', we get the fallacious argument that since a fetus is something both living and human, it is a human being.

Nonetheless, it does seem clear that a fetus has very few of the above family of characteristics, whereas a newborn baby exhibits a much larger proportion of them—and a two-year-old has even more. Note that one traditional anti-abortion argument has centered on pointing out the many ways in which a fetus resembles a baby. They emphasize its development ("It already has ten fingers . . . ") without mentioning its dissimilarities to adults (it still has gills and a tail). They also try to evoke the sort of sympathy on our part that we only feel toward other persons ("Never to laugh . . . or feel the sunshine?"). This all seems to be a relevant way to argue, since its purpose is to persuade us that a fetus satisfies so many of the important features on the list that it ought to be treated as a person. Also note that a fetus near the time of birth satisfies many more of these factors than a fetus in the early months of development. This could provide reason for making distinctions among the different stages of pregnancy, as the U.S. Supreme Court has done.[8]

Historically, the time at which a person has been said to come into existence has varied widely. Muslims date personhood from fourteen days after conception. Some medievals followed Aristotle in placing ensoulment at forty days after conception for a male fetus and eighty days for a female fetus.[9] In European common law since the seventeenth century, abortion was considered the killing of a person only after quickening, the time when a pregnant woman first feels the fetus move on its own. Nor is this variety of opinions surprising. Biologically, a human being develops gradually. We shouldn't expect there to be any specific time or sharp dividing point when a person appears on the scene.

For these reasons I believe our concept of a person is not sharp or decisive enough to bear the weight of a solution to the abortion controversy. To use it to solve that problem is to clarify *obscurum per obscurius*.

NOTES

1. We also have paternalistic laws which keep us from harming our own bodies even when no one else is affected. Ironically, anti-abortion laws were originally designed to protect pregnant women from a dangerous but tempting procedure.

2. Mary Anne Warren, "On the Moral and Legal Status of Abortion," *Monist* 57 (1973), p. 55. [Reprinted above, pp. 217–228.]

3. Baruch Brody, "Fetal Humanity and the Theory of Essentialism," in Robert Baker and Frederick Elliston (eds.), *Philosophy and Sex* (Buffalo, N.Y., 1975) [and the article in this text, pp. 229–240.]

4. Michael Tooley, "Abortion and Infanticide," *Philosophy and Public Affairs* 2 (1971).

5. Paul Ramsey, "The Morality of Abortion," in James Rachels, ed., *Moral Problems* (New York, 1971).

6. John Noonan, "Abortion and the Catholic Church: a Summary History," *Natural Law Forum* 12 (1967), pp. 125–131 [and the article in this text, pp. 210–217.]

7. Wittgenstein has argued against the possibility of so capturing the concept of a game, *Philosophical Investigations* (New York, 1958), §66–71.

8. Not because the fetus is partly a person and so has some of the rights of persons, but rather because of the rights of person-like non-persons.

9. Aristotle himself was concerned, however, with the different question of when the soul takes form. For historical data, see Jimmye Kimmey, "How the Abortion Laws Happened," *Ms.* 1 (April, 1973), pp. 48ff and John Noonan, *loc. cit.*

Legal Issues

UNITED STATES SUPREME COURT

Majority Opinion in Roe v. Wade

[Mr. Justice Blackmun delivered the opinion of the Court.]

. . .

It is . . . apparent that at common law, at the time of the adoption of our Constitution, and throughout the major portion of the nineteenth century, abortion was viewed with less disfavor than under most American statutes currently in effect. Phrasing it another way, a woman enjoyed a substantially broader right to terminate a pregnancy than she does in most States today. At least with respect to the early stage of pregnancy, and very possibly without such a limitation, the opportunity to make this

Reprinted from 410 *United States Reports* 113, Decided January 22, 1973.

choice was present in this country well into the nineteenth century. Even later, the law continued for some time to treat less punitively an abortion procured in early pregnancy. . . .

Three reasons have been advanced to explain historically the enactment of criminal abortion laws in the nineteenth century and to justify their continued existence.

It has been argued occasionally that these laws were the product of a Victorian social concern to discourage illicit sexual conduct. Texas, however, does not advance this justification in the present case, and it appears that no court or commentator has taken the argument seriously. . . .

A second reason is concerned with abortion as a medical procedure. When most criminal abortion laws were first enacted, the procedure was a hazardous one for the woman. This was particularly true prior to the development of antisepsis. Antiseptic techniques, of course, were based on discoveries by Lister, Pasteur, and others first announced in 1867, but were not generally accepted and employed until about the turn of the century. Abortion mortality was high. Even after 1900, and perhaps until as late as the development of antibiotics in the 1940s, standard modern techniques such as dilation and curettage were not nearly so safe as they are today. Thus it has been argued that a state's real concern in enacting a criminal abortion law was to protect the pregnant woman, that is, to restrain her from submitting to a procedure that placed her life in serious jeopardy.

Modern medical techniques have altered this situation. Appellants and various *amici* refer to medical data indicating that abortion in early pregnancy, that is, prior to the end of first trimester, although not without its risk, is now relatively safe. Mortality rates for women undergoing early abortions, where the procedure is legal, appear to be as low as or lower than the rates for normal childbirth. Consequently, any interest of the state in protecting the woman from an inherently hazardous procedure, except when it would be equally dangerous for her to forgo it, has largely disappeared. Of course, important state interests in the area of health and medical standards do remain. The state has a legitimate interest in seeing to it that abortion like any other medical procedure, is performed under circumstances that insure maximum safety for the patient. This interest obviously extends at least to the performing physician and his staff, to the facilities involved, to the availability of after-care, and to adequate provision for any complication or emergency that might arise. The prevalence of high mortality rates at illegal "abortion mills" strengthens, rather than weakens, the state's interest in regulating the conditions under which abortions are performed. Moreover, the risk to the woman increases as her pregnancy continues. Thus the state retains a definite interest in protecting the woman's own health and safety when an abortion is performed at a late stage of pregnancy.

The third reason is the state's interest— some phrase it in terms of duty—in protecting prenatal life. Some of the argument for this justification rests on the theory that a new human life is present from the moment of conception. The state's interest and general obligation to protect life then extends, it is argued, to prenatal life. Only when the life of the pregnant mother herself is at stake, balanced against the life she carries within her, should the interest of the embryo or fetus not prevail. Logically, of course, a legitimate state interest in this area need not stand or fall on acceptance of the belief that life begins at conception or at some other point prior to live birth. In assessing the state's interest, recognition may be given to the less rigid claim that as long as at least *potential* life is involved, the state may assert interests beyond the protection of the pregnant woman alone.

Parties challenging state abortion laws have sharply disputed in some courts the contention that a purpose of these laws, when enacted, was to protect prenatal life. Pointing to the absence of legislative history to support the contention, they claim that most state laws were designed solely to protect the woman. Because medical advances have lessened this concern, at least with respect to abortion in early pregnancy, they argue that with respect to such abortions the laws can no longer be justified by any state interest. There is some scholarly support for this view of original purpose. The few states courts called upon to interpret their laws in the late nineteenth and early twentieth centuries did focus on the state's interest in protecting the woman's health rather than in preserving the embryo and fetus. . . .

The Constitution does not explicitly mention any right of privacy. In a line of decisions, however, going back perhaps as far as *Union Pacific R. Co.* v. *Botsford* (1891), the Court has recognized that a right of personal privacy, or a guarantee of certain areas or zones of privacy, does exist under the Constitution. In varying contexts the Court or individual Justices have indeed found at least the roots of that right in the First Amendment, . . . in the Fourth and Fifth Amerndments . . . in the penumbras of the Bill of Rights . . . in the Ninth Amendment . . . or in the concept of liberty guaranteed by the first section of the Fourteenth Amendment, . . . These decisions make it clear that only personal rights that can be deemed "fundamental" or "implicit in the concept of ordered liberty," . . . are included in this guarantee of personal privacy. They also make it clear that the right has some extension to activities relating to marriage, . . . procreation, . . . contraception, . . . family relationships, . . . and child rearing and education. . . .

This right of privacy, whether it be founded in the Fourteenth Amendment's concept of personal liberty and restrictions upon state action, as we feel it is, or, as the District Court determined, in the Ninth Amendment's reservation of rights to the people, is broad enough to encompass a woman's decision whether or not to terminate her pregnancy. . . .

. . . Appellants and some *amici* argue that the woman's right is absolute and that she is entitled to terminate her pregnancy at whatever time, in whatever way, and for whatever reason she alone chooses. With this we do not agree. Appellants' arguments that Texas either has no valid interest at all in regulating the abortion decision, or no interest strong enough to support any limitation upon the woman's sole determination, is unpersuasive. The Court's decisions recognizing a right of privacy also acknowledge that some state regulation in areas protected by that right is appropriate. As noted above, a state may properly assert important interests in safe guarding health, in maintaining medical standards, and in protecting potential life. At some point in pregnancy, these respective interests become sufficiently compelling to sustain regulation of the factors that govern the abortion decision. The privacy right involved, therefore, cannot be said to be absolute. . . .

We therefore conclude that the right of personal privacy includes the abortion decision, but that this right is not unqualified and must be considered against important state interests in regulation.

We note that those federal and state courts that have recently considered abortion law challenges have reached the same conclusion. . . .

Although the results are divided, most of these courts have agreed that the right of privacy, however based, is broad enough to cover the abortion decision; that the right, nonetheless, is not absolute and is subject to some limitations; and that at some point the state interests as to protection of health, medical standards, and prenatal life, become dominant. We agree with this approach. . . .

The appellee and certain *amici* argue that the fetus is a "person" within the language and meaning of the Fourteenth Amendment. In support of this they outline at length and in detail the well-known facts of fetal development. If this suggestion of personhood is established, the appellant's case, of course, collapses, for the fetus' right to life is then guaranteed specifically by the Amendment. The appellant conceded as much on reargument. On the other hand, the appellee conceded on reargument that no case could be cited that holds that a fetus is a person within the meaning of the Fourteenth Amendment. . . .

All this, together with our observation, *supra,* that throughout the major portion of the nineteenth century prevailing legal abortion practices were far freer than they are today, persuades us that the word "person," as used in the Fourteenth Amendment, does not include the unborn. . . . Indeed, our decision in *United States* v. *Vuitch* (1971), inferentially is to the same effect, for we there would not have indulged in statutory interpretation favorable to abortion in specified circumstances if the necessary consequence was the termination of life entitled to Fourteenth Amendment protection.

. . . As we have intimated above, it is reasonable and appropriate for a state to decide that at some point in time another interest, that of health of the mother or that of potential human life, becomes significantly involved. The woman's privacy is no longer sole and any right of privacy she possesses must be measured accordingly.

Texas urges that, apart from the Fourteenth Amendment, life begins at conception and is present throughout pregnancy, and that, therefore, the state has a compelling interest in protecting that life from and after conception. We need not resolve the difficult question of when life begins. When those trained in the respective disciplines of medicine, philosophy, and theology are unable to arrive at any consensus, the judiciary, at this point in the development of man's knowledge, is not in a position to speculate as to the answer.

It should be sufficient to note briefly the wide divergence of thinking on this most sensitive and difficult question. There has always been strong support for the view that life does not begin until live birth. This was the belief of the Stoics. It appears to be the predominant, though not the unanimous, attitude of the Jewish faith. It may be taken to represent also the position of a large segment of the Protestant community, insofar as that can be ascertained; organized groups that have taken a formal position on the abortion issue have generally regarded abortion as a matter for the conscience of the individual and her family. As we have noted, the common law found greater significance in quickening. Physicians and their scientific colleagues have regarded that event with less interest and have tended to focus either upon conception or upon live birth or upon the interim point at which the fetus becomes "viable," that is, potentially able to live outside the mother's womb, albeit with artificial aid. Viability is usually placed at about seven months (28 weeks) but may occur earlier, even at 24 weeks. . . .

In areas other than criminal abortion the law has been reluctant to endorse any theory that life, as we recognize it, begins before live birth or to accord legal rights to the unborn except in narrowly defined situations and except when the rights are contingent upon live birth. . . . In short, the unborn have never been recognized in the law as persons in the whole sense.

In view of all this, we do not agree that, by adopting one theory of life, Texas may override the rights of the pregnant woman that are at stake. We repeat, however, that the state does have an important and legitimate interest in preserving and protecting the health of the pregnant woman, whether she be a resident of the state or a nonresident who seeks medical consultation and treatment there, and that it has still *another* important and legitimate interest in protecting the potentiality of human life. These interests are separate and distinct. Each grows in substantiality as the woman approaches term and, at a point during pregnancy, each becomes "compelling."

With respect to the state's important and legitimate interest in the health of the mother, the "compelling" point, in the light of present medical knowledge, is at approximately the end of the first trimester. This is so because of the now established medical fact . . . that until the end of the first trimester mortality in abortion is less than mortality in normal childbirth. It follows that, from and after this point, a state may regulate the abortion procedure to the extent that the regulation reasonably relates to the preservation and protection of maternal health. Examples of permissible state regulation in this area are requirements as to the qualifications of the person who is to perform the abortion; as to the licensure of that person; as to the facility in which the procedure is to be performed, that is, whether it must be a hospital or may be a clinic or some other place of less-than-hospital status; as to the licensing of the facility; and the like.

This means, on the other hand, that, for the period of pregnancy prior to this "compelling" point, the attending physician, in consultation with his patient, is free to determine, without regulation by the state, that in his medical judgment the patient's pregnancy should be terminated. If that decision is reached, the judgment may be effectuated by an abortion free of interference by the state.

With respect to the state's important and legitimate interest in potential life, the "compelling" point is at viability. This is so because the fetus then presumably has the capability of meaningful life outside the mother's womb. State regulation protective of fetal life after viability thus has both logical and biological justifications. If the state is interested in protecting fetal life after viability, it may go so far as to proscribe abortion during that period except when it is necessary to preserve the life or health of the mother. . . .

To summarize and repeat:

1. A state criminal abortion statute of the current Texas type, that excepts from criminality only a *lifesaving* procedure on behalf of the mother, without regard to pregnancy stage and without recognition of the other interests involved, is violative of the Due Process Clause of the Fourteenth Amendment.

(a) For the stage prior to approximately the end of the first trimester, the abortion decision and its effectuation must be left to the medical judgment of the pregnant woman's attending physician.

(b) For the stage subsequent to approximately the end of the first trimester, the state, in promoting its interest in the health of the mother, may, if it chooses, regulate the abortion procedure in ways that are reasonably related to maternal health.

(c) For the stage subsequent to viability the state, in promoting its interest in the potential-

ity of human life, may, if it chooses, regulate, and even proscribe, abortion except where it is necessary, in appropriate medical judgment, for the preservation of the life or health of the mother.

2. The state may define the term "physician" . . . to mean only a physician currently licensed by the state, and may proscribe any abortion by a person who is not a physician as so defined.

. . . The decision leaves the state free to place increasing restrictions on abortion as the period of pregnancy lengthens, so long as those restrictions are tailored to the recognized state interests. The decision vindicates the right of the physician to administer medical treatment according to his professional judgment up to the points where important state interests provide compelling justifications for intervention. Up to those points the abortion decision in all its aspects is inherently, and primarily, a medical decision, and basic responsibility for it must rest with the physician. If an individual practitioner abuses the privilege of exercising proper medical judgment, the usual remedies, judicial and intraprofessional, are available. . . .

JOHN HART ELY

The Wages of Crying Wolf: A Comment on Roe v. Wade

Let us not underestimate what is at stake: Having an unwanted child can go a long way toward ruining a woman's life. And at bottom *Roe* signals the Court's judgment that this re-

Reprinted by permission of the Yale Law Journal Company and Fred B. Rothman & Company from *The Yale Law Journal*, Vol. 82, (April 1973), pp. 923–28, 931–33, 935–37, 943, 947.

sult cannot be justified by any good that anti-abortion legislation accomplishes. This surely is an understandable conclusion—indeed it is one with which I agree—but ordinarily the Court claims no mandate to second-guess legislative balances, at least not when the Constitution has designated neither of the values in conflict as entitled to special protection. But even assuming it would be a good idea for the Court to assume this function, *Roe* seems a curious place to have begun. Laws prohibiting the use of "soft" drugs or, even more obviously, homosexual acts between consenting adults can stunt "the preferred life styles"[1] of those against whom enforcement is threatened in very serious ways. It is clear such acts harm no one besides the participants, and indeed the case that the participants are harmed is a rather shaky one. Yet such laws survive,[2] on the theory that there exists a societal consensus that the behavior involved is revolting or at any rate immoral.[3] Of course the consensus is not universal but it is sufficient, and this is what is counted crucial, to get the laws passed and keep them on the books. Whether anti-abortion legislation cramps the life style of an unwilling mother more significantly than anti-homosexuality legislation cramps the life style of a homosexual is a close question. But even granting that it does, the *other* side of the balance looks very different. For there is more than simple societal revulsion to support legislation restricting abortion:[4] Abortion ends (or if it makes a difference, prevents) the life of a human being other than the one making the choice.

The Court's response here is simply not adequate. It agrees, indeed it holds, that after the point of viability (a concept it fails to note will become even less clear than it is now as the technology of birth continues to develop[5]) the interest in protecting the fetus is compelling.[6] Exactly why that is the magic moment is not made clear: Viability, as the Court defines it, is achieved some six to twelve weeks after quickening.[7] (Quickening is the point at which the fetus begins discernibly to move independently of the mother[8] and the point that has historically been deemed crucial—to the extent *any* point between conception and birth has been focused on.[9]) But no, it is *viability* that is constitutionally critical: the Court's defense seems to mistake a definition for a syllogism.

With respect to the State's important and legitimate interest in potential life, the "compelling" point is at viability. This is so because the fetus then presumably has the capacity of meaningful life outside the mother's womb.[10]

With regard to why the state cannot consider this "important and legitimate interest" prior to viability, the opinion is even less satisfactory. The discussion begins sensibly enough: The interest asserted is not necessarily tied to the question whether the fetus is "alive," for whether or not one calls it a living being, it is an entity with the potential for (and indeed the likelihood of) life. But all of arguable relevance that follows are arguments that fetuses (a) are not recognized as "persons in the whole sense" by legal doctrine generally and (b) are not "persons" protected by the Fourteenth Amendment.

To the extent they are not entirely inconclusive, the bodies of doctrine to which the Court adverts respecting the protection of fetuses under general legal doctrine tend to undercut rather than support its conclusion. And the argument that fetuses (unlike, say, corporations) are not "persons" under the Fourteenth Amendment fares little better. The Court notes that most constitutional clauses using the word "persons"—such as the one outlining the qualifications for the Presidency—appear to have been drafted with postnatal beings in mind. (It might have added that most of them were plainly drafted with *adults* in mind, but I suppose that wouldn't have helped.) In addition, "the appellee conceded on reargument that no case can be cited that holds that a fetus is a person within the meaning of the Fourteenth Amendment."[11] (The other legal contexts in which the question could have arisen are not enumerated.)

The canons of construction employed here are perhaps most intriguing when they are contrasted with those invoked to derive the constitutional right to an abortion. But in any event, the argument that fetuses lack constitutional rights is simply irrelevant. For it has never been held or even asserted that the state interest needed to justify forcing a person to refrain from an activity, *whether or not that activity is constitutionally protected,* must implicate either the life or the constitutional rights of another person. Dogs are not "persons in the whole sense" nor have they constitutional rights, but that does not mean the state cannot prohibit killing them: It does not even mean the state cannot prohibit killing them in the exercise of the First Amendment right of political protest. Come to think of it, draft cards aren't persons either.

Thus even assuming the Court ought generally to get into the business of second-guessing legislative balances, it has picked a strange case with which to begin. Its purported evaluation of the balance that produced anti-abortion legislation simply does not meet the issue: That the life plans of the mother must, not simply may, prevail over the state's desire to protect the fetus simply does not follow from the judgment that the fetus is not a person. Beyond all that, however, the Court has no business getting into that business.

Were I a legislator I would vote for a statute very much like the one the Court ends up drafting. I hope this reaction reflects more than the psychological phenomenon that keeps bombardiers sane—the fact that it is somehow easier to "terminate" those you cannot see—and am inclined to think it does: that the mother, unlike the unborn child, has begun to imagine a future for herself strikes me as morally quite significant. But God knows I'm not *happy* with that resolution. Abortion is too much like infanticide on the one hand, and too much like contraception on the other, to leave one comfortable with any answer; and the moral issue it poses is as fiendish as any philosopher's hypothetical.[12]

Of course, the Court often resolves difficult moral questions, and difficult questions yield controversial answers. I doubt, for example, that most people would agree that letting a drug peddler go unapprehended is morally preferable to letting the police kick down his door without probable cause. The difference, of course, is that the Constitution, which legitimates and theoretically controls judicial intervention, has some rather pointed things to say about this choice. There will of course be difficult questions about the applicability of its language to specific facts, but at least the document's special concern with one of the values in conflict is manifest. It simply says nothing, clear or fuzzy, about abortion.[13]

The matter cannot end there, however. The Burger Court, like the Warren Court before it, has been especially solicitous of the right to travel from state to state, demanding a compelling state interest if it is to be inhibited.[14] Yet nowhere in the Constitution is such a right mentioned. It is, however, as clear as such things can be that this right was one the framers intended to protect, most specifically[15] by the Privileges and Immunities Clause of Article IV.[16] The right is, moreover, plausibly inferable from the system of government, and the citizen's role therein, contemplated by the Constitution.[17] The Court in *Roe* suggests an inference of neither sort—from the intent of the framers, or from the governmental system contemplated by the Constitution—in support of the constitutional right to an abortion.

. . .

The Court reports that some amici curiae argued for an unlimited right to do as one wishes with one's body. This theory holds, for me at any rate, much appeal. However, there would have been serious problems with its invocation in this case. In the first place, more than the mother's own body is involved in a decision to have an abortion; a fetus may not be a "person in the whole sense," but it is certainly not nothing. Second, it is difficult to find a basis for thinking that the theory was meant to be given constitutional sanction: Surely it is no part of the "privacy" interest the Bill of Rights suggests.

[I]t is not clear to us that the claim . . . that one has an unlimited right to do with one's body as one pleases bears a close relationship to the right of privacy. . . .[18]

Unfortunately, having thus rejected the amici's attempt to define the bounds of the general constitutional right of which the right to an abortion is a part, on the theory that the general right described has little to do with privacy, the Court provides neither an alternative definition nor an account of why *it* thinks privacy is involved. It simply announces that the right to privacy "is broad enough to encompass a woman's decision whether or not to terminate her pregnancy." Apparently this conclusion is thought to derive from the passage that immediately follows it:

The detriment that the State would impose upon the pregnant woman by denying this choice altogether is apparent. Specific and direct harm medically diagnosable even in early pregnancy may be involved. Maternity, or additional offspring, may force upon the woman a distressful life and future. Psychological harm may be imminent. Mental and physical health may be taxed by child care. There is also the distress, for all concerned, associated with the unwanted child, and there is the problem of bringing a child into a family already unable, psychologically and otherwise, to care for it. In other cases, as in this one, the additional difficulties and continuing stigma of unwed motherhood may be involved.[19]

All of this is true and ought to be taken very seriously. But it has nothing to do with privacy in the Bill of Rights sense or any other the Constitution suggests.[20] I suppose there is nothing to prevent one from using the word "privacy" to mean the freedom to live one's life without governmental interference. But the Court obviously does not so use the term.[21] Nor could it, for such a right is at stake in *every* case. Our life styles are constantly limited, often seriously, by governmental regulation; and while many of us would prefer less direction, granting that desire the status of a preferred constitutional right would yield a system of "government" virtually unrecognizable to us and only slightly more recognizable to our forefathers.[22] The Court's observations concerning the serious, life-shaping costs of having a child prove what might to the thoughtless have seemed unprovable: That even though a human life, or a potential human life, hangs in the balance, the moral dilemma abortion poses is so difficult as to be heartbreaking. What they fail to do is even begin to resolve that dilemma so far as our governmental system is concerned by associating either side of the balance with a value inferable from the Constitution.

.   .   .

Of course a woman's freedom to choose an abortion is part of the "liberty" the Fourteenth

Amendment says shall not be denied without due process of law, as indeed is anyone's freedom to do what he wants. But "due process" generally guarantees only that the inhibition be procedurally fair and that it have some "rational" connection—though plausible is probably a better word—with a permissible governmental goal.[23] What is unusual about *Roe* is that the liberty involved is accorded a far more stringent protection, so stringent that a desire to preserve the fetus's existence is unable to overcome it—a protection more stringent, I think it fair to say, than that the present Court accords the freedom of the press explicitly guaranteed by the First Amendment.[24] What is frightening about *Roe* is that this super-protected right is not inferable from the language of the Constitution, the framers' thinking respecting the specific problem in issue, any general value derivable from the provisions they included, or the nation's governmental structure. Nor is it explainable in terms of the unusual political impotence of the group judicially protected vis-à-vis the interest that legislatively prevailed over it. And that, I believe —the predictable early reaction to *Roe* notwithstanding ("more of the same Warren-type activism"[25])—is a charge that can responsibly be leveled at no other decision of the past twenty years. At times the inferences the Court has drawn from the values the Constitution marks for special protection have been controversial, even shaky, but never before has its sense of an obligation to draw one been so obviously lacking.

.   .   .

I do wish "Wolf!" hadn't been cried so often. When I suggest to my students that *Roe* lacks even colorable support in the constitutional text, history, or any other appropriate source of constitutional doctrine, they tell me they've heard all that before. When I point out they haven't heard it before from *me,* I can't really blame them for smiling. . . .

To the public the *Roe* decision must look very much like the New York Legislature's recent liberalization of its abortion law. Even in the unlikely event someone should catch the public's ear long enough to charge that the wrong institution did the repealing, they have heard that "legalism" before without taking to the streets. Nor are the political branches, and this of course is what really counts, likely to take up the cry very strenuously: The sighs of relief as this particular albatross was cut from the legislative and executive necks seemed to me audible. Perhaps I heard wrong—I live in the Northeast, indeed not so very far from Hyannis Port. It is even possible that a constitutional amendment will emerge, though that too has happened before without serious impairment of the Position of the Institution. But I doubt one will: *Roe v. Wade* seems like a durable decision.

It is, nevertheless, a very bad decision. Not because it will perceptibly weaken the Court—it won't; and not because it conflicts with either my idea of progress or what the evidence suggests is society's—it doesn't. It is bad because it is bad constitutional law, or rather because it is *not* constitutional law and gives almost no sense of an obligation to try to be.

NOTES

1. 93 S. Ct. at 759 (Douglas, J., concurring).
2. *Cf.* Poe v. Ullman, 367 U.S. 497, 551–53 (1961), (Harlan, J., dissenting), *quoted* in part in Griswold v. Connecticut, 381 U.S. 479, 499 (1965) (Goldberg, J., concurring), distinguishing laws proscribing homosexual acts (even those performed in the home) as not involving the "right" at stake in those cases.
3. *See, e.g.,* Poe v. Ullman, 367 U.S. 497, 545–46 (Harlan, J., dissenting).
4. Nor is the Court's conclusion that early abortion does not present serious physical risk to the woman involved shared by all doctors.
5. It defines viability so as not to exclude the possibility of artificial support, 93 S. Ct. at 730, and later indicates its awareness of the continuing development of artificial wombs. *Id.* at 731. It gives no sign of having considered the implications of that combination for the trimester program the Constitution is held to mandate, however.
6. Albeit not so compelling that a state is permitted to honor it at the expense of the mother's health.
7. *See* 93 S. Ct. at 716.
8. *Id.*
9. *Id.* at 716–20.
10. *Id.* at 732. *See also id.* at 730:
11. *Id.* at 728–29 (footnote omitted).
12. Some of us who fought for the right to abortion did so with a divided spirit. We have always felt that the decision to abort was a human tragedy to be accepted only because an unwanted pregnancy was even more tragic.

13. Of course the opportunity to have an abortion should be considered part of the "liberty" protected by the Fourteenth Amendment.
14. *See, e.g.,* Dunn v. Blumstein, 405 U.S. 330 (1972); Shapiro v. Thompson, 394 U.S. 618 (1969).
15. *See also* Edwards v. California, 314 U.S. 160 (1941).
16. *See* United States v. Wheeler, 254 U.S. 281, 294 (1920); Slaughterhouse Cases, 83 U.S. (16 Wall.) 36, 75 (1872); U.S. Arts. Confed. art. IV; 3 M. Farrand, The Records of the Federal Convention of 1787, at 112 (1911); *cf.* The Federalist, No. 42, at 307 (Wright ed. 1961).
17. *See* Crandall v. Nevada, 73 U.S. (6 Wall.) 35 (1867); C. Black, Structure and Relationship in Constitutional Law (1969). The Court seems to regard the opportunity to travel *outside* the United States as merely an aspect of the "liberty" that under the Fifth and Fourteenth Amendments cannot be denied without due process. *See* Zemel v. Rusk, 381 U.S. 1, 14 (1965). *Cf.* p. 935 *infra*. [In original text.]
18. 93 S. Ct. at 727.
19. 93 S. Ct. at 727.² *See also id.* at 757 (Douglas, J., concurring).
20. It might be noted that most of the factors enumerated also apply to the inconvenience of having an unwanted two-year-old, or a senile parent, around. Would the Court find the constitutional right of privacy invaded in those situations too? I find it hard to believe it would; even if it did, of course, it would not find a constitutional right to "terminate" the annoyance—presumably because "real" persons are now involved. *But cf.* p. 926 *supra* & note 48 *supra*. [In original text.] But what about ways of removing the annoyance that do not involve "termination"? Can they really be matters of constitutional entitlement?
21. *But cf.* 93 S. Ct. at 758–59 (Douglas, J., concurring).
22. *Cf.* Katz v. United States, 389 U.S. 347, 350–51 (1967).
23. Even this statement of the demands of "substantive due process" is too strong for many Justices and commentators, who deny that any such doctrine should exist. *See, e.g.,* pp. 937–38 *infra*. [In original text.]
24. *See* Branzburg v. Hayes, 408 U.S. 665 (1972).
25. See, e.g., Abortion, The New Republic, Feb. 10, 1973, at 9; Stone, *supra* note 22. [In original text.]

SUGGESTED READINGS FOR CHAPTER 5

Books and Articles

Annas, George J. "Abortion and the Supreme Court: Round Two." *Hastings Center Report* 6 (October, 1976), 15–17.

Beauchamp, Tom L., ed. *Ethics and Public Policy.* Englewood Cliffs, N.J.: Prentice-Hall, 1975. Chap. 6.

Bok, Sissela, *et al.* "The Unwanted Child: Caring for the Fetus Born Alive After an Abortion." *Hastings Center Report* 6 (October, 1976), pp. 10–15.

Callahan, Daniel. *Abortion: Law, Choice and Morality*. New York: Macmillan, 1970.

Feinberg, Joel, ed. *The Problem of Abortion*. Belmont, Calif.: Wadsworth Publishing Company, 1973.

Finnis, John. "The Rights and Wrongs of Abortion: A Reply to Judith Thomson." *Philosophy and Public Affairs* 2 (Winter, 1973), 117–145.

Foot, Philippa. "The Problem of Abortion and the Doctrine of Double Effect." *Oxford Review* 5 (1967). Reprinted in Rachels, James, ed. *Moral Problems*. 2nd edition. New York: Harper & Row, 1975. Pp. 59–70.

Granfield, David. *The Abortion Decision*. Garden City, N.Y.: Doubleday Image Books, 1971.

Hare, R. M. "Abortion and the Golden Rule." *Philosophy and Public Affairs* 4 (Spring, 1975), 201–222.

Noonan, John T., Jr., ed. *The Morality of Abortion: Legal and Historical Perspectives*. Cambridge, Mass.: Harvard University Press, 1970.

Perkins, Robert L., ed. *Abortion: Pro and Con*. Cambridge, Mass.: Schenkman Publishing Co., 1974.

Ramsey, Paul. "The Morality of Abortion." In Labby, Daniel H., ed. *Life or Death: Ethics and Options*. Seattle: University of Washington Press, 1968. Pp. 60–93. Reprinted, with revisions, in Rachels, James, ed. *Moral Problems*. 2nd edition. New York: Harper & Row, 1975. Pp. 37–58.

Thomson, Judith Jarvis. "Rights and Deaths." *Philosophy and Public Affairs* 2 (Winter, 1973), 146–159.

Tooley, Michael. "Abortion and Infanticide." *Philosophy and Public Affairs* 2 (Fall, 1972), 37–65.

Tribe, Laurence H. "Toward a Model of Roles in the Due Process of Life and Law." *Harvard Law Review* 87 (November, 1973), 1–53.

U.S., Supreme Court. *Danforth v. Planned Parenthood of Missouri. Supreme Court Reporter* 96 (1976), 2831–2857.

Bibliographies

Clouser, K. Danner, and Zucker, Arthur, eds. *Abortion and Euthanasia: An Annotated Bibliography*. Philadelphia: Society for Health and Human Values, 1974.

Sollitto, Sharmon, and Veatch, Robert M., comps. *Bibliography of Society, Ethics and the Life Sciences*. Hastings-on-Hudson, N.Y.: Institute of Society, Ethics and the Life Sciences. Updated periodically. See under "Abortion."

Walters, LeRoy, ed. *Bibliography of Bioethics*. Vols. 1- . Detroit: Gale Research Co. Issued annually. See under "Abortion," "Selective Abortion" and "Therapeutic Abortion."

6.
The Definition and Determination of Death

Chapter 5 surveyed some biological aspects of early human development and explored the ethical problem of abortion. The next two chapters will focus on conceptual and ethical issues at the end of human life.

RECENT COMPLICATIONS IN THE DEFINITION OF DEATH

Until approximately twenty years ago the definition of death seemed relatively clear and unambiguous. Most persons would have accepted, without question, the following definition from *Black's Law Dictionary:*

[Death is:] The cessation of life; the ceasing to exist; defined by physicians as a total stoppage of the circulation of the blood, and a cessation of the animal and vital functions consequent thereon, such as respiration, pulsation, etc.[1]

Two recent biomedical developments have tended to complicate the definition of death. The first is the widespread and increasing use of new devices for the prolongation of life, particularly the artificial respirator. With the aid of such devices respiration and heartbeat can be sustained indefinitely, even if the patient is in a comatose state. Indeed, in many cases vital functions can be sustained long after all electrical activity in the brain has ceased. Thus, a simple reliance on the traditional criteria of blood circulation and respiration may no longer be possible in cases where certain types of artificial life-support systems are employed.

A second development which has pointed up the need for a more adequate definition of death is the increasing use of cadaver organs for transplantation. Two divergent interests can be identified in the transplantation situation. On the one hand, patients want to be assured that no novel definition will allow for the removal of organs from still living persons. On the other hand, the prospects for successful transplant are improved if an organ can be removed from a cadaver immediately after death has occurred.

In response to these developments, an Ad Hoc Committee of the Harvard Medical School published in 1968 a report entitled "A Definition of Irreversible Coma." Although this document has subsequently been criticized on numerous grounds, it has been primarily responsible for setting the parameters of the current debate on the definition of death.

LEVELS OF DISCUSSION IN THE DEFINITION AND DETERMINATION OF DEATH

Three distinct levels in the discussion of death can be identified: (1) the basic philosophical concept of death; (2) physiological standards for recognizing death; and (3) methods for determining whether the physiological standards have been fulfilled in a particular case.[2]

The Basic Philosophical Concept of Death. This first category refers to general concepts, or definitions, of death. These concepts of death are frequently based on particular theories of human personhood and are generally not testable through the use of empirical measurements. Three philosophical concepts of death are noted in the Veatch essay in this chapter: the loss of the capacity for rationality, the loss of the capacity to experience, and the loss of the capacity for social interaction. A further concept of death, which has been adopted by some philosophical and religious traditions, is the departure of the soul from the body.

Physiological Standards. Unlike the basic concepts of death, these standards focus on the functioning of specific bodily systems or organs. In most cases empirical tests are available for verifying that the standards have, or have not, been fulfilled. The traditional physiological standard for recognizing death has been the (irreversible) loss of circulatory and/or respiratory function. Since the advent of artificial respirators, this standard has sometimes been limited to the (irreversible) loss of *spontaneous* circulatory and/or respiratory function. Several recently developed physiological standards focus primary attention on the central nervous system —the brain and spinal cord. Among these standards are the (irreversible) loss of the following functions: reflex activity mediated through the brain or spinal cord; electrical activity in the cerebral neocortex; and/or cerebral blood flow. Both the traditional and the more recently developed standards can be employed either individually or in combination.

Methods for Determining the Fulfillment of Standards. This third level of discussion is closely related to the second but refers to specific means for testing whether the physiological standards have been fulfilled. These testing methods frequently change in response to technological advances. In addition, it is possible in some cases to apply several alternative tests to a single standard. For example, the loss of circulatory function can be determined either by taking the patient's pulse or by recording an electrocardiogram. Testing methods which are employed to determine the fulfillment of other standards include the use of electroencephalography to measure electrical activity in the neocortex and the injection of radioactive tracers into the circulatory system for detecting cerebral blood flow.

There is obviously a close correlation between the second and third levels of discussion outlined above, the general standards and the specific testing methods. However, the relationship between the first level, basic concepts of death, and the other two levels is a matter of debate. It seems likely that there are correlations between particular concepts of death and particular physiological standards for recognizing death. A stronger and more controversial claim would be that one's concept of death either influences or determines one's choice of a physiological standard for the recognition of death.

CONFLICTING PROPOSALS FOR THE DETERMINATION OF DEATH

The report of the Harvard Ad Hoc Committee discusses three primary physiological standards for recognizing "irreversible coma," which the Committee calls "a new criterion for death"[3]: (1) unreceptivity and unresponsivity; (2) no spontaneous muscular movements or spontaneous breathing; and (3) no reflexes. A confirmatory standard is the absence of cerebral function, as indicated by a flat electroencephalogram.

The essays by Jonas and Veatch represent sharply divergent responses to the position of the Harvard Ad Hoc Committee. Jonas criticizes the Ad Hoc Committee for attempting to draw a sharp line between life and death when in fact, according to Jonas, life often shades imperceptibly into death. He also rejects the Committee's requirement of *spontaneous* respiration, arguing that artificially sustained life is nonetheless life. In addition, Jonas regards the loss of central nervous system function—even the total loss of brain function—as irrelevant to the question of *defining* death. In his view, the current emphasis on whole-brain or cerebral function is based on an unhealthy mind-body dualism. Jonas' essay thus reflects a return to traditional physiological standards for recognizing death and a refusal to adjust those standards merely because of medicine's new ability to maintain respiratory function and to measure electrical activity in the brain.

A second perspective on the Harvard Ad Hoc Committee criteria is presented by Robert Veatch, who argues that the Committee did not go far enough in the direction of brain death. In his view, the irreversible loss of functioning in the highest region of the brain—the cerebral neocortex—is the primary physiological standard for the recognition of death. Other central nervous system functions, such as the mediation of spinal or brain-stem reflexes or the activation of spontaneous respiration, are on this view irrelevant to the question of life and death. Veatch's viewpoint thus represents the polar opposite of Jonas's position and rejects, as well, many of the standards proposed by the Harvard Ad Hoc Committee.

As the preceding paragraphs make clear, there is a close correlation between the topics of this chapter and the succeeding chapter. Indeed, some borderline cases can be analyzed *either* as cases of determining death (Chapter 6) *or* as cases involving the prolongation of life or euthanasia (Chapter 7), depending upon the physiological standard chosen. For example, Jonas and the Harvard Ad Hoc Committee would classify as "alive" a spontaneously breathing individual with a continuously flat electroencephalogram. Therefore, any decision concerning appropriate medical care for the individual would be a decision about whether to prolong the life of a patient. In contrast, the physiological standard proposed by Robert Veatch—electrical activity in the cerebral neocortex—would lead to the categorization of the same individual as "already dead." Thus, logically speaking, the questions of prolonging life and euthanasia could not arise.

LEGAL APPROACHES TO THE DEFINITION AND DETERMINATION OF DEATH

The issue of criteria for the determination of death has been raised in several American court cases involving organ transplantation. In one civil action a plaintiff charged that his brother's heart had been removed without the family's consent and before the patient had died.[4] In another type of case, defendants charged with murder or manslaughter have argued that surgical removal of the victim's heart for transplantation, not the injury inflicted by the defendant, was the immediate cause of the patient's death.[5] Several states have also enacted statutes which adopt rather divergent criteria for the definition or determination of death.

Capron and Kass recommend the legislative route of policy formulation as preferable to judicial responses to cases which happen to reach the courts. They criticize the earliest death statutes, enacted by Kansas and Maryland, for seeming to propose two alternative "definitions" of death, a respiratory-circulatory definition and a brain-oriented definition. In general, Capron and Kass argue that death legislation should seek to set physiological standards for the recognition of death rather than attempting to define death or to prescribe methods for testing whether the physiological standards have been fulfilled. The authors also propose a model statute which includes two physiological standards, a respiratory-circulatory standard for patients who are not on artificial respirators and a brain-oriented standard for respirator-assisted patients.

It should be noted, in conclusion, that there is no *necessary* connection between the general recommendations of Capron and Kass and their proposal of specific standards for a model statute. One could accept the authors' view concerning the role of legislatures in setting physiological standards for the recognition of death, without committing oneself to the two standards which the authors themselves adopt. Thus, any of the standards discussed in this chapter can, in principle, and may, in fact, be adopted by legislatures in the near or distant future.

L. W.

NOTES

1. *Black's Law Dictionary*, revised 4th edition, 1968, p. 488.
2. Similar distinctions are developed by Alexander M. Capron and Leon R. Kass in the final selection of this chapter. The categories designated by Capron and Kass as "general physiological standards" and "operational criteria" have been combined under the single heading "physiological standards."
3. Pp. 257–258 in this chapter.
4. City of Richmond, Law and Equity Court, *Tucker's Administrator v. Lower,* No. 2831, May 25, 1972.
5. See, for example, the cases discussed by Linda Ekstrom Stanley, "The Law of Homicide: Does It Require a Definition of Death?" *Wake Forest Law Review* 11 (June, 1975), especially pp. 253–255.

THE AD HOC COMMITTEE[1]

A Definition of Irreversible Coma

Our primary purpose is to define irreversible coma as a new criterion for death. There are two reasons why there is need for a definition: (1) Improvements in resuscitative and supportive measures have led to increased efforts to save those who are desperately injured. Sometimes these efforts have only partial success so that the result is an individual whose heart continues to beat but whose brain is irreversibly damaged. The burden is great on patients who suffer permanent loss of intellect, on their families, on the hospitals, and on those in need of hospital beds already occupied by these comatose patients. (2) Obsolete criteria for the definition of death can lead to controversy in obtaining organs for transplantation.

Irreversible coma has many causes, but *we are concerned here only with those comatose individuals who have no discernible central nervous system activity*. If the characteristics can be defined in satisfactory terms, translatable into action—and we believe this is possible—then several problems will either disappear or will become more readily soluble.

More than medical problems are present. There are moral, ethical, religious, and legal issues. Adequate definition here will prepare the way for better insight into all of these matters as well as for better law than is currently applicable.

Reprinted by permission of the author and the publisher from "A Definition of Irreversible Coma," a report of the Ad Hoc Committee of the Harvard Medical School, *Journal of the American Medical Association*, Vol. 205, No. 6 (August 1968), pp. 337–340. Copyright 1968, American Medical Association.

CHARACTERISTICS OF IRREVERSIBLE COMA

An organ, brain or other, that no longer functions and has no possibility of functioning again is for all practical purposes dead. Our first problem is to determine the characteristics of a *permanently* nonfunctioning brain.

A patient in this state appears to be in deep coma. The condition can be satisfactorily diagnosed by points 1, 2, and 3 to follow. The electroencephalogram (point 4) provides confirmatory data, and when available it should be utilized. In situations where for one reason or another electroencephalographic monitoring is not available, the absence of cerebral function has to be determined by purely clinical signs, to be described, or by absence of circulation as judged by standstill of blood in the retinal vessels, or by absence of cardiac activity.

1. *Unreceptivity and Unresponsitivity.* There is a total unawareness to externally applied stimuli and inner need and complete unresponsiveness—our definition of irreversible coma. Even the most intensely painful stimuli evoke no vocal or other response, not even a groan, withdrawal of a limb, or quickening of respiration.

2. *No Movements or Breathing.* Observations covering a period of at least one hour by physicians is adequate to satisfy the criteria of no spontaneous muscular movements or spontaneous respiration or response to stimuli such as pain, touch, sound, or light. After the patient is on a mechanical respirator, the total absence of spontaneous breathing may be established by turning off the respirator

for three minutes and observing whether there is any effort on the part of the subject to breathe spontaneously. (The respirator may be turned off for this time provided that at the start of the trial period the patient's carbon dioxide tension is within the normal range, and provided also that the patient had been breathing room air for at least 10 minutes prior to the trial.)

3. *No reflexes.* Irreversible coma with abolition of central nervous system activity is evidenced in part by the absence of elicitable reflexes. The pupil will be fixed and dilated and will not respond to a direct source of bright light. Since the establishment of a fixed, dilated pupil is clear-cut in clinical practice, there should be no uncertainty as to its presence. Ocular movement (to head turning and to irrigation of the ears with ice water) and blinking are absent. There is no evidence of postural activity (decerebrate or other). Swallowing, yawning, vocalization are in abeyance. Corneal and pharyngeal reflexes are absent.

As a rule the stretch of tendon reflexes cannot be elicited; i.e., tapping the tendons of the biceps, triceps, and pronator nuscles, quadriceps and gastrocnemius muscles with the reflex hammer elicits no contraction of the respective muscles. Plantar or noxious stimulation gives no response.

4. *Flat Electroencephalogram.* Of great confirmatory value is the flat or isoelectric EEG. We must assume that the electrodes have been properly applied, that the apparatus is functioning normally, and that the personnel in charge is competent. We consider it prudent to have one channel of the apparatus used for an electrocardiogram. This channel will monitor the ECG so that, if it appears in the electroencephalographic leads because of high resistance, it can be readily identified. It also establishes the presence of the active heart in the absence of the EEG. We recommend that another channel be used for a noncephalic lead. This will pick up space-borne or vibration-borne artifacts and identify them. The simplest form of such a monitoring noncephalic electrode has two leads over the dorsum of the hand, preferably the right hand, so the ECG will be minimal or absent. Since one of the requirements of this state is that there be no muscle activity, these two dorsal hand electrodes will not be bothered by muscle artifact. The apparatus should be run at standard gains $10\mu v/mm$, $50\mu v/5$ mm. Also it should be isoelectric at double this standard gain which is $5\mu v/5$ mm or $25\mu v/5$ mm. At least ten full minutes of recording are desirable, but twice that would be better.

It is also suggested that the gains at some point be opened to their full amplitude for a brief period (5 to 100 seconds) to see what is going on. Usually in an intensive care unit artifacts will dominate the picture, but these are readily identifiable. There shall be no electroencephalographic response to noise or to pinch.

All of the above tests shall be repeated at least 24 hours later with no change.

The validity of such data as indications of irreversible cerebral damage depends on the exclusion of two conditions: hypothermia (temperature below 90 F [32.2 C]) or central nervous system depressants, such as barbiturates.

OTHER PROCEDURES

The patient's condition can be determined only by a physician. When the patient is hopelessly damaged as defined above, the family and all colleagues who have participated in major decisions concerning the patient, and all nurses involved, should be so informed. Death is to be declared and *then* the respirator turned off. The decision to do this and the responsibility for it are to be taken by the physician-in-charge, in consultation with one or more physicians who have been directly involved in the case. It is unsound and undesirable to force the family to make the decision.

LEGAL COMMENTARY

The legal system of the United States is greatly in need of the kind of analysis and recommendations for medical procedures in cases of irreversible brain damage as described. At present, the law of the United States, in all 50 states and in the federal courts, treats the question of human death as a question of fact to be decided in every case. When any doubt exists, the courts seek medical expert testimony concerning the time of death of the particular individual involved. However, the law makes the assumption that the medical criteria for determining death are settled and not in doubt among physicians. Furthermore, the law assumes that the traditional method among physicians for determination of death is to ascertain the absence of all vital signs. To this extent, *Black's Law Dictionary* (fourth edition, 1951) defines death as

The cessation of life; the ceasing to exist; *defined by physicians* as a total stoppage of the circulation of the blood, and a cessation of the animal and vital functions consequent thereupon, such as respiration, pulsation, etc. [italics added].

In the few modern court decisions involving a definition of death, the courts have used the concept of the total cessation of all vital signs. Two cases are worthy of examination. Both involved the issue of which one of two persons died first.

In *Thomas vs Anderson,* (96 Cal App 2d 371, 211 P 2d 478) a California District Court of Appeal in 1950 said, ''In the instant case the question as to which of the two men died first was a question of fact for the determination of the trial court . . .''

The appellate court cited and quoted in full the definition of death from *Black's Law Dictionary* and concluded, '' . . . death occurs precisely when life ceases and does not occur until the heart stops beating and respiration ends. Death is not a continuous event and is an event that takes place at a precise time.''

The other case is *Smith vs Smith* (229 Ark, 579, 317 SW 2d 275) decided in 1958 by the Supreme Court of Arkansas. In this case the two people were husband and wife involved in an auto accident. The husband was found dead at the scene of the accident. The wife was taken to the hospital unconscious. It is alleged that she ''remained in coma due to brain injury'' and died at the hospital 17 days later. The petitioner in court 'tried to argue that the two people died simultaneously. The judge writing the opinion said the petition contained a ''quite unusual and unique allegation.'' It was quoted as follows:

That the said Hugh Smith and his wife, Lucy Coleman Smith, were in an automobile accident on the 19th day of April, 1957, said accident being instantly fatal to each of them at the same time, although the doctors maintained a vain hope of survival and made every effort to revive and resuscitate said Lucy Coleman Smith until May 6th, 1957, when it was finally determined by the attending physicians that their hope of resuscitation and possible restoration of human life to the said Lucy Coleman Smith was entirely vain, and

That as a matter of modern medical science, your petitioner alleges and states, and will offer the Court competent proof that the said Hugh Smith, deceased, and said Lucy Coleman Smith, deceased, lost their power to will at the same instant, and that their demise as earthly human beings occurred at the same time in said automobile accident, neither of them ever regaining any consciousness whatsoever.

The court dismissed the petition as a *matter of law*. The court quoted *Black's* definition of death and concluded

Admittedly, this condition did not exist, and as a matter of fact, it would be too much of a strain of credulity for us to believe any evidence offered to the effect that Mrs. Smith was dead, scientifically or otherwise, unless the conditions set out in the definition existed.

Later in the opinion the court said, ''Likewise, we take judicial notice that one breathing, though unconscious, is not dead.''

''Judicial notice'' of this definition of death means that the court did not consider that definition open to serious controversy; it considered the question as settled in responsible scientific and medical circles. The judge thus makes proof of uncontroverted facts unnecessary so as to prevent prolonging the trial with unnecessary proof and also to prevent fraud being committed upon the court by quasi ''scientists'' being called into court to controvert settled scientific principles at a price. Here, the Arkansas Supreme Court considered the definition of death to be a settled, scientific, biological fact. It refused to consider the plaintiff's offer of evidence that ''modern medical science'' might say otherwise. In simplified form, the above is the state of the law in the United States concerning the definition of death.

In this report, however, we suggest that responsible medical opinion is ready to adopt new criteria for pronouncing death to have occurred in an individual sustaining irreversible coma as a result of permanent brain damage. If this position is adopted by the medical community, it can form the basis for change in the current legal concept of death. No statutory change in the law should be necessary since the law treats this question essentially as one of fact to be determined by physicians. The only circumstance in which it would be necessary that legislation be offered in the various states to define "death" by law would be in the event that great controversy were engendered surrounding the subject and physicians were unable to agree on the new medical criteria.

It is recommended as a part of these procedures that judgment of the existence of these criteria is solely a medical issue. It is suggested that the physician in charge of the patient consult with one or more other physicians directly involved in the case before the patient is declared dead on the basis of these criteria. In this way, the responsibility is shared over a wider range of medical opinion, thus providing an important degree of protection against later questions which might be raised about the particular case. It is further suggested that the decision to declare the person dead, and then to turn off the respirator, be made by physicians not involved in any later effort to transplant organs or tissue from the deceased individual. This is advisable in order to avoid any appearance of self-interest by the physicians involved.

It should be emphasized that we recommend the patient be declared dead before any effort is made to take him off a respirator, if he is then on a respirator. This declaration should not be delayed until he has been taken off the respirator and all artificially stimulated signs have ceased. The reason for this recommendation is that in our judgment it will provide a greater degree of legal protection to those involved. Otherwise, the physicians would be turning off

the respirator on a person who is, under the present strict, technical application of law, still alive.

COMMENT

Irreversible coma can have various causes: cardiac arrest; asphyxia with respiratory arrest; massive brain damage; intracranial lesions, neoplastic or vascular. It can be produced by other encephalopathic states such as the metabolic derangements associated, for example, with uremia. Respiratory failure and impaired circulation underlie all of these conditions. They result in hypoxia and ischemia of the brain.

From ancient times down to the recent past it was clear that, when the respiration and heart stopped, the brain would die in a few minutes; so the obvious criterion of no heart beat as synonymous with death was sufficiently accurate. In those times the heart was considered to be the central organ of the body; it is not surprising that its failure marked the onset of death. This is no longer valid when modern resuscitative and supportive measures are used. These improved activities can now restore "life" as judged by the ancient standards of persistent respiration and continuing heart beat. This can be the case even when there is not the remotest possibility of an individual recovering consciousness following massive brain damage. In other situations "life" can be maintained only by means of artificial respiration and electrical stimulation of the heart beat, or in temporarily by-passing the heart, or, in conjunction with these things, reducing with cold the body's oxygen requirement.

In an address, "The Prolongation of Life," (1957),[2] Pope Pius XII raised many questions; some conclusions stand out: (1) In a deeply unconscious individual vital functions may be maintained over a prolonged period only by extraordinary means. Verification of the moment of death can be determined, if at all, only by a physician. Some have suggested that the moment of death can be determined, if at all, only by a physician. Some have suggested that the moment of death is the moment when irreparable and overwhelming brain damage occurs. Pius XII acknowledged that it is not "within the competence of the Church" to determine this. (2) It is incumbent on the physician to take all reasonable, ordinary means of restoring the spontaneous vital functions and consciousness, and to employ such extraordinary means as are available to him to this end. It is not obligatory, however, to continue to use extraordinary means indefinitely in hopeless cases. "But normally one is held to use only ordinary means—according to circumstances of persons, places, times, and cultures—that is to say, means that do not involve any grave burden for oneself or another." It is the church's view that a time comes when resuscitative efforts should stop and death be unopposed.

SUMMARY

The neurological impairment to which the terms "brain death syndrome" and "irreversible coma" have become attached indicates diffuse disease. Function is abolished at cerebral, brain-stem, and often spinal levels. This should be evident in all cases from clinical examination alone. Cerebral, cortical, and thalamic involvement are indicated by a complete absence of receptivity of all forms of sensory stimulation and a lack of response to stimuli and to inner need. The term "coma" is used to designate this state of unreceptivity and unresponsitivity. But there is always coincident paralysis of brain-stem and basal ganglionic mechanisms as manifested by an abolition of all postural reflexes, including induced decerebrate postures; a complete paralysis of respiration; widely dilated, fixed pupils; paralysis of ocular movements; swallowing; phonation; face and tongue muscles. Involvement of spi-

nal cord, which is less constant, is reflected usually in loss of tendon reflex and all flexor withdrawal or nocifensive reflexes. Of the brain-stem-spinal mechanisms which are conserved for a time, the vasomotor reflexes are the most persistent, and they are responsible in part for the paradoxical state of retained cardiovascular function, which is to some extent independent of nervous control, in the face of widespread disorder of cerebrum, brain stem, and spinal cord.

Neurological assessment gains in reliability if the aforementioned neurological signs persist over a period of time, with the additional safeguards that there is no accompanying hypothermia or evidence of drug intoxication. If either of the latter two conditions exist, interpretation of the neurological state should await the return of body temperature to normal level and elimination of the intoxicating agent. Under any other circumstances, repeated examinations over a period of 24 hours or longer should be required in order to obtain evidence of the irreversibility of the condition.

NOTES

1. The Ad Hoc Committee includes Henry K. Beecher, MD, *chairman;* Raymond D. Adams, MD; A. Clifford Barger, MD; William J. Curran, LLM, SMHyg; Derek Denny-Brown, MD; Dana L. Farnsworth, MD; Jordi Folch-Pi, MD; Everett I. Mendelsohn, PhD; John P. Merrill, MD; Joseph Murray, MD; Ralph Potter, ThD; Robert Schwab, MD; and William Sweet, MD.

2. Pius XII: The Prolongation of Life, *Pope Speaks* 4:393–398 (No. 4) 1958.

HANS JONAS

Against the Stream: Comments on the Definition and Redefinition of Death

The by now famous "Report of the *Ad Hoc* Committee of the Harvard Medical School to Examine the Definition of Brain Death" advocates the adoption of "irreversible coma as a new definition of death."[1] The report leaves no doubt of the practical reasons "why there is need for a definition," naming these two: relief of patient, kin, and medical resources from the burdens of indefinitely prolonged coma; and removal of controversy on obtaining organs for transplantation. On both counts, the new definition is designed to give the physician the right to terminate the treatment of a condition which not only cannot be improved by such treatment, but whose mere prolongation by it is utterly meaningless to the patient himself. The last consideration, of course, is ultimately the only valid rationale for termination (and for termination only!) and must support all the others. It does so with regard to the reasons mentioned under the first head, for the relief of the patient means automatically also that of his family, doctor, nurses, apparatus, hospital space, and so on. But the other reason—freedom for organ use— has possible implications that are not equally covered by the primary rationale, which is the patient himself. For with this primary rationale (the senselessness of mere vegetative function) the Report has strictly speaking defined not death, the ultimate state, itself, but a criterion for permitting it to take place unopposed—e.g., by turning off the respirator. The Report, however, purports by that criterion to have defined death itself, declaring it on its evidence as already given, not merely no longer to be opposed. But if "the patient is declared dead on the basis of these criteria," i.e., if the comatose individual is not a patient at all but a corpse, then the road to other uses of the definition, urged by the second reason, has been opened in principle and will be taken in practice, unless it is blocked in good time by a special barrier. What follows is meant to reinforce what I called "my feeble attempt" to help erect such a barrier on theoretical grounds.

My original comments of 1968 on the then newly proposed "redefinition of death"[2] . . . were marginal to the discussion of "experimentation on human subjects," which has to do with the living and not the dead. They have since, however, drawn fire from within the medical profession, and precisely in connection with the second of the reasons given by the Harvard Committee why a new definition is wanted, namely, the *transplant* interest, which my kind critics felt threatened by my layman's qualms and lack of understanding. Can I take this as corroborating my initial suspicion that this *interest,* in spite of its notably muted expression in the Committee Report, was and is the major motivation behind the definitional effort? I am confirmed in this suspicion when I hear Dr. Henry K. Beecher, author of the Committee's Report (and its Chairman), ask elsewhere: "Can society afford to discard the tissues and organs of the hopelessly unconscious patient when they could be used to restore the otherwise hopelessly ill, but still salvageable individual?"[3] In any case, the tenor and passion of the discussion which my initial polemic provoked from my medical friends left no doubt where the surgeon's interest in the definition lies. I contend that, pure as this interest, viz., to save other lives, is in itself, its intrusion into the *theoretical* attempt to define death makes the attempt impure; and the Harvard Committee should never have allowed

Hans Jonas, *Philosophical Essays: From Ancient Creed To Technological Man* © 1974, pp. 132–140. Reprinted by permission of Prentice-Hall, Inc., Englewood Cliffs, New Jersey.

itself to adulterate the purity of its scientific case by baiting it with the prospect of this *extraneous*—though extremely appealing—gain. But purity of theory is not my concern here. My concern is with certain practical consequences which under the urgings of that extraneous interest can be drawn from the definition and would enjoy its full sanction, once it has been officially accepted. Doctors would be less than human if certain formidable advantages of such possible consequences would not influence their judgment as to the theoretical adequacy of a definition that yields them—just as I freely admit that my shudder at one aspect of those consequences, and at the danger of others equally sanctioned by that definition, keeps my theoretical skepticism in a state of extreme alertness.

· · ·

I had to answer three charges à propos of the pertinent part of my *Daedalus* essay: that my reasoning regarding "cadaver donors" counteracts sincere life-saving efforts of physicians; that I counter precise scientific facts with vague philosophical considerations; and that I overlook the difference between death of "the organism as a whole" and death of "the whole organism," with the related difference between spontaneous and externally induced respiratory and other movements.

I plead, of course, guilty to the first charge for the case where the cadaver status of the donor is in question, which is precisely what my argument is about. The use of the term "cadaver donor" here simply begs the question, to which only the third charge (see below) addresses itself.

As to the charge of vagueness, it might just be possible that it vaguely reflects the fact that mine is an argument—a precise argument, I believe—*about* vagueness, viz., the vagueness of a condition. Giving intrinsic vagueness its due is not being vague. Aristotle observed that it is the mark of a well-educated man not to insist on greater precision in knowledge than the subject admits, e.g., the same in politics as in mathematics. Reality of certain kinds—of which the life-death spectrum is perhaps one—may be imprecise in itself, or the knowledge obtainable of it may be. To acknowledge such a

state of affairs is more adequate to it than a precise definition, which does violence to it. I am challenging the undue precision of a definition and of its practical application to an imprecise field.

The third point—which was made by Dr. Otto Guttentag—is highly relevant and I will deal with it step by step.

a. The difference between "organism as a whole" and "whole organism" which he has in mind is perhaps brought out more clearly if for "whole organism" we write "every and all parts of the organism." If this is the meaning, then I have been speaking throughout of "death of the organism as a whole," not of "death of the whole organism"; and any ambiguity in my formulations can be easily removed. Local subsystems—single cells or tissues—may well continue to function locally, i.e., to display biochemical activity for themselves (e.g., growth of hair and nails) for some time after death, without this affecting the definition of death by the larger criteria of the whole. But respiration and circulation do not fall into this class, since the effect of their functioning, though performed by subsystems, extends through the total system and insures the functional preservation of its other parts. Why else prolong them artificially in prospective "cadaveric" organ donors (e.g., "maintain renal circulation of cadaver kidneys in situ") except to keep those other parts "in good shape"—viz., alive—for eventual transplantation? The comprehensive system thus sustained is even capable of continued overall metabolism when intravenously fed, and then, presumably, of diverse other (e.g. glandular) functions as well—in fact, I suppose, of pretty much everything not involving neural control. There are stories of comatose patients lingering on for months with those aids; the metaphor of the "human vegetable" recurring in the debate (strangely enough, sometimes in support of redefining death—as if "vegetable" were not an instance of life!) say as much. In short, what is here kept going by various artifices must—with the caution due in this twilight zone—be equated with "the organism as a whole" named in the classical definition of death—much more so, at least, than with any mere, separable part of it.

b. Nor, to my knowledge, does that older definition specify that the functioning whose "irreversible cessation" constitutes death must be spontaneous and does not count for life when artificially induced and sustained (the implications for therapy would be devastating). Indeed, "irreversible" cessation can have a twofold reference: to the function itself or only to the spontaneity of it. A cessation can be irreversible with respect to spontaneity but still reversible with respect to the activity as such—in which case the reversing external agency must continuously substitute for the lost spontaneity. This is the case of the respiratory movements and heart contractions in the comatose. The distinction is not irrelevant, because if we could do for the disabled brain—let's say, the lower nerve centers only—what we can do for the heart and lungs, viz., *make* it work by the continuous input of some external agency (electrical, chemical, or whatever), we would surely do so and not be finicky about the resulting function lacking spontaneity: the functioning as such would matter. Respirator and stimulator could then be turned off, because the nerve center presiding over heart contractions (etc.) has again taken over and returned *them* to being "spontaneous"—just as systems presided over by circulation had enjoyed spontaneity of function when the circulation was only nonspontaneously active. The case is wholly hypothetical, but I doubt that a doctor would feel at liberty to pronounce the patient dead on the ground of the nonspontaneity at the cerebral source, when it can be *made* to function by an auxiliary device.

The purpose of the foregoing thought-experiment was to cast some doubt (a layman's, to be sure) on the seeming simplicity of the spontaneity criterion. With the stratification and interlocking of functions, it seems to me, organic spontaneity is distributed over many levels and loci—any superordinated level enabling its subordinates to be naturally spontaneous, be its own action natural or artificial.

c. The point with irreversible coma as defined by the Harvard group, of course, is precisely that it is a condition which precludes reactivation of any part of the brain in *every* sense. We then have an "organism as a whole" minus the brain, maintained in some partial state of life so long as the respirator and other artifices are at work. And here the question is not: has the patient died? but: how should he—still a patient—be dealt with? Now *this* question must be settled, surely not by a definition of death, but by a definition of man and of what life is human. That is to say, the question cannot be answered by decreeing that death has already occurred and the body is therefore in the domain of things; rather it is by holding, e.g., that it is humanly not justified—let alone, demanded—to artificially prolong the life of a brainless body. This is the answer I myself would advocate. On that philosophical ground, which few will contest, the physician can, indeed should, turn off the respirator and let the "definition of death" take care of itself by what then inevitably happens. (The later utilization of the corpse is a different matter I am not dealing with here, though it too resists the comfortable patness of merely utilitarian answers.) The decision to be made, I repeat, is an axiological one and not already made by clinical fact. It begins when the diagnosis of the condition has spoken: it is not diagnostic itself. Thus, as I have pointed out before, no redefinition of death is needed; only, perhaps, a redefinition of the physician's presumed duty to prolong life under all circumstances.

d. But, it might be asked, is not a definition of death made into law the simpler and more precise way than a definition of medical ethics (which is difficult to legislate) for sanctioning the same practical conclusion, while avoiding the twilight of value judgment and possible legal ambiguity? It would be, if it really sanctioned the same conclusion, and no more. But it sanctions indefinitely more: it opens the gate to a whole range of other possible conclusions, the extent of which cannot even be foreseen, but some of which are disquietingly close at hand. The point is, if the comatose patient is by definition dead, he is a patient no more but a corpse, with which can be done whatever law or custom or the deceased's will or next of kin permit and sundry interests urge doing with a corpse. This includes—why not?—the protracting of the inbetween state, for which we must find a new name ("simulated life"?) since that of "life" has been preempted by the new definition of death, and extracting from it all the profit we can. There are many. So far the "redefiners" speak of no more than keeping the respirator going until the transplant organ is to be removed, then turning it off, then beginning to cut into the "cadaver," this being the end of it—which sounds innocent enough. But why must it be the end? Why turn the respirator off? Once we are assured that we are dealing with a cadaver, there are no logical reasons against (and strong pragmatic reasons for) going on with the artificial "animation" and keeping the "deceased's" body on call, as a bank for life-fresh organs, possibly also as a plant for manufacturing hormones or other biochemical compounds in demand. I have no doubts that methods exist or can be perfected which allow the natural powers for the healing of surgical wounds by new tissue growth to stay "alive" in such a body. Tempting also is the idea of a self-replenishing blood bank. And that is not all. Let us not forget research. Why shouldn't the most wonderful surgical and grafting experiments be conducted on the complaisant subject-nonsubject, with no limits set to daring? why not immunological explorations, infection with diseases old and new, trying out of drugs? We have the active cooperation of a functional organism declared to be dead; we have, that is, the advantages of the living donor without the disadvantages imposed by his rights and interests (for a corpse has none). What a boon for medical instruction, for anatomical and physiological demonstration and practicing on so much better material than the inert cadavers otherwise serving in the dissection room! What a chance for the apprentice to learn *in vivo,* as it were, how to amputate a leg, without his mistakes mattering! And so on, into the wide open field. After all, what is advocated is "the full utilization of modern means to maximize the value of cadaver organs." Well, this is it.

Come, come, the members of the profession will say, nobody is thinking of this kind of thing. Perhaps not; but I have just shown that one *can* think of them. And the point is that the proposed definition of death has removed any reasons not to think of them and, once thought of, not to do them when found desirable (and the next of kin are agreeable). We must remember that what the Harvard group offered was not a definition of irreversible coma as a rationale for breaking off sustaining action, but a definition of death by the criterion of irreversible coma as a rationale for conceptually transposing the patient's body to the class of dead things, *regardless* of whether sustaining action is kept up or broken off. It would be hypocritical to deny that the redefinition amounts to an antedating of the accomplished fact of death (compared to conventional signs that may outlast it); that it was motivated not by exclusive concern with the patient but with certain extraneous interests in mind (organ donorship mostly named so far); and that the actual use of the general license it grants is implicity anticipated. But no matter what particular use is or is not anticipated at the moment, or even anathematized—it would be naive to think that a line can be drawn anywhere for such uses when strong enough interests urge them, seeing that the definition (which is absolute, not graded) negates the very principle for drawing a line. (Given the ingenuity of medical science, in which I have great faith, I am convinced that the "simulated life" can eventually be made to comprise practically every extraneural activity of the human body; and I would not even bet on its never comprising *some* artificially activated neural functions as well: which would be awkward for the argument of nonsensitivity, but still under the roof of that of nonspontaneity.)

e. Now my point is a very simple one. It is this. We do not know with certainty the borderline between life and death, and a definition cannot substitute for knowledge. Moreover, we have sufficient grounds for suspecting that the artificially supported condition of the comatose patient may still be one of life, however reduced—i.e., for doubting that, even with the brain function gone, he is completely dead. In this state of marginal ignorance and doubt the only course to take is to lean over backward toward the side of possible life. It follows that interventions as I described should be regarded on a par with vivisection and on no account be performed on a human body in that equivocal or threshold condition. And the definition that allows them, by stamping as unequivocal what at best is equivocal, must be rejected. But mere rejection in discourse is not enough. Given the pressure of the—very real and very worthy—medical interests, it can be predicted that the permission it implies in theory will be irresistible in practice, once the definition is installed in official authority. Its becoming so installed must therefore be resisted at all cost. It is the only thing that still can be resisted; by the time the practical conclusions beckon, it will be too late. It is a clear case of *principiis obsta*.

The foregoing argumentation was strictly on the plane of common sense and ordinary logic. Let me add, somewhat conjecturally, two philosophical observations.

I see lurking behind the proposed definition of death, apart from its obvious pragmatic motivation, a curious remnant of the old soul-body dualism. Its new apparition is the dualism of brain and body. In a certain analogy to the former it holds that the true human person rests in (or is represented by) the brain, of which the rest of the body is a mere subservient tool. Thus, when the brain dies, it is as when the soul departed: what is left are "mortal remains." Now nobody will deny that the cerebral aspect is decisive for the human quality of the life of the organism that is man's. The position I advanced acknowledges just this by recommending that with the irrecoverable total loss of brain function one should not hold up the naturally ensuing death of the rest of the organism. But it is no less an exaggeration of the cerebral aspect as it was of the conscious soul, to deny the extracerebral body its essential share in the identity of the person. The body is as uniquely the body of this brain and no other, as the brain is uniquely the brain of this body and no other. What is under the brain's central control, the bodily total, is as individual, as much "myself," as singular to my identity (fingerprints!), as noninterchangeable, as the controlling (and reciprocally controlled) brain itself. My identity is the identity of the whole organism, even if the higher functions of personhood are seated in the brain. How else could a man love a woman and not merely her brains? How else could we lose ourselves in the aspect of a face? Be touched by the delicacy of a frame? It's this person's, and no one else's. Therefore, the body of the comatose, so long as —even with the help of art—it still breathes, pulses, and functions otherwise, must still be considered a residual continuance of the subject that loved and was loved, and as such is still entitled to some of the sacrosanctity accorded to such a subject by the laws of God and men. That sacrosanctity decrees that it must not be used as a mere means.

My second observation concerns the morality of our time, to which our "redefiners" pay homage with the best of intentions, which have their own subtle sophistry. I mean the prevailing attitude toward death, whose faintheartedness they indulge in a curious blend with the toughmindedness of the scientist. The Catholic Church had the guts to say: under these circumstances let the patient die—speaking of the patient alone and not of outside interests (society's, medicine's, etc.). The cowardice of modern secular society which shrinks from death as an unmitigated evil needs the assurance (or fiction) that he is already dead when the decision is to be made. The responsibility of a value-laden decision is replaced by the mechanics of a value-free routine. Insofar as the redefiners of death—by saying "he is already dead"—seek to allay the scruples about turning the respirator off, they cater to this modern cowardice which has forgotten that death has its own fitness and dignity, and that a man has a right to be let die. Insofar as by saying so they seek to provide an even better conscience about keeping the respirator on and freely utilizing the body thus arrested on the threshold of life and death, they serve the ruling pragmatism of our time which will let no ancient fear and trembling interfere with the relentless expanding of the realm of sheer thinghood and unrestricted utility. The "splendor and misery" of our age dwells in that irresistible tide.

NOTES

1. See the first essay in this chapter.

2. Jonas's essay, "Philosophical Reflections on Experimenting with Human Subjects," was orginally published in *Daedalus* 98 (2): 219–247, Spring, 1969
3. See Chapter 9, p. 399.

ROBERT M. VEATCH

The Whole-Brain-Oriented Concept of Death: An Outmoded Philosophical Formulation

Debate over the past five years between holders of concepts of death which focus on the brain and those who focus on the more traditional heart and lungs has created a situation wherein defenders of the neurological concepts of death have not been forced to be particularly precise in specifying the meaning of terms. The seemingly endless prolongation of cellular and organ functioning (in what can be appropriately called human corpses) has been brought about by new death-assaulting technologies giving rise to a new and inhuman form of existence. While the potential for use of human organs for therapeutic transplantation should never justify the adoption of a new understanding of what is essentially significant to human life and death, it may require a philosophically responsible clarification of imprecise use of these terms adequate only in a time when little morally critical was at stake. These developments have led to an infatuation with the neurologically oriented concepts, which have made the more traditional heart-and-lung definition of death appear totally inadequate and outmoded. The thesis of this article, however, is that the time has come when crude formulations of the so-called "brain definition of death" can no longer by tolerated.

Holders of the brain-oriented concept of death would probably grant that the only practical problem with the more traditional concept, which focuses on the heart and lungs, is that it will in special occasions produce false positive tests for human life. In these rare cases, individuals who should be considered dead are labeled alive because heart and lung function continues even though brain function may have permanently and irreversibly ceased. Traditional moralists, however, or at least those who tend to hold a more rigorous, life-preserving position regarding moral obligation to an individual human being, have followed the principle of erring in the direction of following the morally safer course. Thus, in this case Hans Jonas (1969) has argued that unless one can be certain of philosophical (technical uncertainty is not being considered here) foundations of the more limited brain-oriented concept, one should opt for the false positive judgment of continuing life, rather than running the moral risk of a false positive pronouncement of death.

The holders of the brain-oriented concept, however, have apparently satisfied themselves that there is no significant risk of making the philosophical mistake of considering a man

Reprinted with permission of Alan R. Liss, Inc. from *Journal of Thanatology*, Vol. 3, No. 1 (1975), pp. 13–17, 20–30.

dead because his brain function has ceased when, in fact, the correct moral judgment would be that the individual is still alive although brain function has irreversibly ceased.

This article attempts to turn the tables on the holders of the concept of death which focuses upon the function of the whole brain and asks them precisely the same question that they have put to holders of the more traditional heart-and-lung-oriented concepts. Since they have opted for a system which would eliminate the rare false positive pronouncement of life, we consider it fair to ask whether the whole-brain concept of death might also lead to conditions in which there would be a false positive judgment that life continues. Is it then possible that there could be a condition wherein portions of the brain retain their normal functioning and yet for all practical purposes the individual should, according to our philosophical understanding of the nature of man, be pronounced dead? In this article, I argue that this indeed is the case, that our concept of death must be further refined, and our technical criteria for death must be modified accordingly so that our concept and criteria most accurately reflect our understanding of what is essentially significant to the nature of man.

PRELIMINARY PHILOSOPHICAL ASSUMPTIONS

THE CONCEPT OF DEATH IS TOTALLY A PHILOSOPHICAL AND IN NO WAY A TECHNICAL-MEDICAL ISSUE

In order to make the argument of this article, it will be necessary to assume a great deal of the debate about the definition of death which has taken place over the past few years. The first major document in this debate is the report of the Ad Hoc Committee to Examine the Definition of Brain Death (1968). It is crucial for philosophical understanding of this debate to realize that this committee did not in any sense offer a new definition of death or even a new definition of brain death. It merely offered, as the title of the report states, criteria for irreversible coma. In no place in the com-

mittee's report did it argue that irreversible coma measured by the criteria it presented is to be equated with brain death and, in turn, that brain death is to be equated with death of the whole human being. In 1968, the distinction between the technical measures of the irreversible loss of a body function and the much more philosophical or moral judgment about the nature of life and death was not clear. This distinction has been made increasingly clear over the years which followed. I have argued previously (Veatch, 1972) that the criteria for loss of a body function must be kept radically separate from the philosophical argumentation. This distinction is also emphasized in a report of the Research Group on Death and Dying of the Institute of Society, Ethics and the Life Sciences, which reviewed the Harvard Criteria for Death (1972). In this article, I shall keep this distinction clear by using the term *concept* when referring to a philosophical understanding of that which is essentially significant to man's nature, while using the term *criteria* in reference to technical measures of the capacity of a body organ or organ system to function. It should be clear that the validity of a "concept" is to be tested philosophically, while "criteria" are to be verified by the empirical methods of biomedical science.

DEATH MAY BE FORMALLY DEFINED AS THE IRREVERSIBLE LOSS OF THAT WHICH IS CONSIDERED TO BE ESSENTIALLY SIGNIFICANT TO THE NATURE OF MAN

The distinction between the technical measures of criteria for loss of a body function and the philosophical argumentation needed for a concept of death can be seen if one begins with a completely formal definition of death. I propose such a formal definition:

Death is the irreversible loss of that which is essentially significant to the nature of man.

Death, as the term is used in the present debate, is not in any sense a biological statement of cessation of cellular respiration or functioning, as the term *death* might be used in referring to the death of a plant or non-human animal. When we say that an amoeba has died, we mean that cellular respiration has ceased, or mobility of the cellular protoplasm has ceased, and nothing more. When we speak of human death, however, we mean something radically different. We are making a practical statement with policy implications. We are saying that it is now appropriate to behave toward the individual in a different way. It is now appropriate to stop certain medical treatments which could not justifiably have been stopped previously. It is appropriate to begin burial ritual and for the deceased's friends and family to begin the mourning process. It might, under certain circumstances, be appropriate to remove vital non-paired organs where this would be inappropriate prior to pronouncing death. An individual's will may be read and an estate transferred to others. If the individual is a holder of public office, say, the president of the United States, the vice president would assume the office of the president. Thus, human death is a social and moral concept quite beyond the biological. It may still be appropriate to talk about the death of an individual's cells or even an organ in the more narrow biological sense, but the only reason the definition of death receives any attention at all in the realm of public policy is that the term summarizes and legitimates what might be called "death behavior," a radically different set of social relationships and actions.

The formal definition of death given here reveals that that formal definition can be given substantive content only by further philosophical analysis. It is necessary to reach some understanding about what is essentially significant to the nature of man. This can never be determined by biological investigation, but only by philosophical or theological reflection.

. . .

THE ESSENTIALLY SIGNIFICANT TO THE NATURE OF MAN

The Harvard Committee had as its objective, if we are to believe its title, the examination of the definition of brain death. Yet, the title of its report clearly indicates that what the committee did was attempt to provide criteria for irreversible coma. Whether the "death" of the brain can be equated without remainder to the state of irreversible coma is in large part a scientific, empirical question. In the per-

spective of the years since the Harvard report was written, however, it seems on the surface that there may well be a great difference between the death of the entire brain and the state of irreversible coma. This forces us to be much more precise about exactly what in the functioning of the brain is of critical importance. Exploration of this question is the purpose of this and the following sections of the article. First, we shall attempt to gain a clearer understanding of what is so essentially significant to the nature of man that its loss is called death and appropriately initiates death behavior.

CAPACITY TO INTEGRATE BODILY FUNCTION

. . . If we are speaking of the death of the organism as a whole, and not simply the death of isolated cells, organs, or organ systems, it at first seems plausible to consider the complex integrating capacity of an organism as that which is essential to it. If this is the case, then the loss of that integrating capacity could appropriately be equated to the organism's death. From what we know of the integrating capacity of the human body, the brain is far and away the dominant locus of this capacity. To be sure, the spinal cord and peripheral nerves are also important, but these do not really provide integration. The spinal reflex at most provides a primitive and pale imitation of integrating function. The mysterious integrating capacity of the nervous system, which has fascinated man and been conceptualized so influentially by Claude Bernard is, by comparison, so much more grand as to make the difference between a simple animal and the human organism.

It seems reasonable from what we think we know about the brain to relate this concept of integrating capacity to the whole brain. If this is what is seen as essentially significant to man, then the examination of the whole brain for signs of functioning may be a plausible test for death of the person.

Yet, the simple equation of the brain death to "irreversible coma" by the Harvard Committee should give us pause. Was it really this integrating capacity the committee members had in mind? If so, why did they substitute the term *irreversible coma?* Henry Beecher, the committee's chairman, writing elsewhere (1970) makes clear which functions he deems essential to man, and he does not seem to include all of the brain's functions. He clearly believes that a man is dead when he irreversibly loses his:

personality, his conscious life, his uniqueness, his capacity for remembering, judging, reasoning, acting, enjoying, worrying, and so on.

Dr. Beecher goes on to argue:

We have proof that these and other functions reside in the brain. . . . It seems clear that when the brain no longer functions, when it is destroyed, so also is the individual destroyed; he no longer exists as a person; he is dead.

Certainly this conclusion follows from what we know about the brain, but there is a fundamental error in the argument. We have suggested that the practical problem with the more conservative heart-and-lung-oriented concepts is that they occasionally produce false positive tests for life. If the argument is to be made for brain-oriented criteria at all (and we have already argued this is a difficult but possible case to make), then certainly that argument must be subject to the same criticism. The functions mentioned by Beecher and summarized by the term *irreversible coma* certainly are in the brain, but clearly do not exhaust the brain's functions. Focusing on the destruction of the whole brain may include additional non-essential functions, just as focusing on the heart and lungs did. The decision will rest upon the plausibility of functions, such as integrating capacity, being centered in the whole brain when contrasted with other more anatomically limited characteristics.

THE CAPACITY FOR RATIONALITY

The list of characteristics includes man's ability to reason. The Latin name for our species clearly implies that reasoning capacity is somehow an essential characteristic. Could it be that it is reasoning capacity, rather than integrating capacity, which is essential? I believe not. Our considered moral judgments about those members of the species who do not have any capacity for reasoning is that they are still to be considered living in a very real way. They are still to have human rights, protected by both moral and positive law.

The baby lacking a language, a culture, and a capacity to reason certainly is living in a human sense in spite of the fact that he has never executed the reasoning function. One might, of course, argue that the baby has the potential for reasoning—the capacity for future reasoning. In this sense, he is included in the human living. But what of those afflicted with senile dementia, the mentally retarded, the apparently permanently psychotic? They also lack a capacity for rationality and in some cases will never regain that capacity. Yet, it is clear that they are still living in a meaningful sense of the term. In fact, one of the great dangers of moving to any brain-oriented concept of death is that it might place us on an evolutionary course, a "slippery slope" leading to the eventual exclusion of certain individuals who lack a certain quality of life from the category of the human. Unless this tendency can be avoided, the dangers of movement to brain-oriented concepts may well exceed the moral right-making tendencies. Whatever may be our propensity to see rationality as the pinnacle of man's functioning, it must not be the characteristic which is essential to consider him living. We must look elsewhere.

THE CAPACITY TO EXPERIENCE

Most of the other functions mentioned in lists of essentially human characteristics—consciousness, capacity for remembering, enjoying, worrying, acting voluntarily—characterize man as an experiential animal. Experience is here taken in the broadest sense. Man experiences cognitively and emotionally. He cathects, he comprehends, he experiences through sense organs and through much more complex experiential modes. It seems clear that a human who has some vestige of consciousness, some capacity to experience in this broadest sense could never be considered dead. To be sure, his life may not be on the highest plane. It may be limited to a blurred vision of reality and stunted emotional experience, but it is nevertheless life of a form sufficiently human to be protected. Death behavior for such an individual is inappropriate.

THE CAPACITY FOR SOCIAL INTERACTION

While man may be experiential, he is also a social creature. At least in the Western tradition, man's capacity to relate to fellow man is fundamental. Is it meaningful to speak of a living human who lacks the capacity for social interaction? We must make clear that we are not at all saying that actual social interaction must take place for a creature to be human. We are not even saying that such interaction has ever taken place. To say this would place man's existence at the mercy of his fellow man. The cruel treatment of a baby who has been abandoned in a room with no human interaction should not define that baby out of existence. Presumably the capacity for social interaction nevertheless remains.

What is the relationship between the capacity for experience and the capacity for social interaction? It appears that they may be synonymous. It is conceivable that a condition could exist which would differentiate the two capacities. But to be able to experience—but not experience others—would certainly be a bizarre form of existence. In practical terms, it would appear to be impossible. If it is the case that capacity to experience and capacity to experience others are coterminous, then we need pursue the matter no further. For practical purposes this seems to be sufficient. We conclude, then, that if we abandon the more traditional concepts of death (those focusing on the departure of the soul or the irreversible cessation of fluid flow) we may well find it more plausible to opt for a concept focusing on the irreversible loss of the capacity for experience or social interaction, rather than the irreversible loss of integrating capacity of the body. If this is the case, the implications for the whole-brain-oriented criteria for death are great.

Before exploring those criteria, there must be one final comment about that which is essential to the nature of man. Is it simply capacity for experience and social interaction per se, or must there also be some embodiment of the capacity? Consider the bizarre and purely hypothetical case in which all of the information of the human brain were transferred to a piece of magnetic tape together with sufficient sensory inputs and outputs to permit some form of rudimentary experiential and social function. Would the erasing of that tape be tantamount to murder? The thought is so novel that perhaps we cannot even conceive clearly of the philosophical significance of the question. It seems quite possible that our concept of the essential must include some embodiment. Man is, after all, something more than a sophisticated computer. At least in the Western tradition the body is an essential element, not something from which man escapes in liberation. If this is the case, then the essential element is embodied capacity for experience and social interaction.

PROBLEMS WITH THE WHOLE-BRAIN-ORIENTED CRITERIA OF DEATH

Our methodology at this point will be to begin by reviewing the criteria for brain death as outlined by the Harvard report and defined and endorsed by the Research Group on Death and Dying of the Institute of Society, Ethics and the Life Sciences. I shall attempt to determine the functions implied as being morally significant which are being tested by the various criteria of the Harvard report. I shall then extend the analysis by examining other brain foci, the functions of which might constitute the essentially significant in the nature of man.*

The Harvard Committee, in proposing the criteria, and the Institute's Research Group, in

---

*It is important to distinguish between criteria which are apparently closely and directly linked to functions considered essentially significant to living and criteria which are more remote and less direct. The most crucial example is the criterion of spontaneous respiration. The observation of spontaneous movement of respiratory muscles might be a direct criterion for the observation of spontaneous respiratory function. On the other hand, it might be an indirect criterion for the irreversible loss of consciousness. It is crucial to distinguish between these two types of criteria. We do not want to rule out a criterion apparently linked to a function that we might decide to be non-essential to human living, when, in fact, that criterion is really an indirect empirical measure of some functions which we indeed can consider to be significant.

endorsement of the criteria, simply failed to deal with the apparent gap between criteria for irreversible coma on the one hand and criteria for complete cessation of brain function on the other. Although empirically the two sets of criteria may be the same, they certainly represent different ranges of function. And there is no theoretical reason why the criteria should be identical, nor is there any clarification given in the reports as to which set of functions is of concern.

BRAIN-MEDIATED REFLEXES

The first criterion for irreversible coma I shall examine will be the absence of brain-mediated reflexes. The Harvard criteria for irreversible coma indicate that there should be no central nervous system reflexes present which are routed through the brain. The contraction of the pupil in response to light is given as the typical case. In later writings, Henry Beecher (1970), the chairman of that committee, makes clear that one must exclude spinal cord reflexes in applying this test. The presence of a spinal reflex arc in a decapitated corpse, according to this view, should not be considered a test for the presence of life. The problem which the committee members did not face, however, is whether a brain reflex, such as the pupillary reflex, should not similarly be excluded. The difference between these reflexes and spinal reflexes is simply that they are mediated through the lower brain stem, rather than the spinal cord.

I shall assume for purposes of this discussion that these brain reflexes are used directly as criteria for irreversible cessation of brain function. That is to say, it is the functioning of the brain stem and the ability to dilate and contract the pupil which are considered significant, and the reflex arc is not considered to be some indirect measure of some other brain function. If we can make this assumption, it seems very doubtful that the ability to contract and dilate the pupil and to execute any other reflex arc which happens to pass through the brain stem is in any way a significant sign of human living. If we can exclude a withdrawal reflex, which

might be elicited by pricking an extremity with a pin, as being insignificant in the diagnosis of living, it seems that the same argument must apply to brain stem reflexes. The ability to maintain nerve circuitry to carry out one of these reflexes does not really add significantly to man's integrating capacity. Certainly it does not directly measure capacity to experience or interact socially.

SPONTANEOUS RESPIRATION, OR BREATHING

Another criterion in the Harvard report is the observation of the presence of spontaneous respiration, or breathing. The technique used is to turn off any artificial respiratory device for a period of three minutes and make observations. The moral question which is raised by this criterion is somewhat more difficult than the presence of brain-mediated reflexes. We have a societally dictated belief that a respiring individual is living. The holder of whole-brain-oriented criteria, however, has made the moral decision that artificial respiration is not a sufficient indicator of human life. Now the same question must be asked with regard to spontaneous respiration. Is the presence of the ability to respire spontaneously essentially significant to man? The question is not merely a philosophical one. Recently, Brierley et al. (1971) reported two cases in which comatose individuals respired spontaneously for long periods of time, four months in one case, and five months in the other. The individuals apparently had no higher brain function, as indicated by repeated isoelectric electroencephalogram. There was generalized necrosis within the neocortex when examined macroscopically and microscopically after cessation of spontaneous respiration.

Those individuals with spontaneous respiration are capable of a continued existence closely related to biological life as seen in plants and other animal species (the ability to respire, together with ability to carry out some rudimentary circulatory and excretory function, is the minimal essential characteristic of non-human biological life). The view that man is closely related to the animal species is a very modern one, growing in part out of Darwinian evolutionary theory. Nevertheless, there are serious problems with this approach. To view man as essentially a respiratory creature is to ignore most of the faculties which philosophers and anthropologists have considered essential to the species. It ignores man's rational capacity, his ability to experience emotion, and to reflect upon that feeling systematically. It ignores his capacity for consciousness and memory, which gives rise to the systematic organization of experience and, in turn, gives rise to purposes, actions, and the eventual building of language and culture.

It should be clear that no philosophical *or* scientific argument can be definitive beyond the appeal to that which is reasonable or "obvious upon reflection." The claim I make, however, is that one who would see the experiential and social function of man as essential to his nature would not find spontaneous respiration a sufficient indicator of human life.

It may be that the criterion of spontaneous respiration incorporated into the Harvard criteria is an indirect measure of one of these functions (the experiential or social). The committee may have taken the position, for instance, that consciousness is the essential characteristic of the nature of man: the absence of spontaneous respiration is the only criterion which assures the loss of the future capacity for consciousness. The Harvard Comitttee, however, was established to determine criteria for brain death, not for the irreversible loss of consciousness. It appears that in the absence of any arguments in the report to the contrary, its authors incorporated the criterion of spontaneous respiration as a direct measure of a function of a part of the brain (i.e., the lower brain center which is responsible for spontaneous respiratory function). If that was their intention, they have indeed given a measure of functioning of a part of the whole brain. But they have not necessarily given a criterion for diagnosing the presence of a living person any more significant than spontaneous beating of a heart supported by artificial oxygenation.

UNRECEPTIVITY AND UNRESPONSIVITITY

The third criterion of irreversible coma, according to the Harvard Report, is the presence of unreceptivity and unresponsivity: "there is a total unawareness to externally applied stimuli and inner need and complete unresponsiveness." It is incontrovertible that were either receptivity or responsiveness present, the individual would be alive whether the concept of death being used is the irreversible loss of integrating function or the irreversible loss of experiential and social interaction capacity. What is confusing, however, is that the report's authors state explicitly that this characteristic of total unawareness is their *definition* of irreversible coma. In effect, they are saying that one of the four criteria for diagnosing irreversible coma is the presence of irreversible coma. The criterion would be more plausible had they claimed that complete unreceptivity and unresponsiveness were their definition of "coma"; however, they make the confusing claim that it is their definition of *irreversible* coma. One wonders whether that can be maintained empirically with any normal understanding of the meaning of the words.

In any case, we are left with unreceptivity and unresponsiveness (i.e., coma, but surely not necessarily irreversible coma) as a criterion of irreversible coma. We are left wondering, however, whether the committee is really interested in criteria for complete loss of the capacity for consciousness and experiential and social functioning, or criteria for complete loss of all brain function. In the preceding paragraph of the report the authors claim that the criteria for irreversible coma are "characteristics of a *permanently* nonfunctioning brain," implying that they are seeking the latter in spite of their avowed purpose. There can be no doubt that with receptivity and responsiveness, the person is not dead—whether integrating (whole-brain-oriented) function or experiential (more narrow neurological) function is the underlying concept. The question remains, however, whether the parts of the brain may retain the capacity for function in the presence of unreceptivity and unresponsiveness and even apparently permanent unreceptivity and unresponsiveness. The answer cannot come from these gross behavioral observations alone. The condition of the patient/corpse described by Brierley et al. (1971), however, implies that some parts of the brain may indeed retain that capacity.

Thus far, we have seen that the criteria of the Harvard report are not particularly helpful in resolving the underlying philosophical debate about which concept of death is justifiable. In principle, they could not be, for the concept of death is independent of the verification of criteria. The fourth criterion, however, suggests the existence of scientific techniques for confirming the absence of experiential and social function in spite of ongoing lower brain activity which continues to carry out complex integrating functions.

FLAT ELECTROENCEPHALOGRAM

The flat electroencephalogram is proposed by the Harvard report as being of "great confirmatory value" for the diagnosis of irreversible coma. While the justification of this claim rests both on the definition of irreversible coma and empirical tests, I suggest, based on my understanding of the available data, that this claim must be questioned. On the one hand, the claim may be a simple one—that an EEG with some activity is incontrovertible evidence that there is some brain function. The flat EEG confirms the existence of a permanently non-functioning brain.

The problem, however, is one we have faced before. Is the EEG measuring whole-brain function or something more limited? From the scientific evidence, the EEG apparently measures simply the presence of neocortical electrical activity. If this is true, it is quite possible that some brain activity could remain in the presence of a flat electroencephalogram. There are two implications. If one is interested in a concept of death such as integrating capacity, which is oriented to the whole brain, it is quite possible (as Brierley et al. [1971] reported) that a flat EEG would be present with brain activity remaining. Thus, while EEG activity refutes the cessation of the functioning of the whole brain, the absence of EEG reading does not necessarily mean the absence of brain function.

More significant for our purposes, if EEG measures only neocortical activity and one chooses a concept of death which is oriented more to functions centered in that portion of the brain, the EEG may not be a confirmatory test, but the central one. The use of tests centered on lower brain function may well be irrelevant (or at least indirect) ones for the irreversible loss of consciousness and experiential and social functions. Thus, the EEG may be the most important test. Whether or not this is true will depend upon empirical tests.

One argument against sole reliance on the EEG would be doubt of its empirical validity. The evidence thus far seems very convincing, however. Silverman et al. (1970) report 2,642 comatose patients with isoelectric EEGs none of whom recovered (except three influenced by CNS depressants and thus excluded from the data). The Institute's report which endorsed the Harvard criteria was aware of this, but chose not to pursue its implications because the authors wanted to avoid the critical question of the alternative concepts of death which are being tested for by the proposed criteria.

The implication is clear. If an integrating function or related concept which is oriented to the whole brain is maintained, the EEG alone is not sufficient for a diagnosis of death and is of only limited confirmatory value. If, however, an experiential and social interaction concept of death is held, or a related one oriented to more narrow brain functions apparently localized in the neocortex, then the EEG does not confirm at all. It is the definitive test. The 2,642 cases are quite persuasive. Perhaps they are so convincing that reasonable doubt of their validity for diagnosing irreversible loss of experiential capacity is removed. If this is the case, the adoption of this criterion for death will still depend upon the adoption of the related concept.

THE SIGNIFICANT PORTIONS OF THE CORTEX

There is one final step in the clarification of the concepts of death related to brain function which go beyond the older, more simplistic whole-brain-oriented concepts. If the EEG measures neocortical function, it presumably may measure any neocortical activity. Yet, we have concluded that experiential and social integrating function is the essential element in the nature of man the loss of which is to be called death. Once again the danger of false positive diagnosis of living must be raised. The neocortical cells and nerve circuits responsible for experiential and social integrating function are certainly complex. They would have to include some sensory portions of the cortex, as well as the limbic system and other areas responsible for emotion. Yet, is it not theoretically possible that some cortical cells could retain viability and yet the person would be dead in the sense we have discussed? What, for instance, if only motor cortex cells continued to survive through some freak preservation of blood supply to a small area of the cortex or some theoretical artificial perfusion? Whether or not the EEG would be present and whether the existence of only this kind of cortical activity could be distinguished are empirical questions. At the philosophical level, however, for one who sees the essence of man to be an embodied experiential and social capacity, the presence of viable motor cells would be of no more significance than the presence of the spinal or cranial reflex arc. Thus, the concept of death being dealt with cannot be reduced without remainder to the criterion of a flat EEG. The irreversible loss of these essential functions may be compatible with the presence of some form of EEG reading. Whether empirical tests can be made to make such a distinction and whether such solely motor cell capacity could ever exist are beyond this discussion.

The problem of doubt returns once again—this time with doubt between the older, broader whole-brain-oriented integrating function and the more limited experiential function. As for myself, the case for the concept of man which sees his experiential and social functioning as central is persuasive. The debate about the competing philosophical concepts is complex, much more complex than the original proponents of the older and more naive concept of brain death ever realized. While I personally favor the more limited experiential concept and am now convinced of the empirical validity of the related EEG criterion, I am not convinced that a philosophical issue so complex requires universal conformity. I would thus favor a law which recognizes the complexity of the debate

and permits the patient or the patient's agent to choose among the plausible death concepts: those related to body fluid flow (heart and lung oriented), to integrating capacity (whole brain oriented), or experiential and social interaction capacity (neocortically oriented).

Never should the choice be in the hands of another private citizen left to act upon his own without due process even if that private citizen happens to be a physician. If there is to be restriction of individual freedom at all (as there must be in extreme cases), the state must be the agent establishing restrictions, restrictions which would be applied uniformly. . . .

My objective in this discussion has been to push beyond the older, simpler whole-brain-oriented concept of death, which is now often used in the literature without careful definition, to obtain more precise usage of terms. Whether a person dies when he loses functions which have a primary locus in the whole brain, in a part of the brain, or in some other organs, it is the person who dies. The choice of the concept of death will require a more precise philosophical choice among these alternatives and the use of criteria for death will, in turn, depend upon those philosophical choices.

REFERENCES

Ad Hoc Committee of the Harvard Medical School to Examine the Definition of Brain Death (1968). "A definition of irreversible coma." *Journal of the American Medical Association,* 205:337–40.

Beecher, Henry K. (1970). "The new definition of death: some opposing views." Paper presented at the American Association for the Advancement of Science, Annual Meeting, Symposium on Meaning of Death. December 27–29.

Brierley, J. B., et al. (1971). "Neocortical death after cardiac arrest." *Lancet,* September 11, pp. 560–65.

Institute of Society, Ethics and the Life Sciences, Task Force on Death and Dying (1972). "Refinements in criteria for the determination of death." *Journal of the American Medical Association,* 221:48–53.

Jonas, Hans (1969). "Philosophical reflections on human experimentation." *Daedalus,* 98 (2):219–47.

Silverman, D., et al. (1970). "Irreversible coma associated with electrocerebral silence." *Neurology*, 20:525–33.

Veatch, Robert M. (1972). "Brain death: welcome definition or dangerous judgment?" *Hastings Center Report*, 2 (5):10–13.

Legal Approaches

ALEXANDER M. CAPRON AND LEON R. KASS

A Statutory Definition of the Standards for Determining Human Death: An Appraisal and a Proposal

In recent years, there has been much discussion of the need to refine and update the criteria for determining that a human being has died.[1] In light of medicine's increasing ability to maintain certain signs of life artificially and to make good use of organs from newly dead bodies, new criteria of death have been proposed by medical authorities.[2] Several states have enacted or are considering legislation to establish a statutory "definition of death," at the prompting of some members of the medical profession who apparently feel that existing, judicially-framed standards might expose physicians, particularly transplant surgeons, to civil or criminal liability.[3] Although the leading statute in this area[4] appears to create more problems than it resolves, some legislation may be needed for the protection of the public as well as the medical profession, and, in any

Reprinted with permission of University of Pennsylvania Law Review and Fred B. Rothman & Company from *University of Pennsylvania Law Review*, Vol. 121, No. 1 (November 1972), pp. 87–88, 102–118.

event, many more states will probably be enacting such statutes in the near future. . . .

WHAT CAN AND SHOULD BE LEGISLATED?

Arguments both for and against the desirability of legislation "defining" death often fail to distinguish among the several different subjects that might be touched on by such legislation. As a result, a mistaken impression may exist that a single statutory model is, and must be, the object of debate. An appreciation of the multiple meanings of a "definition of death" may help to refine the deliberations.

Death, in the sense the term is of interest here, can be defined purely formally as the transition, however abrupt or gradual, between the state of being alive and the state of being dead.[5] There are at least four levels of "definitions" that would give substance to this formal notion; in principle, each could be the subject of legislation: (1) the basic concept or idea; (2) general physiological standards; (3) operational criteria; and (4) specific tests or procedures.[6]

The *basic concept* of death is fundamentally a philosophical matter. Examples of possible "definitions" of death at this level include "permanent cessation of the integrated functioning of the organism as a whole," "departure of the animating or vital principle," or "irreversible loss of personhood." These abstract definitions offer little concrete help in the practical task of determining whether a person has died but they may very well influence how one goes about devising standards and criteria.

In setting forth the *general physiological standard(s)* for recognizing death, the definition moves to a level which is more medico-technical, but not wholly so. Philosophical issues persist in the choice to define death in terms of organ systems, physiological functions, or recognizable human activities, capacities, and conditions. Examples of possible general standards include "irreversible cessation of spontaneous respiratory and/or circulatory functions," "irreversible loss of spontaneous brain functions," "irreversible loss of the ability to respond or communicate," or some combination of these.

Operational criteria further define what is meant by the general physiological standards. The absence of cardiac contraction and lack of movement of the blood are examples of traditional criteria for "cessation of spontaneous circulatory functions," whereas deep coma, the absence of reflexes, and the lack of spontaneous muscular movements and spontaneous respiration are among criteria proposed for "cessation of spontaneous brain functions" by the Harvard Committee.

Fourth, there are the *specific tests and procedures* to see if the criteria are fulfilled. Pulse, heart beat, blood pressure, electrocardiogram, and examination of blood flow in the retinal vessels are among the specific tests of cardiac contraction and movement of the blood. Reaction to painful stimuli, appearance of the pupils and their responsiveness to light, and observation of movement and breathing over a specified time period are among specific tests

of the "brain function" criteria enumerated above.

There appears to be general agreement that legislation should not seek to "define death" at either the most general or the most specific levels (the first and fourth). In the case of the former, differences of opinion would seem hard to resolve, and agreement, if it were possible, would provide little guidance for practice. In the case of the latter, the specific tests and procedures must be kept open to changes in medical knowledge and technology. Thus, arguments concerning the advisability and desirability of a statutory definition of death are usually confined to the two levels we have called "standards" and "criteria," yet often without any apparent awareness of the distinction between them. The need for flexibility in the face of medical advance would appear to be a persuasive argument for not legislating any specific operational criteria. Moreover, these are almost exclusively technical matters, best left to the judgment of physicians. Thus, the kind of "definition" suitable for legislation would be a definition of the general physiological standard or standards. Such a definition, while not immutable, could be expected to be useful for a long period of time and would therefore not require frequent amendment.

There are other matters that could be comprehended in legislation "defining" death. The statute could specify who (and how many) shall make the determination. In the absence of a compelling reason to change past practices, this may continue to be set at "a physician,"[7] usually the doctor attending a dying patient or the one who happens to be at the scene of an accident. Moreover, the law ought probably to specify the "time of death." The statute may seek to fix the precise time when death may be said to have occurred, or it may merely seek to define a time that is clearly after "the precise moment," that is, a time when it is possible to say "the patient is dead," rather than "the patient has just now died." If the medical procedures used in determining that death has occurred call for verification of the findings after a fixed period of time (for example, the Harvard Committee's recommendation that the tests be repeated after twenty-four hours), the statute could in principle assign the "moment of death" to either the time when the criteria were first met or the time of verification. The former has been the practice with the traditional criteria for determining death.

Finally, legislation could speak to what follows upon the determination. The statute could be permissive or prescriptive in determining various possible subsequent events, including especially the pronouncement and recording of the death, and the use of the body for burial or other purposes.[8] It is our view that these matters are best handled outside of a statute which has as its purpose to "define death."

PRINCIPLES GOVERNING THE FORMULATION OF A STATUTE

In addition to carefully selecting the proper degree of specificity for legislation, there are a number of other principles we believe should guide the drafting of a statute "defining" death. First, the phenomenon of interest to physicians, legislators, and laymen alike is human death. Therefore, the statute should concern the death of a human being, not the death of his cells, tissues or organs, and not the "death" or cessation of his role as a fully functioning member of his family or community. This point merits considerable emphasis. There may be a proper place for a statutory standard for deciding when to turn off a respirator which is ventilating a patient still clearly alive, or, for that matter, to cease giving any other form of therapy. But it is crucial to distinguish this question of "when to allow to die?" from the question with which we are here concerned, namely, "when to declare dead?" Since very different issues and purposes are involved in these questions, confusing the one with the other clouds the analysis of both. The problem of determining when a person is dead is difficult enough without its being tied to the problem of whether physicians, or anyone else, may hasten the death of a terminally-ill patient, with or without his consent or that of his relatives, in order to

minimize his suffering or to conserve scarce medical resources. Although the same set of social and medical conditions may give rise to both problems, they must be kept separate if they are to be clearly understood.

Distinguishing the question "is he dead?" from the question "should he be allowed to die?" also assists in preserving continuity with tradition, a second important principle. By restricting itself to the "is he dead?" issue, a revised "definition" permits practices to move incrementally, not by replacing traditional cardiopulmonary standards for the determination of death but rather by supplementing them. These standards are, after all, still adequate in the majority of cases, and are the ones that both physicians and the public are in the habit of employing and relying on. The supplementary standards are needed primarily for those cases in which artificial means of support of comatose patients render the traditional standards unreliable.

Third, this incremental approach is useful for the additional and perhaps most central reason that any new means for judging death should be seen as just that and nothing more—a change in method dictated by advances in medical practice, but not an alteration of the meaning of "life" and "death." By indicating that the various standards for measuring death relate to a single phenomenon legislation can serve to reduce a primary source of public uneasiness on this subject. Once it has been established that certain consequences—for example, burial, autopsy, transfer of property to the heirs, and so forth—follow from a determination of death, definite problems would arise if there were a number of "definitions" according to which some people could be said to be "more dead" than others.

There are, of course, many instances in which the law has established differing definitions of a term, each framed to serve a particular purpose. One wonders, however, whether it does not appear somewhat foolish for the law to offer a number of arbitrary definitions of a natural phenomenon such as death. Nevertheless, legislators might seek to identify a series of points during the process of dying, each of which might be labelled "death" for certain purposes. Yet so far as we know, no arguments have been presented for special purpose standards except in the area of organ transplantation. Such a separate "definition of death," aimed at increasing the supply of viable organs, would permit physicians to declare a patient dead before his condition met the generally applicable standards for determining death if his organs are of potential use in transplantation. The adoption of a special standard risks abuse and confusion, however. The status of prospective organ donor is an arbitrary one to which a person can be assigned by relatives[9] or physicians and is unrelated to anything about the extent to which his body's functioning has deteriorated. A special "definition" of death for transplantation purposes would thus need to be surrounded by a set of procedural safeguards that would govern not only the method by which a person is to be declared dead but also those by which he is to be classified as an organ donor. Even more troublesome is the confusion over the meaning of death that would probably be engendered by multiple "definitions." Consequently, it would be highly desirable if a statute on death could avoid the problems with a special "definition." Should the statute happen to facilitate organ transplantation, either by making more organs available or by making prospective donors and transplant surgeons more secure in knowing what the law would permit, so much the better.

If however, more organs are needed for transplantation than can be legally obtained, the question whether the benefits conferred by transplantation justify the risks associated with a broader "definition" of death should be addressed directly rather than by attempting to subsume it under the question "what is death?" Such a direct confrontation with the issue could lead to a discussion about the standards and procedures under which organs might be taken from persons near death, or even those still quite alive, at their own option[10] or that of relatives, physicians, or representatives of the state. The major advantage of keeping the issues separate is not, of course, that this will facilitate transplantation, but that it will remove a present source of concern: it is unsettling to contemplate that as you lie slowly dying physicians are free to use a more "lenient" standard to declare you dead if they want to remove your organs for transplantation into other patients.

Fourth, the standards for determining death ought not only to relate to a single phenomenon but should also be applied uniformly to all persons. A person's wealth or his "social utility" as an organ donor should not affect the way in which the moment of his death is determined.

Finally, while there is a need for uniformity of application at any one time, the fact that changes in medical technology brought about the present need for "redefinition" argues that the new formulation should be flexible. As suggested in the previous section, such flexibility is most easily accomplished if the new "definition" confines itself to the general standards by which death is to be determined and leaves to the continuing exercise of judgment by physicians the establishment and application of appropriate criteria and specific tests for determining that the standards have been met.

THE KANSAS STATUTE

The first attempt at a legislative resolution of the problems discussed here was made in 1970 when the State of Kansas adopted "An Act relating to and defining death."[11] The Kansas statute has received a good deal of attention; similar legislation was enacted in the spring of 1972 in Maryland and is presently under consideration in a number of other jurisdictions.[12] The Kansas legislation, which was drafted in response to developments in organ transplantation and medical support of dying patients, provides "alternative definitions of death,"[13] set forth in two paragraphs. Under the first, a person is considered "medically and legally dead" if a physician determines "there is the absence of spontaneous respiratory and cardiac function and . . . attempts at resuscitation are considered hopeless."[14] In the second "definition," death turns on the absence of spontaneous brain function if during "reasonable attempts" either to "maintain or restore spontaneous circulatory or respiratory function," it appears that "further attempts at resuscitation or supportive maintenance will not succeed."[15] The purpose of the latter "definition" is made clear by the final sentence paragraph:

Death is to be pronounced before artificial means of supporting respiratory and circulatory function are terminated and *before any vital organ is removed for the purpose of transplantation.*[16]

The primary fault with this legislation is that it appears to be based on, or at least gives voice to, the misconception that there are two separate phenomena of death. This dichotomy is particularly unfortunate because it seems to have been inspired by a desire to establish a special definition for organ transplantation, a definition which physicians would not, however, have to apply, in the draftsman's words, "to prove the irrelevant deaths of most persons."[17] Although there is nothing in the Act itself to indicate that physicians will be less concerned with safeguarding the health of potential organ donors, the purposes for which the Act was passed are not hard to decipher, and they do little to inspire the average patient with confidence that his welfare (including his not being prematurely declared dead) is of as great concern to medicine and the State of Kansas as is the facilitation of organ transplantation.[18] As Professor Kennedy cogently observes, "public disquiet [over transplantation] is in no way allayed by the existence in legislative form of what appear to be alternative definitions of death."[19] One hopes that the form the statute takes does not reflect a conclusion on the part of the Kansas legislature that death occurs at two distinct points during the process of dying.[20] Yet this inference can be derived from the Act, leaving upon the prospect "that X at a certain stage in the process of dying can be pronounced dead, whereas Y, having arrived at the same point, is not said to be dead."[21]

The Kansas statute appears also to have attempted more than the "definition" of death, or rather, to have tried to resolve related questions by erroneously treating them as matters of "definition." One supporter of the statute praises it, we think mistakenly, for this reason: "Intentionally, the statute extends to these questions: When can a physician avoid attempting resuscitation? When can he terminate resuscitative efforts? When can he discontinue artificial maintenance?"[22] To be sure, "when the patient is dead" is one obvious answer to these questions, but by no means the only one. As indicated above, we believe that the question "when is the patient dead?" needs to be distinguished and treated separately from the questions "when may the doctor turn off the respirator?" or "when may a patient—dying yet still alive—be allowed to die?"

A STATUTORY PROPOSAL

As an alternative to the Kansas statute we propose the following:

A person will be considered dead if in the announced opinion of a physician, based on ordinary standards of medical practice, he has experienced an irreversible cessation of spontaneous respiratory and circulatory functions. In the event that artificial means of support preclude a determination that these functions have ceased, a person will be considered dead if in the announced opinion of a physician, based on ordinary standards of medical practice, he has experienced an irreversible cessation of spontaneous brain functions. Death will have occurred at the time when the relevant functions ceased.

This proposed statute provides a "definition" of death confined to the level of *general physiological standards,* and it has been drafted in accord with the five principles set forth above in section V. First, the proposal speaks in terms of the *death* of a *person.* The determination that a person has died is to be based on an evaluation of certain vital bodily functions, the permanent absence of which indicates that he is no longer a living human being. By concentrating on the death of a human being as a whole, the statute rightly disregards the fact that some cells or organs may continue to "live" after this point, just as others may have ceased functioning long before the determination of death. This statute would leave for resolution by other means the question of when the absence or deterioration of certain capacities, such as the ability to communicate, or functions, such as the cerebral, indicates that a person may or should be allowed to die without further medical intervention.

Second, the proposed legislation is predicated upon the single phenomenon of death. Moreover, it applies uniformly to all persons,[23] by specifying the circumstances under which each of the standards is to be used rather than leaving this to the unguided discretion of physicians. Unlike the Kansas law, the model statute does not leave to arbitrary decision a choice between two apparently equal yet different "alternative definitions of death."[24] Rather, its second standard is applicable only when "artificial means of support preclude" use of the first. It does not establish a separate kind of death, called "brain death." In other words, the proposed law would provide two standards gauged by different functions, for measuring different manifestations of the same phenomenon. If cardiac and pulmonary functions have ceased, brain functions cannot continue; if there is no brain activity and respiration has to be maintained artificially, the same state (*i.e.*, death) exists. Some people might prefer a single standard, one based either on cardiopulmonary or brain functions. This would have the advantage of removing the last trace of the "two deaths" image, which any reference to alternative standards may still leave. Respiratory and circulatory indicators, once the only touchstone, are no longer adequate in some situations. It would be possible, however, to adopt the alternative, namely that death is *always* to be established by assessing spontaneous brain functions. Reliance only on brain activity, however, would represent a sharp and unnecessary break with tradition. Departing from continuity with tradition is not only theoretically unfortunate in that it violates another principle of good legislation suggested previously, but also practically very difficult, since most physicians customarily employ cardiopulmonary tests for death and would be slow to change, especially when the old tests are easier to perform, more accessible and acceptable to the lay public, and perfectly adequate for determining death in most instances.

Finally, by adopting standards for death in terms of the cessation of certain vital bodily functions but not in terms of the specific criteria or tests by which these functions are to be measured, the statute does not prevent physicians from adapting their procedures to changes in medical technology.

A basic substantive issue remains: what are the merits of the proposed standards? For ordinary situations, the appropriateness of the traditional standard, "an irreversible cessation of spontaneous respiratory and circulatory functions," does not require elaboration. Indeed, examination by a physician may be more a formal than a real requirement in determining that most people have died. In addition to any obvious injuries, elementary signs of death such as absence of heartbeat and breathing, cold skin, fixed pupils, and so forth, are usually sufficient to indicate even to a layman that the accident victim, the elderly person who passes away quietly in the night, or the patient stricken with a sudden infarct has died. The difficulties arise when modern medicine intervenes to sustain a patient's respiration and circulation. . . . The indicators of brain damage appear reliable, in that studies have shown that patients who fit the Harvard criteria have suffered such extensive damage that they do not recover. Of course, the task of the neurosurgeon or physician is simplified in the common case where an accident victim has suffered such gross, apparent injuries to the head that it is not necessary to apply the Harvard criteria in order to establish cessation of brain functioning.

The statutory standard, "irreversible cessation of spontaneous brain functions," is intended to encompass both higher brain activities and those of the brainstem. There must, of course, also be no spontaneous respiration; the second standard is applied only when breathing is being artificially maintained. The major emphasis placed on brain functioning, although generally consistent with the common view of what makes man distinctive as a living creature, brings to the fore a basic issue: What aspects of brain function should be decisive? The question has been reframed by some clinicians in light of their experience with patients who have undergone what they term "neocortical death" (that is, complete destruction of higher brain capacity, demonstrated by a flat E.E.G.). "Once neocortical death has been unequivocally established and the possibility of any recovery of consciousness and intellectual activity [is] thereby excluded, . . . although [the] patient breathes spontaneously, is he or she alive?"[25] While patients with irreversible brain damage from cardiac arrest seldom survive more than a few days, cases have recently been reported of survival for up to two and one-quarter years.[26] Nevertheless, though existence in this state falls far short of a full human life, the very fact of spontaneous respiration, as well as coordinated movements and reflex activities at the brainstem and spinal cord levels, would exclude these patients from the scope of the statutory standards.[27] The condition of "neocortical death" may well be a proper justification for interrupting all forms of treatment and allowing these patients to die, but this moral and legal problem cannot and should not be settled by "defining" these people "dead."

The legislation suggested here departs from the Kansas statute in its basic approach to the problem of "defining" death: the proposed statute does not set about to establish a special category of "brain death" to be used by transplanters. Further, there are a number of particular points of difference between them. For example, the proposed statute does not speak of persons being "medically and legally dead," thus avoiding redundancy and, more importantly, the mistaken implication that the "medical" and "legal" definitions could differ. Also, the proposed legislation does not include the provision that "death is to be pronounced before" the machine is turned off or any organs removed. Such a *modus operandi,* which was incorporated by Kansas from the Harvard Committee's report, may be advisable for physicians on public relations grounds, but it has no place in a statute "defining" death. The proposed statute already provides that "Death

will have occurred at the time when the relevant functions ceased." If supportive aids, or organs, are withdrawn after this time, such acts cannot be implicated as having caused death. The manner in which, or exact time at which, the physician should articulate his finding is a matter best left to the exigencies of the situation, to local medical customs or hospital rules, or to statutes on the procedures for certifying death or on transplantation if the latter is the procedure which raises the greatest concern of medical impropriety. The real safeguard against doctors killing patients is not to be found in a statute "defining" death. Rather, it inheres in physicians' ethical and religious beliefs, which are also embodied in the fundamental professional ethic of *primum non nocere* and are reinforced by homicide and "wrongful death" laws and the rules governing medical negligence applicable in license revocation proceedings or in private actions for damages.

. . .

CONCLUSION

Changes in medical knowledge and procedures have created an apparent need for a clear and acceptable revision of the standards for determining that a person has died. Some commentators have argued that the formulation of such standards should be left to physicians. The reasons for rejecting this argument seem compelling: the "definition of death" is not merely a matter for technical expertise, the uncertainty of the present law is unhealthy for society and physicians alike, there is a great potential for mischief and harm through the possibility of conflict between the standards applied by some physicians and those assumed to be applicable by the community at large and its legal system, and patients and their relatives are made uneasy by physicians apparently being free to shift around the meaning of death without any societal guidance. Accordingly, we conclude the public has a legitimate role to play in the formulation and adoption of such standards. This Article has proposed a model statute which bases a determination of death primarily on the traditional standard of final respiratory and circulatory cessation; where the artificial maintenance of these functions precludes the use of such a standard, the statute authorizes that death be determined on the basis of irreversible cessation of spontaneous brain functions. We believe the legislation proposed would dispel public confusion and concern and protect physicians and patients, while avoiding the creation of "two types of death," for which the statute on this subject first adopted in Kansas has been justly criticized. The proposal is offered not as the ultimate solution to the problem, but as a catalyst for what we hope will be a robust and well-informed public debate over a new "definition." Finally, the proposed statute leaves for future resolution the even more difficult problems concerning the conditions and procedures under which a decision may be reached to cease treating a terminal patient who does not meet the standards set forth in the statutory "definition of death."

NOTES

1. *See, e.g.,* P. Ramsey, The Patient as Person 59–119 (1970); Louisell, *Transplantation; Existing Legal Constraints,* in Ethics in Medical Progress: With Special Reference to Transplantation 91–92 (G. Wolstenholme & M. O'Connor eds. 1966) [hereinafter cited as Medical Progress]; *Discussion* of Murray, *Organ Transplantation: The Practical Possibilities,* in *id.* 68 (comments of Dr. G. E. Schreiner), 71 (comments of Dr. M. F. A. Woodruff); Wasmuth & Stewart, *Medical and Legal Aspects of Human Organ Transplantation,* 14 Clev.–Mar. L. Rev 442 (1965); Beecher, *Ethical Problems Created by the Hopelessly Unconscious Patient,* 278 New Eng. J. Med 1425 (1968); Wasmuth, *The Concept of Death,* 30 Ohio St. L. J. 32 (1969); Note, *The Need for a Redefinition of "Death,"* 45 Chi.–Kent L. Rev. 202 (1969).

2. *See, e.g.,* Ad Hoc Committee of the Harvard Medical School to Examine the Definition of Brain Death, *A Definition of Irreversible Coma,* 205 J.A.M.A. 337 (1968) [hereinafter cited as *Irreversible Coma*]; *Discussion* of Murray, *Organ Transplantation: The Practical Possibilities,* in Medical Progress, *supra* note 1, 15 69–74 (remarks of Drs. G. P. J. Alexandre, R. Y. Calne, J. Hamburger, J. E. Murray, J. P. Revillard & G. E. Schreiner); *When Is a Patient Dead?,* 204 J.A.M.A. 1000 (1968) (editorial); *Updating the Definition of Death,* Med. World News, Apr. 28, 1967, at 47. . . .

3. *See, e.g.,* Taylor, *A Statutory Definition of Death in Kansas,* 215 J.A.M.A. 296 (1971) (letter to the editor), in which the principal draftsman of the Kansas statute states that the law was believed necessary to protect transplant surgeons against the risk of "a criminal charge, for the existence of a resuscitated heart in another body should be

excellent evidence that the donor was not dead [under the "definition" of death then existing in Kansas] until the operator excised the heart.". . . The specter of civil liability was raised in *Tucker v. Lower,* a recent action brought by the brother of a heart donor against the transplantation team at the Medical College of Virginia. . . .

4. Kan. Stat. Ann. § 77–202 (Supp. 1971); see notes 11–24 *infra* & accompanying text for a discussion of this statute.

5. For a debate on the underlying issues see Morison, *Death; Process or Event?* 173 Science 694 (1970); Kass, *Death as an Event: A Commentary on Robert Morison,* 173 Science 698 (1971).

6. To our knowledge, this delineation of four levels has not been made elsewhere in the existing literature on this subject. Therefore, the terms "concept," "standard," "criteria," and "tests and procedures" as used here bear no necessary connection to the ways in which others may use these same terms, and in fact we recognize that in some areas of discourse, the term "standards" is more, rather than less, operational and concrete than "criteria"—just the reverse of our ordering. Our terminology was selected so that the category we call "criteria" would correspond to the level of specificity at which the Ad Hoc Harvard Committee framed its proposals, which it called and which are widely referred to as the *"new criteria"* for determining death. We have attempted to be consistent in our use of these terms throughout this Article. Nevertheless, our major purpose here is not to achieve public acceptance of our terms, but to promote awareness of the four different levels of a "definition" of death to which the terms refer.

7. Cf. Uniform Anatomical Gift Act § 7(b).

8. If . . . sound procedures for stating death are agreed to and carried out, then theologians and moralists and every other thoughtful person should agree with the physicians who hold that it is *then* permissible to maintain circulation of blood and supply of oxygen in the corpse of a donor to preserve an *organ* until it can be used in transplantation. Whether one gives the body over for decent burial, performs an autopsy, gives the cadaver for use in medical education, or uses it as a "vital organ bank" are all alike procedures governed by decent respect for the bodies of deceased men and specific regulations that ensure this. The ventilation and circulation of organs for transplant raises no question not already raised by these standard procedures. None are life-and-death matters. P. Ramsey, The Patient as Person 72 (1970).

9. Uniform Anatomical Gift Act § 2(c). For example, if a special standard were adopted for determining death in potential organ donors, relatives of a dying patient with limited financial means might feel substantial pressure to give permission for his organs to be removed in order to bring to a speedier end the care given the patient.

10. *See, e.g.,* Blachly, *Can Organ Transplantation Provide an Altruistic-Expiatory Alternative to Suicide?,* 1 Life-Threatening Behavior 6 (1971); Scribner, *Ethical Problems of Using Artificial Organs to Sustain Human Life,* 10 Trans. Am. Soc. Artif. Internal Organs 209, 211 (1964) (advocating legal guidelines to permit voluntary euthanasia for purpose of donating organs for transplantation).

11. Law of Mar. 17, 1970, ch. 378, [1970] Kan. Laws 994 (codified at Kan. Stat. Ann. § 77–202 (Supp. 1971)). It provides in full:

A person will be considered medically and legally dead if, in the opinion of a physician, based on ordinary standards of medical practice, there is the absence of spontaneous brain function; and if based on ordinary standards of medical practice, during reasonable attempts to either maintain or restore spontaneous circulatory or respiratory function in the absence of aforesaid brain function, it appears that further attempts at resuscitation or supportive maintenance will not succeed, death will have occurred at the time when these conditions first coincide. Death is to be pronounced before artificial means of supporting respiratory and circulatory function are terminated and before any vital organ is removed for purposes of transplantation.

These alternative definitions of death are to be utilized for all purposes in this state, including the trials of civil and criminal cases, any laws to the contrary notwithstanding.

12. . . . In the Maryland law, which is nearly identical to its Kansas progenitor, the phrase "in the opinion of a physician" was deleted from the first paragraph, and the phrase "and because of a known disease or condition" was added to the second paragraph following "ordinary standards of medical practice." Maryland Sessions Laws ch. 693 (1972). Interestingly, Kansas and Maryland were also among the first states to adopt the Uniform Anatomical Gift Act in 1968, even prior to its official revision and approval by the National Conference of Commissioners on Uniform State Laws.

13. Note 11 *supra*.

14. *Id.* In using the term "hopeless," the Kansas legislature apparently intended to indicate that the "absence of spontaneous respiratory and cardiac function" must be irreversible before death is pronounced. In addition to being rather roundabout, this formulation is also confusing in that it might be taken to address the "when to allow to die?" question as well as the "is he dead?" question. *See* note 22 *infra* and accompanying text.

15. Note 11 *supra*.

16. *Id.* (emphasis added).

17. Taylor, *supra* note 3 at 296.

18. Cf. Kass, *A Caveat on Transplants,* The Washington Post, Jan. 14, 1968, § B, at 1, col. 1.

19. Kennedy, *The Kansas Statute on Death: An Appraisal,* 285 New Eng. J. Med. 947 (1971).

20. General use of the term "resuscitation" might suggest the existence of a common notion that a person can die once, be revived (given life again), and then die again at a later time—in the other words, that death can occur at two or more distinct points in time. But resuscitation only restores life "from *apparent* death or unconsciousness." Webster's Third New International Dictionary 1937 (1966) (emphasis added). The proposed statute, text accompanying note 24 infra, takes account of the possibility of resuscitation by providing that death occurs only when there has been an *irreversible* cessation of the relevant vital bodily functions. Cf. 3 M. Houts & I. H. Haut, Courtroom Medicine § 1.01 (3)(d) (1971):

"The ability to resuscitate patients after apparent death, coupled with observations that in many cases the restoration was not to a state of consciousness, understanding and intellectual functioning, but merely to a decerebrate, vegetative existence, and with advances in neurology that have brought greater, though far from complete, understanding of the functions of the nervous system, has drawn attention to the role of the nervous system in maintaining life."

21. Kennedy, *op. cit.*

22. Mills, *The Kansas Death Statute; Bold and Innovative,* 285 New Eng. J. Med. 968 (1971).

23. Differences in the exact mode of diagnosing death will naturally occur as a result of differing circumstances under which the physician's examination is made. Thus, the techniques employed with an automobile accident victim lying on the roadside at night may be less sophisticated than those used with a patient who has been receiving treatment in a well-equipped hospital.

24. Kan. Stat. Ann. § 77–202 (Supp. 1971).

25. Brierley, Adams, Graham & Simpsom, *Neocortical Death After Cardiac Arrest,* 2 Lancet 560, 565 (1971) [hereinafter cited as Brierley]. In addition to a flat (isoelectric) electroencephalogram, a "neuropathological examination of a biopsy specimen . . . from the posterior half of a cerebral hemisphere" provides further confirmation. *Id.* The editors of a leading medical journal question "whether a state of cortical death can be diagnosed clinically." Editorial, *Death of a Human Being,* 2 Lancet 590 (1971). Cf. note 14 *supra* [original text].

26. Brierley and his colleagues report two cases of their own in which the patients each survived in a comatose condition for five months after suffering cardiac arrest before dying of pulmonary complications. They also mention two unreported cases of a Doctor Lewis, in one of which the patient survived for 2¼ years. Brierley, *supra* note 25, at 565.

27. The exclusion of patients without neocortical function from the category of death may appear somewhat arbitrary in light of our disinclination to engage in a philosophical discussion of the basic concepts of human "life" and "death." *See* text accompanying notes 5–6 *supra.* Were the "definition" contained in the proposed statute a departure from what has traditionally been meant by "death," such a conceptual discussion would clearly be in order. But, as this Article has tried to demonstrate, our intention has been more modest: to provide a clear restatement of the traditional understanding in terms which are useful in light of modern medical capabilities and practices. . . .

A philosophical examination of the essential attributes of being "human" might lead one to conclude that persons who, for example, lack the mental capacity to communicate in any meaningful way, should be regarded as "not human" or "dead." It would nevertheless probably be necessary and prudent to treat the determination of that kind of "death" under special procedures until such time as medicine is able routinely to diagnose the extent and irreversibility of the loss of the "central human capacities" (however defined) with the same degree of assurance now possible in determining that death has occurred. Consequently, even at the conceptual level, we are inclined to think that it is best to distinguish the question "is he dead?" from such questions as "should he be allowed to die?" and "should his death be actively promoted?"

SUGGESTED READINGS FOR CHAPTER 6

Books and Articles

Beauchamp, Tom L., and Perlin, Seymour, eds. *Ethical Issues in Death and Dying.* Englewood Cliffs, N.J.: Prentice-Hall, 1978.

Beecher, Henry K. "After the 'Definition of Irreversible Coma'." *New England Journal of Medicine* 281 (November 6, 1969), 1070–1071.

Beecher, Henry K. "Ethical Problems Created by the Hopelessly Unconscious Patient." *New England Journal of Medicine* 278 (June 27, 1968), 1425–1430.

Black, Peter McL. "Three Definitions of Death." *Monist* 60 (January, 1977), 136–146.

Brierley, J. B., *et al.* "Neocortical Death after Cardiac Arrest." *Lancet* 2 (September 11, 1971), 560–565.

California Medical Association, Committee on Evolving Trends in Society Affecting Life. *Death and Dying: Determining and Defining Death–A Compilation of Definitions, Selected Readings, and Bibliography.* San Francisco: California Medical Association, 1975.

Conference of Royal Colleges and Faculties of the United Kingdom. "Diagnosis of Brain Death." *Lancet* 2 (November 13, 1976), 1069–1070.

Gaylin, Willard. "Harvesting the Dead." *Harper's* 249 (September, 1974), 23–28+.

Harp, James R. "Criteria for the Determination of Death." *Anesthesiology* 40 (April, 1974), 391–397.

Institute of Society, Ethics and the Life Sciences, Task Force on Death and Dying. "Refinements in Criteria for the Determination of Death." *Journal of the American Medical Association* 221 (July 3, 1972), 48–53.

Jennett, Bryan. "The Donor Doctor's Dilemma: Observations on the Recognition and Management of Brain Death." *Journal of Medical Ethics* 1 (July, 1975), 63–66.

Morison, Robert, and Kass, Leon. "Death—Process or Event?" *Science* 173 (August 20, 1971), 694–702.

Ramsey, Paul. *The Patient as Person.* New Haven: Yale University Press, 1970. Chap. 2.

Skegg, P. D. G. "Irreversibly Comatose Individuals: 'Alive' or 'Dead'?" *Cambridge Law Journal* 33 (April, 1974), 130–144.

"Study Suggests New, Less Rigid Criteria for Declaring Death." *Medical World News* 16 (January 27, 1975), 26–27.

Van Till, H. A. H. "Diagnosis of Death in Comatose Patients under Resuscitation Treatment: A Critical Review of the Harvard Report." *American Journal of Law and Medicine* 2 (Summer, 1976), 1–40.

Veatch, Robert M. *Death, Dying, and the Biological Revolution.* New Haven: Yale University Press, 1976. Chaps. 1 and 2.

Bibliographies

Sollitto, Sharmon, and Veatch, Robert M., comps. *Bibliography of Society, Ethics and the Life Sciences.* Hastings-on-Hudson, N.Y.: Institute of Society, Ethics and the Life Sciences. Periodically updated. See under "Defining Death."

Walters, LeRoy, ed. *Bibliography of Bioethics.* Vols. 1– . Detroit: Gale Research Co. Issued annually. See under "Brain Death" and "Determination of Death."

7.
Euthanasia and the Prolongation of Life

The previous chapter examined concepts of death and standards for recognizing when death has occurred. The present chapter considers ethical issues in the treatment of living persons who are seriously or terminally ill. In the discussion of these issues a variety of words and phrases have been employed, including "death with dignity," "euthanasia," "the prolongation of life," and "allowing to die." As we shall see, alternative ways of conceptualizing the topic of this chapter are sometimes correlated with divergent ethical perspectives.

GENERAL CONCEPTUAL AND ETHICAL QUESTIONS

Three major conceptual issues frequently arise in discussions of euthanasia and the prolongation of life: (1) the distinction between killing and allowing to die; (2) the distinction between "voluntary" and "involuntary" decisions concerning death; and (3) the proper usage of the term "euthanasia."

The killing/allowing-to-die debate includes two subquestions: Is it possible to draw a clear *logical* distinction between actions and omissions? and, Even if such a distinction can be drawn, is it *morally* relevant? Several commentators, among them George P. Fletcher, Robert Veatch, and the American Medical Association, assert that a meaningful logical distinction can be drawn between killing and allowing to die. Three major arguments are adduced in support of the distinction:

1. Ordinary language: Speakers of English regularly distinguish between "causing harm" and "permitting harm to occur." Most English-speakers would classify allowing to die as an example of the latter category.

2. Naturalness and artificiality: Not employing artificial means of prolonging life is equivalent to allowing natural death to occur.

3. Causation: In cases where a patient dies following nontreatment the proximate cause of death is the patient's disease, not nontreatment.

James Rachels, on the other hand, argues that the cessation of treatment in terminal cases is "the intentional termination of the life of one human being by another" and, more generally, that letting a patient die is an action, not merely an omission. He therefore concludes that no clear conceptual distinction between killing and allowing to die can be sustained.

On the second subquestion, the moral relevance of the killing/allowing to-die distinction, there is a measure of agreement between Rachels and his opponents. Neither side accepts a simple correlation between the killing/allowing-to-die distinction and the wrong/right distinction. For example, Rachels and Fletcher agree that certain omissions are morally (or legally) blameworthy. Even the AMA statement (cited by Rachels) implicitly recognizes the moral accountability of physicians for some types of omissions by carefully circumscribing the conditions in which the cessation of treatment is considered to be justified: only extraordinary means may be withheld and then only in cases in which there is irrefutable evidence that biological death is imminent. On the other hand, both the AMA statement and Veatch seem to regard the killing of a patient, even for humane reasons, as morally wrong; thus, in their view there is a close connection between killing (a patient) and morally wrong action. Rachels obviously disagrees.

The distinction between "voluntary" and "involuntary" decisions about death is less controversial; however, the term "involuntary" may be ambiguous. Voluntary decisions about death are those in which a competent adult patient requests or gives informed consent to a particular course of medical treatment or nontreatment. In contrast, the term "involuntary" is generally applied to situations in which the patient—because of age, mental impairment, or unconsciousness—is not competent to give informed consent to life-death decisions and where the decision is reached by others in the absence of the patient's ability to consent.

The third conceptual issue identified above is perhaps the most controversial: What is the proper usage of the term "euthanasia"? *Webster's Third New International Dictionary* (Unabridged) provides two definitions of the term: (1) "an easy death or means of inducing one"; and (2) "the act or practice of painlessly putting to death persons suffering from incurable conditions or diseases." Two features of these definitions may be noted. Both seem to employ the language of acting rather than refraining to act, or killing rather than allowing to die. The second definition suggests that the action is performed by a party other than the patient.

If Webster's definitions reflect common usage, then the paradigm case of euthanasia is the active termination of a suffering patient's life by a second party. If the termination is requested or consented to by the patient, then the action is called "voluntary euthanasia." In cases where the patient is not mentally competent to give consent, the action is termed "involuntary euthanasia."

Some commentators, including Rachels and Joseph Fletcher[1], have proposed that the concept of euthanasia should properly include cases in which a patient is *allowed to die*. This proposal is perhaps correlated with its advocates' conviction that there is no clear logical or ethical distinction between killing and allowing to die. On this view, the paradigm case of euthanasia described above is an instance of "active" or "positive" eithanasia, while the act of allowing a patient to die is called "passive" or "negative" euthanasia. The combination of this distinction with the voluntary/involuntary distinction yields four subtypes of euthanasia, which can be represented diagrammatically as follows:

	Voluntary	Involuntary
Active	Voluntary Active	Involuntary Active
Passive	Voluntary Passive	Involuntary Passive

Other commentators, including the American Medical Association, Arthur Dyck[2], and probably George Fletcher, would reject this proposed usage of the euthanasia concept on both logical and ethical grounds. Their conceptualization can be diagrammed approximately as follows:

	Voluntary	Involuntary
Euthanasia	Voluntary Euthanasia	Involuntary Euthanasia

	Voluntary	Involuntary
Allowing to Die	Voluntary Allowing to Die	Involuntary Allowing to Die

In the remaining sections of this introduction, the term euthanasia will be employed in the restricted sense suggested by the second definition in Webster's unabridged dictionary, i.e., it will refer only to the termination of a patient's life by a second party. Other phrases—for example, refusal of treatment, withholding of treatment, or cessation of treatment—will be applied to situations not involving euthanasia in the strict sense.

DECISIONS BY COMPETENT ADULTS

This section focuses on voluntary decisions by patients and carries forward the discussion of informed consent and refusal of treatment which began in Chapter 4. It is also reminiscent of Joel Feinberg's essay on liberty in Chapter 1 and the emphasis on the right of self-determination identified in the introduction to Chapter 2.

Life and death decisions are frequently presented as dilemmas for medical professionals: What are the moral obligations of the physician or nurse to the dying patient? Robert Veatch argues that, at least in the case of competent adult patients, this way of posing the question is misguided. According to Veatch, the primary issue is that of the patient's rights, particularly his or her right to refuse life-prolonging treatment. Implicit in Veatch's analysis is the question whether there are moral limits to such a right, that is, whether a patient would be morally obligated to undergo a low-risk, life-saving treatment which offered a high probability of success.

A tangible way for patients to express their wishes concerning terminal care is provided by the so-called "Living Will" developed by the Euthanasia Educational Council. This document, which is technically a declaration of intention rather than a will, requests that in case of apparently irreversible illness no "artificial means" or "heroic measures" be employed to prolong the signer's life. Although the "Living Will" focuses primary attention on the right to refuse treatment, its allusion to pain-killing medication (e.g., morphine) which may also "hasten the moment of death" indicates one of the practical difficulties in maintaining a clear distinction between killing and allowing to die.

In the essays of Yale Kamisar and Glanville Williams one is clearly confronted with the issue of mercy-killing, or euthanasia. Williams argues that the case for voluntary euthanasia in the terminal stages of painful diseases is based on two values. The first is liberty; that is, Williams, like Veatch, places a high value on patient autonomy but, unlike Veatch, extends the sphere of patient self-determination to include the right to have one's life directly terminated. The second value espoused by Williams is the prevention of cruelty, which is closely related to the principles of beneficence identified in the introduction to Chapter 2.

Kamisar raises three primary objections to voluntary euthanasia: (1) the diagnosis that a patient's disease is "incurable" may be mistaken, or a cure for the disease may be discovered; (2) the "voluntary" character of decisions by seriously ill patients is open to question; and (3) programs of voluntary euthanasia are likely to be the opening wedge for proposed programs of involuntary euthanasia. Kamisar is prepared to concede that in individual, extreme cases voluntary euthanasia could be morally justified. His essay can therefore be interpreted as a rule-utilitarian argument against both the general practice of euthanasia and the legalization of the practice. (See the discussion of rule-utilitarianism in Paul Taylor's essay in Chapter 1.)

It is conceivable that some of Kamisar's objections to voluntary euthanasia could also be raised against the refusal of life-saving treatment. Medical diagnoses could be equally mistaken in treatment-refusal cases. Similarly, the voluntary character of a seriously ill patient's decision to refuse treatment might be open to question, particularly if the patient were pressured by family or society to assert his or her "right to die."

DECISIONS ABOUT INFANTS AND INCOMPETENTS

In recent years the question of appropriate treatment for handicapped newborn infants and seriously ill, comatose patients has become a matter of intense public concern. Interest in this question has been stimulated in part by a series of dramatic cases, including the "Quinlan case" and the "Johns Hopkins case." In the latter case an infant born with Down's Syndrome (monogolism) and an intestinal blockage was denied corrective surgery and allowed to die at the parents' request.

Decisions about the treatment of infants and comatose patients are of necessity made by parties other than the patients themselves. They are thus *involuntary* decisions in the sense proposed above. Until now, the public debate has centered primarily on the issue of allowing patients to die (by the withholding or cessation of treatment) rather than on the active termination of life, although Rachels, Kamisar, and Williams devote some attention to the latter issue as well.

Three major ethical positions on the treatment of handicapped infants and comatose patients can be distinguished. The first position would argue that the life of every infant and incompetent patient should be saved, if medically possible. As Duff and Campbell point out, a policy of maximal treatment was in fact followed during the 1960's for newborns suffering from a severe defect of the spinal cord (meningomyelocele). This first position excludes both euthanasia and allowing to die. The primary justifications for this position are, negatively, that no one should be authorized to make life-death decisions on behalf of another and, positively, that every patient, regardless of his or her condition, has an overriding right to life.

A second position would make the decision about treatment on the basis of the patient's projected long-term welfare. In this case a proxy for the patient seeks to make an anticipatory judgment concerning the quality of life which the patient is likely to enjoy, as balanced against the suffering which the patient is likely to endure. Richard McCormick and the New Jersey Supreme Court both espouse this patient-oriented standard: McCormick stresses the importance of the infant's "potentiality for human relationships," while the court considers what Karen Quinlan *would* decide about her medical treatment if she could decide.

A third position would allow decisions concerning the treatment of infants and the incompetent to be determined, or at least strongly influenced, by familial and broader social considerations. If the patient's continued existence would be likely to undermine a marriage, adversely affect other family members, or claim an undue share of society's scarce medical resources, then a decision to allow the patient to die would be morally approved. A benefit-harm calculus underlies this third position, as it did the second. However, factors other than patient benefit are also included in the calculus. Without explicitly opting for this third position, Duff and Campbell report that some parents include familial considerations in their decision to allow a severely handicapped newborn infant to die.

In addition to discussing some of the ethical issues involved in involuntary life-death decisions, the New Jersey Supreme Court proposes a public-policy mechanism for making such decisions. The court seems reluctant to entrust sole decisionmaking power to the patient's family or physician. It therefore recommends consultation by the physician with other individuals and groups, including, for example, discussion of difficult cases with interprofessional hospital-based ethics committees. According to the court, such broad-based local review would protect physicians as well as patients and their families and would, in most cases, obviate the need for formal judicial review.

L.W.

NOTES

1. Joseph Fletcher, "Ethics and Euthanasia," in Robert H. Williams, ed., *To Live and to Die: When, Why and How* (New York: Springer-Verlag, 1973), pp. 113–122.

2. Arthur J. Dyck, "An Alternative to the Ethic of Euthanasia," in Williams, ed., *ibid.*, pp. 98–112.

JAMES RACHELS

Active and Passive Euthanasia

The distinction between active and passive euthanasia is thought to be crucial for medical ethics. The idea is that it is permissible, at least in some cases, to withhold treatment and allow a patient to die, but it is never permissible to take any direct action designed to kill the patient. This doctrine seems to be accepted by most doctors, and it endorsed in a statement adopted by the House of Delegates of the American Medical Association on December 4, 1973:

The intentional termination of the life of one human being by another—mercy killing—is contrary to that for which the medical profession stands and is contrary to the policy of the American Medical Association.

The cessation of the employment of extraordinary means to prolong the life of the body when there is irrefutable evidence that biological death is imminent is the decision of the patient and/or his immediate family. The advice and judgment of the physician should be freely available to the patient and/or his immediate family.

However, a strong case can be made against this doctrine. In what follows I will set out some of the relevant arguments, and urge doctors to reconsider their views on this matter.

To begin with a familiar type of situation, a patient who is dying of incurable cancer of the throat is in terrible pain, which can no longer be satisfactorily alleviated. He is certain to die within a few days, even if present treatment is continued, but he does not want to go on living for those days since the pain is unbearable. So

he asks the doctor for an end to it, and his family joins in the request.

Suppose the doctor agrees to withhold treatment, as the conventional doctrine says he may. The justification for his doing so is that the patient is in terrible agony, and since he is going to die anyway, it would be wrong to prolong his suffering needlessly. But now notice this. If one simply withholds treatment, it may take the patient longer to die, and so he may suffer more than he would if more direct action were taken and a lethal injection given. This fact provides strong reason for thinking that, once the initial decision not to prolong his agony has been made, active euthanasia is actually preferable to passive euthanasia, rather than the reverse. To say otherwise is to endorse the option that leads to more suffering rather than less, and is contrary to the humanitarian impulse that prompts the decision not to prolong his life in the first place.

Part of my point is that the process of being "allowed to die" can be relatively slow and painful, whereas being given a lethal injection is relatively quick and painless. Let me give a different sort of example. In the United States about one in 600 babies is born with Down's syndrome. Most of these babies are otherwise healthy—that is, with only the usual pediatric care, they will proceed to an otherwise normal infancy. Some, however, are born with congenital defects such as intestinal obstructions that require operations if they are to live. Sometimes, the parents and the doctor will decide not to operate, and let the infant die. Anthony Shaw describes what happens then.

. . . When surgery is denied [the doctor] must try to keep the infant from suffering while natural forces

Reprinted with permission from *The New England Journal of Medicine,* Vol. 292, No. 2 (Jan. 9, 1975), pp. 78–80.

sap the baby's life away. As a surgeon whose natural inclination is to use the scalpel to fight off death, standing by and watching a salvageable baby die is the most emotionally exhausting experience I know. It is easy at a conference, in a theoretical discussion, to decide that such infants should be allowed to die. It is altogether different to stand by in the nursery and watch as dehydration and infection wither a tiny being over hours and days. This is a terrible ordeal for me and the hospital staff—much more so than for the parents who never set foot in the nursery.[1]

I can understand why some people are opposed to all euthanasia, and insist that such infants must be allowed to live. I think I can also understand why other people favor destroying these babies quickly and painlessly. But why should anyone favor letting "dehydration and infection wither a tiny being over hours and days?" The doctrine that says that a baby may be allowed to dehydrate and wither, but may not be given an injection that would end its life without suffering, seems so patently cruel as to require no further refutation. The strong language is not intended to offend, but only to put the point in the clearest possible way.

My second argument is that the conventional doctrine leads to decisions concerning life and death made on irrelevant grounds.

Consider again the case of the infants with Down's syndrome who need operations for congenital defects unrelated to the syndrome to live. Sometimes, there is no operation, and the baby dies, but when there is no such defect, the baby lives on. Now, an operation such as that to remove an intestinal obstruction is not prohibitively difficult. The reason why such operations are not performed in these cases is, clearly, that the child has Down's syndrome and the parents and doctor judge that because of that fact it is better for the child to die.

But notice that this situation is absurd, no matter what view one takes of the lives and potentials of such babies. If the life of such an infant is worth preserving, what does it matter if it needs a simple operation? Or, if one thinks

1. Shaw A.: 'Doctor, Do We Have a Choice?' *The New York Times Magazine,* January 30, 1972, p. 54.

it better that such a baby should not live on, what difference does it make that it happens to have an unobstructed intestinal tract? In either case, the matter of life and death is being decided on irrelevant grounds. It is the Down's syndrome, and not the intestines, that is the issue. The matter should be decided, if at all, on that basis, and not be allowed to depend on the essentially irrelevant question of whether the intestinal tract is blocked.

What makes this situation possible, of course, is the idea that when there is an intestinal blockage, one can "let the baby die," but when there is no such defect there is nothing that can be done, for one must not "kill" it. The fact that this idea leads to such results as deciding life or death on irrelevant grounds is another good reason why the doctrine should be rejected.

One reason why so many people think that there is an important moral difference between active and passive euthanasia is that they think killing someone is morally worse than letting someone die. But is it? Is killing, in itself, worse than letting die? To investigate this issue, two cases may be considered that are exactly alike except that one involves killing whereas the other involves letting someone die. Then, it can be asked whether this difference makes any difference to the moral assessments. It is important that the cases be exactly alike, except for this one difference, since otherwise one cannot be confident that it is this difference and not some other that accounts for any variation in the assessments of the two cases. So, let us consider this pair of cases:

In the first, Smith stands to gain a large inheritance if anything should happen to his six-year-old cousin. One evening while the child is taking his bath, Smith sneaks into the bathroom and drowns the child, and then arranges things so that it will look like an accident.

In the second, Jones also stands to gain if anything should happen to his six-year-old cousin. Like Smith, Jones sneaks in planning to drown the child in his bath. However, just as he enters the bathroom Jones sees the child slip and hit his head, and fall face down in the water. Jones is delighted; he stands by, ready to push the child's head back under if it is necessary, but it is not necessary. With only a little thrashing about, the child drowns all by himself, "accidentally," as Jones watches and does nothing.

Now Smith killed the child, whereas Jones "merely" let the child die. That is the only difference between them. Did either man behave better, from a moral point of view? If the difference between killing and letting die were in itself a morally important matter, one should say that Jones's behavior was less reprehensible than Smith's. But does one really want to say that? I think not. In the first place, both men acted from the same motive, personal gain, and both had exactly the same end in view when they acted. It may be inferred from Smith's conduct that he is a bad man, although that judgment may be withdrawn or modified if certain further facts are learned about him—for example, that he is mentally deranged. But would not the very same thing be inferred about Jones from his conduct? And would not the same further considerations also be relevant to any modification of this judgment? Moreover, suppose Jones pleaded, in his own defense, "After all, I didn't do anything except just stand there and watch the child drown. I didn't kill him; I only let him die." Again, if letting die were in itself less bad than killing, this defense should have at least some weight. But it does not. Such a "defense" can only be regarded as a grotesque perversion of moral reasoning. Morally speaking, it is no defense at all.

Now it may be pointed out, quite properly, that the cases of euthanasia with which doctors are concerned are not like this at all. They do not involve personal gain or the destruction of normal healthy children. Doctors are concerned only with cases in which the patient's life is of no further use to him, or in which the patient's life has become or will soon become a terrible burden. However, the point is the same in these cases: the bare difference between killing and letting die does not, in itself, make a moral difference. If a doctor lets a patient die, for humane reasons, he is in the same moral position as if he had given the patient a lethal injection for humane reasons. If his decision was wrong—if, for example, the patient's illness was in fact curable—the decision would be equally regrettable no matter which method was used to carry it out. And if the doctor's decision was the right one, the method used is not in itself important.

The AMA policy statement isolates the crucial issue very well; the crucial issue is "the intentional termination of the life of one human being by another." But after identifying this issue, and forbidding "mercy killing," the statement goes on to deny that the cessation of treatment is the intentional termination of a life. This is where the mistake comes in, for what is the cessation of treatment, in these circumstances, if it is not "the intentional termination of the life of one human being by another?" Of course it is exactly that, and if it were not, there would be no point to it.

Many people will find this judgment hard to accept. One reason, I think, is that it is very easy to conflate the question of whether killing is, in itself, worse than letting die, with the very different question of whether most actual cases of killing are more reprehensible than most actual cases of letting die. Most actual cases of killing are clearly terrible (think, for example, of all the murders reported in the newspapers), and one hears of such cases every day. On the other hand, one hardly ever hears of a case of letting die, except for the actions of doctors who are motivated by humanitarian reasons. So one learns to think of killing in a much worse light than of letting die. But this does not mean that there is something about killing that makes it in itself worse than letting die, for it is not the bare difference between killing and letting die that makes the difference in these cases. Rather, the other factors—the murderer's motive of personal gain, for example, contrasted with the doctor's humanitarian motivation—account for different reactions to the different cases.

I have argued that killing is not in itself any worse than letting die; if my contention is right, it follows that active euthanasia is not any worse than passive euthanasia. What arguments can be given on the other side? The most common, I believe, is the following:

"The important difference between active and passive euthanasia is that, in passive euthanasia, the doctor does not do anything to bring about the patient's death. The doctor does nothing, and the patient dies of whatever ills already afflict him. In active euthanasia, however, the doctor does something to bring about the patient's death: he kills him. The doctor who gives the patient with cancer a lethal injection has himself caused his patient's death; whereas if he merely ceases treatment, the cancer is the cause of the death."

A number of points need to be made here. The first is that it is not exactly correct to say that in passive euthanasia the doctor does nothing, for he does do one thing that is very important: he lets the patient die. "Letting someone die" is certainly different, in some respects, from other types of action—mainly in that it is a kind of action that one may perform by way of not performing certain other actions. For example, one may let a patient die by way of not giving medication, just as one may insult someone by way of not shaking his hand. But for any purpose of moral assessment, it is a type of action nonetheless. The decision to let a patient die is subject to moral appraisal in the same way that a decision to kill him would be subject to moral appraisal: it may be assessed as wise or unwise, compassionate or sadistic, right or wrong. If a doctor deliberately let a patient die who was suffering from a routinely curable illness, the doctor would certainly be to blame for what he had done, just as he would be to blame if he had needlessly killed the patient. Charges against him would then be appropriate. If so, it would be no defense at all for him to insist that he didn't "do anything." He would have done something very serious indeed, for he let his patient die.

Fixing the cause of death may be very important from a legal point of view, for it may determine whether criminal charges are brought against the doctor. But I do not think that this notion can be used to show a moral difference between active and passive euthanasia. The reason why it is considered bad to be the cause of someone's death is that death is regarded as a great evil—and so it is. However, if it has been decided that euthanasia—even passive euthanasia—is desirable in a given case, it has also been decided that in this instance death is no greater an evil than the patient's continued existence. And if this is true, the usual reason for not wanting to be the cause of someone's death simply does not apply.

Finally, doctors may think that all of this is only of academic interest—the sort of thing that philosophers may worry about but that has no practical bearing on their own work. After all, doctors must be concerned about the legal consequences of what they do, and active euthanasia is clearly forbidden by the law. But even so, doctors should also be concerned with the fact that the law is forcing upon them a moral doctrine that may well be indefensible, and has a considerable effect on their practices. Of course, most doctors are not now in the position of being coerced in this matter, for they do not regard themselves as merely going along with what the law requires. Rather, in statements such as the AMA policy statement that I have quoted, they are endorsing this doctrine as a central point of medical ethics. In that statement, active euthanasia is condemned not merely as illegal but as "contrary to that for which the medical profession stands," whereas passive euthanasia is approved. However, the preceding considerations suggest that there is really no moral difference between the two, considered in themselves (there may be important moral differences in some cases in their *consequences,* but, as I pointed out, these differences may make active euthanasia, and not passive euthanasia, the morally preferable option). So, whereas doctors may have to discriminate between active and passive euthanasia to satisfy the law, they should not do any more than that. In particular, they should not give the distinction any added authority and weight by writing it into official statements of medical ethics.

GEORGE P. FLETCHER

Prolonging Life: Some Legal Considerations

I

Much of what follows is an exercise in conceptual analysis. It is an effort to devise a test for determining which of two competitive schemes—that for acts or that for omissions—should apply in analyzing a given question of responsibility for the death of another. It is significant inquiry, if only to add a word to the discussion of the ponderous legal quandaries of physicians who care for terminal patients. The problem is also of wider significance for the theory of tort and criminal liability. The area of liability for omissions bristles with moral, analytic and institutional puzzles. In the course of this inquiry, we shall confront some of these problems and others we shall catalogue in passing.

II

The question is posed: Is the physicians' discontinuing aid to a terminal patient an act or omission? To be sure, the choice of legal track does not yield radically different results. For some omissions, physicians are liable in much the same way as they are for unpermitted operations and negligent treatment. One need only consider the following turn of events. Doctor Brown is the family doctor of the Smith family and has been for several years. Tim Smith falls ill with pneumonia. Brown sees him once or twice at the family home and administers the necessary therapy. One evening, upon receiving a telephone call from the Smith family that Tim is in a critical condition, Dr. Brown decides that he should prefer to remain at his bridge game than to visit the sick child. Brown fails to render aid to the child; it is clear that Brown would be liable criminally and civilly if death should ensue. That he has merely omitted to act, rather than asserted himself in-

Reprinted with permission of Fred B. Rothman and Co. from *Washington Law Review*, Vol. 42 (1967), pp. 999, 1004–1016.

tentionally to end life, is immaterial in assessing his criminal and civil liability. Of course, the doctor would not be under an obligation to respond to the call of a stranger who said that he needed help. But there is a difference between a stranger and someone who has placed himself in the care of a physician. The factor of reliance and reasonable expectation that the doctor will render aid means that the doctor is legally obligated to do so.[1] His failure to do so is then tantamount to an intentional infliction of harm. As his motive, be it for good or ill, is irrelevant in analyzing his liability for assertive killing, his motive is also irrelevant in analyzing his liability for omitting to render aid when he is obligated to do so.

Thus, it makes no difference whether a doctor omits to render aid because he prefers to continue playing bridge or if he does so in the hope that the patient's misery will come quickly to a natural end. A doctor may be criminally and civilly liable either for intentionally taking life or for omitting to act and thus permitting death to occur. However, the sources of these two legal proscriptions are different. And this difference in the source of the law may provide the key for the analysis of the doctor's liability in failing to prolong life in the case discussed at the outset of this article. That a doctor may not actively kill is an application of the general principle that no man may actively kill a fellow human being. In contrast, the principle that a doctor may not omit to render aid to a patient justifiably relying upon him is a function of the special relationship that exists between doctor and patient. Thus, in analyzing the doctor's legal duty to his patient, one must take into consideration whether the question involved is an act or an omission. If it is an act, the relationship between the doctor and patient is irrelevant. If it is an omission, the relationship is all controlling.

With these points in mind, we may turn to an analysis of specific aspects of the medical decision not to prolong life. The first problem is to isolate the relevant medical activity. The recurrent pattern includes: stopping cardiac resuscitation, turning off a respirator, a pacemaker or a kidney machine, and removing the tubes and devices used with these life-sustaining machines. The initial decision of classification determines the subsequent legal analysis of the case. If turning off the respirator is an ''act'' under the law, then it is unequivocally forbidden: it is on a par with injecting air into the patient's veins. If, on the other hand, it is classified as an ''omission,'' the analysis proceeds more flexibly. Whether it would be forbidden as an omission would depend on the demands imposed by the relationship between doctor and patient.

There are gaps in the law; and we are confronted with one of them. There is simply no way to focus the legal authorities to determine whether the process of turning off the respirator is an act or an omission. That turning off the respirator takes physical movement need not be controlling. There might be ''acts'' without physical movement, as, for example, if one should sit motionless in the driver's seat as one's car heads toward an intended victim. Surely that would be an act causing death; it would be first-degree murder regardless of the relationship between the victim and his assassin. Similarly, there might be cases of omissions involving physical exertion, perhaps even the effort required to turn off the respirator. The problem is not whether there is or there is not physical movement; there must be another test.

That other test, I should propose, is whether on all the facts we should be inclined to speak of the activity as one that causes harm or one merely that permits harm to occur. The usage of the verbs ''causing'' and ''permitting'' corresponds to the distinction in the clear cases between acts and omissions. If a doctor injects air into the veins of a suffering patient, he causes harm. On the other hand, if the doctor fails to stop on the highway to aid a stranger

injured in an automobile accident, he surely permits harm to occur, and he might be morally blameworthy for that; but as the verb ''cause'' is ordinarily used, his failing to stop is not the cause of the harm.[2]

As native speakers of English, we are equipped with linguistic sensitivity for the distinction between causing harm and permitting harm to occur. That sensitivity reflects a common sense perception of reality; and we should employ it in classifying the hard cases arising in discussions of the prolongation of life. Is turning off the respirator an instance of causing death or permitting death to occur? If the patient is beyond recovery and on the verge of death, one balks at saying that the activity causes death. It is far more natural to speak of the case as one of permitting death to occur. It is significant that we are inclined to refer to the respirator as a means for prolonging life; we would not speak of insulin shots for a diabetic in the same way. The use of the term ''prolongation of life'' builds on the same perception of reality that prompts us to say that turning off the respirator is an activity permitting death to occur, rather than causing death. And that basic perception is that using the respirator interferes artificially in the pattern of events. Of course, the perception of the natural and of the artificial is a function of time and culture. What may seem artificial today, may be a matter of course in ten years. Nonetheless, one *does* perceive many uses of the respirator today as artificial prolongations of life. And that perception of artificiality should be enough to determine the legal classification of the case. Because we are prompted to refer to the activity of turning off the respirator as activity permitting death to occur, rather than causing death, we may classify the case as an omission, rather than as an act.

To clarify our approach, we might consider this scenario. A pedestrian D notices that a nearby car, parked with apparently inadequate brakes, is about to roll down hill. P's house is parked directly in its path. D rushes to the front of the car and with effort he is able to arrest its movement for a few minutes. Though he feels able to hold back the car for several more minutes (time enough perhaps to give warning of the danger), he decides that he has had enough; and he steps to one side, knowing full well that his quarry will roll squarely into P's front yard. That is precisely what it does. What are P's rights against D? Again, the problem is whether the defendant's behavior should be treated as an act or as an omission. If it is act, he is liable for trespass against P's property. If it is an omission, the law of trespass is inapplicable; and the problem devolves into a search for a relationship between P and D that would impose on D the duty to prevent this form of damage to P's property. Initially, one is inclined to regard D's behavior as an act bringing on harm. Like the physician's turning off a respirator, his stepping aside represents physical exertion. Yet as in the physician's case, we are led to the opposite result by asking whether under the circumstances D caused the harm or merely permitted it to occur. Surely, a newspaper account would employ the latter description; D let the car go, he permitted it to roll on, but he is no more a causal factor than if he had not initially intervened to halt its forward motion. We deny D's causal contribution for reasons akin to those in the physician's case. In both instances, other factors are sufficient in themselves to bring on the harmful result. As the car's brakes were inadequate to hold it on the hill, so the patient's hopeless condition brought on his death. With sufficient causal factors present, we can imagine the harm's occurring without the physician's or the pedestrian's contribution. And thus we are inclined to think of the behavior of each as something less than a causal force.[3]

One might agree that as a matter of common sense, we can distinguish between causing harm and permitting harm to occur and yet balk at referring to the way people ordinarily describe phenomena in order to solve hard problems of legal policy. After all, what if people happen to describe things differently? Would that mean that we would have to devise different answers to the same legal problems? To vindicate a resort to common sense notions and linguistic usage as a touchstone for separating acts from omissions, we must clarify the interlacing of these three planes of the problem: (1) the distinction between acts and omissions,

(2) the ordinary usage of the terms "causing" and "permitting" and (3) resorting in cases of omissions, but not in cases of acts, to the relationship between the agent and his victim in setting the scope of the agent's duties. The question uniting the second and third variables is this: Is there good reason for being guided by the relationship between the parties in cases where the agent has permitted harm to occur, but not in cases where the agent has intentionally and directly caused harm to a stranger? To answer this question, we need to turn in some detail to the function of causal judgments in analyzing liability, whereupon we may clarify the link between the first and second variables of the analysis, namely between the category of omissions and the process of permitting harm to occur.

Ascribing liability for tortious and criminal harm may be looked upon as a two-stage process. The first stage is the isolation of a candidate for liability. In virtually all dimensions of the law of crimes and torts, we rely upon the concept of causation to separate from the mass of society those individuals who might prove to be liable for the proscribed harm. Upon reducing the number of potentially liable parties to those that have caused the harm, the final stage of analysis demands an evaluation of the facts under the apt rules of liability, *e.g.*, those prescribing negligence and proximate cause as conditions for liability.

The one area of the law where one has difficulty isolating candidates for liability is the area of omissions. When others have stood by and permitted harm to occur, we either have too many candidates for liability or we have none at all. A helpless old woman succumbs to starvation. Many people knew of her condition and did nothing; the postman, her hired nurse, her daughter, the bill collector, the telephone operator—each of them allowed her to die. Could we say, on analogy to causing death, that permitting the death to occur should serve as the criterion for selecting these people as candidates for liability? If we say that all of them are candidates for liability, then the burden falls to the criteria of fault to decide which of them, if any, should be liable for wrongful death and criminal homicide. The problem is whether the criteria of fault are sufficiently sensitive to resolve the question of liability. What kinds of questions should we ask in assessing fault? Did each voluntarily omit to render aid? Did any one of them face a particular hazard in doing so? Were any of them in a particularly favorable position to avert the risk of death? If these are the questions we must ask in assessing fault and affixing liability, we are at a loss to discriminate among the candidates for liability. Each acted voluntarily with knowledge of the peril; none faced personal hazard in offering assistance; and their capacities to avert the risk were equal. Thus, we may use the concept of permitting as we do the notion of causation to narrow the field to those who should be judged on criteria of fault. But if we do, the criteria of fault are useless (at least in the type of case sketched here) for discriminating among the candidates.

One wonders why this is so. In the arena of caused harms, one may have a large number of candidates for liability. The conventional test of causing harm sweeps wide in encompassing all those but for whose contribution the harm would not have occured. Yet the criteria of liability—reasonableness of risk, ambit of risk, proximate cause—are effective in further reducing the field to those we might fairly hold liable. The reason is that each causal agent is chargeable with a different risk that loss of the given kind would occur. The risks differ in quantum and scope. Some bear a remote relationship to the harm; others seem reasonable in light of other circumstances. These differences in the posture of each causal agent toward the risk of harm enable us to assess their individual fault with some sensitivity.

In contrast, those who permit harm to occur do not bear individualized responsibility for the risk of harm. Their status derives not from the creation of the risk, but merely from knowledge that the risk exists and from the opportunity to do something about it. One could speak of the likelihood that each could avert the harm. And in some cases, this approach might be useful; a doctor's failing to render aid to a man lying in the street is more egregious than a layman's turning the other way. Yet in the general run of case—the starvation of the old woman discussed above, the Kitty Genovese incident[4]—the risks assignable to passive bystanders are of the same murky order: each could have done something but did not.

. . .

Affixing liability fairly in cases of omission requires a more sensitive filtering mechanism prior to the application of the traditional criteria of personal fault. The concept of permitting harm sweeps too wide; and the criteria of personal fault tend to be of little avail in narrowing the field. Thus one can understand the role of the relationship between the parties as a touchstone of liability. Legal systems, both common law and Continental, have resorted to the relationship between the parties as a device for narrowing the field to those individuals whose liability may be left to depend on personal fault. According to the conventional rules, the old woman's nurse and daughter are candidates potentially liable for permitting death to occur. Liability would rest on personal fault, primarily on the voluntariness of each in omitting to render aid. Thus the conventional rules as to when one has a duty to render aid fulfill the same function as the causal inquiry in its domain: these rules, like the predication of causation, isolate individuals whose behavior is then scrutinized for the marks of negligent and intentional wrongdoing.

By demonstrating the parallel between the causal concept in cases of acts and the relationship between the parties in cases of omissions, we have come a long way in support of our thesis. We have shown that in cases of permitting harm to occur, one is required to resort to the relationship between the parties in order fairly to select those parties whose liability should turn on criteria of personal fault. In the absence of a causal judgment, with its attendant assignment of differentiated responsibility for the risk of harm, one can proceed only by asking: Is this the kind of relationship, e.g., parent-child, doctor-patient, in which one person ought to help another? And on grounds ranging from common decency to contract, one derives individual duties to render aid when needed.

One step of the argument remains: the conclusion that cases of permitting harm are instances of omissions, not of acts. This is a step that turns not so much on policy and analysis, as on acceptance of the received premises of the law of homicide. One of these premises is that acting intentionally to cause death is unconditionally prohibited: the relationship between the defendant and his victim is irrelevant. One may resort to the relationship between the parties only in cases of omissions indirectly resulting in harm.[5] With these two choices and no others, the logic of classification is ineluctable. Cases of permitting harm, where one must have recourse to the relationship between the parties, cannot be classified as cases of acts: to do so would preclude excusing the harm on the ground that the relationship between the parties did not require its avoidance. Thus, to permit recourse to relationship of the parties, one must treat cases of permitting harm as cases of omissions.

To complete our inquiry, we need attend to an asymmetry in the analysis of causing and permitting. As Professors Hart and Honore have shown,[6] some omissions may be the causes of harm. And thus, the category of causing harm includes some cases of omitting as well as all cases of acting to bring on harm. Suppose, for example, that an epileptic regularly takes pills to avert a seizure. Yet on one occasion he omits to take the pills in the hope that he is no longer required to. He has a seizure. The cause of his seizure is clear: he omitted to take the prescribed pill. In the same way, a physician failing to give a diabetic patient a routine shot of insulin would be the cause of harm that might ensue. The taking of the pill and the giving of the shot are the expected state of affairs. They represent normality, and their omission, abnormality. Because we anticipate the opposite, the omission explains what went wrong, why our expectations were not realized. In contrast, if pills to avert epileptic seizures had just been devised, we would not say as to someone who had never taken the pills

that his failure to do so had brought on his attack. In that case, our expectations would be different, the omission to take pills would not represent an abnormality, and the anticipated omission would not be a satisfying causal explanation of the attack.[7]

A doctor's failure to give his diabetic patient an insulin shot is a case warranting some attention. By contemporary standards, insulin shots, unlike mechancial respirators, do not interfere artificially in the course of nature; because the use of insulin is standard medical practice, we would not describe its effect as one of prolonging life. We would not say that withholding the shot permits death; it is a case of an omission causing harm. With the prohibition against causing death, one should not have to refer to the doctor-patient relationship to determine the criminality of the doctor's omission. Yet in fact, common law courts would ground a conviction for omitting to give the shot on the doctor's duty to render aid to his patient—a duty derived from the doctor-patient relationship. Thus we encounter an apparent inconsistency: a case of causing in which one resorts to the relationship of the parties to determine criminality. We can reconcile the case with our thesis by noting that cases of omissions causing harm possess the criteria —regularity of performance and reliance—that give rise to duties of care. The doctor is clearly under a duty to provide his patient with an insulin shot if the situation demands it. And the duty is so clear precisely because one expects an average doctor in the 1960s to use insulin when necessary; this is the same expectation that prompts us to say that his failure to give the shot would be the cause of his patient's death.

That an omission can on occasion be the cause of harm prompts us slightly to reformulate our thesis. We cannot say that causing harm may serve as the criterion for an act as opposed to an omissions because some instances of causation are omissions. But we may claim with undiminished force that permitting harm to occur should be sufficient for classification as an omission. Upon analysis, we find that our thesis for distinguishing acts from omissions survives only in part; it works for some omissions, but not for all. Yet, so far as the stimulus of this investigation is concerned, the problem of physicians permitting death to come to their terminal patients, the thesis continues to hold: permitting a patient to die is a case in which one appropriately refers to the relationship of the parties to set the scope of the physician's legal duty to his patient; in this sense it functions as an omission in legal analysis.

III

By permitting recourse to the doctor-patient relationship in fixing the scope of the doctor's duties to his patient, we have at least fashioned the concepts of the common law to respond more sensitively to the problems of the time. We have circumvented the extravagant legal conclusion that a physician's turning off a kidney machine or a respirator is tantamount to murder. Yet one critical inquiry remains. How does shunting the analysis into the track of legal omissions actually affect the physician's flexibility in the operating room? We say that his duties are determined by his relationship with his patient; specifically, it is the consensual aspect of the relationship that is supposed to control the leeway of the physician. Yet there is some question as to where the control actually resides.

To take a clear case, let us suppose that prior to the onset of a terminal illness, the patient demands that his physician do everything to keep him alive and breathing as long as possible. And the physician responds, "Even if you have a flat EEG reading and there is no chance of recovery?" "Yes," the patient replies. If the doctor agrees to this bizarre demand, he becomes obligated to keep the respirator going indefinitely. Happily, cases of this type do not occur in day-to-day medical practice. In the average case, the patient has not given a thought to the problem; and his physician is not likely to alert him to it. The problem then is whether there is an implicit understanding between physician and patient as to how the physician should proceed in the last stages of a

terminal illness. But would there be an implicit understanding about what the physician should do if the patient is in a coma and dependent on a mechanical respirator? This is not the kind of thing as to which the average man has expectations. And if he did, they would be expectations that would be based on the customary practices of the time. If he had heard about a number of cases in which patient had been sustained for long periods of time on respirators, he might (at least prior to going into the coma) expect that he would be similarly sustained.

Thus, the analysis leads us along the following path. The doctor's duty to prolong life is a function of his relationship with his patient; and in the typical case, that relationship devolves into the patient's expectations of the treatment he will receive. Those expectations, in turn, are a function of the practices prevailing in the community at the time, and practices in the use of respirators to prolong life are no more and no less than what doctors actually do in the time and place. Thus, we have come full circle. We began the inquiry by asking: Is it legally permissible for doctors to turn off respirators used to prolong the life of doomed patients? And the answer after our tortuous journey is simply: It all depends on what doctors customarily do. The law is sometimes no more precise than that.

The conclusion of our circular journey is that doctors are in a position to fashion their own law to deal with cases of prolongation of life. By establishing customary standards, they may determine the expectations of their patients and thus regulate the understanding and the relationship between doctor and patient. And by regulating that relationship, they may control their legal obligations to render aid to doomed patients.

Thus the medical profession confronts the challenge of developing humane and sensitive customary standards for guiding decisions to prolong the lives of terminal patients. This is not a challenge that the profession may shirk. For the doctor's legal duties to render aid derive from his relationship with the patient. That relationship, along with the expectations implicit in it, is the responsibility of the individual doctor and the individual patient. With respect to problems not commonly discussed by the doctor with his patient, particularly the problems of prolonging life, the responsibility for the patient's expectations lies with the medical profession as a whole.

NOTES

1. Other relationships of reliance giving rise to duties of care are those of carrier and passenger, innkeeper and guest, ship captain and seaman, school master and pupil. W. PROSSER, TORTS 337 (3d ed. 1964).

2. For the sake of exposition, the thesis is put simply at this stage; it receives some adjustment below. *See* text at pp. 299–300.

3. This conclusion is supported by the German theory of conditions *(Bedingungstheorie)*, which holds that a factor is not casual if one can imagine the same sequence of events in the absence of that factor. H. L. A. HART & A. M. HONORE, CAUSATION IN THE LAW 391–92 (1959).

4. Thirty-eight people in New York City watched and listened as Kitty Genovese was murdered outside their apartment building, 198 NATION 602–04 (1964).

5. E.g., Rex v. Smith, 2 Car & P. 448, 172 E.R. 203 (Gloucester Assizes 1826) (The analysis of criminality of D for failing to care for an idiot brother turns on whether keeping the brother locked up was an act or omission. Finding the latter, the court held that the defendant bore no duty to aid his brother and directed an acquittal). . . .

6. H. L. A. HART & A. M. HONORE, CAUSATION IN THE LAW 35–36 (1959).

7. The relationship between expectations and causation is developed more fully in HART & HONORE, *ibid.*, ch. 2.

Decisions by Competent Adults

ROBERT M. VEATCH

Choosing Not to Prolong Dying

Lucy Morgan is a 94-year-old patient being maintained in a nursing home. Some years ago she suffered a severe cerebral hemorrhage. She is blind, largely deaf, and often in a semi-conscious state. Mrs. Morgan is an educated woman, the wife of the former president of Antioch College. About four years ago she wrote an essay, entitled, "On Drinking the Hemlock," in which she pleaded for a dignified and simple way to choose to die. Now she, like thousands of other patients in hospitals, rest homes, and bedrooms throughout the world,

is having her dying prolonged. What, before the biological revolution with its technological gadgetry, would have been a short and peaceful exit is now often drawn out for months or years by the unmitigated and sometimes merciless intervention of penicillin, pacemakers, polygraphs, tubes, tetracycline and transplantation.

Technology's new possibilities have created chaos in the care of the dying. What happens to Mrs. Morgan and others like her depends upon the medical and nursing staffs of the institutions in which these patients are confined. One patient may be mercilessly probed and primed with infusions so that dying is prolonged end-

Reprinted by permission from *Medical Dimensions* magazine, December 1972. Copyright © 1972, MBA Communications, Inc.

lessly, while another in a similar condition may have heroic treatment stopped so that the process of dying may proceed uninterrupted, whether or not permission for the withdrawal has been given. A third patient may, with or without his consent, have an air embolism injected into a vein.

THE ISSUES AT STAKE

Before examining some of the policies being proposed, we should get the issues straight. Lawyers and moralists make three distinctions in discussing euthanasia and the choice not to prolong dying. First, there may be legal and moral differences between directly killing the terminal patient and allowing him to die. In one study, fifty-nine percent of the physicians in two West Coast hospitals said that they would practice what was called "negative euthanasia" if it were legal, while twenty-seven percent said that they would practice positive euthanasia.

Euthanasia has become a terribly confused term in the discussion. In some cases, it is taken literally to mean simply a good death; in others it is limited to the more narrow direct or positive killing of the terminal patient. In light of this confusion, it seems wise to ban the term from the debate entirely.

The legality of directly ending a patient's life is highly questionable, to say the least. Legal cases are very rare. The one decision which is particularly relevant is in the case of Dr. Hermann N. Sander, a New Hampshire physician who entered into the chart of a cancer patient that he had injected air into the patient's blood stream. He admitted that his purpose was to end suffering and pain and the jury returned a verdict for the defendant. But the critical factor in the case was the pathologist's testimony that he could not establish the cause of death with certainty. Thus the jury was not condoning "mercy killing." According to Curran and Shapiro in *Law, Medicine and Forensic Science,* "The general rule in the United States is that one who either kills one suffering from a fatal or incurable disease, even with the consent of that party, or who provides that party

with the means of suicide, is guilty of either murder or manslaughter." It is safe to say that no lawyer would advise his medical clients that they would not be prosecuted if they practiced positive euthanasia.

On the other hand, the cessation of treatment may be a different matter morally if not legally. It is well known that a competent patient has the right to refuse even lifesaving treatment. To my knowledge, there are no cases in which a physician has been brought to trial for stopping the treatment of a terminal patient. It seems most unlikely that he would be guilty of either moral or legal offense if a competent patient had ordered the treatment ended. If he had done so without the patient's instructions, however, the charge, presumably, would be abandonment. The legal status of ceasing to treat or omitting treatment is very much in doubt especially when a competent patient has not specifically refused treatment.

At the moral level, some recognize the difference between killing and omitting or ceasing treatment. Others insist that this kind of distinction is mere semantics, because in either case the result is that the patient dies. Yet, if we were given the choice of turning off a respirator to allow a terminal patient to die or actively injecting an embolism, almost all of us would choose the first act, at least barring some extenuating circumstances which changed the moral calculations, such as the presence of extreme intractable pain and suffering.

There are two kinds of cases in which the distinction would make an actual difference. The first is when the prognosis had been in error and merely ceasing certain treatment could result in continued living, while active killing would result in death. The second involves the possibility of actual abuse. In any case, the physician should not be put in a position to dispose of unwanted patients. It is argued that for practical, if not moral, reasons, we need to separate active killing from cessation and omission of treatment, recognizing that many physicians favor the latter but not the former. It becomes expedient, then, to adopt a policy which would cover virtually all cases, minimize the chances for error, and be acceptable to a broader public.

It is a sad commentary on the tradition of medical ethics that the question of euthanasia is almost always raised in terms of what the medical professional should decide to do for a terminal patient: Should *he* treat; should *he* omit treatment; should *he* stop treatment; should *he* inject the embolism? Yet, there is another perspective: that of the patient. While the legal and moral status of killing and allowing a patient to die may be dubious, the principle of the right to refuse treatment is well recognized. It is morally and legally sound to emphasize the role of the patient as decision-maker when he is legally competent. Of course, this still leaves open cases when the patient is not legally competent, but at least we have a moral and legal foundation from which to form a policy. The next step would be to decide upon an appropriate agent for the legally incompetent patient.

PATIENT ADVOCATE

First priority should go to an agent whom the patient, while competent, would be permitted to appoint expressly for this purpose. When this has not been done, the next of kin should have both the rights and responsibilities to determine what is in the patient's interest. While the potential for abuse exists, the next of kin is in the best position to know the patient's personal values and beliefs upon which treatment-refusing decisions must be based. There would still be the established possibility of going to court to overturn the judgment of the next of kin in case he was acting maliciously or choosing not to prolong the patient's living rather than his dying. But the choice to refuse some death-prolonging treatment should not, in and of itself, be taken as evidence of immoral or illegal activity. In that rare case where no relatives are available, a court-appointed guardian might provide the best safeguard of the patient's interests.

ORDINARY AND EXTRAORDINARY MEANS

A second distinction that must be clarified in a policy permitting the choice not to prolong dying is the difference between ordinary and extraordinary means. These terms have three meanings: usual vs. unusual treatment, useful vs. useless treatment, and simply imperative vs. elective treatment. The Catholic tradition as summarized by Pope Pius XII is: "Normally one is held to use only ordinary means—according to circumstances of persons, places, times and culture—that is to say, means that do not involve any grave burden for oneself or another." Clearly, defining what is ordinary according to the circumstances named will make the distinction a difficult one. We can circumvent this entire quagmire simply by focusing on the moral principle of the right to refuse treatment as a basis for policy. This does not mean that it will always be moral to refuse treatment, but if patient freedom and dignity are to be central to policy decision, we may have to recognize that patients are entitled to make their own decisions and, therefore, to refuse even those treatments which are thought to be usual or useful. This might be the case when, for instance, a patient faces a lifetime hemodialysis regimen for chronic nephritis. Recently, such a patient decided that the thought of being attached by tubes for 16 to 24 hours a week for the rest of his life was an unbearable and dehumanizing possibility. He chose, we think morally and legally, to cease the dialysis treatment.

ALLOWING TO LIVE AND ALLOWING TO DIE

Third, it is important to distinguish between the choice not to prolong dying and the choice not to prolong living. Two closely related cases which I have encountered recently reveal the difference. In the first, a baby was born with trisomy-18 and severe respiratory distress as well as gross CNS anomalies. He would not live no matter what heroic procedures were attempted. A second case was that of a Mongoloid infant who had been born with esophageal atresia. The choice of the parents to refuse corrective surgery for the atresia was, in fact, the choice that the quality of life as a Mongoloid would not be satisfactory either for the infant or his parents. On the other hand, the choice to cease respiration for the trisomy-18 baby was made when there was nothing that man could do to save the infant's life.

Any policy which is adopted must come to terms with these distinctions, for it may be morally and legally acceptable to reject an unusually heroic and probably useless procedure but wrong, at least morally, to refuse a simple IV when it would lead relatively painlessly to many years of normal healthy life. It may be wrong to decide that someone else's life is not worth living but acceptable to recognize that even the forces of modern science are not able to cope with some diseases.

WHAT SHOULD OUR POLICY BE?

Some authorities say that we cannot adopt a systematic policy which would permit the choice not to prolong dying. The physician's duty, they feel, is to preserve life. When some treatment can be offered, even for a patient who is almost certainly going to die, that treatment *must* be offered. Even if this view is correct, it is utopian and one which few clinicians would be able to accept if taken literally as a practical way of dealing with death. We must stop the heroic procedures at some point. If the only course available for a patient in his last days is to fly him and the medical team around the country to try some newly devised experimental surgery, at least some will say that morally we are not required to proceed or, in fact, that it would be wrong to proceed. At some time, the decision must be made that the dying process has been tampered with long enough and that there is nothing more that man can or should do.

PHYSICIAN *AD HOC* DECISION-MAKING

Four policy alternatives are currently being debated. The first is the defense of the status quo: We should have no policy at all. In fact, right now we do have a policy—the individual physician decides, on an *ad hoc* basis at the moment when the patient is in a terminal condition, if and when treatment should be given. This is sometimes done in consultation with other members of the medical team, members of the family, and the clergyman, but, for the most part, the real decision rests in the doctor's hands.

A strong case can be made for the present policy. At least ideally, if not in practice, the physician knows the patient's condition and is committed to his best interest. Every doctor is aware that each medical case is unique, and to develop more systematic decision-making procedures could be very dangerous. Nevertheless, it seems to me that the present policy is the second worst of all possible alternatives. We have already seen that about half of the physicians in one study would exercise the choice not to prolong life if it were clearly made legal. There is also a difference of opinion among patients. A random pairing of patient and physician views would mean that if the physician is making the decision, in many cases the patient who would not want the dying prolonged will have this done against his wishes; another patient who desperately desires the last heroic operation will not receive it.

It may be even worse. There may be systematic differences between the medical professionals and the laymen. Many physicians claim that their special ethical duty is to preserve life. If the physicians have different ethical principles or even if they merely have different ethical judgments about what benefits the patient, it creates a terrible dilemma.

Even if physician and patient would reach the identical conclusion, the patient's freedom and dignity in matters most directly affecting his own living and dying would still be infringed upon. All of these objections have led to the search for other methods of decision-making.

THE PROFESSIONAL COMMITTEE

In an attempt to take the burden off the shoulders of the individual physician, a growing number of hospitals now use committees of physicians to decide who should receive the last bed in the intensive care unit or the scarce and expensive hemodialysis treatment. The committee eliminates some of the random biases which an individual physician might have either in favor of excessively heroic intervention or inadequate treatment. Yet, is it right that a patient whose position is at one extreme or the other should have his own views moderated? Particulary if there are systematic differences between the professional and lay communities? Even the committee structure would impose upon many patients views which they find unacceptable.

This serious drawback to the committee must be added to the more obvious problem—that with the committee-making structure one loses the primary advantage of decision-making by the individual physician. While, hopefully, he would know some details of the patient's life and values, we cannot hope that this would hold true for the committee. Even more significantly, the committee mechanism perpetuates the view that the medical professional by his training has somehow acquired expertise in making the moral judgment about when it is no longer appropriate to prolong dying. If the committee structure is the alternative, perhaps we should stay with the status quo and let the individual physician make the choice unhindered and unguided.

PERSONAL LETTERS

Other alternatives are beginning to appear. The Euthanasia Educational Fund has drafted a letter which an individual might address to his family physician, clergyman or lawyer. It directs that "if the time comes when I can no longer take part in decisions for my own future, [and] if there is no reasonable expectation of my recovery from physical or mental disability, I request that I be allowed to die and not be kept alive by artificial means or heroic measures." This "living will" makes no pretense of being legally binding. It merely gives guidance to the physician and others concerned. It also frees the physician from having to guess what the patient's wishes might be.

The instructions are extremely vague, however, and while useful for general guidance, do not go very far in removing the difficulties of earlier proposals. For example, "reasonable expectation" and "artificial means or heroic measures" beg for clarification, and it is the reader of the will who will have to interpret. For this reason, we know of two physicians who have drafted very specific letters as instruction for their own terminal care. One instructs "in the event of a cerebral accident other than a subarachnoid hemorrhage, I want no treatment of any kind until it is clear that I will be able to think effectively. . . . In the event of subarachnoid hemorrhage, use your own judgment in the acute state. . . ." The other directs that there be no artificial respiration "to prolong my life if I had lost the ability to breathe for more than two or three (not five or six) minutes." While possibly more specific than the "living will," these instructions may not be of much help to the layman. He simply does not have the technical knowledge to be so precise.

In either case, the idea of a letter pre-addressed to one's personal physician assumes that one has a personal physician. This, unfortunately, is not always the case. Also required is that one be dying in the care of the physician to whom the letter is sent. Carrying the letter in a wallet might help, but certainly will not do much to relieve the anxiety of the potentially dying patient. Even if one assumes that a personal physician will be caring for the dying patient, the letter still requires trust and understanding. This can no longer be assumed, but if such a relationship does exist, the need for the letter decreases in proportion.

LEGISLATION TO PERMIT DEATH WITH DIGNITY

All of these problems have instigated legislative proposals which would give clearer procedures for the decision not to prolong dying. In 1969 a bill patterned after the British euthanasia legislative proposal was introduced into the Idaho legislature. It explicitly included both "positive" and "negative" actions and received very little support in this country. Rep. Walter Sackett, himself a physician, has placed several proposals before the Florida legislature. One bill, which was introduced in 1970 but did not pass, would have permitted an individual to execute a document specifying that "his life shall not be prolonged beyond the point of a meaningful existence." If the patient himself cannot execute the document, the bill provided that the person of the next degree of kinship could. While this bill would have eliminated some of the problems of other proposals, the vagueness of the term "meaningful existence" is its critical flaw. The physician on the case presumably would be forced to determine whether or not the patient's life could ever again be meaningful.

A third type of legislation, to be based on the already existing right of the patient to refuse treatment, is worthy of consideration as a public policy. In cases where the patient is not competent, some agent must make the decision on the patient's behalf—that is an unpleasant reality of life. It seems to me that an agent appointed by the patient while competent should have first priority, then the next of kin, and finally, in the rare case where the patient has no relatives, a court-appointed agent.

The physician would thus be protected from having to make a non-medical, moral judgment about what is right for the patient. At the same time, the patient and his family would be able to fulfill their rights and obligations to look after the patient's welfare. Anything short of this will deprive the patient of life, liberty and probably happiness as well.

These four types of policy proposals will be receiving much more attention in the next few months. None of them is a panacea; each raises serious moral and public policy questions. But the chaos generated by biomedical technology's assault on death demands new policy clarification. That new policy will be forthcoming soon. It must be.

EUTHANASIA EDUCATIONAL COUNCIL

A Living Will

TO MY FAMILY, MY PHYSICIAN, MY LAWYER, MY
CLERGYMAN; TO ANY MEDICAL FACULTY IN
WHOSE CARE I HAPPEN TO BE; TO ANY
INDIVIDUAL WHO MAY BECOME RESPONSIBLE
FOR MY HEALTH, WELFARE OR AFFAIRS

Death is as much a reality as birth, growth, maturity and old age—it is the one certainty of life. If the time comes when I, _____ _____ can no longer take part in decisions for my own future, let this statement stand as an expression of my wishes, while I am still of sound mind.

If the situation should arise in which there is no reasonable expectation of my recovery from physical or mental disability, I request that I be allowed to die and not be kept alive by artificial means or "heroic measures". I do not fear death itself as much as the indignities of deterioration, dependence and hopeless pain. I, therefore, ask that medication be mercifully administered to me to alleviate suffering even though this may hasten the moment of death.

This request is made after careful consideration. I hope you who care for me will feel morally bound to follow its mandate. I recognize that this appears to place a heavy responsibility upon you, but it is with the intention of relieving you of such responsibility and of placing it upon myself in accordance with my strong convictions, that this statement is made.

Signed _____

Date _____

Witness _____

Witness _____

Copies of this request have been given to _____

_____

_____

_____

Published April 1974 and reprinted with permission of the Euthanasia Educational Council, New York.

YALE KAMISAR

Some Nonreligious Views Against Proposed "Mercy-killing" Legislation

A recent book, Glanville Williams' *The Sanctity of Life and the Criminal Law,* once again brings to the fore the controversial topic of euthanasia, more popularly known as "mercy killing." In keeping with the trend of the euthanasia movement over the past generation, Williams concentrates his efforts for reform on the *voluntary* type of euthanasia, for example, the cancer victim begging for death; as opposed to the *involuntary variety,* that is, the case of the congenital idiot, the permanently insane or the senile. . . .

The Law On The Books condemns all mercy-killings.[1] That this has a substantial deterrent effect, even its harshest critics admit. Of course, it does not stamp out all mercy-killings, just as murder and rape provisions do not stamp out all murder and rape, but presumably it does impose a substantially greater responsibility on physicians and relatives in a euthanasia situation and turns them away from significantly more doubtful cases than would otherwise be the practice under any proposed euthanasia legislation to date. When a mercy-killing occurs, however, The Law In Action is as malleable as The Law On The Books is uncompromising. The high incidence of failures to indict, acquittals, suspended sentences and reprieves lend considerable support to the view that—

If the circumstances are so compelling that the defendant ought to violate the law, then they are compelling enough for the jury to violate their oaths. The law does well to declare these homicides unlawful. It does equally well to put no more than the sanction of an oath in the way of an acquittal.[2]

Reprinted with permission of the author and the publisher from *Minnesota Law Review,* Vol. 42, No. 6 (May 1958).

The complaint has been registered that "the prospect of a sentimental acquittal cannot be reckoned as a certainty."[3] Of course not. The defendant is not always *entitled* to a sentimental acquittal. The few American convictions cited for the proposition that the present state of affairs breeds "inequality" in application may be cited as well for the proposition that it is characterized by elasticity and flexibility. In any event, if inequality of application suffices to damn a particular provision of the criminal law, we might as well tear up all our codes—beginning with the section on chicken-stealing. . . .

The existing law on euthanasia is hardly perfect. But if it is not too good, neither, as I have suggested, is it much worse than the rest of the criminal law. At any rate, the imperfections of the existing law are not cured by Williams' proposal. Indeed, I believe adoption of his views would add more difficulties than it would remove.

Williams strongly suggests that "euthanasia can be condemned only according to a religious opinion."[4] He tends to view the opposing camps as Roman Catholics versus Liberals. Although this has a certain initial appeal to me, a non-Catholic and a self-styled liberal, I deny that this is the only way the battle lines can, or should, be drawn. I leave the religious arguments to the theologians. I share the view that "those who hold the faith may follow its precepts without requiring those who do not hold it to act as if they did."[5] But I do find substantial utilitarian obstacles on the high road to euthanasia.

As an ultimate philosophical proposition, the case for voluntary euthanasia is strong. Whatever may be said for and against suicide generally, the appeal of death is immeasurably greater when it is sought not for a poor reason or just any reason, but for "good cause," so to speak; when it is invoked not on behalf of a "socially useful" person, but on behalf of, for example, the pain-racked "hopelessly incurable" cancer victim. *If* a person is *in fact* (1) presently incurable, (2) beyond the aid of any respite which may come along in his life expectancy, suffering (3) intolerable and (4) unmitigable pain and of a (5) fixed and (6) rational desire to die, I would hate to have to argue that the hand of death should be stayed. But abstract propositions and carefully formed hypotheticals are one thing; specific proposals designed to cover everyday situations are something else again.

In essence, Williams' specific proposal is that death be authorized for a person in the above situation "by giving the medical practitioner a wide discretion and trusting to his good sense."[6] This, I submit, raises too great a risk of abuse and mistake to warrant a change in the existing law. That a proposal entails risk of mistake is hardly a conclusive reason against it. But neither is it irrelevant. Under any euthanasia program the consequences of mistake, of course, are always fatal. As I shall endeavor to show, the incidence of mistake of one kind or another is likely to be quite appreciable. If this indeed be the case, unless the need for the authorized conduct is compelling enough to override it, I take it the risk of mistake *is* a conclusive reason against such authorization. I submit too, that the possible radiations from the proposed legislation, *e.g.,* involuntary euthanasia of idiots and imbeciles (the typical "mercy-killings" reported by the press) and the emergence of the legal precedent that there are lives not "worth living," give additional cause to pause.

I see the issue, then, as the need for voluntary euthanasia versus (1) the incidence of mistake and abuse; and (2) the danger that legal machinery initially designed to kill those who are a nuisance to themselves may someday engulf those who are a nuisance to others.

The "freedom to choose a merciful death by euthanasia" may well be regarded . . . "as a special area of civil liberties". . . . The civil liberties angle is definitely a part of Professor Williams' approach:

> If the law were to remove its ban on euthanasia, the effect would merely be to leave this subject to the individual conscience. This proposal would . . . be easy to defend, as restoring personal liberty in a field in which men differ on the question of conscience. . . .
>
> On a question like this there is surely everything to be said for the liberty of the individual.[7]

I am perfectly willing to accept civil liberties as the battlefield, but issues of "liberty" and "freedom" mean little until we begin to pin down *whose* "liberty" and "freedom" and for *what* need and at *what* price. . . .

I am more concerned about the life and liberty of those who would needlessly be killed in the process or who would irrationally choose to partake of the process. Williams' price on behalf of those who are *in fact* "hopeless incurables" and *in fact* of a fixed and rational desire to die is the sacrifice of (1) some few, who, though they know it not, because their physicians know it not, need not and should not die; (2) others, probably not so few, who, though they go through the motions of "volunteering," are casualties of strain, pain or narcotics to such an extent that they really know not what they do. My price on behalf of those who, despite appearances to the contrary, have some relatively normal and reasonably useful life left in them, or who are incapable of making the choice, is the lingering on for awhile of those who, if you will, *in fact* have no desire and no reason to linger on. . . .

THE "CHOICE"

Under current proposals to establish legal machinery, elaborate or otherwise, for the administration of a quick and easy death, it is not enough that those authorized to pass on the question decide that the patient, in effect, is "better off dead." The patient must concur in this opinion. Much of the appeal in the current proposal lies in this so-called "voluntary" attribute.

But is the adult patient really in a position to concur? Is he truly able to make euthanasia a "voluntary" act? There is a good deal to be said, is there not, for Dr. Frohman's pithy comment that the "voluntary" plan is supposed to be carried out "only if the victim is both sane and crazed by pain."[8]

By hypothesis, voluntary euthanasia is not to be resorted to until narcotics have long since been administered and the patient has developed a tolerance to them. *When,* then, does the patient make the choice? While heavily drugged? Or is narcotic relief to be withdrawn for the time of decision? But if heavy dosage no longer deadens pain, indeed, no longer makes it bearable, how overwhelming is it when whatever relief narcotics offer is taken away, too?

"Hypersensitivity to pain after analgesia has worn off is nearly always noted."[9] Moreover, "the mental side-effects of narcotics, unfortunately for anyone wishing to suspend them temporarily without unduly tormenting the patient, appear to outlast the analgesic effect" and "by many hours."[10] The situation is further complicated by the fact that "a person in terminal stages of cancer who had been given morphine steadily for a matter of weeks would certainly be dependent upon it physically and would probably be addicted to it and react with the addict's response."[11]

The narcotics problem aside, Dr. Benjamin Miller, who probably has personally experienced more pain than any other commentator on the euthanasia scene, observes:

Anyone who has been severely ill knows how distorted his judgment became during the worst moments of the illness. Pain and the toxic effect of disease, or the violent reaction to certain surgical procedures may change our capacity for rational and courageous thought.[12]

If, say, a man in this plight were a criminal defendant and he were to decline the assistance of counsel would the courts hold that he had "intelligently and understandingly waived the benefit of counsel?"[13]

Undoubtedly, some euthanasia candidates will have their lucid moments. How they are to be distinguished from fellow-sufferers who do not, or how these instances are to be distinguished from others when the patient is exercising an irrational judgment is not an easy matter. Particularly is this so under Williams' proposal, where no specially qualified persons, psychiatrically trained or otherwise, are to assist in the process.

Assuming, for purposes of argument, that the occasion when a euthanasia candidate possesses a sufficiently clear mind can be ascertained and that a request for euthanasia is then made, there remain other problems. The mind of the pain-racked may occasionally be clear, but is it not also likely to be uncertain and variable? This point was pressed hard by the great physician, Lord Horder, in the House of Lords debates:

During the morning depression he [the patient] will be found to favour the application under this Bill, later in the day he will think quite differently, or will have forgotten all about it. The mental clarity with which noble Lords who present this Bill are able to think and to speak must not be thought to have any counterpart in the alternating moods and confused judgments of the sick man.[14]

The concept of "voluntary" in voluntary euthanasia would have a great deal more substance to it if, as is the case with voluntary admission statutes for the mentally ill, the patient retained the right to reverse the process within a specified number of days after he gives written notice of his desire to do so—but unfortunately this cannot be. The choice here, of course, is an irrevocable one.

The likelihood of confusion, distortion or vacillation would appear to be serious drawbacks to any voluntary plan. Moreover, Williams' proposal is particularly vulnerable in this regard, since, as he admits, by eliminating the fairly elaborate procedure of the American and English Societies' plans, he also eliminates a time period which would furnish substantial evidence of the patient's settled intention to avail himself of euthanasia.[15] But if Williams does not always choose to slug it out, he can box neatly and parry gingerly:

[T]he problem can be exaggerated. Every law has to face difficulties in application, and these difficulties are not a conclusive argument against a law if it has a beneficial operation. The measure here proposed is designed to meet the situation where the patient's consent to euthanasia is clear and incontrovertible. The physician, conscious of the need to protect himself against malicious accusations, can devise his own safeguards appropriate to the circumstances; he would normally be well advised to get the patient's consent in writing, just as is now the practice before operations. Sometimes the patient's consent will be particularly clear because he will have expressed a desire for ultimate euthanasia while he is still clear-headed and before he comes to be racked by pain; if the expression of desire is never revoked, but rather is reaffirmed under the pain, there is the best possible proof of full consent. If, on the other hand, there is no such settled frame of mind, and if the physician chooses to administer euthanasia when the patient's mind is in a variable state, he will be walking in the margin of the law and may find himself unprotected.[16]

If consent is given at a time when the patient's condition has so degenerated that he has become a fit candidate for euthanasia, when, if ever, will it be "clear and incontrovertible?" Is the suggested alternative of consent in advance a satisfactory solution? Can such a consent be deemed an informed one? Is this much different from holding a man to a prior statement of intent that if such and such an employment opportunity would present itself he would accept it, or if such and such a young woman were to come along he would marry her? Need one marshal authority for the proposition that many an "iffy" inclination is disregarded when the actual facts are at hand?

Professor Williams states that where a pre-pain desire for "ultimate euthanasia" is "reaffirmed" under pain, "there is the best possible proof of full consent." Perhaps. But what if it is alternately renounced and reaffirmed under pain? What if it is neither affirmed or renounced? What if it is only renounced? Will a physician be free to go ahead on the ground that the prior desire was "rational," but the present desire "irrational"? Under Williams' plan, will not the physician frequently "be walking in the margin of the law" —just as he is now? Do we really accomplish much more under this proposal than to put the euthanasia principle on the books?

Even if the patient's choice could be said to be "clear and incontrovertible," do not other difficulties remain? Is this the kind of choice, assuming that it can be made in a fixed and rational manner, that we want to offer a gravely ill person? Will we not sweep up, in the process, some who are not really tired of life, but think others are tired of them; some who do not really want to die, but who feel they should not live on, because to do so when there looms the legal alternative of euthanasia is to do a selfish or a cowardly act? Will not some feel an obligation to have themselves "eliminated" in order that funds allocated for their terminal care might be better used by their families, or, financial worries aside, in order to relieve their families of the emotional strain involved?

It would not be surprising for the gravely ill person to seek to inquire of those close to him whether he should avail himself of the legal alternative of euthanasia. Certainly, he is likely to wonder about their attitude in the matter. It is quite possible, is it not, that he will not exactly be gratified by any inclination on their part—however noble their motives may be in fact—that he resort to the new procedure? At this stage, the patient-family relationship may well be a good deal less than it ought to be. . . .

And what of the relatives? If their views will not always influence the patient, will they not at least influence the attending physician? Will a physician assume the risks to his reputation, if not his pocketbook, by administering the *coup de grace* over the objection—however irrational—of a close relative? Do not the relatives, then, also have a "choice?" Is not the decision on their part to do nothing and say nothing *itself* a "choice?" In many families there will be some, will there not, who will consider a stand against euthanasia the only proof of love, devotion and gratitude for past events? What of the stress and strife if close relatives differ—as they did in the famous *Sander* case—over the desirability of euthanatizing the patient?

. . .

At such a time, members of the family are not likely to be in the best state of mind, either, to make this kind of decision. Financial stress and conscious or unconscious competition for the family's estate aside:

The chronic illness and persistent pain in terminal carcinoma may place strong and excessive stresses upon the family's emotional ties with the patient. The family members who have strong emotional attachment to start with are most likely to take the patient's fears, pains and fate personally. Panic often strikes them. Whatever guilt feelings they may have toward the patient emerge to plague them.

If the patient is maintained at home, many frustrations and physical demands may be imposed on the family by the advanced illness. There may develop extreme weakness, incontinence and bad odors. The pressure of caring for the individual under these circumstances is likely to arouse a resentment and, in turn, guilt feelings on the part of those who have to do the nursing.[17]

Nor should it be overlooked that while Professor Williams would remove the various procedural steps and the various personnel contemplated in the American and English Bills and bank his all on the "good sense" of the general practitioner, no man is immune to the fear, anxieties and frustrations engendered by the apparently helpless, hopeless patient. Not even the general practitioner:

Working with a patient suffering from a malignancy causes special problems for the physician. First of all, the patient with a malignancy is most likely to engender anxiety concerning death, even in the doctor. And at the same time, this type of patient constitutes a serious threat or frustration to medical ambition. As a result, a doctor may react more emotionally and less objectively than in any other area of medical practice. . . . His deep concern may make him more pessimistic than is necessary. As a result of the feeling of frustration in his wish to help, the doctor may have moments of annoyance with the patient. He may even feel almost inclined to want to avoid this type of patient.[18]

.   .   .

Putting aside the problem of whether the good sense of the general practitioner warrants dispensing with other personnel, there still remain the problems posed by *any* voluntary euthanasia program: the aforementioned considerable pressures on the patient and his family. Are these the kind of pressures we want to inflict on any person, let alone a very sick person? Are these the kind of pressures we want to impose on any family, let alone an emotionally-shattered family? And if so, why are they not also proper considerations for the crippled, the paralyzed, the quadruple amputee, the iron lung occupant and their families?

Might it not be said of the existing ban on euthanasia, as Professor Herbert Wechsler has said of the criminal law in another connection:

It also operates, and perhaps more significantly, at anterior stages in the patterns of conduct, the dark shadow of organized disapproval eliminating from the ambit of consideration alternatives that might otherwise present themselves in the final competition of choice.[19]

THE "HOPELESSLY INCURABLE" PATIENT AND THE FALLIBLE DOCTOR

Professor Williams notes as "standard argument" the plea that "no sufferer from an apparently fatal illness should be deprived of his life because there is always the possibility that the diagnosis is wrong, or else that some remarkable cure will be discovered in time."[20]

Until the euthanasia societies of England and America had been organized and a party decision reached, shall we say, to advocate euthanasia only for incurables on their request, Dr. Abraham L. Wolbarst, one of the most ardent supporters of the movement, was less troubled about putting away "insane or defective people [who] have suffered mental incapacity and tortures of the mind for many years" than he was about the "incurables".[21] He recognized the "difficulty involved in the decision as to incurability" as one of the "doubtful aspects of euthanasia."

Doctors are only human beings, with few if any supermen among them. They make honest mistakes, like other men, because of the limitations of the human mind.[22]

He noted further that "it goes without saying that, in recently developed cases with a possibility of cure, euthanasia should not even be considered," that "the law might establish a limit of, say, ten years in which there is a chance of the patient's recovery."[23]

Dr. Benjamin Miller [has a more personal interest in the problem of euthanasia.] He himself was left to die the death of a "hopeless" tuberculosis victim only to discover that he was suffering from a rare malady which affects the lungs in much the same manner but seldom kills. Five years and sixteen hospitalizations later, Dr. Miller dramatized his point by recalling the last diagnostic clinic of the brilliant Richard Cabot, on the occasion of his official retirement:

He was given the case records [complete medical histories and results of careful examinations] of two patients and asked to diagnose their illnesses. . . . The patients had died and only the hospital pathologist knew the exact diagnosis beyond doubt, for he had seen the descriptions of the postmortem findings. Dr. Cabot, usually very accurate in his diagnosis, that day missed both.

The chief pathologist who had selected the cases was a wise person. He had purposely chosen two of the most deceptive to remind the medical students and young physicians that even at the end of a long and rich experience one of the greatest diagnosticians of our time was still not infallible.[24]

Richard Cabot was the John W. Davis, the John Lord O'Brian, of his profession. When one reads the account of his last clinic, one cannot help but think of how fallible the *average* general practitioner must be, how fallible the *young doctor just starting practice* must be —and this, of course, is all that some small communities have in the way of medical care— how fallible the *worst* practitioner, young or old, must be. If the range of skill and judgment among licensed physicians approaches the wide gap between the very best and the very worst members of the bar—and I have no reason to think it does not—then the minimally competent physician is hardly the man to be given the responsibility for ending another's life. Yet, under Williams' proposal at least, the marginal physician, as well as his more distinguished brethren, would have legal authorization to make just such decisions. Under Williams' proposal, euthanatizing a patient or two would all be part of the routine day's work.

. . .

Faulty diagnosis is only one ground for error. Even if the diagnosis is correct, a second ground for error lies in the possibility that some measure of relief, if not a full cure, may come to the fore within the life expectancy of the patient. Since Glanville Williams does not deign this objection to euthanasia worth more than a passing reference,[25] it is necessary to turn elsewhere to ascertain how it has been met.

One answer is:

It must be little comfort to a man slowly coming apart from multiple sclerosis to think that, fifteen years from now, death might not be his only hope.[26]

To state the problem this way is of course, to avoid it entirely. How do we know that fifteen *days* or fifteen *hours* from now, "death might not be [the incurable's] only hope?"

A second answer is:

[N]o cure for cancer which might be found 'tomorrow' would be of any value to a man or women 'so far advanced in cancerous toxemia as to be an applicant for euthanasia'.[27]

As I shall endeavor to show, this approach is a good deal easier to formulate than it is to apply. For one thing, it presumes that we know today *what* cures will be found tomorrow. For another, it overlooks that if such cases can be said to exist, the patient is likely to be *so far* advanced in cancerous toxemia as to be no longer capable of understanding the step he is taking and hence *beyond* the stage when euthanasia ought to be administered.

A generation ago, Dr. Haven Emerson, then President of the American Public Health Association, made the point that "no one can say today what will be incurable tomorrow. No one can predict what disease will be fatal or permanently incurable until medicine becomes stationary and sterile." Dr. Emerson went so far as to say that "to be at all accurate we must drop altogether the term 'incurables' and substitute for it some such term as 'chronic illness'."[28]

That was a generation ago. Dr. Emerson did not have to go back more than a decade to document his contention. Before Banting and

Best's insulin discovery, many a diabetic had been doomed. Before the Whipple-Minot-Murphy liver treatment made it a relatively minor malady, many a pernicious anemia sufferer had been branded "hopeless." Before the uses of sulfanilimide were disclosed, a patient with widespread streptococcal blood poisoning was a condemned man.[29]

Today, we may take even that most resolute disease, cancer, and we need look back no further than the last decade of research in this field to document the same contention.

. . .

True, many types of cancer still run their course virtually unhampered by man's arduous efforts to inhibit them. But the number of cancers coming under some control is ever increasing. With medicine attacking on so many fronts with so many weapons who would bet a man's life on when and how the next type of cancer will yield, if only just a bit?

. . .

VOLUNTARY V. INVOLUNTARY EUTHANASIA

Ever since the 1870s, when what was probably the first euthanasia debate of the modern era took place, most proponents of the movement—at least when they are pressed—have taken considerable pains to restrict the question to the plight of the unbearably suffering incurable who *voluntarily seeks* death while most of their opponents have striven equally hard to frame the issue in terms which would encompass certain involuntary situations as well, *e.g.*, the "congenital idiots," the "permanently insane," and the senile.

Glanville Williams reflects the outward mood of many euthanasiasts when he scores those who insist on considering the question from a broader angle:

The [English Society's] bill [debated in the House of Lords in 1936 and 1950] excluded any question of compulsory euthanasia, even for hopelessly defective infants. Unfortunately, a legislative proposal is not assured of success merely because it is worded

in a studiously moderate and restrictive form. The method of attack, by those who dislike the proposal, is to use the 'thin edge of the wedge' argument. . . . There is no proposal for reform on any topic, however conciliatory and moderate, that cannot be opposed by this dialectic.[30]

Why was the bill "worded in a studiously moderate and restrictive form?" If it were done as a matter of principle, if it were done in recognition of the ethico-moral-legal "wall of separation" which stands between voluntary and compulsory "mercy-killings," much can be said for the euthanasiasts' lament about the methods employed by the opposition. But if it were done as a matter of political expediency—with great hopes and expectations of pushing through a second and somewhat less restrictive bill as soon as the first one had sufficiently "educated" public opinion and next a third still less restrictive bill—what standing do the euthanasiasts then have to attack the methods of the opposition? No cry of righteous indignation could ring more hollow, I would think, than the protest from those utilizing the "wedge" principle themselves that their opponents are making the wedge objection.

. . .

The boldness and daring which characterizes most of Glanville Williams' book dims perceptibly when he comes to involuntary euthanasia proposals. As to the senile, he states:

At present the problem has certainly not reached the degree of seriousness that would warrant an effort being made to change traditional attitudes toward the sanctity of life of the aged. Only the grimmest necessity could bring about a change that, however cautious in its approach, would probably cause apprehension and deep distress to many people, and inflict a traumatic injury upon the accepted code of behaviour built up by two thousand years of the Christian religion. It may be however, that as the problem becomes more acute it will itself cause a reversal of generally accepted values.[31]

To me, this passage is the most startling one in the book. On page 348 Williams invokes "traditional attitudes towards the sanctity of life" and "the accepted code of behaviour built up by two thousand years of the Christian religion'' to check the extension of euthanasia to the senile, but for 347 pages he had been merrily rolling along debunking both. Substitute ''cancer victim'' for ''the aged'' and Williams' passage is essentially the argument of many of his *opponents* on the voluntary euthanasia question.

The unsupported comment that ''the problem [of senility] has certainly not reached the degree of seriousness'' to warrant euthanasia is also rather puzzling, particularly coming as it does after an observation by Williams on the immediately preceding page that ''it is increasingly common for men and women to reach an age of 'second childishness and mere oblivion,' with a loss of almost all adult faculties except that of digestion.''[32]

How ''serious'' does a problem have to be to warrant a change in these ''traditional attitudes''? If, as the statement seems to indicate, ''seriousness'' of a problem is to be determined numerically, the problem of the cancer victim does not appear to be as substantial as the problem of the senile. For example, taking just the 95,837 first admissions to ''public prolonged-care hospitals'' for mental diseases in the United States in 1955, 23,561—or one fourth—were cerebral arteriosclerosis or senile brain disease cases.[33] I am not at all sure that there are 20,000 cancer victims per year who die *unbearably painful* deaths. Even if there were, I cannot believe that among their ranks are some 20,000 per year who, when still in a rational state, so long for a quick and easy death that they would avail themselves of legal machinery for euthanasia.

If the problem of the incurable cancer victim ''has reached the degree of seriousness that would warrant an effort being made to change traditional attitudes toward the sanctity of life,'' as Williams obviously thinks it has, then so has the problem of senility. In any event, the senility problem will undoubtedly soon reach even Williams' requisite degree of seriousness:

A decision concerning the senile may have to be taken within the next twenty years. The number of old people are increasing by leaps and bounds. Pneumonia, 'the old man's friend' is now checked by antibiotics. The effects of hardship, exposure, starvation and accident are now minimized. Where is this leading us? . . . What of the drooling, helpless, disorientated old man or the doubly incontinent old woman lying log-like in bed? Is it here that the real need for euthanasia exists?[34]

If, as Williams indicates, ''seriousness'' of the problem is a major criterion for euthanatizing a category of unfortunates, the sum total of mentally deficient persons would appear to warrant high priority, indeed.

When Williams turns to the plight of the ''hopelessly defective infants,'' his characteristic vim and vigor are, as in the senility discussion, conspicuously absent:

While the Euthanasia Society of England has never advocated this, the Euthanasia Society of America did include it in its original program. The proposal certainly escapes the chief objection to the similar proposal for senile dementia: it does not create a sense of insecurity in society, because infants cannot, like adults, feel anticipatory dread of being done to death if their condition should worsen. Moreover, the proposal receives some support on eugenic grounds, and more importantly on humanitarian grounds—both on account of the parents, to whom the child will be a burden all their lives, and on account of the handicapped child itself. (It is not, however, proposed that any child should be destroyed against the wishes of its parents.) Finally, the legalization of euthanasia for handicapped children would bring the law into closer relation to its practical administration, because juries do not regard parental mercy-killing as murder. For these various reasons the proposal to legalize humanitarian infanticide is put forward from time to time by individuals. They remain in a very small minority, and the proposal may at present be dismissed as politically insignificant.[35]

It is understandable for a reformer to limit his present proposals for change to those with a real prospect of success. But it is hardly reassuring for Williams to cite the fact that only ''a very small minority'' has urged euthanasia for ''hopelessly defective infants'' as the *only* reason for not pressing for such legislation now. If, as Williams sees it, the only advantage voluntary euthanasia has over the involuntary variety lies in the organized movements on its behalf, that advantage can readily be wiped out.

In any event, I do not think that such "a very small minority" has advocated "humanitarian infanticide." Until the organization of the English and American societies led to a concentration on the voluntary type, and until the by-products of the Nazi euthanasia program somewhat embarrassed, if only temporarily, most proponents of involuntary euthanasia, about as many writers urged one type as another. Indeed, some euthanasiasts have taken considerable pains to demonstrate the superiority of defective infant euthanasia over incurably ill euthanasia.

As for dismissing euthanasia of defective infants as "politically insignificant," the only poll that I know of which measured the public response to both types of euthanasia revealed that *45 percent favored euthanasia for defective infants under certain conditions while only 37.3 percent approved euthanasia for the incurably and painfully ill under any conditions.*[36] Furthermore, of those who favored the mercy killing cure for incurable adults, some 40 percent would require only family permission or medical board approval, but not the patient's permission.[37]

Nor do I think it irrelevant that while public resistance caused Hitler to yield on the adult euthanasia front, the killing of malformed and idiot children continued unhindered to the end of the war, the definition of "children" expanding all the while.[38] Is it the embarrassing experience of the Nazi euthanasia program which has rendered destruction of defective infants presently "politically insignificant"? If so, is it any more of a jump from the incurably and painfully ill to the unorthodox political thinker than it is from the hopelessly defective infant to the same "unsavory character?" Or is it not so much that the euthanasiasts are troubled by the Nazi experience as it is that they are troubled that the public is troubled by the Nazi experience?

I read Williams' comments on defective infants [as arguments] for the proposition that there are some very good reasons for euthanatizing defective infants, but the time is not yet ripe. When will it be? When will the proposal become politically significant? After a voluntary euthanasia law is on the books and public opinion is sufficiently "educated?"

Williams' reasons for not extending euthanasia—once we legalize it in the narrow "voluntary" area—to the senile and the defective are much less forceful and much less persuasive than his arguments for legalizing voluntary euthanasia in the first place. I regard this as another reason for not legalizing voluntary euthanasia in the first place.

. . .

A FINAL REFLECTION

There have been and there will continue to be compelling circumstances when a doctor or relative or friend will violate The Law On The Books and, more often than not, receive protection from The Law In Action. But this is not to deny that there are other occasions when The Law On The Books operates to stay the hand of all concerned, among them situations where the patient is in fact (1) presently incurable, (2) beyond the aid of any respite which may come along in his life expectancy, suffering (3) intolerable and (4) unmitigable pain and of a (5) fixed and (6) rational desire to die. That any euthanasia program may only be the opening wedge for far more objectionable practices, and that even within the bounds of a "voluntary" plan such as Williams' the incidence of mistake or abuse is likely to be substantial, are not much solace to one in the above plight.

It may be conceded that in a narrow sense it is an "evil" for such a patient to have to continue to suffer—if only for a little while. But in a narrow sense, long-term sentences and capital punishment are "evils," too.[39] If we can justify the infliction of imprisonment and death by the state "on the ground of the social interests to be protected"[40] then surely we can similarly justify the postponement of death by the state. The objection that the individual is thereby treated not as an "end" in himself but only as a "means" to futher the common good was, I think, aptly disposed of by Holmes long ago. "If a man lives in society, he is likely to find himself so treated."[41]

NOTES

1. In Anglo-American jurisprudence a "mercy-killing" is murder. In theory, neither good motive nor consent of the victim is relevant. See, *e.g.,* 2 Burdick, Law of Crimes §§ 422, 447 (1946); Miller, Criminal Law 55, 172 (1934); Perkins, Criminal Law 721 (1957); 1 Wharton, Criminal Law and Procedure § 194 (Anderson 1957); Orth, *Legal Aspects Relating to Euthanasia,* 2 Md. Med. J. 120 (1953) (symposium on euthanasia); 48 Mich. L. Rev. 1199 (1950); Anno., 25 A.L.R. 1007 (1923).

In a number of countries, *e.g.,* Germany, Norway, Switzerland, a compassionate motive and/or "homicide upon request" operate to reduce the penalty. See generally Helen Silving's valuable comparative study, *supra* note 7 [in original text]. However, apparently only Uruguayan law completely immunizes a homicide characterized by both of the above factors. *Id.* at 369 and n. 21. The Silving article only contains an interesting and fairly extensive comparative study of assisted suicide and the degree to which it is treated differently from a direct "mercy-killing." In this regard see also Friedman, *Suicide, Euthanasia and the Law,* 85 Med. Times 681 (1957).

2. Curtis, It's Your Law 95 (1954).

3. Williams, *The Sanctity of Life and the Criminal Law* (1957), p. 328.

4. *Id.* at 312.

5. Wechsler and Michael, *A Rationale of the Law of Homicide: I,* 37 Columbia L. Rev. 740 (1937).

6. Williams, p. 339.

7. *Id.* at 341, 346.

8. Frohman, *Vexing Problems In Forensic Medicine: A Physician's View,* 31 N.Y.U.L. Rev. 1215, 1222 (1956).

9. Goodman and Gilman, The Pharmacological Basis of Therapeutics 235 (2d ed. 1955).

10. Sharpe, *Medication As A Threat To Testamentary Capacity,* 35 N.C.L. Rev. 380, 392 (1957) and medical authorities cited therein.

11. *Id.* at 384.

12. Miller, *Why I Oppose Mercy Killings,* Woman's Home Companion, June 1950, pp. 38, 103.

13. Moore v. Michigan, 355 U.S. 155, 161 (1957).

14. 103 House of Lords Debates (5th ser.) 466, 492–93 (1936).

15. Williams, pp. 343–44.

16. *Id.* at 344.

17. Zarling, *Psychological Aspects of Pain in Terminal Malignancies,* in Management of Pain in Cancer, 211–12 (Schiffrin, ed., 1956).

18. *Id.* at 213–14.

19. Wechsler, *The Issues of the Nuremberg Trial,* 62 Pol. Sci. Q. 11, 16 (1947).

20. Williams, p. 318.

21. Wolbarst, *Legalize Euthanasia!,* 94 The Forum 330, 332 (1935). *But see* Wolbarst, *The Doctor Looks at Euthanasia,* 149 Medical Record, 354 (1939).

22. Wolbarst, *Legalize Euthanasia!,* 94 The Forum 330, 331 (1935).

23. *Id.* at 332.

24. Miller, *supra* note 12, at 39.

25. See Williams, p. 318.

26. *Pro & Con: Shall We Legalize "Mercy Killing"?,* Readers Digest, Nov. 1938, pp. 94, 96.

27. James, *Euthanasia–Right or Wrong?,* Survey Graphic, May, 1948, pp. 241, 243; Wolbarst, *The Doctor Looks at Euthanasia,* 149 Medical Record, 354, 355 (1939).

28. Emerson, *Who Is Incurable? A Query and Reply,* N.Y. Times, Oct. 22, 1933, § 8, p. 5, col. 1.

29. *Ibid.,* Miller, *supra* note 12, at 39.

30. Williams, pp. 333–34.

31. Williams, p. 348.

32. *Id.* at 347.

33. U.S. Dep't of Health, Education and Welfare, Patients in Mental Institutions 1955, Part II, Public Hospital for the Mentally Ill 21. Some 13,972 were cerebral arteriosclerosis cases; 9,589 had senile brain diseases.

34. Banks, *Euthanasia,* 26 Bull. N.Y. Acad. Med. 297, 305 (1950).

35. Williams, pp. 349–50.

36. *The Fortune Quarterly Survey:* IX, Fortune, July 1937, pp. 96, 106.

37. *The Fortune Quarterly Survey,* note 36, *supra,* at 106.

38. Mitscherlich and Mielke, Doctors of Infamy 114 (1949).

39. Perhaps this would not be true if the only purpose of punishment was to reform the criminal. But whatever *ought to be* the case, this obviously *is not.* "If it were, every prisoner should be released as soon as it appears clear that he will never repeat his offence, and if he is incurable he should not be punished at all." Holmes, The Common Law 42 (1881).

40. Michael and Adler, Crime, Law and Social Science 351 (1933).

41. Holmes, The Common Law 44 (1881).

GLANVILLE WILLIAMS

"Mercy-killing" Legislation—A Rejoinder

I welcome Professor Kamisar's reply to my argument for voluntary euthanasia, because it is on the whole a careful, scholarly work, keeping to knowable facts and accepted human values. It is, therefore, the sort of reply that can be rationally considered and dealt with. In this short rejoinder I shall accept most of Professor Kamisar's valuable footnotes, and merely submit that they do not bear out his conclusion.

The argument in favour of voluntary euthanasia in the terminal stages of painful diseases is quite a simple one, and is an application of two values that are widely recognised. The first value is the prevention of cruelty. Much as men differ in their ethical assessments, all agree that cruelty is an evil—the only difference of opinion residing in what is meant by cruelty. Those who plead for the legalization of euthanasia think that it is cruel to allow a human being to linger for months in the last stages of agony, weakness and decay, and to refuse him his demand for merciful release. There is also a second cruelty involved —not perhaps quite so compelling, but still worth consideration: the agony of the relatives in seeing their loved one in his desperate plight. Opponents of euthanasia are apt to take a cynical view of the desires of relatives, and this may sometimes be justified. But it cannot be denied that a wife who has to nurse her husband through the last stages of some terrible disease may herself be so deeply affected by the experience that her health is ruined, either mentally or physically. Whether the situation can be eased for such a person by voluntary euthanasia I do not know; probably it depends very much on the individuals concerned, which is as much as to say that no solution in terms of a general regulatory law can be satisfactory. The conclusion should be in favour of individual discretion.

The second value involved is that of liberty. The criminal law should not be invoked to repress conduct unless this is demonstrably necessary on social grounds. What social interest is there in preventing the sufferer from choosing to accelerate his death by a few months? What positive value does his life still possess for society, that he is to be retained in it by the terrors of the criminal law?

And, of course, the liberty involved is that of the doctor as well as that of the patient. It is the doctor's responsibility to do all he can to prolong worth-while life, or, in the last resort, to ease his patient's passage. If the doctor honestly and sincerely believes that the best service he can perform for his suffering patient is to accede to his request for euthanasia, it is a grave thing that the law should forbid him to do so.

This is the short and simple case for voluntary euthanasia, and, as Kamisar admits, it cannot be attacked directly on utilitarian grounds. Such an attack can only be by finding possible evils of an indirect nature. These evils, in the view of Professor Kamisar, are (1) the difficulty of ascertaining consent, and arising out of that the danger of abuse; (2) the risk of an incorrect diagnosis; (3) the risk of administering euthanasia to a person who could later have been cured by developments in medical knowledge; (4) the "wedge" argument.

Before considering these matters, one preliminary comment may be made. In some parts of his Article Kamisar hints at recognition of the fact that a practice of mercy-killing exists among the most reputable of medical practitioners. Some of the evidence for this will be found in my book.[1] In the first debate in the House of Lords, Lord Dawson admitted the fact, and claimed that it did away with the need

Reprinted with permission of the author and the publisher from *Minnesota Law Review,* Vol. 43, No. 1 (1958).

1. The Sanctity of Life and the Criminal Law 334–39 (1957).

for legislation. In other words, the attitude of conservatives is this: let medical men do mercy-killing, but let it continue to be called murder, and be treated as such if the legal machinery is by some unlucky mischance made to work; let us, in other words, take no steps to translate the new morality into the concepts of the law. I find this attitude equally incomprehensible in a doctor, as Lord Dawson was, and in a lawyer, as Professor Kamisar is. Still more baffling does it become when Professor Kamisar seems to claim as a virtue of the system that the jury can give a merciful acquittal in breach of their oaths. The result is that the law frightens some doctors from interposing, while not frightening others—though subjecting the braver group to the risk of prosecution and possible loss of liberty and livelihood. Apparently, in Kamisar's view, it is a good thing if the law is broken in a proper case, because that relieves suffering, but also a good thing that the law is there as a threat in order to prevent too much mercy being administered; thus, whichever result the law has is perfectly right and proper. It is hard to understand on what moral principle this type of ethical ambivalence is to be maintained. If Kamisar does approve of doctors administering euthanasia in some clear cases, and of juries acquitting them if they are prosecuted for murder, how does he maintain that it is an insuperable objection to euthanasia that diagnosis may be wrong and medical knowledge subsequently extended?

However, the references to merciful acquittals disappear after the first few pages of the Article, and thenceforward the argument develops as a straight attack on euthanasia. So although at the beginning Kamisar says that he would hate to have to argue against mercy-killing in a clear case, in fact he does proceed to argue against it with some zest.

·   ·   ·

Kamisar's first objection, under the heading of ''The Choice,'' is that there can be no such thing as truly voluntary euthanasia in painful and killing diseases. He seeks to impale the advocates of euthanasia on an old dilemma. Either the victim is not yet suffering pain, in which case his consent is merely an uninformed and anticipatory one—and he cannot bind himself by contract to be killed in the future—or he is crazed by pain and stupified by drugs, in which case he is not of sound mind. I have dealt with this problem in my book; Kamisar has quoted generously from it, and I leave the reader to decide. As I understand Kamisar's position, he does not really persist in the objection. With the laconic ''Perhaps,'' he seems to grant me, though unwillingly, that there are cases where one can be sure of the patient's consent. But having thus abandoned his own point, he then goes off to a different horror, that the patient may give his consent only in order to relieve his relatives of the trouble of looking after him.

On this new issue, I will return Kamisar the compliment and say: ''Perhaps.'' We are certainly in an area where no solution is going to make things quite easy and happy for everybody, and all sorts of embarrassments may be conjectured. But these embarrassments are not avoided by keeping to the present law: we suffer from them already. If a patient, suffering pain in a terminal illness, wishes for euthanasia partly because of this pain and partly because he sees his beloved ones breaking under the strain of caring for him, I do not see how this decision on his part, agonizing though it may be, is necessarily a matter of discredit either to the patient himself or to his relatives. The fact is that, whether we are considering the patient or his relatives, there are limits to human endurance.

The author's next objection rests on the possibility of mistaken diagnosis. . . . I agree with him that, before deciding on euthanasia in any particular case, the risk of mistaken diagnosis would have to be considered. Everything that is said in the Article would, therefore, be most relevant when the two doctors whom I propose in my suggested measure come to consult on the question of euthanasia; and the possibility of mistake might most forcefully be brought before the patient himself. But have these medical questions any real relevance to the legal discussion?

Kamisar, I take it, notwithstanding his wide reading in medical literature, is by training a lawyer. He has consulted much medical opinion in order to find arguments against changing the law. I ought not to object to this, since I have consulted the same opinion for the opposite purpose. But what we may well ask ourselves is this: is it not a trifle bizarre that we should be doing it at all? Our profession is the law, not medicine; how does it come about that lawyers have to examine medical literature to assess the advantages and disadvantages of a medical practice?

If the import of this question is not immediately clear, let me return to my imaginary State of Ruritania. Many years ago, in Ruritania as elsewhere, surgical operations were attended with great risk. Pasteur had not made his discoveries, and surgeons killed as often as they cured. In this state of things, the legislature of Ruritania passed a law declaring all surgical operations to be unlawful in principle, but providing that each specific type of operation might be legalized by a statute specially passed for the purpose. The result is that, in Ruritania, as expert medical opinion sees the possibility of some new medical advance, a pressure group has to be formed in order to obtain legislative approval for it. Since there is little public interest in these technical questions, and since, moreover, surgical operations are thought in general to be inimical to the established religion, the pressure group has to work for many years before it gets a hearing. When at last a proposal for legalization is seriously mooted, the lawyers and politicians get to work upon it, considering what possible dangers are inherent in the new operation. Lawyers and politicians are careful people, and they are perhaps more prone to see the dangers than the advantages in a new departure. Naturally they find allies among some of the more timid or traditional or less knowledgeable members of the medical profession, as well as among the priesthood and the faithful. Thus it is small wonder that whereas appendicectomy has been practised in civilised countries since the beginning of the present century, a proposal to

legalize it has still not passed the legislative assembly of Ruritania.

It must be confessed that on this particular matter the legal prohibition has not been an unmixed evil for the Ruritanians. During the great popularity of the appendix operation in much of the civilised world during the twenties and thirties of this century, large numbers of these organs were removed without adequate cause, and the citizens of Ruritania have been spared this inconvenience. On the other hand, many citizens of that country have died of appendicitis, who would have been saved if they had lived elsewhere. And whereas in other countries the medical profession has now learned enough to be able to perform this operation with wisdom and restraint, in Ruritania it is still not being performed at all. Moreover, the law has destroyed scientific inventiveness in that country in the forbidden fields.

Now, in the United States and England we have no such absurd general law on the subject of surgical operations as they have in Ruritania. In principle, medical men are left free to exercise their best judgment, and the result has been a brilliant advance in knowledge and technique. But there are just two—or possibly three—operations which are subject to the Ruritanian principle. These are abortion, euthanasia, and possibly sterilization of convenience. In these fields we, too, must have pressure groups, with lawyers and politicians warning us of the possibility of inexpert practitioners and mistaken diagnosis, and canvassing medical opinion on the risk of an operation not yielding the expected results in terms of human happiness and the health of the body politic. In these fields we, too, are forbidden to experiment to see if the foretold dangers actually come to pass. Instead of that, we are required to make a social judgment on the probabilities of good and evil before the medical profession is allowed to start on its empirical tests.

This anomaly is perhaps more obvious with abortion than it is with euthanasia. Indeed, I am prepared for ridicule when I describe euthanasia as a medical operation. Regarded as surgery it is unique, since its object is not to save or prolong life but the reverse. But euthanasia has another object which it shares with many surgical operations—the saving of pain. And it is now widely recognised, as Lord Dawson said in the debate in the House of Lords, that the saving of pain is a legitimate aim of medical practice. The question whether euthanasia will effect a net saving of pain and distress is, perhaps, one that can be only finally answered by trying it. But it is obscurantist to forbid the experiment on the ground that until it is performed we cannot certainly know its results. Such an attitude, in any other field of medical endeavor, would have inhibited progress.

The argument based on mistaken diagnosis leads into the argument based on the possibility of dramatic medical discoveries. Of course, a new medical discovery which gives the opportunity of remission or cure will almost at once put an end to mercy-killings in the particular group of cases for which the discovery is made. On the other hand, the discovery cannot affect patients who have already died from their disease. The argument based on mistaken diagnosis is therefore concerned only with those patients who have been mercifully killed just before the discovery becomes available for use. The argument is that such persons may turn out to have been ''mercy–killed'' unnecessarily, because if the physician had waited a bit longer they would have been cured. Because of this risk for this tiny fraction of the total number of patients, patients who are dying in pain must be left to do so, year after year, against their entreaty to have it ended.

Just how real is the risk? When a new medical discovery is claimed, some time commonly elapses before it becomes tested sufficiently to justify large-scale production of the drug, or training in the techniques involved. This is a warning period when euthanasia in the particular class of case would probably be halted anyway. Thus it is quite probable that when the new discovery becomes available, the euthanasia process would not in fact show any mistakes in this regard.

Kamisar says that in my book I ''did not deign this objection to euthanasia more than a passing reference.'' I still do not think it is worth any more than that.

The author advances the familiar but hardly convincing argument that the quantitative need for euthanasia is not large. As one reason for this argument, he suggests that not many patients would wish to benefit from euthanasia, even if it were allowed. I am not impressed by the argument. It may be true, but it is irrelevant. So long as there are *any* persons dying in weakness and grief who are refused their request for a speeding of their end, the argument for legalizing euthanasia remains. Next, the Article suggests that there is no great need for euthanasia because of the advances made with pain-killing drugs. . . . In my book, recognising that medical science does manage to save many dying patients from the extreme of physical pain, I pointed out that it often fails to save them from an artificial, twilight existence, with nausea, giddiness, and extreme restlessness, as well as the long hours of consciousness of a hopeless condition. A dear friend of mine, who died of cancer of the bowel, spent his last months in just this state, under the influence of morphine, which deadened pain, but vomiting incessantly, day in and day out. The question that we have to face is whether the unintelligent brutality of such an existence is to be imposed on one who wished to end it.

. . .

The last part of the Article is devoted to the ancient ''wedge'' argument which I have already examined in my book. It is the trump card of the traditionalist, because no proposal for reform, however strong the arguments in favour, is immune from the wedge objection. In fact, the stronger the arguments in favour of a reform, the more likely it is that the traditionalist will take the wedge objection—it is then the only one he has. C. M. Cornford put the argument in its proper place when he said that the wedge objection means this, that you should not act justly today, for fear that you may be asked to act still more justly tomorrow.

We heard a great deal of this type of argument in England in the nineteenth century, when it was used to resist almost every social and economic change. In the present century we have had less of it, but (if I may claim the hospitality of these columns to say so) it seems still to be accorded an exaggerated importance in American thought. When lecturing on the law of torts in an American university a few years ago, I suggested that just as compulsory liability insurance for automobiles had spread practically through the civilised world, so we should in time see the law of tort superseded in this field by a system of state insurance for traffic accidents, administered independently of proof of fault. The suggestion was immediately met by one student with a horrified reference to "creeping socialism." That is the standard objection made by many people to any proposal for a new department of state activity. The implication is that you must resist every proposal, however admirable in itself, because otherwise you will never be able to draw the line. On the particular question of socialism, the fear is belied by the experience of a number of countries which have extended state control of the economy without going the whole way to socialistic state regimentation.

Kamisar's particular bogey, the racial laws of Nazi Germany, is an effective one in the democratic countries. Any reference to the Nazis is a powerful weapon to prevent change in the traditional taboo on sterilization as well as euthanasia. The case of sterilization is particularly interesting on this; I dealt with it at length in my book, though Kamisar does not mention its bearing on the argument. When proposals are made for promoting voluntary sterilization on eugenic and other grounds, they are immediately condemned by most people as the thin end of a wedge leading to involuntary sterilization; and then they point to the practices of the Nazis. Yet a more persuasive argument pointing in the other direction can easily be found. Several American states have sterilization laws, which for the most part were originally drafted in very wide terms, to cover desexualisation as well as sterilization, and authorizing involuntary as well as voluntary operations. This legislation goes back long before the Nazis; the earliest statute

was in Indiana in 1907. What has been its practical effect? In several states it has hardly been used. A few have used it, but in practice they have progressively restricted it until now it is virtually confined to voluntary sterilization. This is so, at least, in North Carolina, as Mrs. Woodside's study strikingly shows. In my book I summed up the position as follows:

The American experience is of great interest because it shows how remote from reality in a democratic community is the fear—frequently voiced by Americans themselves—that voluntary sterilization may be the 'thin end of the wedge,' leading to a large-scale violation of human rights as happened in Nazi Germany. In fact, the American experience is the precise opposite—starting with compulsory sterilization, administrative practice has come to put the operation on a voluntary footing.

But it is insufficient to answer the "wedge" objection in general terms; we must consider the particular fears to which it gives rise. Kamisar professes to fear certain other measures that the Euthanasia societies may bring up if their present measure is conceded to them. Surely, these other measures, if any, will be debated on their merits? Does he seriously fear that anyone in the United States is going to propose the extermination of people of a minority race or religion? Let us put aside such ridiculous fancies and discuss practical politics.

The author is quite right in thinking that a body of opinion would favour the legalization of the involuntary euthanasia of hopelessly defective infants, and some day a proposal of this kind may be put forward. The proposal would have distinct limits, just as the proposal for voluntary euthanasia of incurable sufferers has limits. I do not think that any responsible body of opinion would now propose the euthanasia of insane adults, for the perfectly clear reason that any such practice would greatly increase the sense of insecurity felt by the borderline insane and by the large number of insane persons who have sufficient understanding on this particular matter.

Kamisar expresses distress at a concluding remark in my book in which I advert to the possibility of old people becoming an overwhelming burden on mankind. I share his feeling that there are profoundly disturbing possibilities here; and if I had been merely a propagandist, intent upon securing agreement for a specific measure of law reform, I should have done wisely to have omitted all reference to this subject. Since, however, I am merely an academic writer, trying to bring such intelligence as I have to bear on moral and social issues, I deemed the topic too important and threatening to leave without a word. I think I have made it clear, in the passages cited, that I am not for one moment proposing any euthanasia of the aged in present society; such an idea would shock me as much as it shocks Kamisar and would shock everybody else. Still, the fact that we may one day have to face is that medical science is more successful in preserving the body than in preserving the mind. It is not impossible that, in the foreseeable future, medical men will be able to preserve the mindless body until the age, say, of 1000, while the mind itself will have lasted only a tenth of that time. What will mankind do then? It is hardly possible to imagine that we shall establish huge hospital-mausolea where the aged are kept in a kind of living death. Even if it is desired to do this, the cost of the undertaking may make it impossible.

This is not an immediately practical problem, and we need not yet face it. The problem of maintaining persons afflicted with senile dementia is well within our economic resources as the matter stands at present. Perhaps some barrier will be found to medical advance which will prevent the problem becoming more acute. Perhaps, as time goes on, and as the alternatives become more clearly realised, men will become more resigned to human control over the mode of termination of life. Or the solution may be that after the individual has reached a certain age, or a certain degree of decay, medical science will hold its hand, and allow him to be carried off by natural causes. But what if these natural causes are themselves painful? Would it not be better kindness to substitute human agency?

In general, it is enough to say that we do not have to know the solutions to these problems. The only doubtful moral question on which we have to make an immediate decision in relation to involuntary euthanasia is whether we owe a moral duty to terminate the life of an insane person who is suffering from a painful and incurable disease. Such a person is left unprovided for under the legislative proposal formulated in my book. The objection to any system of involuntary euthanasia of the insane is that it may cause a sense of insecurity. It is because I think that the risk of this fear is a serious one that a proposal for the reform of the law must leave the insane out.

RAYMOND S. DUFF
AND A. G. M. CAMPBELL

Moral and Ethical Dilemmas in the Special-Care Nursery

Between 1940 and 1970 there was a fifty-eight per cent decrease in the infant death rate in the United States.[1] This reduction was related in part to the application of new knowledge to the care of infants. Neonatal mortality rates in hospitals having infant intensive-care units have been about one-half those reported in hospitals without such units.[2] There is now evidence that in many conditions of early infancy the long-term morbidity may also be reduced.[3] Survivors of these units may be healthy, and their parents grateful, but some infants continue to suffer from such conditions as chronic cardiopulmonary disease, short-bowel-syndrome or various manifestations of brain damage; others are severely handicapped by a myriad of congenital malformations that in previous times would have resulted in early death. Recently, both lay and professional persons have expressed increasing concern about the quality of life for these severely impaired survivors and their families.[4,5] Many pediatricians and others are distressed with the long-term results of pressing on and on to save life at all costs and in all circumstances. Eliot Slater[6] stated, "If this is one of the consequences of the sanctity-of-life ethic, perhaps our formulation of the principle should be revised."

The experiences described in this communication document some of the grave moral and ethical dilemmas now faced by physicians and families. They indicate some of the problems in a large special-care nursery where medical technology has prolonged life and where

Reprinted with permission from *The New England Journal of Medicine,* Vol. 289, No. 25 (Oct. 25, 1973), pp. 890–894.

"informed" parents influence the management decisions concerning their infants.

BACKGROUND AND METHODS

The special-care nursery of the Yale-New Haven Hospital not only serves an obstetric service for over 4000 live births annually but also acts as the principal referral center in Connecticut for infants with major problems of the newborn period. From January 1, 1970, through June 30, 1972, 1615 infants born at the Hospital were admitted, and 556 others were transferred for specialized care from community hospitals. During this interval, the average daily census was 26, with a range of 14 to 37.

For some years the unit has had a liberal policy for parental visiting, with the staff placing particular emphasis on helping parents adjust to and participate in the care of their infants with special problems. By encouraging visiting, attempting to create a relaxed atmosphere within the unit, exploring carefully the special needs of the infants, and familiarizing parents with various aspects of care, it was hoped to remove much of the apprehension—indeed, fear—with which parents at first view an intensive-care nursery.[7] At any time, parents may see and handle their babies. They commonly observe or participate in most routine aspects of care and are often present when some infant is critically ill or moribund. They may attend, as they choose, the death of their own infant. Since an average of two to three deaths occur each week and many infants are critically ill for long periods, it is obvious that the concentrated, intimate social interactions between personnel, infants and parents in an emotionally charged atmosphere often make the work of the staff very difficult and demanding. However, such participation and recognition of parents' rights to information about their infant appear to be the chief foundations of "informed consent" for treatment.

Each staff member must know how to cope with many questions and problems brought up by parents, and if he or she cannot help, they must have access to those who can. These requirements can be met only when staff members work closely with each other in all the varied circumstances from simple to complex, from triumph to tragedy. Formal and informal meetings take place regularly to discuss the technical and family aspects of care. As a given problem may require, some or all of several persons (including families, nurses, social workers, physicians, chaplains and others) may convene to exchange information and reach decisions. Thus, staff and parents function more or less as a small community in which a concerted attempt is made to ensure that each member may participate in and know about the major decisions that concern him or her. However, the physician takes appropriate initiative in final decision making, so that the family will not have to bear that heavy burden alone.

For several years, the responsibilities of attending pediatrician have been assumed chiefly by ourselves, who, as a result, have become acquainted intimately with the problems of the infants, the staff, and the parents. Our almost constant availability to staff, private pediatricians and parents has resulted in the raising of more and more ethical questions about various aspects of intensive care for critically ill and congenitally deformed infants. The penetrating questions and challenges, particularly of knowledgeable parents (such as physicians, nurses, or lawyers), brought increasing doubts about the wisdom of many of the decisions that seemed to parents to be predicated chiefly on technical considerations. Some thought their child had a right to die since he could not live well or effectively. Others thought that society should pay the costs of care that may be so destructive to the family economy. Often, too, the parents' or siblings' rights to relief from the seemingly pointless, crushing burdens were

important considerations. It seemed right to yield to parent wishes in several cases as physicians have done for generations. As a result, some treatments were withheld or stopped with the knowledge that earlier death and relief from suffering would result. Such options were explored with the less knowledgeable parents to ensure that their consent for treatment of their defective children was truly informed. As Eisenberg[8] pointed out regarding the application of technology, "At long last, we are beginning to ask, not *can* it be done, but *should* it be done?" In lengthy, frank discussions, the anguish of the parents was shared, and attempts were made to support fully the reasoned choices, whether for active treatment and rehabilitation or for an early death.

To determine the extent to which death resulted from withdrawing or with-holding treatment, we examined the hospital records of all children who died from January 1, 1970, through June 30, 1972.

RESULTS

In total, there were 299 deaths; each was classified in one of two categories; deaths in Category 1 resulted from pathologic conditions in spite of the treatment given; 256 (86 per cent) were in this category. Of these, 66 per cent were the result of respiratory problems or complications associated with extreme prematurity (birth weight under 1000 g). Congenital heart disease and other anomalies accounted for an additional 22 per cent (Table 1).

TABLE 1. PROBLEMS CAUSING DEATH IN CATEGORY 1.

Problem	No. of Deaths	Percentage
Respiratory	108	42.2
Extreme prematurity	60	23.4
Heart disease	42	16.4
Multiple anomalies	14	5.5
Other	32	12.5
Totals	256	100.0

Deaths in Category 2 were associated with severe impairment, usually from congenital disorders (Table 2): 43 (14 per cent) were in this group. These deaths or their timing was associated with discontinuance or withdrawal of treatment. The mean duration of life in Category 2 (table 3) was greater than that in Category 1. This was the result of a mean life of 55 days for eight infants who became chronic cardiopulmonary cripples but for whom prolonged and intensive efforts were made in the hope of eventual recovery. They were infants who were dependent on oxygen, digoxin and diuretics, and most of them had been treated for the idiopathic respiratory-distress syndrome with high oxygen concentrations and positive-pressure ventilation.

TABLE 2. PROBLEMS ASSOCIATED WITH DEATH IN CATEGORY 2.

Problem	No. of Deaths	Percentage
Multiple anomalies	15	34.9
Trisomy	8	18.6
Cardiopulmonary	8	18.6
Meningomyelocele	7	16.3
Other central-nervous-system defects	3	7.0
Short-bowel syndrome	2	4.6
Totals	43	100.0

Some examples of management choices in Category 2 illustrate the problems. An infant with Down's syndrome and intestinal atresia, like the much-publicized one at Johns Hopkins Hospital,[9] was not treated because his parents thought that surgery was wrong for their baby and themselves. He died seven days after birth. Another child had chronic pulmonary disease after positive-pressure ventilation with high oxygen concentrations for treatment of severe idiopathic respiratory-distress syndrome. By five months of age, he still required 40 per cent oxygen to survive, and even then, he was chronically dyspneic and cyanotic. He also suffered from cor pulmonale, which was difficult to control with digoxin and diuretics. The nurses, parents and physicians considered it cruel to continue, and yet difficult to stop. All were attached to this child, whose life they had tried so hard to make worthwhile. The family had endured high expenses (the hospital bill exceeding $15,000), and the strains of the illness were believed to be threatening the marriage bonds and to be causing sibling behavioral disturbances. Oxygen supplementation was stopped, and the child died in about three hours. The family settled down and 18 months later had another baby, who was healthy.

TABLE 3. SELECTED COMPARISONS OF 256 CASES IN CATEGORY 1 AND 43 IN CATEGORY 2.

Attribute	Category 1	Category 2
Mean length of life	4.8 days	7.5 days
Standard deviation	8.8	34.3
Range	1–69	1–150
Portion living for < 2 days	50.0%	12.0%

A third child had meningomyelocele, hydrocephalus and major anomalies of every organ in the pelvis. When the parents understood the limits of medical care and rehabilitation, they believed no treatment should be given. She died at five days of age.

We have maintained contact with most families of children in Category 2. Thus far, these families appear to have experienced a normal mourning for their losses. Although some have exhibited doubts that the choices were correct, all appear to be as effective in their lives as they were before this experience. Some claim that their profoundly moving experience has provided a deeper meaning in life, and from this they believe they have become more effective people.

Members of all religious faiths and atheists were participants as parents and as staff in these experiences. There appeared to be no relation between participation and a person's religion. Repeated participation in these troubling events did not appear to reduce the worry of the staff about the awesome nature of the decisions.

DISCUSSION

That decisions are made not to treat severely defective infants may be no surprise to those familiar with special-care facilities. All laymen and professionals familiar with our nursery appeared to set some limits upon their application of treatment to extend life or to investigate a pathologic process. For example, an experienced nurse said about one child, "We lost him several weeks ago. Isn't it time to quit?" In another case, a house officer said to a physician investigating an aspect of a child's disease, "For this child, don't you think it's time to turn off your curiosity so you can turn on your kindness?" Like many others, these children eventually acquired the "right to die."

Arguments among staff members and families for and against such decisions were based on varied notions of the rights and interests of defective infants, their families, professionals and society. They were also related to varying ideas about prognosis. Regarding the infants, some contended that individuals should have a right to die in some circumstances such as anencephaly, hydranencephaly, and some severely deforming and incapacitating conditions. Such very defective individuals were considered to have little or no hope of achieving meaningful "humanhood."[10] For example, they have little or no capacity to love or be loved. They are often cared for in facilities that have been characterized as "hardly more than dying bins,"[11] an assessment with which, in our experience, knowledgeable parents (those who visited chronic-care facilities for placement of their children) agreed. With institutionalized well children, social participation may be essentially nonexistent, and maternal deprivation severe; this is known to have an adverse, usually disastrous, effect upon the child.[12] The situation for the defective child is probably worse, for he is restricted socially both by his need for care and by his defects. To escape "wrongful life,"[13] a fate rated as worse than death, seemed right. In this regard, Lasagna[14] notes, "We may, as a society, scorn the civilizations that slaughtered their infants, but our present treatment of the retarded is in some ways more cruel."

Others considered allowing a child to die wrong for several reasons. The person most involved, the infant, had no voice in the decision. Prognosis was not always exact, and a few children with extensive care might live for months, and occasionally years. Some might survive and function satisfactorily. To a few

persons, withholding treatment and accepting death was condemned as criminal.

Families had strong but mixed feelings about management decisions. Living with the handicapped is clearly a family affair, and families of deformed infants thought there were limits to what they could bear or should be expected to bear. Most of them wanted maximal efforts to sustain life and to rehabilitate the handicapped; in such cases, they were supported fully. However, some families, especially those having children with severe defects, feared that they and their other children would become socially enslaved, economically deprived, and permanently stigmatized, all perhaps for a lost cause. Such a state of "chronic sorrow" until death has been described by Olshansky.[15] In some cases, families considered the death of the child right both for the child and for the family. They asked if that choice could be theirs or their doctors.

As Feifel has reported,[16] physicians on the whole are reluctant to deal with the issues. Some, particularly specialists based in the medical center, gave specific reasons for this disinclination. There was a feeling that to "give up" was disloyal to the cause of the profession. Since major research, teaching and patient-care efforts were being made, professionals expected to discover, transmit and apply knowledge and skills; patients and families were supposed to co-operate fully even if they were not always grateful. Some physicians recognized that the wishes of families went against their own, but they were resolute. They commonly agreed that if they were the parents of very defective children, withholding treatment would be most desirable for them. However, they argued that aggressive management was indicated for others. Some believed that allowing death as a management option was euthanasia and must be stopped for fear of setting a "poor ethical example" or for fear of personal prosecution or damage to their clinical departments or to the medical center as a whole. Alexander's report on Nazi Germany[17] was cited in some cases as providing justification for pressing the effort to combat disease. Some persons were concerned about the loss through death of "teaching material." They feared the training of professionals for the care of defective children in the future and the advancing of the state of the art would be compromised. Some parents who became aware of this concern thought their children should not become experimental subjects.

Practicing pediatricians, general practitioners and obstetricians were often familiar with these families and were usually sympathetic with their views. However, since they were more distant from the special-care nursery than the specialists of the medical center, their influence was often minimal. As a result, families received little support from them, and tension in community-medical relations was a recurring problem.

Infants with severe types of meningomyelocele precipitated the most controversial decisions. Several decades ago, those who survived this condition beyond a few weeks usually became hydrocephalic and retarded, in addition to being crippled and deformed. Without modern treatment, they died earlier.[18] Some may have been killed or at least not resuscitated at birth.[19] From the early 1960's, the tendency has been to treat vigorously all infants with meningomyelocele. As advocated by Zachary[20] and Shurtleff,[21] aggressive management of these children became the rule in our unit as in many others. Infants were usually referred quickly. Parents routinely signed permits for operation though rarely had they seen their children's defects or had the nature of various management plans and their respective prognoses clearly explained to them. Some physicians believed that parents were too upset to understand the nature of the problems and the options for care. Since they believed informed consent had no meaning in these circumstances, they either ignored the parents or simply told them that the child needed an operation on the back as the first step in correcting several defects. As a result, parents often felt completely left out while the activities of care proceeded at a brisk pace.

Some physicians experienced in the care of these children and familiar with the impact of such conditions upon families had early reservations about this plan of care.[22] More recently, they were influenced by the pessimistic appraisal of vigorous management schemes in some cases.[5] Meningomyelocele, when treated vigorously, is associated with higher survival rates,[21] but the achievement of satisfactory rehabilitation is at best difficult and usually impossible for almost all who are severely affected. Knowing this, some physicians and some families[23] decide against treatment of the most severely affected. If treatment is not carried out, the child's condition will usually deteriorate from further brain damage, urinary-tract infections and orthopedic difficulties, and death can be expected much earlier. Two thirds may be dead by three months, and over 90 per cent by one year of age. However, the quality of life during that time is poor, and the strains on families are great, but not necessarily greater than with treatment.[24] Thus, both treatment and nontreatment constitute unsatisfactory dilemmas for everyone, especially for the child and his family. When maximum treatment was viewed as unacceptable by families and physicians in our unit, there was a growing tendency to seek early death as a management option, to avoid that cruel choice of gradual, often slow, but progressive deterioration of the child who was required under these circumstances in effect to kill himself. Parents and the staff then asked if his dying needed to be prolonged. If not, what were the most appropriate medical responses?

Is it possible that some physicians and some families may join in a conspiracy to deny the right of a defective child to live or to die? Either could occur. Prolongation of the dying process by resident physicians having a vested interest in their careers has been described by Sudnow.[25] On the other hand, from the fatigue of working long and hard some physicians may give up too soon, assuming that their cause is lost. Families, similarly, may have mixed motives. They may demand death to obtain relief from the high costs and the tensions inherent in suffering, but their sense of guilt in this thought may produce the opposite demand, perhaps in violation of the sick person's rights. Thus, the challenge of deciding what course to take can be most tormenting for the family and the physician. Unquestionably, not facing the issue would appear to be the easier course, at least temporarily; no doubt many patients, families, and physicians decline to join in an effort to solve the problems. They can readily assume that what is being done is right and sufficient and ask no questions. But pretending there is no decision to be made is an arbitrary and potentially devastating decision of default. Since families and patients must live with the problems one way or another in any case, the physician's failure to face the issues may constitute a victimizing abandonment of patients and their families in times of greatest need. As Lasagna[14] pointed out, "There is no place for the physician to hide."

Can families in the shock resulting from the birth of a defective child understand what faces them? Can they give truly "informed consent" for treatment or withholding treatment? Some of our colleagues answer no to both questions. In our opinion, if families regardless of background are heard sympathetically and at length and are given information and answers to their questions in words they understand, the problems of their children as well as the expected benefits and limits of any proposed care can be understood clearly in practically all instances. Parents *are* able to understand the implications of such things as chronic dyspnea, oxygen dependency, incontinence, paralysis, contractures, sexual handicaps and mental retardation.

Another problem concerns who decides for a child. It may be acceptable for a person to reject treatment and bring about his own death. But it is quite a different situation when others are doing this for him. We do not know how often families and their physicians will make just decisions for severely handicapped children. Clearly, this issue is central in evaluation of the process of decision making that we have described. But we also ask, if these parties cannot make such decisions justly, who can?

We recognize great variability and often much uncertainty in prognoses and in family capacities to deal with defective newborn infants. We also acknowledge that there are limits of support that society can or will give to assist handicapped persons and their families. Severely deforming conditions that are associated with little or no hope of a functional existence pose painful dilemmas for the laymen and professionals who must decide how to cope with severe handicaps. We believe the burdens of decision making must be borne by families and their professional advisers because they are most familiar with the respective situations. Since families primarily must live with and are most affected by the decisions, it therefore appears that society and the health professions should provide only general guidelines for decision making. Moreover, since variations between situations are so great, and the situations themselves so complex, it follows that much latitude in decision making should be expected and tolerated. Otherwise, the rules of society or the policies most convenient for medical technologists may become cruel masters of human beings instead of their servants. Regarding any "allocation of death"[26] policy we readily acknowledge that the extreme excesses of Hegelian "rational utility" under dictatorships must be avoided.[17] Perhaps it is less recognized that the uncontrolled application of medical technology may be detrimental to individuals and families. In this regard, our views are similar to those of Waitzkin and Stoeckle.[27] Physicians may hold excessive power over decision making by limiting or controlling the information made available to patients or families. It seems appropriate that the profession be held accountable for presenting fully all management options and their expected consequences. Also, the public should be aware that professionals often face conflicts of interest that may result in decisions against individual preferences.

What are the legal implications of actions like those described in this paper? Some persons may argue that the law has been broken, and others would contend otherwise. Perhaps more than anything else, the public and professional silence on a major social taboo and some common practices has been broken further. That seems appropriate, for out of the ensuing dialogue perhaps better choices for patients and families can be made. If working out these dilemmas in ways such as those we suggest is in violation of the law, we believe the law should be changed.

REFERENCES

1. Wegman M. E.: "Annual summary of vital statistics —1970." *Pediatrics* 48:979–983, 1971.

2. Swyer P. R.: "The regional organization of special care for the neonate." *Pediatr. Clin. North. Am.* 17:761–776, 1970.

3. Rawlings G., Reynold E.O.R., Stewart A., et. al.: "Changing prognosis for infants of very low birth weight." *Lancet* 1:516–519, 1971.

4. Freeman E.: "The god committee." *New York Times Magazine,* May 21, 1972, pp. 84–90.

5. Lorber J.: "Results of treatment of mye-lomeningocele." *Dev. Med. Child. Neurol.* 13:279–303, 1971.

6. Slater E.: "Health service or sickness service." *Br. Med. J.* 4:734–736, 1971.

7. Klaus M.H., Kennell J.H.: "Mothers separated from their newborn infants." *Pediatr. Clin. North. Am.* 17:1015–1037, 1970.

8. Eisenberg, L.: "The human nature of human nature." *Science* 176:123–128, 1972.

9. Report of the Joseph P. Kennedy Foundation International Symposium on Human Rights, Retardation and Research, Washington, DC, The John F. Kennedy Center for the Performing Arts, October 16, 1971.

10. Fletcher J.: "Indicators of humanhood: a tentative profile of man," *The Hastings Center Report,* Vol. 2, No. 5, November, 1972, pp. 1–4.

11. Freeman H.E., Brim O.G. Jr., Williams G.: "New dimensions of dying," *The Dying Patient.* Edited by O.G. Brim Jr. New York, Russell Sage Foundation, 1970, pp. xiii–xxvi.

12. Spitz R.A.: "Hospitalism: an inquiry into the genesis of psychiatric conditions in early childhood." *Psychoanal. Study Child.* 1:53–74, 1945.

13. Engelhardt H.T. Jr.: "Euthanasia and children: the injury of continued existence." *J. Pediatr.* 83:170–171, 1973.

14. Lasagna L.: *Life, Death and the Doctor.* New York, Alfred A. Knopf, 1968.

15. Olshansky S.: "Chronic sorrow: a response to having a mentally defective child." *Soc. Casework* 43: 190–193, 1962.

16. Feifel H.: "Perception of death." *Ann. NY Acad. Sci.* 164:669–677, 1969.

17. Alexander L.: "Medical science under dictatorship." *N. Engl. J. Med.* 241:39–47, 1949.

18. Laurence K.M. and Tew B.J.: "Natural history of spina bifida cystica and cranium bifidum cysticum: major central nervous system malformations in South Wales." Part IV. *Arch. Dis. Child* 46: 127–138, 1971.

19. Forrest D.M.: "Modern trends in the treatment of spina bifida: early closure in spina bifida: results and problems." *Proc. R. Soc. Med.* 60: 763–767, 1967.

20. Zachary R.B.: "Ethical and social aspects of treatment of spina bifida." *Lancet* 2:274–276, 1968.

21. Shurtleff D.B.: "Care of the myelodysplastic patient." *Ambulatory Pediatrics.* Edited by M. Green, R. Haggerty. Philadelphia, W.B. Saunders Company, 1968, pp. 726–741.

22. Matson D.D.: "Surgical treatment of mye-lomeningocele." *Pediatrics* 42:225–227, 1968.

23. MacKeith R.C.: "A new look at spina bifida aperta." *Dev. Med. Child. Neurol.* 13:277–278, 1971.

24. Hide D.W., Williams H.P., Ellis H.L.: "The outlook for the child with a myelomeningocele for whom early surgery was considered inadvisable." *Dev. Med. Child. Neurol.* 14:304–307, 1972.

25. Sudnow D.: *Passing On.* Englewood Cliffs, New Jersey, Prentice Hall, 1967.

26. Manning B.: "Legal and policy issues in the allocation of death," *The Dying Patient.* Edited by O.G. Brim Jr. New York, Russell Sage Foundation, 1970, pp. 253–274.

27. Waitzkin H., Stoeckle J.D.: "The communication of information about illness." *Adv. Psychosom. Med.* 8:180–215, 1972.

RICHARD A. McCORMICK

To Save or Let Die: The Dilemma of Modern Medicine

On February 24, the son of Mr. and Mrs. Robert H. T. Houle died following court-ordered emergency surgery at Maine Medical Center. The child was born February 9, horribly deformed. His entire left side was malformed; he had no left eye, was practically without a left ear, had a deformed left hand; some of his vertebrae were not fused. Furthermore, he was afflicted with a tracheal esophageal fistula and could not be fed by mouth. Air leaked into his stomach instead of going to the lungs, and fluid from the stomach pushed up into the lungs. As Dr. Andre Hellegers recently noted, "It takes little imagination to think there were further internal deformities" (*Obstetrical and Gynecological News,* April 1974).

As the days passed, the condition of the child deteriorated. Pneumonia set in. His reflexes became impaired and because of poor circulation, severe brain damage was suspected. The tracheal esophageal fistula, the immediate threat to his survival, can be corrected with relative ease by surgery. But in view of the associated complications and deformities, the parents refused their consent to surgery on "Baby Boy Houle." Several doctors in the Maine Medical Center felt differently and took the case to court. Maine Superior Court Judge David G. Roberts ordered the surgery to be performed. He ruled: "At the moment of live birth there does exist a human being entitled to the fullest protection of the law. The most basic right enjoyed by every human being is the right to life itself."

"MEANINGFUL LIFE"

Instances like this happen frequently. In a recent issue of the *New England Journal of Medicine,* Drs. Raymond S. Duff and A. G. M. Campbell[1] reported on 299 deaths in the special-care nursery of the Yale-New Haven Hospital between 1970 and 1972. Of these, 43 (14%) were associated with discontinuance of treatment for children with multiple anomalies, trisomy, cardiopulmonary crippling, meningomyelocele, and other central nervous system defects. After careful consideration of each of these 43 infants, parents and physicians in a group decision concluded that the prognosis for "meaningful life" was extremely poor or hopeless, and therefore rejected further treatment. The abstract of the Duff-Campbell report states: "The awesome finality of these decisions, combined with a potential for error in prognosis, made the choice agonizing for families and health professionals. Nevertheless, the issue has to be faced, for not to decide is an arbitrary and potentially devastating decision of default."

In commenting on this study in the *Washington Post* (October 28, 1973), Dr. Lawrence K. Pickett, chief-of-staff at the Yale-New Haven Hospital, admitted that allowing hopelessly ill patients to die "is accepted medical practice." He continued: "This is nothing new. It's just being talked about now."

It has been talked about, it is safe to say, at least since the publicity associated with the famous "Johns Hopkins Case"[2] some three years ago. In this instance, an infant was born with Down syndrome and duodenal atresia. The blockage is reparable by relatively easy surgery. However, after consultation with spiritual advisors, the parents refused permission for this corrective surgery, and the child died by starvation in the hospital after 15 days. For to feed him by mouth in this condition would have killed him. Nearly everyone who has commented on this case has disagreed with the decision.

It must be obvious that these instances—and they are frequent—raise the most agonizing

Reprinted with permission of the author and the publisher from *Journal of the American Medical Association,* Vol. 229, No. 8 (July 1974), pp. 172–176. Copyright 1974, American Medical Association.

and delicate moral problems. The problem is best seen in the ambiguity of the term "hopelessly ill." This used to and still may refer to lives that cannot be saved, that are irretrievably in the dying process. It may also refer to lives that can be saved and sustained, but in a wretched, painful, or deformed condition. With regard to infants, the problem is, which infants, if any, should be allowed to die? On what grounds or according to what criteria, as determined by whom? Or again, is there a point at which a life that can be saved is not "meaningful life," as the medical community so often phrases the question? . . .

Thus far, the ethical discussion of these truly terrifying decisions has been less than fully satisfactory. Perhaps this is to be expected since the problems have only recently come to public attention. In a companion article to the Duff-Campbell report,[1] Dr. Anthony Shaw[3] of the Pediatric Division of the Department of Surgery, University of Virginia Medical Center, Charlottesville, speaks of solutions "based on the circumstances of each case rather than by means of a dogmatic formula approach." Are these really the only options available to us? Shaw's statement makes it appear that the ethical alternatives are narrowed to dogmatism (which imposes a formula that prescinds from circumstances) and pure concretism (which denies the possibility or usefulness of any guidelines).

ARE GUIDELINES POSSIBLE?

Such either-or extremism is understandable. It is easy for the medical profession, in its fully justified concern with the terrible concreteness of these problems and with the issue of who makes these decisions, to trend away from any substantive guidelines. As *Time* remarked in reporting these instances: "Few, if any, doctors are willing to establish guidelines for determining which babies should receive lifesaving surgery or treatment and which should not" (*Time,* March 25, 1974). On the other hand, moral theologians, in their fully justified concern to avoid total normlessness and arbitrariness wherein the right is "discovered," or really "created," only in and by brute decision, can easily be insensitive to the moral relevance of the raw experience, of the conflicting tensions and concerns provoked through direct cradleside contact with human events and persons.

But is there no middle course between sheer concretism and dogmatism? I believe there is. Dr. Franz J. Ingelfinger,[4] editor of the *New England Journal of Medicine,* in an editorial on the Duff-Campbell-Shaw articles, concluded, even if somewhat reluctantly: "Society, ethics, institutional attitudes and committees can provide the broad guidelines, but the onus of decision-making ultimately falls on the doctor in whose care the child has been put." Similarly, Frederick Carney of Southern Methodist University, Dallas, and the Kennedy Institute . . . stated of these cases: "What is obviously needed is the development of substantive standards to inform parents and physicians who must make such decisions" (*Washington Post,* March 20, 1974).

"Broad guidelines," "substantive standards." There is the middle course, and it is the task of a community broader than the medical community. A guideline is not a slide rule that makes the decision. It is far less than that. But it is far more than the concrete decision of the parents and the physician, however seriously and conscientiously this is made. It is more like a light in a room, a light that allows the individual objects to be seen in the fullness of their context. Concretely, if there are certain infants that we agree ought to be saved in spite of illness or deformity, and if there are certain infants that we agree should be allowed to die, then there is a line to be drawn. And if there is a line to be drawn, there ought to be some criteria, even if very general, for doing this. Thus, if nearly every commentator has disagreed with the Hopkins decision, should we not be able to distill from such consensus some general wisdom that will inform and guide future decisions? I think so.

This task is not easy. Indeed, it is so harrowing that the really tempting thing is to run from it. The most sensitive, balanced, and penetrating study of the Hopkins case that I have seen is that of the University of Chicago's James Gustafson.[2] Gustafson disagreed with the decision of the Hopkins physicians to deny surgery to the mongoloid infant. In summarizing his dissent, he notes: "Why would I draw the line on a different side of mongolism than the physicians did? While reasons can be given, one must recognize that there are intuitive elements, grounded in beliefs and profound feelings, that enter into particular judgments of this sort." He goes on to criticize the assessment made of the child's intelligence as too simplistic, and he proposes a much broader perspective on the meaning of suffering than seemed to have operated in the Hopkins decision. I am in full agreement with Gustafson's reflections and conclusions. But ultimately, he does not tell us where he would draw the line or why, only where he would *not,* and why.

This is very helpful already, and perhaps it is all that can be done. Dare we take the next step, the combination and analysis of such negative judgments to extract from them the positive criterion or criteria inescapably operative in them? Or more startlingly, dare we *not* if these decisions are already being made? Gustafson is certainly right in saying that we cannot always establish perfectly rational accounts and norms for our decisions. But I believe we must never cease trying, in fear and trembling to be sure. Otherwise, we have exempted these decisions in principle from the one critique and control that protects against abuse. Exemption of this sort is the root of all exploitation whether personal or political. Briefly, if we must face the frightening task of making quality-of-life judgments—and we must—then we must face the difficult task of building criteria for these judgments.

FACING RESPONSIBILITY

What has brought us to this position of awesome responsibility? Very simply, the sophistication of modern medicine. Contemporary resuscitation and life-sustaining devices have brought a remarkable change in the state of the question. Our duties toward the care and preservation of life have been traditionally stated in terms of the use of ordinary and extraordinary means. For the moment and for purposes of brevity, we may say that, morally speaking, ordinary means are those whose use does not entail grave hardships to the patient. Those that would involve such hardship are extraordinary. Granted the relativity of these terms and the frequent difficulty of their application, still the distinction has had an honored place in medical ethics and medical practice. Indeed, the distinction was recently reiterated by the House of Delegates of the American Medical Association in a policy statement. After disowning intentional killing (mercy killing), the AMA statement continues: "The cessation of the employment of extraordinary means to prolong the life of the body when there is irrefutable evidence that biological death is imminent is the decision of the patient and/or his immediate family. The advice and judgment of the physician should be freely available to the patient and/or his immediate family" (*JAMA* 227:728, 1974).

This distinction can take us just so far—and thus the change in the state of the question. The contemporary problem is precisely that the question no longer concerns only those for whom "biological death is imminent" in the sense of the AMA statement. Many infants who would have died a decade ago, whose "biological death was imminent," can be saved. Yesterday's failures are today's successes. Contemporary medicine with its team approaches, staged surgical techniques, monitoring capabilities, ventilatory support systems, and other methods, can keep almost anyone alive. This has tended gradually to shift the problem from the means to reverse the dying process to the quality of the life sustained and preserved. The questions, "Is this means too hazardous or difficult to use" and "Does this measure only prolong the patient's dying," while still useful and valid, now often become "Granted that we can easily save the life, what kind of life are we saving?" This is a quality-of-life judgment. And we fear it. And certainly we should. But with increased power goes increased responsibility. Since we have the power, we must face the responsibility.

A RELATIVE GOOD

In the past, the Judeo-Christian tradition has attempted to walk a balanced middle path between medical vitalism (that preserves life at any cost) and medical pessimism (that kills when life seems frustrating, burdensome, "useless"). Both of these extremes root in an identical idolatry of life—an attitude that, at least by inference, views death as an unmitigated, absolute evil, and life as the absolute good. The middle course that has structured Judeo-Christian attitudes is that life is indeed a basic and precious good, but a good to be preserved precisely as the condition of other values. It is these other values and possibilities that found the duty to preserve physical life and also dictate the limits of this duty. In other words, life is a relative good, and the duty to preserve it a limited one. These limits have always been stated in terms of the *means* required to sustain life. But if the implications of this middle position are unpacked a bit, they will allow us, perhaps, to adapt to the type of quality-of-life judgment we are now called on to make without tumbling into vitalism or a utilitarian pessimism.

A beginning can be made with a statement of Pope Pius XII[5] in an allocution to physicians delivered November 24, 1957. After noting that we are normally obliged to use only ordinary means to preserve life, the Pontiff stated: "A more strict obligation would be too burdensome for most men and would render the attainment of the higher, more important good too difficult. Life, death, all temporal activities are in fact subordinated to spiritual ends." Here it would be helpful to ask two questions. First, what are these spiritual ends, this "higher, more important good?" Second, how is its attainment rendered too difficult by insisting on the use of extraordinary means to preserve life?

The first question must be answered in terms of love of God and neighbor. This sums up briefly the meaning, substance and consummation of life from a Judeo-Christian perspective. What is or can easily be missed is that these two loves are not separable. St. John wrote: "If any man says 'I love God' and hates his brother, he is a liar. For he who loves not his brother, whom he sees, how can he love God whom he does not see?" (1 John 4:20–21). This means that our love of neighbor is in some very real sense our love of God. The good our love wants to do Him and to which He enables us, can be done only for the neighbor, as Karl Rahner has so forcefully argued. It is in others that God demands to be recognized and loved. If this is true, it means that, in Judeo-Christian perspective, the meaning, substance, and consummation of life is found in human *relationships,* and the qualities of justice, respect, concern, compassion, and support that surround them.

Second, how is the attainment of this "higher, more important (than life) good" rendered "too difficult" by life-supports that are gravely burdensome? One who must support his life with disproportionate effort focuses the time, attention, energy, and resources of himself and others not precisely on relationships, but on maintaining the condition of relationships. Such concentration easily becomes overconcentration and distorts one's view of and weakens one's pursuit of the very relational goods that define our growth and flourishing. The importance of relationships gets lost in the struggle for survival. The very Judeo-Christian meaning of life is seriously jeopardized when undue and unending effort must go into its maintenance.

I believe an analysis similar to this is implied in traditional treatises on preserving life. The illustrations of grave hardship (rendering the means to preserve life extraordinary and non-obligatory) are instructive, even if they are outdated in some of their particulars. Older moralists often referred to the hardship of moving to another climate or country. As the late Gerald Kelly, SJ,[6] noted of this instance: "They (the classical moral theologians) spoke of other inconveniences, too: e.g., of moving to another climate or another country to preserve one's life. For people whose lives were, so to speak, rooted in the land, and whose native town or village was as dear as life itself, and for whom, moreover, travel was always difficult and often dangerous—for such people, moving to another country or climate was a truly great hardship, and more than God would demand as a 'reasonable' means of preserving one's health and life.''

Similarly, if the financial cost of life-preserving care was crushing, that is, if it would create grave hardships for oneself or one's family, it was considered extraordinary and non-obligatory. Or again, the grave inconvenience of living with a badly mutilated body was viewed, along with other factors (such as pain in preanesthetic days, uncertainty of success), as constituting the means extraordinary. Even now, the contemporary moralist, M. Zalba, SJ,[7] states that no one is obliged to preserve his life when the cost is ''a most oppressive convalescence'' (*molestissima convalescentia*).

THE QUALITY OF LIFE

In all of these instances—instances where the life could be saved—the discussion is couched in terms of the means necessary to preserve life. But often enough it is the kind of, the quality of the life thus saved (painful, poverty-stricken and deprived, away from home and friends, oppressive) that establishes the means as extraordinary. *That* type of life would be an excessive hardship for the individual. It would distort and jeopardize his grasp on the overall meaning of life. Why? Because, it can be argued, human relationships—which are the very possibility of growth in love of God and neighbor—would be so threatened, strained, or submerged that they would no longer function as the heart and meaning of the individual's life as they should. Something other than the ''higher, more important good'' would occupy first place. Life, the condition of other values and achievements, would usurp the place of these and become itself the ultimate value. When that happens, the value of human life has been distorted out of context. . . .

Can these reflections be brought to bear on the grossly malformed infant? I believe so. Obviously there is a difference between having a terribly mutilated body as the result of surgery, and having a terribly mutilated body from

birth. There is also a difference between a long, painful, oppressive convalescence resulting from surgery, and a life that is from birth one long, painful, oppressive convalescence. Similarly, there is a difference between being plunged into poverty by medical expenses and being poor without ever incurring such expenses. However, is there not also a similarity? Can not these conditions, whether caused by medical intervention or not, equally absorb attention and energies to the point where the ''higher, more important good'' is simply too difficult to attain? It would appear so. Indeed, is this not precisely why abject poverty (and the systems that support it) is such an enormous moral challenge to us? It simply dehumanizes.

Life's potentiality for other values is dependent on two factors, those external to the individual, and the very condition of the individual. The former we can and must change to maximize individual potential. That is what social justice is all about. The latter we sometimes cannot alter. It is neither inhuman nor unchristian to say that there comes a point where an individual's condition itself represents the negation of any truly human—ie, relational—potential. When that point is reached, is not the best treatment no treatment? I believe that the *implications* of the traditional distinction between ordinary and extraordinary means point in this direction.

In this tradition, life is not a value to be preserved in and for itself. To maintain that would commit us to a form of medical vitalism that makes no human or Judeo-Christian sense. It is a value to be preserved precisely as a condition for other values, and therefore insofar as these other values remain attainable. Since these other values cluster around and are rooted in human relationships, it seems to follow that life is a value to be preserved only insofar as it contains some potentiality for human relationships. When in human judgment this potentiality is totally absent or would be, because of the condition of the individual, totally subordinated to the mere effort for survival, that life can be said to have achieved its potential.

HUMAN RELATIONSHIPS

If these reflections are valid, they point in the direction of a guideline that may help in decisions about sustaining the lives of grossly deformed and deprived infants. That guideline is the potential for human relationships associated with the infant's condition. If that potential is simply nonexistent or would be utterly submerged and undeveloped in the mere struggle to survive, that life has achieved its potential. There are those who will want to continue to say that some terribly deformed infants may be allowed to die *because* no extraordinary means need be used. Fair enough. But they should realize that the term "extraordinary" has been so relativized to the condition of the patient that it is this condition that is decisive. The means is extraordinary because the infant's condition is extraordinary. And if that is so, we must face this fact head-on—and discover the substantive standard that allows us to say this of some infants, but not of others.

Here several caveats are in order. First, this guideline is not a detailed rule that preempts decisions; for relational capacity is not subject to mathematical analysis but to human judgment. However, it is the task of physicians to provide some more concrete categories or presumptive biological symptoms for this human judgment. For instance, nearly all would very likely agree that the anencephalic infant is without relational potential. On the other hand, the same cannot be said of the mongoloid infant. The task ahead is to attach relational potential to presumptive biological symptoms for the gray area between such extremes. In other words, individual decisions will remain the anguishing onus of parents in consultation with physicians.

Second, because this guideline is precisely that, mistakes will be made. Some infants will be judged in all sincerity to be devoid of any meaningful relational potential when that is actually not quite the case. This risk of error should not lead to abandonment of decisions; for that is to walk away from the human scene. Risk of error means only that we must proceed with great humility, caution, and tentativeness. Concretely, it means that if err we must at times, it is better to err on the side of life—and therefore to tilt in that direction.

Third, it must be emphasized that allowing some infants to die does not imply that "some lives are valuable, others not" or that "there is such a thing as a life not worth living." Every human being, regardless of age or condition, is of incalculable worth. The point is not, therefore, whether this or that individual has value. Of course he has, or rather *is* a value. The only point is whether this undoubted value has any potential at all, in continuing physical survival, for attaining a share, even if reduced, in the "higher, more important good." This is not a question about the inherent value of the individual. It is a question about whether this worldly existence will offer such a valued individual any hope of sharing those values for which physical life is the fundamental condition. Is not the only alternative an attitude that supports mere physical life as long as possible with every means?

Fourth, this whole matter is further complicated by the fact that this decision is being made for someone else. Should not the decision on whether life is to be supported or not be left to the individual? Obviously, wherever possible. But there is nothing inherently objectionable in the fact that parents with physicians must make this decision at some point for infants. Parents must make many crucial decisions for children. The only concern is that the decision not be shaped out of the utilitarian perspectives so deeply sunk into the consciousness of the contemporary world. In a highly technological culture, an individual is always in danger of being valued for his function, what he can do, rather than for who he is.

It remains, then, only to emphasize that these decisions must be made in terms of the child's good, this alone. But that good, as fundamentally a relational good, has many dimensions. Pius XII,[5] in speaking of the duty to preserve life, noted that this duty "derives from well-ordered charity, from submission to the Creator, from social justice, as well as from devotion towards his family.'' All of these considerations pertain to that "higher, more important good.'' If that is the case with the duty to preserve life, then the decision not to preserve life must likewise take all of these into account in determining what is for the child's good.

Any discussion of this problem would be incomplete if it did not repeatedly stress that it is the pride of the Judeo-Christian tradition that the weak and defenseless, the powerless and unwanted, those whose grasp on the goods of life is most fragile—that is, those whose potential is real but reduced—are cherished and protected as our neighbor in greatest need. Any application of a general guideline that forgets this is but a racism of the adult world profoundly at odds with the gospel, and eventually corrosive of the humanity of those who ought to be caring and supporting as long as that care and support has human meaning. It has meaning as long as there is hope that the infant will, in relative comfort, be able to experience our caring and love. For when this happens, both we and the child are sharing in that "greater, more important good.''

Were not those who disagreed with the Hopkins decision saying, in effect, that for the infant, involved human relationships were still within reach and would not be totally submerged by survival? If that is the case, it is potential for relationships that is at the heart of these agonizing decisions.

REFERENCES

1. Duff S, Campbell AGM: "Moral and ethical dilemmas in the special-care nursery." *N Engl J Med* 289:890–894, 1973.

2. Gustafson JM: "Mongolism, parental desires, and the right to life." *Perspect Biol Med* 16:529–559, 1973.

3. Shaw A: "Dilemmas of 'informed' consent in children." *N Engl J Med* 289:885–890, 1973.

4. Ingelfinger F: "Bedside ethics for the hopeless case." *N Engl J Med* 289:914, 1973.

5. Pope Pius XII: *Acta Apostolicae Sedis* 49:1031–1032, 1957.

6. Kelly G: *Medico-Moral Problems*. St. Louis, Catholic Hospital Association of the United States and Canada, 1957, p 132.

7. Zalba, M: *Theologiae Moralis Summa*. Madrid, La Editorial Catolica, 1957, vol 2, p 71.

NEW JERSEY SUPREME COURT

In the Matter of Karen Quinlan, An Alleged Incompetent

[The opinion of the Court was delivered by Hughes, Chief Justice.]

The central figure in this tragic case is Karen Ann Quinlan, a New Jersey resident. At the age of 22, she lies in a debilitated and allegedly moribund state at Saint Clare's Hospital in Denville, New Jersey. The litigation has to do, in final analysis, with her life—its continuance or cessation—and the responsibilities, rights,

Reprinted from 70 *New Jersey Reports* 10. Decided March 31, 1976.

and duties, with regard to any fateful decision concerning it, of her family, her guardian, her doctors, the hospital, the State through its law enforcement authorities, and finally the courts of justice. . . .

The matter is of transcendent importance, involving questions related to the definition and existence of death, the prolongation of life through artificial means developed by medical technology undreamed of in past generations of the practice of the healing arts; the impact of such durationally indeterminate and artificial life prolongation on the rights of the incompetent, her family and society in general; the bearing of constitutional right and the scope of judicial responsibility, as to the appropriate response of an equity court of justice to the extraordinary prayer for relief of the plaintiff. Involved as well is the right of the plaintiff, Joseph Quinlan, to guardianship of the person of his daughter.

. . .

THE FACTUAL BASE

An understanding of the issues in their basic perspective suggests a brief review of the factual base developed in the testimony and documented in greater detail in the opinion of the trial judge. *In re Quinlan*, 137 *N.J. Super.* 227 (Ch. Div. 1975).

On the night of April 15, 1975, for reasons still unclear, Karen Quinlan ceased breathing for at least two 15-minute periods. She received some ineffectual mouth-to-mouth resuscitation from friends. She was taken by ambulance to Newton Memorial Hospital. There she had a temperature of 100 degrees, her pupils were unreactive and she was unresponsive even to deep pain. The history at the time of her admission to that hospital was essentially incomplete and uninformative.

Three days later, Dr. Morse examined Karen at the request of the Newton admitting physician, Dr. McGee. He found her comatose with evidence of decortication, a condition relating to derangement of the cortex of the brain causing a physical posture in which the upper extremities are flexed and the lower extremities are extended. She required a respirator to assist her breathing. Dr. Morse was unable to obtain an adequate account of the circumstances and events leading up to Karen's admission to the Newton Hospital. Such initial history or etiology is crucial in neurological diagnosis. Relying as he did upon the Newton Memorial records and his own examination, he concluded that prolonged lack of oxygen in the bloodstream, anoxia, was identified with her condition as he saw it upon

first observation. When she was later transferred to Saint Clare's Hospital she was still unconscious, still on a respirator and a tracheotomy had been performed. On her arrival Dr. Morse conducted extensive and detailed examinations. An electroencephalogram (EEG) measuring electrical rhythm of the brain was performed and Dr. Morse characterized the result as "abnormal but it showed some activity and was consistent with her clinical state." Other significant neurological tests, including a brain scan, an angiogram, and a lumbar puncture were normal in result. Dr. Morse testified that Karen has been in a state of coma, lack of consciousness, since he began treating her. He explained that there are basically two types of coma, sleep-like unresponsiveness and awake unresponsiveness. Karen was originally in a sleep-like unresponsive condition but soon developed "sleep-wake" cycles, apparently a normal improvement for comatose patients occurring within three to four weeks. In the awake cycle she blinks, cries out and does things of that sort but is still totally unaware of anyone or anything around her.

Dr. Morse and other expert physicians who examined her characterized Karen as being in a "chronic persistent vegetative state." Dr. Fred Plum, one of such expert witnesses, defined this as a "subject who remains with the capacity to maintain the vegetative parts of neurological function but who . . . no longer has any cognitive function."

Dr. Morse, as well as the several other medical and neurological experts who testified in this case, believed with certainty that Karen Quinlan is not "brain dead." They identified the Ad Hoc Committee of Harvard Medical School report . . . as the ordinary medical standard for determining brain death, and all of them were satisfied that Karen met none of the criteria specified in that report and was therefore not "brain dead" within its contemplation.

. . .

Because Karen's neurological condition affects her respiratory ability (the respiratory system being a brain stem function) she requires a respirator to assist her breathing.

From the time of her admission to Saint Clare's Hospital Karen has been assisted by an MA-1 respirator, a sophisticated machine which delivers a given volume of air at a certain rate and periodically provides a "sigh" volume, a relatively large measured volume of air designed to purge the lungs of excretions. Attempts to "wean" her from the respirator were unsuccessful and have been abandoned.

The experts believe that Karen cannot now survive without the assistance of the respirator; that exactly how long she would live without it is unknown; that the strong likelihood is that death would follow soon after its removal, and that removal would also risk further brain damage and would curtail the assistance the respirator presently provides in warding off infection.

It seemed to be the consensus not only of the treating physicians but also of the several qualified experts who testified in the case, that removal from the respirator would not conform to medical practices, standards and traditions.

The further medical consensus was that Karen in addition to being comatose is in a chronic and persistent "vegetative" state, having no awareness of anything or anyone around her and existing at a primitive reflex level. Although she does have some brain stem function (ineffective for respiration) and has other reactions one normally associates with being alive, such as moving, reacting to light, sound and noxious stimuli, blinking her eyes, and the like, the quality of her feeling impulses is unknown. She grimaces, makes stereotyped cries and sounds and has chewing motions. Her blood pressure is normal.

Karen remains in the intensive care unit at Saint Clare's Hospital, receiving 24-hour care by a team of four nurses characterized, as was the medical attention, as "excellent." She is nourished by feeding by way of a nasalgastro tube and is routinely examined for infection, which under these circumstances is a serious life threat. The result is that her condition is considered remarkable under the unhappy circumstances involved.

Karen is described as emaciated, having suffered a weight loss of at least 40 pounds, and undergoing a continuing deteriorative process.

Her posture is described as fetal-like and grotesque; there is extreme flexion-rigidity of the arms, legs and related muscles and her joints are severely rigid and deformed.

From all of this evidence, and including the whole testimonial record, several basic findings in the physical area are mandated. Severe brain and associated damage, albeit of uncertain etiology, has left Karen in a chronic and persistent vegetative state. No form of treatment which can cure or improve that condition is known or available. As nearly as may be determined, considering the guarded area of remote uncertainties characteristic of most medical science predictions, she can *never* be restored to cognitive or sapient life. Even with regard to the vegetative level and improvement therein (if such it may be called) the prognosis is extremely poor and the extent unknown if it should in fact occur.

She is debilitated and moribund and although fairly stable at the time of argument before us (no new information having been filed in the meanwhile in expansion of the record), no physician risked the opinion that she could live more than a year and indeed she may die much earlier. Excellent medical and nursing care so far has been able to ward off the constant threat of infection, to which she is peculiarly susceptible because of the respirator, the tracheal tube and other incidents of care in her vulnerable condition. Her life accordingly is sustained by the respirator and tubal feeding, and removal from the respirator would cause her death soon, although the time cannot be stated with more precision.

. . .

We have adverted to the "brain death" concept and Karen's disassociation with any of its criteria, to emphasize the basis of the medical decision made by Dr. Morse. When plaintiff and his family, finally reconciled the certainty of Karen's impending death, requested the withdrawal of life support mechanisms, he demurred. His refusal was based upon his conception of medical standards, practice and ethics described in the medical testimony, such as in the evidence given by another neurologist, Dr. Sidney Diamond, a witness for the State. Dr. Diamond asserted that no physician would have failed to provide respirator support at the outset, and none would interrupt its life-saving course thereafter, except in the case of cerebral death. In the latter case, he thought the respirator would in effect be disconnected from one already dead, entitling the physician under medical standards and, he thought, legal concepts, to terminate the supportive measures. We note Dr. Diamond's distinction of major surgical or transfusion procedures in a terminal case not involving cerebral death, such as here:

The subject has lost human qualities. It would be incredible, and I think unlikely, that any physician would respond to a sudden hemorrhage, massive hemorrhage or a loss of all her defensive blood cells, by giving her large quantities of blood. I think that . . . major surgical procedures would be out of the question even if they were known to be essential for continued physical existence.

This distinction is adverted to also in the testimony of Dr. Julius Korein, a neurologist called by plaintiff. Dr. Korein described a medical practice concept of "judicious neglect" under which the physician will say:

Don't treat this patient any more, . . . it does not serve either the patient, the family, or society in any meaningful way to continue treatment with this patient.

Dr. Korein also told of the unwritten and unspoken standard of medical practice implied in the foreboding initials DNR (do not resuscitate), as applied to the extraordinary terminal case:

Cancer, metastatic cancer, involving the lungs, the liver, the brain, multiple involvements, the physician may or may not write: Do not resuscitate. . . . [I]t could be said to the nurse: if this man stops breathing don't resuscitate him. . . . No physician that I know personally is going to try and resuscitate a man riddled with cancer and in agony and he stops breathing. They are not going to put him on a respirator. . . . I think that would be the height of misuse of technology.

While the thread of logic in such distinctions may be elusive to the non-medical lay mind, in

relation to the supposed imperative to sustain life at all costs, they nevertheless relate to medical decisions, such as the decision of Dr. Morse in the present case. We agree with the trial court that that decision was in accord with Dr. Morse's conception of medical standards and practice.

. . .

CONSTITUTIONAL AND LEGAL ISSUES

THE RIGHT OF PRIVACY[1]

It is the issue of the constitutional right of privacy that has given us most concern, in the exceptional circumstances of this case. Here a loving parent, *qua* parent and raising the rights of his incompetent and profoundly damaged daughter, probably irreversibly doomed to no more than a biologically vegetative remnant of life, is before the court. He seeks authorization to abandon specialized technological procedures which can only maintain for a time a body having no potential for resumption or continuance of other than a "vegetative" existence.

We have no doubt, in these unhappy circumstances, that if Karen were herself miraculously lucid for an interval (not altering the existing prognosis of the condition to which she would soon return) and perceptive of her irreversible condition, she could effectively decide upon discontinuance of the life-support apparatus, even if it meant the prospect of natural death. To this extent we may distinguish [*John F. Kennedy Memorial Hosp. v. Heston*], . . . which concerned a severely injured young woman (Delores Heston), whose life depended on surgery and blood transfusion; and who was in such extreme shock that she was unable to express an informed choice (although the Court apparently considered the case as if the patient's own religious decision to resist transfusion were at stake), but most importantly a patient apparently salvable to long life and vibrant health;—a situation not at all like the present case.

We have no hesitancy in deciding, in the instant diametrically opposite case, that no external compelling interest of the State could compel Karen to endure the unendurable, only to vegetate a few measurable months with no realistic possibility of returning to any semblance of cognitive or sapient life. We perceive no thread of logic distinguishing between such a choice on Karen's part and a similar choice which, under the evidence in this case, could be made by a competent patient terminally ill, riddled by cancer and suffering great pain; such a patient would not be resuscitated or put on a respirator in the example described by Dr. Korein, and *a fortiori* would not be kept *against his will* on a respirator.

· · ·

The claimed interests of the State in this case are essentially the preservation and sanctity of human life and defense of the right of the physician to administer medical treatment according to his best judgment. In this case the doctors say that removing Karen from the respirator will conflict with their professional judgment. The plaintiff answers that Karen's present treatment serves only a maintenance function; that the respirator cannot cure or improve her condition but at best can only prolong her inevitable slow deterioration and death; and that the interests of the patient, as seen by her surrogate, the guardian, must be evaluated by the court as predominant, even in the face of an opinion *contra* by the present attending physicians. Plaintiff's distinction is significant. The nature of Karen's care and the realistic chances of her recovery are quite unlike those of the patients discussed in many of the cases where treatments were ordered. In many of those cases the medical procedure required (usually a transfusion) constituted a minimal bodily invasion and the chances of recovery and return to functioning life were very good. We think that the State's interest *contra* weakens and the individual's right to privacy grows as the degree of bodily invasion increases and the prognosis dims. Ultimately there comes a point at which the individual's rights overcome the State interest. It is for that reason that we believe Karen's choice, if she were competent to make it, would be vindicated by the law. Her prognosis is extremely poor—she will never resume cognitive life. And the bodily invasion is very great—she requires 24 hour intensive nursing care, antibiotics, the assistance of a respirator, a catheter and feeding tube.

Our affirmation of Karen's independent right of choice, however, would ordinarily be based upon her competency to assert it. The sad truth, however, is that she is grossly incompetent and we cannot discern her supposed choice based on the testimony of her previous conversations with friends, where such testimony is without sufficient probative weight. 137 *N.J. Super.* at 260. Nevertheless we have concluded that Karen's right of privacy may be asserted on her behalf by her guardian under the peculiar circumstances here present.

If a putative decision by Karen to permit this non-cognitive, vegetative existence to terminate by natural forces is regarded as a valuable incident of her right of privacy, as we believe it to be, then it should not be discarded solely on the basis that her condition prevents her conscious exercise of the choice. The only practical way to prevent destruction of the right is to permit the guardian and family of Karen to render their best judgment, subject to the qualifications hereinafter stated, as to whether she would exercise it in these circumstances. If their conclusion is in the affirmative this decision should be accepted by a society the overwhelming majority of whose members would, we think, in similar circumstances, exercise such a choice in the same way for themselves or for those closest to them. It is for this reason that we determine that Karen's right of privacy may be asserted in her behalf, in this respect, by her guardian and family under the particular circumstances presented by this record.

· · ·

THE MEDICAL FACTOR

Having declared the substantive legal basis upon which plaintiff's rights as representative of Karen must be deemed predicated, we face and respond to the assertion on behalf of defendants that our premise unwarrantably offends prevailing medical standards. We thus turn to consideration of the medical decision supporting the determination made below, conscious of the paucity of pre-existing legislative and judicial guidance as to the rights and liabilities therein involved.

A significant problem in any discussion of sensitive medical-legal issues is the marked, perhaps unconscious, tendency of many to distort what the law is, in pursuit of an exposition of what they would like the law to be. Nowhere is this barrier to the intelligent resolution of legal controversies more obstructive than in the debate over patient rights at the end of life. Judicial refusals to order lifesaving treatment in the face of contrary claims of bodily self-determination or free religious exercise are too often cited in support of a preconceived "right to die," even though the patients, wanting to live, have claimed no such right. Conversely, the assertion of a religious or other objection to lifesaving treatment is at times condemned as attempted suicide, even though suicide means something quite different in the law. [Byrn, "Compulsory Lifesaving Treatment For The Competent Adult," 44 *Fordham L. Rev.* 1 (1975)].

Perhaps the confusion there adverted to stems from mention by some courts of statutory or common law condemnation of suicide as demonstrating the state's interest in the preservation of life. We would see, however, a real distinction between the self-infliction of deadly harm and a self-determination against artificial life support or radical surgery, for instance, in the face of irreversible, painful and certain imminent death. The contrasting situations mentioned are analogous to those continually faced by the medical profession. When does the institution of life-sustaining procedures, ordinarily mandatory, become the subject of medical discretion in the context of administration to persons *in extremis?* And when does the withdrawal of such procedures, from such persons already supported by them, come within the orbit of medical discretion? When does a determination as to either of the foregoing contingencies court the hazard of civil or criminal liability on the part of the physician or institution involved?

The existence and nature of the medical dilemma need hardly be discussed at length, portrayed as it is in the present case and complicated as it has recently come to be in view of the dramatic advance of medical technology. The dilemma is there, it is real, it is constantly resolved in accepted medical practice without

attention in the courts, it pervades the issues in the very case we here examine. The branch of the dilemma involving the doctor's responsibility and the relationship of the court's duty was thus conceived by Judge Muir:

Doctors . . . to treat a patient, must deal with medical tradition and past case histories. They must be guided by what they do know. The extent of their training, their experience, consultation with other physicians, must guide their decision-making processes in providing care to their patient. The nature, extent and duration of care by societal standards is the responsibility of a physician. The morality and conscience of our society places this responsibility in the hands of the physician. What justification is there to remove it from control of the medical profession and place it in the hands of the courts? [137 *N.J. Super.* at 259].

Such notions as to the distribution of responsibility, heretofore generally entertained, should however neither impede this Court in deciding matters clearly justiciable nor preclude a re-examination by the Court as to underlying human values and rights. Determinations as to these must, in the ultimate, be responsive not only to the concepts of medicine but also to the common moral judgment of the community at large. In the latter respect the Court has a non-delegable judicial responsibility.

Put in another way, the law, equity and justice must not themselves quail and be helpless in the face of modern technological marvels presenting questions hitherto unthought of. Where a Karen Quinlan, or a parent, or a doctor, or a hospital, or a State seeks the process and response of a court, it must answer with its most informed conception of justice in the previously unexplored circumstances presented to it. That is its obligation and we are here fulfilling it, for the actors and those having an interest in the matter should not go without remedy.

. . .

The medical obligation is related to standards and practice prevailing in the profession. The physicians in charge of the case, as noted above, declined to withdraw the respirator. That decision was consistent with the proofs

. . . [in the lower court] as to the then existing medical standards and practices. Under the law as it then stood, Judge Muir was correct in declining to authorize withdrawal of the respirator.

However, in relation to the matter of the declaratory relief sought by plaintiff as representative of Karen's interests, we are required to reevaluate the applicability of the medical standards projected in the court below. The question is whether there is such internal consistency and rationality in the application of such standards as should warrant their constituting an ineluctable bar to the effectuation of substantive relief for plaintiff at the hands of the court. We have concluded not.

In regard to the foregoing it is pertinent that we consider the impact on the standards both of the civil and criminal law as to medical liability and the new technological means of sustaining life irreversibly damaged.

The modern proliferation of substantial malpractice litigation and the less frequent but even more unnerving possibility of criminal sanctions would seem, for it is beyond human nature to suppose otherwise, to have bearing on the practice and standards as they exist. The brooding presence of such possible liability, it was testified here, had no part in the decision of the treating physicians. As did Judge Muir, we afford this testimony full credence. But we cannot believe that the stated factor has not had a strong influence on the standards, as the literature on the subject plainly reveals. (See footnote 2, *infra*). Moreover our attention is drawn not so much to the recognition by Drs. Morse and Javed of the extant practice and standards but to the widening ambiguity of those standards themselves in their application to the medical problems we are discussing.

The agitation of the medical community in the face of modern life prolongation technology and its search for definitive policy are demonstrated in the large volume of relevant professional commentary.[2]

The wide debate thus reflected contrasts with the relative paucity of legislative and judicial guides and standards in the same field. The medical profession has sought to devise guidelines such as the ''brain death'' concept of the

Harvard Ad Hoc Committee mentioned above. But it is perfectly apparent from the testimony we have quoted of Dr. Korein, and indeed so clear as almost to be judicially noticeable, that humane decisions against resuscitative or maintenance therapy are frequently a recognized *de facto* response in the medical world to the irreversible, terminal, pain-ridden patient, especially with familial consent. And these cases, of course, are far short of ''brain death.''

We glean from the record here that physicians distinguish between curing the ill and comforting and easing the dying; that they refuse to treat the curable as if they were dying or ought to die, and that they have sometimes refused to treat the hopeless and dying as if they were curable. In this sense, as we were reminded by the testimony of Drs. Korein and Diamond, many of them have refused to inflict an undesired prolongation of the process of dying on a patient in irreversible condition when it is clear that such ''therapy'' offers neither human nor humane benefit. We think these attitudes represent a balanced implementation of a profoundly realistic perspective on the meaning of life and death and that they respect the whole Judeo-Christian tradition of regard for human life. No less would they seem consistent with the moral matrix of medicine, ''to heal,'' very much in the sense of the endless mission of the law, ''to do justice.''

Yet this balance, we feel, is particularly difficult to perceive and apply in the context of the development by advanced technology of sophisticated and artificial life-sustaining devices. For those possibly curable, such devices are of great value, and, as ordinary medical procedures, are essential. Consequently, as pointed out by Dr. Diamond, they are necessary because of the ethic of medical practice. But in light of the situation in the present case (while the record here is somewhat hazy in distinguishing between ''ordinary'' and ''extraordinary'' measures), one would have to think that the use of the same respirator or like support could be considered ''ordinary'' in the context of the possibly curable patient but "extraordinary" in the context of the forced sustaining by cardio-respiratory processes of an irreversibly doomed patient. And this dilemma is sharpened in the face of the malpractice and criminal action threat which we have mentioned.

. . .

There must be a way to free physicians, in the pursuit of their healing vocation, from possible contamination by self-interest or self-protection concerns which would inhibit their independent medical judgments for the well-being of their dying patients. We would hope that this opinion might be serviceable to some degree in ameliorating the professional problems under discussion.

A technique aimed at the underlying difficulty (though in a somewhat broader context) is described by Dr. Karen Teel, a pediatrician and a director of Pediatric Education, who writes in the *Baylor Law Review* under the title "The Physician's Dilemma: A Doctor's View: What The Law Should Be." Dr. Teel recalls:

Physicians, by virtue of their responsibility for medical judgments are, partly by choice and partly by default, charged with the responsibility of making ethical judgments which we are sometimes ill-equipped to make. We are not always morally and legally authorized to make them. The physician is thereby assuming a civil and criminal liability that, as often as not, he does not even realize as a factor in his decision. There is little or no dialogue in this whole process. The physician assumes that his judgment is called for and, in good faith, he acts. Someone must and it has been the physician who has assumed the responsibility and the risk.

I suggest that it would be more appropriate to provide a regular forum for more input and dialogue in individual situations and to allow the responsibility of these judgments to be shared. Many hospitals have established an Ethics Committee composed of physicians, social workers, attorneys, and theologians, . . . which serves to review the individual circumstances of ethical dilemma and which has provided much in the way of assistance and safeguards for patients and their medical caretakers. Generally, the authority of these committees is primarily restricted to the hospital setting and their official status is more that of an advisory body than of an enforcing body.

The concept of an Ethics Committee which has this kind of organization and is readily accessible to those persons rendering medical care to patients, would be, I think, the most promising direction for further study at this point. . . .

[This would allow] some much needed dialogue regarding these issues and [force] the point of exploring all of the options for a particular patient. It diffuses the responsibility for making these judgments. Many physicians, in many circumstances, would welcome this sharing of responsibility. I believe that such an entity could lend itself well to an assumption of a legal status which would allow courses of action not now undertaken because of the concern for liability. [27 *Baylor L. Rev.* 6, 8–9 (1975)].

The most appealing factor in the technique suggested by Dr. Teel seems to us to be the diffusion of professional responsibility for decision, comparable in a way to the value of multi-judge courts in finally resolving on appeal difficult questions of law. Moreover, such a system would be protective to the hospital as well as the doctor in screening out, so to speak, a case which might be contaminated by less than worthy motivations of family or physician. In the real world and in relationship to the momentous decision contemplated, the value of additional views and diverse knowledge is apparent.

. . .

And although the deliberations and decisions which we describe would be professional in nature they should obviously include at some stage the feelings of the family of an incompetent relative. Decision-making within health care if it is considered as an expression of a primary obligation of the physician, *primum non nocere,* should be controlled primarily within the patient-doctor-family relationship, as indeed was recognized by Judge Muir in his supplemental opinion of November 12, 1975.

If there could be created not necessarily this particular system but some reasonable counterpart, we would have no doubt that such decisions, thus determined to be in accordance with medical practice and prevailing standards, would be accepted by society and by the courts, at least in cases comparable to that of Karen Quinlan.

The evidence in this case convinces us that the focal point of decision should be the prognosis as to the reasonable possibility of return to cognitive and sapient life, as distinguished from the forced continuance of that biological vegetative existence to which Karen seems to be doomed.

In summary of the present Point of this opinion, we conclude that the state of the pertinent medical standards and practices which guided the attending physicians in this matter is not such as would justify this Court in deeming itself bound or controlled thereby in responding to the case for declaratory relief established by the parties on the record before us.

ALLEGED CRIMINAL LIABILITY

Having concluded that there is a right of privacy that might permit termination of treatment in the circumstances of this case, we turn to consider the relationship of the exercise of that right to the criminal law. We are aware that such termination of treatment would accelerate Karen's death. The County Prosecutor and the Attorney General stoutly maintain that there would be criminal liability for such acceleration. Under the statutes of this State, the unlawful killing of another human being is criminal homicide. *N.J.S.A.* 2A:113–1, 2, 5. We conclude that there would be no criminal homicide in the circumstances of this case. We believe, first, that the ensuing death would not be homicide but rather expiration from existing natural causes. Secondly, even if it were to be regarded as homicide, it would not be unlawful.

These conclusions rest upon definitional and constitutional bases. The termination of treatment pursuant to the right of privacy is, within the limitations of this case, *ipso facto* lawful. Thus, a death resulting from such an act would not come within the scope of the homicide statutes proscribing only the unlawful killing of another. There is a real and in this case determinative distinction between the unlawful taking of the life of another and the ending of artificial life-support systems as a matter of self-determination.

. . .

2. *See, e.g.,* Downing, *Euthanasia and the Right to Death* (1969); St. John-Stevas, *Life, Death and the Law* (1961); Williams, *The Sanctity of Human Life and the Criminal Law* (1957); Appel, "Ethical and Legal Questions Posed by Recent Advances in Medicine," 205 *J. A. M. A.* 513 (1968); Cantor, "A Patient's Decision To Decline Life-Saving Medical Treatment: Bodily Integrity Versus The Preservation Of Life," 26 *Rutgers L.Rev.* 228 (1973); Claypool, "The Family Deals with Death," 27 *Baylor L. Rev.* 34 (1975); Elkinton, "The Dying Patient, The Doctor and The Law," 13 *Vill. L. Rev.* 740 (1968); Fletcher, "Legal Aspects of the Decision Not to Prolong Life," 203 *J. A. M. A.* 65 (1968); Foreman, "The Physician's Criminal Liability for the Practice of Euthanasia," 27 *Baylor L. Rev.* 54 (1975); Gurney, "Is There A Right To Die?—A Study of the Law of Euthanasia," 3 *Cumb.-Sam. L. Rev.* 235 (1972); Mannes, "Euthanasia vs. The Right To Life," 27 *Baylor L. Rev.* 68 (1975); Sharp & Crofts, "Death with Dignity and The Physician's Civil Liability," 27 *Baylor L. Rev.* 86 (1975); Sharpe & Hargest, "Lifesaving Treatment for Unwilling Patients," 36 *Fordham L. Rev.* 695 (1968); Skegg, "Irreversibly Comatose Individuals: 'Alive' or 'Dead'?" 33 *Camb. L.J.* 130 (1974); Comment, "The Right to Die," 7 *Houston L. Rev.* 654 (1970); Note, "The Time Of Death—A Legal, Ethical and Medical Dilemma," 18 *Catholic Law.* 243 (1972); Note, "Compulsory Medical Treatment: The State's Interest Re-evaluated," 51 *Minn. L. Rev.* 293 (1966).

SUGGESTED READINGS
FOR CHAPTER 7

Books and Articles

Beauchamp, Tom L., and Perlin, Seymour, eds. *Ethical Issues in Death and Dying.* Englewood Cliffs, N.J.: Prentice-Hall, 1978.

Behnke, John A., and Bok, Sissela, eds. *The Dilemma of Euthanasia.* Garden City, N.Y.: Doubleday Anchor, 1975.

Bok, Sissela. "Personal Directions for Care at the End of Life." *New England Journal of Medicine* 295 (August 12, 1976), 367–369.

California. "Natural Death Act." *Health and Safety Code,* Division 7, Part 1, Chapter 3.9.

Cantor, Norman. "A Patient's Decision to Decline Life-Saving Medical Treatment: Bodily Integrity versus the Preservation of Life." *Rutgers Law Review* 26 (Winter, 1972), 228–264.

Downing, A. B. *Euthanasia and the Right to Die.* New York: Humanities Press, 1970.

Dyck, Arthur. "An Alternative to the Ethic of Euthanasia." In Williams, Robert H., ed. *To Live and To Die: When, Why, and How.* New York: Springer-Verlag, 1973. Pp. 98–112.

Fletcher, Joseph. "Ethics and Euthanasia." In Williams, Robert H., ed. *To Live and To Die: When, Why, and How.* New York: Springer-Verlag, 1973. Pp. 113–122.

Gustafson, James M. "Mongolism, Parental Desires, and the Right to Life." *Perspectives in Biology and Medicine* 16 (Summer, 1973), 529–557.

Hare, R. M. "Euthanasia: A Christian View." *Philosophic Exchange* 2 (Summer, 1975), 43–52.

Kohl, Marvin, ed. *Beneficent Euthanasia.* Buffalo: Prometheus Books, 1975.

Massachusetts General Hospital, Clinical Care Committee. "Optimum Care for Hopelessly Ill Patients." *New England Journal of Medicine* 295 (August 12, 1976), 362–364.

Ramsey, Paul. "On (Only) Caring for the Dying." In his *The Patient as Person.* New Haven: Yale University Press, 1970. Pp. 113–164.

Robertson, John A., and Fost, Norman. "Passive Euthanasia of Defective Newborn Infants: Legal Considerations." *Journal of Pediatrics* 88 (May, 1976), 883–889.

Shaw, Anthony. "Dilemmas of 'Informed Consent' in Children." *New England Journal of Medicine* 289 (October 25, 1973), 885–890.

Veatch, Robert M. *Death, Dying and the Biological Revolution.* New Haven: Yale University Press, 1976.

Bibliographies

Clouser, K. Danner, and Zucker, Arthur, eds. *Abortion and Euthanasia: An Annotated Bibliography.* Philadelphia: Society for Health and Human Values, 1974.

Sollitto, Sharmon, and Veatch, Robert M., comps. *Bibliography of Society, Ethics and the Life Sciences.* Hastings-on-Hudson, N.Y.: Institute of Society, Ethics and the Life Sciences, 1976. Updated periodically. See under "Death and Dying."

Walters, LeRoy, ed. *Bibliography of Bioethics.* Vols. 1-. Detroit: Gale Research Co. Issued annually. See under "Active Euthanasia," "Allowing to Die," "Euthanasia," "Living Wills," "Prolongation of Life," "Treatment Refusal," "Voluntary Euthanasia," and "Withholding Treatment."

8.

The Allocation of Scarce Medical Resources

As medicine has expanded its services, a problem has accompanied this expansion: scarce resources have often become even scarcer. This scarcity is not simply one of expensive equipment and medicine. Highly specialized practitioners, artificial organs, blood for the treatment of hemophilia, donors for organ transplant operations, and research facilities are all in scarce supply. The basic *economic problem* is how these scarce resources may be most efficiently allocated, in the light of economic facts and predictions, in order to satisfy human needs and desires. The basic *ethical problem* is one of distributive justice: by what policies can we ensure justice in the distribution of available resources? These are not two entirely separate problems, of course. Rather, we should say that there is both an economic dimension and an ethical dimension to the problem of allocation.

The problem is further divisible into two levels, macroallocation and microallocation. At the macroallocation level, decisions are made concerning how much shall be expended for medical resources in society, as well as how it is to be distributed. Such decisions are taken by Congress, state legislatures, health organizations, private foundations, and health insurance companies. At the microallocation level, decisions are taken by particular hospital staffs or doctors concerning who shall obtain whatever resources are available. Problems at both of these levels are dicussed in this chapter.

THE PROBLEM OF MACROALLOCATION

Macroallocation decisions have recently assumed an increasing significance for the distribution of health resources, largely because federal funds and foundation grants now support the bulk of ongoing medical research and specialized treatment. Local and national health planning has also taken on added significance. There are two dimensions to such planning: (1) How much in the way of the total available money and resources should be allotted to biomedical research and clinical practice? (2) Of the amount allotted to biomedicine, how much should go to which specific projects (e.g., how much to cancer research, how much to preventive medicine, and how much to the production of expensive machines used in treatment facilities)? In order to answer such questions, one must take account both of competing medical needs and of competing nonmedical domestic needs (such as expenditures for food, housing, education, and welfare), as well as considering the needs of persons in other countries (such as the need of hundreds of thousands of food-starved people in other nations).

Ethical questions of distributive justice arise at every point in such deliberations. Consider the following examples. That there is an unequal distribution of economic resources among individual nations and among persons within these nations is a fact none would deny. But what, if anything, should be done about this inequality of distribution? Do the richer nations of the world have a moral obligation to provide more medical resources to other nations than they now provide? Should more of our own tax dollars be spent for medical purposes, and if so on what medical items? Should we distribute these medical benefits in a different way than we now distribute them? Do disadvantaged or especially needy persons have a "right" to a disproportionate amount of the available resources?

In order to answer such question, we need to determine what constitutes an economically just system of distribution. Since there are competing systems of distribution, we must decide which are the fairest. Here practical considerations such as whether the poor should receive more medical resources than they now do, whether more hospitals should be located in rural regions, and whether all citizens should have an equal amount of money expended on them each year regardless of need are all involved. In order to answer such questions in a principled rather than arbitrary way, we must resort to principles of distributive justice. Most societies use different principles of distribution in different contexts. In the United States, for example, unemployment and welfare payments are distributed on the basis of *need* (and to some extent on the basis of previous length of employment); jobs and promotions are in many sectors awarded (distributed) on the basis of demonstrated *achievement and merit;* the higher incomes of wealthy professionals are allowed (distributed) on the grounds of superior *effort or merit or social contribution* (or perhaps all three); and, at least theoretically, the opportunity for elementary and secondary education is distributed *equally to all* citizens.

The different ways of distributing resources—of which the above are instances—may be concisely stated as principles of distributive justice (a list roughly corresponding to Gene Outka's in this chapter):

1. To each person an equal share.
2. To each person according to individual need.
3. To each person according to individual effort.
4. To each person according to societal contribution.
5. To each person according to merit (individual ability).

The ethical problems of macroallocation are largely those of deciding which of these principles, if any, are the proper ones to use in distributing medical goods and services, and under what conditions they should be employed. It is noteworthy, however, that this list is not a complete one for purposes of macroallocation. The above five principles pertain largely to individuals rather than to institutions or branches of government. The principle of utility—to take one obvious example—is more frequently used for purposes of allocations to institutions. Consider a community hospital as illustrative of this point. The hospital must compete with other community institutions for tax dollars, but once that allocation has been made (perhaps using the principle of utility), hospital supplies and space may be allocated to individuals (perhaps on the basis of need).

A different, but especially urgent, issue is whether allocation for *preventive* medicine should take priority over allocation for *crisis* medicine. From one perspective, the prevention of disease by the alteration of unsanitary environments and by the provision of health information is cheaper and more efficient in raising health levels and saving lives than is crisis medicine (in the form of surgery, kidney dialysis, intensive care units, etc.). But from another perspective, a concentrated preventive approach is morally unsatisfactory if it would lead to the neglect of needy persons who could directly benefit from the resources of crisis medicine—

even if the preventive approach is more efficient in the long run in preventing disease and maintaining health. At least two aspects of this problem are apparent here. First, there is the problem of weighing maximum cost-efficiency against the costly needs of individuals. Second, there is the problem of allocation priorities when some choice must be made between preventive medicine and crisis medicine.

Finally, the question of a right to a certain level of health care is at least loosely connected to these problems of distributive justice, since it is one aspect of the moral problem of how health care should be distributed.[1] In this context a "right" is understood as an *entitlement* to some measure of health care, and not simply as a *benefit*.[2] One might support the idea of a right to *equal access* to health care, as Outka does. This approach makes a direct appeal to principles (1) and (2) in the preceding list for its justification. On the other hand, one might reject the language of equal access, as Charles Fried does, while favoring the notion of a right to a *decent minimum* of health care. (Fried's proposal is not to be understood as a right to the best possible care, since the best available treatments are often prohibitively expensive and sometimes are luxuries rather than necessities.) This decent minimum proposal cannot be directly derived from any single one of the above distributive principles. This may be because, when fully elaborated, any such proposal will make an appeal to several of the principles, or it may be because the right to health care is independent of any such scheme of principles. The decent minimum proposal is especially interesting because it raises the theoretical and practical problem of whether one can consistently, fairly, and unambiguously structure a public policy which recognizes a right to have primary human needs for health care met, but without thereby incorporating a right to exotic and intolerably expensive forms of treatment.

THE PROBLEM OF MICROALLOCATION

The outstripping of supply by demand has raised an acute microallocation problem for both ethicists and hospital administrators: Who shall receive medical resources, and who shall be denied them? In the case of certain disease treatments and medical equipment, the problems are especially acute, for here the question is, "Who shall live when not everyone can live?" Unlike contractual arrangements between patients and physicians, this question is not decided *by* the patient but *for* the patient by others. And there is direct competition between individuals for life itself, just as there is in the proverbial case of a lifeboat where some must go overboard in order that the others stay afloat. Biomedical examples requiring decisions of allocation include hemodialysis machines and both kidneys and hearts donated for transplantation. Here ethicists are called upon to construct acceptable criteria for choosing the set of patients who will live at the expense of those who will die unless treatment is provided.

To almost all who have written on this subject of scarce resources, it has seemed that reliance purely on the moral intuitions of attending physicians is insufficient, though this was often the system used for hemodialysis selection and is perhaps still the most widespread practice. While it is generally accepted that there must be an initial screening in order to determine medically acceptable patients, all further screening of those who pass the first stage must be based on nonmedical criteria. In the hope of finding a more satisfactory ethical basis for making such decisions, three prominent positions have been advanced.

1. *Complex criteria systems* Some authors have argued that a cluster of criteria should determine allocation decisions. Generally the argument has not so much been that satisfaction of one or more of these criteria is necessary in order to justify receiving treatment, but that, depending upon available resources, those who satisfy the most criteria (a quantitative consideration), especially the most important criteria (a qualitative consideration), ought to receive treatment. Possible criteria for selection include (a) medical acceptability (capacity to benefit from treatment, without complicating ailments), (b) ability to contribute either financially or perhaps experimentally as a subject of research, (c) age and life expectancy, and (d) past and potential future contributions of the patient to society. Some of these criteria are strictly utilitarian (e.g., the appeal to potential future contributions), while others appear to be deontological (e.g., the equal treatment of medical equals and the appeal to past social contributions). Those who support the use of complex criteria systems usually argue that such a system has the weight of both principles of justice and utility behind it; but there is widespread disagreement concerning the appropriateness and relative importance, if any, of these criteria. (Complex criteria systems are defended in the article by Nicholas Rescher.)

2. *Random selection systems.* Other ethicists have argued either that complex criteria systems are inherently unworkable and in all likelihood discriminatory or that such judgments reduce persons to their social roles, violate human dignity, are personally damaging to those patients on whom a negative judgment is rendered, and jeopardize the physician/patient relationship. They have argued instead either for a natural random selection system ("first come, first served") or for a formal random selection system, such as a lottery. They generally argue for such systems on the grounds that they preserve human dignity, while best implementing principles of fairness and equality of opportunity—in this case equality of opportunity for life itself. Such deontological considerations are buttressed by the claim that possible favoritism in the choice both of criteria for selection and of patients is eliminated by random procedures. (Random selection systems are defended in the article by James Childress.)

3. *No-treatment systems.* A minority, but nonetheless somewhat influential, view is that since the ethical context is one in which some must be selected to die and in which none can save himself except by intentionally allowing another to die, we ought not to select at all. Instead, treatment should be given to none, because none should live when not all can. This answer, which may seem highly implausible, is more promising when thought of as analogous to the sinking lifeboat circumstance. Some have argued that since none can be saved in such situations unless an innocent life is taken, and since it is always morally wrong to take the life of another innocent party, it would be wrong here as well. One may, of course, challenge the analogy to the lifeboat case, as well as the claim that another life is being taken by the person whose life is being saved. (A line of argument generally favorable to no-treatment systems is found in a book by Edmond Cahn, which Childress discusses.)

Whether one is considering the problem of macroallocation or the problem of microallocation, the inevitability of choice ought to be apparent. These are not moral dilemmas that can be put aside to be answered later. We have been and will be continuing for many years to operate on principles and systems which implicitly or explicitly provide an answer to the ethical questions. But are they the best answers?

T. L. B.

NOTES

1. It might be held that human rights (to health care) require the use of certain distributive principles. On the other hand, it might be held that certain distributive principles confer human rights (to health care). The problem of whether rights *or* principles of distributive justice have priority cannot be considered here.

2. Feinberg's article on ''Rights'' in Chapter 1 might be consulted at this point.

GENE OUTKA

Social Justice and Equal Access to Health Care[1]

I want to consider the following question. Is it possible to understand and to justify morally a societal goal which increasing numbers of people, including Americans, accept as normative? The goal is: the assurance of comprehensive health services for every person irrespective of income or geographic location. Indeed, the goal now has almost the status of a platitude. Currently in the United States politicians in various camps give it at least verbal endorsement (see, e.g., Nixon, 1972:1; Kennedy, 1972:234–252). I do not propose to examine the possible sociological determinants in this emergent consensus. I hope to show that whatever these determinants are, one may offer a plausible case in defense of the goal on reasonable grounds. To demonstrate why appeals to the goal get so successfully under our skins, I shall have recourse to a set of conceptions of social justice. Some of the standard conceptions, found in a number of writings on justice, will do (these writings include Bedau, 1971; Hospers, 1961:416–468; Lucas, 1972; Perelman, 1963; Rescher, 1966; Ryan, 1916; Vlastos, 1962). By reflecting on them it seems to me a prima facie case can be established, namely, that every person in the entire resident population should have equal access to health care delivery.

The case is prima facie only. I wish to set aside as far as possible a related question which comes readily enough to mind. In the world of "suboptimal alternatives," with the constraints for example which impinge on the government as it makes decisions about resource

Reprinted with permission of the publisher from the *Journal of Religious Ethics*, Vol. 2, No. 1 (Spring 1974), pp. 11–32.

allocation, what is one to say? What criteria should be employed? Paul Ramsey, in *The Patient as Person* (1970:240), thinks that the large question of how to choose between medical and other societal priorities is "almost, if not altogether, incorrigible to moral reasoning." Whether it is or not is a matter which must be ignored for the present. One may simply observe in passing that choices are unavoidable nonetheless, as Ramsey acknowledges, even where the government allows them to be made by default, so that in some instances they are determined largely by which private pressure groups prove to be dominant. In any event, there is virtue in taking up one complicated question at a time and we need to get the thrust of the case for equal access before us. It is enough to observe now that Americans attach an obviously high priority to organized health care.

.   .   .

Which then among the standard conceptions of social justice appear to be particularly relevant or irrelevant? Let us consider the following five:

I. To each according to his merit or desert.

II To each according to his societal contribution.

III. To each according to his contribution in satisfying whatever is freely desired by others in the open marketplace of supply and demand.

IV. To each according to his needs.

V. Similar treatment for similar cases.

In general I shall argue that the first three of these are less relevant because of certain distinctive features which health crises possess. I shall focus on crises here not because I think preventive care is unimportant (the opposite is true), but because the crisis situation shows most clearly the special significance we attach to medical treatment as an institutionalized activity or social practice, and the basic purpose we suppose it to have.

I

To each according to his merit or desert. Meritarian conceptions, above all perhaps, are grading ones: advantages are allocated in accordance with amounts of energy expended or kinds of results achieved. What is judged is particular conduct which distinguishes persons from one another and not only the fact that all the parties are human beings. Sometimes a competitive aspect looms large.

In certain contexts it is illuminating to distinguish between efforts and achievements. In the case of efforts one characteristically focuses on the individual: rewards are based on the pains one takes. Some have supposed, for example, that entry into the kingdom of heaven is linked more directly to energy displayed and fidelity shown than to successful results attained.

To assess achievements is to weigh actual performance and productive contributions. The academic prize is awarded to the student with the highest grade-point average, regardless of the amount of midnight oil he or she burned in preparing for the examinations. Sometimes we may exclaim, "it's just not fair," when person X writes a brilliant paper with little effort while we are forced to devote more time with less impressive results. But then our complaint may be directed against differences in innate ability and talent which no expenditure of effort altogether removes.

After the difference between effort and achievement, and related distinctions, have been acknowledged, what should be stressed I think is the general importance of meritarian or desert criteria in the thinking of most people about justice. These criteria may serve to illuminate a number of disputes about the justice of various practices and institutional arrangements in our society. It may help to explain, for instance, the resentment among the working class against the welfare system. However

wrongheaded or self-deceptive the resentment often is, particularly when directed toward those who want to work but for various reasons beyond their control cannot, at its better moments it involves in effect an appeal to desert considerations. "Something for nothing" is repudiated as unjust; benefits should be proportional (or at least related) to costs; those who can make an effort should do so, whatever the degree of their training or significance of their contribution to society; and so on. So, too, persons deserve to have what they have labored for; unless they infringe on the works of others their efforts and achievements are justly theirs.

. . .

I would simply hold now (1) that the idea of justice is not exhaustively characterized by the notion of desert, even if one agrees that the latter plays an important role; and (2) that the notion of desert is especially ill-suited to play an important role in the determination of policies which should govern a system of health care.

Why is it so ill-suited? Here we encounter some of the distinctive features which it seems to me health crises possess. Let me put it in this way. Health crises seem non-meritarian because they occur so often for reasons beyond our control or power to predict. They frequently fall without discrimination on the (according-to-merit) just and unjust, i.e., the virtuous and the wicked, the industrious and the slothful alike.

While we may believe that virtues and vices cannot depend upon natural contingencies, we are bound to admit, it seems, that many health crises do. It makes sense therefore to say that we are equal in being randomly susceptible to these crises. Even those who ascribe a prominent role to desert acknowledge that justice has also properly to do with pleas of "But I could not help it" (Lucas, 1972:321). One seeks to distinguish such cases from those acknowledged to be praiseworthy or blameworthy. Then it seems unfair as well as unkind to discriminate among those who suffer health crises on the basis of their personal deserts. For it would be odd to maintain that a newborn child deserves his hemophilia or the tumor afflicting her spine.

These considerations help to explain why the following rough distinction is often made. Bernard Williams, for example, in his discussion of "equality in unequal circumstances," identifies two different sorts of inequality, inequality of merit and inequality of need, and two corresponding goods, those earned by effort and those demanded by need (1971:126–137). Medical treatment in the event of illness is located under the umbrella of need. He concludes: "Leaving aside preventive medicine, the proper ground of distribution of medical care is ill health: this is a necessary truth" (1971:127). An irrational state of affairs is held to obtain if those whose needs are the same are treated unequally, when needs are the ground of the treatment. One might put the point this way. When people are equal in the relevant respects—in this case when their needs are the same and occur in a context of random, undeserved susceptibility—that by itself is a good reason for treating them equally (see also Nagel, 1973:354).

In many societies, however, a second necessary condition for the receipt of medical treatment exists de facto: the possession of money. This is not the place to consider the general question of when inequalities in wealth may be regarded as just. It is enough to note that one can plausibly appeal to all of the conceptions of justice we are embarked in sorting out. A person may be thought to be entitled to a higher income when he works more, contributes more, risks more, and not simply when he needs more. We may think it fair that the industrious should have more money than the slothful and the surgeon more than the tobacconist. The difficulty comes in the misfit between the reasons for differential incomes and the reasons for receiving medical treatment. The former may include a pluralistic set of claims in which different notions of justice must be meshed. The latter are more monistically focused on needs, and the other no-

tions not accorded a similar relevance. Yet money may nonetheless remain as a causally necessary condition for receiving medical treatment. It may be the power to secure what one needs. The senses in which health crises are distinctive may then be insufficiently determinative for the policies which govern the actual availability of treatment. The nearly automatic links between income, prestige, and the receipt of comparatively higher quality medical treatment should then be subjected to critical scrutiny. For unequal treatment of the rich ill and the poor ill is unjust if, again, needs rather than differential income constitute the ground of such treatment.

Suppose one agrees that it is important to recognize the misfit between the reasons for differential incomes and the reasons for receiving medical treatment, and that therefore income as such should not govern the actual availability of treatment. One may still ask whether the case so far relies excessively on "pure" instances where desert considerations are admittedly out of place. That there are such pure instances, tumors afflicting the spine, hemophilia, and so on, is not denied. Yet it is an exaggeration if we go on and regard all health crises as utterly unconnected with desert. Note for example that Williams leaves aside preventive medicine. And if in a cool hour we examine the statistics, we find that a vast number of deaths occur each year due to causes not always beyond our control, e.g., automobile accidents, drugs, alcohol, tobacco, obesity, and so on. In some final reckoning it seems that many persons (though crucially, not all) have an effect on, and arguably a responsibility for, their own medical needs. Consider the following bidders for emergency care: (1) a person with a heart attack who is seriously overweight; (2) a football hero who has suffered a concussion; (3) a man with lung cancer who has smoked cigarettes for forty years; (4) a 60 year old man who has always taken excellent care of himself and is suddenly stricken with leukemia; (5) a three year old girl who has swallowed poison left out carelessly by her parents; (6) a 14 year old boy who has been beaten without provocation by a gang and suffers brain damage and recurrent attacks of uncontrollable terror; (7) a college student who has slashed his wrists (and not for the first time) from a psychological need for attention; (8) a woman raised in the ghetto who is found unconscious due to an overdose of heroin.

These cases help to show why the whole subject of medical treatment is so crucial and so perplexing. They attest to some melancholy elements in human experience. People suffer in varying ratios the effects of their natural and undeserved vulnerabilities, the irresponsibility and brutality of others, and their own desires and weaknesses. In some final reckoning then desert considerations seem not irrelevant to many health crises. The practical applicability of this admission, however, in the instance of health care delivery, appears limited. We may agree that it underscores the importance of preventive health care by stressing the influence we sometimes have over our medical needs. But if we try to foster such care by increasing the penalties for neglect, we normally confine ourselves to calculations about incentives. At the risk of being denounced in some quarters as censorious and puritanical, perhaps we should for example levy far higher taxes on alcohol and tobacco and pump the dollars directly into health care programs rather than (say) into highway building. Yet these steps would by no means lead necessarily to a demand that we correlate in some strict way a demonstrated effort to be temperate with the receipt of privileged medical treatment as a reward. Would it be feasible to allocate the additional tax monies to the man with leukemia before the overweight man suffering a heart attack on the ground of a difference in desert? At the point of emergency care at least, it seems impracticable for the doctor to discriminate between these cases, to make meritarian judgments at the point of catastrophe. And the number of persons who are in need of medical treatment for reasons utterly beyond their control remains a datum with tenacious relevance. There are those who suffer the ravages of a tornado, are handicapped by a genetic defect, beaten without provocation, etc. A commitment to the basic purpose of medical care and to the institutions for achieving it involves the recognition of this persistent state of affairs.

II

To each according to his societal contribution. This conception gives moral primacy to notions such as the public interest, the common good, the welfare of the community, or the greatest good of the greatest number. Here one judges the social consequences of particular conduct. The formula can be construed in at least two ways (Rescher, 1966:79–80). It may refer to the interest of the social group considered collectively, where the group has some independent life all its own. The group's welfare is the decisive criterion for determining what constitutes any member's proper share. Or the common good may refer only to an aggregation of distinct individuals and considered distributively.

Either version accords such a primacy to what is socially advantageous as to be unacceptable not only to defenders of need, but also, it would seem, of desert. For the criteria of effort and achievement are often conceived along rather individualistic lines. The pains an agent takes or the results he brings about deserve recompense, whether or not the public interest is directly served. No automatic harmony then is necessarily assumed between his just share as individually earned and his proper share from the vantage point of the common good. Moreover, the test of social advantage *simpliciter* obviously threatens the agapeic concern with some mimimal consideration due each person which is never to be disregarded for the sake of long-range social benefits. No one should be considered as *merely* a means or instrument.

The relevance of the canon of social productiveness to health crises may accordingly also be challenged. Indeed, such crises may cut against it in that they occur more frequently to those whose comparative contribution to the general welfare is less, e.g., the aged, the disabled, children.

Consider for example Paul Ramsey's persuasive critique of social and economic criteria for the allocation of a single scarce medical resource. He begins by recounting the imponderables which faced the widely-discussed "public committee" at the Swedish Hospital in Seattle when it deliberated in the early 1960's. The sparse resource in this case was the kidney machine. The committee was charged with the responsibility of selecting among patients suffering chronic renal failure those who were to receive dialysis. Its criteria were broadly social and economic. Considerations weighed included age, sex, marital status, number of dependents, income, net worth, educational background, occupation, past performance and future potential. The application of such criteria proved to be exceedingly problematic. Should someone with six children always have priority over an artist or composer? Were those who arranged matters so that their families would not burden society to be penalized in effect for being provident? And so on. Two critics of the committee found "a disturbing picture of the bourgeoisie sparing the bourgeoisie" and observed that "the Pacific Northwest is no place for a Henry David Thoreau with bad kidneys" (quoted in Ramsey, 1970:248).

The mistake, Ramsey believes, is to introduce criteria of social worthiness in the first place. In those situations of choice where not all can be saved and yet all need not die, "the equal right of every human being to live, and not relative personal or social worth, should be the ruling principle" (1970:256). The principle leads to a criterion of "random choice among equals" expressed by a lottery scheme or a practice of "first-come, first-served." Several reasons stand behind Ramsey's defense of the criterion of random choice. First, a religious belief in the equality of persons before God leads intelligibly to a refusal to choose between those who are dying in any way other than random patient selection. Otherwise their equal value as human beings is threatened. Second, a moral primacy is ascribed to survival over other (perhaps superior) interests persons may have, in that it is the condition of everything else. ". . . Life is a value incommensurate with all others, and so not negotiable by bartering one man's worth against another's" (1970:256). Third, the entire enterprise of estimating a person's social worth is viewed with final skepticism. ". . . We have no way of knowing how really and truly to estimate a man's societal worth or his worth to others or to himself in unfocused social situations in the ordinary lives of men in their communities" (1970:256). This statement, incidentally, appears to allow something other than randomness in *focused* social situations; when, say, a President or Prime Minister and the owner of the local bar rush for the last place in the bomb shelter, and the knowledge of the former can save many lives. In any event, I have been concerned with a restricted point to which Ramsey's discussion brings illustrative support. The canon of social productiveness is notoriously difficult to apply as a workable criterion for distributing medical services to those who need them.

One may go further. A system of health care delivery which treats people on the basis of the medical care required may often go against (at least narrowly conceived) calculations of societal advantage. For example, the health care needs of people tend to rise during that period of their lives, signaled by retirement, when their incomes and social productivity are declining. More generally:

> Some 40 to 50 percent of the American people—the aged, children, the dependent poor, and those with some significant chronic disability are in categories requiring relatively large amounts of medical care but with inadequate resources to purchase such care. (Somers, 1971a:20)

If one agrees, for whatever reasons, with the agapeic judgment that each person should be regarded as irreducibly valuable, then one cannot succumb to a social productiveness criterion of human worth. Interests are to be equally considered even when people have ceased to be, or are not yet, or perhaps never will be, public assets.

III

To each according to his contribution in satisfying whatever is freely desired by others in the open marketplace of supply and demand. Here we have a test which, though similar to the preceding one, concentrates on what is desired de facto by certain segments of the community rather than the community as a whole, and on the relative scarcity of the service rendered. It is tantamount to the canon of supply and demand as espoused by various laissez-faire theoreticians (cf. Rescher, 1966:80–81). Rewards should be given to those who by virtue of special skill, prescience, risk-taking, and the like discern what is desired and are able to take the requisite steps to bring satisfaction. A surgeon, it may be argued, contributes more than a nurse because of the greater training and skill required, burdens borne, and effective care provided, and should be compensated accordingly. So too perhaps, a star quarter-back on a pro-football team should be remunerated even more highly because of the rare athletic prowess needed, hazards involved, and widespread demand to watch him play.

This formula does not then call for the weighing of the value of various contributions, and tends to conflate needs and wants under a notion of desires. It also assumes that a prominent part is assigned to consumer free-choice. The consumer should be at liberty to express his preferences, and to select from a variety of competing goods and services. Those who resist many changes currently proposed in the organization and financing of health care delivery in the U.S.A.—such as national health insurance—often do so by appealing to some variant of this formula.

Yet it seems health crises are often of overriding importance when they occur. They appear therefore not satisfactorily accommodated to the context of a free marketplace where consumers may freely choose among alternative goods and services.

To clarify what is at stake in the above contention, let us examine an opposing case. Robert M. Sade, M.D., published an article in *The New England Journal of Medicine* entitled "Medical Care as a Right: A Refutation" (1971). He attacks programs of national health insurance in the name of a person's right to select one's own values, determine how they may be realized, and dispose of them if one chooses without coercion from other men. The values in question are construed as economic ones in the context of supply and demand. So we read:

In a free society, man exercises his right to sustain his own life by producing economic values in the form of goods and services that he is, or should be, free to exchange with other men who are similarly free to trade with him or not. The economic values produced, however, are not given as gifts by nature, but exist only by virtue of the thought and effort of individual men. Goods and services are thus owned as a consequence of the right to sustain life by one's own physical and mental effort. (1971:1289)

Sade compares the situation of the physician to that of the baker. The one who produces a loaf of bread should as owner have the power to dispose of his own product. It is immoral simply to expropriate the bread without the baker's permission. Similarly, "medical care is neither a right nor a privilege: it is a service that is provided by doctors and others to people who wish to purchase it" (1971:1289). Any coercive regulation of professional practices by the society at large is held to be analogous to taking the bread from the baker without his consent. Such regulation violates the freedom of the physician over his own services and will lead inevitably to provider-apathy.

The analogy surely misleads. To assume that doctors autonomously produce goods and services in a fashion closely akin to a baker is grossly oversimplified. The baker may himself rely on the agricultural produce of others, yet there is a crucial difference in the degree of dependence. Modern physicians depend on the achievements of medical technology and the entire scientific base underlying it, all of which is made possible by a host of persons whose salaries are often notably less. Moreover, the amount of taxpayer support for medical research and education is too enormous to make any such unqualified case for provider-autonomy plausible.

· · ·

For much of the way, then, an appeal to supply and demand and consumer choice is not quite fitting. It neglects the issue of the value of various contributions. And it fails to allow for the recognition that medical treatments may be overridingly desired. In contexts of catastrophe at any rate, when life itself is threatened, most persons (other than those who are apathetic or seek to escape from the terrifying prospects) cannot take medical care to be merely one option among others.

IV

To each according to his needs. The concept of needs is sometimes taken to apply to an entire range of interests which concern a person's "psycho-physical existence" (Outka, 1972:esp. 264-265). On this wide usage, to attribute a need to someone is to say that the person lacks what is thought to conduce to his or her "welfare"—understood in both a physiological sense (e.g., for food, drink, shelter, and health) and a psychological one (e.g., for continuous human affection and support).

Yet even in the case of such a wide usage, what the person lacks is typically assumed to be basic. Attention is restricted to recurrent considerations rather than to every possible individual whim or frivolous pursuit. So one is not surprised to meet with the contention that a preferable rendering of this formula would be: "to each according to his essential needs" (Perelman, 1963:22). This contention seems to me well taken. It implies, for one thing, that basic needs are distinguishable from felt needs or wants. For the latter may encompass expressions of personal preference unrelated to considerations of survival or subsistence, and sometimes artifically generated by circumstances of rising affluence in the society at large.

Essential needs are also typically assumed to be given rather than acquired. They are not constituted by any action for which the person is responsible by virtue of his or her distinctively greater effort. It is almost as if the designation "innocent" may be linked illuminatingly to need, as retribution, punishment, and so on, are to desert, and in complex ways, to freedom. Thus essential needs are likewise distinguishable from deserts. Where needs are unequal, one thinks of them fortuitously distributed; as part, perhaps, of a kind of "natural lottery" (see Rawls, 1971:e.g., 104). So very often the advantages of health and the burdens of illness, for example, strike one as arbitrary effects of the lottery. It seems wrong to say that a newborn child deserves as a reward all of his faculties when he has done nothing in particular which distinguishes him from another newborn who comes into the world deprived of one or more of them. Similarly, though crudely, many religious believers do not look on natural events as personal deserts. They are not inclined to pronounce sentences such as "That evil person with incurable cancer got what he deserved." They are disposed instead to search for some distinction between what they may call the conditions of finitude on the one hand and sin and moral evil on the other. If the distinction is "ultimately" invalid, in this life it seems inscrutably so. Here and now it may be usefully drawn. Inequalities in the need for medical treatment are taken, it appears, to reflect the conditions of finitude more than anything else.

One can even go on to argue that among our basic or essential needs, the case of medical treatment is conspicuous in the following sense. While food and shelter are not matters about which we are at liberty to please ourselves, they are at least predictable. We can plan, for instance, to store up food and fuel for the winter. It may be held that responsibility increases along with the power to predict. If so, then many health crises seem peculiarly random and uncontrollable. Cancer, given the present state of knowledge at any rate, is a contingent disaster, whereas hunger is a steady threat. Who will need serious medical care, and when, is then perhaps a classic example of uncertainty.

. . .

Justice has properly to do with pleas of "But I could not help it." It seeks to distinguish such cases from those acknowledged to be praiseworthy or blameworthy. The formula "to each according to his needs" is one cogent way of identifying the moral relevance of these pleas. To ignore them may be thought to be unfair as well as unkind when they arise from the deprivation of some essential need. The move to confine the notion of justice wholly to desert considerations is thereby resisted as well. Hence we may say that sometimes "questions of social justice arise just because people are unequal in ways they can do very little to change and . . . only by attending to these inequalities can one be said to be giving their interests equal consideration" (Benn, 1971:164).

V

Similar treatment for similar cases. This conception is perhaps the most familiar of all. Certainly it is the most formal and inclusive one. It is frequently taken as an elementary appeal to consistency and linked to the universalizability test. One should not make an arbitrary exception on one's own behalf, but rather should apply impartially whatever standards one accepts. The conception can be fruitfully applied to health care questions and I shall assume its relevance. Yet as literally interpreted, it is necessary but not sufficient. For rightly or not, it is often held to be as compatible with no positive treatment whatever as with active promotion of other peoples' interests, as long as all are equally and impartially included. Its exponents sometimes assume such active promotion without demonstrating clearly how this is built into the conception itself. Moreover, it may obscure a distinction which we have seen agapists and others make: between equal consideration and identical treatment. Needs may differ and so treatments must, if benefits are to be equalized.

I have placed this conception at the end of the list partly because it moves us, despite its formality, toward practice. Let me suggest briefly how it does so. Suppose first of all one agrees with the case so far offered. Suppose, that is, it has been shown convincingly that a need-conception of justice applies with greater relevance than the earlier three when one reflects about the basic purpose of medical care. To treat one class of people differently from another because of income or geographic location should therefore be ruled out, because such reasons are irrelevant. (The irrelevance is conceptual, rather than always, unfortunately, causal.) In short, all persons should have equal access, "as needed, without financial, geo-

graphic, or other barriers, to the whole spectrum of health services" (Somers and Somers, 1972a:122).

Suppose however, secondly, that the goal of equal access collides on some occasions with the realities of finite medical resources and needs which prove to be insatiable. That such collisions occur in fact it would be idle to deny. And it is here that the practical bearing of the formula of similar treatment for similar cases should be noticed. Let us recall Williams' conclusion: "the proper ground of distribution of medical care is ill health: this is a necessary truth." While I agree with the essentials of his argument—for all the reasons above—I would prefer, for practical purposes, a slightly more modest formulation. Illness is the proper ground for the *receipt* of medical care. However, the *distribution* of medical care in less-than-optimal circumstances requires us to face the collisions. I would argue that in such circumstances the formula of similar treatment for similar cases may be construed so as to guide actual choices in the way most compatible with the goal of equal access. The formula's allowance of no positive treatment whatever may justify exclusion of entire classes of cases from priority list. Yet it forbids doing so for irrelevant or arbitrary reasons. So (1) if we accept the case for equal access, but (2) if we simply cannot, physically cannot, treat all who are in need, it seems more just to discriminate by virtue of categories of illness, for example, rather than between the rich ill and poor ill. All persons with a certain rare, non-communicable disease would not receive priority, let us say, where the costs were inordinate, the prospects for rehabilitation remote, and for the sake of equalized benefits to many more. Or with Ramsey we may urge a policy of random patient selection when one must decide between claimants for a medical treatment unavailable to all. Or we may acknowledge that any notion of "comprehensive benefits" to which persons should have equal access is subject to practical restrictions which will vary from society to society depending on resources at a given time. Even in a country as affluent as the United States there will surely always be items excluded, e.g., perhaps over-the-counter drugs, some teenage orthodontia, cosmetic surgery, and the like (Somers and Somers, 1972b:182). Here too the formula of similar treatment for similar cases may serve to modify the application of a need-conception of justice in order to address the insatiability-problem and limit frivolous use. In all of the foregoing instances of restriction, however, the relevant feature remains the illness, discomfort, etc. itself. The goal of equal access then retains its prima facie authoritativeness. It is imperfectly realized rather than disregarded.

VI

These latter comments lead on to the question of institutional implications. I cannot aim here of course for the specificity rightly sought by policy-makers. My endeavor has been conceptual elucidation. While the ethicist needs to be apprised about the facts, he or she does not, qua ethicist, don the mantle of the policy-expert. In any case, only rarely does anyone do both things equally well. Yet cross-fertilization is extremely desirable. For experts should not be isolated from the wider assumptions their recommendations may reflect. I shall merely list some of the topics which would have to be discussed at length if we were to get clear about the implications. Examples will be limited to the current situation in the United States.

Anyone who accepts the case for equal access will naturally be concerned about de facto disparities in the availability of medical treatment. Let us consider two relevant indictments of current American practice. They appear in the writings not only of those who attack indiscriminately a system seen to be governed only by the appetite for profit and power, but also of those who denounce in less sweeping terms and espouse more cautiously reformist positions. The first shortcoming has to do with the maldistribution of supply. Per capita ratios of physicians to populations served vary, sometimes notoriously, between affluent suburbs and rural and inner city areas.

This problem is exacerbated by the distressing data concerning the greater health needs of the poor. Chronic disease, frequency and duration of hospitalization, psychiatric disorders, infant death rates, etc.—these occur in significantly larger proportions to lower income members of American society (Appel, 1970; Hubbard, 1970). A further complication is that "the distribution of health insurance coverage is badly skewed. Practically all the rich have insurance. But among the poor, about two-thirds have none. As a result, among people aged 25 to 64 who die, some 45 to 50 per cent have neither hospital nor surgical coverage" (Somers, 1971a:46). This last point connects with a second shortcoming frequently cited. Even those who are otherwise economically independent may be shattered by the high cost of a "catastrophic illness" (see some eloquent examples in Kennedy, 1972).

Proposals for institutional reforms designed to overcome such disparities are bound to be taken seriously by any defender of equal access. What he or she will be disposed to press for, of course, is the removal of any double standard or "two class" system of care. The viable procedures for bringing this about are not obvious, and comparisons with certain other societies (for relevant alternative models) are drawn now with perhaps less confidence (see Anderson, 1973). One set of commonly discussed proposals includes (1) incentive subsidies to physicians, hospitals, and medical centers to provide services in regions of poverty (to overcome in part the unwillingness—to which no unique culpability need be ascribed—of many providers and their spouses to work and live in grim surroundings); (2) licensure controls to avoid comparatively excessive concentrations of physicians in regions of affluence; (3) a period of time (say, two years) in an underserved area as a requirement for licensing; (4) redistribution facilities which allow for population shifts.

A second set of proposals is linked with health insurance itself. While I cannot venture into the intricacies of medical economics or comment on the various bills for national health insurance presently inundating Congress, it may be instructive to take brief note of one proposal in which, once more, the defender of equal access is bound to take an interest (even if he or she finally rejects it on certain practical grounds). The precise details of the proposal are unimportant for our purposes (for one much-discussed version, see Feldstein, 1971). Consider this crude sketch. Each citizen is (in effect) issued a card by the government. Whenever "legitimate" medical expenses (however determined for a given society) exceed, say, 10 per cent of his or her annual taxable income, the card may be presented so that additional costs incurred will be paid for out of general tax revenues. The reasons urged on behalf of this sort of arrangement include the following. In the case of medical care there is warrant for proportionately equalizing what is spent from anyone's total taxable income. This warrant reflects the conditions, discussed earlier, of the natural lottery. Insofar as the advantages of health and the burdens of illness are random and undeserved, we may find it in our common interest to share risks. A fixed percentage of income attests to the misfit, also mentioned previously, between the reasons for differential total income and the reasons for receiving medical treatment. If money remains a causally necessary condition for receiving medical treatment, then a way must be found to place it in the hands of those who need it. The card is one such means. It is designed effectively to equalize purchasing power. In this way it seems to accord nicely with the goal of equal access. On the other side, the requirement of initial out-of-pocket expenses—sufficiently large in comparison to average family expenditures on health care—is designed to discourage frivolous use and foster awareness that medical care is a benefit not to be simply taken as a matter of course. It also safeguards against an excessively large tax burden while providing universal protection against the often disastrous costs of serious illnesses. Whether 10 per cent is too great a chunk for the very poor to pay, and whether by itself the proposal will feed price inflation and neglect of preventive medicine are questions which would have to be answered.

Another kind of possible institutional reform will also greatly interest the defender of equal access. This has to do with the "design of health care systems" or "care settings." The prevalent setting in American society has always been "fee-for-service." It is left up to each person to obtain the requisite care and to pay for it as he or she goes along. Because costs for medical treatment have accelerated at such an alarming rate, and because the sheer diffusion of energy and effort so characteristic of American medical practice leaves more and more people dissatisfied, alternatives to fee-for-service have been considered of late with unprecedented seriousness. The alternative care setting most widely discussed is prepaid practice, and specifically the "health maintenance organization" (HMO). Here one finds "an organized system of care which accepts the responsibility to provide or otherwise assure comprehensive care to a defined population for a fixed periodic payment per person or per family . . ." (Somers, 1971b:v). The best-known HMO is the Kaiser-Permanente Medical Care Program (see also Garfield, 1971). Does the HMO serve to realize the goal of equal access more fully? One line of argument in its favor is this. It is plausible to think that equal access will be fostered by the more economical care setting. HMO's are held to be less costly per capita in at least two respects: hospitalization rates are much below the national average; and less often noted, physician manpower is as well. To be sure, one should be sensitive to the corruptions in each type of setting. While fee-for-service has resulted in a suspiciously high number of surgeries (twice as many per capita in the United States as in Great Britain), the HMO physician may more frequently permit the patient's needs to be overridden by the organization's pressure to economize. It may also be more difficult in an HMO setting to provide for close personal relations between a particular physician and a particular patient (something commended, of course, on all sides). After such corruptions are allowed for, the data seem encouraging to such an extent that a defender of equal access will certainly support the repeal of any law which limits the development of prepaid practice, to approve of "front aid" subsidies for HMO's to increase their number overall and achieve a more equitable distribution throughout the country, and so on. At a minimum, each care setting should be available in every region. If we assume a common freedom to choose between them, each may help to guard against the peculiar temptations to which the other is exposed.

To assess in any serious way proposals for institutional reform such as the above is beyond the scope of this paper. We would eventually be led, for example, into the question of whether it is consistent for the rich to pay more than the poor for the same treatment when, again, needs rather than income constitute the ground of the treatment (Ward, 1973), and from there into the tangled subject of the "ethics of redistribution" in general (see, e.g., Benn and Peters, 1965:155–178; de Jouvenal, 1952). Other complex issues deserve to be considered as well, e.g., the criteria for allocation of limited resources,[2] and how conceptions of justice apply to the providers of health care.[3]

Those committed to self-conscious moral and religious reflection about subjects in medicine have concentrated, perhaps unduly, on issues about care of individual patients (as death approaches, for instance). These issues plainly warrant the most careful consideration. One would like to see in addition, however, more attention paid to social questions in medical ethics. To attend to them is not necessarily to leave behind all of the matters which reach deeply into the human condition. Any detailed case for institutional reforms, for example, will be enriched if the proponent asks soberly whether certain conflicts and certain perplexities allow for more than partial improvements and provisional resolutions. Can public and private interests ever be made fully to coincide by legislative and administrative means? Will the commitment of a physician to an individual patient and the commitment of the legislator to the "common good" ever be harmonized in every case? Our anxiety may be too intractable. Our fear of illness and of dying may be so pronounced and immediate that we will seize the nearly automatic connections between privilege, wealth, and power if we can. We will do everything possible to have our kidney machines even if the charts make it clear that many more would benefit from mandatory immunization at a fraction of the cost. And our capacity for taking in rival points of view may be too limited. Once we have witnessed tangible suffering, we cannot just return with ease to public policies aimed at statistical patients. Those who believe that justice is the pre-eminent virtue of institutions and that a case can be convincingly made on behalf of justice for equal access to health care would do well to ponder such conflicts and perplexities. Our reforms might then seem, to ourselves and to others, less abstract and jargon-filled in formulation and less sanguine and piecemeal in substance. They would reflect a greater awareness of what we have to confront.

NOTES

1. Much of the research for this paper was done during the Fall Term, 1972–73, when I was on leave in Washington, D.C. I am very grateful for the two appointments which made this leave possible: as Service Fellow, Office of Special Projects, Health Services and Mental Health Administration, Department of Health, Education, and Welfare; and as Visiting Scholar, Kennedy Institute, Georgetown University.

2. The issue of priorities is at least threefold: (1) between improved medical care and other social needs, e.g., to restrain auto accidents and pollution; (2) between different sorts of medical treatments for different illnesses, e.g., prevention vs. crisis intervention and exotic treatments; (3) between persons all of whom need a single scarce resource and not all can have it, e.g., Ramsey's discussion of how to decide among those who are to receive dialysis.

3. What sorts of appeals to justice might be cogently made to warrant, for instance, the differentially high income physicians receive? Here are three possibilities: (1) the greater skill and responsibility involved should be rewarded proportionately, i.e., one should attend to considerations of *desert;* (2) there should be *compensation* for the money invested for education and facilities in order to restore circumstances of approximate equality (this argument, while a common one in medical circles, would need to consider that medical education is received in part at public expense and that the modern physician is the highest paid professional in the country); (3) the difference should benefit the least advantaged more than an alternative arrangement where disparities are less. We prefer a society where the medical profession flourishes and everyone has a longer life expectancy to one where everyone is poverty-stricken with a shorter life expectancy ("splendidly equalized destitution"). Yet how are we to ascertain the minimum degree of differential income required for the least advantaged members of the society to be better off?

Discussions of "justice and the interests of providers" are, I think, badly needed. Physicians in the United States have suffered a decline in prestige for various reasons, e.g., the way many used Medicare to support and increase their own incomes. Yet one should endeavor to assess their interests fairly. A concern for professional autonomy is clearly important, though one may ask whether adequate attention has been paid to the distinction between the imposition of cost-controls from outside and interference with professional medical judgments. One may affirm the former, it seems, and still reject—energetically—the latter.

REFERENCES

Anderson, Odin. *Health Care: Can There Be Equity? The United States, Sweden and England.* New York: Wiley, 1973.

Appel, James Z. "Health care delivery." Pp. 141–166 in Boisfeuillet Jones (ed.), *The Health of Americans.* Englewood Cliffs, N.J.: Prentice-Hall, Inc., 1970.

Bedau, Hugo A. "Radical egalitarianism." Pp. 168–180 in Hugo A. Bedau (ed.), *Justice and Equality.* Englewood Cliffs, N.J.: Prentice-Hall, Inc., 1971.

Benn, Stanley I. "Egalitarianism and the equal consideration of interests." Pp. 152–167 in Hugo A. Bedau (ed.), *Justice and Equality.* Englewood Cliffs, N.J.: Prentice-Hall, Inc., 1971.

Benn, Stanley I. and Richard S. Peters. *The Principles of Political Thought.* New York: The Free Press, 1965.

de Jouvenel, Bertrand. *The Ethics of Redistribution.* Cambridge: University Press, 1952.

Feldstein, Martin S. "A new approach to national health insurance." *The Public Interest* 23 (Spring 1971):93–105.

Garfield, Sidney R. "Prevention of dissipation of health services resources." *American Journal of Public Health* 61:1499–1506, 1971.

Hicks, Nancy. "Nation's doctors move to police medical care." Pp. 1, 52 in *New York Times,* Sunday, October 28, 1973.

Honoré, A. M. "Social justice." Pp. 61–94 In Robert S. Summers (ed.), *Essays in Legal Philosophy.* Oxford: Basil Blackwell, 1968.

Hospers, John. *Human Conduct.* New York: Harcourt, Brace and World, Inc., 1961.

Hubbard, William N. "Health knowledge." Pp. 93–120 in Boisfeuillet Jones (ed.), *The Health of Americans.* Englewood Cliffs, N.J.: Prentice-Hall, Inc., 1970.

Kennedy, Edward M. *In Critical Condition: The Crisis in America's Health Care.* New York: Simon and Schuster, 1972.

Lucas, J. R. "Justice." *Philosophy* 47, No. 181 (July 1972):229–248.

Nagel, Thomas. "Equal treatment and compensatory discrimination." *Philosophy and Public Affairs* 2, No. 4 (Summer 1973): 348–363.

Nixon, Richard M. "President's message on health care system." Document No. 92–261 (March 2, 1972). House of Representatives, Washington, D.C.

Outka, Gene. *Agape: An Ethical Analysis.* New Haven and London: Yale University Press, 1972.

Perelman, Ch. *The Idea of Justice and the Problem of Argument.* Trans. John Petrie. London: Routledge and Kegan Paul, 1963.

Ramsey, Paul. *The Patient as Person.* New Haven and London: Yale University Press, 1970.

Rawls, John. *A Theory of Justice.* Cambridge, Mass.: Harvard University Press, 1971.

Rescher, Nicholas. *Distributive Justice.* Indianapolis: The Bobbs-Merrill Company, Inc., 1966.

Ryan, John A. *Distributive Justice.* New York: The Macmillan Company, 1916.

Sade, Robert M. "Medical care as a right: a refutation." *The New England Journal of Medicine* 285 (December 1971):1288–1292.

Schultze, Charles L., Edward R. Fried, Alice M. Rivlin and Nancy H. Teeters. *Setting National Priorities: The 1973 Budget.* Washington, D.C.: The Brookings Institution, 1972.

Somers, Anne R. *Health Care in Transition: Directions for the Future.* Chicago: Hospital Research and Educational Trust, 1971.

——— (ed.). *The Kaiser-Permanente Medical Care Program.* New York: The Commonwealth Fund, 1971.

Somers, Anne R. and Herman M. Somers. "The organization and financing of health care: issues and directions for the future." *American Journal of Orthopsychiatry* 42 (January 1972): 119–136.

——— and ———. "Major issues in national health insurance." *Milbank Memorial Fund Quarterly* 50, No. 2, Part 1 (April 1972):177–210.

Vlastos, Gregory. "Justice and equality." Pp. 31–72 in Richard B. Brandt (ed.), *Social Justice.* Englewood Cliffs, N.J.: Prentice-Hall, Inc., 1962.

Ward, Andrew. "The idea of equality reconsidered." *Philosophy* 48 (January 1973):85–90.

Williams, Bernard A. O. "The idea of equality." Pp. 116–137 in Hugo A. Bedau (ed.), *Justice and Equality.* Englewood Cliffs, N.J.: Prentice-Hall, Inc., 1971.

CHARLES FRIED

Equality and Rights in Medical Care

In this article I present arguments intended to support the following conclusions:

1. To say there is a right to health care does not imply a right to equal access, a right that whatever is available to any shall be available to all.

2. The slogan of equal access to the best health care available is just that, a dangerous slogan which could be translated into reality only if we submitted either to intolerable government controls of medical practice or to a thoroughly unreasonable burden of expense.

3. There is sense to the notion of a right to a decent standard of care for all, dynamically defined, but still not dogmatically equated with the best available.

4. We are far from affording such a standard to many of our citizens and that is profoundly wrong.

5. One of the major sources of the exaggerated demands for equality are the pretensions, inflated claims, inefficiencies, and guildlike, monopolistic practices of the health professions.

I. BACKGROUND

The notion of some kind of a right to health care is not likely to be found in any but the most recent writings, not to mention legislation. After all, even the much more well-established institution of free, universal public education has not achieved the status of a federal constitutional right, is not a constitutional right by the law of many states, and stands as a right more as an inference from the practices and legislation of states, counties, and municipalities. The federal constitutional litigation regarding rights in that area has been restricted to the provision *equally* of whatever public education is in fact provided. So it should not be surprising that the notion of a right to health care is

Reprinted with permission of the author from *Hastings Center Report,* Vol. 6 (February 1976), pp. 29–34.

something of a novelty. Moreover, it is only fairly recently that health care could deliver a product which was as unambiguously beneficial as elementary schooling. Nevertheless, if one looks to the laws, practices, and understandings of states, counties, and municipalities, one sees growing up through the last century, and certainly in the twentieth century, an understanding which might be thought of as the inchoate recognition of a right to health care. Indeed, there are those who might say that such an inchoate recognition might be discerned as far back as Elizabethan England.

As one considers this progress, one should not misrepresent history, for in that history lies an important lesson. For the progress may represent not simply a progress in our ideas of social justice, but a progress in what medicine could do. The fact is that the increasingly general provision of medical care may be correlated as well with what medical care could accomplish as with any changing social doctrines. What could medicine accomplish a hundred or even fifty years ago? It is well known that the improvements in health that were wrought in those days were largely the result of improved sanitation, working conditions, diet, and the like. Beyond that, specifically medical ministrations could do very little. They could provide ease, amenities, relief, but rarely a cure. So society may be forgiven if it did not provide elaborate medical care to the poor until recently, since provision of medical care in essence would have meant simply the provision of amenities and placebos. And since society appeared little concerned to assure the amenities to its poor generally, it is no great surprise that it had scant inclination to provide these amenities to the sick poor.

The detailed history of the extension of medical care to the poor, and indeed to those who were not poor but lived in out-of-the-way places, has yet to be written. The emergence of a notion of a right to health care and the embodiment of such a notion in legislation and court decisions must also await difficult historical research. Nevertheless, it is worth noting that, at least in American public discourse, the idea of a right to medical care developed into something which had the appearance of inevitability only recently, in what might be called the intermediate, perhaps golden, age of modern medicine. This was a period when advances in treating acute illness, advances such as the antibiotics, could really make a large difference in prolonging life or restoring health; but the most elaborate technologies which may make only marginal improvements in situations previously thought to be hopeless had not yet been generally developed. In this recent "Golden Age" we could unambiguously afford a notion of a general right to medical care because there were a number of clear successes available to medicine, and these successes were not unduly costly. Having conquered the infectious diseases, medical science has undertaken the degenerative diseases, the malignant neoplasms, and the diseases of unknown etiology; and one must say that the ratio between expense and benefit has become exponentially more unfavorable. So it is really only now that the notion of a right to health care poses acute analytical and social problems. It is for that reason that neither history nor legal analysis will much illuminate our future course. What we do now will be a matter of our choosing, and for this reason careful analysis of the notion of a right to health care is crucial.

II. EQUALITY AND RIGHTS: ANALYTICAL DISTINCTIONS

First, something should be said by way of at least informal definition of this term "right." A right is more than just an interest that an individual might have, a state of affairs or a state of being which an individual might prefer. A claim of right invokes entitlements; and when we speak of entitlements, we mean not those things which it would be nice for people to have, or which they would prefer to have, but which they must have, and which if they do not

have they may demand, whether we like it or not. Although I would not want to say that a right is something we must recognize "no matter what," nevertheless a right is something we must accord unless _____ and what we put in to fill in the unless clause should be tightly confined and specific.

This notion of rights has interesting and not altogether obvious relations to the concept of equality, and confusions about those relations are very likely to lead to confused arguments about the very area before us—rights to health care and equality in respect to health care.

First, it should be noted that equality itself may be considered a right. Thus, a person can argue that he is not necessarily entitled to any particular thing—whether it be income, or housing, or education, or health care—but that he is entitled to equality in respect to that thing, so that whatever anyone gets he should get, too. And this is a nice example of my previous proposition about the notion of rights generally. For to recognize a right to equality may very well be—I suppose it often is—contrary to many other policies that we may have, and particularly contrary to attempts to attain some kind of efficiency. Yet, by the very notion of rights, if there is a right to equality, then granting equality cannot depend on whether or not it is efficient to do so.

Second, there is the relation between rights and equality which runs the other way, too: to say that a class of persons, or all persons, have a certain right implies that they all have that right equally. If it is said that all persons within the jurisdiction of the United States have a constitutionally protected right to freedom of speech, whatever that may mean, one thing seems clear: that this right should not depend on what it is one wants to say, who one is, and the like. Indeed, if the government against whom this right is protected were to make such distinctions, for instance, subjecting to constraints the speech of "irresponsible persons," that would be the exact concept of denial of freedom of speech to those persons.

These relations between the notion of right and of equality suggest the great importance of being very clear and precise about how a particular right is conceived: confusions in this regard are rampant in respect to health, and are the source of much pointless controversy. But because the point is quite general, let me first take an example from another area. If we were sloppy in our thinking about what the right of freedom of speech is—and many people are as sloppy about that as they are about their definition of the rights in the area which is our immediate concern—if we were sloppy about that definition, we might, for instance, consider that there has been a denial of right because some people have access to radio or television in getting their ideas across, while others have only the street-corner soapbox to broadcast their views. Indeed, there are those who might find it unjust that even on the soapbox the timid or inarticulate are much less effective than the bold or eloquent. All of these disparities, of course, may or may not be regrettable but they have nothing to do with freedom of speech as a right, given the premise that there is a right to free speech and that this right must be an equal right. It seems clear to me that it is very different from the right to be heard, believed, admired, and applauded. The right to speak freely is just that: a right to be free of constraints and impositions on whatever speaking one might wish to do, should you be able to find someone to listen.

Now this analogy is offered as more than a distant irrelevance. Is it not very similar to many things that are said in the area of health? For analogous to the claim that the right to freedom of speech really implies a right to be heard by the multitude, is the notion that whatever rights might exist in respect to health care are rights to health, rather than to health *care*. And of course the claim is equally absurd in both instances. We may sensibly guarantee that all will be equally free of constraints on the speaking they wish to do, but we should not guarantee that all will be equally effective in getting their views across. Similarly, we may or may not choose to guarantee all equality of access to health care, but we cannot possibly guarantee to all equality of health.

Consider how these clarifications operate upon the historical development I alluded to at the beginning of this analysis. The right whose recognition might be said to have been implicit in social practices throughout the past hundred years was a right not to health care as such, nor yet a right to health, but rather a right to a certain standard of health care, which was defined in terms of what medicine could reasonably do for people. It is this notion which has become so difficult in our present situation, where the apparatus of medicine has become so much more elaborate, pretentious, and costly than it was in earlier times.

Bringing together the historical and the analytical sides, we might conclude that our present dilemma comes from the fact that there are very many expensive things that medicine can do which might possibly help. And if we commit ourselves to the notion that there is a right to whatever health care might be available, we do indeed get ourselves into a difficult situation where overall national expenditure on health must reach absurd proportions—absurd in the sense that far more is devoted to health at the expense of other important social goals than the population in general wants. Indeed, more is devoted to health than the population wants relative not only to important social goals—for example, education or housing—but relative to all the other things which people would like to have money left over to pay for. And if we recognize that it would be absurd to commit our society to devote more than a certain proportion of our national income to health, while at the same time recognizing a "right to health care," we might then be caught on the other horn of the dilemma. For we might then be required to say that because a right to health care implies a right to equality of health care, then we must limit, we must lower the quality of the health care that might be purchased by some lest our commitment to equality require us to provide such care to all and thus carry us over a reasonable budget limit.

Consider the case of the artificial heart. It seems to me not too fanciful an assumption that such a device is technically feasible within a reasonable time, and likely to be hugely expensive both in terms of its actual implantation and in terms of the subsequent care required by those benefiting from the device. Now if the right to health care is taken to mean the right to whatever health care is available to anybody, and if this entails that it is a right to an equal enjoyment of whatever care anyone else enjoys, then what are we to do with respect to the artificial heart? Might we decide not to develop such a device? Though the development and experimental use of it involves an entirely tolerable burden, the general provision of the artificial heart would be an intolerable burden, and since if we provide it to any we must provide it to all, therefore perhaps we should provide it to none.

This solution seems to me both uncomfortable and unstable. For surely there is something odd, if not perverse, about foregoing research on such devices, not because the research might fail, but because it might succeed. Might not this research then go on under some kinds of private auspices if such a governmental decision were made? Would we then go further and forbid even private research, rather than simply refusing to fund it? I can well imagine the next step, where artificial heart research and implantation would become like abortion or sex change operations in the old days: something one went to Sweden or Denmark for. Nor is a lottery device for distributing a limited number of artificial hearts likely to be more stable or satisfactory. For there, too, would we forbid people to go outside the lottery? Would it be a crime to cross national boundaries with the intent of obtaining an artificial heart? The example makes a general point about instituting an all-inclusive "right to health care," with the necessary concomitant of an equal right to whatever health care is available. For if we really instituted such a right and limited the provision of health care to a reasonable level, we would have to institute as well a degree of stringent state control, which it is both unlikely we can achieve and undesirable for us even to try to achieve. There is something that goes very deeply against the grain about any scheme which prohibits scientists from making discoveries which no one claims are harmful as such, but which will cause trouble because we can't give them to everybody. There is something which goes against the grain in a system which might forbid individual doctors to render a service, not because it is harmful, but because its benefits are not available to all.

Or take a much less dramatic case—dental care. It is said that ordinary basic prophylactic care is so lacking for tens of millions of our citizens that quite unnecessarily they do not have their own teeth while still in their prime. I take it that to provide the kind of elaborate dental care deployed on affluent suburban families to rural populations, and to all even poorer urban dwellers, would be a prodigiously expensive undertaking, one that would cost each of us quite heavily. But if we followed the slogan, "The best available made available to all," that is what is meant. My guess is the American people would not want to bear this burden and that as a form of transfer payment the poor would prefer just to have the money to spend on other things. But this shows the dangerousness of slogans, for perhaps the greatest part of the dental damage could be remedied at far less cost by fluoridation and by relatively routine care provided by a type of modestly trained person who is only now beginning to exist. Care of this sort can be afforded and should be provided. But this would mean abandoning the concept of equality and accepting the fact that the poor would be getting less elaborate care than those who are not poor.

Now it might be said that I am exaggerating. The case put forward is the British National Health Service, which is alleged to provide a model of high level care at reasonable costs with equality for all. But I would caution planners and enthusiasts from drawing too much from this example. The situation in Great Britain is very different in many ways. The country is smaller and more homogeneous. Moreover, even in Great Britain there are disparities between the care available between urban and rural areas; there are long waits for so-called "elective procedures"; and there is a small but significant and distinguished private sector outside of National Health which is the focus of great controversy and rancor. Finally, Great

Britain is a country where a substantial portion of the citizenry is committed to the socialist ideal of equalizing incomes and nationalizing the provisions of all vital services. Surely this is a very different situation from that in the United States. Indeed, it may be that the cry for equality of access to health care bears to a general yearning for social equality much the same relation that the opposition to fetal research bears to the opposition to abortion. In each case it is a very large ideological tail wagging a relatively small and confused dog.

My point is analytical. My point is that apart from a rather general commitment to equality and, indeed, to state control of the allocation and distribution of resources, to insist on the right to health care, where that right means a right to equal access, is an anomaly. For as long as our society considers that inequalities of wealth and income are morally acceptable—acceptable in the sense that the system that produces these inequalities is in itself not morally suspect—it is anomalous to carve out a sector like health care and say that *there* equality must reign.

III. TOWARDS A BETTER DEFINITION OF THE RIGHTS INVOLVED

After all, is health care so special? Is it different from education, housing, food, legal assistance? In respect to all of these things, we recognize in our society a right, whose enjoyment may not be made wholly dependent upon the ability to pay. But just as surely in respect to all these things, we do not believe that this right entails equality of enjoyment, so that whatever diet one person or class of persons enjoys must be enjoyed by all. The argument, put forward for instance by some members of the Labor Party in Great Britain, that the independent schools in that country should be abolished because they offer a level of education better than that available in state schools, is an argument which would be found strange and repellent in the United States. Rather, in all of these areas—education, hous-

ing, food, legal assistance—there obtains a notion of a decent, fair standard, such that when this standard is satisfied all that exists in the way of *rights* has been accorded. And it is necessarily so; were we to insist on equality all the way up, that is, past this minimum, we would have committed ourselves to a political philosophy which I take it is not the dominant one in our society.

Is health care different? Everything that can be said about health care is true of food and is at least by analogy true of education, housing, and legal assistance. The real task before us is not, therefore, I think, to explain why there must be complete equality in medicine, but the more subtle and perilous task of determining the decent minimum in respect to health which accords with sound ethical judgments, while maintaining the virtues of freedom, variety, and flexibility which are thought to flow from a mixed system such as ours. The decent minimum should reflect some conception of what constitutes tolerable life prospects in general. It should speak quite strongly to things like maternal health and child health, which set the terms under which individuals will compete and develop. On the other hand, techniques which will offer some remote relief from conditions that rarely strike in the prime of life, and which strike late in the life because something must, might be thought of as too esoteric to be part of the concept of minimum decent care.

On the other hand, the notion of a decent minimum should include humane and, I would say, worthy surroundings of care for those whom we know we are not going to be able to treat. Here, it seems to me, the emphasis on technology and the attention of highly trained specialists is seriously mistaken. Not only is it unrealistic to imagine that such fancy services can be provided for everyone "as a right," but there is serious doubt whether these kinds of services are what most people really want or can benefit from.

In the end, I will concede very readily that the notion of minimum health care, which it does make sense for our society to recognize as a right, is itself an unstable and changing notion. As my initial historical remarks must have suggested, the concept of a decent minimum is always relative to what is available over all, and what the best which is available might be. I suppose (to revert to my parable of the artificial heart) that if we allowed an artificial heart to be developed under private auspices and to be available only to those who could pay for it, or who could obtain it from specialized eleemosynary institutions, then the time might well come when it would have been so perfected that it would be a reasonable component of what one would consider minimum decent care. And the process of arriving at this new situation would be a process imbued with struggle and political controversy. But since I do not believe in utopias or final solutions, a resolution of the problem of the right to health care having these kinds of tensions within it neither worries me nor leads me to suspect that I am on the wrong track. To my mind, the right track consists in indentifying what it is that health care can and cannot provide, in identifying also the cost of health care, and then in deciding how much of this health care, what level of health care, we are ready to underwrite as a floor for our citizenry.

IV. PRACTICAL PROPOSALS

Although the process of defining the decent minimum is inherently a political process, there is a great deal which analysis and research can do to make the process rational and satisfactory. Much of this is a negative service, clearing away misconceptions and fallacies. For instance, as I have already argued, to state that our objective is to provide the best medical care for all, regardless of the ability to pay, must be shown up for the misleading slogan that it is. But there are more subtle misconceptions as well. The most pervasive of these deal with the situation of the medical profession.

Many observers look at the medical profession, its history of resistance to social change, and the fact that doctors as a profession enjoy the highest incomes of any group in the nation —somewhere around $50,000 a year on the average—and they draw their own conclusions. They draw the conclusion that therefore what is needed is necessarily more regulation. They look at the oversupply of surgeons in this country. They note the obvious fact of over-recourse to surgery which seems to result, and they conclude that what is needed is more government regulation. For instance, the problems of supply would be met by a kind of doctors' draft, requiring service in underserviced rural areas. Now I would, for a moment, suggest that we consider some alternative explanations and alternative reforms. Perhaps, after all, the irrationalities in the supply of medical personnel, together with the high incomes earned, are the result not of market forces run wild, but the result of a guild system as tight and self-protective as any we know. It is, perhaps an irony that the medical profession, having persuaded the public of the necessity of strictly limiting entry into the profession, having persuaded the public of the indispensability of highly trained specialists, is now faced with the threat of a kind of doctors' draft to make these rare specialists available to all. Perhaps clearer thinking might indicate that many of the things which highly paid and highly trained doctors do might be done by an army of less pretentious persons.

It is well known, of course, that doctors' fees as such represent the smaller portion of the total health care budget, so it might be thought that I am taking aim at an obvious, vulnerable, and somewhat irrelevant target. Yet this is not so. Though the fees of doctors represent the smaller portion of the medical budget, doctors themselves control almost all of the decisions —from the decision about hospitalization, to the decision whether to prescribe drugs by brand or generic name—which do influence the total cost of medical care. And it is in this respect that doctors have resisted most attempts to make their behavior rational and cost-effective. In general, it is said that this is because no doctor would sacrifice the individual interests of his patient, and this may be a sincere claim. But a certain skepticism is in order. What choice do the patients have to choose more economical systems of delivery?

What doctor, for that matter, even gives his patient the choice between a brand and a generic prescription drug?

But it is in the choice of delivery systems themselves that the consumer is most restricted. Most consumers do not have the choice between a variety of delivery systems from prepaid group plans to the present individual fee-for-service system, with each plan costing what it really costs. If the consumer did have this choice, we might soon find out whether the alleged advantages of the fee-for-service system were something the consumer was willing to pay for. But of course we will never find this out if we are committed to underwrite, out of general revenues, the cost of this most expensive possible delivery system. "The best available to all." That is what we tend to do today for those groups whose medical care we do underwrite. The result is that we are trying to drive down the cost of this most expensive delivery system not by changing its organization but by bureaucratic control. What if, instead, each person were assured a certain amount of money to purchase medical services as he chose? If the restrictive practices of the profession itself could be avoided, would this not help a vast variety of delivery systems to grow up, all competing for the consumer's federally assured dollar? And then those who would want what might be considered as fancier or more individualized services could get them, provided only that they were willing to pay more for them.

Finally, there is a feature of our modern situation which is responsible for the present crisis in health care, and for the impossible dilemma posed by the promise of a right to health care. This is a feature of the society and the culture as a whole. I refer to our culture's inability to face and cope with the persistent facts of illness, old age, and death. Because we are little able to come to terms with the hazards which illness proposes, because the old are a burden and an embarrassment, because we pretend that death does not exist, we employ elaborate ruses to put these things out of the ambit of our ordinary lives. The reason why we hospitalize so much more than is rationally required surely goes beyond the vagaries of the health insurance system. Is it not also the result of the fact that the ill are an embarrassment to us, and that we seek to put them away, so we do not have to care for them, while assuaging our consciences that those "best qualified" to care for them are doing so? And in order that the ruse will work, we greatly overstate what it is that these "qualified" people can do for the ill. Needless to say, they are our willing accomplices in this piece of deception. So it is with the mentally retarded, the aged, and the dying. All of these persons are defined as having an abnormal condition not only justifying but requiring their isolation from us and their care in the hands of "specialists." Perhaps it is time that we recognize that this is part of the neurosis of our age. And of course, those whom we hire to perform our proper human role toward the sick, the old, and the dying can get away with charging a very high price for relieving us of our ordinary human obligations. But is this medical care?

Finally, to avoid misunderstanding, a general theoretic point must be made. My argument must sound harsh and callous—unfeelingly, if not unerringly economic. I have elsewhere argued that it is of the essence of the physician's role and of the patient's expectations that the doctor faced with the patient's need will do everything in his power to alleviate that need.* I believe that. I believe that for the individual physician to do less than his best because of some economic calculation of equity or efficiency is a breach of trust. The doctor in his dealings with his patient must not act like a bureaucrat, policy maker, or legislator. But policy makers, voters, and legislators must think in different terms. It is monstrous if an individual doctor thinks like a budget officer when he cares for his patient in need; but it is chaotic and incoherent if budget officers and voters making general policy think like doctors at the bedside.

*In my book, *Medical Experimentation: Personal Integrity and Social Policy* (Amsterdam and New York: Associated Scientific Publishers/Elsevier, 1974).

LEON R. KASS

The Pursuit of Health and the Right to Health

THE PURSUIT OF HEALTH

The foregoing inquiry into the nature of health [Chapter 3*] though obviously incomplete and in need of refinement, has, I hope, accomplished two things: first, to make at least plausible the claim that somatic health is a finite and intelligible norm, which is the true goal of medicine; and second, by displaying something of the character of healthiness, to provide a basis for considering how it might be better attained. *Curiously, it will soon become apparent that even if we have found the end of medicine, we may have to go beyond medicine in order to find the best means for attaining it.*

Though health is a natural norm, and though nature provides us with powerful inborn means of preserving and maintaining a well-working wholeness, it is wrong to assume that health is the simply given and spontaneous condition of human beings, and unhealth the result largely of accident or of external invasion. In the case of non-human animals, such a view could perhaps be defended. Other animals instinctively eat the right foods (when available) and act in such a way as to maintain their naturally given state of health and vigor. Other animals do not overeat, undersleep, knowingly ingest toxic substances, or permit their bodies to fall into disuse through sloth, watching television and riding in automobiles, transacting business, or writing articles about health. For us human beings, however, even a healthy nature must be nurtured, and maintained by effort and discipline if it is not to become soft and weak and prone to illness, and certain excesses and stresses must be avoided if this softness is not to spawn overt unhealth and disease. One

*This essay is a continuation of the essay in Chapter 3 by Dr. Kass. The essays may, however, be read separately.-Eds.

Reprinted with permission of the publisher and Leon R. Kass from *The Public Interest*, No. 40, Summer 1975. Copyright © 1975 by National Affairs, Inc.

should not, of course, underestimate the role of germs and other hostile agents working from without; but I strongly suspect that the germ theory of disease has been oversold, and that the state of "host resistance," and in particular of the immunity systems, will become increasingly prominent in our understanding of both health and disease.

Once the distinction is made between health nurture and maintenance, on the one hand, and disease prevention and treatment, on the other, it becomes immediately clear that bodily health does not depend only on the body and its parts. It depends decisively on the psyche with which the body associates and cooperates. A few examples will make this clear, if it is not already obvious. Some disorders of body are caused, at least in part, by disorders of soul (psyche); the range goes from the transitory bodily effects of simple nervousness and tension headaches, through the often severe somatic symptoms of depression (e.g., weight loss, insomnia, constipation, impotence), to ulcers and rheumatoid arthritis. Other diseases are due specifically to some aspect of the patient's way of life: cirrhosis in alcoholics, hepatitis in drug addicts, special lung diseases in coal miners, venereal disease in prostitutes.

But the dependence goes much farther than these obvious psycho-and socio-somatic interactions. In a most far-reaching way, our health is influenced by our temperament, our character, our habits, our whole way of life. This fact was once better appreciated than it is today.

In a very early discussion of this question, in the Platonic dialogue *Charmides*, Socrates criticizes Greek physicians for foolishly neglecting the whole when attempting to heal a part. He argues that "just as one must not attempt to cure the eyes without the head or the head without the body, so neither the body without the soul.'' In fact, one must care "first and most'' for the soul if one intends the body to be healthy. If the soul is moderate and sensible, it will not be difficult to effect health in the body; if not, health will be difficult to procure. Greek medicine fails, it is charged, because men try to be physicians of health and of moderation separately.

Socrates does not say that excellence of soul and excellence of body are one and the same; indeed, health is clearly distinguished from moderation. Rather, the claim is that health is at least in large part affected by or dependent upon virtue, that being well in body has much to do with living well, with good habits not only of body but of life.

Now Socrates certainly knew, perhaps better than we, that accident and fortune can bring harm and ill health even to well-ordered bodies and souls. He knew about inborn diseases and seasonal maladies and wounds sustained in battle. He knew that health, though demanding care and discipline and requiring a certain control of our bodily desires, was no sure sign of virtue—and that moderation is not all of virtue. He knew too, as we know, human beings whose healthiness was the best thing about them, and he knew also that to be preoccupied with health is either a sign or a cause of a shrunken human life. Yet he also knew what we are today altogether too willing to forget— that *we are in an important way responsible for our own state of health,* that carelessness, gluttony, drunkenness, and sloth take some of their wages in illness. At a deeper level, he knew that there was a connection between the fact that the human soul aspires beyond mere self-preservation, and the fact that men, unlike animals, can make themselves sick and feverish. He knew, therefore, that health in human beings depends not only on natural gifts, but also on taming and moderating the admirable yet dangerous human desire to live better than sows and squirrels.

Today we are beginning again to consider that Socrates was possibly right, that our way of life is a major key to our sickness and our health. I would myself guess that well more than half the visits to American doctors are occasioned by deviations from health for which the patient, or his way of life, is in some important way responsible. Most chronic lung diseases, much cardiovascular disease, most cirrhosis of the liver, many gastrointestinal disorders (from indigestion to ulcers), numerous muscular and skeletal complaints (from low back pain to flat feet), venereal disease, nutritional deficiencies, obesity and its consequences, and certain kinds of renal and skin infections are in large measure self-induced or self-caused—and contributed to by smoking, overeating, excessive drinking, eating the wrong foods, inadequate rest and exercise, and poor hygiene. To these conditions must be added the results of trauma—including automobile accidents—in which drunkenness plays a leading part, and suicide attempts, as well as accidental poisonings, drug abuse, and many burns. I leave out of the reckoning the as yet poorly studied contributions to unhealth of all varieties made by the special stresses of modern urban life.

There are even indications that cancer is in some measure a disease of how we live, even beyond the clear correlations of lung cancer with smoking and of cancer of the cervix with sexual promiscuity and poor sexual hygiene. If the incidence of each kind of cancer could be reduced to the level at which it occurs in the population in which its incidence is lowest, there would be 90 per cent less cancer. Recent studies show that cancers of all sorts—not only cancers clearly correlated with smoking and drinking—occur less frequently among the clean-living Mormons and Seventh-Day Adventists.

The foregoing, it will be noted, speaks largely about disease and unhealth, and about the role of our excesses and deficiencies in bringing them about. Unfortunately, we know less about what contributes to healthiness, as nearly all epidemiological studies have been studies of disease. But in the last few years, there have appeared published reports of a most fascinating and important series of epidemiological studies on *health,* conducted by Dean Lester Breslow and his colleagues at the UCLA School of Public Health. Having first developed a method for quantifying, albeit crudely, one's state of health and well-functioning, they investigated the effect of various health practices on physical health status. They have discovered, empirically, seven independent "rules" for good health, which correlate very well with healthiness, and also with longevity. People who follow all seven rules are healthier and live longer than those who follow six, six more than five, and so on, in perfect order. Let me report two of their more dramatic findings: The physical health status of those over 75 who followed all the "rules" was about the same as those aged 35-44 who followed fewer than three; and a person who follows at least six of the seven rules has an 11-year longer life expectancy at age 45 than someone who has followed less than four. Moreover, these differences in health connected with health practices persisted at all economic levels, and, except at the very lowest incomes, appeared largely independent of income.[1]

The seven "rules" are: 1) Don't smoke cigarettes. 2) Get seven hours of sleep. 3) Eat breakfast. 4) Keep your weight down. 5) Drink moderately. 6) Exercise daily. 7) Don't eat between meals. ("Visit your doctor" is not on the list, though I must confess that I cannot find out if this variable was investigated.) It seems that Socrates, and also Grandmother, may have been on the right track.

One feels, I must admit, a bit foolish, in the latter half of the twentieth century, which boasts the cracking of the genetic code, kidney machines, and heart transplants, to be suggesting the quaint formula, "Eat right, exercise, and be moderate, for tomorrow you will be healthy." But quaint formulas need not have been proven false to be ignored, and we will look far more foolish if Breslow and his colleagues are onto something which, in our sophistication, we choose to overlook.

IMPLICATIONS FOR POLICY

What might all this point to for medicine and for public policy regarding health? Let me try to sketch in outline the implications of the preceding sections, which, as a point of departure, I would summarize in this way: Health and

only health is the doctor's proper business; but health, understood as well-working wholeness, is not the business only of doctors. Health is, in different ways, everyone's business, and it is best pursued if everyone regards and minds his *own* business—each of us his own health, the doctor the health of his patient, public health officials and legislators the health of the citizens.

With respect to the medical profession itself, there is a clear need to articulate and delimit the physician's domain and responsibilities, to protect against both expansion and contraction. The more obvious and perhaps greater danger seems to be expansion, given the growing technological powers that can serve non-therapeutic ends and the rising demands that these powers be used for non-medical ends. The medical profession must take the initiative in establishing and policing the necessary boundaries.

. . .

But the greatest difficulty is how to protect the boundaries of the medical domain against unreasonable *external* demands for expansion. The public's misperception of medicine is ultimately more dangerous than the doctor's misperception of himself. The movement towards consumer control of medicine, the call for doctors to provide "therapy" for social deviants and criminal offenders, and the increasing governmental regulation of medical practice all run the risk of transforming the physician into a mere public servant, into a technician or helper for hire. Granted, the doctor must not be allowed to be a tyrant. But neither must he become a servant. Rather, he must remain a leader and a teacher. The community must respect the fact that medicine is an art and that the doctor is a man of expert knowledge, deserving more than an equal voice in deciding what his business is. Though one may rightly suspect *some* of the motives behind the medical profession's fear of governmental intrusion, one must acknowledge the justice of at least this concern: Once the definition of health care and the standards of medical practice are made by outsiders—and the National Health Insurance schemes all tend in this direction—the physician becomes a mere technician.

THE CASE FOR HEALTH MAINTENANCE

Yet if the medical profession wants to retain the right to set its own limits, it must not only improve its immunity against foreign additions to its domain, but must also work to restore its own wholeness. The profession must again concern itself with health, with wholeness, with well-working, and not only with the cure of disease. The doctor must attend to health maintenance, and not only treatment or even prevention of specific diseases. . . .

I am not saying that doctors should cease to be concerned about disease, or that they should keep us in hospitals and clinics until we become fully healthy. I do suggest, however, that physicians should be more interested than they are in finding ways to keep us from their doors. Though medicine must remain in large part restorative and remedial, greater attention to healthy functioning and to regimens for becoming and remaining healthy could be very salutary, even toward the limited goal of reducing the incidence of disease. Little intelligence and imagination have thus far been expended by members of the profession, or by health insurance companies, to devise incentive schemes that would reward such a shift in emphasis (e.g., that would reward financially both patient and physician if the patient stays free of the need for his services). . . .

Moving beyond implications for the relation between doctor and patient to those for medical research, I would emphasize the importance of epidemiological research on *healthiness*. We need to devise better indices of healthiness than mortality and morbidity statistics, which, I have argued, are in fact not indices of *health* at all. The studies like those of Breslow and his collaborators are a step in the right direction and should be encouraged. Only with better measures of healthiness can we really evaluate the results of our various health practices and policies.

We also need large-scale epidemiological research into health maintenance, to learn more about what promotes, and what undermines, health. More sophisticated studies in nutrition, bodily exercise, rest and sleep, relaxation, and responses to stress could be very useful, as could expanded research into personal habits of health and hygiene and their effects on general healthiness, overall resistance to disease, and specific resistance to specific diseases. We need to identify and learn about healthy subgroups in the community, like the Mormons, and to discover what accounts for their success.

All of these things are probably obvious, and most of them have been championed for years by people in the fields of public health and preventive medicine—though they too have placed greater emphasis on disease prevention than on health maintenance. Their long-ignored advice is finally beginning to be heeded, with promising results. For example, a recent study reports a surprising downturn (after a 25-year climb) in the death rate from heart attacks among middle-aged men, attributed in part to changes in smoking and eating habits and to new treatments for high blood pressure. Yet this approach will always seem banal and pedestrian in comparison with the glamorous and dramatic style of high-technology therapeutics, with the doctor locked in combat with overt disease, displaying his marvelous and magical powers. My high regard for these powers cannot stifle the question whether the men who first suggested adding chlorine to drinking water or invented indoor plumbing didn't contribute more to healthiness than the Nobel Prize winners in Medicine and Physiology who discovered the chemical wonders of enzyme structure or of vision. It might be worthwhile to consider by what kinds of incentives and rewards the National Institutes of Health or the AMA might encourage more and better research into health maintenance and disease prevention.

FOSTERING RESPONSIBILITY

Yet as has been repeatedly emphasized, doctors and public health officials have only limited power to improve our health. Health is not a commodity which can be delivered. Medicine can help only those who help themselves. Discovering what will promote and maintain health is only half the battle; we must also find ways to promote and inculcate good health habits and to increase personal responsibility for health. This is, no doubt, the most fundamental and also the most difficult task. It is but one more instance of that age-old challenge: how to get people to do what is good for them without tyrannizing them. The principles of freedom and of wisdom do not always—shall I say, do not very often—lead in the same direction.

Since this is not a new difficulty, we do have some experience in how to think about it. Consider the problem of getting people to obey the law. Policemen and judges are clearly needed to handle the major crimes and criminals, but it would be foolish to propose, and dangerous to provide, even that degree of police surveillance and interference required to prevent only the most serious lawbreaking. But though justice is the business of the policeman and the judge, it is not their business alone. Education—at home, in schools, in civic and religious institutions—can "teach" law-abidingness far better than policemen can, and where the former is successful, there is less need of the latter.

Yet even without considering the limitations of this analogy, the limits of the power of teachers—and of policemen as well—to produce law abidingness are all too apparent. And when one considers that fear of immediate, identifiable punishment probably deters lawbreaking more than fear of unhealth deters sloth and gluttony, we see that we face no simple task. The wages of poor health habits during youth are only paid much later, so much later that it is difficult to establish the relation of cause and effect, let alone make it vivid enough to influence people's actions. If it isn't likely to rain for 20 years, few of us are likely to repair our leaky roofs.

This is not a counsel of despair. On the contrary, I am much impressed with the growing interest in health and health education in recent years, including the greater concern for proper nutrition, adequate exercise, dental hygiene, and the hazards of smoking, and the evidence

that, at least among some groups, this attention is bearing fruit. Nevertheless, when we consider the numerous impediments to setting in order our lives and our communities, I think we should retain a healthy doubt about just how healthy we Americans are likely, as a community, to become.

This skepticism is rather lacking in most political pronouncements and policies regarding health. Making unwarranted inferences from medicine's past successes against *infectious* disease, being excessively impressed with the technological brilliance of big hospital medicine, mobilizing crusades and crash programs against cancer and heart disease, the health politicians speak as if more money, more targeted research, better distribution of services, more doctors and hospitals, and bigger and better cobalt machines, lasers, and artificial organs will bring the medical millennium to every American citizen. Going along with all this is a lack of attention to health maintenance and patient responsibility. While it would surely be difficult for the federal government to teach responsibility, we should not be pleased when its actions in fact discourage responsibility.

A RIGHT TO HEALTH?

One step in this direction is the growing endorsement of the so-called right to health, beyond the already ambiguous and dubious right to health care. A recent article argued thus:

The right to *health* is a fundamental right. It expresses the profound truth that a person's autonomy and freedom rest upon his ability to function physically and psychologically. It asserts that no other person can, with moral justification, deprive him of that ability. The right to *health care* or the right to *medical care*, on the other hand, are qualified rights. They flow from the fundamental right, but are implemented in institutions and practices only when such are possible and reasonable and only when other rights are not thereby impeded.[2]

If the right to health means only the right not to have one's health destroyed by another, then it is a reasonable but rather impotent claim in the health care arena; the right to health care or medical care could hardly flow from a right to health, unless the right to health meant also and mainly the right to become and to be kept healthy. But if health is what we say it is, it is an unlikely subject of a right in either sense. Health is a state of being, not something that can be given, and only in indirect ways something that can be taken away or undermined by other human beings. It no more makes sense to claim a right to health than a right to wisdom or courage. These excellences of soul and of body require natural gift, attention, effort, and discipline on the part of each person who desires them. To make my health someone else's duty is not only unfair; it is to impose a duty impossible to fulfill. Though I am not particularly attracted by the language of rights and duties in regard to health, I would lean much more in the direction, once traditional, of saying that health is a *duty,* that one has an obligation to preserve one's own health. The theory of a right to health flies in the face of good sense, serves to undermine personal responsibility, and, in addition, places obligation where it cannot help but be unfulfillable.

THE "KIDNEY-MACHINE" LEGISLATION

Similarly, the amendment to the Medicare legislation which provides payment for "kidney-machine" treatment for all in need, at a cost of from $10,000 to $40,000 per patient, is, for all its good intentions, a questionable step. First of all, it establishes the principle that the federal government is the savior of last resort—or, as is more likely at this price tag, the savior of first resort—for specific persons with specific diseases. In effect, the government has said that it is in the national interest for the government to pay, disease by disease, life by life, for life-saving measures for all its citizens. The justice of providing benefits of this magnitude solely to people with kidney disease has been loudly questioned, and hemophilia organizations are pressing for government financing of equally expensive treatment. Others have called attention to the impossible financial burden that the just extension of this coverage

would entail. Finally, this measure gives governmental endorsement, in a most dramatic and visible way, to the high-cost, technological, therapy-oriented approach to health. This approach has been challenged, on the basis of a searching analysis of this kidney-machine legislation, in a report by a panel of the Institute of Medicine of the National Academy of Sciences, which, with admirable self-restraint, comments: "One wonders how many billions of dollars the nation would now be spending on iron lungs if research for the cure of polio had not been done."[3]

This is not to say that, in the special case of the kidney machines under the special circumstances in which the legislation was passed, a persuasive case was not made on the other side. Clearly, it was hoped that perfection of kidney transplantation or future prevention of kidney disease would make this high-cost insurance obsolete before too long. Moreover, no one wishes to appear to be, or indeed to be, callous about the loss of life, especially preventable and premature loss of life. Still, the dangers of the kidney machine legislation must be acknowledged.

One might even go so far as to suggest that prudent and wise legislators and policy makers must in the future resist (in a way that no private doctor should be permitted to resist) the temptation to let compassion for individual calamities and general sentimentality rule in these matters. Pursuing the best health policy for the American people—that is, a policy to encourage and support the best possible health for the American people—may indeed mean not taking certain measures that would prevent known deaths. Only by focusing on health and how one gets it, and by taking a more long-range view, can our health policy measure up in deed to its good intentions.

IS NATIONAL HEALTH INSURANCE GOOD FOR HEALTH?

The proposals for a National Health Insurance seem also to raise difficulties of this sort, and more. Medical care is certainly very expensive, and therefore, for this reason alone, not equally available to all. The economic problems are profound and genuine, and there are few dispassionate observers who are not convinced that something needs to be done. Many technical questions have been debated and discussed, including the range of coverage and the sources of financing, and organized medicine has voiced its usual concern regarding governmental interference, a concern which I have already indicated I share in regard to the delimitation of the doctor's role and the scope of health care. But some of the most serious issues have received all too little attention.

The proposals for National Health Insurance take for granted the wisdom of our current approaches to the pursuit of health, and thereby insure that in the future we will get more of the same. These proposals will simply make available to the non-insured what the privately insured now get: a hospital-centered, highly technological, disease-oriented, therapy-centered medical care. The proposals have entirely ignored the question of whether what we now do in health is what we should be doing. They not only endorse the status quo, but fail to take advantage of the rare opportunity which financial crises provide to reexamine basic questions and directions. The irony is that real economizing in health care is probably possible only by radically re-orienting the pursuit of health.

One cannot help getting the impression that it is economic *equality,* not health, and not even economizing, that is the primary aim of these proposals. At a recent seminar in which I participated, an official of HEW informally expressed irritation at those who are questioning whether the so-called health care delivery system is really making us healthier, and suggested that their main goal was to undermine liberal programs enacted in recent years. Yet this official went on to say that even if the evidence conclusively showed that all the government's health programs in no way actually improved health, the programs ought to be continued for their extra-medical—i.e., social and economic—benefits. For myself, I confess that I would prefer as my public health official the cold-hearted, even mean-sprited fellow who is interested in health and who knows how to promote it.

All the proposals for National Health Insurance embrace, without qualification, the no-fault principle. They therefore choose to ignore, or to treat as irrelevant, the importance of personal responsibility for the state of one's health. As a result, they pass up an opportunity to build both positive and negative inducements into the insurance payment plan, by measures such as refusing or reducing benefits for chronic respiratory disease care to persons who continue to smoke.

There are, of course, complicated questions of justice raised here, and even to suggest that the sick ever be in any way blamed or penalized flies in the face of current custom and ways of thinking. Yet one need not be a Calvinist or a Spartan to see merit in the words of a wise physician, Robert S. Morison, writing on much the same subject:

In the perspectives of today, cardiovascular illness in middle age not only runs the risk of depriving families of their support, or society of certain kinds of services; it increasingly places on society the obligation to spend thousands of dollars on medical care to rescue an individual from the results of a faulty living pattern. Under these conditions, one wonders how much longer we can go on talking about a right to health without some balancing talk about the individual's responsibility to keep healthy.

I am told that Thorstein Veblen used to deplore the fact that in California they taxed the poor to send the rich to college. One wonders how he would react to a system which taxes the virtuous to send the improvident to hospital.[4]

But even leaving aside questions of justice, and looking only at the pursuit of health, one has reason to fear that the new insurance plan, whichever one it turns out to be, may actually contribute to a worsening rather than an improvement in our nation's health, especially if there is no balancing program to encourage individual responsibility for health maintenance.

One final word. Despite all that I have said, I would also emphasize that health, while a good, cannot be the greatest good, either for an individual or for a community. Politically, an excessive preoccupation with health can conflict with the pursuit of other important social and economic goals (e.g., when cancerphobia leads to government regulations that unreasonably restrict industrial activity or personal freedom). But more fundamentally, it is not mere life, nor even a healthy life, but rather a good and worthy life for which we must aim. And while poor health may weaken our efforts, good health alone is an insufficient condition or sign of a worthy human life. Indeed, though there is no such thing as being too healthy, there is such a thing as being too concerned about health. To be preoccupied with the body is to neglect the soul, for which we should indeed care "first and most," and more than we now do. We must strike a proper balance, a balance that can only be furthered if the approach to health also concentrates on our habits of life.

NOTES

1. Nedra B. Belloc and Lester Breslow, "Relationship of Physical Health Status and Health Practices," *Preventive Medicine 1* (1972), pp. 409–421; and Nedra B. Belloc, "Relationship of Health Practices and Mortality," *Preventive Medicine 2* (1973), pp. 67–81.

2. Philip R. Lee and Albert R. Jonsen, editorial: "The Right to Health Care," *American Review of Respiratory Disease,* Vol. 109 (1974), pp. 591–92 (italics in orginal). Dr. Lee is a former Assistant Secretary for Health at HEW.

3. *Disease by Disease Toward National Health Insurance?* (Washington, D.C., Institute of Medicine-National Academy of Sciences, 1973).

4. R. S. Morison, "Rights and Responsibilities: Redressing the Uneasy Balance," *The Hastings Center Report,* Vol. 4, No. 2 (April 1974), p. 4.

Microallocation

NICHOLAS RESCHER

The Allocation of Exotic Medical Lifesaving Therapy

I. THE PROBLEM

Technological progress has in recent years transformed the limits of the possible in medical therapy. However, the elevated state of sophistication of modern medical technology has brought the economists' classic problem of scarcity in its wake as an unfortunate side product. The enormously sophisticated and complex equipment and the highly trained teams of experts requisite for its utilization are scarce resources in relation to potential demand. The administrators of the great medical institutions that preside over these scarce resources thus come to be faced increasingly with the awesome choice: *Whose life to save?*

A (somewhat hypothetical) paradigm example of this problem may be sketched within the following set of definitive assumptions: We suppose that persons in some particular medically morbid condition are "mortally afflicted": It is virtually certain that they will die within a short time period (say ninety days). We assume that some very complex course of treatment (e.g., a heart transplant) represents a

Reprinted with permission of the author and the publisher from *Ethics,* Vol. 79, No. 3 (April 1969), pp. 173–86. Copyright 1969 by The University of Chicago Press.

substantial probability of life prolongation for persons in this mortally afflicted condition. We assume that the facilities available in terms of human resources, mechanical instrumentalities, and requisite materials (e.g., hearts in the case of a heart transplant) make it possible to give a certain treatment—this "exotic (medical) lifesaving therapy," or ELT for short—to a certain, relatively small number of people. And finally we assume that a substantially greater pool of people in the mortally afflicted condition is at hand. The problem then may be formulated as follows: How is one to select within the pool of afflicted patients the ones to be given the ELT treatment in question; how to select those "whose lives are to be saved"? Faced with many candidates for an ELT process that can be made available to only a few, doctors and medical administrators confront the decision of who is to be given a chance at survival and who is, in effect, to be condemned to die.

As has already been implied, the "heroic" variety of spare-part surgery can pretty well be assimilated to this paradigm. One can foresee the time when heart transplantation, for example, will have become pretty much a routine medical procedure albeit on a very limited basis, since a cardiac surgeon with the technical competence to transplant hearts can operate at best a rather small number of times each week and the elaborate facilities for such operations will most probably exist on a modest scale. Moreover, in "spare-part" surgery there is always the problem of availability of the "spare parts" themselves. A report in one British newspaper gives the following picture: "Of the 150,000 who die of heart disease each year [in the U.K.], Mr. Donald Longmore, research surgeon at the National Heart Hospital [in London] estimates that 22,000 might be eligible for heart surgery. Another 30,000 would need heart and lung transplants. But there are probably only between 7,000 and 14,000 potential donors a year."[1] Envisaging this situation in which at the very most something like one in four heart-malfunction victims can be saved, we clearly confront a problem in ELT allocation.

A perhaps even more drastic case in point is afforded by long-term haemodialysis, an ongoing process by which a complex device—an "artificial kidney machine"—is used periodically in cases of chronic renal failure to substitute for a non-functional kidney in "cleaning" potential poisons from the blood. Only a few major institutions have chronic haemodialysis units, whose complex operation is an extremely expensive proposition. For the present and the foreseeable future the situation is that "the number of places available for chronic haemodialysis is hopelessly inadequate."[2]

The traditional medical ethos has insulated the physician against facing the very existence of this problem. When swearing the Hippocratic Oath, he commits himself to work for the benefit of the sick in "whatsoever house I enter."[3] In taking this stance, the physician substantially renounces the explicit choice of saving certain lives rather than others. Of course, doctors have always in fact had to face such choices on the battlefield or in times of disaster, but there the issue had to be resolved hurriedly, under pressure, and in circumstances in which the very nature of the case effectively precluded calm deliberation by the decision maker as well as criticism by others. In sharp contrast, however, cases of the type we have postulated in the present discussion arise predictably, and represent choices to be made deliberately and "in cold blood."

It is, to begin with, appropriate to remark that this problem is not fundamentally a medical problem. For when there are sufficiently many afflicted candidates for ELT then—so we may assume—there will also be more than enough for whom the purely medical grounds for ELT allocation are decisively strong in any individual case, and just about equally strong throughout the group. But in this circumstance a selection of some afflicted patients over and against others cannot *ex hypothesi* be made on the basis of purely medical considerations.

The selection problem, as we have said, is in substantial measure not a medical one. It is a problem *for* medical men, which must somehow be solved by them, but that does not make it a medical issue—any more than the problem of hospital building is a medical issue. As a problem it belongs to the category of philosophical problems—specifically a problem of moral philosophy or ethics. Structurally, it bears a substantial kinship with those issues in this field that revolve about the notorious whom-to-save-on-the-lifeboat and whom-to-throw-to-the-wolves-pursuing-the-sled questions. But whereas questions of this just-indicated sort are artificial, hypothetical, and far-fetched, the ELT issue poses a *genuine* policy question for the responsible administrators in medical institutions, indeed a question that threatens to become commonplace in the foreseeable future.

Now what the medical administrator needs to have, and what the philosopher is presumably *ex officio* in a position to help in providing, is a body of *rational guidelines* for making choices in these literally life-or-death situations. This is an issue in which many interested parties have a substantial stake, including the responsible decision maker who wants to satisfy his conscience that he is acting in a reasonable way. Moreover, the family and associates of the man who is turned away—to say nothing of the man himself—have the right to an acceptable explanation. And indeed even the general public wants to know that what is being done is fitting and proper. All of these interested parties are entitled to insist that a reasonable code of operating principles provides a defensible rationale for making the life-and-death choices involved in ELT.

II. THE TWO TYPES OF CRITERIA

Two distinguishable types of criteria are bound up in the issue of making ELT choices. We shall call these *Criteria of Inclusion* and *Criteria of Comparison,* respectively. The distinction at issue here requires some explanation. We can think of the selection as being made by a two-stage process: (1) the selection from among all possible candidates (by a suitable screening process) of a group to

be taken under serious consideration as candidates for therapy, and then (2) the actual singling out, within this group, of the particular individuals to whom therapy is to be given. Thus the first process narrows down the range of comparative choice by eliminating *en bloc* whole categories of potential candidates. The second process calls for a more refined, case-by-case comparison of those candidates that remain. By means of the first set of criteria one forms a selection group; by means of the second set, an actual selection is made within this group.

Thus what we shall call a "selection system" for the choice of patients to receive therapy of the ELT type will consist of criteria of these two kinds. Such a system will be acceptable only when the reasonableness of its component criteria can be established.

III. ESSENTIAL FEATURES OF AN ACCEPTABLE ELT SELECTION SYSTEM

To qualify as reasonable, an ELT selection must meet two important "regulative" requirements: it must be *simple* enough to be readily intelligible, and it must be *plausible,* that is, patently reasonable in a way that can be apprehended easily and without involving ramified subtleties. Those medical administrators responsible for ELT choices must follow a modus operandi that virtually all the people involved can readily understand to be acceptable (at a reasonable level of generality, at any rate). Appearances are critically important here. It is not enough that the choice be made in a *justifiable* way; it must be possible for people—*plain* people—to "see" (i.e., understand without elaborate teaching or indoctrination) that *it is justified,* insofar as any mode of procedure can be justified in cases of this sort.

One "constitutive" requirement is obviously an essential feature of a reasonable selection system: all of its component criteria—those of inclusion and those of comparison alike—must be reasonable in the sense of being *rationally defensible.* The ramifications of this requirement call for detailed consideration. But one of its aspects should be noted without further ado: it must be *fair* —it must treat relevantly like cases alike, leaving no room for "influence" or favoritism, etc.

IV. THE BASIC SCREENING STAGE: CRITERIA OF INCLUSION (AND EXCLUSION)

Three sorts of considerations are prominent among the plausible criteria of inclusion/exclusion at the basic screening stage: the constituency factor, the progress-of-science factor, and the prospect-of-success factor.

A. THE CONSTITUENCY FACTOR

It is a "fact of life" that ELT can be available only in the institutional setting of a hospital or medical institute or the like. Such institutions generally have normal clientele boundaries. A veterans' hospital will not concern itself primarily with treating non-veterans, a children's hospital cannot be expected to accommodate the "senior citizen," an army hospital can regard college professors as outside its sphere. Sometimes the boundaries are geographic—a state hospital may admit only residents of a certain state. (There are, of course, indefensible constituency principles—say race or religion, party membership, or ability to pay; and there are cases of borderline legitimacy, e.g., sex.[4]) A medical institution is justified in considering for ELT only persons within its own constituency, provided this constituency is constituted upon a defensible basis. Thus the haemodialysis selection committee in Seattle "agreed to consider only those applications who were residents of the state of Washington. . . . They justified this stand on the grounds that since the basic research . . . had been done at . . . a state-supported institution —the people whose taxes had paid for the research should be its first beneficiaries."[5]

While thus insisting that constituency considerations represent a valid and legitimate factor in ELT selection, I do feel there is much to be said for minimizing their role in life-or-death cases. Indeed a refusal to recognize them at all is a significant part of medical tradition, going back to the very oath of Hippocrates. They represent a departure from the ideal arising with the institutionalization of medicine, moving it away from its original status as an art practiced by an individual practitioner.

B. THE PROGRESS-OF-SCIENCE FACTOR

The needs of medical research can provide a second valid principle of inclusion. The research interests of the medical staff in relation to the specific nature of the cases at issue is a significant consideration. It may be important for the progress of medical science—and thus of potential benefit to many persons in the future—to determine how effective the ELT at issue is with diabetics or persons over sixty or with a negative Rh factor. Considerations of this sort represent another type of legitimate factor in ELT selection.

A very definitely *borderline* case under this head would revolve around the question of a patient's willingness to pay, not in monetary terms, but in offering himself as an experimental subject, say by contracting to return at designated times for a series of tests substantially unrelated to his own health, but yielding data of importance to medical knowledge in general.

C. THE PROSPECT-OF-SUCCESS FACTOR

It may be that while the ELT at issue is not without *some* effectiveness in general, it has been established to be highly effective only with patients in certain specific categories (e.g., females under forty of a specific blood type). This difference in effectiveness—in the absolute or in the probability of success—is (we assume) so marked as to constitute virtually a difference in kind rather than in degree. In this case, it would be perfectly legitimate to adopt the general rule of making the ELT at issue available only or primarily to persons in this substantial-promise-of-success category. (It is on grounds of this sort that young children and persons over fifty are generally ruled out as candidates for haemodialysis.)

We have maintained that the three factors of constituency, progress of science, and prospect of success represent legitimate criteria of inclusion for ELT selection. But it remains to examine the considerations which legitimate them. The legitimating factors are in the final analysis practical or pragmatic in nature. From the practical angle it is advantageous—indeed to some extent necessary—that the arrangements governing medical institutions should embody certain constituency principles. It makes good pragmatic and utilitarian sense that progress-of-science considerations should be operative here. And, finally, the practical aspect is reinforced by a whole host of other considerations—including moral ones—in supporting the prospect-of-success criterion. The workings of each of these factors are of course conditioned by the ever-present element of limited availability. They are operative only in this context, that is, prospect of success is a legitimate consideration at all only because we are dealing with a situation of scarcity.

V. THE FINAL SELECTION STAGE: CRITERIA OF SELECTION

Five sorts of elements must, as we see it, figure primarily among the plausible criteria of selection that are to be brought to bear in further screening the group constituted after application of the criteria of inclusion: the relative-likelihood-of-success factor, the life-expectancy factor, the family role factor, the potential-contributions factor, and the services-rendered factor. The first two represent the *biomedical* aspect, the second three the *social* aspect.

A. THE RELATIVE-LIKELIHOOD-OF-SUCCESS FACTOR

It is clear that the relative likelihood of success is a legitimate and appropriate factor in making a selection within the group of qualified patients that are to receive ELT. This is obviously one of the considerations that must count very significantly in a reasonable selection procedure.

The present criterion is of course closely related to item *C* of the preceding section. There we were concerned with prospect-of-success considerations categorically and *en bloc*. Here at present they come into play in a

particularized case-by-case comparison among individuals. If the therapy at issue is not a once-and-for-all proposition and requires ongoing treatment, cognate considerations must be brought in. Thus, for example, in the case of a chronic ELT procedure such as haemodialysis it would clearly make sense to give priority to patients with a potentially reversible condition (who would thus need treatment for only a fraction of their remaining lives).

B. THE LIFE-EXPECTANCY FACTOR

Even if the ELT is "successful" in the patient's case he may, considering his age and/or other aspects of his general medical condition, look forward to only a very short probable future life. This is obviously another factor that must be taken into account.

C. THE FAMILY ROLE FACTOR

A person's life is a thing of importance not only to himself but to others—friends, associates, neighbors, colleagues, etc. But his (or her) relationship to his immediate family is a thing of unique intimacy and significance. The nature of his relationship to his wife, children, and parents, and the issue of their financial and psychological dependence upon him, are obviously matters that deserve to be given weight in the ELT selection process. Other things being anything like equal, the mother of minor children must take priority over the middle-aged bachelor.

D. THE POTENTIAL FUTURE-CONTRIBUTIONS FACTOR (PROSPECTIVE SERVICE)

In "choosing to save" one life rather than another, "the society," through the mediation of the particular medical institution in question —which should certainly look upon itself as a trustee for the social interest—is clearly warranted in considering the likely pattern of future *services to be rendered* by the patient (adequate recovery assumed), considering his age, talent, training, and past record of performance. In its allocations of ELT, society "invests" a scarce resource in one person as against another and is thus entitled to look to the probable prospective "return" on its investment.

It may well be that a thoroughly egalitarian society is reluctant to put someone's social contribution into the scale in situations of the sort at issue. One popular article states that "the most difficult standard would be the candidate's value to society," and goes on to quote someone who said: "You can't just pick a brilliant painter over a laborer. The average citizen would be quickly eliminated."[6] But what if it were not a brilliant painter but a brilliant surgeon or medical researcher that was at issue? One wonders if the author of the *obiter dictum* that one "can't just pick" would still feel equally sure of his ground. In any case, the fact that the standard is difficult to apply is certainly no reason for not attempting to apply it. The problem of ELT selection is inevitably burdened with difficult standards.

Some might feel that in assessing a patient's value to society one should ask not only who if permitted to continue living can make the greatest contribution to society in some creative or constructive way, but also who by dying would leave behind the greatest burden on society in assuming the discharge of their residual responsibilities.[7] Certainly the philosophical utilitarian would give equal weight to both these considerations. Just here is where I would part ways with orthodox utilitarianism. For—though this is not the place to do so—I should be prepared to argue that a civilized society has an obligation to promote the furtherance of positive achievements in cultural and related areas even if this means the assumption of certain added burdens.[8]

E. THE PAST SERVICES-RENDERED FACTOR (RETROSPECTIVE SERVICE)

A person's services to another person or group have always been taken to constitute a valid basis for a claim upon this person or group —of course a moral and not necessarily a legal claim. Society's obligation for the recognition and reward of services rendered—an obligation whose discharge is also very possibly conducive to self-interest in the long run—is thus another factor to be taken into account. This should be viewed as a morally necessary correlative of the previously considered factor of *prospective* service. It would be morally indefensible of society in effect to say: "Never mind about services you rendered yesterday— it is only the services to be rendered tomorrow that will count with us today." We live in very future-oriented times, constantly preoccupied in a distinctly utilitarian way with future satisfactions. And this disinclines us to give much recognition to past services. But parity considerations of the sort just adduced indicate that such recognition should be given *on grounds of equity*. No doubt a justification for giving weight to services rendered can also be attempted along utilitarian lines. ("The reward of past services rendered spurs people on to greater future efforts and is thus socially advantageous in the long-run future.") In saying that past services should be counted "on grounds of equity"—rather than "on grounds of utility"—I take the view that even if this utilitarian defense could somehow be shown to be fallacious, I should still be prepared to maintain the propriety of taking services rendered into account. The position does not rest on a utilitarian basis and so would not collapse with the removal of such a basis.[9]

As we have said, these five factors fall into three groups: the biomedical factors *A* and *B*, the familial factor *C*, and the social factors *D* and *E*. With items *A* and *B* the need for a detailed analysis of the medical considerations comes to the fore. The age of the patient, his medical history, his physical and psychological condition, his specific disease, etc., will all need to be taken into exact account. These biomedical factors represent technical issues: they call for the physicians' expert judgment and the medical statisticians' hard data. And they are ethically uncontroversial factors— their legitimacy and appropriateness are evident from the very nature of the case.

Greater problems arise with the familial and social factors. They involve intangibles that are difficult to judge. How is one to develop subcriteria for weighing the relative social contributions of (say) an architect or a librarian or a mother of young children? And they involve highly problematic issues. (For example, should good moral character be rated a plus and bad a minus in judging services rendered?) And there is something strikingly unpleasant in grappling with issues of this sort for people brought up in times greatly inclined towards maxims of the type "Judge not!" and "Live and let live!" All the same, in the situation that concerns us here such distasteful problems must be faced, since a failure to choose to save some is tantamount to sentencing all. Unpleasant choices are intrinsic to the problem of ELT selection; they are of the very essence of the matter.[10]

But is reference to all these factors indeed inevitable? The justification for taking account of the medical factors is pretty obvious. But why should the social aspect of services rendered and to be rendered be taken into account at all? The answer is that they must be taken into account not from the *medical* but from the *ethical* point of view. Despite disagreement on many fundamental issues, moral philosophers of the present day are pretty well in consensus that the justification of human actions is to be sought largely and primarily—if not exclusively—in the principles of utility and of justice.[11] But utility requires reference of services to be rendered and justice calls for a recognition of services that have been rendered. Moral considerations would thus demand recognition of these two factors. (This, of course, still leaves open the question of whether the point of view provides a valid basis of action: Why base one's actions upon moral principles? —or, to put it bluntly—Why be moral? The present paper is, however, hardly the place to grapple with so fundamental an issue, which has been canvassed in the literature of philosophical ethics since Plato.)

VI. MORE THAN MEDICAL ISSUES ARE INVOLVED

An active controversy has of late sprung up in medical circles over the question of whether non-physician laymen should be given a role in ELT selection (in the specific context of chronic haemodialysis). One physician writes: "I think that the assessment of the candidates should be made by a senior doctor on the [dialysis] unit, but I am sure that it would be helpful to him—both in sharing responsibility and in avoiding personal pressure—if a small unnamed group of people [presumably including laymen] officially made the final decision. I visualize the doctor bringing the data to the group, explaining the points in relation to each case, and obtaining their approval of his order of priority."[12]

Essentially this procedure of a selection committee of laymen has for some years been in use in one of the most publicized chronic dialysis units, that of the Swedish Hospital of Seattle, Washington.[13] Many physicians are apparently reluctant to see the choice of allocation of medical therapy pass out of strictly medical hands. Thus in a recent symposium on the "Selection of Patients for Haemodialysis,"[14] Dr. Ralph Shakman writes: "Who is to implement the selection? In my opinion it must ultimately be the responsibility of the consultants in charge of the renal units . . . I can see no reason for delegating this responsibility to lay persons. Surely the latter would be better employed if they could be persuaded to devote their time and energy to raise more and more money for us to spend on our patients."[15] Other contributors to this symposium strike much the same note. Dr. F. M. Parsons writes: "In an attempt to overcome . . . difficulties in selection some have advocated introducing certain specified lay people into the discussions. Is it wise? I doubt whether a committee of this type can adjudicate as satisfactorily as two medical colleagues, particularly as successful therapy involves close cooperation between doctor and patient."[16] And Dr. M. A. Wilson writes in the same symposium: "The suggestion has been made that lay panels should select individuals for dialysis from among a group who are medically suitable. Though this would relieve the doctor-in-charge of a heavy load of responsibility, it would place the burden on those who have no personal knowledge and have to base their judgments on medical or social reports. I do not believe this would result in better decisions for the group or improve the doctor-patient relationship in individual cases."[17]

But no amount of flag waving about the doctor's facing up to his responsibility—or prostrations before the idol of the doctor-patient relationship and reluctance to admit laymen into the sacred precincts of the conference chambers of medical consultations—can obscure the essential fact that ELT selection is not a wholly medical problem. When there are more than enough places in an ELT program to accommodate all who need it, then it will clearly be a medical question to decide who does have the need and which among these would successfully respond. But when an admitted gross insufficiency of places exists, when there are ten or fifty or one hundred highly eligible candidates for each place in the program, then it is unrealistic to take the view that purely medical criteria can furnish a sufficient basis for selection. The question of ELT selection becomes serious as a phenomenon of scale—because, as more candidates present themselves, strictly medical factors are increasingly less adequate as a selection criterion precisely because by numerical category-crowding there will be more and more cases whose "status is much the same" so far as purely medical considerations go.

The ELT selection problem clearly poses issues that transcend the medical sphere because—in the nature of the case—many residual issues remain to be dealt with once *all* of the medical questions have been faced. Because of this there is good reason why laymen as well as physicians should be involved in the selection process. Once the medical considerations have been brought to bear, fundamental social issues remain to be resolved. The instrumentalities of ELT have been created through the social investment of scarce resources, and the interests of the society deserve to play a role in their utilization. As representatives of their social interests, lay opinions should function to complement and supplement medical views once the proper arena of medical considerations is left behind.[18] Those physicians who have urged the presence of lay members on selection panels can, from this point of view, be recognized as having seen the issue in proper perspective.

One physician has argued against lay representation on selection panels for haemodialysis as follows: "If the doctor advises dialysis and the lay panel refuses, the patient will regard this as a death sentence passed by an anonymous court from which he has no right of appeal."[19] But this drawback is not specific to the use of a lay panel. Rather, it is a feature inherent in every *selection* procedure, regardless of whether the selection is done by the head doctor of the unit, by a panel of physicians, etc. No matter who does the selecting among patients recommended for dialysis, the feelings of the patient who has been rejected (and knows it) can be expected to be much the same, provided that he recognizes the actual nature of the choice (and is not deceived by the possibly convenient but ultimately poisonous fiction that because the selection was made by physicians it was made entirely on medical grounds).

In summary, then, the question of ELT selection would appear to be one that is in its very nature heavily laden with issues of medical research, practice, and administration. But it will not be a question that can be resolved on solely medical grounds. Strictly social issues of justice and utility will invariably arise in this area —questions going outside the medical area in whose resolution medical laymen can and should play a substantial role.

VII. THE INHERENT IMPERFECTION (NON-OPTIMALITY) OF ANY SELECTION SYSTEM

Our discussion to this point of the design of a selection system for ELT has left a gap that is a very fundamental and serious omission. We have argued that five factors must be taken into substantial and explicit account:

A. *Relative likelihood of success.* Is the chance of the treatment's being "successful" to be rated as high, good, average, etc.?[20]

B. *Expectancy of future life*. Assuming the "success" of the treatment, how much longer does the patient stand a good chance (75 per cent or better) of living—considering his age and general condition?

C. *Family role*. To what extent does the patient have responsibilities to others in his immediate family?

D. *Social contributions rendered*. Are the patient's past services to his society outstanding, substantial, average, etc.?

E. *Social contributions to be rendered*. Considering his age, talents, training, and past record of performance, is there a substantial probability that the patient will—*adequate recovery being assumed*—render in the future services to his society that can be characterized as outstanding, substantial, average, etc.?

This list is clearly insufficient for construction of a reasonable selection system, since that would require not only *that these factors be taken into account* (somehow or other), but —going beyond this—would specify *a specific set of procedures for taking account of them*. The specific procedures that would constitute such a system would have to take account of the interrelationship of these factors (e.g., *B* and *E*), and to set out exact guidelines as to the relevant weight that is to be given to each of them. This is something our discussion has not as yet considered.

In fact, I should want to maintain that there is no such thing here as a single rationally superior selection system. The position of affairs seems to me to be something like this: (1) It is necessary (for reasons already canvassed) to *have* a system, and to have a system that is rationally defensible, and (2) to be rationally defensible, this system must take the factors *A–E* into substantial and explicit account. But (3) the exact manner in which a rationally defensible system takes account of these factors cannot be fixed in any one specific way on the basis of general considerations. Any of the variety of ways that give *A–E* "their due" will be acceptable and viable. One cannot hope to find

within this range of workable systems some one that is *optimal* in relation to the alternatives. There is no one system that does "the (uniquely) best"—only a variety of systems that do "as well as one can expect to do" in cases of this sort.

The situation is structurally very much akin to that of rules of partition of an estate among the relations of a decedent. It is important *that there be* such rules. And it is reasonable that spouse, children, parents, siblings, etc., be taken account of in these rules. But the question of the exact method of division—say that when the decedent has neither living spouse nor living children then his estate is to be divided, dividing 60 per cent between parents, 40 per cent between siblings versus dividing 90 per cent between parents, 10 per cent between siblings—cannot be settled on the basis of any general abstract considerations of reasonableness. Within broad limits, a *variety* of resolutions are all perfectly acceptable—so that no one procedure can justifiably be regarded as "the (uniquely) best" because it is superior to all others.[21]

VIII. A POSSIBLE BASIS FOR A REASONABLE SELECTION SYSTEM

Having said that there is no such thing as *the optimal* selection system for ELT, I want now to sketch out the broad features of what I would regard as *one acceptable* system.

The basis for the system would be a point rating. The scoring here at issue would give roughly equal weight to the medical considerations (*A* and *B*) in comparison with the extramedical considerations (*C*=family role, *D*=services rendered, and *E*=services to be rendered), also giving roughly equal weight to the three items involved here (*C, D,* and *E*). The result of such a scoring procedure would provide the essential *starting point* of our ELT selection mechanism. I deliberately say "starting point" because it seems to me that one should not follow the results of this scoring in an *automatic* way. I would propose that the actual selection should only be guided but not actually be dictated by this scoring procedure, along lines now to be explained.

The detailed procedure I would propose—not of course as optimal (for reasons we have seen), but as eminently acceptable—would combine the scoring procedure just discussed with an element of chance. The resulting selection system would function as follows:

1. First the criteria of inclusion of Section IV above would be applied to constitute a *first phase selection group*—which (we shall suppose) is substantially larger than the number n of persons who can actually be accommodated with ELT.

2. Next the criteria of selection of Section V are brought to bear via a scoring procedure of the type described in Section VIII. On this basis a *second phase selection group* is constituted which is only *somewhat* larger—say by a third or a half—than the critical number n at issue.

3. If this second phase selection group is relatively homogeneous as regards rating by the scoring procedure—that is, if there are no really major disparities within this group (as would be likely if the initial group was significantly larger than n)—then the final selection is made by *random* selection of n persons from within this group.

This introduction of the element of chance—in what could be dramatized as a "lottery of life and death"—must be justified. The fact is that such a procedure would bring with it three substantial advantages.

First, as we have argued above (in Section VII), any acceptable selection system is inherently non-optimal. The introduction of the element of chance prevents the results that life-and-death choices are made by the automatic application of an admittedly imperfect selection method.

Second, a recourse to chance would doubtless make matters easier for the rejected patient and those who have a specific interest in him. It would surely be quite hard for them to accept his exclusion by relatively mechanical application of objective criteria in whose implementation subjective judgment is involved.

But the circumstances of life have conditioned us to accept the workings of chance and to tolerate the element of luck (good or bad): human life is an inherently contingent process. Nobody, after all, has an absolute right to ELT—but most of us would feel that we have "every bit as much right" to it as anyone else in significantly similar circumstances. The introduction of the element of chance assures a like handling of like cases over the widest possible area that seems reasonable in the circumstances.

Third (and perhaps least), such a recourse to random selection does much to relieve the administrators of the selection system of the awesome burden of ultimate and absolute responsibility.

These three considerations would seem to build up a substantial case for introducing the element of chance into the mechanism of the system for ELT selection in a way limited and circumscribed by other weightier considerations, along some such lines as those set forth above.[22]

It should be recognized that this injection of *man-made* chance supplements the element of *natural* chance that is present inevitably and in any case (apart from the role of chance in singling out certain persons as victims for the affliction at issue). As F. M. Parsons has observed: "any vacancies [in an ELT program—specifically haemodialysis] will be filled immediately by the first suitable patients, even though their claims for therapy may subsequently prove less than those of other patients refused later."[23] Life is a chancy business and even the most rational of human arrangements can cover this over to a very limited extent at best.

NOTES

1. Christine Doyle, "Spare-Part Heart Surgeons Worried by Their Success," *Observer*, May 12, 1968.

2. J. D. N. Nabarro, "Selection of Patients for Haemodialysis," *British Medical Journal* (March 11,

1967), p. 623. Although several thousand patients die in the U.K. each year from renal failure—there are about thirty new cases per million of population—only 10 per cent of these can for the foreseeable future be accommodated with chronic haemodialysis. Kidney transplantation—itself a very tricky procedure—cannot make a more than minor contribution here. As this article goes to press, I learn that patients can be maintained in home dialysis at an operating cost about half that of maintaining them in a hospital dialysis unit (roughly an $8,000 minimum). In the United States, around 7,000 patients with terminal uremia who could benefit from haemodialysis evolve yearly. As of mid-1968, some 1,000 of these can be accommodated in existing hospital units. By June 1967, a world-wide total of some 120 patients were in treatment by home dialysis. (Data from a forthcoming paper, "Home Dialysis," by C. M. Conty and H. V. Murdaugh. See also R. A. Baillod *et al.,* "Overnight Haemodialysis in the Home," *Proceedings of the European Dialysis and Transplant Association,* VI [1965], 99 ff.).

3. For the Hippocratic Oath see *Hippocrates: Works* (Loeb ed.; London, 1959), I, p. 298.

4. Another example of borderline legitimacy is posed by an endowment "with strings attached," e.g., "In accepting this legacy the hospital agrees to admit and provide all needed treatment for any direct descendant of myself, its founder."

5. Shana Alexander, "They Decide Who Lives, Who Dies," *Life,* LIII (November 9, 1962), 102–25 (see p. 107).

6. Lawrence Lader, "Who Has the Right To Live?" *Good Housekeeping* (January 1968), p. 144.

7. This approach could thus be continued to embrace the previous factor, that of family role, the preceding item (*C*).

8. Moreover a doctrinaire utilitarian would presumably be willing to withdraw a continuing mode of ELT such as haemodialysis from a patient to make room for a more promising candidate who came to view at a later stage and who could not otherwise be accommodated. I should be unwilling to adopt this course, partly on grounds of utility (with a view to the demoralization of insecurity), partly on the non-utilitarian ground that a "moral commitment" has been made and must be honored.

9. Of course the difficult question remains of the relative weight that should be given to prospective and retrospective service in cases where these factors conflict. There is good reason to treat them on a par.

10. This in the symposium on "Selection of Patients for Haemodialysis," *British Medical Journal* (March 11, 1967), pp. 622–24. F. M. Parsons writes: "But other forms of selecting patients [distinct from first come, first served] are suspect in my view if they imply evaluation of man by man. What criteria could be used? Who could justify a claim that the life of a mayor would be more valuable than that of the humblest citizen of his borough? Whatever we may think as individuals none of us is indispensable." But having just set out this hard-line view he immediately backs away from it: "On the other hand, to assume that there was little to choose between Alexander Fleming and Adolf Hitler . . . would be nonsense, and we should be naive if we were to pretend that we could not be influenced by their achievements and characters if we had to choose between the two of them. Whether we like it or not we cannot escape the fact that this kind of selection for long-term

haemodialysis will be required until very large sums of money become available for equipment and services [so that *everyone* who needs treatment can be accommodated]."

11. The relative fundamentality of these principles is, however, a substantially disputed issue.

12. J. D. N. Nabarro, *op. cit.,* p. 622.

13. See Shanna Alexander, *op. cit.*

14. *British Medical Journal* (March 11, 1967), pp. 622–24.

15. *Ibid.,* p. 624. Another contributor writes in the same symposium, "The selection of the few [to receive haemodialysis] is proving very difficult—a true 'Doctor's Dilemma'—for almost everybody would agree that this must be a medical decision, preferably reached by consultation among colleagues" (Dr. F. M. Parsons, *ibid.,* p. 623).

16. "Selection of Patients for Haemodialysis." *op. cit.* (n. 10 above), p. 623.

17. Dr. Wilson's article concludes with the perplexing suggestion—wildly beside the point given the structure of the situation at issue—that "the final decision will be made by the patient." But this contention is only marginally more ludicrous than Parson's contention that in selecting patients for haemodialysis "gainful employment in a well chosen occupation is necessary to achieve the best results" since "only the minority wish to live on charity" (*ibid.*).

18. To say this is of course not to deny that such questions of applied medical ethics will invariably involve a host of medical considerations—it is only to insist that extramedical considerations will also invariably be at issue.

19. M. A. Wilson, "Selection of Patients for Haemodialysis," *op. cit.,* p. 624.

20. In the case of an ongoing treatment involving complex procedure and dietary and other mode-of-life restrictions—and chronic haemodialysis definitely falls into this category—the patient's psychological makeup, his willpower to "stick with it" in the face of substantial discouragements—will obviously also be a substantial factor here. The man who gives up, takes not his life alone, but (figuratively speaking) also that of the person he replaced in the treatment schedule.

21. To say that acceptable solutions can range over broad limits is *not* to say that there are no limits at all. It is an obviously intriguing and fundamental problem to raise the question of the factors that set these limits. This complex issue cannot be dealt with adequately here. Suffice it to say that considerations regarding precedent and people's expectations, factors of social utility, and matters of fairness and sense of justice all come into play.

22. One writer has mooted the suggestion that: "Perhaps the right thing to do, difficult as it may be to accept, is to select [for haemodialysis] from among the medical and psychologically qualified patients on a strictly random basis" (S. Gorovitz, "Ethics and the Allocation of Medical Resources." *Medical Research Engineering,* V [1966], p. 7). Outright random selection would, however, seem indefensible because of its refusal to give weight to considerations which, under the circumstances, *deserve* to be given weight. The proposed procedure of superimposing a certain degree of randomness upon the rational-choice criteria would seem to combine the advantages of the two without importing the worst defects of either.

23. "Selection of Patients for Haemodialysis," *op. cit.,*

p. 623. The question of whether a patient for chronic treatment should ever be terminated from the program (say if he contracts cancer) poses a variety of difficult ethical problems with which we need not at present concern ourselves. But it does seem plausible to take the (somewhat anti-utilitarian) view that a patient should not be terminated simply because a "better qualified" patient comes along later on. It would seem that quasi-contractual relationship has been created through established expectations and re-ciprocal understandings, and that the situation is in this regard akin to that of the man who, having undertaken to sell his house to one buyer, cannot afterward unilaterally undo this arrangement to sell it to a higher bidder who "needs it worse" (thus maximizing the over-all utility).

JAMES F. CHILDRESS

Who Shall Live When Not All Can Live?

Who shall live when not all can live? Although this question has been urgently forced upon us by the dramatic use of artificial internal organs and organ transplantations, it is hardly new. George Bernard Shaw dealt with it in "The Doctor's Dilemma":

SIR PATRICK. Well, Mr. Savior of Lives: which is it to be? that honest decent man Blenkinsop, or that rotten blackguard of an artist, eh?

RIDGEON. It's not an easy case to judge, is it? Blenkinsop's an honest decent man; but is he any use? Dubedat's a rotten blackguard; but he's a genuine source of pretty and pleasant and good things.

SIR PATRICK. What will he be a source of for that poor innocent wife of his, when she finds him out?

RIDGEON. That's true. Her life will be a hell.

SIR PATRICK. And tell me this. Suppose you had this choice put before you: either to go through life and find all the pictures bad but all the men and women good, or go through life and find all the pictures good and all the men and women rotten. Which would you choose?[1]

A significant example of the distribution of scarce medical resources is seen in the use of penicillin shortly after its discovery. Military officers had to determine which soldiers would be treated—those with venereal disease or those wounded in combat?[2] In many respects

such decisions have become routine in medical circles. Day after day physicians and others make judgments and decisions "about allocations of medical care to various segments of our population, to various types of hospitalized patients, and to specific individuals,"[3] for example, whether mental illness or cancer will receive the higher proportion of available funds. Nevertheless, the dramatic forms of "Scarce Life-Saving Medical Resources" (hereafter abbreviated as SLMR) such as hemodialysis and kidney and heart transplants have compelled us to examine the moral questions that have been concealed in many routine decisions. I do not attempt in this paper to show how a resolution of SLMR cases can help us in the more routine ones which do not involve a conflict of life with life. Rather I develop an argument for a particular method of determining who shall live when not all can live. No conclusions are implied about criteria and procedures for determining who shall receive medical resources that are not directly related to the preservation of life (e.g. corneal transplants) or about standards for allocating money and time for studying and treating certain diseases.

Just as current SLMR decisions are not totally discontinuous with other medical decisions, so we must ask whether some other

Reprinted with permission of the publisher from *Soundings*, Vol. 53, No 4 (Winter 1970), pp. 339–55.

cases might, at least by analogy, help us develop the needed criteria and procedures. Some have looked at the principles at work in our responses to abortion, euthanasia, and artificial insemination.[4] Usually they have concluded that these cases do not cast light on the selection of patients for artificial and transplanted organs. The reason is evident: in abortion, euthanasia, and artificial insemination, there is no conflict of life with life for limited but indispensable resources (with the possible exception of therapeutic abortion). In current SLMR decisions, such a conflict is inescapable, and it makes them so morally perplexing and fascinating. If analogous cases are to be found, I think that we shall locate them in moral conflict situations.

ANALOGOUS CONFLICT SITUATIONS

An especially interesting and pertinent one is *U.S. v. Holmes.*[5] In 1841 an American ship, the *William Brown,* which was near Newfoundland on a trip from Liverpool to Philadelphia, struck an iceberg. The crew and half the passengers were able to escape in the two available vessels. One of these, a longboat, carrying too many passengers and leaking seriously, began to founder in the turbulent sea after about twenty-four hours. In a desperate attempt to keep it from sinking, the crew threw overboard fourteen men. Two sisters of one of the men either jumped overboard to join their brother in death or instructed the crew to throw them over. The criteria for determining who should live were "not to part man and wife, and not to throw over any women." Several hours later the others were rescued. Returning to Philadelphia, most of the crew disappeared, but one, Holmes, who had acted upon orders from the mate, was indicted, tried, and convicted on the charge of "unlawful homicide."

We are interested in this case from a moral rather than a legal standpoint, and there are several possible responses to and judgments about it. Without attempting to be exhaustive I shall sketch a few of these. The judge contended that lots should have been cast, for in such conflict situations, there is no other procedure "so consonant both to humanity and to justice." Counsel for Holmes, on the other hand, maintained that the "sailors adopted the only principle of selection which was possible in an emergency like theirs,—a principle more humane than lots."

Another version of selection might extend and systematize the maxims of the sailors in the direction of "utility"; those are saved who will contribute to the greatest good for the greatest number. Yet another possible option is defended by Edmond Cahn in *The Moral Decision.* He argues that in this case we encounter the "morals of the last days." By this phrase he indicates than an apocalyptic crisis renders totally irrelevant the normal differences between individuals. He continues,

In a strait of this extremity, all men are reduced—or raised, as one may choose to denominate it—to members of the genus, mere congeners and nothing else. Truly and literally, all were "in the same boat," and thus none could be saved separately from the others. I am driven to conclude that otherwise—that is, if none sacrifice themselves of free will to spare the others—they must all wait and die together. For where all have become congeners, pure and simple, no one can save himself by killing another.[6]

Cahn's answer to the question "who shall live when not all can live" is "none" unless the voluntary sacrifice by some persons permits it.

Few would deny the importance of Cahn's approach although many, including this writer, would suggest that it is relevant mainly as an affirmation of an elevated and, indeed, heroic or saintly morality which one hopes would find expression in the voluntary actions of many persons trapped in "borderline" situations involving a conflict of life with life. It is a maximal demand which some moral principles impose on the individual in the recognition that self-preservation is not a good which is to be defended at all costs. The absence of this saintly or heroic morality should not mean, however, that everyone perishes. Without making survival an absolute value and without justifying all means to achieve it, we can maintain that simply letting everyone die is irresponsible. This charge can be supported from several different standpoints, including society at large as well as the individuals involved. Among a group of self-interested individuals, none of whom volunteers to relinquish his life, there may be better and worse ways of determining who shall survive. One task of social ethics, whether religious or philosophical, is to propose relatively just institutional arrangements within which self-interested and biased men can live. The question then becomes: which set of arrangements—which criteria and procedures of selection—is most satisfactory in view of the human condition (man's limited altruism and inclination to seek his own good) and the conflicting values that are to be realized?

There are several significant differences between the *Holmes* and SLMR cases, a major one being that the former involves *direct* killing of another person, while the latter involves only *permitting* a person to die when it is not possible to save all. Furthermore, in extreme situations such as *Holmes,* the restraints of civilization have been stripped away, and something approximating a state of nature prevails, in which life is "solitary, poor, nasty, brutish and short." The state of nature does not mean that moral standards are irrelevant and that might should prevail, but it does suggest that much of the matrix which normally supports morality has been removed. Also, the necessary but unfortunate decisions about who shall live and die are made by men who are existentially and personally involved in the outcome. Their survival too is at stake. Even though the institutional role of sailors seems to require greater sacrificial actions, there is obviously no assurance that they will adequately assess the number of sailors required to man the vessel or that they will impartially and objectively weigh the common good at stake. As the judge insisted in his defense of casting lots in the *Holmes* case: "In no other than this [casting lots] or some like way are those having equal rights put upon an equal footing, and in no other way is it possible to guard against partiality and oppression, violence, and conflict." This difference should not be exaggerated since self-interest, professional pride, and the like obviously affect the

outcome of many medical decisions. Nor do the remaining differences cancel *Holmes'* instructiveness.

CRITERIA OF SELECTION FOR SLMR

Which set of arrangements should be adopted for SLMR? Two questions are involved: Which standards and criteria should be used? and, Who should make the decision? The first question is basic, since the debate about implementation, e.g., whether by a lay committee or physician, makes little progress until the criteria are determined.

We need two sets of criteria which will be applied at two different stages in the selection of recipients of SLMR. First, medical criteria should be used to exclude those who are not "medically acceptable." Second, from this group of "medically acceptable" applicants, the final selection can be made. Occasionally in current American medical practice, the first stage is omitted, but such an omission is unwarranted. Ethical and social responsibility would seem to require distributing these SLMR only to those who have some reasonable prospect of responding to the treatment. Furthermore, in transplants such medical tests as tissue and blood typing are necessary, although they are hardly fully developed.

"Medical acceptability" is not as easily determined as many non-physicians assume since there is considerable debate in medical circles about the relevant factors (e.g., age and complicating diseases). Although ethicists can contribute little or nothing to this debate, two proposals may be in order. First, "medical acceptability" should be used only to determine the group from which the final selection will be made, and the attempt to establish fine degrees of prospective response to treatment should be avoided. Medical criteria, then, would exlude some applicants but would not serve as a basis of comparison between those who pass the first stage. For example, if two applicants for dialysis were medically acceptable, the physicians would *not* choose the one with the *better* medical prospects. Final selection would be made on other grounds.

Second, psychological and environmental factors should be kept to an absolute minimum and should be considered only when they are without doubt critically related to medical acceptability (e.g., the inability to cope with the requirements of dialysis which might lead to suicide).[7]

The most significant moral questions emerge when we turn to the final selection. Once the pool of medically acceptable applicants has been defined and still the number is larger than the resources, what other criteria should be used? How should the final selection be made? First, I shall examine some of the difficulties that stem from efforts to make the final selection in terms of social value; these difficulties raise serious doubts about the feasibility and justifiability of the utilitarian approach. Then I shall consider the possible justification for random selection or chance.

Occasionally criteria of social worth focus on past contributions but most often they are primarily future-oriented. The patient's potential and probable contribution to the society is stressed, Although this obviously cannot be abstracted from his present web of relationships (e.g., dependents) and occupational activities (e.g., nuclear physicist). Indeed, the magnitude of his contribution to society (as an abstraction) is measured in terms of these social roles, relations, and functions. Enough has already been said to suggest the tremendous range of factors that affect social value or worth.[8] Here we encounter the first major difficulty of this approach: How do we determine the relevant criteria of social value?

The difficulties of quantifying various social needs are only too obvious. How does one quantify and compare the needs of the spirit (e.g., education, art, religion), political life, economic activity, technological development? Joseph Fletcher suggests that "some day we may learn how to 'quantify' or 'mathematicate' or 'computerize' the value problem in selection, in the same careful and thorough way that diagnosis has been."[9] I am not convinced that we can ever quantify values, or that we should attempt to do so. But even if the

various social and human needs, in principle, could be quantified, how do we determine how much weight we will give to each one? Which will have priority in case of conflict? Or even more basically, in the light of which values and principles do we recognize social "needs"?

One possible way of determining the values which should be emphasized in selection has been proposed by Leo Shatin.[10] He insists that our medical decisions about allocating resources are already based on an unconscious scale of values (usually dominated by material worth). Since there is really no way of escaping this, we should be self-conscious and critical about it. How should we proceed? He recommends that we discover the values that most people in our society hold and then use them as criteria for distributing SLMR. These values can be discovered by attitude or opinion surveys. Presumably if fifty-one percent in this testing period put a greater premium on military needs than technological development, military men would have a greater claim on our SLMR than experimental researchers. But valuations of what is significant change, and the student revolutionary who was denied SLMR in 1970 might be celebrated in 1990 as the greatest American hero since George Washington.

Shatin presumably is seeking criteria that could be applied nationally, but at the present, regional and local as well as individual prejudices tincture the criteria of social value that are used in selection. Nowhere is this more evident than in the deliberations and decisions of the anonymous selection committee of the Seattle Artificial Kidney Center where such factors as church membership and Scout leadership have been deemed significant for determining who shall live.[11] As two critics conclude after examining these criteria and procedures, they rule out "creative nonconformists, who rub the bourgeoisie the wrong way but who historically have contributed so much to the making of America. The Pacific Northwest is no place for a Henry David Thoreau with bad kidneys."[12]

Closely connected to this first problem of determining social values is a second one. Not only is it difficult if not impossible to reach agreement on social values, but it is also rarely easy to predict what our needs will be in a few years and what the consequences of present actions will be. Furthermore it is difficult to predict which persons will fulfill their potential function in society. Admissions committees in colleges and universities experience the frustrations of predicting realization of potential. For these reasons, as someone has indicated, God might be a utilitarian, but we cannot be. We simply lack the capacity to predict very accurately the consequences which we then must evaluate. Our incapacity is never more evident than when we think in societal terms.

Other difficulties make us even less confident that such an approach to SLMR is advisable. Many critics raise the spectre of abuse, but this should not be overemphasized. The fundamental difficulty appears on another level: the utilitarian approach would in effect reduce the person to his social role, relations, and functions. Ultimately it dulls and perhaps even eliminates the sense of the person's transcendence, his dignity as a person which cannot be reduced to his past or future contribution to society. It is not at all clear that we are willing to live with these implications of utilitarian selection. Wilhelm Kolff, who invented the artificial kidney, has asked: "Do we really subscribe to the principle that social standing should determine selection? Do we allow patients to be treated with dialysis only when they are married, go to church, have children, have a job, a good income and give to the Community Chest?"[13]

The German theologian Helmut Thielicke contends that any search for "objective criteria" for selection is already a capitulation to the utilitarian point of view which violates man's dignity.[14] The solution is not to let all die, but to recognize that SLMR cases are "borderline situations" which inevitably involve guilt. The agent, however, can have courage and freedom (which, for Thielicke, come from justification by faith) and can

go ahead anyway and seek for criteria for deciding the question of life or death in the matter of the artificial kidney. Since these criteria are . . . questionable, necessarily alien to the meaning of human

existence, the decision to which they lead can be little more than that arrived at by casting lots.[15]

The resulting criteria, he suggests, will probably be very similar to those already employed in American medical practice.

He is most concerned to preserve a certain *attitude* or *disposition* in SLMR—the sense of guilt which arises when man's dignity is violated. With this sense of guilt, the agent remains "sound and healthy where it really counts."[16] Thielicke uses man's dignity only as a judgmental, critical, and negative standard. It only tells us how all selection criteria and procedures (and even the refusal to act) implicate us in the ambiguity of the human condition and its metaphysical guilt. This approach is consistent with his view of the task of theological ethics: "to teach us how to understand and endure—not 'solve'—the borderline situation."[17] But ethics, I would contend, can help us discern the factors and norms in whose light relative, discriminate judgments can be made. Even if all actions in SLMR should involve guilt, some may preserve human dignity to a greater extent than others. Thielicke recognizes that a decision based on any criteria is "little more than that arrived at by casting lots." But perhaps selection by chance would come the closest to embodying the moral and nonmoral values that we are trying to maintain (including a sense of man's dignity).

THE VALUES OF RANDOM SELECTION

My proposal is that we use some form of randomness or chance (either natural, such as "first come, first served," or artificial, such as a lottery) to determine who shall be saved. Many reject randomness as a surrender to nonrationality when responsible and rational judgments can and must be made. Edmond Cahn criticizes "Holmes' judge" who recommended the casting of lots because, as Cahn puts it, "the crisis involves stakes too high for gambling and responsibilities too deep for destiny."[18] Similarly, other critics see randomness as a surrender to "non-human" forces which necessarily vitiates human values. Sometimes these values are identified with the process of decision-making (e.g., it is important to have persons rather than impersonal forces determining who shall live). Sometimes they are identified with the outcome of the process (e.g., the features such as creativity and fullness of being which make human life what it is are to be considered and respected in the decision). Regarding the former, it must be admitted that the use of chance seems cold and impersonal. But presumably the defenders of utilitarian criteria in SLMR want to make their application as objective and impersonal as possible so that subjective bias does not determine who shall live.

Such criticisms, however, ignore the moral and nonmoral values which might be supported by selection by randomness or chance. A more important criticism is that the procedure that I develop draws the relevant moral context too narrowly. That context, so the argument might run, includes the society and its future and not merely the individual with his illness and claim upon SLMR. But my contention is that the values and principles at work in the narrower context may well take precedence over those operative in the broader context both because of their weight and significance and because of the weaknesses of selection in terms of social worth. As Paul Freund rightly insists, ''The more nearly total is the estimate to be made of an individual, and the more nearly the consequence determines life and death, the more unfit the judgment becomes for human reckoning. . . . Randomness as a moral principle deserves serious study.''[19] Serious study would, I think, point toward its implementation in certain conflict situations, primarily because it preserves a significant degree of *personal dignity* by providing *equality* of opportunity. Thus it cannot be dismissed as a ''non-rational'' and ''non-human'' procedure without an inquiry into the reasons, including human values, which might justify it. Paul Ramsey stresses this point about the *Holmes* case:

Instead of fixing our attention upon ''gambling'' as the solution—with all the frivolous and often corrupt associations the word raises in our minds—we

should think rather of *equality* of opportunity as the ethical substance of the relations of those individuals to one another that might have been guarded and expressed by casting lots.[20]

The individual's personal and transcendent dignity, which on the utilitarian approach would be submerged in his social role and function, can be protected and witnessed to by a recognition of his equal right to be saved. Such a right is best preserved by procedures which establish equality of opportunity. Thus selection by chance more closely approximates the requirements established by human dignity than does utilitarian calculation. It is not infallibly just, but it is preferable to the alternatives of letting all die or saving only those who have the greatest social responsibilities and potential contribution.

This argument can be extended by examining values other than individual dignity and equality of opportunity. Another basic value in the medical sphere is the relationship of trust between physician and patient. Which selection criteria are most in accord with this relationship of trust? Which will maintain, extend, and deepen it? My contention is that selection by randomness or chance is preferable from this standpoint too.

Trust, which is inextricably bound to respect for human dignity, is an attitude of expectation about another. It is not simply the expectation that another will perform a particular act, but more specifically that another will act toward him in certain ways—which will respect him as a person. As Charles Fried writes:

Although trust has to do with reliance on a disposition of another person, it is reliance on a disposition of a special sort: the disposition to act morally, to deal fairly with others, to live up to one's undertakings, and so on. Thus to trust another is first of all to expect him to accept the principle of morality in his dealings with you, to respect your status as a person, your personality.[21]

This trust cannot be preserved in life-and-death situations when a person expects decisions about him to be made in terms of his social worth, for such decisions violate his status as a person. An applicant rejected on grounds of inadequacy in social value or virtue would have reason for feeling that his ''trust'' had been betrayed. Indeed, the sense that one is being viewed not as an end in himself but as a means in medical progress or the achievement of a greater social good is incompatible with attitudes and relationships of trust. We recognize this in the billboard which was erected after the first heart transplants: "Drive Carefully. Christiaan Barnard Is Watching You." The relationship of trust between the physician and patient is not only an instrumental value in the sense of being an important factor in the patient's treatment. It is also to be endorsed because of its intrinsic worth as a relationship.

Thus the related values of individual dignity and trust are best maintained in selection by chance. But other factors also buttress the argument for this approach. Which criteria and procedures would men agree upon? We have to suppose a hypothetical situation in which several men are going to determine for themselves and their families the criteria and procedures by which they would want to be admitted to and excluded from SLMR if the need arose.[22] We need to assume two restrictions and then ask which set of criteria and procedures would be chosen as the most rational and, indeed, the fairest. The restrictions are these: (1) The men are *self-interested*. They are interested in their own welfare (and that of members of their families), and this, of course, includes survival. Basically, they are not motivated by altruism. (2) Furthermore, they are *ignorant* of their own talents, abilities, potential, and probable contribution to the social good. They do not know how they would fare in a competitive situation, e.g., the competition for SLMR in terms of social contribution. Under these conditions which institution would be chosen— letting all die, utilitarian selection, or the use of chance? Which would seem the most rational? the fairest? By which set of criteria would they want to be included in or excluded from the list of those who will be saved? The rational choice in this setting (assuming self-interest and ignorance of one's competitive success) would be random selection or chance since this alone provides equality of opportunity. A possible response is that one would prefer to take a "risk" and therefore choose the utilitarian approach. But I think not, especially since I add-

ed that the participants in this hypothetical situation are choosing for their children as well as for themselves; random selection or chance could be more easily justified to the children. It would make more sense for men who are self-interested but uncertain about their relative contribution to society to elect a set of criteria which would build in equality of opportunity. They would consider selection by chance as relatively just and fair.[23]

An important psychological point supplements earlier arguments for using chance or random selection. The psychological stress and strain among those who are rejected would be greater if the rejection is based on insufficient social worth than if it is based on chance. Obviously stress and strain cannot be eliminated in these borderline situations, but they would almost certainly be increased by the opprobrium of being judged relatively "unfit" by society's agents using society's values. Nicholas Rescher makes this point very effectively:

A recourse to chance would doubtless make matters easier for the rejected patient and those who have a specific interest in him. It would surely be quite hard for them to accept his exclusion by relatively mechanical application of objective criteria in whose implementation subjective judgment is involved. But the circumstances of life have conditioned us to accept the workings of chance and to tolerate the element of luck (good or bad): human life is an inherently contingent process. Nobody, after all, has an absolute right to ELT [Exotic Lifesaving Therapy]—but most of us would feel that we have "every bit as much right" to it as anyone else in significantly similar circumstances.[24]

Although it is seldom recognized as such, selection by chance is already in operation in practically every dialysis unit. I am not aware of any unit which removes some of its patients from kidney machines in order to make room for later applicants who are better qualified in terms of social worth. Furthermore, very few people would recommend it. Indeed, few would even consider removing a person from a kidney machine on the grounds that a person better qualified *medically* had just applied. In a discussion of the treatment of chronic renal failure by dialysis at the University of Virginia Hospital Renal Unit from November 15, 1965 to November 15, 1966, Dr. Harry Abram writes: "Thirteen patients sought treatment but were not considered because the program had reached its limit of nine patients."[25] Thus, in practice and theory, natural chance is accepted at least within certain limits.

My proposal is that we extend this principle (first come, first served) to determine who among the medically acceptable patients shall live or that we utilize artificial chance such as a lottery or randomness. "First come, first served" would be more feasible than a lottery since the applicants make their claims over a period of time rather than as a group at one time. This procedure would be in accord with at least one principle in our present practices and with our sense of individual dignity, trust, and fairness. Its significance in relation to these values can be underlined by asking how the decision can be justified to the rejected applicant. Of course, one easy way of avoiding this task is to maintain the traditional cloak of secrecy, which works to a great extent because patients are often not aware that they are being considered for SLMR in addition to the usual treatment. But whether public justification is instituted or not is not the significant question; it is rather what reasons for rejection would be most acceptable to the unsuccessful applicant. My contention is that rejection can be accepted more readily if equality of opportunity, fairness, and trust are preserved, and that they are best preserved by selection by randomness or chance.

This proposal has yet another advantage since it would eliminate the need for a committee to examine applicants in terms of their social value. This onerous responsibility can be avoided.

Finally, there is a possible indirect consequence of widespread use of random selection which is interesting to ponder, although I do *not* adduce it as a good reason for adopting random selection. It can be argued, as Professor Mason Willrich of the University of Virginia Law School has suggested, that SLMR cases would practically disappear if these scarce resources were distributed randomly rather than on social worth grounds. Scarcity would no longer be a problem because the holders of economic and political power would make certain that they would not be excluded by a random selection procedure; hence they would help to redirect public priorities or establish private funding so that life-saving medical treatment would be widely and perhaps universally available.

In the framework that I have delineated, are the decrees of chance to be taken without exception? If we recognize exceptions, would we not open Pandora's box again just after we had succeeded in getting it closed? The direction of my argument has been against any exceptions, and I would defend this as the proper way to go. But let me indicate one possible way of admitting exceptions while at the same time circumscribing them so narrowly that they would be very rare indeed.

An obvious advantage of the utilitarian approach is that occasionally circumstances arise which make it necessary to say that one man is practically indispensable for a society in view of a particular set of problems it faces (e.g., the President when the nation is waging a war for survival). Certainly the argument to this point has stressed that the burden of proof would fall on those who think that the social danger in this instance is so great that they simply cannot abide by the outcome of a lottery or a first come, first served policy. Also, the reason must be negative rather than positive; that is, we depart from chance in this instance not because we want to take advantage of this person's potential contribution to the improvement of our society, but because his immediate loss would possibly (even probably) be disastrous (again, the President in a grave national emergency). Finally, social value (in the negative sense) should be used as a standard of exception in dialysis, for example, only if it would provide a reason strong enough to warrant removing another person from a kidney machine if all machines were taken. Assuming this strong reluctance to remove anyone once the commitment has been made to him, we would be willing to put this patient ahead of another applicant for a vacant machine only if we would be willing (in circumstances in which all machines are being used) to vacate a machine by removing someone from it. These restrictions would make an exception almost impossible.

While I do not recommend this procedure of recognizing exceptions, I think that one can defend it while accepting my general thesis about selection by randomness or chance. If it is used, a lay committee (perhaps advisory, perhaps even stronger) would be called upon to deal with the alleged exceptions since the doctors or others would in effect be appealing the outcome of chance (either natural or artificial). This lay committee would determine whether this patient was so indispensable at this time and place that he had to be saved even by sacrificing the values preserved by random selection. It would make it quite clear that exception is warranted, if at all, only as the "lesser of two evils." Such a defense would be recognized only rarely, if ever, primarily because chance and randomness preserve so many important moral and nonmoral values in SLMR cases.

NOTES

1. George Bernard Shaw, *The Doctor's Dilemma* (New York, 1941), pp. 132–133.

2. Henry K. Beecher, "Scarce Resources and Medical Advancement," *Daedalus* (Spring 1969), pp. 279–280.

3. Leo Shatin, "Medical Care and the Social Worth of a Man," *American Journal of Orthopsychiatry*, 36 (1967), 97.

4. Harry S. Abram and Walter Wadlington, "Selection of Patients for Artificial and Transplanted Organs," *Annals of Internal Medicine*, 69 (September 1968), 615–620.

5. *United States v. Holmes* 26 Fed. Cas. 360 (C.C.E.D. Pa. 1842). All references are to the text of the trial as reprinted in Philip E. Davis, ed., *Moral Duty and Legal Responsibility: A Philosophical-Legal Casebook* (New York, 1966), pp. 102–118.

6. *The Moral Decision* (Bloomington, Ind., 1955), p. 71.

7. For a discussion of the higher suicide rate among dialysis patients than among the general population and an interpretation of some of the factors at work, see H. S. Abram, G. L. Moore, and F. B. Westervelt, "Suicidal Behavior in Chronic Dialysis Patients," *American Journal of Psychiatry* (in press). This study shows that even "if one does not include death through not following the regimen

the incidence of suicide is still more than 100 times the normal population."

8. I am excluding from consideration the question of the ability to pay because most of the people involved have to secure funds from other sources, public or private, anyway.

9. Joseph Fletcher, "Donor Nephrectomies and Moral Responsibility," *Journal of the American Medical Women's Association*, 23 (Dec. 1968), p. 1090.

10. Leo Shatin, op. cit., pp. 96–101.

11. For a discussion of the Seattle selection committee, see Shana Alexander, "They Decide Who Lives, Who Dies," *Life*, 53 (Nov. 9, 1962), 102. For an examination of general selection practices in dialysis see "Scarce Medical Resources," *Columbia Law Review*, 69:620 (1969) and Harry S. Abram and Walter Wadlington, op. cit.

12. David Sanders and Jesse Dukeminier, Jr., "Medical Advance and Legal Lag: Hemodialysis and Kidney Transplantation," *UCLA Law Review*, 15:367 (1968) 378.

13. "Letters and Comments," *Annals of Internal Medicine*, 61 (Aug. 1964), 360. Dr. G. E. Schreiner contends that "if you really believe in the right of society to make decisions on medical availability on these criteria you should be logical and say that when a man stops going to church or is divorced and loses his job, he ought to be removed from the programme and somebody else who fulfills these criteria substituted. Obviously no one faces up to this logical consequence" (G. E. W. Wolstenholme and Maeve O'Connor, eds. *Ethics in Medical Progress: With Special Reference to Transplantation*, A Ciba Foundation Symposium [Boston, 1966], p. 127).

14. Helmut Thielicke, "The Doctor as Judge of Who Shall Live and Who Shall Die," *Who Shall Live?* ed. by Kenneth Vaux (Philadelphia, 1970), p. 172.

15. Ibid., pp. 173–174.

16. Ibid., p. 173.

17. Thielicke, *Theological Ethics*, Vol. I, *Foundations* (Philadelphia, 1966), p. 602.

18. Cahn, op. cit., p. 71.

19. Paul Freund, "Introduction," *Daedalus* (Spring 1969), xiii.

20. Paul Ramsey, *Nine Modern Moralists* (Englewood Cliffs, N.J., 1962), p. 245.

21. Charles Fried, "Privacy," In *Law, Reason, and Justice*, ed. by Graham Hughes (New York, 1969), p. 52.

22. My argument is greatly dependent on John Rawls's version of justice as fairness, which is a reinterpretation of social contract theory. Rawls, however, would probably not apply his ideas to "borderline situations." See "Distributive Justice: Some Addenda," *Natural Law Forum*, 13 (1968), 53. For Rawls's general theory, see "Justice as Fairness," *Philosophy, Politics and Society* (Second Series), ed. by Peter Laslett and W. G. Runciman (Oxford, 1962), pp. 132–157 and his other essays on aspects of this topic.

23. Occasionally someone contends that random selection may reward vice. Leo Shatin (op. cit., p. 100) insists that random selection "would reward socially disvalued qualities by giving their bearers the same special medical care opportunities as those received by the bearers of socially valued qualities. Personally I do not favor such a method." Obviously society must engender certain qualities in its members, but not all of its institutions must be devoted to that purpose. Furthermore, there are strong

reasons, I have contended, for exempting SLMR from that sort of function.

24. Nicholas Rescher, "The Allocation of Exotic Medical Lifesaving Therapy," *Ethics,* 79 (April 1969), 184. He defends random selection's use only after utilitarian and other judgements have been made. If there are no "major disparities" in terms of utility, etc., in the second stage of selection, then final selection could be made randomly. He fails to give attention to the moral values that random selection might preserve.

25. Harry S. Abram, M. D., "The Psychiatrist, the Treatment of Chronic Renal Failure, and the Prolongation of Life: II" *American Journal of Psychiatry* 126:157–167 (1969), 158.

SUGGESTED READINGS
FOR CHAPTER 8

Books and Articles

Arrow, Kenneth J., *et al.* "Government Decision Making and the Preciousness of Life." In Tancredi, Laurence R., ed. *Ethics of Health Care*. Washington: National Academy of Sciences, 1974. Pp. 33–64

Branson, Roy, and Veatch, Robert M., eds. *Ethics and Health Policy*. Cambridge, Mass.: Ballinger Publishing Co., 1976.

Childress, James, and Fletcher, Joseph. "Who Has First Claim on Health Care Resources?" *Hastings Center Report* 5 (August, 1975), pp. 13–15.

"Due Process in The Allocation of Scarce Lifesaving Medical Resources." *Yale Law Journal* 84 (July, 1975), 1734–1749.

Fein, Rashi. "On Achieving Access and Equity in Health Care." *Milbank Memorial Fund Quarterly* 50 (October, 1972), 157–190.

Feinberg, Joel. *Social Philosophy*. Englewood Cliffs, N.J.: Prentice-Hall, 1973. Chap. 7.

Fried, Charles. "Rights and Health Care—Beyond Equity and Efficiency." *New England Journal of Medicine* 293 (July 31, 1975), 241–245.

Fuchs, Victor. *Who Shall Live*? New York: Basic Books, 1974.

Hiatt, Howard H. "Protecting the Medical Commons: Who Is Responsible?" *New England Journal of Medicine* 293 (July 31, 1975), 235–241.

Jonsen, Albert R. "The Totally Implantable Artificial Heart." *Hastings Center Report* 3 (November, 1973), 1–4.

Katz, Jay, and Capron, Alexander M. *Catastrophic Diseases: Who Decides What? A Psychological and Legal Analysis* . . . New York: Russell Sage Foundation, 1975.

Ramsey, Paul. *The Patient as Person*. New Haven: Yale University Press, 1970. Chap. 7.

Rescher, Nicholas. *Distributive Justice*. Indianapolis: Bobbs-Merrill, 1966.

"Scarce Medical Resources." *Columbia Law Review* (April, 1969), 620–692.

"World Famine and Lifeboat Ethics." *Soundings* 59 (Spring, 1976). Special issue.

Young, Robert. "Some Criteria for Making Decisions Concerning the Distribution of Scarce Medical Resources." *Theory and Decision* 6 (November, 1975), 439–455.

Bibliographies

Sollitto, Sharmon, and Veatch, Robert M., comps. *Bibliography of Society, Ethics and the Life Sciences*. Hastings-on-Hudson, N.Y.: Institute of Society, Ethics and the Life Sciences. Updated periodically. See under "Scarce Medical Resources, Transplantation, and Hemodialysis."

Walters, LeRoy, ed. *Bibliography of Bioethics*. Vols. 1- . Detroit: Gale Research Co. Issued annually. See under "Resource Allocation," and "Selection for Treatment."

Part V

HUMAN EXPERIMENTATION

9.
General Issues in Experimentation

Chapter 4 discussed a series of ethical problems which arise in the professional-patient relationship. In parallel fashion the present chapter explores several general ethical issues raised by human experimentation.

CONCEPTUAL QUESTIONS

The definition of "human experimentation" (or "research involving human subjects") can perhaps be best approached by way of considering the concepts of "therapy" and "experimentation." In the biomedical and behavioral fields "therapy" refers to a class of activities designed solely to benefit an individual or all members of a group. Therapy can take several forms: it can be a treatment for a disease, or it can be diagnostic or even preventive measures. In contrast, "experimentation," or "research," refers to a class of scientific activities designed to develop or contribute to generalizable knowledge. Examples of experimentation are the comparative study of alternative methods for training pigeons and the laboratory analysis of a chemical reaction. "Human experimentation," then, is experimentation (or research) which involves human subjects.

Two subtypes of human experimentation can be identified. (1) *Therapeutic* experimentation, as the phrase suggests, is closely akin to therapy. However, unlike therapy, which is designed *solely* to benefit a patient, therapeutic experimentation has a dual purpose: it is performed *primarily* for the benefit of the patient-subject; at the same time, the intervention is undertaken in a controlled way, so that the knowledge gained from the study can be applied to other contexts or to future subjects and patients. An example of therapeutic experimentation is a controlled trial which compares the relative effectiveness of two anticancer drugs administered to cancer patients. (2) *Nontherapeutic* experimentation, on the other hand, is performed primarily for the purpose of gaining new knowledge, not for the benefit of the subject. For example, healthy human volunteers frequently participate in the early phases of drug testing, when the safety of new drugs for human use is being evaluated. (Charles Fried's essay in this chapter discusses the therapeutic-non-therapeutic distinction at greater length.)

THE MORAL JUSTIFICATION OF HUMAN EXPERIMENTATION

In the literature which discusses human experimentation, including the codes of ethics, surprisingly little attention is paid to the moral justification for involving human subjects in experimentation. This silence is particularly striking when one considers that the traditional ethic of medicine has been exclusively a patient-benefit ethic. The motto *primum non nocere* (do no harm) has generally been interpreted to mean "Do nothing which is not intended for the direct benefit of the patient.'' What reasons can be given for deviating in any way from therapy, as that term was defined above?

The major justification for human experimentation is the utilitarian argument that the social benefits to be gained from such experimentation are very great or, conversely, that the harms resulting from the cessation of such investigations would be extremely grave. In his essay in this chapter Robert Marston notes that the therapeutic value of many reputed "therapies" is in fact unknown. He therefore recommends carefully controlled studies of both traditional and newly-developed therapies to establish their relative effectiveness. In Marston's view, the only alternative to a plague of medically induced illnesses is the wide-scale use of experimentation with human subjects. On a more positive note, Marston asserts that nontherapeutic experiments of the past, for example, Walter Reed's studies of yellow fever, have produced significant social benefits.

A second approach to the justification of human experimentation is more deontological in character and focuses on requirements of justice. Proponents of the justice argument note that every person currently alive is the beneficiary of past human experimentation. To be more specific, the willingness of past human volunteers to take part in studies of antibiotics (like penicillin) and vaccines (like the polio vaccine) contributes to the health of all of us. According to this view, it is unfair for us to reap the benefits of past experimentation without making a reciprocal contribution to the alleviation of disability and disease.

Hans Jonas vigorously challenges both of these proposed justifications. In answer to the utilitarian justification, he argues that while human experimentation generally contributes to medical progress, most research involving human subjects is not *essential* to the well-being or survival of the human species. According to Jonas, progress, even medical progress, is "an optional goal, not an unconditional commitment." On this view, only a national health emergency or a similar "clear and present danger" would provide a sufficient justification for human experimentation.

Jonas also rejects the argument that participation in human experimentation by beneficiaries of past experimentation is a requirement of justice. In his view, most volunteers of the past, including investigators involved in auto-experimentation, performed acts of altruism and moral heroism. If we of the present owe any debt to the past, it is a debt of gratitude to these bygone heroes, not an obligation to society required by a principle of justice. Jonas' dismissal of the justice argument reemphasizes his view that human experimentation is in most cases an optional rather than an essential human activity.

A presupposition of Jonas' position on the justification of human experimentation is that individual human rights—for example, the right to be free from invasions of one's body and the right to consent—are supremely important. Jonas also regards all nontherapeutic research involving human subjects as an infringement of the individual's "primary inviolability," or in Kantian terms, as the use of a person as a means rather than an end. Because of this primary commitment to protecting the rights, dignity, and inviolability of the individual, Jonas is unwilling to accept ordinary social benefits as a sufficient justification for human experimentation.

One additional justification, not explicitly mentioned by Marston or Jonas, is sometimes advanced in support of research involving human subjects. Investigators, it is asserted, should be free to decide what kinds of research they will perform and how they wish to conduct that research. According to this view, the freedom of scientific inquiry should be protected from outside interference, unless there are strong reasons for overriding the presumption of freedom. Thus, if an investigator can find human subjects who are willing to take part in his proposed research, he or she should generally be allowed to proceed with the research. Critics of this freedom-of-inquiry position reply that there is a significant difference between the freedom to do research and the freedom to involve human subjects in research. In addition, they argue that the knowledge differential between most investigators and most subjects is so great that some paternalistic intervention by society is justified, if only to ensure that the consent of prospective subjects is adequately informed.

EXPERIMENTAL DESIGN

If human experimentation as a practice can be justified in certain circumstances, then one can proceed to consider certain rules or principles which should be applied to the conduct of experimentation. Many of these principles have been developed in the various codes of research ethics, beginning with the Nuremberg Code. Perhaps the most prominent principle discussed in the codes is the informed consent requirement. However, the codes also devote significant attention to the proper design of experiments and to the minimization of risks to subjects.

The requirement of adequate experimental design is end-oriented or utilitarian in character. The central aim of this requirement is to ensure that human experimentation will be conducted efficiently, that is, in a way that maximizes the amount of information gained from exposing human subjects to the minimum amount of risk. From this general principle flow several specific requirements. First, as David Rutstein notes, studies which are so poorly designed that they cannot possibly produce reliable data should not be performed at all. The codes of research ethics add a second principle, that research involving humans should be based upon prior laboratory and animal studies. A third principle is perhaps the obverse side of the first; all studies which involve human subjects should be carefully controlled, so that the biases of the investigator do not vitiate experimental results. Fourth, careful methods of statistical analysis should be employed in interpreting the data derived from human research, so that the greatest possible benefit is derived from each study.

These formal principles do not, in themselves, set standards for maximum levels of anticipated harm, minimum levels of anticipated benefit, or appropriate ratios of benefit to harm. However, the questions of benefit and harm seem to be directly relevant to the discussion of adequate experimental design. A maximum level of anticipated harm is suggested in the Nuremberg Code: in general, "No experiment should be conducted where there is *a priori* reason to believe that death or disabling injury will occur." A minimum limit of anticipated benefit is advocated by Rutstein, who argues that no "trivial" experiments should be performed. As for the benefit-harm ratio, both the codes and Rutstein stipulate that the anticipated benefits of a proposed study should be proportionate to the risk of harm to human subjects.

One type of controlled study—the randomized clinical trial—has been the topic of rather intense debate. In this experimental design, ill patients are allocated on a random basis to one of two or more alternative treatments; the relative efficacy of the treatments is then determined by closely monitoring the progress of patient-subjects assigned to each treatment. The technique of randomization is chosen to avoid investigator bias in selecting subjects for various treatments and to cancel out unknown variables. (The essays by Thomas Chalmers and Charles Fried propose several principles for the ethical conduct of randomized clinical trials.)

INFORMED CONSENT

Since the Nuremberg trials, no aspect of human experimentation has received greater attention than the issue of consent. In the Nuremberg Code itself consent is discussed in the first and longest article. Given the context of the Nuremberg judgment, it is not surprising that the emphasis there was on subjects' consent being truly voluntary and uncoerced. Subsequently, in judicial decisions dealing with therapy rather than experimentation, the term "informed consent" was coined, to give equal attention to the disclosure of all facts that would be material to a free and knowledgeable decision. In parallel fashion, several codifications of research ethics, including the Helsinki Declaration, have gradually developed the concept of informed consent in the context of experimentation.

Each component of the concept raises its own issues. The "information" aspect of informed consent may refer to an investigator making "reasonable" disclosures, or it may contemplate that the prospective subjects actually comprehend what they have been told as well. The consent component refers to an uncoerced decision to take part in the already disclosed and comprehended procedure or project, but this leaves open the question whether voluntariness is to be judged by objective standards (of an average person) or subjective standards that refer solely to a particular individual.[1]

A variety of justifications or rationales for the informed-consent requirement have been advanced. According to Paul Ramsey, "The principle of informed consent is the cardinal *canon of loyalty* joining men together in medical practice and investigation." In Ramsey's discussion of informed consent it becomes clear that he regards the informed-consent principle as a deontological check on any effort to justify human experimentation solely on a utilitarian basis. A more legally-oriented approach is presented by Charles Fried, who views informed consent against the backdrop of legal doctrines concerning battery and negligence. The law of battery protects patients and subjects against unauthorized touching, while the law of negligence holds investigators liable for injuries inflicted by procedures which deviate from standard and accepted medical practice.[2] Although utilitarian justifications for the informed-consent requirement can be developed—for example, the premise that it encourages self-scrutiny by the investigator[3]—deontological or procedural justifications have predominated both in the relevant court decisions and in the general literature which discusses the ethics of human experimentation.

Chalmers, Fried, and Ingelfinger discuss several special problems in the application of the informed-consent requirement. Chalmers raises the question: How much information should be disclosed to participants in randomized clinical trials? His answer and Fried's differ. Chalmers argues that patient-subjects should not be informed that their treatment will be allocated on a random basis; he also suggests that to disclose the preliminary results of a randomized clinical trial to prospective subjects would render impossible the completion of the trial. In contrast, Fried emphasizes the investigator's duty to provide full information to subjects concerning both the fact of randomization and the progress of the trial. Franz Ingelfinger's editorial acknowledges the value of informed consent as an ideal but questions whether either adequate comprehension or free choice is often achieved in practice.

The requirements of adequate research design and reasonably free and sufficiently informed consent are generally regarded as *necessary* conditions of ethically-acceptable human experimentation. However, it is not clear that these two conditions are *sufficient* to justify proposed research involving human subjects. One might wish to add a justice requirement, that the risks and benefits of research should be fairly allocated among different social classes and ethnic groups. Some commentators, including Charles Fried,[4] have proposed a fourth requirement which is also based on considerations of justice: in their view, all subjects who accept the risks of research for the sake of society should also receive equitable compensation for injuries sustained in the course of their participation in that research.

SOCIAL CONTROL

The issue of social control raises procedural rather than substantive questions. The various alternative mechanisms of social control are established as means for ensuring, insofar as possible, that human experimentation is conducted in accordance with basic ethical principles and requirements.

In the final essay of this chapter Bernard Barber describes some of the social-control mechanisms which have been developed to regulate human experimentation in the United States. Against this backdrop Barber presents data gathered by himself and his colleagues in a 1970 survey of investigator's attitudes and practices. His conclusion: at the time of the survey, existing institutional mechanisms for the social control of human experimentation were failing to provide adequate protection for many human subjects. The task of translating ethical principles into research practice continues to present a significant challenge to researchers and policymakers alike.

L. W.

NOTES

1. Alexander M. Capron, "Informed Consent in Catastrophic Disease Research and Treatment," *University of Pennsylvania Law Review* 123 (December, 1974), pp. 404–418.

2. See Charles Fried, *Medical Experimentation: Personal Integrity and Social Policy* (New York: American Elsevier, 1974), pp. 14–25.

3. Capron, *op. cit.,* pp. 371–374.

4. Fried, *op. cit.,* pp. 399–449 in this chapter.

The Nuremberg Code

The great weight of the evidence before us is to the effect that certain types of medical experiments on human beings, when kept within reasonably well-defined bounds, conform to the ethics of the medical profession generally. The protagonists of the practice of human experimentation justify their views on the basis that such experiments yield results for the good of society that are unprocurable by other methods or means of study. All agree, however, that certain basic principles must be observed in order to satisfy moral, ethical and legal concepts.

1. The voluntary consent of the human subject is absolutely essential.

This means that the person involved should have legal capacity to give consent; should be so situated as to be able to exercise free power of choice, without the intervention of any element of force, fraud, deceit, duress, overreaching, or other ulterior form of constraint or coercion; and should have sufficient knowledge and comprehension of the elements of the subject matter involved as to enable him to make an understanding and enlightened decision. This latter element requires that before the acceptance of an affirmative decision by the experimental subject there should be made known to him the nature, duration, and purpose of the experiment; the method and means by which it is to be conducted; all inconveniences and hazards reasonably to be expected; and the effects upon his health or person which may possibly come from his participation in the experiment.

The duty and responsibility for ascertaining the quality of the consent rests upon each individual who initiates, directs or engages in the experiment. It is a personal duty and responsibility which may not be delegated to another with impunity.

2. The experiment should be such as to yield fruitful results for the good of society, unprocurable by other methods or means of study, and not random and unnecessary in nature.

3. The experiment should be so designed and based on the results of animal experimentation and a knowledge of the natural history of the disease or other problem under study that the anticipated results will justify the performance of the experiment.

4. The experiment should be so conducted as to avoid all unnecessary physical and mental suffering and injury.

5. No experiment should be conducted where there is an *a priori* reason to believe that death or disabling injury will occur; except, perhaps, in those experiments where the experimental physicians also serve as subjects.

6. The degree of risk to be taken should never exceed that determined by the humanitarian importance of the problem to be solved by the experiment.

7. Proper preparations should be made and adequate facilities provided to protect the experimental subject against even remote possibilities of injury, disability, or death.

8. The experiment should be conducted only by scientifically qualified persons. The highest degree of skill and care should be required through all stages of the experiment of those who conduct or engage in the experiment.

9. During the course of the experiment the human subject should be at liberty to bring the experiment to an end if he has reached the physical or mental state where continuation of the experiment seems to him to be impossible.

From *Trials of War Criminals Before the Nuremberg Military Tribunals Under Control Council Law No. 10,* Vol. II, Nuremberg, October 1946-April 1949.

10. During the course of the experiment the scientist in charge must be prepared to terminate the experiment at any stage, if he has probable cause to believe, in the exercise of the good faith, superior skill and careful judgment

WORLD MEDICAL ASSOCIATION 405

required of him that a continuation of the experiment is likely to result in injury, disability, or death to the experimental subject.

WORLD MEDICAL ASSOCIATION

Declaration of Helsinki*

INTRODUCTION

It is the mission of the medical doctor to safeguard the health of the people. His or her knowledge and conscience are dedicated to the fulfillment of this mission.

The Declaration of Geneva of The World Medical Association binds the doctor with the words. ''The health of my patient will be my first consideration,'' and the International Code of Medical Ethics declares that, ''Any act or advice which could weaken physical or mental resistance of a human being may be used only in his interest.''

The purpose of biomedical research involving human subjects must be to improve diagnostic, therapeutic and prophylactic procedures and the understanding of the aetiology and pathogenesis of disease.

In current medical practice most diagnostic, therapeutic or prophylactic procedures involve hazards. This applies *a fortiori* to biomedical research.

Medical progress is based on research which ultimately must rest in part on experimentation involving human subjects.

In the field of biomedical research a fundamental distinction must be recognized between medical research in which the aim is essentially diagnostic or therapeutic for a patient, and medical research, the essential object of which is purely scientific and without direct diagnostic or therapeutic value to the person subjected to the research.

Special caution must be exercised in the conduct of research which may affect the environment, and the welfare of animals used for research must be respected.

Because it is essential that the results of laboratory experiments be applied to human beings to further scientific knowledge and to help suffering humanity, The World Medical Association has prepared the following recommendations as a guide to every doctor in biomedical research involving human subjects. They should be kept under review in the future. It must be stressed that the standards as drafted are only a guide to physicians all over the world. Doctors are not relieved from criminal, civil and ethical responsibilities under the laws of their own countries.

I. BASIC PRINCIPLES

1. Biomedical research involving human subjects must conform to generally accepted scientific principles and should be based on adequately performed laboratory and animal experimentation and on a thorough knowledge of the scientific literature.

2. The design and performance of each experimental procedure involving human sub-

*Recommendations guiding medical doctors in biomedical research involving human subjects.

Adopted by the 18th World Medical Assembly, Helsinki, Finland, 1964, and revised by the 29th World Medical Assembly, Tokyo, Japan, October 1975. Reprinted with permission of the World Medical Association, Inc. from the ''Declaration of Helsinki,'' revised edition.

jects should be clearly formulated in an experimental protocol which should be transmitted to a specially appointed independent committee for consideration, comment and guidance.

3. Biomedical research involving human subjects should be conducted only by scientifically qualified persons and under the supervision of a clinically competent medical person. The responsibility for the human subject must always rest with a medically qualified person and never rest on the subject of research, even though the subject has given his or her consent.

4. Biomedical research involving human subjects cannot legitimately be carried out unless the importance of the objective is in proportion to the inherent risk to the subject.

5. Every biomedical research project involving human subjects should be preceded by careful assessment of predictable risks in comparison with foreseeable benefits to the subject or to others. Concern for the interests of the subject must always prevail over the interests of science and society.

6. The right of the research subject to safeguard his or her integrity must always be respected. Every precaution should be taken to respect the privacy of the subject and to minimize the impact of the study on the subject's physical and mental integrity and on the personality of the subject.

7. Doctors should abstain from engaging in research projects involving human subjects unless they are satisfied that the hazards involved are believed to be predictable. Doctors should cease any investigation if the hazards are found to outweigh the potential benefits.

8. In publication of the results of his or her research, the doctor is obliged to preserve the accuracy of the results. Reports of experimentation not in accordance with the principles laid down in this Declaration should not be accepted for publication.

9. In any research on human beings, each potential subject must be adequately informed of the aims, methods, anticipated benefits and potential hazards of the study and the discomfort it may entail. He or she should be informed that he or she is at liberty to abstain from participation in the study and that he or she is free to withdraw his or her consent to participation at any time. The doctor should then obtain the subject's freely-given informed consent, preferably in writing.

10. When obtaining informed consent for the research project the doctor should be particularly cautious if the subject is in a dependent relationship to him or her or may consent under duress. In that case the informed consent should be obtained by a doctor who is not engaged in the investigation and who is completely independent of this official relationship.

11. In case of legal incompetence, informed consent should be obtained from the legal guardian in accordance with national legislation. Where physical or mental incapacity makes it impossible to obtain informed consent, or when the subject is a minor, permission from the responsible relative replaces that of the subject in accordance with national legislation.

12. The research protocol should always contain a statement of the ethical considerations involved and should indicate that the principles enunciated in the present Declaration are complied with.

II. MEDICAL RESEARCH COMBINED WITH PROFESSIONAL CARE (CLINICAL RESEARCH)

1. In the treatment of the sick person, the doctor must be free to use a new diagnostic and therapeutic measure, if in his or her judgement it offers hope of saving life, reestablishing health or alleviating suffering.

2. The potential benefits, hazards and discomfort of a new method should be weighed against the advantages of the best current diagnostic and therapeutic methods.

3. In any medical study, every patient—including those of a control group, if any—should be assured of the best proven diagnostic and therapeutic method.

4. The refusal of the patient to participate in a study must never interfere with the doctor-patient relationship.

5. If the doctor considers it essential not to obtain informed consent, the specific reasons for this proposal should be stated in the experimental protocol for transmission to the independent committee (I, 2).

6. The doctor can combine medical research with professional care, the objective being the acquisition of new medical knowledge, only to the extent that medical research is justified by its potential diagnostic or therapeutic value for the patient.

III. NON-THERAPEUTIC BIOMEDICAL RESEARCH INVOLVING HUMAN SUBJECTS (NON-CLINICAL BIOMEDICAL RESEARCH)

1. In the purely scientific application of medical research carried out on a human being, it is the duty of the doctor to remain the protector of the life and health of that person on whom biomedical research is being carried out.

2. The subjects should be volunteers—either healthy persons or patients for whom the experimental design is not related to the patient's illness.

3. The investigator or the investigating team should discontinue the research if in his/her or their judgement it may, if continued, be harmful to the individual.

4. In research on man, the interest of science and society should never take precedence over considerations related to the well-being of the subject.

Moral Justification

ROBERT Q. MARSTON

Medical Science, the Clinical Trial, and Society

. . .The need for scientific knowledge is intensified today because doctors have never before been in a position to produce so much positive good on one hand, or harm on the other, through the double-edged potency of their therapeutic weapons. However, the issue is not altogether a modern one. According to Dr. William Rowe, the Emperor Napoleon Bonaparte once said "I do not want two dis-

From an unpublished address presented at the dedication ceremonies for the McLeod Nursing Building and the Jordan Medical Education Building at the University of Virginia, Charlottesville, Va., November 10, 1972.

eases, one nature-made, one doctor-made."[1] Napoleon's pointed comment was sharper than he could possibly have known. The march of medical knowledge in the intervening years has expanded immeasurably the possibility of "doctor-made" disease.

René Dubos spelled out some of the specifics of the potential dangers from the tools of medical science in these words "who could have dreamt a generation ago that hypervitaminosis would become a common form of nutritional disease in the Western world?. . . and the use of x-rays would be held responsible for the increase in certain types of cancer? That the introduction of detergents in various synthetics would increase the incidence of allergy. . . that advances in chemotherapy and other therapeutic procedures would create a new staphylococcus pathology?. . . that patients with all forms of iatrogenic diseases would occupy such a large number of beds in the modern hospital?"[2]

This very progress is the compelling reason for continuing and close examination of the relations between medical science and clinical trials—and other research involving human subjects. We are dealing with a dynamic, ever-changing base of substantive knowledge. Sometimes the progress of a research project itself moves the state of knowledge so rapidly that serious and involved ethical problems arise concerning the continuation of that same experiment.

For example, in Sir Austin Bradford Hill's article, "Medical Ethics and Controlled Trials," he described the complex situation which arose in a trial of long-term therapy using anticoagulants in cerebrovascular disease. He relates, "In previous uncontrolled studies there was a distinct if inconclusive suggestion in favor of their [anticoagulants] use, and sufficient indeed, to make a trial difficult. Yet when put to the test of a controlled trial, with the comparison of a fully treated group and a group given a dose insufficient to interfere with the clotting mechanism, it not only appeared that no protection was afforded against the recurrence of cerebrovascular accident, but there was a small but definite risk of cerebral hemorrhage in the fully treated cases. Here we have an instance—and by no means unique—of the wheel turning full circle. At the start of the trial was it ethical to withhold the treatment? At its end, was it ethical to give it? It is very easy to be wise (and critical) after the event; the problem is to be wise (and ethical) before the event."[3]

Any discussion of the benefits of scientific investigation involving the use of human subjects brings to mind a graduate of [the University of Virginia's] School of Medicine, Walter Reed, who received his M.D. degree at the age of seventeen. He became a national hero because of his contribution to the control of yellow fever. Every school child knows the story of how the construction of the Panama Canal was stopped because of devastation from yellow fever. In 1900, Walter Reed and his associates discovered that yellow fever is transmitted to a non-immune individual by means of a bite of a mosquito that had previously fed on the blood of someone sick with this disease.[4] What is not always remembered about this event is the serious ethical question that was raised by Dr. Reed's experiments. At that time, it was not known that experimental animals could be given the disease; therefore, human studies were necessary. Army volunteers were both exposed to infected mosquitoes and given subcutaneous injections of virulent material. The subjects were aware of the risk, indeed, Dr. Lazear, the group's entomologist and bacteriologist, died after an accidental bite. None of the individuals living normally in non-risk areas could have been expected to benefit themselves from these experiments. It is highly unlikely that the experiments would have been permitted under today's guidelines. And yet the social benefits were great, the experiments were well designed and the moral implications were seriously considered at the time, and the results are part of our national history.

In shocking contrast is the example from American history of the result of treatment by unverified methods. The central figure is Dr. Benjamin Rush. His conduct in earlier epidemics of yellow fever was described by Dr. William Bean as "especially tragic because Rush treated literally hundreds of victims of the disease. His purging and bleeding became almost a routine premortal ceremony—the heroic aspects of Benjamin Rush, his many ideas about mental health, his signing of the Declaration of Independence, have made us forget the harm he did. His willingness to follow the guttering candle of ignorance, his dogmatic conviction that he was right, his consummate ability to fool himself consistently helped to kill an unmeasured plenty of his patients in Philadelphia. That his motives were pure and serene constitutes another example of the unlimited capacity of man to fool himself."[5]

Let me turn from the past to focus on the essential need for research involving human beings. There are several obvious reasons why such research must be carried on. First, in many instances, there may not be a suitable animal model. Second, even if such an animal model exists, there always comes a time at which the test must be carried out in man. Even when the situation is as clearcut as it was when it became possible to prevent the death of experimentally infected mice by treatment with penicillin, it still was necessary to test the antibiotic in man. Medical history is full of examples in which the promise of animal experimentation failed to hold up in humans, or in which the results in man exceeded those that would have been predicted from animal experimentation. Finally, and most relevant to this discussion, is the need to test definitively in humans the procedures and therapies which are already part of the practice of medicine. The potency of modern procedures and therapies is such that the experimental method is often the only effective way to determine if their benefits are outweighed by undue hazard.

The late Dr. George James, known as an advocate for reform in health services, stated the problem well in one of his last talks: "In the discussion of ethical considerations relating to clinical research," Dr. James said, "the rights of the unborn generations to benefit from the fruits of the research must also be weighed. It can be debated that no man today has the free and moral right to condemn his grandchildren to the same perils of disease to which he is exposed by virtue of the present lack of effective scientific information, and his failure to participate in a search for it. It would help greatly to educate the population about this principle if the defects in our present medical armamentarium are to be made evident."[6]

Dr. Archibald L. Cochrane has pointed out in his recently published book titled "Effectiveness and Efficiency" that the United Kingdom's National Health Service has in the main achieved its goal to make health services available and accessible to the entire population at a cost that individuals could afford. However, he said the impact of the program on the health of the people of Great Britain was limited by the scientific base. In Dr. Cochrane's words, "There is a strong suggestion that the increase in input since the start of the [National Health Service] has not been matched by any marked increase in output in the 'cure' section. In the illustrative examples there were strong suggestions of inefficient use of effective therapies, and considerable use of ineffective ones."[7] A major theme in his book underlines the necessity of undertaking appropriate randomized clinical trials as a primary means for building the scientific base.

There are several key areas in which the equivalent of Benjamin Rush's well intended but disastrous actions occur or may occur today. I have already quoted from Bradford Hill concerning the use of anticoagulants in the prevention of stroke. We have recently concluded scientific studies in the use of oral antidiabetics to control diabetes from which it has been possible to identify an increased risk from the use of such drugs. Studies concerning the side effects of smallpox inoculation, balanced against the need for such inoculations in this country, have led to a modification in recommendations concerning the use of smallpox vaccine.

Each branch of medicine has similar examples demonstrating the role of ignorance as a dominant deterrent in the achievement of effective health programs.

Objective data on the hazards of medical practice are scarce. Such studies as we have can be over-interpreted in either direction. But let me give one example.

Gardner and Cluff have found in their review of prospective studies of adverse reaction in hospital patients that "with certain exceptions, the percentage of patients with untoward reactions to drugs in the hospital has ranged between 10 and 18 percent despite the wide variety of institutions and investigational methods."[8] Even when one accepts the fact that serious disease justifies measures that increase the risk of adverse reactions, these figures are sufficiently high for concern.

We stand today at a point at which there is a need and opportunity to strengthen markedly the scientific basis of medicine to the advantage of all. However, the need and opportunity exist at the time when (1) there is a trend back to "trial and error medicine;" (2) there is a failure to recognize even in the health professions, as well as the public at large, the need for and the value of randomized clinical trials, and (3) there is increasing concern about the welfare of individuals involved as subjects in research. When all is said and done, there are really three ways for determining what actions to take in disease prevention, treatment or rehabilitation. First, is the logical extension of fundamental knowledge to its application in man—the movement from scientific theory to scientific practice. Increasingly in the future actions on this basis must be coupled with the practical demonstration of their effectiveness. . . .

The second basis for making decisions is the empirical use of the results of experience, the experience of colleagues and teachers. Medicine has been particularly dependent on this type of wisdom and will be in the future. This accumulated wisdom may serve both patient and doctor well. However, it is a transient type of wisdom. It is the best that one can do under the circumstances, weighing all of the factors, but subject to modification when and if adequate information becomes available.

The third mechanism for making decisions is exemplified by the controlled clinical trial. Because such research tends to be long-term, difficult and expensive, the clinical trial is less understood and appreciated than the dramatic results of penicillin or a new vaccine. Further, the large clinical trial tends often to be unrewarding in a professional sense to the individual investigators who make up the scientific team. Although it is incompletely understood and incompletely applied, the clinical trial is the type of research on which we will become increasingly dependent as time goes on. . . .

REFERENCES

1. Quoted in "Iatrogenic Disease," William S. Rowe, *The Medical Journal of Australia,* September 13, 1969, Vol. 2, p. 560.

2. Forepage—*The Complications of Modern Medical Practices,* David M. Spain, 1963.

3. "Medical Ethics and Controlled Trials," Sir Austin Bradford Hill, *The British Medical Journal,* No. 5337, p. 1043, April 20, 1963.

4. Reed, W.; Carroll, J., and Agramonte, A.: "Etiology of Yellow Fever: An Additional Note." *The Journal of the American Medical Association.* Vol. 36, 431–440, Feb. 16, 1901.

5. William B. Bean, *The Archives of Internal Medicine,* Vol. 117, p. 1, 1966.

6. "Clinical Research in Achieving the Right to Health," Dr. George James, *The Annals of the New York Academy of Sciences,* Vol. 169, p. 301.

7. Cochrane, A. L.: *Effectiveness and Efficiency,* 1971, p. 67.

8. Pierce Gardner and Leighton E. Cluff: "The Epidemiology of Adverse Drug Reactions. A Review and Perspective." *The Johns Hopkins Medical Journal,* Vol. 126, p. 77.

HANS JONAS

Philosophical Reflections on Experimenting with Human Subjects

Experimenting with human subjects is going on in many fields of scientific and technological progress. It is designed to replace the over-all instruction by natural, occasional experience with the selective information from artificial, systematic experiment which physical science has found so effective in dealing with inanimate nature. Of the new experimentation with man, medical is surely the most legitimate; psychological, the most dubious; biological (still to come), the most dangerous. I have chosen here to deal with the first only, where the case *for* it is strongest and the task of adjudicating conflicting claims hardest. . . .

THE PECULIARITY OF HUMAN EXPERIMENTATION

Experimentation was originally sanctioned by natural science. There it is performed on inanimate objects, and this raises no moral problems. But as soon as animate, feeling beings become the subjects of experiment, as they do in the life sciences and especially in medical research, this innocence of the search for knowledge is lost and questions of conscience arise. The depth to which moral and religious sensibilities can become aroused over these questions is shown by the vivisection issue. Human experimentation must sharpen the issue as it involves ultimate questions of personal dignity and sacrosanctity. One profound difference between the human experiment and the physical (beside that between animate and inanimate, feeling and unfeeling nature) is this: The physical experiment employs small-scale, artificially devised substitutes for that about which knowledge is to be obtained, and the experimenter extrapolates

Reprinted with permission of George Braziller, Inc. from *Experimentation with Human Subjects* by Paul A. Freund (ed.). Copyright © 1969, 1970 by the American Academy of Arts and Sciences.

from these models and simulated conditions to nature at large. Something deputizes for the "real thing"—balls rolling down an inclined plane for sun and planets, electric discharges from a condenser for real lightning, and so on. For the most part, no such substitution is possible in the biological sphere. We must operate on the original itself, the real thing in the fullest sense, and perhaps affect it irreversibly. No simulacrum can take its place. Especially in the human sphere, experimentation loses entirely the advantage of the clear division between vicarious model and true object. Up to a point, animals may fulfill the proxy role of the classical physical experiment. But in the end man himself must furnish knowledge about himself, and the comfortable separation of noncommittal experiment and definitive action vanishes. An experiment in education affects the lives of its subjects, perhaps a whole generation of schoolchildren. Human experimentation for whatever purpose is always *also* a responsible, nonexperimental, definitive dealing with the subject himself. And not even the noblest purpose abrogates the obligations this involves.

This is the root of the problem with which we are faced: Can both that purpose and this obligation be satisfied? If not, what would be a just compromise? Which side should give way to the other? The question is inherently philosophical as it concerns not merely pragmatic difficulties and their arbitration, but a genuine conflict of values involving principles of a high order. May I put conflict in these terms. On principle, it is felt, human beings *ought* not to be dealt with in that way (the "guinea pig" protest); on the other hand, such dealings are increasingly urged on us by considerations, in turn appealing to principle, that claim to override those objections. Such a claim must be carefully assessed, especially when it is swept along by a mighty tide. Putting the matter thus, we have already made one important assumption rooted in our "Western" cultural tradition: The prohibitive rule is, to that way of thinking, the primary and axiomatic one; the permissive counter-rule, as qualifying the first, is secondary and stands in need of justification. We must justify the infringement of a primary inviolability, which needs no justification itself; and the justification of its infringement must be by values and needs of a dignity commensurate with those to be sacrificed.

. . .

HEALTH AS A PUBLIC GOOD

The cause invoked [for medical experimentation] is health and, in its more critical aspect, life itself—clearly superlative goods that the physician serves directly by curing and the researcher indirectly by the knowledge gained through his experiments. There is no question about the good served nor about the evil fought —disease and premature death. But a good to whom and an evil to whom? Here the issue tends to become somewhat clouded. In the attempt to give experimentation the proper dignity (on the problematic view that a value becomes greater by being "social" instead of merely individual), the health in question or the disease in question is somehow predicated on the social whole, as if it were society that, in the persons of its members, enjoyed the one and suffered the other. For the purposes of our problem, public interest can then be pitted against private interest, the common good against the individual good. Indeed, I have found health called a national resource, which of course it is, but surely not in the first place.

In trying to resolve some of the complexities and ambiguities lurking in these conceptualizations, I have pondered a particular statement, made in the form of a question, which I found in the *Proceedings* of the earlier *Daedalus* conference: "Can society afford to discard the tissues and organs of the hopelessly unconscious patient when they could be used to restore the otherwise hopelessly ill, but still salvageable individual?" And somewhat later:

"A strong case can be made that society can ill afford to discard the tissues and organs of the hopelessly unconscious patient; they are greatly needed for study and experimental trial to help those who can be salvaged."[1] I hasten to add that any suspicion of callousness that the "commodity" language of these statements may suggest is immediately dispelled by the name of the speaker, Dr. Henry K. Beecher, for whose humanity and moral sensibility there can be nothing but admiration. But the use, in all innocence, of this language gives food for thought. Let me, for a moment, take the question literally. "Discarding" implies proprietary rights—nobody can discard what does not belong to him in the first place. Does society then own my body? "Salvaging" implies the same and, moreover, a use-value to the owner. Is the life-extension of certain individuals then a public interest? "Affording" implies a critically vital level of such an interest—that is, of the loss or gain involved. And "society" itself—what is it? When does a need, an aim, an obligation become social? Let us reflect on some of these terms.

WHAT SOCIETY CAN AFFORD

"Can Society afford . . . ?" Afford what? To let people die intact, thereby withholding something from other people who desperately need it, who in consequence will have to die too? These other, unfortunate people indeed cannot afford not to have a kidney, heart, or other organ of the dying patient, on which they depend for an extension of their lease on life; but does that give them a right to it? And does it oblige society to procure it for them? What is it that *society* can or cannot afford—leaving aside for the moment the question of what it has a *right* to? It surely can afford to lose members through death; more than that, it is built on the balance of death and birth decreed by the order of life. This is too general, of course, for our question, but perhaps it is well to remember. The specific question seems to be whether society can afford to let some people die whose death might be deferred by particular means if these were authorized by society. Again, if it is merely a question of what society can or cannot afford, rather than of what it ought or ought not to do, the answer must be: Of course, it can. If cancer, heart disease, and other organic, non-contagious ills, especially those tending to strike the old more than the young, continue to exact their toll at the normal rate of incidence (including the toll of private anguish and misery), society can go on flourishing in every way.

Here, by contrast, are some examples of what, in sober truth, society cannot afford. It cannot afford to let an epidemic rage unchecked; a persistent excess of deaths over births, but neither—we must add—too great an excess of births over deaths; too low an average life expectancy even if demographically balanced by fertility, but neither too great a longevity with the necessitated correlative dearth of youth in the social body; a debilitating state of general health; and things of this kind. These are plain cases where the whole condition of society is critically affected, and the public interest can make its imperative claims. The Black Death of the Middle Ages was a *public* calamity of the acute kind; the life-sapping ravages of endemic malaria or sleeping sickness in certain areas are a public calamity of the chronic kind. Such situations a society as a whole can truly not "afford," and they may call for extraordinary remedies, including, perhaps, the invasion of private sacrosanctities.

This is not entirely a matter of numbers and numerical ratios. Society, in a subtler sense, cannot "afford" a single miscarriage of justice, a single inequity in the dispensation of its laws, the violation of the rights of even the tiniest minority, because these undermine the moral basis on which society's existence rests. Nor can it, for a similar reason, afford the absence or atrophy in its midst of compassion and of the effort to alleviate suffering—be it widespread or rare—one form of which is the effort to conquer disease of any kind, whether "socially" significant (by reason of number) or not. And in short, society cannot afford the absence among its members of *virtue* with its readiness for sacrifice beyond defined duty. Since its presence—that is to say, that of personal idealism—is a matter of grace and not of decree, we have the paradox that society depends for its existence on intangibles of nothing less than a religious order, for which it can hope, but which it cannot enforce. All the more must it protect this most precious capital from abuse.

For what objectives connected with the medico-biological sphere should this reserve be drawn upon—for example, in the form of accepting, soliciting, perhaps even imposing the submission of human subjects to experimentation? We postulate that this must be not just a worthy cause, as any promotion of the health of anybody doubtlessly is, but a cause qualifying for transcendent social sanction. Here one thinks first of those cases critically affecting the whole condition, present and future, of the community we have illustrated. Something equivalent to what in the political sphere is called "clear and present danger" may be invoked and a state of emergency proclaimed, thereby suspending certain otherwise inviolable prohibitions and taboos. We may observe that averting a disaster always carries greater weight than promoting a good. Extraordinary danger excuses extraordinary means. This covers human experimentation, which we would like to count, as far as possible, among the extraordinary rather than the ordinary means of serving the common good under public auspices. Naturally, since foresight and responsibility for the future are of the essence of institutional society, averting disaster extends into long-term prevention, although the lesser urgency will warrant less sweeping licenses.

SOCIETY AND THE CAUSE OF PROGRESS

Much weaker is the case where it is a matter not of saving but of improving society. Much of medical research falls into this category. As stated before, a permanent death rate from heart failure or cancer does not threaten society. So long as certain statistical ratios are maintained, the incidence of disease and of disease-induced mortality is not (in the strict sense) a "social" misfortune. I hasten to add that it is not therefore less of a human misfortune, and the call for relief issuing with silent eloquence from each victim and all potential victims is of no lesser dignity. But it is misleading to equate the fundamentally human response to it with what is owed to society: it is owed by man to man—and it is thereby owed by society to the individuals as soon as the adequate ministering to these concerns outgrows (as it progressively does) the scope of private spontaneity and is made a public mandate. It is thus that society assumes responsibility for medical care, research, old age, and innumerable other things not originally of the public realm (in the original "social contract"), and they become duties toward "society" (rather than directly toward one's fellow man) by the fact that they are socially operated.

Indeed, we expect from organized society no longer mere protection against harm and the securing of the conditions of our preservation, but active and constant improvement in all the domains of life: the waging of the battle against nature, the enhancement of the human estate—in short, the promotion of progress. This is an expansive goal, one far surpassing the disaster norm of our previous reflections. It lacks the urgency of the latter, but has the nobility of the free, forward thrust. It surely is worth sacrifices. It is not at all a question of what society can afford, but of what it is committed to, beyond all necessity, by our mandate. Its trusteeship has become an established, ongoing, institutionalized business of the body politic. As eager beneficiaries of its gains, we now owe to "society," as its chief agent, our individual contributions toward its *continued pursuit*. I emphasize "continued pursuit." Maintaining the existing level requires no more than the orthodox means of taxation and enforcement of professional standards that raise no problems. The more optional goal of pushing forward is also more exacting. We have this syndrome: Progress is by our choosing an acknowledged interest of society, in which we have a stake in various degrees; science is a necessary instrument of progress; research is a necessary instrument of science; and in medical science experimentation on human subjects is a necessary instrument of research. There-

fore, human experimentation has come to be a societal interest.

The destination of research is essentially melioristic. It does not serve the preservation of the existing good from which I profit myself and to which I am obligated. Unless the present state is intolerable, the melioristic goal is in a sense gratuitous, and this not only from the vantage point of the present. Our descendants have a right to be left an unplundered planet; they do not have a right to new miracle cures. We have sinned against them, if by our doing we have destroyed their inheritance—which we are doing at full blast; we have not sinned against them, if by the time they come around arthritis has not yet been conquered (unless by sheer neglect). And generally, in the matter of progress, as humanity had no claim on a Newton, a Michelangelo, or a St. Francis to appear, and no right to the blessings of their unscheduled deeds, so progress, with all our methodical labor for it, cannot be budgeted in advance and its fruits received as a due. Its coming-about at all and its turning out for good (of which we can never be sure) must rather be regarded as something akin to grace.

THE MELIORISTIC GOAL, MEDICAL RESEARCH, AND INDIVIDUAL DUTY

Nowhere is the melioristic goal more inherent than in medicine. To the physician, it is not gratuitous. He is committed to curing and thus to improving the power to cure. Gratuitous we called it (outside disaster conditions) as a *social* goal, but noble at the same time. Both the nobility and the gratuitousness must influence the manner in which self-sacrifice for it is elicited, and even its free offer accepted. Freedom is certainly the first condition to be observed here. The surrender of one's body to medical experimentation is entirely outside the enforceable "social contract."

Or can it be construed to fall within its terms —namely, as repayment for benefits from past experimentation that I have enjoyed myself? But I am indebted for these benefits not to society, but to the past "martyrs," to whom society is indebted itself, and society has no right to call in my personal debt by way of adding new to its own. Moreover, gratitude is not an enforceable social obligation; it anyway does not mean that I must emulate the deed. Most of all, if it was wrong to exact such sacrifice in the first place, it does not become right to exact it again with the plea of the profit it has brought me. If, however, it was not exacted, but entirely free, as it ought to have been, then it should remain so, and its precedence must not be used as a social pressure on others for doing the same under the sign of duty.

. . .

THE "CONSCRIPTION" OF CONSENT

. . .The mere issuing of the appeal, the calling for volunteers, with the moral and social pressures it inevitably generates, amounts even under the most meticulous rules of consent to a sort of *conscripting*. And some soliciting is necessarily involved. . . . And this is why "consent," surely a non-negotiable minimum requirement, is not the full answer to the problem. Granting then that soliciting and therefore some degree of conscripting are part of the situation, who may conscript and who may be conscripted? Or less harshly expressed: Who should issue appeals and to whom?

The naturally qualified issuer of the appeal is the research scientist himself, collectively the main carrier of the impulse and the only one with the technical competence to judge. But his being very much an interested party (with vested interests, indeed, not purely in the public good, but in the scientific enterprise as such, in "his" project, and even in his career) makes him also suspect. The ineradicable dialectic of this situation—a delicate incompatibility problem—calls for particular controls by the research community and by public authority that we need not discuss. They can mitigate, but not eliminate the problem. We have to live with the ambiguity, the treacherous impurity of everything human.

SELF-RECRUITMENT OF THE COMMUNITY

To whom should the appeal be addressed? The natural issuer of the call is also the first

natural addressee: the physician-researcher himself and the scientific confraternity at large. With such a coincidence—indeed, the noble tradition with which the whole business of human experimentation started—almost all of the associated legal, ethical, and metaphysical problems vanish. If it is full, autonomous identification of the subject with the purpose that is required for the dignifying of his serving as a subject—here it is; if strongest motivation—here it is; if fullest understanding—here it is; if freest decision—here it is; if greatest integration with the person's total, chosen pursuit—here it is. With the fact of self-solicitation the issue of consent in all its insoluble equivocality is bypassed *per se*. Not even the condition that the particular purpose be truly important and the project reasonably promising, which must hold in any solicitation of others, need be satisfied here. By himself, the scientist is free to obey his obsession, to play his hunch, to wager on chance, to follow the lure of ambition. It is all part of the "divine madness" that somehow animates the ceaseless pressing against frontiers. For the rest of society, which has a deep-seated disposition to look with reverence and awe upon the guardians of the mysteries of life, the profession assumes with this proof of its devotion the role of a self-chosen, consecrated fraternity, not unlike the monastic orders of the past, and this would come nearest to the actual, religious origins of the art of healing.

. . .

"IDENTIFICATION" AS THE PRINCIPLE OF RECRUITMENT IN GENERAL

If the properties we adduced as the particular qualifications of the members of the scientific fraternity itself are taken as general criteria of selection, then one should look for additional subjects where a maximum of identification, understanding, and spontaneity can be expected—that is, among the most highly motivated, the most highly educated, and the least "captive" members of the community. From this naturally scarce resource, a descending order of permissibility leads to greater abundance and ease of supply, whose use should become proportionately more hesitant as the exculpating criteria are relaxed. An inversion of normal "market" behavior is demanded here—namely, to accept the lowest quotation last (and excused only by the greatest pressure of need); to pay the highest price first.

The ruling principle in our considerations is that the "wrong" of reification can only be made "right" by such authentic identification with the cause that it is the subject's as well as the researcher's cause—whereby his role in its service is not just permitted by him, but *willed*. That sovereign will of his which embraces the end as his own restores his personhood to the otherwise depersonalizing context. To be valid it must be autonomous and informed. The latter condition can, outside the research community, only be fulfilled by degrees; but the higher the degree of the understanding regarding the purpose and the technique, the more valid becomes the endorsement of the will. A margin of mere trust inevitably remains. Ultimately, the appeal for volunteers should seek this free and generous endorsement, the appropriation of the research purpose into the person's own scheme of ends. Thus, the appeal is in truth addressed to the one, mysterious, and sacred source of any such generosity of the will— "devotion," whose forms and objects of commitment are various and may invest different motivations in different individuals. The following, for instance, may be responsive to the "call" we are discussing: compassion with human suffering, zeal for humanity, reverence for the Golden Rule, enthusiasm for progress, homage to the cause of knowledge, even longing for sacrificial justification (do not call that "masochism," please). On all these, I say, it is defensible and right to draw when the research objective is worthy enough; and it is a prime duty of the research community (especially in view of what we called the "margin of trust") to see that this sacred source is never abused for frivolous ends. For a less than adequate cause, not even the freest, unsolicited offer should be accepted.

THE RULE OF THE "DESCENDING ORDER" AND ITS COUNTER-UTILITY SENSE

We have laid down what must seem to be a forbidding rule to the number-hungry research industry. Having faith in the transcendent potential of man, I do not fear that the "source" will ever fail a society that does not destroy it— and only such a one is worthy of the blessings of progress. But "elitistic" the rule is (as is the enterprise of progress itself), and elites are by nature small. The combined attribute of motivation and information, plus the absence of external pressures, tends to be socially so circumscribed that strict adherence to the rule might numerically starve the research process. This is why I spoke of a descending order of permissibility, which is itself permissive, but where the realization that it is a *descending* order is not without pragmatic import. Departing from the august norm, the appeal must needs shift from idealism to docility, from high-mindedness to compliance, from judgment to trust. Consent spreads over the whole spectrum. I will not go into the casuistics of this penumbral area. I merely indicate the principle of the order of preference: The poorer in knowledge, motivation, and fredom of decision (and that, alas, means the more readily available in terms of numbers and possible manipulation), the more sparingly and indeed reluctantly should the reservoir be used, and the more compelling must therefore become the countervailing justification.

Let us note that this is the opposite of a social utility standard, the reverse of the order by "availability and expendability": The most valuable and scarcest, the least expendable elements of the social organism, are to be the first candidates for risk and sacrifice. It is the standard of *noblesse oblige;* and with all its counterutility and seeming "wastefulness," we feel a rightness about it and perhaps even a higher "utility," for the soul of the community lives by this spirit.[2] It is also the opposite of what the day-to-day interests of research clamor for, and for the scientific community to honor it will mean that it will have to fight a strong temptation to go by routine to the readiest sources of supply—the suggestible, the ignorant, the dependent, the "captive" in various senses.[3] I do not believe that heightened resistance here must cripple research, which cannot be permitted; but it may indeed slow it down by the smaller numbers fed into experimentation in consequence. This price—a possibly slower rate of progress—may have to be paid for the preservation of the most precious capital of higher communal life.

EXPERIMENTATION ON PATIENTS

So far we have been speaking on the tacit assumption that the subjects of experimentation are recruited from among the healthy. To the question "Who is conscriptable?" the spontaneous answer is: Least and last of all the sick—the most available of all as they are under treatment and observation anyway. That the afflicted should not be called upon to bear additional burden and risk, that they are society's special trust and the physician's trust in particular—these are elementary responses of our moral sense. Yet the very destination of medical research, the conquest of disease, requires at the crucial stage trial and verification on precisely the sufferers from the disease, and their total exemption would defeat the purpose itself. In acknowledging this inescapable necessity, we enter the most sensitive area of the whole complex, the one most keenly felt and most searchingly discussed by the practitioners themselves. No wonder, it touches the heart of the doctor-patient relation, putting its most solemn obligations to the test. There is nothing new in what I have to say about the ethics of the doctor-patient relation, but for the purpose of confronting it with the issue of experimentation some of the oldest verities must be recalled.

THE FUNDAMENTAL PRIVILEGE OF THE SICK

In the course of treatment, the physician is obligated to the patient and to no one else. He is not the agent of society, nor of the interests of medical science, nor of the patient's family, nor of his co-sufferers, or future sufferers from the same disease. The patient alone counts when he is under the physician's care. By the simple law of bilateral contract (analogous, for example, to the relation of lawyer to client and its "conflict of interest" rule), the physician is bound not to let any other interest interfere with that of the patient in being cured. But manifestly more sublime norms than contractual ones are involved. We may speak of a sacred trust; strictly by its terms, the doctor is, as it were, alone with his patient and God.

There is one normal exception to this—that is, to the doctor's not being the agent of society vis-à-vis the patient, but the trustee of his interests alone: the quarantining of the contagious sick. This is plainly not for the patient's interest, but for that of others threatened by him. (In vaccination, we have a combination of both: protection of the individual and others.) But preventing the patient from causing harm to others is not the same as exploiting him for the advantage of others. And there is, of course, the abnormal exception of collective catastrophe, the analogue to a state of war. The physician who desperately battles a raging epidemic is under a unique dispensation that suspends in a nonspecifiable way some of the structures of normal practice, including possibly those against experimental liberties with his patients. No rules can be devised for the waiving of rules in extremities. And as with the famous shipwreck examples of ethical theory, the less said about it the better. But what is allowable there and may later be passed over in forgiving silence cannot serve as a precedent. We are concerned with non-extreme, non-emergency conditions where the voice of principle can be heard and claims can be adjudicated free from duress. We have conceded that there are such claims, and that if there is to be medical advance at all, not even the superlative privilege of the suffering and the sick can be kept wholly intact from the intrusion of its needs. About this least palatable, most disquieting part of our subject, I have to offer only groping, inconclusive remarks.

THE PRINCIPLE OF "IDENTIFICATION" APPLIED TO PATIENTS

On the whole, the same principles would seem to hold here as are found to hold with "normal subjects": motivation, identification, understanding on the part of the subject. But it is clear that these conditions are peculiarly difficult to satisfy with regard to a patient. His physical state, psychic preoccupation, dependent relation to the doctor, the submissive attitude induced by treatment—everything connected with his condition and situation makes the sick person inherently less of a sovereign person than the healthy one. Spontaneity of self-offering has almost to be ruled out; consent is marred by lower resistance or captive circumstance, and so on. In fact, all the factors that make the patient, as a category, particularly accessible and welcome for experimentation at the same time compromise the quality of the responding affirmation that must morally redeem the making use of them. This, in addition to the primacy of the physician's duty, puts a heightened onus on the physician-researcher to limit his undue power to the most important and defensible research objectives and, of course, to keep persuasion at a minimum.

Still, with all the disabilities noted, there is scope among patients for observing the rule of the "descending order of permissibility" that we have laid down for normal subjects, in vexing inversion of the utility order of quantitative abundance and qualitative "expendability." By the principle of this order, those patients who most identify with and are cognizant of the cause of research—members of the medical profession (who after all are sometimes patients themselves)—come first; the highly motivated and educated, also least dependent, among the lay patients come next; and so on down the line. An added consideration here is seriousness of condition, which again operates in inverse proportion. Here the profession must fight the tempting sophistry that the hopeless case is expendable (because in prospect already expended) and therefore especially usable; and generally the attitude that the poorer the chances of the patient the more justifiable his recruitment for experimentation (other than for his own benefit). The opposite is true.

NONDISCLOSURE AS A BORDERLINE CASE

Then there is the case where ignorance of the subject, sometimes even of the experimenter, is of the essence of the experiment (the "double blind"-control group-placebo syndrome). It is said to be a necessary element of the scientific process. Whatever may be said about its ethics in regard to normal subjects, especially volunteers, it is an outright betrayal of trust in regard to the patient who believes that he is receiving treatment. Only supreme importance of the objective can exonerate it, without making it less of a transgression. The patient is definitely wronged even when not harmed. And ethics apart, the practice of such deception holds the danger of undermining the faith in the *bona fides* of treatment, the beneficial intent of the physician—the very basis of the doctor-patient relationship. In every respect, it follows that concealed experiment on patients—that is, experiment under the guise of treatment—should be the rarest exception, at best, if it cannot be wholly avoided.

This has still the merit of a borderline problem. The same is not true of the other case of necessary ignorance of the subject—that of the unconscious patient. Drafting him for non-therapeutic experiments is simply and unqualifiedly impermissible; progress or not, he must never be used, on the inflexible principle that utter helplessness demands utter protection.

When preparing this paper, I filled pages with a casuistics of this harrowing field, but then scrapped most of it, realizing my dilettante status. The shadings are endless, and only the physician-researcher can discern them properly as the cases arise. Into his lap the decision is thrown. The philosophical rule, once it has admitted into itself the idea of a sliding scale, cannot really specify its own application. It can only impress on the practitioner a general maxim or attitude for the exercise of his judgment and conscience in the concrete occasions of his work. In our case, I am afraid, it means making life more difficult for him.

It will also be noted that, somewhat at variance with the emphasis in the literature, I have not dwelt on the element of "risk" and very little on that of "consent." Discussion of the first is beyond the layman's competence; the emphasis on the second has been lessened because of its equivocal character. It is a truism to say that one should strive to minimize the risk and to maximize the consent. The more demanding concept of "identification," which I have used, includes "consent" in its maximal or authentic form, and the assumption of risk is its privilege.

NO EXPERIMENTS ON PATIENTS UNRELATED TO THEIR OWN DISEASE

Although my ponderings have, on the whole, yielded points of view rather than definite prescriptions, premises rather than conclusions, they have led me to a few unequivocal yeses and noes. The first is the emphatic rule that patients should be experimented upon, if at all, *only* with reference to *their disease*. Never should there be added to the gratuitousness of the experiment as such the gratuitousness of service to an unrelated cause. This follows simply from what we have found to be the *only* excuse for infracting the special exemption of the sick at all—namely, that the scientific war on disease cannot accomplish its goal without drawing the sufferers from disease into the investigative process. If under this excuse they become subjects of experiment, they do so *because,* and only because, of *their* disease.

This is the fundamental and self-sufficient consideration. That the patient cannot possibly benefit from the unrelated experiment therapeutically, while he might from experiment related to his condition, is also true, but lies beyond the problem area of pure experiment. I am in any case discussing nontherapeutic experimentation only, where *ex hypothesi* the patient does not benefit. Experiment as part of therapy—that is, directed toward helping the subject himself—is a different matter altogether and raises its own problems but hardly philosophical ones. As long as a doctor can say, even if only in his own thought: "There is no known cure for your condition (or: You have responded to none); but there is promise in a new treatment still under investigation, not quite tested yet as to effectiveness and safety; you will be taking a chance, but all things considered, I judge it in your best interest to let me try it on you"—as long as he can speak thus, he speaks as the patient's physician and may err, but does not transform the patient into a sub-

ject of experimentation. Introduction of an untried therapy into the treatment where the tried ones have failed is not "experimentation on the patient."

Generally, and almost needless to say, with all the rules of the book, there is something "experimental" (because tentative) about every individual treatment, beginning with the diagnosis itself; and he would be a poor doctor who would not learn from every case for the benefit of future cases, and a poor member of the profession who would not make any new insights gained from his treatments available to the profession at large. Thus, knowledge may be advanced in the treatment of any patient, and the interest of the medical art and all sufferers from the same affliction as well as the patient himself may be served if something happens to be learned from his case. But his gain to knowledge and future therapy is incidental to the *bona fide* service to the present patient. He has the right to expect that the doctor does nothing to him just in order to learn.

In that case, the doctor's imaginary speech would run, for instance, like this: "There is nothing more I can do for you. But you can do something for me. Speaking no longer as your physician but on behalf of medical science, we could learn a great deal about future cases of this kind if you would permit me to perform certain experiments on you. It is understood that you yourself would not benefit from any knowledge we might gain; but future patients would." This statement would express the purely experimental situation, assumedly here with the subject's concurrence and with all cards on the table. In Alexander Bickel's words: "It is a different situation when the doctor is no longer trying to make [the patient] well, but is trying to find out how to make others well in the future."[4]

But even in the second case, that of the nontherapeutic experiment where the patient does not benefit, at least the patient's own disease is enlisted in the cause of fighting that disease, even if only in others. It is yet another thing to say or think: "Since you are here—in the hospital with its facilities—anyway, under our care and observation anyway, away from your job (or, perhaps, doomed) anyway, we wish to profit from your being available for some other research of great interest we are presently engaged in.'' From the standpoint of merely medical ethics, which has only to consider risk, consent, and the worth of the objective, there may be no cardinal difference between this case and the last one. I hope that the medical reader will not think I am making too fine a point when I say that from the standpoint of the subject and his dignity there is a cardinal difference that crosses the line between the permissible and the impermissible, and this by the same principle of ''identification'' I have been invoking all along. Whatever the rights and wrongs of any experimentation on any patient —in the one case, at least that residue of identification is left him that it is his own affliction by which he can contribute to the conquest of that affliction, his own kind of suffering which he helps to alleviate in others; and so in a sense it is his own cause. It is totally indefensible to rob the unfortunate of this intimacy with the purpose and make his misfortune a convenience for the furtherance of alien concerns.

. . .

CONCLUSION

. . . I wish only to say in conclusion that if some of the practical implications of my reasonings are felt to work out toward a slower rate of progress, this should not cause too great dismay. Let us not forget that progress is an optional goal, not an unconditional commitment, and that its tempo in particular, compulsive as it may become, has nothing sacred about it. Let us also remember that a slower progress in the conquest of disease would not threaten society, grievous as it is to those who have to deplore that their particular disease be not yet conquered, but that society would indeed be threatened by the erosion of those moral values whose loss, possibly caused by too ruthless a pursuit of scientific progress, would make its most dazzling triumphs not worth having. Let us finally remember that it cannot be the aim of progress to abolish the lot of mortality. Of some ill or other, each of us will die. Our mortal condition is upon us with its harshness but also its wisdom—because without it there would not be the eternally renewed promise of the freshness, immediacy, and eagerness of youth; nor would there be for any of us the incentive to number our days and make them count. With all our striving to wrest from our mortality what we can, we should bear its burden with patience and dignity.

NOTES

1. *Proceedings of the Conference on the Ethical Aspects of Experimentation on Human Subjects,* November 3–4, 1967 (Boston, Massachusetts; hereafter called *Proceedings*), pp. 50–51.

2. Socially, everyone is expendable relatively—that is, in different degrees; religiously, no one is expendable absolutely: The ''image of God'' is in all. If it can be enhanced, then not by anyone being expended, but by someone expending himself.

3. This refers to captives of circumstance, not of justice. Prison inmates are, with respect to our problem, in a special class. If we hold to some idea of guilt, and to the supposition that our judicial system is not entirely at fault, they may be held to stand in a special debt to society, and their offer to serve—from whatever motive—may be accepted with a minimum of qualms as a means of reparation.

4. *Proceedings,* p. 33.

DAVID D. RUTSTEIN

The Ethical Design of Human Experiments

This analysis of the ethical considerations governing human experiments is based on the assumption that it is ethical under carefully controlled conditions to study on human beings mechanisms of health and disease and to test new drugs, biological products, procedures, methods, and instruments that give promise of improving the health of human beings, of preventing or treating their diseases, or postponing their untimely deaths. Without such an assumption, there can be no systematic method of medical advance. Progress would have to depend on the surreptitious, illegal, or unsupervised research and testing of new modes of prevention and treatment of disease. The ethical standards of such irregular activities would certainly be at a far lower level than can be guaranteed when the testing of new methods of treatment is openly practiced.

Proceeding on that assumption, how can one design experiments upon human beings that will yield the desired scientific information and yet avoid or keep ethical contraindications to a minimum? This question is asked in the belief that in the design of the experiment itself many ethical dilemmas may be resolved. Attention must be given to the ways an experiment can be designed to maintain its scientific validity, meet ethical requirements, and yet yield the necessary new knowledge.

Let us concentrate on laying out new guidelines that might lead to the solution of ethical problems rather than on focusing our attention on the difficulties that these problems present. The ethical requirements that have created the

Reprinted with permission of George Braziller, Inc. from *Experimentation with Human Subjects* by Paul A. Freund (ed.). Copyright © 1969, 1970 by the American Academy of Arts and Sciences.

most difficulty are obtaining informed consent from the potential subject; the need for the subject to derive a health benefit from the experiment; and keeping the risk to the subject as small as possible. Such questions are important and relevant because ethical considerations are paramount when experiments are to be performed on human subjects. It is the thesis of this essay that in the design of a human experiment it is mandatory to select those experimental conditions, subjects, and methods of measurement that impose the fewest ethical constraints. Such an approach will not cause the ethical problems of human experiments to disappear. If a definitive attempt is made, during the planning stages of an experiment on human beings, to keep the ethical as well as scientific criteria in mind, it is possible often to perform the necessary research to yield the desired information.

SCIENTIFICALLY UNSOUND STUDIES ARE UNETHICAL

It may be accepted as a maxim that a poorly or improperly designed study involving human subjects—one that could not possibly yield scientific facts (that is, reproducible observations) relevant to the question under study—is by definition unethical. Moreover, when a study is in itself scientifically invalid, all other ethical considerations become irrelevant. There is no point in obtaining "informed consent" to perform a useless study. A worthless study cannot possibly benefit anyone, least of all the experimental subject himself. Any risk to the patient, however small, cannot be justified. In essence, the scientific validity of a study on human beings is in itself an ethical principle.

. . .

ASKING THE RIGHT QUESTION

The design of an experiment depends at first on the question asked by the investigator. Some questions are in themselves unethical. One cannot ask whether plague bacilli are more virulent in human beings when injected into the bloodstream than when they are sprayed into the throat. One may obtain hints as to the answer to such a question by epidemiologic comparison of the spread of pneumonic plague (spread from the lungs into the air) and bubonic plague (spread by insect bite). Anecdotal information on the spread of plague can also be obtained through the study of laboratory accidents. But a deliberate experiment to answer this question cannot be performed.

The human experiments performed by the Nazis during World War II horrified the world because they were designed to answer unethical questions. "How long can a human being survive in ice cold water?" will, it is to be hoped, never again be a question to be answered by a scientific experiment. Thus, as a first step in the design of any human experiment, we must first be sure that the question itself is an ethical one.

Moreover, an unethical experiment can sometimes be converted into an ethical one by rephrasing the question. In drug testing, for example, it is not ethical to design an experiment to answer the question: "Is treatment of the disease with the new drug more effective than no treatment at all?" In answering such a question, the patients in the control group would literally have to receive "no treatment" and that is completely unacceptable. Instead, if the patients in the control group are given the best possible current treatment of the disease, we may now ask an ethical question: "Is treatment with the new drug more effective than the generally accepted treatment for this particular disease?"

We faced this problem in the design of the United States–United Kingdom Cooperative Rheumatic Fever Study, which was concerned with measuring the relative effectiveness of cortisone and ACTH in the treatment of that disease.[1] We could not give rheumatic fever patients in the control group "no treatment." We would have had to go so far as to prohibit bed rest, which itself may be helpful to rheumatic fever patients, because patients in bed have a slower heart rate. Instead, we asked the question: "Is treatment with ACTH or cortisone better, worse, or the same as the best generally accepted drug treatment for this disease?"

Our control group, in addition to all the other non-specific treatments which the treated groups also received, were given large doses of aspirin—the generally accepted drug treatment of the time. A question that compares the new treatment with the most effective of the time is not only ethical, but it is also the most practical question. If the new treatment is to replace the generally accepted treatment, it must be demonstrated clearly to be better.

With a question framed in that way, one may obtain consent from the patient by explaining that he will receive either the best treatment of the time or the new drug. It is made clear that, although promising in animal and other experiments, the new drug has not yet been shown in human experiments to be better, worse, or the same as the generally accepted treatment. Most patients will accept these alternatives. The investigator himself would be reassured that he has done the best for his patient's health and safety, while evaluating a more promising remedy for his disease.

. . .

THE ETHICS OF CONTROLLED HUMAN EXPERIMENTATION

Controls are essential in such human experiments as the testing of a drug or a surgical procedure. In order to evaluate new therapy, it is necessary to identify those additional benefits of the new remedy which exceed the improvement that might be expected in the course of the natural history of the disease. To be sure, in a disease such as human rabies, which is practically 100 per cent fatal, controlled observations are not needed because any recovery of treated patients is an obvious benefit. Acute leukemia and virulent tumors such as reticulum-cell sarcoma are other examples of diseases whose natural history is one of immutable progression to death and where benefit can be identified without a controlled experiment.

Most diseases do not fall into such a clearcut category. Even diseases such as cancer of the breast have such a variable course that one is not certain to this moment if surgery prolongs the life of the patient suffering from this disease. The variability of the disease from patient to patient makes it difficult, if not impossible, to evaluate the additional effectiveness of the surgical remedy without a controlled study.

Controlled studies also keep the investigator from leaving the world of reality. The enthusiastic research worker often concentrates on whether the new treatment seems to work. Psychologically, he is apt to pay less attention to possible harmful effects of the new treatment. The result of this attitude is documented repeatedly by the myriad of treatments that make the headlines and promise miraculous cures on the front pages of our best newspapers, only to be completely discarded a few years later. This phenomenon is not without its harmful effects. The definite, albeit limited, benefits of established treatments are often cast aside in favor of the dramatic new, but as yet unproven method of treatment for a human disease. For example, before the advent of the sulfa drugs and antibiotics, there were fairly effective procedures that alleviated and at times cured urinary-tract infection. When these new therapeutic agents became available, some physicians concentrated on intensive therapy with one of the new agents and often felt that it was no longer necessary to practice many of the important details of treatment that had been given in the past. Now, after several decades, there is a gradual return to a more balanced regimen of treatment that places each of the antibiotics in proper perspective in the total treatment of urinary-tract infection. In such situations, a controlled study that is properly performed permits a clean comparison of the helpful and harmful effects of the new treatment and of the older established method of therapy. If, in addition, circumstances permit the ethical use of a placebo control, information can also be obtained about the natural history of the disease.

One might ask whether it is unethical not to perform a controlled human experiment. The Pasteur experiment with rabies vaccine is classic. Controlled human experimentation was completely unknown when Pasteur first tested his new vaccine on those Russian *muzhiks* who were bitten by rabid wolves. All were given the vaccine and all recovered. The result was so dramatic and so electrifying that further experimentation seemed unnecessary. When it was later learned, however, that the chances were relatively low of developing this uniformly fatal disease—human rabies—even after a bite from a known rabid animal, and that the vaccine itself causes paralysis which is not infrequently fatal, it became important to determine whether the vaccine really does more good than harm.

But it became impossible to do a controlled experiment on rabies vaccine. After the general acceptance of the treatment, if a controlled experiment were to be performed, and if a subject in the control group developed rabies, the experimenter might not only be sued for malpractice, but might even be deemed criminally culpable for not having given the patient the "accepted treatment of the time." This same situation is now developing in the estimation of the benefits of heart transplantation and in measuring the value of intensive-care units in the treatment of heart attacks from coronary disease.

In hospitals where heart transplantation is performed, there are many more eligible recipients than donors. It would be relatively easy to randomize the procedure and measure the effectiveness of this new operation. Whenever a heart from a human donor became available, a random selection could be made among all of the eligible recipients. Those not selected would then comprise a control group whose course and outcome could be compared with those of the recipients of a transplanted heart.

The same situation obtains in the treatment of heart attacks from coronary disease in intensive-care units. There is as yet no published control study demonstrating the effectiveness of intensive care in the treatment of acute myocardial infarction. Once again, a control study is possible because in any one center the numbers eligible for care may far exceed the available facilities. A randomly allocated control study would provide the precise information that is needed to estimate the value of this procedure. Instead, we are already beginning to hear ex-cathedra statements of the effectiveness of intensive-care units that are unsupported by the required scientific evidence.

Even up to the present moment, many patients suffer severe discomfort or are permanently harmed from treatments whose validity has been based on uncontrolled observations. Thousands of hypertensive patients in the 1930's and '40's were subjected to extensive surgery for the removal of their thoracolumbar sympathetic nervous system in the belief that the progress of the disease would be arrested. The treatment is no longer used.

Would this problem have been resolved had controlled studies been performed by means of random allocation in which half of the patients would have had sham operations? In an analogous situation when uncontrolled evidence suggested that the internal mammary artery operation might be helpful in the treatment of angina pectoris, Dr. Henry Beecher recommended a study in which the patients in the control groups would be given a sham operation.[2] He indicated that a far smaller total number of human subjects would have been needed and a definitive answer could be obtained by such a procedure. Although scientifically sound, I do not believe that it is ethical to perform sham operations on human subjects because of the operative risk and the lack of potential benefit to the patient. Instead, controlled studies could have been performed with the randomly allocated control patients being given the best medical treatment of the time together with a period of bed rest similar to that of the surgical convalescent.

The history of diseases of unknown etiology is replete with serially accepted and discarded fads of treatment. Peptic ulcer is an example. The Sippy rigid alkali and milk diet became the Meulengracht meat diet and in time became a bland diet with enough alkali to relieve the patient's symptoms. The short-circuiting surgical operation of gastro-enterostomy changed to one for removal of a large portion of the acid-secreting part of the stomach—partial gastrectomy—and then to the less traumatic procedure of removing the nerve supply to the stomach and upper intestine—vagotomy. Along the way, a procedure for freezing the stomach was introduced, then discarded, not because the fad had worn itself out, but because it was obviously harmful. All these treatments might or might not have been accompanied with psychiatric therapy. To this day, the treatment of peptic ulcer, as is the case of many diseases of unknown etiology, is an art with little solid scientific support.

In essence, a new treatment of a disease may be better, worse, or the same as the generally accepted one. The controlled clinical trial has not only been effective in rejecting useless treatments, but perhaps even more helpful in recognizing a harmful therapy, such as the anticoagulant treatment of cerebral thrombosis. That treatment was earning growing acceptance until, in a controlled clinical trial, it was recognized that cerebral hemorrhage was a more frequent complication in the group treated with anticoagulants than among the patients in the control group.[3] The trial was terminated.

One may conclude that if the question under study is an ethical one, and if the design of the study is sound, taking both the scientific and the ethical constraints into consideration, controlled studies when indicated impose fewer ethical problems than uncontrolled human experiments.

. . .

MODERN DESIGN OF HUMAN EXPERIMENTS

The advent of the electronic computer has increased the efficiency of biomedical research and, in turn, has had its ethical implications. In the days of collecting laboratory measurements on the smoked drum, it was easier to collect data than to analyze them. Indeed, final interpretation of experiments was often delayed for months as data were collated and analyzed by hand tabulations, often made by the investigator himself in odd moments between the pressing needs of laboratory duties and teaching. Rarely was the analysis of data given priority over his other activities. At the top of the list was the next experiment, the gross results of which were eagerly anticipated while the detailed analysis was again postponed.

As a result of these traditional limitations on data handling and processing, and with the increasing complexity of our understanding of biological systems, there has been a growing tendency to design experiments in simplified systems where at any one time a few variables can be measured with great precision. This method of research has yielded a great deal of generally applicable biological knowledge. But because the systems of the human body are so complex and the new simplified approach to research so remote from them, the research results have become less and less applicable to the solution of problems of human health and disease. Indeed, the clinical problem that may have originally inspired the research program may often be forgotten as the scientist concentrates on further and further detailed study of his simplified system. As a corollary, when such clinical investigation became more remote from human subjects, fewer ethical problems were created.

With the advent of the electronic computer, the underlying situation was completely reversed. The revolution in data handling and processing has now made it much easier to analyze and interpret than to collect scientific data. The analysis of scientific data, if the experiment's design is sound, should now take relatively little time and effort. Indeed, the immediate availability of an analysis of the data of an experiment should permit the scientist to concentrate on the significance of the experimental results. The scientist now has the time to take into consideration the results of this last experiment so as to plan better the next one.

More importantly, clinical experimentation no longer need be limited to the study of a few variables at any one time in simplified systems.

Experiments can presently be designed to study the complex interrelationships of many variables at the same time. For example, instead of studying the salt and water metabolism of the kidney as if it were completely independent of all the other functions of this organ, it is now possible to study total organ function. Indeed, computer handling of data makes it feasible to study total body functions. Furthermore, with on-line data collection and analysis in real time, it is feasible, for example, to build into a physiologic experiment many contingent measurements depending upon what happens in the earlier stages of the experiment. With such study design, medical research can deal more directly with complex systems in the human subject. Moreover, because the research system is closer to that of the human being, the experimental results should be more easily applicable to the improvement of health and the prevention and treatment of human disease.

This modern method of research—with its more complicated design and more intensive and thorough study of each human subject—is uncovering new ethical questions: How long can one safely run a particular experiment on a patient with a certain disease? How much blood may be collected for research purposes over a specified period of time and how frequently may the experiment be repeated? Will a particularly long continued intensive experiment interfere with the best treatment of the patient? It is clear that more comprehensive clinical experiments requiring more intensive scientific planning will also demand more careful attention to the protection of the human subject. Moreover, now that more complete experiments can be performed, human subjects must not be "wasted" in trivial experiments. This is not to say that simple but complete and penetrating experiments should not be performed. It is a plea for more meticulous planning based on modern technology, computer facilities, and biostatistical consultation to yield more applicable experimental results without increasing the risk to the human subject. It will force us to ask the question: "Is it ethical to perform *limited experiments* if, with more careful planning and with no increased risk to the patient, much more valuable information could be collected of more immediate applicability to patients, including the subject himself?"

. . .

If we can agree that scientific medical research can continue to serve ethically as the basis for medical progress, there is an immediate need to re-examine the design of human experiments from both the scientific and ethical points of view; to reshape the design of human experiments and take advantage of new technology; to increase, improve, make more relevant the data collected in human experiments, and yet, at the same time, strengthen the ethical principles of medical research.

NOTES

1. "A Joint Report: The Treatment of Acute Rheumatic Fever in Children. A Cooperative Clinical Trial of ACTH, Cortisone, and Aspirin," *Circulation,* Vol. II (1955), pp. 343–77; *British Medical Journal,* Vol. 1 (1955), pp. 555–74.

2. H. K. Beecher, "Surgery as Placebo—A Quantitative Study of Bias," *Journal of the American Medical Association,* Vol. 176 (1961), pp. 1102–1107.

3. A. B. Hill, J. Marshall, and D. A. Shaw, "A Controlled Clinical Trial of Long-Term Anticoagulant Therapy in Cerebrovascular Disease," *Quarterly Journal of Medicine,* Vol. 29, New Series (1960), pp. 597–609.

THOMAS C. CHALMERS

The Ethics of Randomization as a Decision-Making Technique, and the Problem of Informed Consent

. . .

. . . "Do no harm while nature heals" was the motto of my father who practiced medicine at the end of the nineteenth and early part of the twentieth century. This was a relatively easy course for him to follow in those days when the only effective medicines were digitalis and morphine, and life-threatening treatments such as major surgery were just beginning to be used. Nowadays the busy physician makes several decisions a week which are critical to the life and health of his patient. Whether alone or with consultations, he makes these decisions by means of so-called clinical judgement, a subtle distillation of his personal experience and the knowledge that he has been able to glean from the medical literature.

The major danger in basing action on personal experience is the unavoidable excess influence of the most recent experience. The last case or two, especially if dramatically successful, or unsuccessful, cannot help but have more influence on the next decision than those cases encountered in the more distant past. As an aside I should like to suggest that the older clinician is the more able decision maker not only because he has had more experience, but also because a growing defect in memory for recent events allows him to give a more equal weight to his experiences, no matter when they occurred.

The second important component of clinical judgement is a knowledge of the medical literature, both basic and clinical. Unfortunately

From *Report of the Fourteenth Conference of Cardiovascular Training Grant Program Directors, National Heart Institute* (Washington, D.C.: U.S. Department of Health, Education, and Welfare, 1967).

basic research has, almost by definition, little immediate application to the treatment of patients. The practicing physician must be able to evaluate and rely on the clinical medicine literature when he treats patients, and he must be ready to defend his decisions by referring to the articles written by his peers or to his own research experience. When the treatment is symptomatic, it probably makes little difference what the physician does. The potent factor is his interest in his patient. However, when the treatment is life-threatening, as with major surgery or other drastic regimens, then the physician and his patient are in trouble because the clinical literature is so notoriously unscientific. By this I mean that the conclusions of the authors are seldom borne out by the data. Less than 20 percent of the clinical trials reported in the medical literature are controlled, and unfortunately the more drastic and dangerous the therapy the less are controls employed. The major defect in most reports of new therapies is the complete inability of the author or the reader to separate out the effects of the treatment under study from the effects of selection of patients for that treatment. In addition, the physician attempting to decide about life-threatening therapies rarely considers another important selection factor, the multiple variables that determine whether a series of patients is written up or not, and whether a paper is accepted for publication or not. So the final reported series may represent a very small and unidentifiable sub-group of the total number of patients presenting with the disorder under study, and it is next to impossible to apply that information correctly in making decisions about individual members of the total population with that disease.

It is clear by now that I am trying to develop a case for the controlled clinical trial in the initial investigation of a life-threatening therapy. A carefully constructed protocol will contain a randomization procedure by which clearly defined patients are assigned to the new or conventional therapy. In that case the relative efficacy of the new treatment and the population to which it can be applied can be clearly determined. If the new treatment turns out to be best, the patients assigned to that will have been the lucky ones. If the new treatment is comparatively bad, the controls will be the lucky ones. In either case, the patients will be carefully treated and may thus do better than those who are not studied at all.

. . .

From the scientific standpoint, there is no doubt about the need for controlled trials of all new procedures which may on the average be more harmful than helpful. Yet in the last 30 years any number of new procedures have been introduced, only to be discarded or modified many years later when the slow process of individual clinical experience suggested that they were actually dangerous, or at least not as effective as the original proponents had thought. It is unlikely that total ignorance of scientific methodology is the reason for the great scarcity of well-controlled trials of new therapies in clinical medicine. It is more likely that those who introduced and publicized the new methods felt that it was unethical to withhold the possibility of benefit from any available patients, and that they certainly had to decide who was suitable for the operation according to their best clinical judgement rather than according to some very un-doctor-like randomization procedure. To me it seems clear that to randomize patients into a group receiving the new therapy being evaluated, and a group receiving the standard therapy, whether it be a similar treatment or no treatment, depending on what is currently accepted for the disease, is much more ethical and is much more in the interest of the individual patients than is treatment of consecutive selected patients as if the new therapy had already been established; or conversely, the withholding of a new therapy from a group of patients as if it had already been proven to be ineffective.

Three problems remain to be discussed with regard to this discussion of randomization: when to start, what to tell the patients, and when to stop.

One often hears experienced clinical investigators insist that a randomized controlled trial should never be started until the techniques of the new therapy have been worked out in a preliminary group of patients. I am convinced that from the ethical standpoint this is very dangerous reasoning. New therapeutic procedures are always changed and are usually improved by experience with the first few patients. However, it is extremely difficult for the investigators not to acquire enthusiasm, or the opposite emotional response, when they have tried out the new therapy in a consecutive series of patients. If they have worked out a good dosage regimen or what they consider an effective operative procedure, they are almost by definition convinced that the new treatment has enough merit so that they cannot ethically deprive a control group from receiving it. Or they might prematurely discard a new treatment because of poor results, when in fact a randomized control group might have done much worse. So I believe that it is important to randomize from the very first patient not only to protect future patients but also to protect the first patients, who should have a chance to fall into the control group when the new treatment may well be ineffective because of the inexperience of the person who is applying it. The control patient can always be removed from that group and placed in the experimental group if and when the new treatment seems to be superior to the old.

The second problem has to do with the obtaining of informed consent in therapeutic trials in life-threatening procedures. There can be no argument against the requirement that the investigating physician must obtain completely informed consent from patients taking part in trials which are done for the sake of research and from which they do not necessarily have more to gain than to lose. But I believe that the situation is somewhat different when randomization is carried out because the physician does not know which therapy is better for the individual patients. There are two potent arguments against informing patients with a life-threatening disease that the decision about whether or not he should have a life-threatening operation will be made by chance rather than by clinical judgement. (1) It is not in the best interest of the patients because it seems

likely that 9 out of 10 would refuse these studies, and therefore the operation, if so informed. If they were in their right senses, they would find a doctor who thought he knew which was the better treatment, or they would conclude that if the differences were so slight that such a trial had to be carried out, they would prefer to take their chances on no operation. Assuming that there is a 50 percent chance that the operation will prove to be effective, then half the patients who were scared out of the operation by having been asked for their informed consent, would have been mistreated. Furthermore, it is probable that a very sick patient needs to have complete confidence in the fact that his doctor has the knowledge to make the right decisions with regard to his care. In the course of a traumatic illness the loss of that confidence may do great harm to the patient. It is a rare patient who could be expected to be objective enough about his own serious illness to welcome the fact that his physician has enough knowledge to avoid decisions based on ignorance.

The second argument against informing patients that the decision to operate or not will be based on randomization lies in the fact that it is not customary in the ordinary practice of medicine to inform patients of all the details with regard to how decisions are made in their treatment. Few patients would be saved by established surgical procedures if the physician and surgeon had to recount in every detail the complications of the operation. The most vigorous advocates of portacaval shunt surgery would be able to do no more operations if they were required to explain to each patient that of the 50 reports in the literature the only controlled studies showed no effects, and all of the enthusiastic reports were totally uncontrolled. The physician must assume some responsibility for making decisions in the best interest of his patients.

Although in my opinion the physician may withhold information from the patient about the exact details of how decisions are made in a randomized study, he must inform the patient of the pros and cons of each therapeutic maneuver under consideration, and he must assure the patient that he will not carry out any therapy that he knows to be wrong. He must inform the patient that he is taking part in a study of a procedure that has not yet been established as efficacious. In other words, the patient should know that he is taking part in a research project and should be free to refuse to take part. And it should go without saying that all physicians concerned in a randomized study must be convinced that the knowledge necessary to make a decision [about] that patient is not available.

This brings me to the third problem, and to me the most serious one, that must be faced by the physician concerned with the ethics of controlled trials, namely how one makes the decision about when to stop the trial, when a decision should be made to treat all patients according to the apparent results of the trial. The biostatistician tells us that we must determine from the variability before we start the trial what a reasonable number of experiences would be, and that usually we should not stop until there is less than a 10 or 15 percent chance that we are missing a real difference, or less than a 5 percent chance that the difference we might have demonstrated is a true one and not one due to chance. This is entirely reasonable from the standpoint of the application of the conclusion to future patients. The conclusion can be reached either by the fixed sample technique with occasional peeking by a disinterested person, or by the sequential analysis technique. Either way one should be reasonably sure before stopping a study that the conclusion would be valid and not reversed by further experience. One owes this to the patients who were randomized into the less favorable treatment, if there is a difference.

But what about the rights of the patient who enters a study at a time when one treatment is leading the other, but when the study is being continued because the difference is not significant? One can easily argue that since the difference is not significant, the result can be reversed by further experience. But one can also argue that the welfare of that one patient is more assured if he receives the treatment that is ahead rather than the one that is currently behind in the evaluation. In other words, randomization could be unfair to him because he might be assigned to a treatment that has a less than 50 percent chance of being shown to be the correct one. This argument can then be reduced to the ridiculous by pointing out that the first patient in a study makes it more or less likely that one treatment will come out ahead. The situation is not analogous to the oft-quoted coin flipping rule that the results of previous flips do not influence the next one. In the case of the controlled trial the result of each comparison adds to the evidence for or against the superiority of one or the other treatment. To this problem I can see no solution, and I would appreciate consideration by this group of the argument that if one considers solely the welfare of the individual patient one can never do a controlled trial.

The fact that the investigator is also the patient's physician requires that he tell the subject of the investigation which treatment is ahead. In situations in which both the disease and the treatment are life-threatening, it is unlikely that the patient would consent to be assigned to the treatment that is less likely to prove effective

In summary, I should like to present you for discussion three conclusions: (1) In the gradual evolution of our knowledge with regard to the prevention and treatment of disease the controlled clinical trial is by far the most effective way of saving people from the misapplication of dangerous and ineffective treatments. (2) We now know how to design scientifically precise and reliable trials of all preventive and therapeutic maneuvers. (3) Currently there are serious ethical and legal barriers to the conduct of any but the most insignificant trials.

PAUL RAMSEY

Consent as a Canon of Loyalty

. . .

One need not read very far in medical ethics —and especially not in the literature concerning medical experimentation or the ethical "codes" that have been formulated since the medical cases at the Nuremberg trials—without realizing that medical ethics has not its sole basis in the overall benefits to be produced. It is not a consequence-ethics alone. It is not solely a teleological ethics, to use the language of philosophy. It is not even an ethics of the "greatest possible medical benefits for the greatest possible number" of people. That calculus too easily comes to mean the "greatest possible medical benefits regardless of the number" of patients who without their proper consent may be made the subjects of promising medical investigations. Medical ethics is not solely a benefit-producing ethics even in regard to the individual patient, since he should not always be helped without his will.

As stated in the *Ethical Guidelines for Organ Transplantation* of the American Medical Association,[1] so also of medical experimentation involving human subjects: "Man participates in these procedures: he is the patient in them; or he performs them. All mankind is the ultimate beneficiary of them." Observe that the respect in which man is the patient and man the performer of medical care or medical investigation (the relation between doctor and patient/subject) places an independent moral limit upon the fashion in which the rest of mankind can be made the ultimate beneficiary of these procedures. In the language of philosophy, a deontological dimension or test holds chief place in medical ethics, beside teleological considerations. That is to say, there must be a determination of the rightness or wrongness of the action and not only of the good to be obtained in medical care or from medical investigation.

A crucial element in answer to the question, What constitutes right action in medical practice? is the requirement of a reasonably free and adequately informed consent. In current medical ethics, this is a chief *canon of loyalty* (as I shall call it) between the man who is patient/subject and the man who performs medical investigational procedures. Physicians discuss the consent-requirement just as ethicists discuss fairness- or justice-claims: these tests must be satisfied along with the benefits (the "good") obtained.

. . .

THE ETHICS OF CONSENT

Hopefully while not exceeding an ethicist's putative competence or trespassing upon the competence of medical men, I wish to undertake an analysis of the consent-requirement itself. The principle of an informed consent is a statement of the fidelity between the man who performs medical procedures and the man on whom they are performed. Other aspects of medical ethics—for example, the requirement of a good experimental design and of professional skill at least as good as is customary in ordinary medical practice—treat the man as a purely passive subject or patient. These are also the requirements that hold for an ethical experiment upon animals. But any human being is more than a patient or experimental subject; he is a *personal* subject—every bit as

Reprinted with permission of the publisher from *The Patient as Person* (New Haven, Conn.: Yale University Press, 1970), pp. 2, 5, 6, 8–11.

much a man as the physician-investigator. Fidelity is between man and man in these procedures. Consent expresses or establishes this relationship, and the requirement of consent sustains it. Fidelity is the bond between consenting man and consenting man in these procedures. The principle of an informed consent is the cardinal *canon of loyalty* joining men together in medical practice and investigation. In this requirement, faithfulness among men—the faithfulness that is normative for all the covenants or moral bonds of life with life—gains specification for the primary relations peculiar to medical practice.

Consent as a canon of loyalty can best be exhibited by a paraphrase of Reinhold Niebuhr's celebrated defense of democracy on both positive and negative grounds: "Man's capacity for justice makes democracy possible; man's propensity to injustice makes democracy necessary."[2] Man's capacity to become joint adventurers in a common cause makes the consensual relation possible; man's propensity to overreach his joint adventurer even in a good cause makes consent necessary. In medical experimentation the common cause of the consensual relation is the advancement of medicine and benefit to others. In therapy and in diagnostic or therapeutic investigations, the common cause is some benefit to the patient himself; but this is still a joint venture in which patient and physician can say and ideally should both say, "I cure."

Therefore, I suggest that men's capacity to become joint adventurers in a common cause makes possible a consent to enter the relation of patient to physician or of subject to investigator. This means that *partnership* is a better term than *contract* in conceptualizing the relation between patient and physician or between subject and investigator. The fact that these pairs of people are joint adventurers is evident from the fact that consent is a continuing and a repeatable requirement. We can legitimately appeal to permissions presumably granted by or implied in the original contract only to the extent that these are not incompatible with the demands of an ongoing partnership sustained by an actual or implied *present* consent and terminable by any present or future dissent from it. For this to be at all a human enterprise—a covenantal relation between the man who performs these procedures and the man who is patient in them—the latter must make a reasonably free and an adequately informed consent. Ideally, he must be constantly engaged in doing so. This is basic to the cooperative enterprise in which he is one partner.

.   .   .

The foregoing paragraphs describe the basis of the requirement that experimentation involving human subjects should be undertaken only when an informed consent has been secured. There are enormous problems, of course, in knowing how to subsume cases under this moral regulation expressive of respect for the man who is the subject in medical investigations no less than in applying this same moral regulation expressive of the meaning of medical care. What is and what is not a mature and informed consent is a preciously subtle thing to determine. Then there are questions about how to apply this rule arising from those sorts of medical research in which the patient's knowing enough to give an informed consent may alter the findings sought; and there is debate about whether the use of prisoners or medical students in medical experimentation, or paying the participants, would not put them under too much duress for them to be said to consent freely even if fully informed. Despite these ambiguities, however, to obtain an understanding consent is a minimum obligation of a common enterprise and in a practice in which men are committed to men in definable respects. The *faithfulness*-claims which every man, simply by being a man, places upon the researcher are the morally relevant considerations. This is the ground of the consent-rule in medical practice, though obviously medical practice has also its consequence-features.

Indeed, precisely because there are unknown future benefits and precisely because the results of the experimentation may be believed to be so important as to be overriding, this rule governing medical experimentation upon human beings is needed to ensure that for the sake of those consequences no man shall be degraded and treated as a thing or as an animal in order that good may come of it. In this age of research medicine it is not only that medical benefits are attained by research but also that a man rises to the top in medicine by the success and significance of his research. The likelihood that a researcher would make a mistake in departing from a generally valuable rule of medical practice because he is biased toward the research benefits of permitting an "exception" is exceedingly great. In such a seriously important moral matter, this should be enough to rebut a policy of being open to future possible exceptions to this canon of medical ethics. On grounds of the faithfulness-claims alone, we must surely say that future experience will provide no morally significant exception to the requirement of an informed consent—although doubtless we may learn a great deal more about the meaning of this particular canon of loyalty, and how to apply it in new situations with greater sensitivity and refinement—or we may learn more and more how to practice violations of it.

Doubtless medical men will always be learning more and more about the specific meaning which the requirement of an informed consent has in practice. Or they could learn more and more how to violate or avoid this requirement. But they are not likely to learn that it more and more does not govern the ethical practice of medicine. It is, of course, impossible to demonstrate that there could be *no* exceptions to this requirement. But with regard to unforeseeable future possibilities or apparently unique situations that medicine may face, there is this rule-assuring, principle-strengthening, and practice-upholding rule to be added to the requirement of an informed consent. *In the grave moral matters of life and death, of maiming or curing, of the violation of persons or their bodily integrity, a physician or experimenter is more liable to make an error in moral judgment if he adopts a policy of holding himself open to the possibility that there may be significant, future permissions to ignore the principle of the consent than he is if he holds this requirement of an informed consent always relevant and applicable.* If so, he ought as a practical matter to regard the consent-principle as closed to further morally significant alteration or exception. In this way he braces himself to respect the personal subject while he treats him as patient or tries procedures on him as an experimental subject for the good of mankind.

The researcher knows that his judgment will generally be biased by the fact that he strongly desires one of the consequences (the rapid completion of his research for the good of mankind) which he could hope to attain by breaking or avoiding the requirement of an informed consent. This, too, should strengthen adherence in practice to the principle of consent. If every doer loves his deed more than it ought to be loved, so every researcher his research— and, of course, its promise of future benefits for mankind. The investigator should strive, as Aristotle suggested, to hit the mean of moral virtue or excellence by "leaning against" the excess or the defect to which he knows himself, individually or professionally, and mankind generally in a scientific age, to be especially inclined. To assume otherwise would be to assume an equally serene rationality on the part of men in all moral matters. It would be to assume that a man is as able to sustain good moral judgment and to make a proper choice with a strong interest in results obtainable by violating the requirement of an informed consent as he would be if he had no such interest.

Thus the principle of consent is a canon of loyalty expressive of the faithfulness-claims of persons in medical care and investigation. Let us grant that we cannot theoretically rule out the possibility that there can be exceptions to this requirement in the future. This, as least, is conceivable in extreme examples. It is not logically impossible. Still this is a rule of the highest human loyalty that ought not in practice to be held open to significant future revision. To say this concerning the there and then of some future moral judgment would mean here and now to weaken the protection of coadventurers from violation and self-violation in the common cause of medical care and the advancement of medical science. The material and spiritual pressures upon investigators in this age of research medicine, the collective bias in the direction of successful research, the propensities of the scientific mind toward the consequences alone are all good reasons—even if they are not all good moral reasons—for strengthening the requirement of an informed consent. This helps to protect coadventurers in the cause of medicine from harm and from harmfulness. This is the edification to be found in the thought that man's propensity to over-reach a joint adventurer even in a good cause makes consent necessary.

This negative aspect of the ethics of medical research is essential even if only because the constraints of the consent-requirement serve constantly to drive our minds back to the positive meaning or warrant for this principle in the man who is the patient and the man who performs these procedures. An informed consent alone exhibits and establishes medical practice and investigation as a voluntary association of free men in a common cause. The negative constraint of the consent-requirement serves its positive meaning. It directs our attention always upon the man who is the patient in all medical procedures and a partner in all investigations, and away from that celebrated "non-patient," the future of medical science. Thus consent lies at the heart of medical care as a joint adventure between patient and doctor. It lies at the heart of man's continuing search for cures to all man's diseases as a great human adventure that is carried forward jointly by the investigator and his subjects. Stripped of the requirement of a reasonably free and an adequately informed consent, experimentation and medicine itself would speedily become inhumane.

No one today would propose to eliminate the consent-requirement directly, but this can be done more subtly, or by indirection. Even while retaining it, the consent-requirement can be effectively annulled, or transformed into a disappearing, powerless guideline, simply by writing into it a "quantity-of-benefits-to-come"-exception clause. Thus we could make ourselves ready to override or avoid the consent-requirement in view of future good to be achieved. To do this is to make ourselves conditionally willing to use a subject in medical investigations as a mere means.

·   ·   ·

NOTES

1. Report of the Judicial Council, E. G. Shelley, M.D., Chairman, and approved by the House of Delegates of the American Medical Association, June 1968.

2. *The Children of Light and the Children of Darkness* (New York: Scribner's, 1949), p. xi.

FRANZ J. INGELFINGER

Informed (But Uneducated) Consent

The trouble with informed consent is that it is not educated consent. Let us assume that the experimental subject, whether a patient, a volunteer, or otherwise enlisted, is exposed to a completely honest array of factual detail. He is told of the medical uncertainty that exists and that must be resolved by research endeavors, of the time and discomfort involved, and of the tiny percentage risk of some serious consequences of the test procedure. He is also reassured of his rights and given a formal, quasilegal statement to read. No exculpatory language is used. With his written signature, the subject then caps the transaction, and whether he sees himself as a heroic martyr for the sake of mankind, or as a reluctant guinea pig dragooned for the benefit of science, or whether, perhaps, he is merely bewildered, he obviously has given his "informed consent." Because established routines have been scrupulously observed, the doctor, the lawyer, and the ethicist are content.

But the chances are remote that the subject really understands what he has consented to—in the sense that the responsible medical investigator understands the goals, nature, and hazards of his study. How can the layman comprehend the importance of his perhaps not receiving, as determined by the luck of the draw, the highly touted new treatment that his roommate will get? How can he appreciate the sensation of living for days with a multi-lumen intestinal tube passing through his mouth and pharynx? How can he interpret the information that an intravascular catheter and radiopaque dye injection have an 0.01 per cent probability of leading to a dangerous thrombosis or cardiac arrhythmia? It is moreover quite unlikely that any patient-subject can see himself accurately within the broad context of the situation, to weigh the inconveniences and hazards that he will have to undergo against the improvements that the research project may bring to the management of his disease in general and to his own case in particular. The difficulty that the public has in understanding information that is both medical and stressful is exemplified by [a] report [in the *New England Journal of Medicine*, August 31, 1972, page 433]—only half the families given genetic counseling grasped its impact.

Nor can the information given to the experimental subject be in any sense totally complete. It would be impractical and probably unethical for the investigator to present the nearly endless list of all possibile contingencies; in fact, he may not himself be aware of every untoward thing that might happen. Extensive detail, moreover, usually enhances the subject's confusion. Epstein and Lasagna showed that comprehension of medical information given to untutored subjects is inversely correlated with the elaborateness of the material presented.[1] The inconsiderate investigator, indeed, conceivably could exploit his authority and knowledge and extract "informed consent" by overwhelming the candidate-subject with information.

Ideally, the subject should give his consent freely, under no duress whatsoever. The facts are that some element of coercion is instrumental in any investigator-subject transaction. Volunteers for experiments will usually be influenced by hopes of obtaining better grades, earlier parole, more substantial egos, or just mundane cash. These pressures, however, are but fractional shadows of those enclosing the patient-subject. Incapacitated and hospitalized because of illness, frightened by strange and impersonal routines, and fearful for his health and perhaps life, he is far from exercising a free power of choice when the person to whom he anchors all his hopes asks,

Reprinted with permission from *The New England Journal of Medicine*, Vol. 287, No. 9, pp. 465–466, Aug. 31, 1972.

"Say, you wouldn't mind, would you, if you joined some of the other patients on this floor and helped us to carry out some very important research we are doing?" When "informed consent" is obtained, it is not the student, the destitute bum, or the prisoner to whom, by virtue of his condition, the thumb screws of coercion are most relentlessly applied; it is the most used and useful of all experimental subjects, the patient with disease.

When a man or woman agrees to act as an experimental subject, therefore, his or her consent is marked by neither adequate understanding nor total freedom of choice. The conditions of the agreement are a far cry from those visualized as ideal. Jonas would have the subject identify with the investigative endeavor so that he and the researcher would be seeking a common cause: "Ultimately, the appeal for volunteers should seek . . . free and generous endorsement, the appropriation of the research purpose into the person's [i.e., the subject's] own scheme of ends."[2] For Ramsey, "informed consent" should represent a "covenantal bond between consenting man and consenting man [that] makes them . . . joint adventurers in medical care and progress."[3] Clearly, to achieve motivations and attitudes of this lofty type, an educated and understanding, rather than merely informed, consent is necessary.

Although it is unlikely that the goals of Jonas and of Ramsey will ever be achieved, and that human research subjects will spontaneously volunteer rather than be "conscripted,"[2] efforts to promote educated consent are in order. In view of the current emphasis on involving "the community" in such activities as regional planning, operation of clinics, and assignment of priorities, the general public and its political leaders are showing an increased awareness and understanding of medical affairs. But the orientation of this public interest in medicine is chiefly socioeconomic. Little has been done to give the public a basic understanding of medi-

cal research and its requirements not only for the people's money but also for their participation. The public, to be sure, is being subjected to a bombardment of sensation-mongering news stories and books that feature "breakthroughs," or that reveal real or alleged exploitations—horror stories of Nazi-type experimentation on abused human minds and bodies. Muckraking is essential to expose malpractices, but unless accompanied by efforts to promote a broader appreciation of medical research and its methods, it merely compounds the difficulties for both the investigator and the subject when "informed consent" is solicited.

The procedure currently approved in the United States for enlisting human experimental subjects has one great virtue: patient-subjects are put on notice that their management is in part at least an experiment. The deceptions of the past are no longer tolerated. Beyond this accomplishment, however, the process of obtaining "informed consent," with all its regulations and conditions, is no more than elaborate ritual, a device that, when the subject is uneducated and uncomprehending, confers no more than the semblance of propriety on human experimentation. The subject's only real protection, the public as well as the medical profession must recognize, depends on the conscience and compassion of the investigator and his peers.

REFERENCES

1. Epstein, L. C., Lasagna, L.: "Obtaining informed consent: form or substance." *Arch Intern Med* 123:682–688, 1969.
2. Jonas, H: "Philosophical reflections on experimenting with human subjects." *Daedalus* 98:219–247, Spring, 1969.
3. Ramsey, P: "The ethics of a cottage industry in an age of community and research medicine." *N Engl J Med* 284:700–706, 1971.

CHARLES FRIED

Informed Consent and Medical Experimentation

GENERAL LEGAL PRINCIPLES APPLIED TO MEDICAL EXPERIMENTATION[1]

At the outset we must distinguish between therapeutic and non-therapeutic experimentation.[2] Experimentation is clearly non-therapeutic when it is carried out on a person solely to obtain information of use to others, and in no way to treat some illness that the experimental subject might have. Experimentation is therapeutic when a therapy is tried with the sole view of determining the best way of treating that patient. There is a sense, as a number of commentators have observed, in which so far as there is more or less uncertainty about the best way to proceed in the patient's case, treatment is often experimental.[3] Also what is learned in treating one patient will be of use in treating others. This may be so, but it in no way obscures the distinction between therapeutic and non-therapeutic research, since therapeutic research is carried out only and only so far as that subject's interests require. Any benefits to others are incidental to this dominant goal. These are clear cases at the extreme.

There are in practice large numbers of gradations in between. Much research is mainly therapeutic, in the sense that the patients' interests are foremost, but nevertheless things may be done which are not dictated solely by the need to treat that patient: tests may be continued even after all the information needed to determine the best treatment of the particular patient has already been completed; or substances may be injected for a period or in doses not strictly necessary for the cure of that patient, but with the motive of developing in-

formation of use to others.[4] Moving in from the clear case at the other extreme, that of non-therapeutic research, it must be recognized that persons who become research subjects in non-therapeutic experimentation may often be the beneficiaries of a degree of medical attention which they might not otherwise enjoy, and which thus redounds to their benefit.[5] And there are all possible degrees and gradations in between.

NON-THERAPEUTIC EXPERIMENTATION[6]

No special doctrines apply to non-therapeutic experimentation. Indeed, to the extent that the experimentation is non-therapeutic, the fact that it is being carried out by doctors should be entirely irrelevant. The usual privileges under which doctors work, and the usual special doctrines according to which the liabilities of doctors are judged should not be applicable, since they proceed from the premise that the doctor must be given considerable latitude as he works in the presumed interests of his patient. But that is not the case in non-therapeutic research. The doctor confronts his subject simply as a scientist.

In general, the law imposes a strict duty of disclosure, wherever an individual with a great deal to lose is exposed to a risk or is asked to relinquish rights by someone with considerably greater knowledge.[7] And this is true, whether the relation is one of buyer and seller or involves some public interest. Persons selling cosmetics,[8] automobiles[9] or pharmaceuticals[10] are required to make full disclosures of all the hazards involved in the products they sell. But policemen seeking damaging admissions from suspects are also required to issue a warning of constitutional rights and to offer legal assistance before those rights are waived.[11] There is no reason why the case should be any different where a researcher asks an experimental subject to risk his health.

Reprinted with permission of the publisher from *Medical Experimentation: Personal Integrity and Social Policy* (New York: American Elsevier Publishing Co., Inc., 1974), pp. 25–36.

Indeed the case might be made that the developing doctrines of strict liability would argue for the imposition of liability without fault, and regardless of disclosures for harm occasioned in the course of non-therapeutic experimentation.[12] In general, it is coming to be believed that those who are in a better position to appreciate the risks of a course of conduct, who are in a better position to insure against those risks or otherwise spread their cost to the broadest group of beneficiaries, and finally whose responsible decisions in evaluating the propriety of the risks we can influence by imposing upon them the costs of those decisions, should be strictly liable (that is liable without fault) for the risks that their conduct imposes.[13] These conditions are amply met in the case of non-therapeutic experimentation. Finally, if the financial pressures of caring for and compensating subjects injured in non-therapeutic experiments meant that experimenters exercised greater caution and carefully evaluated the benefits to be expected from the research, this would be a highly desirable consequence. It is for this reason that a number of commentators have suggested either strict liability for non-therapeutic experimentation or some form of compulsory medical experimentation insurance. In either case the experimental subject would be assured of proper medical care as well as compensatory payments for any injuries he suffers in the experiment. Since most subjects of non-therapeutic experimentation are either idealistic persons for whom the small amounts of compensation are not a significant inducement, or disadvantaged persons for whom the small compensation acts as an all too significant inducement, this added responsibility would seem fair and appropriate.

THERAPEUTIC EXPERIMENTATION

Legal decisions and commentators have always stated that a practitioner is only justified in using "accepted remedies," unless his patient specifically consents to the use of an "experimental" remedy.[14] This statement has seemed reactionary and unreasonable to doctors, but if one puts it in the context of general doctrine one might say that its teeth are quite effectively drawn. General principles require the consent of the patient to any therapy, usual or unusual. It is just that as the therapy moves away from the standard and the accepted, the need for explicit consent, full disclosure of risks and alternatives, becomes more acute, and more likely to pose an issue. The doctor who prescribes an accepted remedy, under the principles set forth so far, might have a good defense to the claim that he should have told his client about alternative, untried or experimental remedies.[15]

The obligation to advise the patient of alternative therapies does not extend to all the hypothetical, untried or experimental remedies that various researchers are in the process of developing. Where, however, the therapy used is itself experimental, then this fact and the existence of either alternatives or professional doubts become material facts, which like all material facts should be disclosed. Beyond this, where the experimentation is truly and exclusively therapeutic, there are no particular legal constraints that do not apply to the practice of medicine generally.[16] It is simply that the implication of those general doctrines may take on a special coloring in this context.

MIXED THERAPEUTIC AND NON-THERAPEUTIC RESEARCH: THE PROBLEM OF THE RANDOMIZED CLINICAL TRIAL

The kind of medical experimentation which causes the greatest legal and ethical perplexities is what might be called mixed therapeutic and non-therapeutic experimentation: The patient is indeed being treated for a particular illness, and a serious effort is being made to cure him. The systems of treatment, however, are not chosen solely with the view to curing the particular patient of his particular ills. Rather, the treatment takes place in the context of an experiment or a research program to test new procedures, or to compare the efficacy of various established procedures.[17] Nor is it the case that this research purpose is limited to carefully reporting the results of treatments in particular cases. Rather, therapies are tried, continued or varied, and patients are assigned to treatment categories partially in response to the needs of the research design, i.e. not exclusively by considering the particular patient's needs at the particular time. Usually it will be the case that there is genuine doubt about which is the best treatment, or the best treatment modality, so that the doctors participating in the experiment do not believe they are compromising the interests of their patients.[18] Or where this is not completely true, it is often the case that no serious nor irreversible harms or risk are imposed in pursuing the research design rather than pursuing singlemindedly the interests of the particular patient. The clearest case, and the one which is the focus of our concern in this essay, is the randomized clinical trial (RCT), in which patients are assigned to treatment categories by some randomizing device, with the thought that in this way any bias of the experimenter and any unsuspected interfering factor can be eliminated by the statistical method used.[19] And generally it is said that the alternative therapies between which patients are randomized both have a great deal to recommend them, so that there is no real sense in which one or the other group is being deliberately disadvantaged—at least until the results of the experiments are in.[20]

What is the legal status of experimentation having both therapeutic and non-therapeutic aspects? Since there is a general obligation to obtain consent to a therapy, and since that obligation becomes more exigent as the treatment to be used departs from the ordinary and the accepted, there is at least the legal obligation to obtain consent for the use of the treatment contemplated, with full disclosure of the expected benefits and hazards. This much is straightforward, and not peculiar to the area of mixed therapeutic and non-therapeutic experimentation and RCTs. Moreover, as we have seen, a number of courts have insisted that the disclosure made in obtaining consent include a disclosure of the existence and characteristics of alternative therapies.[21] Certainly if the therapy proposed is experimental in the sense of innovative, this fact along with some description of more traditional alternatives should be part of the disclosure.

The crucial question, and one as to which there is no decided case, asks whether it is also necessary to disclose first that an experiment is being conducted, and second and more delicately the nature of the experiment and the experimental design.

Specifically, in the case of the RCT must the doctor disclose the fact that the patient's therapy will be determined by a randomizing procedure rather than by an individualized judgement on the part of the physician? Some physicians active in mixed therapeutic and non-therapeutic experimentation have argued that it is both unnecessary and undesireable to make this last disclosure.[22] It is undesirable because some patients might be scared off, withdraw from the experiment and seek help elsewhere. It is also undesirable because of those patients who, while remaining in the experiment, might be caused such a degree of distress and anxiety that it would interfere with their cure. The disclosure of randomization is argued to be unnecessary since the medical evidence regarding the alternative treatments will often be evenly balanced (that is why the experiment is being conducted—to help resolve the doubts) so that it is in no way inaccurate to tell the patient that medical opinion is divided on the best therapy, and that the patient will receive the best available therapy according to current medical judgements. To tell the patient that he is being randomized, on this view, would add nothing of relevance regarding the expected outcome of his treatment, and thus nothing of relevance to his choice whether or not to consent to the treatment.

There are no authoritative decisions holding that consent in the absence of a disclosure that the patient is being randomized or that his treatment is being determined by reference to factors other than his individual concerns is invalid consent because of incomplete disclosure. The general principle holds that a person must be given all material information relating to the proposed therapy. But is the fact of randomization, or of the existence of an experiment such material information? The information would seem to deal rather with the way in which the therapy is chosen than with the characteristics of the therapy itself. Nevertheless, it would seem that most patients would consider the information regarding the choice mechanism as highly relevant,[23] and would feel that they had been "had" upon discovering that they had received or not received surgery because of a number in a random number table. But does this sentiment create a duty; does it mean, for instance, that consent to the treatment was ineffective and the participating doctors are guilty of a battery?

Though there is no authoritative decision to point to, there are analogies from other areas of law which would suggest that full candid disclosure should include disclosure of randomization. The very fact that the doctor acts in the dual capacity of therapist and researcher, and that his role as researcher to some degree does or may influence his decisions as a therapist, would argue that the fullest disclosure of all the circumstances relating to that dual role, and to the basis on which functions are exercised and decisions made would be required.[24] If the relation were not that of doctor and patient, but of lawyer and client,[25] or of trustee and beneficiary of a trust fund,[26] or of a director or officer of a corporation and the corporation,[27] there would be a strict duty to disclose the existence of any interest which the fiduciary has that may conflict with or influence the exercise of his functions in his fiduciary capacity. The fiduciary owes a duty of strict and unreserved loyalty to his client.[28]

Imagine the case of a lawyer for a public defender organization who has agreed to participate in a foundation sponsored research project on sentencing. As part of the research protocol his decision as to whether to plead certain categories of offenders guilty or to go to trial is determined at random. This is intended to discover how that decision affects the eventual outcome of the case at the time of sentencing and parole. His clients are not told that this is how the lawyer's "advice" as to plea is determined.[29]

The law of conflict of interests and of fiduciary relations clearly provides that the fiduciary may not pursue activities that either do in fact conflict with the exercise of his judgements as a fiduciary, or might conflict with or influence the exercise of his judgement, or

might appear to do so, without the explicit consent of his client.[30] And if the consent is obtained other than on the basis of the fullest disclosure of all facts not only which the fiduciary deems relevant but which he knows his client might consider relevant, the disclosure is incomplete, the consent is fraudulently obtained, and the fiduciary is in breach of his fiduciary relationship.[31] There is no reason why the doctor should not be held to be in a fiduciary relationship to his patient, and therefore why the same fiduciary obligations that obtain for a lawyer, a money manager, a corporation executive or director should not obtain for a doctor.[32]

However the issue of informing patients of the fact of randomization might be resolved, it would seem that there is a continuing duty on the part of the patient's physician to inform himself about the progress of the experiment and to inform his patient about any significant new information coming out of the experiment that might bear on the patient's choice to remain in the study or to seek other types of therapy.[33] This is an important issue in RCTs involving long term courses of treatment. If patients abandon one alternative on the basis of early, inconclusive results, no definitive conclusion can be drawn from the trial. Failure to make continuing disclosures and to offer continuing options to the patient in the light of developing information may not constitute the tort of battery, however, since there may be no physical contact requiring a new consent. The wrong which is done to the patient would be in the nature of negligent practice, and as to that the determinative standard is the standard of practice of a respected segment of the profession. The physician who does not keep his patient continuously informed may argue that to do so would interfere with the experiment, and he might find experts to testify that such continuing disclosure in the course of an experiment is not thought to be good practice.[34] The argument should not be accepted uncritically since the practice which the doctor in the case of an RCT would refer to would not be traditional therapeutic practice, but rather the practice of experimentation itself. Indeed it would seem that the doctrine of the case, holding that a physician had a duty to inform his patient that his broken leg was not healing properly and that there was another method of treatment available in a nearby city which was more likely to result in cure,[35] is equally applicable to the case of a participant in an RCT who has been assigned to a treatment category which, as the experiment progresses and the data comes in, appears to be the less successful treatment. Nor would the device, by which only a supervising committee and not the patient's physician has access to the results of the experiment for a determined period of time,[36] insulate the physician from the consequences of this doctrine.[37]

NOTES

1. See generally, J. Katz, *Experimentation with Human Beings* (1972); Berger, "Reflections on Law and Experimental Medicine," 15 *U.C.L.A. L. Rev.* 436 (1968); Freund, "Ethical Problems in Human Experimentation," 273 *N. Eng. J. Med.* 687 (1965), Hirsh, "The Medico-Legal Framework for Medical Research" in *New Dimensions in Legal and Ethical Concepts for Human Research,* 169 *Annals N. Y. Acad. Sci.* (1970) [hereinafter cited as *Annals*]; Jaffe, "Law as a System of Control," in 98 *Daedalus, Ethical Aspects of Experimentation with Human Subjects* (1969) [issue cited hereinafter as *Daedalus*]; Kaplan, "Experimentation—An Articulation of a New Myth," 46 *Neb. L. Rev.* 87 (1967); Note, 75 *Harv. L. Rev.* 1445 (1962); Note, 20 *Stan. L. Rev.* 99 (1967); Note, *Syr. L. Rev.* 1067 (1973).
2. See Halushka v. University of Saskatchewan, 53 D.L.R. 2d 436 (1965); Hyman v. Jewish Chronic Disease Hosp., 42 Misc. 2d 427, 248 N.Y.S. 2d 245 (Sup. Ct. 1964), rev'd per curiam, 21 App. Div. 2d 495, 251 N.Y.S. 2d 818, rev'd 15 N.Y. 2d 317, 206 N.E. 2d 338, 258 N.Y.S. 2d 397 (1965); USDHEW, *NIH, Institutional Guide to DHEW Policy on Protection of Human Subjects* (1971) [hereinafter cited as *NIH*]; Capron, "The Law of Genetic Therapy," in Katz, supra note 1, at 574; Grad, "Regulation of Clinical Research by the State," in *Annals;* "Symposium," 36 *Fordham L. Rev.* 673 (1968).
3. See Fortner v. Koch, 272 Mich. 273, 261 N.W. 762 (1835); Freund, "Legal Frameworks for Human Experimentation," in *Daedalus;* Grad, supra; Katz, supra.
4. See *NIH,* at 6.
5. This was argued in defense of the experiments in Hyman v. Jewish Chronic Disease Hospital discussed in Katz, supra, chapter 1.
6. See authorities cited supra note 1.

7. See generally, W. Prosser, *Torts* § 99 (4th ed., 1971); Calabresi, "Toward A Test for Strict Liability in Torts," 81 *Yale L. J.,* 1055 (1972).
8. Larsen v. General Motors Corp., 391 F. 2d 495 (8th Cir. 1968); Witt v. Chrysler Corp., 15 Mich. App. 576, 167 N.W. 2d 100 (1969), Blitzstein v. Ford Motor Co., 288 F. 2d 738 (5th Cir. 1961).
9. Crotty v. Shartenberg's-New Haven, Inc., 147 Conn. 460, 162 A. 2d 513 (1960) (hair remover); Reynolds v. Sun Ray Drug Company, 135 N.J.L. 475, 52 A. 2d 666 (Ct. Err. & App. 1947) (lipstick); Esborg v. Bailey Drug Co., 61 Wash. 2d 347, 378 P. 2d 298 (1963) (hair tint).
10. Martin v. Bengue, Inc., 25 N.J. 359, 136 A. 2d 626 (1957); Marcus v. Specific Pharmaceuticals, 82 N.Y.S. 2d 194 (N.Y. Sup. Ct. 1948); Halloran v. Parke, Davis & Co., 245 App. Div. 727, 280 N.Y.S. 58 (1935).
11. Miranda v. Arizona, 384 U.S. 436 (1966).
12. See Calabresi, "Reflections on Medical Experimentation" in *Daedalus;* Freund, in *Daedalus;* Havighurst, "Compensating Persons Injured in Human Experimentation" 169 *Science* 153 (1970); Note, "Medical Experimentation Insurance" 70 *Colum. L. Rev.* 965 (1970); cf. Ehrenzweig "Compulsory Hospital-Accident Insurance: A Needed First Step Toward the Displacement of Liability for Medical Malpractice" 31 *U. Chi. L. Rev.* 279 (1964); R. Keeton, "Compensation for Medical Accidents" 121 *U. Pa. L. Rev.* 590 (1973); Note, "Medical Malpractice Litigation: Some Suggested Improvements and a Possible Alternative" 18 *U. Fla. L. Rev.* 623 (1966).
13. Calabresi, *The Cost of Accidents: An Economic and Legal Analysis* (1970).
14. Slater v. Baker, 2 Wils. K.B. 359, 95 Eng. Rep. 860 (1767); Carpenter v. Blake, 60 Barb. N.Y. 488 (1871); Langford v. Kosterlitz, 107 Cal. App. 175, 290 P. 80 (1930); Comment, "Non-Therapeutic Research Involving Human Subjects," 24 *Syr. L. Rev.* 1067 (1973), at 1069–1071.
15. Fortner v. Koch, supra note 3; Curran, "Governmental Regulation of the Use of Human Subjects in Medical Research" in *Daedalus.*
16. There may come a point, of course, where the procedure is so risky, the benefits so uncertain, and the basis of the treatment so speculative that to use it even with consent is tantamount to unprofessional conduct and quackery. The vagueness of the boundary is, of course, a cause for disquiet for practitioners working with new therapies.
17. See authorities collected at Katz, supra note 1, at 376–79; A. L. Cochrane, *Effectiveness and Efficiency* (1972); Chalmers, "Controlled Studies in Clinical Cancer Research," 287 *N. Engl. J. Med.* 75 (July 13, 1972); Shaw and Chalmers, "Ethics in Cooperative Trials" in *Annals;* Veterans Administration Cooperative Study Group, "Effects of Treatment on Morbidity in Hypertension" 213 *J.A.M.A.* 1143 (1970); also reported in Freis et al., *Anti-Hypertensive Therapy–Principles and Practice* (F. Gross, ed. 1966).
18. Chalmers, "The Ethics of Randomization as a Decision Making Technique and the Problem of Informed Consent," in *USDHEW Report of the 14th Annual Conference of Cardiovascular Training Grant Program Directors, National Heart Inst.* (1967); Chalmers, supra; Shaw and Chalmers, supra; Cochrane, supra; Chalmers, "When Should Randomization Begin" *The Lancet* 858 (April 20, 1968); Moore, "Ethical Boundaries in Initial Clinical Trials" in *Daedalus;* Mather et al., "Acute Myocardial Infarction, Home and Hospital Treatment" *B. Med. J.* 334 (August 7. 1971); Rutstein, "The Ethical Design of Human Experimentation" in *Daedalus.*

19. See Chalmers and Cochrane, supra; and see generally *The Quantitative Analysis of Social Problems* (Tufte, ed. 1970); Campbell and Erlebacher, "Regression Artifacts in Quasi-Experimental Design" in *The Disadvantaged Child–Compensatory Education,* vol. 3 (1970).

20. Thus, for instance, in a major RCT of the efficacy of simple as compared to radical mastectomy for cancer of the breast, Sir John Bruce writes: "one of the important ethical necessities before a random clinical is undertaken is a near certainty that none of the treatment options is likely to be so much inferior that harm could accrue to those allocated to it. In the present instance . . . it looked as if the mode of primary treatment made no significant difference, at least in terms of survival." "Operable Cancer of the Breast—A Controlled Clinical Trial," 28 *Cancer* 1443 (1971).

21. See supra note 25 [in original text].

22. See Chalmers, "The Ethics of Randomization as a Decision Making Technique and the Problem of Informed Consent," supra note 18; Chalmers, discussion in *Annals,* at 513–16; Lasagna, "Drug Evaluation Problems in Academia and Other Contexts" in *Annals.*

23. Cf. Alexander, "Psychiatry—Methods and Processes for Investigation of Drugs," in *Annals;* Park et al., "Effects of Informed Consent in Research Patients and Study Results" 145 *J. Nerv. Ment. Dis.* 349 (1967), quoted in Katz, supra note 1, at 690.

24. Freund, supra note 3.

25. See American Bar Association, *Canons of Professional Ethics,* Canon 6, at 11 (1963). Canon 6 states clearly that the lawyer's duty, within the law is "solely" to his client, and should not be influenced by other interests or loyalties.

26. See *Scott on Trusts,* § 2.5, 39–43 (3d. ed. 1967).

27. See Geddes v. Anaconda Copper Co., 254 U.S. 590 (1920) (director); Bingham v. Ditzler, 309 Ill. App. 581, 33 N.E. 939 (1941) (officer).

28. See, e.g., Guth v. Loft, 23 D. Ch. 255, 5 A. 2d 503 (1939); In re Westhall's Estate, 125 N.J. Eq. 340, 5 A. 2d 757 (1939); People v. People's Trust Co., 180 App. Div. 494, 167 N.Y.S. 767 (1917).

29. Professor Paul Freund has suggested that it would be improper for a judge to randomize in sentencing. 273 *N. Engl. J. Med.* 657 (1965). Whatever the objection to this may be, it is quite different from the objections I raise in my hypothetical cases or in medical practice. The convicted criminal is not the client of the judge and the judge does not owe him an undivided duty of loyalty. Indeed it is his job to consider social interests in sentencing the individual, and the randomized experiment may be a way of doing this.

30. See, e.g., In re Schummer's Will, 206 N.Y.S. 113, 210 App. Div. 296 (1924); affirmed In re Schummer's Estate, 154 N.E. 600, 243 N.Y. 548 (1926); In re Westhall's Estate, 5 A. 2d 757, 125 N.J. Eq. 551 (1939); Bearse v. Styler, 34 N.E. 2d 672, 309 Mass. 288 (1941).

31. See, e.g., Goodwin v. Agassiz, 186 N.E. 659, 283 Mass. 358 (1933); Daily v. Superior Court, 4 Cal. App. 2d 127, 40 P. 2d 936 (1935); Christensen v. Christensen, 327 Ill. 448,158 N.E. 706 (1927).

32. Hammonds v. Aetna Cas. & Sur. Co., 237 F. Supp. 96 (N.D. Ohio 1965); motion denied, 243 F. Supp. 79 (1965); Stafford v. Schultz, 42 Cal. 2d 767, 270 P. 2d 1 (1954); Lockett v. Goodill, 71 Wash. 2d 654, 430 P. 2d 589 (1967).

33. See supra notes 45 and 46 [in original text] and accompanying text.

34. E.g., Chalmers, "Controlled Studies in Clinical Cancer Research," 287 *N. Engl. J. Med.* 75 (July 13, 1972); Shaw and Chalmers, "Ethics in Cooperative Trials," in *Annals;* cf. V. A. Cooperative Study Group, supra note 17.

35. Tvedt v. Haugen, 70 N.D. 338, 294 N.W. 183 (1940).

36. Chalmers, "Controlled Studies in Clinical Cancer Research" supra note 17.

37. The position I propose here is supported by Zeisel, "Reducing the Hazards of Human Experimentation through Modifications in Research Design," in *Annals.* See also Rutstein, "The Ethical Design of Human Experimentation" in *Daedalus.*

BERNARD BARBER

The Ethics of Experimentation with Human Subjects

The power, scope and funding of biomedical research have expanded enormously in the past 40 years. So also, inevitably, has clinical research with human subjects. That expansion has led in the past decade to widespread reflection on what is increasingly perceived as a new social problem: the abuse of human subjects of medical experimentation. In particular it is alleged that human subjects are not always protected from undue risk and do not always have the opportunity to voluntarily give their adequately informed consent to participation in experiments.

A social problem is defined in part by the concern it arouses, and this one has clearly aroused concern. Members of the medical profession itself led the way, with increasing numbers of journal articles, books and seminars on the issues. The public has become aroused, largely through popular accounts of dramatic incidents—genuine scandals in certain cases—involving the violation of the dignity and rights of patients. And the Federal Government has moved to protect human subjects, potential or actual. Beginning in 1966 the National Institutes of Health, the Food and Drug Administration and the Department of Health, Education, and Welfare have issued increasingly detailed regulations governing experimentation with human subjects in projects they support, which means in most of the biomedical research done in the country. In 1974 a National Commission for the Protection of Human Subjects of Biomedical and Behavioral

Reprinted with permission of the author and the publisher from *Scientific American*, Vol. 234, No. 2 (February 1976), pp. 25, 27–31. Copyright © 1976 by Scientific American, Inc. All rights reserved.

Research was established to advise the Department of Health, Education, and Welfare, and it is to be replaced by a long-term National Advisory Council that is to deal with the same issues.

The regulations, commissions and councils and the very fact of interference in medical activities by outsiders are viewed by many investigators as being onerous and even dangerous. On the other hand, many outsiders believe far more social control is required. The debate on the issue has been conducted without much reference to objective evidence. In 1970 our Research Group on Human Experimentation undertook two studies of investigators' attitudes and practices. On the basis of our results I would argue that there is indeed inadequate ethical concern among biomedical investigators, that it is reflected in excessively risky procedures and that better internal and external controls are essential.

. . .

Our national survey questionnaire was answered by 293 teaching and non-teaching hospitals and other research institutions that, our analysis showed, constituted a nationally representative sample of all such institutions. Those who filled out the questionnaire were generally themselves active researchers and members of their institution's review committee, set up to pass on research proposals. We asked the investigators to give us their response to six simulated proposals such as those that might come before a review committee. The proposals were detailed research protocols designed to measure the degree of the investigators' concern about informed consent and their willingness to approve of studies involving various levels of risk. We could be confident that the protocols were "hypothetical-actual" rather than "hypothetical-fantastic" because we constructed them with careful attention to the research literature, checked them with specialists and pretested them with a dozen chiefs of research at medical centers, who found them to be convincingly real.

One protocol described a study of chromosome breakage in users of hallucinogenic drugs; blood samples (for chromosomes) and urine samples (for evidence of drug use) were to be taken, at no risk but also without notification of the experimental purpose, from students routinely visiting the university health center. Another protocol proposed that the thymus gland, which is a component of the immune system, be removed unnecessarily from a random sample of children undergoing heart surgery; the objective was to learn the effect of the thymectomy on the survival of an experimental skin graft made at the same time. The other protocols dealt with a random test of alternative treatments for a congenital heart defect in children; with an evaluation of the efficacy of a new drug for severe depression (placebos were given to some patients); with a study of lung function in patients kept under unnecessarily prolonged anesthesia after undergoing a routine hernia repair, and with an investigation of the effect of radioactive calcium on bone metabolism in children. . . .

The answers to the thymectomy, anesthesia and radioactive-calcium protocols in particular gave us measures of the respondents' attitudes toward the balancing of risks and benefits. A clear pattern emerged. In the case of the high-risk thymectomy, for example, 72 percent of the respondents said the project should not be approved no matter how high the probability was that it would establish the efficacy of thymectomy in promoting transplant survival. On the other hand, 28 percent of the respondents said they would approve the experiment; 6 percent said they would approve it even if the chance of significant results was no better than one in 10. . . . Similarly, 54 percent were against doing the calcium study at all—but 14 percent said they would approve it even if the

odds were only one in 10 that it would lead to an important medical discovery. Our basic finding was that whereas the majority of the investigators were what we called "strict" with regard to balancing risks against benefits, a significant minority were "permissive," that is, they were much more willing to accept an unsatisfactory risk-benefit ratio.

The same general pattern of a strict majority and a permissive minority emerged from our second study, in which we interviewed 350 investigators actively engaged in research with human subjects. The investigators were at institutions to which we gave the synthetic names University Hospital and Research Center and Community and Teaching Hospital. The institutions were picked (by a technique known as cluster analysis) as being representative of two kinds of medical center that do considerable amounts of research. The interviewees told us about 424 different studies involving human subjects, and for each study they estimated the risk for subjects, the potential benefit for subjects, the potential benefit for future patients and the potential scientific importance of the study. It was reassuring to find that the investigators considered that only 56 percent of the clinical investigations graded for risk and benefits involved any risk for the subjects. We went on, however, to cross-tabulate the estimated risks and benefits . . . and we concluded that in 18 percent of the studies the risk was not adequately counterbalanced by the benefits. We called those studies the "less favorable" ones, and we proceeded to classify them further according to their potential benefits for other patients or for medical science. Even when these compensating justifications were taken into account, tabulation revealed a "least favorable" category of studies in which the poor immediate risk-benefit ratio was not compensated for by possible future benefits. These "least favorable" investigations constituted 8 percent of the investigations in our analysis.

The concept of informed consent is a troublesome one. The investigator wants to have enough subjects and is afraid of scaring them off. Patients are likely to be concerned about their own condition, may feel powerless with respect to the physician or hospital and often have difficulty understanding medical language or concepts. Even established medical procedures can have somewhat unpredictable consequences, so that physicians feel there is a limit to how completely "informed" a patient can be. The fact remains that regulations of Government funding agencies and most institutions now require that the human subject of an experiment (or his guardian, in the case of small children and mentally incompetent patients) understand that something is being done (or some treatment is being withheld) for reasons other than immediate therapeutic ones; the subject or guardian must be informed of any risks and must give consent voluntarily.

With regard to informed consent, our questionnaires and interviews again revealed a minority with "permissive" views and practices, although that minority was smaller than it was for unfavorable risk-benefit ratios. For example, 23 percent of the questionnaire respondents said they would approve the chromosome-break proposal, which presented the informed-consent issue clearly and in effect by itself. The situation was more complex in the heart-defect protocol. Here other dubious elements competed with the fact that the investigator would not inform the parents that his decision whether or not to operate would be a random one, not based on therapeutic considerations. Only 12 percent of our respondents said they would approve of the study without requiring any revisions, but only 65 percent specifically mentioned the lack of informed consent as a problem.

The best available research evidence on informed consent comes from a study conducted by Bradford H. Gray, who was then a graduate student at Yale University, at a distinguished university hospital and research center (not the one in our interview study). With the consent of the responsible investigator, Gray interviewed 51 women who were the subjects in a study of the effects of a new labor-inducing drug. Although the women had signed a con-

sent form, often in the hectic course of the admitting procedure or in the labor room itself, 20 of them (39 percent) learned only from Gray's interview, which was held after the drug infusion had been started or even after the delivery, that they were the subjects of research. Among those who did know, most of them did not understand at least one aspect of the study: that there might be hazards, that it was a double-blind experiment, that they would be subjected to special monitoring and test procedures or that they were not required to participate; four of the women said they would have refused to participate if they had known there was any choice. Many of the women had been referred for the study by their private physician, but instead of being informed that an experimental drug was to be administered they were told that it would be a "new" drug; they trusted their doctor and assumed that "new" meant "better."

How does it happen that the treatment of human subjects is sometimes less than ethical, even in some of the most respected university-hospital centers? We think the abuses can be traced to defects in the training of physicians and in the screening and monitoring of research by review committees, and also to a fundamental tension between investigation and therapy. We have data bearing on each of these causative factors.

It is in medical school that the profession's central and most serious concerns are presumably given time and place and that its basic knowledge and values are instilled. Yet the evidence from our interviews shows that there is not much training in research ethics in medical school. Of the more than 300 investigators who responded to questions in this area, only 13 percent reported they had been exposed in medical school to part of a course, a seminar or even a single lecture devoted to the ethical issues involved in experimentation with human subjects; only one respondent said he had taken an entire course dealing with the issues. Another 13 percent reported that the subject had come to their attention when, as students, they did practice procedures on one another; for 24 percent it was in the course of experiments with animals; 34 percent remembered discussion of ethical issues in specific research projects. One or more of these learning experiences were reported by 43 percent of the respondents—but the remaining 57 percent reported not a single such experience. The figures were about the same whether the investigators were graduates of elite U.S. medical schools, other U.S. schools or foreign schools. The figures were a little better, however, for those who had graduated since 1950 than for older investigators.

What little ethics training there is is apparently not very effective: the investigators who reported having learned something about research ethics were only slightly less permissive in response to protocols presenting the risk-benefit issue than those who reported no such experiences. It would appear that both the amount and the quality of medical-school training in the ethics of research could be improved. In this connection it is worth remembering that the many physicians who are not engaged in investigation at all also need some background in experimentation ethics, if only so they can evaluate requests that they direct their patients toward a colleague's research project.

Scientific "peer review" is a keystone of scientific inquiry, operating implicitly in many ways and explicitly in the case of professional journals, grant-awarding committees and many institutional reviewing boards such as the "tissue committees" that assess the results of surgery in hospitals. Ethical peer review of experimentation with human beings should be the counterpart of scientific peer review, but until the mid-1960's such activity received limited support among biomedical researchers. Even after 1966, when the NIH mandated ethical peer review for all its grantees, effective review did not become universal. Our questionnaire went to hospitals and other research centers that had filed with the NIH formal assurances that the required institutional review committee had been established, but 10 percent of the respondents said their institution's committee reviewed only proposals for outside funds and 5 percent reported that only formal proposals to the NIH were reviewed. The two institutions in our interview study were among the 85 percent that stated they were reviewing all re-

search proposals, and yet 8 percent of our interviewees volunteered the information that at least one of their own investigations with human subjects had not been reviewed.

How effective are the review committees in handling the protocols that do come before them? Our questionnaire respondents told us that in 34 percent of the institutions the committees had never required any revisions, rejected any proposals or had any proposals withdrawn in anticipation of rejection for ethical reasons; 31 percent reported revisions, 32 percent outright rejections and 19 percent withdrawals. Either some of these committees have very few ethical problems coming before them or they are ineffective. Gray's study in an institution with an active and strong committee suggests that they are ineffective rather than underworked. The committee whose performance he examined found relatively few proposals that did not need some kind of modification, and he thinks "a record of few actions by committees is an indication that their members are indifferent or that their standards are loose."

The peer-review groups seemed weak in other ways. In some institutions there was no face-to-face discussion among the reviewers. Only 22 percent of the committees had members from outside the institution, something that was then recommended and has since been mandated by the Department of Health, Education, and Welfare. In practically none of the institutions was there continuous monitoring of studies that were approved, although this was even then required by Government regulations. In general ethical peer review is hampered by the fact that each committee operates in isolation and must consider every new issue on its own and without benefit of precedent. A case-reporting system, such as operates in the law, would make that unnecessary and would promote both equity among institutions and high standards. The major weakness in the system is the lack of keen interest in and support of the review committees on the part of most working biomedical investigators. Research is their business; research is their mission and predominant interest, not applied ethics or active advocacy of patients' rights.

Most biomedical investigators are, however, interested in taking care of patients and making them well. As a result medical institutions and individual investigators operate today with two powerful sets of values and goals. On the one hand there is the pursuit and advancement of scientific knowledge. On the other there is the provision of humane and effective therapy for patients. Through a broad range of complex interactions these two sets of values and goals are harmonious, even complementary and mutually reinforcing. Occasionally, however, scientific research and humane therapy can be in conflict. When that happens, there is sometimes a tendency to choose the pursuit of knowledge at the expense of the ethical treatment of patients. An irreducible miminum of conflict may be inevitable. The ethical task now is to come as close as possible to that minimum—and to resolve unavoidable conflict in favor of humane therapy.

There is evidence that the enhanced excitement attending scientific achievement and the rewards bestowed on it in recent decades have skewed the decision-making process in many cases of conflict. As our data show, the medical schools have been largely indifferent to training their students in the ethics of research. Moreover, their record in peer review has been inferior to that of other institutions. Answers to our questionnaire showed they were less likely than other research centers to have set up a review committee before the NIH required one, less likely to have one that met the first NIH guidelines in 1966, less likely to have a committee that reviews all clinical research and less likely to include on their committee medical or nonmedical members from outside the institution. Medical schools, the Association of American Medical Colleges and professional associations of clinical investigators have been much quicker to seek research funds or to protest funding cuts than to organize seriously for the purpose of studying the ethics of research and making policy in that area.

The same emphasis on the pursuit of knowledge rather than on ethics is apparent among individual biomedical investigators. Ethical concern for the subjects of their research is not a major factor when they select their collaborators; at least it is not often mentioned as a characteristic they look for in collaborators. Scientific ability is a major concern. When we asked our 350 interview subjects, "What three characteristics do you most want to know about another researcher before entering into a collaborative relationship with him?" 86 percent of the respondents mentioned scientific ability, 45 percent mentioned motivation to work hard and 43 percent mentioned personality. Only 6 percent of them listed anything we could classify as "ethical concern for research subjects."

The tension between investigation and ethical concern is perhaps best illustrated by indications that the struggle for scientific priority and recognition exerts pressure on ethical considerations. Our data show that the social structure of competition and reward is one of the sources of permissive behavior in experimentation with human subjects; the relatively unsuccessful scientist, striving for recognition, was most likely to be permissive both in his approval of hypothetical protocols and in his own investigative work. We divided our respondents into four categories based on the number of papers they had published and the number of times their work had been cited by other workers; the frequency of citation has been shown to be a good measure of scientific excellence. We called the most-cited investigators the "high quality" scientists and those who had published a great deal but were never cited the "extreme mass-producer" scientists. It was the extreme mass-producers who were most often engaged in investigations with less favorable risk-benefit ratios, who approved of the protocols with poorer risk-benefit ratios and who least often expressed awareness of the importance of consent. Caught up in the socially structured competitive system of science, unsuccessful in it but still pursuing the prize of peer recognition, they appear to be more likely to overvalue scientific work as against humane therapy.

It is not only the mass-producers, contending for recognition among peers in their discipline, who are apt to be more permissive. We also weighed the rank achieved by each worker within his own institution against various measures of his effectiveness compared with that of his colleagues. We found that the "underrewarded" investigators tended to be the more permissive. There is also a quite different kind of medical investigator who we think is likely to be pushed toward permissive practices by scientific competition: some of the professionally esteemed, highly successful medical scientists who are engaged in intense competition for priority and recognition in well publicized areas of research. There are not many of those people, and they did not emerge in our sample, although some workers who refused to be interviewed may belong in that category. In the absence of real data we can only point to such evidence as published discussions concerning the worldwide heart-transplant competition of a few years ago, which raised questions about the premature exposure of human subjects to what were then still experimental procedures.

Given the fact that there are ethical defects in current medical-research standards and practices, do the resulting abuses strike particularly, as is often alleged, at certain social groups: at the poor, at children and at institutionalized patients (prisoners in particular)?

The evidence from our interviews with 350 investigators indicates that the poorer patients in hospitals are indeed at a disadvantage as subjects of research. For each of the 424 studies our respondents reported, they told us whether fewer than 50 percent, between 50 and 75 percent or more than 75 percent of the subjects were ward or clinic patients (as opposed to patients in private or semiprivate rooms and under the care of their own physician). We found first of all that ward and clinic patients were more likely to be subjects of experiments. Moreover, when we examined the cases we had previously identified as having "less favorable" and "least favorable" risk-benefit ratios, we found that both categories were almost twice as likely to involve subjects more than three-quarters of whom were ward and clinic

patients as the studies with the more favorable ratios were.

The ward and clinic patients are, of course, vulnerable to that kind of discrimination. They can most readily be channeled into an experimental group by admitting physicians and clerks without interference from a personal physician. They tend to be less knowledgeable about hospitals, more readily intimidated and less likely to understand what they are told about an experimental project, and therefore less likely to be able to withhold their consent or to give genuinely informed consent. In sum, they are the least likely to be able to protect themselves.

Many institutionalized patients are poor and perhaps incompetent, and they may feel completely dependent on the institution's administrators and physicians. Prisoners are a special case: they are institutionalized in an implicitly coercive situation, so that genuinely informed consent may be a logical impossibility. On the other hand, a prison population is by definition a good source of experimental and control subjects living under controllable conditions, and there have been instances where prison studies have been conducted humanely, with good scientific results and apparently with good effect on the prisoners' morale. Experimentation with prisoners is nevertheless subject to grave abuses. Last summer the head of the Food and Drug Administration told a Senate committee that a review of experimentation in 19 prisons revealed abuses ranging from unprofessional supervision of drug tests to inadequate medical care and follow-up treatment.

Children constitute still another special group. Small children cannot give consent for their own participation in experiments; older children, who could, are often not asked. As the Willowbrook incident demonstrated, parents are not always adequately protective of their children's interests. In the case of institutionalized patients, prisoners and children, new regulations of the Department of Health, Education, and Welfare call for special protective committees and procedures. These will only be effective, however, in a context of better ethical training for investigators and more effective peer review.

The ethical problems that attend medical research with human subjects are representative of an entire class of problems created by the impact of professionals and professional power on the general public and on public policy. In the area of research with human subjects the medical investigators are not alone; there is a tendency in other fields too for humane concerns to be left at the laboratory door. Psychologists and sociologists have often been accused of circumventing the requirement for consent and of applying unethical manipulative techniques in their investigations of human behavior, and neither profession has welcomed scrutiny from outsiders or restrictive regulation. The issue goes beyond research ethics, however. Many professions now command knowledge that has great potential usefulness for human welfare but bestows power that can be abused. Because professional power is largely based on knowledge that has not yet diffused to the general public it must to a considerable degree be self-regulated, but because professional power is of such major public consequence it must also be subject to significant public control. The medical-research profession does not have a proud record of self-regulation or acceptance of public controls.

SUGGESTED READINGS FOR CHAPTER 9

Books and Articles

American Psychological Association, Ad Hoc Committee on Ethical Standards in Psychological Research. *Ethical Principles in the Conduct of Research with Human Participants*. Washington, D.C.: American Psychological Association, 1973.

Barber, Bernard, *et al. Research on Human Subjects: Problems of Social Control in Medical Experimentation*. New York: Russell Sage Foundation, 1973.

Beecher, Henry K. *Research and the Individual: Human Studies*. Boston: Little, Brown, 1970.

Blackstone, William T. "The American Psychological Association Code of Ethics for Research Involving Human Participants: An Appraisal." *Southern Journal of Philosophy* 13 (Winter, 1975), 407–418.

Byar, David P. "Randomized Clinical Trials: Perspectives on Some Recent Ideas." *New England Journal of Medicine* 295 (July 8, 1976), 74–80.

Capron, Alexander M. "Informed Consent in Catastrophic Disease Research and Treatment." *University of Pennsylvania Law Review* 123 (December, 1974), 340–438.

Childress, James F. "Compensating Injured Research Subjects: I. The Moral Argument." *Hastings Center Report* 6 (December, 1976), 21–27.

Fost, Norman C. "A Surrogate System for Informed Consent." *Journal of the American Medical Association* 233 (August 18, 1975), 800–803.

Freund, Paul, ed. *Experimentation with Human Subjects*. New York: George Braziller, 1970.

Fried, Charles. *Medical Experimentation: Personal Integrity and Social Policy*. New York: American Elsevier, 1974.

Gray, Bradford H. *Human Subjects in Medical Experimentation*. New York: John Wiley, 1975.

Hershey, Nathan, and Miller, Robert D. *Human Experimentation and the Law*. Germantown, Md.: Aspen Systems, 1976.

Katz, Jay, with Capron, Alexander Morgan, and Glass, Eleanor Swift. *Experimentation with Human Beings*. New York: Russell Sage Foundation, 1972.

Rivlin, Alice M., and Timpane, P. Michael, eds. *Ethical and Legal Issues of Social Experimentation*. Washington, D.C.: Brookings Institution, 1975.

Robertson, John A. "Compensating Injured Research Subjects: II. The Law." *Hastings Center Report* 6 (December, 1976), 29–31.

U.S., Department of Health, Education, and Welfare. "Protection of Human Subjects." *Federal Register* 39 (May 30, 1974), 18914–18920.

Walters, LeRoy. "Some Ethical Issues in Research Involving Human Subjects." *Perspectives in Biology and Medicine* 20 (Winter, 1977), 193–211.

Bibliographies

Sollitto, Sharmon, and Veatch, Robert M., comps. *Bibliography of Society, Ethics and the Life Sciences*. Hastings-on-Hudson, N.Y.: Institute of Society, Ethics and the Life Sciences. Updated periodically. See under "Experimentation and Consent."

Walters, LeRoy, ed. *Bibliography of Bioethics*. Vols. 1– . Detroit: Gale Research Company. Issued annually. See under "Behavioral Research," "Biomedical Research," "Clinical Investigators," and "Human Experimentation."

10.
Experimentation with Specific Subject Groups

Ethical guidelines for human experimentation generally presuppose that the subjects who take part in research are adults who have normal mental capacities and who are not pregnant, not seriously ill, not institutionalized, and not in desperate need of money. Special subject groups who differ in one or more respects from this "normal adult human subject" model include the mentally retarded, the mentally ill, the poor, the critically ill, the dying, the comatose, pregnant women, fetuses, children, and institutionalized persons. In this chapter we examine the ethical issues raised by research involving three of these special subject groups: children, fetuses, and prisoners.

EXPERIMENTATION WITH CHILDREN

The term "child" (or "minor") is frequently applied to humans of widely divergent ages, from one-day-old infants to adolescents on the verge of attaining legal majority. The documents selected for inclusion in this chapter presuppose that the term refers to biologically human beings who either lack completely the capacity to consent (e.g., newborn infants) or who because of their early stage of intellectual development possess only limited capacities of understanding and consent (e.g., five-year-olds). Intellectually speaking, the later stages of childhood gradually shade into adulthood; thus, the ethical issues raised by research involving older groups of children gradually become less similar to those raised by research involving young children and begin to resemble more closely the issues raised by research involving adults.

The general justification for including children in biomedical research is that, physiologically speaking, children are not merely "little adults." For example, many drugs produce totally different effects in adults and children, or even in newborn infants and two-year-olds. Unless carefully controlled studies of pediatric reactions to such drugs are performed, children are likely to receive either ineffective or highly toxic doses of the drugs. Proponents of research on children also emphasize the need for additional data concerning the normal development of children—for instance, data concerning resistance to disease, nutritional needs, and body size and weight.

Therapeutic research, that is, research performed primarily for the benefit of a particular child, is generally thought to raise fewer ethical and legal difficulties than nontherapeutic research. Parents are legally empowered to give proxy consent for pediatric treatment. Since therapeutic research is closely akin to therapy, it is frequently assumed that parents are also authorized to consent to their children's participation in therapeutic research. (This assumption is questioned by some commentators, since therapeutic research, in contrast to therapy, is not directed *solely* to the benefit of patients.)

Should parents also be permitted to give consent for the participation of their children in *nontherapeutic* research? Answers to this question differ. Paul Ramsey adopts the most stringent position on nontherapeutic pediatric research. His argument can be summarized as follows:

1. No nontherapeutic research should be performed without the informed consent of the research subject.

2. Young children are incapable of giving informed consent.

3. Therefore, no nontherapeutic research involving young children should be performed.

A second and somewhat less restrictive position is proposed by Richard McCormick. McCormick suggests that in some cases the risks of nontherapeutic pediatric research may be minimal, while the potential benefits of the research to children as a class may be very great. To this consideration McCormick adds a second, which is premised on the social nature of human beings. In his view, all members of society are mutually interdependent and therefore owe to each other the performance of certain minimal moral duties. Among these duties is the obligation to take part in minimally risky nontherapeutic research which promises great benefit to the society as a whole. Since children, too, are members of the society, they stand under a similar obligation, although they may be too young to recognize the fact. Because children, like adults, *ought to* want to promote the social good, it is in McCormick's view morally legitimate for their parents to consent for them to do so. By implication, then, it is permissible for parents to provide proxy consent for their children's participation in minimally risky nontherapeutic research.

Alexander Capron seeks to develop appropriate public policy guidelines for one type of pediatric research, the clinical testing of drugs. Without committing himself to any particular view on the moral permissibility of nontherapeutic research involving children, Capron explores a series of mechanisms for minimizing the risks of pediatric research and for allocating such risks in an equitable manner.

EXPERIMENTATION WITH HUMAN FETUSES

The definition of the word "fetus" is somewhat less controversial than the definition of "child." With some oversimplification a fetus can be defined as a biologically human organism *in utero* from the moment of fertilization to the time of physical separation from the mother, or a human organism outside the uterus from the moment of fertilization to the time of clear viability. (For a detailed discussion of the major stages in fetal growth see the essay by André Hellegers in Chapter 5.)

From the standpoint of anatomical and physiological development, fetuses are not simply "little children." This difference provides the biomedical basis for a general moral justification of fetal research. Proponents of research involving fetuses argue that new intrauterine diagnostic procedures and therapies cannot be developed apart from such research. In addition, advocates of fetal research note that many therapies are employed to meet the health needs of pregnant women without clear knowledge of their effects on fetal health and development. Carefully controlled studies could help to elucidate the effects of alternative therapies.

In ethical analyses of fetal research a distinction is frequently drawn between two classes of live fetuses: (1) fetuses scheduled to go to term and be born, which will be called "term fetuses" and (2) fetuses either scheduled to be aborted or already aborted, which will be called "abortion fetuses."[1] From an ethical standpoint, term fetuses are virtually equivalent to "little children." The parent or parents anticipate

---

1. These categories were first employed by Hans O. Tiefel, "The Cost of Fetal Research: Ethical Considerations," *New England Journal of Medicine* 294 (January 8, 1976), 85–90.

that the fetus will be born and will develop through childhood to adulthood. The major differences between a child and a term fetus are differences in age, visibility, and degree of physical dependence on a particular person. Thus, the ethical and legal analyses of Ramsey, McCormick, and Capron concerning pediatric research can without difficulty be applied to research involving term fetuses.

Research which involves abortion fetuses raises some additional ethical issues. One of these issues is the problem of *consent*. In the case of term fetuses one can speak of parental proxy consent in an extended sense, since the parents (or parent) generally intend to raise the child and to assume legal responsibility for it. The parental relationship to abortion fetuses differs due to the fact that the parents (or parent) do not anticipate bearing long-term responsibility for the welfare of the fetus or child. On some views of fetal status, the question then arises, "In what sense, if any, can the biological parent(s) of an abortion fetus give proxy consent on behalf of the fetus?" A second type of consent issue arises in cases in which a woman (or both parents) consents to a fetal research procedure in anticipation of abortion. The difficult question in such cases concerns the woman's freedom to change her decision about abortion subsequent to the performance of the research, particularly if the research procedure may have done irreparable harm to the fetus.

The consent issue, in turn, is based on the more fundamental questions of the *status of the fetus* and of one's *moral obligations to the fetus*. These questions were discussed at length in the introduction and readings of Chapter 5 on abortion. In the present chapter Richard Wasserstrom presents four alternative views of fetal status and opts for the view that the fetus represents a "distinctive, relatively unique" category of being. LeRoy Walters, on the other hand, emphasizes the biological continuities between late fetal and early pediatric development.

On the question of our moral obligations toward abortion fetuses, there is also significant disagreement among the authors represented in this chapter. Willard Gaylin and Marc Lappé argue that certain types of research on the fetus *in utero* prior to abortion are morally justified because the research protects term fetuses from possible harm and because the research procedures do far less damage to the fetus than the abortion procedure itself. Wasserstrom raises several ethical objections to research on the fetus in utero but finds research on the nonviable fetus outside the uterus to be ethically acceptable. A third position is advocated by Walters, who proposes a formal-equality principle: in the research context, abortion fetuses and term fetuses should receive equal treatment.

EXPERIMENTATION WITH PRISONERS

It is obvious that prisoners as a group do not differ physiologically from other adults. Thus, the moral justification for research involving prisoners includes no reference to the unique biological properties of this subject group. Nor is there any inherent difference between prisoners and other adults in the capacity to comprehend an explanation of proposed research—the "information" component of informed consent. Rather, the debate concerning prisoner research focuses on the issues of personal and social benefit, justice, and freedom.

Proponents of research involving prisoners argue that such research is highly beneficial both to the research subjects and to society. Some investigators have noted that the experience of participation in research improves the self-image of many prisoner-participants. At the same time, prisoner involvement in various types of nontherapeutic research, for example, the early phases of drug testing, makes a major contribution to the welfare of society. Other advocates of research involving prisoners base their case on deontological arguments concerning freedom and justice. In their view, every adult human being should have a right to determine whether or not he or she will participate in biomedical research. To accord this right to all other social groups but not to prisoners would be to discriminate unjustly against this group. Frank Ayd's essay advances several of the arguments outlined above.

Opponents of prisoner involvement in research frequently concede the social benefit argument. However, they point to past abuses of prisoners in research as evidence that the alleged benefits of research to the subjects have on occasion been mixed with considerable harm. In addition, critics of prison research advance their own arguments based on justice and freedom. It is unjust, they assert, for society to ask prisoners to bear the present disproportionate share of research risks, particularly the risks of nontherapeutic research. As for freedom, opponents of prison research argue that the prison context is coercive—either inherently or as presently constituted—and that voluntary consent by prisoners to participation in research is therefore impossible. (In Chapter 11 Hugo Bedau makes a similar point regarding behavior control in punitive contexts.) The essay by Alexander Capron advances several of these antiresearch arguments and proposes new mechanisms for the social control of research involving prisoners.

L. W.

PAUL RAMSEY

Consent As a Canon of Loyalty with Special Reference to Children in Medical Investigation

From consent as a canon of loyalty in medical practice it follows that children, who cannot give a mature and informed consent, or adult incompetents, should not be made the subjects of medical experimentation unless, other remedies having failed to relieve their grave illness, it is reasonable to believe that the administration of a drug as yet untested or insufficiently tested on human beings, or the performance of an untried operation, may further *the patient's own recovery*.

Now that is not a very elaborate moral rule governing medical practice in the matter of experiments involving children or incompetents as human subjects. It is a good example of the general claims of childhood specified for application in medical care and research. It is also a qualification immediately entailed by the meaning of consent in medical investigations as a joint undertaking between men. Again, one has to be prudent (which does not mean overcautious or scrupulous) in order to know how to care for child-patients in this way. One must know the possible relation of a proposed procedure to the child's own recovery, and also its likely effectiveness compared with other methods that have been or could be tried. These considerations may provide the doctor with necessary and sufficient reason for investigations upon children, perhaps even very hazardous ones. One has to proportion the peril to the diagnostic or therapeutic needs of the child.

Practical medical judgment has undeniable and ominous room for its determinations, since

a "benefit" is whatever is *believed* to be of help to the child. Still the limits this rule imposes on practice are essentially clear; where there is no possible relation to the child's recovery, a child is not to be made a mere object in medical experimentation for the sake of good to come. The likelihood of benefits that could flow from the experiment for many other children is an equally insufficient warrant for child experimentation. The individual child is to be tended in illness or in dying, since he himself is not able to donate his illness or his dying to be studied and worked upon solely for the advancement of medicine. Again, future experience may tell us more about the meaning of this particular rule expressive of loyalty to a human child, and we may learn a great deal more about how to apply it in new situations with greater sensitivity and refinement—or we may learn more and more how to practice violations of it. But we are committed to refraining from morally significant exceptions to this rule defining impermissible medical experimentation upon children.

To experiment on children in ways that are not related to them as patients is already a sanitized form of barbarism; it already removes them from view and pays no attention to the faithfulness-claims which a child, simply by being a normal or a sick or dying child, places upon us and upon medical care. We should expect no morally significant exceptions to this canon of faithfulness to the child. To expect future justifiable exceptions is, in some sense, already to have forgotten the child.

To the layman, the most startling chapters in Dr. M. H. Pappworth's rather too sensational

Reprinted with permission of the publisher from *The Patient as Person* (New Haven, Conn.: Yale University Press, 1970), pp. 11–17.

volume *Human Guinea Pigs*[1] are those in which he catalogues case after case of catheterization, percutaneous biopsy, and other hazardous experiments performed upon children, or upon women and their unborn children, *having no relation to their treatment.* Experts have estimated that catheterization of the right heart causes about one death per one thousand cases; of the left heart, five deaths per one thousand cases; and that the death rate in liver biopsy is from one to three per one thousand.[2] Moreover, a study of 55 deaths from heart catheterization has shown that there is "a close relation between the mortality rate and the patient's age." Deaths from this procedure result with greatest frequency in the first two months of life.[3] A parent is competent to consent for his child, and morally may venture to consent for his child to be subjected to these hazards, if the child is afflicted by a malady that is equally or more dangerous to him and to which the investigational procedure is definitely related. The diagnostic procedure may in fact prove to be of no benefit in the child's own treatment. But no parent is morally competent to consent that his child shall be submitted to hazardous or other experiments having no diagnostic or therapeutic significance for the child himself.

Pappworth's book has been criticized for, among other things, drawing the worst conclusion from the fact that articles in medical journals reporting an experiment often fail to state that consent was obtained or how it was obtained. This may be a valid objection, especially since an indication that a piece of research was funded by the National Institutes of Health now means that a "peer" research committee in the medical center where the experimentation was conducted certified that consent would be obtained. But mention or failure to mention that consent was obtained is surely not the point. Nor is the point merely that, upon reading some of these cases of experiments, even hazardous ones, brought upon children with no relation to their own possible treatment, one has great difficulty understanding how any parent psychologically *could* consent to the procedure. The point is rather

that morally no parent *should* consent—or be asked to consent to any such thing even if he is quite capable of doing so, and even if in fact his informed consent was obtained in all cases where this fact is not mentioned in the reports.

To attempt to consent for a child to be made an experimental subject is to treat a child as not a child. It is to treat him as if he were an adult person who has consented to become a joint adventurer in the common cause of medical research. If the grounds for this are alleged to be the presumptive or implied consent of the child, that must simply be characterized as a violent and a false presumption. Nontherapeutic, nondiagnostic experimentation involving human subjects must be based on true consent if it is to proceed as a human enterprise. No child or adult incompetent can choose to become a participating member of medical undertakings, and no one else on earth should decide to subject these people to investigations having no relation to their own treatment. That is a canon of loyalty to them. This they claim of us simply by being a human child or incompetent. When he is grown, the child may put away childish things and become a true volunteer. This is the meaning of being a volunteer: that a man enter and establish a consensual relation in some joint venture for medical progress—where before he could not, nor could anyone else, "volunteer" him for submission to unknown possible hazards for the sake of good to come.

If the requirement of parents, investigators, and state authorities in regard to their wards is "Never subject children to the unknown possible hazards of medical investigations having no relation to their own treatment," we must understand that the maladies for which the individual needs treatment and protection need not already be resident within the compass of the child's own skin. He can properly be regarded as one of a population, and we can add to the foregoing words: "except in epidemic conditions." Dr. Salk tried his polio vaccine on himself and his own children first. Then it was tested on selected children within a normal population. This involved some risk for the children vaccinated, and for other children as well, that the disease *might* be contracted from the vaccine itself, or that there might be unexpected injurious results. But the normal population of children was already subjected to waves of crippling epidemic summer after summer. A parent consenting for his child to be used in this trial was balancing the risks from the trial against the hazards from polio itself for that same child.

Physician-investigators are often in a quandary in which they are torn between the warrants for giving an experimental drug, and the warrants for withholding it from anyone in order to test it. Neither act seems justified, or both acts are equally warranted, when there is no available remedy and the indications are that a new drug may succeed. This situation also justifies a parent or guardian in consenting for a child, since we are supposing the hazard of the proposed treatment to be less or no greater than the hazard of the disease itself when treated by the established procedures. That would be a medical trial having clear relation to the treatment or protection of the child himself. He is not made, without his consent, the subject of medical investigations of possible benefit only to other children, other patients, or for the future advancement of medical science.

These may have been the circumstances surrounding the field trial of the vaccine for rubella (German measles) made in Taiwan, if this was in epidemic conditions, or in expectation of epidemic conditions, early in 1968 by a medical team from the University of Washington, headed by Dr. Thomas Grayston.[4] The vaccine was given to 3,269 young grade-school boys in the cities of Taipei and Taichung, while roughly an equal number were left unvaccinated for comparison purposes. The latter group were given Salk polio vaccine so that they would derive some benefit from the experience to which they were subjected. This generous "payment" does not alter the moral dilemma of withholding the rubella vaccine from a selected group. Yet there may have been an equipoise between the hazards of contracting rubella or other damage from the vaccine and the hazards of contracting it if not vaccinated. There could have been a likelihood favoring the vaccinated of the two comparison groups.

These considerations, we may suppose, produced the quandary in the conscience of the investigators that was partially relieved by giving the unrelated Salk vaccine to the control group. Such equipose alone would warrant—and it would sufficiently warrant—a parent or guardian in consenting that his child or ward be used for these research purposes. In the face of actual or predictable epidemic conditions, this would be medical investigation having some measurable or immeasurable relation to a child's own treatment or protection, as surely as the catheterization of the heart of a child with congenital heart trouble may be needed in his own diagnosis and treatment; and to this type of treatment a parent may venture to consent in his child's behalf. If no gulf is to be fixed between maladies beneath the skin and diseases afflicting children as members of a population, then the consent-requirement means: "Never submit children to medical investigation not related to their own treatment, except in face of epidemic conditions, endangering also each individual child." This is simply the meaning of the consent-requirement in application, not a "quantity-of-benefit-to-come" exception clause or a violation of this canon of loyalty to child-patients.

Indeed, a stricter construction of the necessary connection between proxy consent and the foreseeable needs of the child would permit the use of only girl children in field trials of rubella vaccine. Rubella is not the most contagious type of measles. The benefit to the subjects used in these trials (which plus the consent of parents legitimated subjecting them to experiment) was mainly to prevent their giving birth to children with congenital malformations should they later contract rubella during pregnancy. Therefore, there was stronger argument for considering only girl children as part of a population in establishing the necessary connection between experiment and "treatment."

More questionable were the earlier trials of the rubella vaccine performed upon the inmates of a retarded children's home in Conway, Arkansas. These subjects were not specially endangered by an epidemic of rubella. Few of the girls among them will ever be able to become part of the population of child-bearing women, or be in danger of pregnancy while in institutions. Using them simply had the advantage that they were segregated from the rest of the population, and any degree of risk to them would not spread to other people, including women of child-bearing age.

If children are incapable of truly consenting to experiments having unknown hazards for the sake of good to come, and if no one else should consent for them in cases unrelated to their own treatment, then medical research and society in general must choose a perhaps more difficult course of action to gain the benefits we seek from medical investigations. Surely it was possible to secure normal adult volunteers to consent to segregate themselves from the rest of the population for the duration of a rubella trial.[5] That method was simply more costly and inconvenient. At the same time, this illustrates the general fact that if we as a society are to proceed to the conquest of diseases, indeed, if we are to teach medical skills with fairness and justice to the poor and the ward patients, and

with no violation of the basic claims of childhood, then there must be far greater encouragement generally in our society of a willingness to engage as joint adventurers for medical progress than has been achieved, or believed morally required by the principle of consent, in the past.

NOTES

1. Boston: Beacon, 1968.
2. Henry K. Beecher, "Medical Research and the Individual," in Daniel H. Labby (ed.), *Life or Death: Ethics and Options* (Seattle: University of Washington Press, 1968), p. 148.
3. Eugene Braunwald, "Deaths Related to Cardiac Catheterization," *Circulation,* Supplement III to vols. 27 and 28 (May 1968), pp. 17–26.
4. *New York Times,* October 17, 1968.
5. *New York Times,* April 5, 1969, reported that a hundred monks and nuns, from both Anglican and Roman Catholic orders, living in enclosed communities, were the voluntary subjects in testing American, British, and Belgian vaccines against German measles. This project was organized and directed by Dr. J. A. Dudgeon of London's Great Ormond Street Hospital for Sick Children.

RICHARD A. McCORMICK

Proxy Consent in the Experimentation Situation

It is widely admitted within the research community that if there is to be continuing and proportionate progress in pediatric medicine, experimentation is utterly essential. This conviction rests on two closely interrelated facts. First, as Alexander Capron has pointed out [1], "Children cannot be regarded simply as 'little people' pharmacologically. Their metabolism, enzymatic and excretory systems, skeletal de-

Reprinted with permission of the author and the publisher from *Perspectives in Biology and Medicine,* Vol. 18, No. 1 (Autumn 1974), pp. 2–20. Copyright 1974 by The University of Chicago Press.

velopment and so forth differ so markedly from adults' that drug tests for the latter provide inadequate information about dosage, efficacy, toxicity, side effects, and contraindications for children." Second, and consequently, there is a limit to the usefulness of prior experimentation with animals and adults. At some point or other experimentation with children becomes necessary.

LEGAL CONSIDERATION

At this point, however, a severe problem arises. The legal and moral legitimacy of experimentation (understood here as procedures involving no direct benefit to the person participating in the experiment) is founded above all on the informed consent of the subject. But in many instances, the young subject is either legally or factually incapable of consent. Furthermore, it is argued, the parents are neither legally nor morally capable of supplying this consent for the child. As Dr. Donald T. Chalkley of the National Institutes of Health puts it: "A parent has no legal right to give consent for the involvement of his child in an activity not for the benefit of that child. No legal guardian, no person standing *in loco parentis,* has that right"[2]. It would seem to follow that infants and some minors are simply out of bounds where clinical research is concerned. Indeed, this conclusion has been explicitly drawn by the well-known ethician Paul Ramsey. He notes: "If children are incapable of truly consenting to experiments having unknown hazards for the sake of good to come, and if no one else should consent for them in cases unrelated to their own treatment, then medical research and society in general must choose a perhaps more difficult course of action to gain the benefits we seek from medical investigations" [3, p. 17].

Does the consent requirement taken seriously exclude all experiments on children? If it does, then children themselves will be the ultimate sufferers. If it does not, what is the moral justification for the experimental procedures? The problem is serious, for, as Ramsey notes, an investigation involving children as subjects is "a prismatic case in which to tell whether we mean to take seriously the consent-requirement" [3, p. 28].

Before concluding with Shirkey that those incompetent of consent are "therapeutic orphans" [4], I should like to explore the notion and validity of proxy consent. More specifically, the interest here is in the question, Can and may parents consent, and to what extent, to experiments on their children where the procedures are nonbeneficial for the child involved? Before approaching this question, it is necessary to point out the genuine if restricted input of the ethician in such matters. Ramsey has rightly pointed up the difference between the ethics of consent and ethics in the consent situation. This latter refers to the meaning and practical applications of the requirement of an informed consent. It is the work of prudence and pertains to the competence and responsibility of physicians and investigators. The former, on the other hand, refers to the principle requiring an informed consent, the ethics of consent itself. Such moral principles are elaborated out of competences broader than those associated with the medical community.

A brief review of the literature will reveal that the question raised above remains in something of a legal and moral limbo. The *Nuremberg Code* states only that "the voluntary consent of the human subject is absolutely essential. This means that the person involved should have legal capacity to give consent" [5]. Nothing specific is said about infants or those who are mentally incompetent. Dr. Leo Alexander, who aided in drafting the first version of the *Nuremberg Code,* explained subsequently that his provision for valid consent from next of kin where mentally ill patients are concerned was dropped by the Nuremberg judges, "probably because [it] did not apply in the specific cases under trial" [3, p. 26; 6]. Be that as it may, it has been pointed out by Beecher [5, p. 231] that a strict observance of Nuremberg's rule 1 would effectively cripple study of mental disease and would simply prohibit all experimentation on children.

The *International Code of Medical Ethics* (General Assembly of the World Medical Assocation, 1949) states simply: "Under no circumstances is a doctor permitted to do anything that would weaken the physical or mental resistance of a human being except from strictly therapeutic or prophylactic indications imposed in the interest of his patient" [5, p. 236]. This statement is categorical and if taken literally means that "young children and the mentally incompetent are categorically excluded from all investigations except those that directly may benefit the subjects" [7]. However, in 1954 the General Assembly of the World Medical Association (in *Principles for Those in Research and Experimentation*) stated: "It should be required that each person who submits to experimentation be informed of the nature, the reason for, and the risk of the proposed experiment. If the patient is irresponsible, consent should be obtained from the individual who is legally responsible for the individual" [5, p. 240]. In the context it is somewhat ambiguous whether this statement is meant to apply beyond experimental procedures that are performed for the patient's good.

The *Declaration of Helsinki* (1964) is much clearer on the point. After distinguishing "clinical research combined with professional care" and "non-therapeutic clinical research," it states of this latter: "Clinical research on a human being cannot be undertaken without his free consent, after he has been fully informed; if he is legally incompetent the consent of the legal guardian should be procured" [5, p. 278]. In 1966 the American Medical Association, in its *Principles of Medical Ethics,* endorsed the Helsinki statement. It distinguished clinical investigation "primarily for treatment" and clinical investigation "primarily for the accumulation of scientific knowledge." With regard to this latter, it noted that "consent, in writing, should be obtained from the subject, or from his legally authorized representative if the subject lacks the capacity to consent." More specifically, with regard to minors or mentally incompetent persons, the AMA statement reads: "Consent, in writing, is given by a legally authorized representative of the subject under circumstances in which an informed and prudent adult would reasonably be expected to volunteer himself or his child as a subject" [5, p. 223].

In 1963, the Medical Research Council of Great Britain issued its *Responsibility in Investigations on Human Subjects* [5, pp. 262 ff.]. Under title of "Procedures Not of Direct Benefit to the Individual" the Council stated: "The situation in respect of minors and mentally subnormal or mentally disordered persons is of particular difficulty. In the strict view of the law parents and guardians of minors cannot give consent on their behalf to any procedures which are of no particular benefit to them and which may carry some risk of harm." Then, after discussing consent as involving a full understanding of "the implications to himself of the procedures to which he was consenting," the Council concluded: "When true consent in this sense cannot be obtained, procedures which are of no direct benefit and which might carry a risk of harm to the subject should not be undertaken." If it is granted that every experiment involves some risk, then the MRC statement would exclude any experiment on children. Curran and Beecher have pointed out [8] that this strict reading of English law is based on the advice of Sir Harvey Druitt, though there is no statute or case law to support it. Nevertheless, it has gone relatively unchallenged.

Statements of the validity of proxy consent similar to those of the *Declaration of Helsinki* and the American Medical Association have been issued by the American Psychological Association [5, pp. 256ff.] and the Food and Drug Administration [5, pp. 299ff.]. The most recent formulation touching on proxy consent is that of the Department of Health, Education, and Welfare in its *Protection of Human Subjects: Policies and Procedures* [9]. In situations where the subject cannot himself give consent, the document refers to "supplementary judgment." It states: "For the purposes of this document, supplementary judgment will refer to judgments made by local committees in addition to the subject's consent (when possible) and that of the parents or legal guardian (where applicable), as to whether or not a subject may participate in clinical research." The DHEW proposed guidelines admit that the law on parental consent is not clear in all respects. Proxy consent is valid with regard to established and generally accepted therapeutic procedures; it is, in practice, valid for therapeutic research. However, the guidelines state that "when research might expose a subject to risk without defined therapeutic benefit or other positive effect on that subject's well-being, parental or guardian consent appears to be insufficient." These statements about validity concern law, in the sense (I would judge) of what would happen should a case determination be provoked on the basis of existing precedent.

After this review of the legal validity of proxy consent and its limitations, the DHEW guidelines go on to draw two ethical conclusions. First, "When the risk of a proposed study is generally considered not significant, and the potential benefit is explicit, the ethical issues need not preclude the participation of children in biomedical research." Presumably, this means that where there is risk, ethical issues do preclude the use of children. However, the DHEW document did not draw this conclusion. Rather, its second ethical conclusion states: "An investigator proposing research activities which expose children to risk must document, as part of the application for support, that the information to be gained can be obtained in no other way. The investigator must also stipulate either that the risk to the subjects will be insignificant or that, although some risk exists, the potential benefit is significant and far outweighs that risk. In no case will research activities be approved which entail substantial risk except in the cases of clearly therapeutic procedures." These proposed guidelines admit, therefore, three levels of risk within the ethical calculus: insignificant risk, some risk, and substantial risk. Proxy consent is, by inference, ethically acceptable for the first two levels but not for the third.

The documents cited move almost imperceptibly back and forth between legal and moral considerations, so that it is often difficult to know whether the major concern is one or the other, or even how the relationship of the legal and ethical is conceived. Nevertheless, it can be said that there has been a gradual move away from the absolutism represented in the *Nuremberg Code* to the acceptance of proxy consent, possibly because the *Nuremberg Code* is viewed as containing, to some extent, elements of a reaction to the Nazi experiments.

Medical literature of the noncodal variety has revealed this same pattern or ambiguity. For instance, writing in the *Lancet,* Dr. R. E. W. Fisher reacted to the reports of the use of children in research procedures as follows: "No medical procedure involving the slightest risk or accompanied by the slightest physical or mental pain may be inflicted on a child for experimental purposes unless there is a reasonable chance, or at least a hope, that the child may benefit thereby" [10]. On the other hand, Franz J. Ingelfinger, editor of the *New England Journal of Medicine,* contends that the World Medical Association's statement ("Under no circumstances . . ." [above]) is an extremist position that must be modified [7]. His suggested modification reads: "Only when the risks are small and justifiable is a doctor permitted. . . ." It is difficult to know from Ingelfinger's wording whether he means small and therefore justifiable or whether "justifiable" refers to the hoped-for benefit. Responses to this editorial were contradictory. N. Baumslag and R. E. Yodaiken state: "In our opinion there are no conditions under which any children may be used for experimentation not primarily designed for their benefit" [11]. Ian Shine, John Howieson, and Ward Griffen, Jr., came to the opposite conclusion: "We strongly support his [Ingelfinger's] proposals provided that one criterion of 'small and justifiable risks' is the willingness of the experimentor to be an experimentee, or to offer a spouse or child when appropriate" [12].

Curran and Beecher had earlier disagreed strongly with the rigid interpretation given the statement of the Medical Research Council through Druitt's influence. Their own conclusion was that "children under 14 may participate in clinical investigation which is not for their benefit where the studies are sound, promise important new knowledge for mankind, and there is no discernible risk" [8, p.81]. The editors of *Archives of Disease in Childhood* recently endorsed this same conclusion, adding only "necessity of informed parental consent" [13]. Discussing relatively minor procedures such as weighing a baby, skin pricks, venipunctures, etc., they contend that "whether or not these procedures are acceptable must depend, it seems to us, on whether the potential gain to others is commensurate with the discomfort to the individual." They see the Medical Research Council's statement as an understandable but exaggerated reaction to the shocking disclosures of the Nazi era. A new value judgment is required in our time, one based on the low risk/benefit ratio.

This same attitude is proposed by Alan M. W. Porter [14]. He argues that there are grounds "for believing that it may be permissible and reasonable to undertake minor procedures on children for experimental purposes with the permission of the parents." The low risk/benefit ratio is the ultimate justification. Interestingly, Porter reports the reactions of colleagues and the public to a research protocol he had drawn up. He desired to study the siblings of children who had succumbed to "cot death." The research involved venipuncture. A pediatric authority told Porter that venipuncture was inadmissible under the Medical Research Council code. Astonished, Porter showed the protocol to the first 10 colleagues he met. The instinctive reaction of nine out of 10 was "Of course you may." Similarly, a professional market researcher asked (for Porter) 10 laymen about the procedure, and all responded that he could proceed. In other words, Porter argues that public opinion (and therefore, presumably, moral common sense) stands behind the low risk/benefit ratio approach to experimentation on children.

This sampling is sufficient indication of the variety of reactions likely to be encountered when research on children is discussed.

THE VIEWS OF ETHICIANS

The professional ethicians who have written on this subject have also drawn rather different conclusions. John Fletcher argues that a middle path between autonomy (of the physician) and heteronomy (external control) must be discovered [15]. The Nuremberg rule "does not take account of exceptions which can be controlled and makes no allowance whatsoever for the exercise of professional judgment." It is clear that Fletcher would accept proxy consent in some instances, though he has not fully specified what these would be.

Thomas J. O'Donnell, S.J., notes that, besides informed consent, we also speak of three other modalities of consent [16]. First, there is presumed consent. Life-saving measures that

are done on an unconscious patient in an emergency room are done with presumed consent. Second, there is implied consent. The various tests done on a person who undergoes a general checkup are done with implied consent, the consent being contained and implied in the very fact of his coming for a checkup. Finally, there is vicarious consent. This is the case of the parent who consents for therapy on an infant. O'Donnell wonders whether these modalities of consent, already accepted in the therapeutic context, can be extended to the context of clinical investigation (and by this he means research not to the direct benefit of the child). It is his conclusion that vicarious consent can be ethically operative "provided it is contained within the strict limits of a presumed consent (on the part of the subject) proper to clinical research and much narrower than the presumptions that might be valid in a therapeutic context." Practically, this means that O'Donnell would accept the validity of vicarious consent only where "danger is so remote and discomfort so minimal that a normal and informed individual would be presupposed to give ready consent." O'Donnell discusses neither the criteria nor the analysis that would set the "strict limits of a presumed consent."

Princeton's Paul Ramsey is the ethician who has discussed this problem at greatest length [3]. He is in clear disagreement with the positions of Fletcher and O'Donnell. Ramsey denies the validity of proxy consent in nonbeneficial (to the child) experiments simply and without qualification. Why? We may not, he argues, submit a child either to procedures that involve any measure of risk of harm or to procedures that involve no harm but simply "offensive touching." "A subject can be wronged without being harmed," he writes. This occurs whenever he is used as an object, or as a means only rather than also as an end in himself. Parents cannot consent to this type of thing, regardless of the significance of the experiment. Ramsey sees the morality of experimentation on children to be exactly what Paul Freund has described as the law on the matter: "The law here is that parents may consent for the child if the invasion of the child's body is for the child's welfare or benefit" [17, 18].

In pursuit of his point, Ramsey argues as follows: "To attempt to consent for a child to be made an experimental subject is to treat a child as not a child. It is to treat him as if he were an adult person who has consented to become a joint adventurer in the common cause of medical research. If the grounds for this are alleged to be the presumptive or implied consent of the child, that must simply be characterized as a violent and a false presumption." Thus, he concludes simply that "no parent is morally competent to consent that his child shall be submitted to hazardous *or other experiments* having no diagnostic or therapeutic significance for the child himself" (emphasis added). Though he does not say so, Ramsey would certainly conclude that a law that tolerates proxy consent to any purely experimental procedure is one without moral warrants, indeed, is immoral because it legitimates (or tries to) treating a human being as a means only.

A careful study, then, of the legal, medical, and ethical literature on proxy consent for non-therapeutic research on children reveals profoundly diverging views. Generally, the pros and cons are spelled out in terms of two important values: individual integrity and societal good through medical benefits. Furthermore, in attempting to balance these two values, this literature by and large either affirms or denies the moral legitimacy of a risk/benefit ratio, what ethicians refer to as a teleological calculus. It seems to me that in doing this, current literature has not faced this tremendously important and paradigmatic issue at its most fundamental level. For instance, Ramsey bases his prohibitive position on the contention that nonbeneficial experimental procedures make an "object" of an individual. In these cases, he contends, parents cannot consent for the individual. Consent is the heart of the matter. If the parents could legitimately consent for the child, then presumably experimental procedures would not make an object of the infant and would be permissible. Therefore, the basic question seems to be, Why cannot the parents provide consent for the child? Why is their consent considered null here while it is accepted when procedures are therapeutic? To say that the child would be treated as as object does not answer this question; it seems that it presupposes the answer and announces it under this formulation.

TRADITIONAL MORAL THEOLOGY

There is in traditional moral theology a handle that may allow us to take hold of this problem at a deeper root and arrive at a principled and consistent position, one that takes account of all the values without arbitrarily softening or suppressing any of them. That handle is the notion of parental consent, particularly the theoretical implications underlying it. If this can be unpacked a bit, perhaps a more satisfying analysis will emerge. Parental consent is required and sufficient for therapy directed at the child's own good. We refer to this as vicarious consent. It is closely related to presumed consent. That is, it is morally valid precisely insofar as it is a reasonable presumption of the child's wishes, a construction of what the child would wish could he consent for himself. But here the notion of "what the child would wish" must be pushed further if we are to avoid a simple imposition of the adult world on the child. Why *would* the child so wish? The answer seems to be that he would choose this if he were capable of choice because he *ought* to do so. This statement roots in a traditional natural-law understanding of human moral obligations.

. . .

The natural-law tradition argues that there are certain identifiable values that we *ought* to support, attempt to realize, and never directly suppress because they are definitive of our flourishing and well-being. It further argues that knowledge of these values and of the prescriptions and proscriptions associated with them is, in principle, available to human reason. This is, they require for their discovery no divine revelation.

MORAL LEGITIMACY OF PROXY CONSENT

What does all this have to do with the moral legitimacy of proxy consent? It was noted that parental (proxy, vicarious) consent is required and sufficient for therapy directed to the child's own good. It was further noted that it is morally valid precisely insofar as it is a reasonable presumption of the child's wishes, a construction of what the child would wish could he do so. Finally, it was suggested that the child *would* wish this therapy because he *ought* to do so. In other words, a construction of what the child *would* wish (presumed consent) is not an exercise in adult capriciousness and arbitrariness, subject to an equally carpicious denial or challenge when the child comes of age. It is based, rather, on two assertions: (*a*) that there are certain values (in this case life itself) definitive of our good and flourishing, hence values that we *ought* to choose and support if we want to become and stay human, and that therefore these are good also for the child; and (*b*) that these "ought" judgments, at least in their more general formulations, are a common patronage available to all men, and hence form the basis on which policies can be built

Specifically, then, I would argue that parental consent is morally legitimate where therapy on the child is involved precisely because we know that life and health are goods for the child, that he *would* choose them because he *ought* to choose the good of life, his own self-preservation as long as this life remains, all things considered, a human good. To see whether and to what extent this type of moral analysis applies to experimentation, we must ask, Are there other things that the child *ought*, as a human being, to choose precisely because and insofar as they are goods definitive of his growth and flourishing? Concretely, *ought* he to choose his own involvement in nontherapeutic experimentation, and to what extent? Certainly there are goods or benefits, at least potential, involved. But are they goods that the child *ought* to choose? Or again, if we can argue that a certain level of involvement in nontherapeutic experimentation is good for the child and therefore that he *ought* to choose it, then there are grounds for saying that parental consent for this is morally legitimate and should be recognized as such.

Perhaps a beginning can be made as follows. To pursue the good that is human life means not only to choose and support this value in one's own case, but also in the case of others when the opportunity arises. In other words, the individual *ought* also to take into account, realize, make efforts in behalf of the lives of others also, for we are social beings and the goods that define our growth and invite to it are goods that reside also in others. It can be good for one to pursue and support this good in others. Therefore, when it factually is good, we may say that one *ought* to do so (as opposed to not doing so). If this is true of all of us up to a point and within limits, it is no less true of the infant. He would choose to do so because he *ought* to do so. Now, to support and realize the value that is life means to support and realize health, the cure of disease, and so on. Therefore, up to a point, this support and realization is good for all of us individually. To share in the general effort and burden of health maintenance and disease control is part of our flourishing and growth as humans. To the extent that it is good for all of us to share this burden, we all *ought* to do so. And to the extent that we *ought* to do so, it is a reasonable construction or presumption of our wishes to say that we would do so. The reasonableness of this presumption validates vicarious consent.

It was just noted that sharing in the common burden of progress in medicine constitutes an individual good for all of us *up to a point*. That qualification is crucially important. It suggests that there are limits beyond which sharing is not or might not be a good. What might be the limits of this sharing? When might it no longer be a good for all individuals and therefore something that all need not choose to do? I would develop the matter as follows.

Adults may donate (*inter vivos*) an organ precisely because their personal good is not to be conceived individualistically but socially, that is, there is a natural order to other human persons which is in the very notion of the human personality itself. The personal being and good of an individual do have a relationship to the being and good of others, difficult as it may be to keep this in a balanced perspective. For this reason, an individual can become (in carefully delimited circumstances) more fully a person by donation of an organ, for by communicating to another of his very being he has more fully integrated himself into the mysterious unity between person and person.

Something similar can be said of participation in nontherapeutic experimentation. It can be an affirmation of one's solidarity and Christian concern for others (through advancement of medicine). Becoming an experimental subject can involve any or all of three things: some degree of risk (at least of complications), pain, and associated inconvenience (e.g., prolonging hospital stay, delaying recovery, etc.). To accept these for the good of others could be an act of charitable concern.

There are two qualifications to these general statements that must immediately be made, and these qualifications explain the phrase "up to a point." First, whether it is personally good for an individual to donate an organ or participate in experimentation is a very circumstantial and therefore highly individual affair. For some individuals, these undertakings could be or prove to be humanly destructive. Much depends on their personalities, past family life, maturity, future position in life, etc. The second and more important qualification is that these procedures become human goods for the donor or subject precisely because and therefore only when they are voluntary, for the personal good under discussion is the good of expressed charity. For these two reasons I would conclude that no one else can make such decisions for an individual, that is, reasonably presume his consent. He has a right to make them for himself. In other words, whether a person *ought* to do such things is a highly individual affair and cannot be generalized in the way the good of self-preservation can be. And if we cannot say of an individual that he ought to do these things, proxy consent has no reasonable presumptive basis.

But are there situations where such considerations are not involved and where the presumption of consent is reasonable, because we may continue to say of all individuals that (other things being equal) they *ought* to be willing? I believe so. For instance, where organ donation is involved, if the only way a young child could be saved were by a blood transfusion from another child, I suspect that few would find such blood donation an unreasonable presumption on the child's wishes. The reason for the presumption is, I believe, that a great good is provided for another at almost no cost to the child. As the scholastics put it, *parum pro nihilo reputatur* ("very little counts for nothing"). For this reason we may say, lacking countervailing individual evidence, that the individual *ought* to do this.

Could the same reasoning apply to experimentation? Concretely, when a particular experiment would involve no discernible risks, no notable pain, no notable inconvenience, and yet hold promise of considerable benefit, should not the child be constructed to wish this in the same way we presume he chooses his own life, because he *ought* to? I believe so. He *ought* to want this not because it is in any way for his own medical good, but because it is not in any realistic way to his harm, and represents a potentially great benefit for others. He *ought* to want these benefits for others.

WHAT THEY OUGHT TO WANT

If this is a defensible account of the meaning and limits of presumed consent where those incompetent to consent are concerned, it means that proxy consent can be morally legitimate in some experimentations. Which? Those that are scientifically well designed (and therefore offer hope of genuine benefit), that cannot succeed unless children are used (because there are dangers involved in interpreting terms such as "discernible" and "negligible," the child should not unnecessarily be exposed to these even minimal risks), that contain no discernible risk or undue discomfort for the child. Here it must be granted that the notions of "discernible risk" and "undue discomfort" are themselves slippery and difficult, and probably somewhat relative. They certainly involve a value judgment and one that is the heavy responsibility of the medical profession (not the moral theologian) to make. For example, perhaps it can be debated whether venipuncture involves "discernible risks" or "undue discomfort" or not. But if it can be concluded that, in human terms, the risk involved or the discomfort is negligible or insignificant, then I believe there are sound reasons in moral analysis for saying that parental consent to this type of invasion can be justified.

Practically, then, I think there are good moral warrants for adopting the position espoused by Curran, Beecher, Ingelfinger, the *Helsinki Declaration*, the *Archives of Disease in Childhood*, and others. Some who have adopted this position have argued it in terms of a low risk/benefit ratio. This is acceptable if properly understood, that is, if "low risk" means for all practical purposes and in human judgment "no realistic risk." If it is interpreted in any other way, it opens the door wide to a utilitarian subordination of the individual to the collectivity. It goes beyond what individuals would want because they *ought* to. For instance, in light of the above analysis, I find totally unacceptable the DHEW statement that "the investigator must also stipulate either that the risk to the subjects will be insignificant, or that *although some risk exists, the potential benefit is significant and far outweighs that risk.* " This goes beyond what all of us, as members of the community, necessarily *ought* to do. Therefore, it is an invalid basis for proxy consent. For analogous reasons, in light of the foregoing analysis I would conclude that parental consent for a kidney transplant from one noncompetent 3-year-old to another is without moral justification.

. . .

These considerations do not mean that all noncompetents (where consent is concerned) may be treated in the same way, that the same presumptions are morally legitimate in all cases. For if the circumstances of the infant or child differ markedly, then it is possible that there are appropriate modifications in our construction of what he *ought* to choose. For instance, I believe that institutionalized infants demand speicial consideration. They are in a situation of peculiar danger for several reasons. First, they are often in a disadvantaged condition physically or mentally so that there is

a temptation to regard them as "lesser human beings." Medical history shows our vulnerability to this type of judgment. Second, as institutionalized, they are a controlled group, making them particularly tempting as research subjects. Third, experimentation in such infants is less exposed to public scrutiny. These and other considerations suggest that there is a real danger of overstepping the line between what we all ought to want and what only the individual might want out of heroic, self-sacrificial charity. If such a real danger exists, then what the infant is construed as wanting beause he *ought* must be modified. He need not *ought to want* if this involves him in real dangers of going beyond this point.

. . .

The editor of the *Journal of the American Medical Association*, Robert H. Moser, in the course of an editorial touching on, among other things, the problem of experimentation, asks whether we are ever justified in the use of children. His answer: "It is an insoluble dilemma. All one can ask is that each situation be studied with consummate circumspection and be approached rationally and compassionately" [19]. If circumspection in each situation is to be truly consummate, and if the approach is to be rational and compassionate, then the situation alone cannot be the decisional guide. If the situation alone is the guide, if everything else is a "dilemma," then the qualities Moser seeks in the situation are in jeopardy, and along with them human rights. One can indeed, to paraphrase Moser, ask more than that each situation be studied. He can ask that a genuine ethics of consent be brought to the situation so that ethics in the consent situation will have some chance of surviving human enthusiasms. And an ethics of consent finds its roots in a solid natural-law tradition which maintains that there are basic values that define our potential as human beings; that we ought (within limits and with qualifications) to choose, support, and never directly suppress these values in our conduct; that we can know, therefore, what others would choose (up to a point) because they ought; and that this knowledge is the basis for a soundly grounded and rather precisely limited proxy consent.

REFERENCES

1. A. Capron. Clin. Res., 21:141, 1973.
2. Med. World News, June 8, 1973, p. 41.
3. P. Ramsey. THE PATIENT AS PERSON. New Haven, Conn.: Yale Univ. Press, 1970.
4. H. Shirkey. J. Pediatr., 72:119, 1968.
5. H. K. Beecher. RESEARCH AND THE INDIVIDUAL. Boston: Little, Brown, 1970.
6. L. Alexander. Dis. Nerv. Syst., 27:62, 1966.
7. F. J. Ingelfinger, N. Engl. J. Med., 288:791, 1973.
8. W. J. Curran and H. K. Beecher. J. Am. Med. Ass., 210:77, 1969.
9. Department of Health, Education, and Welfare. Federal Register, 38:31738, 1973.
10. R. E. W. Fisher. Lancet (Letters), November 7, 1953, p. 993.
11. N. Baumslag and R. W. Yodaiken. N. Engl. J. Med. (Letters), 288:1247, 1973.
12. I. Shine, J. Howieson, and W. Griffen, Jr. N. Engl. J. Med. (Letters), 288:1248, 1973.
13. Editorial. Arch. Dis. Child., 48:751, 1973.
14. A. W. Franklin, A. M. Porter, and D. N. Raine. Br. Med. J., May 19, 1973, p. 402.
15. J. Fletcher. Law Contemp. Probl., 32:620, 1967.
16. T. J. O'Donnell. J. Am. Med. Ass., 227:73, 1974.
17. P. Freund. N. Engl. J. Med., 273:691, 1965.
18. ———. Trial, 2:48, 1966.
19. R. H. Moser. J. Am. Med. Ass., 277:432, 1974.

ALEXANDER M. CAPRON

Legal Considerations Affecting Clinical Pharmacological Studies in Children

The interplay of some basic medical, ethical, and legal precepts presents pediatric pharmacology with an important and difficult problem. For scientific and legal reasons, drugs must be tested for safety and efficacy before being regularly employed in therapy, and this testing has to take account of relevant differences among groups of prospective users based on such population differences as age, race, and sex as well as differences in the manner in which the drug will be used within each population group. Law and medical ethics also require that informed consent be obtained from the subjects on whom drug tests are conducted. Hence if the members of a particular group—such as the pediatric age group—are incapable of giving informed consent, then drugs cannot be tested on them or approved for use in their group.

. . .

Reprinted with permission of the author and Charles B. Slack, Inc. from Clinical Research, Vol. 12, No. 2 (February 1973), pp. 141–150.

SEPARATE TESTS FOR EACH GROUP

Children cannot be regarded simply as "little people" pharmacologically. Their metabolism, enzymatic and excretory systems, skeletal development and so forth differ so markedly from adults' that drug tests for the latter provide inadequate information about dosage, efficacy, toxicity, side effects, and contraindications for children.[1,2] As Dr. Jean Lockhart has stated:

The penalty for ignoring [the] special considerations [which determine choice of drug and drug dosage in children] may be lack of therapeutic response on the one hand or, on the other, severe, drug-induced adverse reactions. The "gray syndrome," probably the most striking example of the latter, is believed caused by the failure of the immature liver to conjugate free chloramphenicol to its glucuronide and failure of the kidneys to rapidly excrete the free chloramphenicol. Novobiocin has been shown to produce hyperbilirubinemia in neonates, presumably due to a conjugation defect. Chloroanilines absorbed through the skin of newborns in hospital nurseries have caused methemoglobinemia.[3]

The Food and Drug regulations reflect this scientific premise by requiring that drug labeling "prescribe, recommend or suggest its use only under the conditions" for which it has been tested and approved.[4]

TESTING REQUIRES "INFORMED CONSENT"

For physicians, the phrase *informed consent* probably conjures up the image of a cumbersome, unnecessary formality (the signing of a printed *Informed Consent Form*) and brings to mind the disastrous consequences for physicians (and their insurance carriers) when this legal formality has not been observed. Yet, behind the informed consent rule lies a fundamental tenet of our society: belief in the concept of individual self-determination regarding any interferences with one's bodily integrity. In recent years, the courts have combined the requirement of intentional choice with the requirement of disclosure as they have come to recognize that the relationship of physician and patient makes it incumbent on the professional to inform the layman fully if the latter is to take an active role in making the decision which nominally has always been his to make. The evolution of the law has thus placed on the physician the unaccustomed and difficult duty "to disclose and explain to the patient as simply as necessary the nature of the ailment, the nature of the proposed treatment, the probability of success or of alternatives, and perhaps the risks of unfortunate results and unforeseen conditions."[5] While this obligation may always seem time-consuming and frequently wasteful, it only serves to underscore the basic concern of society that so far as is possible individuals be exposed only to those risks which they have voluntarily chosen for themselves. Our emphasis on consent reflects not only solicitude for individual human integrity but also a desire to educate individuals about the burdens and costs inherent in the making of choices.

In certain circumstances, the law deviates from the requirement of consent, either by presuming it to exist (for emergency treatment) or by allowing a guardian to substitute his approval for that of a person who is physically or mentally incapable or legally incompetent to give consent. It is by the latter means, of course, that physicians routinely get permission for therapeutic interventions in children who are too young to consent. This does not help us with our difficulty, however, since authoritative commentators such as Sir Harvey Druitt, KCB, author of the legal views expressed in the British Medical Research Council's *Responsibility in Investigations on Human Subjects,* are of the opinion that

> the parent has no legal authority to consent to medical procedures being carried out on his child for the advancement of scientific knowledge or for the benefit of humanity, if those procedures "are of no particular benefit to" the child and "may carry some risk of harm."[6]

Professors Henry Beecher and William Curran of Harvard Medical School argue vigorously that this overstates the actual rule, and that American statutes, medical codes, and cases permit parents to give consent for medical interventions of *no direct* —and in some instances, *no indirect* —benefit to their child. This is certainly one reading of the leading case in this area, *Bonner v. Moran.* [7] The trial court had told the jury in *Bonner* that it could find that no parental approval was necessary for the 15-year-old plaintiff to have given valid consent to donate a skin graft to his cousin if he was "capable of appreciating the nature, extent and consequences of the invasion" (as phrased by the *Restatement of Torts*). The jury found for the doctor-defendant, and on appeal the court reversed. It held that the consent of an "immature colored boy" was not sufficient for an operation on himself that was not for his benefit and that was "so involved in its technique as to require a mature mind to understand precisely what the donor was offering to give."[8] The case was returned to the lower court for a retrial in which the jury was to be instructed that the surgeon was liable unless the boy's mother had given her consent, directly or by implication.

Beecher and Curran argue that "the case does *not* hold that medical procedures cannot be performed on minors where there is no direct benefit to them. On the contrary, it holds that such procedures *can* be legally permitted as long as the parents (or other guardians) consent to the procedure."[6] This casts more weight onto the opinion than it can bear. The actual ground for the overruling is arguably that the boy was simply too immature to understand the complications involved, with the issue of there being no benefits to the boy thrown in as a mere addition. The reasons that the mother might have consented—the newspaper acclaim and scholarship donations—apply equally to show that there were benefits to the boy. Moreover, the case is really one of apparent ratification of the consent of a youngster, rather than of someone else making the choice instead of his making it. The *Bonner* court nowhere suggests that a parent has independent authority to give consent for a "nonbeneficial" intervention in a child who is too young to give any consent or who opposes the intervention. This question remains unsettled.

In other words, *Bonner* is less than definitive, and its singularity only emphasizes that courts have otherwise gone out of their way to avoid having to rule on this question. At first it appeared that some light would be shed on this issue by the disposition of court petitions in Massachusetts in the 1950s requesting permission for the transplantation of a kidney from a healthy child to his ailing twin. Peter Bent Brigham Hospital sought declaratory judgments in a series of such cases because its attorneys advised that the parents could not "legally consent to said operation because it is an invasion of the person of [the well twin] which is allegedly not for his benefit."[9] The court, aided and abetted by the lawyers and physicians involved, avoided this issue, however, by finding that the donor would benefit from losing a kidney because "the risk of emotional disturbance [from loss of his twin would] be reduced." The court went so far as to rule—after shifting the ultimate decision as to risks and benefits back onto the physicians "if [they] decide to perform the operation"—that the operation was "necessary to [the well twin's] future welfare and happiness." A similar result was reached in *Strunk v. Strunk,*[10] in which the court held (1) that it must deal with the personal affairs of a 27-year-old ward of a state hospital who had an I.Q. of 35 "in the same

manner as [he] would if he had his faculties," and (2) that in the exercise of this judgment, it was in his "best interest" to donate a kidney to his ailing 28-year-old brother to avoid what a psychiatrist predicted would otherwise be "an extremely traumatic effect upon him" were the brother to die.

Consequently, despite the almost unquestionable validity of the premise that informed consent is necessary for drug testing in adults, in the case of pediatric experimentation the role and function of informed consent need to be re-evaluated. Rather than undermining the rule by degree, through increasing the scope of exceptions, or by neglect, through allowing experimentation to occur in "inconspicuous" places such as state-run institutions, I would have us inquire whether there are other means of safeguarding the interests which the consent requirement is designed to protect and then analyze who should participate in the exercise and review of whatever means are devised.

MINORS' INABILITY TO CONSENT

. . . There is no certain age at which children (often called *infants* or *minors* by the law) are old enough to give binding consent. The common law fixed the age at 21, but that has been modified by statutory as well as common law exceptions.[11] The American Law Institute, in Section 59 of its *Restatement of the Law of Torts,* presents this as a question of fact rather than law:

If a child . . . is capable of appreciating the nature, extent and consequences of the invasion, his assent prevents the invasion from creating liability, though the assent of the parent, guardian or other person is not obtained or is expressly refused.

Two results may follow from a drug being labelled *Not to be used in children* or *Clinical studies have been insufficient to establish recommendations for use in infants and children.* First, physicians may prescribe the drug despite the warning. Although this action violates the basic premise of our discussion (that drugs must be tested in a group before being used to treat members of the group), this procedure is not unlawful in any criminal or regulatory sense. The FDA [Food and Drug Administration] requires drug manufacturers to file applications before distributing a drug for use in an untested manner, but its regulatory hand does not reach into the physician's office at present. The major restraint on the use of nonapproved drugs is, of course, the physician's potential tort liability.

The second possible result is that drugs which are not approved for use in children will not be prescribed for them. Although this result avoids the hazards associated with the previous alternative, it is viewed as unfair in the medical literature, presumably because some children will be denied treatment which will do them more good than harm and might even save their lives. Although I am in no position to challenge this hypothesis, I should like to question it. In other words, while one must agree that the problem at hand is a genuine one (this flows ineluctably from the validity of the premises), care is needed in defining the problem's dimensions.

A MODEL OF SUCCESSIVE APPROXIMATIONS

It may be possible to get a handle on the issue confronting us by employing a model of successive approximations. Since the nature of the problem probably prevents one from ever arriving at an ideal solution which fits within all the foregoing premises and yet avoids their conclusion, the best solution may be simply to limit the problem by stages rather than to attempt an end run which requires an arbitrary abandonment of the premises themselves.

LIMITING THE PERCEIVED NEED

As a first limitation, reconsider the question posed earlier: how many drugs are there which are not approved for use in children, yet which appear able to offer a significant improvement in the treatment of a disease or disorder occurring in childhood? The need for a new drug must be appraised very critically before it is tested in children. For example, one must ask just how serious is the condition in question if allowed to run its course or if treated in the presently accepted manner? Is the new drug necessary if it offers (merely) a more complete, a swifter, a less painful, or a cheaper cure than is possible now? Is there a need (in terms of numbers affected and severity of the effect) to test the drug immediately, or could tests in children be postponed until more is known about the drug's effects or until our knowledge of the human system gives medicine the tools to simulate a child's reaction to a drug by use of a computer?

LIMITING RISKS

Once the category of drugs at issue has been narrowed, the risks of each must be evaluated. While it is doubtful that it would be possible to state an across-the-board level of risk which could be applied in all situations, certain steps can be taken to limit risks. Most fundamentally, in addition to thorough animal testing, I would suggest that a drug should not be tested in children unless it has been approved for use in adults or (when the disease in question does not occur in adults) has been investigated for toxicity, side effects and contraindications through extensive *Phase One*-type testing in adult volunteers. References in the medical literature to a "reluctance to test drugs in children"[3] appear to reflect this same concern that children be exposed only to the most limited of risks. This is one area in which peer group review committees can play a very positive and important role.

LIMITING THE PARTICIPANTS

As with the questions of need and risks, the question "who should participate in drug tests?" must be answered on two levels. First, one has to formulate general rules about the categories of subjects who are, and are not, acceptable experimental subjects. Then there must be mechanisms (i.e., people and institutions operating according to certain rules) to choose individual subjects by applying the formulations to the groups in question. Here we find ourselves facing again the toughest hurdle on the course: the need to choose subjects for experimentation from among a group whose members are incapable of volunteering themselves. While the previous limiting steps may have made approaching the hurdle a little easier than it might otherwise have been, they have not removed it. Yet, as I have undoubtedly made amply clear, I do not see any legitimate way around this obstacle.

As one way of finessing the problem, some have suggested that only *Phase Two* and *Three* tests (on sick children) but not *Phase One* tests (on normal children) be conducted.[3,12] This alternative raises a number of questions, however. First, would the outcome of such a procedure be an adequate, well-controlled study as required by the FDA? There are sound scientific reasons for conducting *Phase One* investigations, to determine a drug's pharmacological and toxicological effects, free of the complications imposed by disease; there may also be need to conduct placebo studies. If the absence of such steps reduce the certainty of efficacy and safety, this added risk factor must be recognized as an additional cost which has been assumed because normal testing procedures have not been followed. This leads to a second question: is it proper to place additional risks (in drug testing and use) on sick children? A *yes* answer to this question, if carried to its logical end, would suggest that drugs should be tested *only* on the basis of need for an individual child, without formal approval (basically the present state of affairs, which is seen as needing repair). Third, has the dilemma of using children for "nonbeneficial" research actually been avoided? Even with sick children, certain procedures (from placebo studies to various evaluations of the experimental drug's effect) may not be of any direct benefit to the patient-subject; we are still likely to be left with a number of situations in which some testing will be necessary although not beneficial to the pediatric patient-subjects involved.

Who, then, should participate in these studies? First, a limitation: no studies should be done on institutionalized subjects or on other subjects whose freedom is severely limited (unless the disease or disorder occurs only in these subjects). The reasons for this restriction seem obvious; the annals of medicine are replete with examples of the ways in which concern over risks and respect for the subject as a human being slowly erode when investigators rely on this class of subject. While the experiments in the Nazi concentration camps epitomize this phenomenon, there are other less flagrant examples which occurred prior to the German experience and which continue to occur.[13] Recent examples are the study of hepatitis which has been carried out on mentally retarded children for the past 15 years at the Willowbrook State School in Staten Island, New York,[14-16] and the study on untreated syphilis carried out by the Public Health Service since the 1930s in Tuskegee, Alabama.[17] Moreover, if consent is to play a role in the selection mechanism, the representatives of children under physical, mental, or economic constraint are poorly positioned to exercise unfettered choice.

Accepting this broad limitation, what means are available for selecting participants?

1. Selection by Guardian. As was previously stated, the present means of choosing subjects operates on a variation of informed consent model in which the child's guardians (usually his parents) are said to exercise their power of consent for him. This preserves some of the intent of the informed consent system, in that the person given the power is one who presumptively understands and identifies with the child and can therefore be expected to act so as to protect him in a manner similar to the one which he would himself have chosen. Nevertheless, the fundamental purpose of informed consent—to assure that one suffers only those risks he has chosen—is not met by substituted consent, and it would be well to end the charade of *consent* (implying self-choice) for children's participation in research and to speak instead of *selection* or the like.

One result of this perspective is to highlight the fact that putting this power of selection in parents, as we now do, is as much a matter of history or of convenience as it is a matter of principle. There are any number of explanations for this societal allocation of authority: respect for the family and a desire to foster the diversity which it brings; the fitness of giving the power to decide to the same people who created the child and have the duty to support and protect him; the belief that a child cannot be much harmed by parental choices which fall within the range permitted by society and a willingness to bear the risks of harm this allocation entails or a belief that in most cases "harm" would be hard for society to distill and measure anyway; or simply the conclusion that the administrative costs of giving authority to anyone but the parents outweigh the risks for children and for society unless the parents are shown to be unable to exercise their authority adequately. While the authority assigned parents may be framed in terms of a right on their part, such right is far from absolute, howsoever it may be justified in terms of the foregoing or other rationales.

Even if society continues to assume, as a general rule, that parents are the best (in whatever sense) representatives of their children, it may wish to place certain checks on their decisions—for example, by inquiring into the grounds for the decisions. The common law had the habit of taking things at face value, and it seldom probed the background of a decision or agreement, much less the parties' states of mind. Depending on the type of experiment for which the child is being volunteered, properly trained personnel should be employed to analyze the basis of the parents' decision and their motivation so as to rule out cases in which the decision was made on a faulty basis, with a desire to punish or hurt the child, or with other pathological intent. So as to prevent the spectacle of pharmacologists exploiting the economic deprivation (and even desperation) which occurs in our country, no economic incentives should be attached to the system of parental choice, or any incentives should be graduated to make them "wealth-neutral" (a very difficult task). A further danger in using a system of selection based on economic rewards is that "the market" in this situation does not behave according to standard theory because parents' responsiveness to a monetary incentive is based on their own relative need for money, which (in the usual market ratio-nale) is said to reflect society's valuation of their worth, yet cannot similarly be said to reflect society's valuation of the child-subject.

Selection on Basis of Fitness. It is also possible that other persons, perhaps those who work with large numbers of children, would make good selectors for experimentation. While it would be difficult to assure that such persons would act with the level of concern and attention which is normative in the parent-child relationship, their greater familiarity with children might make them more perceptive in identifying those who, for physiological or psychological reasons, would be best suited for testing. It would, of course, be possible to use this method in conjunction with the method of monitored parental selection previously set forth. Those charged with making the decisions could be individuals or groups with varying representation, depending on the expertise that was sought. Their determinations of fitness could be stated in summary form, or through an open, public process. Provided that public confidence existed for the grounds on which the decisions were to be made and for the integrity of the decision-makers—and given both the significance and distasteful nature of the decisions, this is a large assumption —it would probably make little difference whether the deliberations were public or private, since the final outcome would contain the value judgments which inhere in the system as to who is a proper experimental subject. This "rational" process differs from the processes of juries and draft-boards, who operate with broad discretion and need not provide "reasons" for their decisions; the revelation of their processes would probably disturb the public by making clear the value-laden grounds on which they act.

2. *Random Choice.* If we are, in fact, speaking of a definable group and if all members of the group have a roughly equal chance of being afflicted with the diseases which are to be treated in the group, then consideration should also be given to selecting experimental subjects from the group on a random basis. There is something in us which rebels at this notion, but once the field of experiments has been properly

limited this alternative cannot be dismissed out of hand. There are many other situations in which membership in a group imposes obligations in return for sharing in the benefits conferred by membership (such as the availability of improved and adequately tested pharmaceuticals). The drafting of young men into the armed services provides a current example. Although I for one would prefer a system which achieved its ends through voluntary heroism rather than obligatory sacrifice, such a system may not produce enough volunteers and, in the case of children, it makes no sense to speak of volunteerism anyway. One can object to random selection on pragmatic grounds, however, for it fails to distinguish those children who are best suited for testing (although it could be used in combination with the second alternative just discussed), and it may make adverse test sequelae more difficult for the parents to bear than would a more rational system, especially one in which they exercised the decision-making power. Nevertheless, the randomness of the procedure itself is less bothersome than the alternative which many favor of using sick children as test subjects, since to the randomness of being afflicted with the disease and its accompanying suffering would be added the risk of further suffering from a drug whose safety and efficacy are unknown.

Thus far, these alternatives have been discussed entirely in functional terms, but it is obvious that they would bring about important changes in the rights and duties of the various participants: children, parents, investigators, and society. Yet I suspect that what makes one uncomfortable about the second and third alternatives is neither their deliberateness (in the case of selection by fitness) nor their arbitrariness (in the case of random selection), but their allocation of authority to officers of the state. We attempt to protect our liberties by placing limitations on the powers of the state; yet, not always trusting the state to be so self-limiting, we also seek protection by dispersing power as widely as possible and, when it is necessary to place power in the government, by putting as many internal checks on its exercise as possible without disabling the system entirely. These liberty-protecting devices are

enshrined in our constitution, as prohibitions on "involuntary servitude," guarantees of "due process," and the like. While the selective service system has withstood challenge on constitutional grounds,[18-20] any system of drafting children for medical experimentation would certainly be subject to attack,[21] and its necessity would have to be rather compelling for it to be upheld. One interesting aspect of this is that the result desired (conducting adequate tests) might also be achieved through the first alternative, that of giving parents more freedom in volunteering their children for research for the benefit of children generally rather than of their child in particular. And yet our doubts about such a method would probably not be framed in constitutional terms but in terms of private rights (the parents' v. the child's) in civil law terms.[22]

LIMITING DAMAGES

If it is thus possible to formulate a proper class of subjects and a means of administering the rule thus devised—and the alternatives just mentioned probably do not exhaust the field—one must still face the prospect that for all the narrowing of need, risks, and participants there will still be cases in which the results will not match the ideal being sought. These are the cases in which a child-subject suffers an injury, which he will not, of course, have chosen. One way of reducing the incidence of harm is to insist that peer group review committees diligently carry out their duty of monitoring ongoing research so as to assure that adequate measures are always taken to keep the risks within the limits originally approved and to detect and correct deleterious results as quickly and completely as possible.[23] There is nevertheless no assurance that serious injuries can always be prevented.

A partial remedy for this failing is to insist on full compensation to the subject, without regard to the level of diligence and care exercised by the investigator. Despite this description, this proposal should not be confused with the no-fault systems of automobile insurance which are now being enacted in a number of states. In those systems, persons involved in traffic accidents can collect a limited amount (up to $2,000 to $4,000 in most cases) for actual expenses occasioned by the accident (but not for pain and suffering) on simple proof that the accident occured. The theory behind this method of handling accident compensation is that it will reduce the total costs of accidents and that the determination of fault is often too expensive, especially when, in many situations, more than one person is blameworthy to some degree.[24,25] This no-fault method is not easily translatable to the medical sphere, however, because in many medical interventions, and particularly those of an experimental cast, there is often no clear norm, deviation from which can be said to constitute negligence. In experimentation on adults, the cost of the injury has to be borne by the subject, since he chose to expose himself to it (and usually waived his right to recover). If there is a measure of injustice in that instance, there is entirely too much injustice in laying this burden on the child who was selected for (rather than having consented to) the experiment.

Full compensation also makes good sense economically since it treats injuries like the other costs of developing a new drug, which ought to be reflected in the drug's price.[26,27] If the costs of the injury are instead borne by some form of general medical or social insurance, more drug research will take place than is justified by society's economic demands. If insufficient research is undertaken, because the market mechanism cannot adequately collectivize individuals' demands for medical innovations which they as individuals do not anticipate needing, there are better (i.e., more precise, fairer, etc.) methods for stimulating the necessary research than throwing the cost of pharmacological mistakes onto experimental subjects, for them to pass on to society at large on a haphazard basis. . . .

CONCLUSION

Pediatric clinical pharmacology is confronted with the medicolegal dilemma that on the one hand drugs which have not been tested on children either cannot be used to treat them or must be used in a fairly unscientific and risky fashion, and on the other hand the needed drug testing may itself be foreclosed in the pediatric age group if no one is authorized to give informed consent for a child's participation in medical interventions that are not intended to benefit him directly. Although the ideal solution—fully voluntary participation by well-informed subjects who undertake the risks of a drug trial as co-adventurers with the clinical investigators—is not possible in pediatric pharmacology, a *model of successive approximations* may reduce the scope of the problem to more manageable proportions. The model operates by first limiting the perceived need and the risks and then by replacing the concept of substituted informed consent with various modes of choosing the pediatric subjects, such as selection by guardian, by professionals on basis of fitness, or by lot. Finally, the model would attempt to limit the impact of injuries suffered by providing for full compensation to the subjects. The proposed approach is not presented as a panacea for this very difficult problem but as an attempt to encourage legal and medical re-examination of current methods of dealing with the issue.

REFERENCES

1. Food and Drug Administration: Proceedings of a Conference on Pediatric Pharmacology. Washington, US Gov't Ptg Off, 1967.
2. Lowe C. U.: "Pediatrics—proper utilization of children as research subjects." *Ann NY Acad Sci* 169:337–343, 1970.
3. Lockhart J. D.: "The information gap in pediatric drug therapy." *Mod Med* 38:56–68, Nov 16, 1970.
4. 21 CFR § 130.4, 1972.
5. Natanson v Kline, 186 (Kan. 383, 410, 350 P.2d 1093, 1106, *clarified,* 187 Kan. 186, 354 P.2d 670 (1960).
6. Curran W. J., Beecher H. K.: "Experimentation in children." *JAMA* 210:77–81, 1969.
7. 126 F.2d 121 (DC Cir 1941).
8. 126 F.2d at 123.
9. Petition in Foster v Harrison, Mass Sup Jud Court, Suffolk, SS No 68674 Equity, 1957.
10. 445 SW 2d 145 (Ky 1969).
11. *See* Bakker v Welsh, 144 Mich 632 (1906).
12. American Academy of Pediatrics, Committee on Drugs: Drug testing in children—FDA regulations. *Ped* 43:463–465, 1969.
13. Katz J., with Capron A. M., Glass E. S.: *Experimentation with Human Beings.* New York: Russell Sage Foundation, 1972.

14. Krugman S., Giles J. P., Hammond J.: "Viral hepatitis type B (MS-2 strain)—studies on active immunization." *JAMA* 217:41–45, 1971.

15. Editorial: "Prevention of viral hepatitis—mission impossible?" *JAMA* 217:70–71, 1971.

16. Goldby S.: "Experiments at the Willowbrook State School." *Lancet* 1:749, 1971.

17. Heller J.: "Syphilis victims in US study without therapy for 40 years." *NY Times,* Jul 26, 1972, pp. 1,8.

18. Selective Draft Law Cases, 245 US 366 (1918).

19. Lichter v United States, 334 Us 742 (1948).

20. United States v O'Brien, 391 US 367 (1968).

21. *Cf* Black, C. Jr: "Constitutional problems in compulsory national service." *Yale Law Report,* Summer 1967, pp 19–20.

22. *But see* Prince v Massachusetts, 321 US 158 (1944) (limiting parents' authority to make child a "martyr" to religion, a constitutionally based argument).

23. *See* FDA Regulations on Institutional Committee Review of Clinical Investigations of New Drugs in Human Beings, 36 *Federal Register* 5037, 1971, *amending* 21 CFR § 130.3, 1972.

24. Calabresi G.: *The Costs of Accidents.* New Haven: Yale University Press, 1970.

25. Blum W. J., Kalven H. Jr.: *Public Law Perspectives on a Private Law Problem.* Boston: Little, Brown and Co. 1965.

26. Ladimer I.: "Clinical research insurance." *J Chron Dis* 16:1229–1235, 1963.

27. Calabresi G.: "Reflections on medical experimentation in humans." *Daedalus* 98:387–405, 1969.

Experimentation with Fetuses

LEROY WALTERS

Ethical and Public-Policy Issues in Fetal Research

The Commission shall conduct an investigation and study of the nature and extent of research involving living fetuses, the purposes for which such research has been undertaken, and alternative means for achieving such purposes. The Commission shall . . . recommend to the Secretary policies defining the circumstances (if any) under which such research may be conducted or supported.—Public Law 93–348, section 202b

. . .

I. SCOPE AND FOCUS

The legislation which created the Commission clearly focuses attention upon "research involving living fetuses." Thus, this essay will

Reprinted from National Commission for the Protection of Human Subjects of Biomedical and Behavioral Research, *Research on the Fetus: Appendix* (Washington, D.C.: U.S. Department of Health, Education, and Welfare, 1975).

not discuss the problem of research involving the dead fetus, living tissues derived from the dead fetus, or the placenta, fluids, and membranes. As noted below, the term "fetus" will be used in a general rather than a technical sense to apply to the living human conceptus (1) *in utero* from the time of implantation to the time of delivery or abortion and (2) outside the uterus from a point eight days after fertilization to the point at which the organism is viable.

II. DEFINITIONS

A. Fetus: the human conceptus *in utero* from the blastocyst stage to delivery and outside the uterus from the blastocyst stage to the point at which the organism is viable. Beyond this latter point, an extrauterine organism would be designated a "newborn infant."

B. Live or living: possessing at least one of the standard signs of life, namely, heartbeat, respiration, movement, or, in the case of the fetus, pulsation of the umbilical cord.

C. Dead: the state in which the organism as a whole shows none of the standard signs of life (in the absence of artificial life support systems) and is not capable of being resuscitated. Individual tissues and cells may live on after the organism as a whole is dead.

D. Viable: sufficiently mature to be able to continue to live apart from direct connection with the mother, assuming standard neonatal care. I would recommend that for the sake of clarity this term be analyzed into three subcategories:

1. Clearly viable: sufficiently mature to be able to survive in virtually all cases, if no serious illness or malformation is present (suggested estimate: birth weight of 2,300 grams or more).[1]

2. Probably viable: sufficiently mature to possess a 50 percent or greater chance of survival, based on current national averages for fetal survival (suggested estimate: birth weight 1,250 to 2,299 grams).[2]

3. Possibly viable: possessing a 49 percent or less chance of survival, based on current national averages for fetal survival. For the purposes of this definition, the birth weight of a possibly viable fetus must equal or exceed the birth weight of the smallest fetus known to have survived through well documented medical records (1975 estimate: birth weight of 500 to 1,249 grams).[3]

E. Previable or nonviable: weighing less at birth than the smallest recorded surviving fetus[4]; clearly incapable of continuing to live apart from direct connection with the mother, assuming standard neonatal care. A graphic representation of the definitions proposed in D and E, including the suggested estimates, would take the following form:

F. Therapy: the use of established and accepted methods of treatment to meet the needs of a patient.[5]

G. Therapeutic research: the use of treatment methods which are not established and accepted, with the primary *intent* of benefitting the patient receiving the new treatment.[6] (Whether the new treatment *in fact* benefits the patient is an important question but, according to the ethical codes which have addressed the problem of clinical research, it is a secondary question.)

H. Nontherapeutic research: the use of procedures which are not established and accepted methods of treatment with the primary *intent* of gaining scientific knowledge or of benefitting persons other than the experimental subject.[7]

III. MAJOR TYPES OF FETAL RESEARCH

Conceptually, one can distinguish at least the following major categories of fetal research:

1. Research involving live or dead fetuses;

2. Research involving fetuses *in utero* or outside the uterus;

3. Research involving induced abortion or either spontaneous abortion or spontaneous delivery;

4. Research involving previable or viable fetuses;

5. Nontherapeutic or therapeutic (for fetuses) research;

6. Research involving various degrees of risk to fetuses: minimal, moderate or serious.

If one excludes research involving dead fetuses (category 1) and the risk-question (category 6), one is still left with 16 possible combinations of the remaining categories, i.e., 16 distinct types of fetal research. If one includes the three levels of risk noted in category 6, this total rises to 48 potential types of fetal research. . . .

There is, however, a more inductive approach which can be adopted in enumerating

PREVIABLE	POSSIBLY VIABLE	PROBABLY VIABLE	CLEARLY VIABLE
500g	1,250g	2,300g	

the major types of fetal research. One can review reports or survey articles which have appeared in the medical literature during the past 15 years to ascertain what kinds of live-fetus research have in fact been done. . . .

Chronologically speaking, live-fetus research seems to be done most frequently at four stages of fetal life: (1) when the fetus is *in utero* and will remain *in utero* for at least one week; (2) when the fetus is *in utero* and delivery or induced abortion is anticipated within a few hours or days; (3) during an abortion procedure, i.e., after the procedure has begun but while the maternal-feto-placenta unit is still intact; and (4) following the completion of abortion, i.e., after the surgical separation of the fetus from the mother.

From a medical or biological standpoint, one can distinguish the following major types of live-fetus research in the medical literature:

1. Prenatal diagnosis;
2. Intrauterine therapy;
3. Studies of fetal behaviour;
4. Nutrition studies;
5. Studies of placental transfer;
6. Studies of fetal physiology or metabolism;
7. Studies of abortion techniques;
8. Tissue studies;
9. Studies of oxygenation or life-prolongation;
10. Studies of techniques for facilitating delivery.

Certain of these ten research procedures are likely to be correlated with particular chronological stages of fetal life.

In the following paragraphs, I shall briefly describe some of the live-fetus research which has been conducted and reported in the scientific literature of the past 15 years. The studies will be organized according to the four chronological stages noted above.

1. *The fetus in utero more than one week prior to delivery or abortion*

   a. Prenatal diagnosis: The traditional use of x-ray has been supplemented by a series of newer techniques, including amniocentesis[8], ultrasound[9], fetoscopy[10], and fetal blood sampling.[11]

   b. Intrauterine therapy: Intrauterine blood transfusions for Rh incompatibility have

been employed for several years; more recently attempts have been made to treat adrenogenital syndrome,[12] fetal lung immaturity,[13] and a type of acidemia[15] prenatally.

   c. Studies of fetal behavior: Most studies seem to concentrate on fetal response to sound[15], although some studies investigate the effect on the fetus of light and other types of stimuli.[16]

   d. Nutrition studies: Prospective studies involving animals have been performed, but few prospective studies on humans have been done[17]; a major retrospective study has examined the effect of the Dutch "hunger winter" of 1944/45 on fetal development.[18]

   e. Studies of placental transfer: Numerous retrospective studies have been done concerning the effect on the fetus of drugs administered to the mother for therapeutic reasons;[19] several prospective studies of placental transfer have been performed prior to induced abortion, including two rubella-vaccine studies.[20] The prospective studies are performed more than a week prior to induced abortion, so that sufficient time elapses to allow the effect of the experimental procedure on the fetus to become apparent.

2. *The fetus in utero a few hours or days prior to delivery or abortion*

   a. Prenatal diagnosis: Some new techniques of prenatal diagnosis, for example, fetoscopy, have been tested on fetuses prior to abortion.[21]

   b. Nutrition studies: In a study entitled "Response to Starvation in Pregnancy" women scheduled for abortion fasted during an 84-hour period immediately prior to the abortion-procedure.[22]

   c. Studies of placental transfer: In pregnant women nearing the time of delivery, several studies have investigated placental transfer of radioisotopes, ethyl alcohol, or steroids.[23] In cases involving abortion, numerous studies of placental transfer have been performed. Most of these studies begin several hours prior to abortion, at which time an agent is administered to the mother intravenously. The agent, having crossed the placenta, is recovered from the fetus during or following the abortion procedure either by drawing a fetal blood sample or by examining fetal organs. Specific compounds which have been tested in placental transfer studies at the time of abortion include: erythromycin and clindamycin,[24] ^{125}I-glucagon,[25] cortisol,[26] diphenylhydantoin[27], and gentamycin[28].

d. Studies of abortion techniques: For the most part, such studies have concentrated on maternal comfort and safety;[29] recently one study has investigated the mechanism by which fetal death is produced in saline-induced abortion.[30]

e. Studies of techniques for facilitating delivery: In pregnant women nearing the time of delivery, numerous studies have been conducted to test the effect on the fetus of agents which delay or induce the onset of labor[31] and various types of obstetrical anesthesia, e.g., paracervical block.[32]

3. *The fetus during the abortion procedure, while the maternal-feto-placental unit is intact*

a. Placental transfer: During abortion by hysterotomy, studies of placental transfer investigate whether a compound introduced on the fetal side of the placenta crosses the placenta and enters the maternal bloodstream. For example, two studies of fetal circulation and blood volume injected radioactive isotopes into the umbilical vein, then sought to detect the presence of radioactivity in the mother.[33]

b. Studies of fetal physiology or metabolism: In such studies the attachment of the fetus to the placenta and to the mother assures the continuation of fetal circulation. During hysterotomy-procedures various researchers have investi-

gated blood flow within the fetal circulatory system[34] and fetal metabolism of arginine,[35] sulfur,[36] and ^{125}I-glucagon.[37]

4. *The fetus outside the uterus following separation from the mother, i.e., the abortus*[38]

a. Studies of fetal physiology or metabolism: Since the aborted fetus may continue to live for a period of time following abortion by hysterotomy or hysterectomy, it is possible to study certain aspects of fetal physiology even after spontaneous or induced abortion. One study which involved abortion-hysterectomies perfused the pregnant uteri with barium sulfate solution in order to perform angiographic studies of the circulatory system in the uterus and the placenta.[39] Another study decapitated 8 live aborted fetuses, perfused the fetal heads through the carotid arteries, and measured cerebral oxidation of a glucose-substitute.[40]

b. Tissue or organ studies: The removal, or harvesting, of fetal organs or tissues is frequently the final step in studies of fetal metabolism which commenced prior to abortion. In some cases such organs are removed from the still-living organism immediately following the abortion-procedure. Studies which have involved the retrieval of organs from the live abortus include an investigation of biosynthesis in the fetal liver and brain[41] and two projects which examined the enzyme response of the fetal liver.[42]

c. Studies of oxygenation or life-prolongation: Previable aborted fetuses lack the capacity to breathe and to absorb oxygen through the lungs. Several investigators have tested the feasibility of prolonging fetal life by other means of oxygenation. One study placed fetuses in an immersion chamber and sought to discover whether "the skin of a fetus immersed in a oxygen-pressured nutrient could be utilized as an organ of absorption and excretion".[43] Another study serially attached several aborted fetuses to an artificial placenta.[44]

As the foregoing survey makes clear, "fetal research" is not one but many things. Several of the studies noted above were clearly therapeutic in intent, particularly if one considers diagnosis to be a prerequisite of therapy. Other studies were not done for the benefit of the fetuses involved. . . . Since it is nontherapeutic research on fetuses which seems to raise the most serious questions in the public mind, I will concentrate primary attention on the problem of *nontherapeutic* fetal research.

The survey of major types of fetal research also indicates that fetal research involves both fetuses which will come to term and be born and fetuses which will be, are being, or have been aborted. Here again a limitation is in order. . . . I will . . . focus especially on ethical issues involved in research before, during, or after induced abortion. Since abortion is generally performed before fetal viability is clearly achieved, such fetuses will generally be previable or, at most, only possibly-viable.

There are few published discussions of the ethical issues involved in live-fetus research.[45] The few documents which do exist reveal that the Commission is faced with a situation of ethical pluralism. So far as I am able to detect, there exists no national consensus on the question of fetal research.

In my view, four identifiable positions have emerged on the ethics of research involving live (not clearly-viable) fetuses before, during, or after induced abortion:

1. Nontherapeutic fetal research should not be done under any circumstances.

2. Nontherapeutic fetal research should be done only to the extent that such research is permitted on children or on fetuses which will be carried to term.

3. Greater latitude should be allowed for nontherapeutic fetal research than for research on children or on fetuses which will be carried to term. However, certain types of experimental procedures should not be performed, even in nontherapeutic fetal research.

4. Any type of nontherapeutic fetal research may legitimately be performed. . . .

In this section I shall seek to demonstrate that Position 2 is a reasonable ethical position. In the succeeding section I shall attempt to show that such a position could also be translated into a constructive and workable public policy.

One can arrive at Position 2 by extrapolating backward from a position on the ethics of pediatric research. In recent years, some philosophers and ethicists have argued that nontherapeutic research on children who cannot consent should not be performed under any circumstances.[46] However, Richard McCormick has presented what seem to me to be a very cogent argument for including children in certain kinds of no-risk or low-risk nontherapeutic research. McCormick's central thesis is that all members of society owe certain minimal debts to society; among these debts is one's obligation to take part in low-risk biomedical or behavioral research. He concludes that parents should be authorized to consent to a child's taking part in experiments which the child *should* be willing to take part in if the child *could* understand and consent.[47]

If one accepts this position on pediatric research, one can easily extend it to cover the prenatal period in the life of a fetus which will be carried to term and be born. The parent or parents of such a fetus can be expected to have the interests of the fetus in view, just as parents of already-born children normally consider the interests of their offspring. Thus, proxy consent for nontherapeutic research on a fetus prior to birth is both possible and ethically consistent with consent for nontherapeutic pediatric research.

In the case of a fetus which will be aborted or has been aborted, the situation is somewhat more complex. The mother has decided, perhaps for good reason, that the life of the fetus should be terminated. Because she will not be obliged to consider the interests of the child on a long-term basis, she cannot give proxy consent *in the same sense* as the mother or both parents of an already-born child or a fetus-to-be-born. There is, in addition, an inherent difficulty in conceptualizing what "risk" or "harm" might mean when one is speaking of an organism which will shortly die at a previable stage of life. I suggest that it is possible to skirt these difficult problems as well as to be ethically consistent if one adopts the general rule: Nontherapeutic research procedures which are permissible in the case of fetuses which will be carried to term are also permissible in the case of (a) live fetuses which will be aborted and (b) live fetuses which have been aborted.

The fundamental presupposition of the position here advocated is that there is a substantial measure of continuity between previable fetal life and viable fetal life or pediatric life. This continuity cannot, in my view, be conclusively demonstrated by means of factual arguments. However, a proponent of the continuity-thesis can point to a series of considerations which render the thesis at least not implausible. It seems clear, for example, that the living previable fetus has a qualitatively different potential from a living tissue or a living sub-human animal. One notes, too, that Anglo-American law has displayed a certain ambivalence vis-à-vis the previable fetus, according to the fetus some, but not all, of the legal protections enjoyed by children or adults.[48] It can also be argued that in form or general appearance the 12- or 16-week-old previable fetus resembles the viable fetus more closely than it resembles the embryo or blastocyst. Finally, one is struck by both the technology-dependence and the somewhat arbitrary character of the viability watershed: fetuses which twenty years ago would have been correctly classified as previable are now surviving in neonatal intensive-care units; today the immaturity of a single organ system, the lungs, constitutes the major barrier between a 450-gram fetus and viability.

There are strong counterarguments which can be mounted against the continuity-thesis and the ethical position advocated above. I shall briefly mention and comment on two. It might be argued, first, that the right to have a previable fetus aborted is firmly established in American law and that the termination of life is much more harmful to the fetus than *any* experimental procedures—even highly invasive procedures—which might be performed upon it. In response to this argument, one would wish to question whether abortion and fetal research are, indeed, analogous questions and whether the moral justification of abortion entails, as well, the justification of fetal research. In the case of abortion there exists a clear conflict between maternal interests and the developing fetus. The woman alleges a right to be rid of an immediate, serious threat to her previous pattern of life. This right is now guaranteed by the law for the stages of pregnancy prior to fetal viability. In the case of fetal research, however, there is, so far as I can see, no similar clear and immediate conflict between the previable fetus and society at large or any other social group. Thus, it would seem that the proponent of highly-invasive fetal research must build an entirely new case for such research rather than being able to piggyback his or her case on the fact of presumably-lethal abortion procedures.

A second major counterargument to the position taken in this paper is more consequential in character. This argument can be taken in any of several directions. It is asserted, for example, that if fetal research proceeds without limitation, one can expect such research to yield major advances in scientific knowledge or results of great benefit to all future fetuses and premature infants. A narrower and more limited consequentialist claim is that by performing high-risk safety-studies of new procedures on fetuses which will be or have been aborted, one can prevent damage to fetuses which will later be born and who will subsequently bear the stigma of prenatal damage throughout an entire lifetime.

This is a significant argument and deserves to be taken seriously. There are, however, several avenues of reply. It may be noted, first, that many of the benefits promised from fetal research without limitation could also be achieved by research carried on within the ethical guidelines here proposed. Second, it can be argued that the positive consequences of fetal research without limitation, desirable as they seem, are not the only consequences which need to be considered. A comprehensive social-impact statement would take into account, in addition, the possible dehumanizing effects on investigators of their performing highly invasive procedures on still-living fetuses. One would also wish to inquire whether such research would set a precedent for the performance of similar procedures on other classes of human organisms—for example, on newborns who are mortally ill or comatose elderly persons.

The safety-studies objection is perhaps the most difficult one to meet. Negatively, it seems to me that the potential problems of dehumanization and precedent-setting are pertinent to this argument, as well. More positively, if, as I have advocated, children and fetuses are to be involved in low-risk nontherapeutic research for the sake of society, then society would seem to owe such subjects a reciprocal debt. There would inevitably be accidents resulting from low-risk nontherapeutic or higher-risk therapeutic forms of research. In my view, society would have a serious moral obligation to develop programs of compensation and care for a new class of "disabled veterans"—those wounded in the battle against disease.

V. RECOMMENDATIONS FOR A NATIONAL POLICY ON FETAL RESEARCH

Policy-making always involves the setting of priorities, and the priorities one chooses reflect the values one wishes to maximize. Thus, there is always a significant ethical component in the policy-making process.

However, policy-making takes into account certain factors which ethics generally does not. In a pluralistic society it seeks to accommodate a variety of belief-systems and interests rather than elevating the views of any single group to the status of national policy. Policy-making also attempts to achieve maximal continuity with some of the generally-accepted principles within the society. Finally, policy-makers, at their best, seek to ensure that national policies are formulated and expressed in terms that are clearly understandable to the public at large.

In my view, the Commission is in an ideal position to articulate a clear, well-reasoned national policy on fetal research which can become the basis for ongoing discussion and a possible movement toward national consensus. I wish to recommend that the Commission adopt a policy which emphasizes equality of treatment or equal protection for all categories of human subjects. More specifically, I would recommend that the Commission adopt a policy which approximates Position 2 in the foregoing ethical analysis. On the policy-level, this recommendation can be stated in terms of three parallel propositions:

(1) Nontherapeutic research on children should be permitted, if such research involves no risk or only minimal risk to the subjects.

(2) Nontherapeutic research on fetuses which will be carried to term should be permitted, if such research involves no risk or only minimal risk to the subjects.

(3) Nontherapeutic research procedures which are permitted in the case of fetuses which will be carried to term should also be permitted in the case of (a) live fetuses which will be aborted and (b) live fetuses which have been aborted.

A policy developed along the lines suggested has numerous advantages, in my view. I will attempt to list several:

1. It is formal and therefore flexible; it does not prohibit any particular research procedure but establishes a general test which all proposed procedures would be required to meet.

2. It is a mediating policy, which corresponds to moderate positions on the spectrum of current ethical opinion regarding fetal research.

3. The proposed policy is in continuity with past policy-recommendations by the Peel Committee and DHEW concerning research involving the fetus *in utero* in anticipation of abortion. Like these previous policies, it protects the woman's right to change her mind concerning a planned abortion.

4. It obviates the need for a definition of viability, since the same formal guidelines apply to both previable and viable fetuses.

5. It takes into account the sensibilities of the large numbers of persons who object to highly-invasive research on live aborted fetuses.

6. Finally, the proposed policy, if adopted, would permit many valuable types of fetal research to continue. Research involving living tissues from dead fetuses would not be affected in any way by the policy here proposed and could thus continue unabated. Studies of prenatal diagnosis, intrauterine therapy, fetal behavior, placental transfer, fetal physiology or metabolism, oxygenation-techniques, and the facilitation of delivery could all be continued, provided that the various categories of fetuses were treated equally and provided that the nontherapeutic procedures would involve either no risk or only minimal risk to the subjects.

. . .

NOTES

1. The estimates suggested here are based primarily on data contained in two sources. Battaglia, Frederick C., and Lubchenco, Lula O., "A practical classification of newborn infants by weight and gestational age." *Journal of Pediatrics* 71 (2):159–163, August 1967. Hellman, Louis M., and Pritchard, Jack A. *Williams Obstetrics (Fourteenth Edition).* New York: Appleton-Century-Crofts, 1971, p. 1028. The graph developed by Battaglia and Lubchenco, based on 1964 data, suggests that both weight and gestational age may need to be taken into account.

2. Battaglia, Frederick C. and Lubchenco, Lula O. *Op. cit.,* n. 1, p. 161.

3. *Ibid.*

4. Hellman, Louis M., and Pritchard, Jack A. *Op. cit.,* n. 1, p. 1028. See also Avery, Mary Ellen. "Considerations on the definition of viability." *New England Journal of Medicine* 292 (4):206–207, 23 January 1975.

5. Office of the Secretary, Department of Health, Education, and Welfare. "Protection of human subjects." *Federal Register* 39(105):18917 (§46.3b), 30 May 1974.

6. World Medical Association. Declaration of Helsinki (1964). Reprinted by Henry Beecher in *Research and the Individual: Human Studies* (Boston: Little, Brown, 1970), p. 277. American Medical Association. *Ethical Guidelines for Clinical Investigation* (1966). Reprinted in Beecher, *Research and the Individual,* p. 223.

7. *Ibid.*

8. Burton, Barbara K.; Gerby, Albert B.; and Nadler, Henry L. "Present status of intrauterine diagnosis of genetic defects." *American Journal of Obstetrics and Gynecology* 118 (5):718–746, 1 March 1974.

9. Kohorn, Ernest I., and Kaufman, Michael. "Sonar in the first trimester of pregnancy." *Obstetrics and Gynecology* 44 (4):473–483, October 1974.

10. Patrick, J. E.; Perry, J. B.; and Kinch, R. A. H. "Fetoscopy and fetal blood sampling: a percutaneous approach." *American Journal of Obstetrics and Gynecology* 119 (4):539–542, 15 June 1974.

11. Hobbins, John C., and Mahoney, Maurice J. "In utero diagnosis of hemoglobinopathies: technic for obtaining fetal blood." *New England Journal of Medicine* 290(10):1065–1067, 9 May 1974.

12. Frasier, S. Douglas; Weiss, Bennett A.; and Horton, Richard. "Amniotic fluid testosterone: implications for the prenatal diagnosis of congenital adrenal hyperplasia." *Journal of Pediatrics* 84(5):738–741, May 1974.

13. Howie, R. N., and Liggins, G. C. "Prevention of respiratory distress syndrome in premature infants by antepartum glucocorticoid treatment." *In* Villee, Claude A., et al., eds., *Respiratory Distress Syndrome.* New York: Academic Press, 1973, p. 369–380.

14. Ampola, Mary G., et al. "In utero treatment of methylmalonic acidemia with vitamin B^{12}." *Pediatric Research* 8 (4):387, April 1974.

15. Goodlin, Robert C., and Schmidt, William. "Human fetal arousal levels as indicated by heart rate recordings." *American Journal of Obstetrics and Gynecology* 114 (5):613–621, 1 November 1972.

16. Liley, A. W. "The foetus as a personality." *Australian and New Zealand Journal of Psychiatry* 6 (2):99–105, June 1972. Sudman, Einar. "An embrace-reflex observed in a 5-cm human fetus." *Acta Paediatrica Scandinavica* 62(5):547–549, September 1973.

17. Winick, Myron; Brasel, Jo Anne; and Velasco, Elba G. "Effects of prenatal nutrition upon pregnancy risk." *Clinical Obstetrics and Gynecology* 16 (1):184–198, March 1973.

18. Stein, Zena, and Susser, Mervyn. "The Dutch famine, 1944–1945, and the reproductive process. I. Effects on six indices at birth." *Pediatric Research* 9 (2):70–76, February 1975.

19. Carrington, Elsie R. Editorial: "Relationship of stilbestrol exposure in utero to vaginal lesions in adolescence." *Journal of Pediatrics* 85(2), 295–296, August 1974. Forfar, John O. and Nelson, Matilda M. "Epidemiology of drugs taken by pregnant women: drugs that may affect the fetus adversely." *Clinical Pharmacology and Therapeutics* 14 (4,pt.2):632–642, July, August 1973.

20. Bolognese, Ronald J., et al. "Rubella vaccination during pregnancy." *American Journal of Obstetrics and Gynecology* 112(7):903–907, 1 April 1972. Vaheri, Antti, et al. "Isolation of attenuated rubella-vaccine virus from human products of conception and uterine cervix." *New England Journal of Medicine* 286 (20):1071–1074, 18 May 1972.

21. Chang, Henry, et al. "In utero diagnosis of hemoglobinopathies: hemoglobin synthesis in fetal red cells." *New England Journal of Medicine* 290 (19):1067–1068, 9 May 1974.

22. Gray, Bradford H. *Human Subjects in Medical Experimentation: A Sociological Study of the Conduct and Regulation of Clinical Research.* New York: Wiley-Interscience, 1975. p. 56–58.

23. Clavero, Jose A. "Blood flow in the intervillous space and fetal blood flow. I. Normal values in human pregnancies at term." *American Journal of Obstetrics and Gynecology* 116 (3):340–346, 1 June 1973. Idänpään-Heikkilä, Juhana, et al. "Elimination and metabolic effects of ethanol in mother, fetus, and newborn infant." *American Journal of Obstetrics and Gynecology* 112(3):387–393, 1 February 1972. Simmer, Hans H., et al. "On the regulation of estrogen production by cortisol and ACTH in human pregnancy at term." *American Journal of Obstetrics and Gynecology* 119 (3):283–296, 1 June 1974.

24. Philipson, Agneta; Sabath, L. D.; and Charles, David. "Transplacental passage of erythromycin and clin-

damycin." *New England Journal of Medicine* 288 (23):1219–1221, 288 (23):1219–1221, 7 June 1973.

25. Adam, Peter A. J., *et al.* "Human placental barrier to ^{125}I-glucagon early in gestation. " *Journal of Clinical Endocrinology and Metabolism* 34 (5):772–782, May 1972.

26. Murphy, Beverly E. Pearson, *et al.* "Conversion of maternal cortisol to c⌐rtisone during placental transfer to the human fetus." *American Journal of Obstetrics and Gynecology* 118 (4):538–541, 15 February 1974.

27. Mirkin, Bernard L. "Diphenylhydantoin: placental transfer, fetal localization, neonatal metabolism, and possible teratogenic effects." *Journal of Pediatrics* 78 (2):329–337, February 1971.

28. Kauffman, Ralph E.; Morris, John A.; and Azaroff, Daniel L. "Placental transfer and fetal urinary excretion of gentamicin during constant rate maternal infusion." *Pediatric Research* 9 (2):104–107, February 1975.

29. Wentz, Anne C.; Burnett, Lonnie C.; and King, Theodore M. "Methodology in premature pregnancy termination." *Obstetrical and Gynecological Survey* 28 (1):2–19, January 1973; 29 (1):6–42, January 1974.

30. Galen, Robert S., *et al.* "Fetal pathology and mechanism of fetal death in saline-induced abortion: a study of 143 gestations and critical review of the literature." *American Journal of Obstetrics and Gynecology* 120 (3):347–355, 1 October 1974.

31. Nochimson, David J., *et al.* "The effects of ritodrine hydrochloride on uterine activity and the cardiovascular system." *American Journal of Obstetrics and Gynecology* 118(4):523–528, 15 February 1974. Gray, Bradford. *Op. cit.* n. 22, p. 59–65.

32. Freeman, Roger K., *et al.* "Fetal cardiac response to paracervical block anesthesia." *American Journal of Obstetrics and Gynecology* 113(5):583–591, 1 July 1972.

33. Rudolph, Abraham M., *et al.* "Studies on the circulation of the previable human fetus." *Pediatric Research* 5(9):452–465, September 1971. Morris, John A., *et al.* "Measurement of fetoplacental blood volume in the human previable fetus." *American Journal of Obstetrics and Gynecology* 118 (7):927–934, 1 April 1974.

34. Rudolph, Abraham M., *et al. Op. cit.*, n. 35. Morris, J. A.; Haswell, G. L.; and Hustead, R. F. "Research in the human mid-trimester fetus." *Obstetrics and Gynecology* 39(4), 634–635, April 1972.

35. King, Katherine, *et al.* "Differing sensitivity of human fetal receptor sites to arginine-induced insulin and growth hormone release." *Pediatric Research* 7(4):329, April 1973.

36. Gaull, Gerald; Sturman, John A.; and Räihä, Niels C. R. "Development of mammalian sulfur metabolism: absence of cystathionase in human fetal tissues." *Pediatric Research* 6 (6):538–547, June 1972.

37. Adam, Peter A. J., *et al. Op. cit.*, n. 27.

38. This section will not discuss experimentation involving the clearly-viable fetus, which is generally considered to be a newborn infant.

39. Kormano, Martti; Timonen, Henri; and Luukkainen, Tapani. "Microangiographic observations on the uterine and maternal placental vasculature in early human pregnancy." *American Journal of Obstetrics and Gynecology* 120 (1):8013, 1 September 1974.

40. Adam, Peter A. J.; Räihä, Neils; Rabiala, Eeva-Lüsa, *et al.* "Cerebral oxidation of glucose and D-BOH-BUTYRATE by the isolated perfused human fetal head." *Pediatric Research* 7(4):309, April 1973.

41. Sturman, John A., and Gaull, Gerald E. "Polyamine biosynthesis in human fetal liver and brain." *Pediatric Research* 8(4):231–237, April 1974.

42. Kirby, Lorne, and Hahn, Peter. "Enzyme response to prednisolone and dibutryl adenosine 3', 5'-monophosphate in human fetal liver." *Pediatric Research* 8(1):37–41, January 1974. Kirby, Lorne, and Hahn, Peter. "Enzyme induction in human fetal liver." *Pediatric Research* 7(2):75–81, February 1973.

43. Goodlin, Robert C. "Cutaneous respiration in a fetal incubator." *American Journal of Obstetrics and Gynecology* 85(5):571–579, 1 July 1963.

44. Chamberlain, Geoffrey. "An artificial placenta." *American Journal of Obstetrics and Gynecology* 100(5):615–626, 1 March 1968.

45. The major discussions of ethical issues in fetal research are the following:

a. Report of the Advisory Group. *The Use of Fetuses and Fetal Material for Research.* London: Her Majesty's Stationery Office, 1972.

b. Morison, Robert S., and Twiss, Sumner B. "The human fetus as useful research material." *Hastings Center Report* 3 (2):8–10, April 1973.

c. National Institutes of Health, Department of Health, Education, and Welfare. "Protection of human subjects: policies and procedures." *Federal Register* 38 (221): 31738–31749, 16 November 1973.

d. Walters, LeRoy. "Ethical issues in experimentation on the human fetus." *Journal of Religious Ethics* 2 (1):33–54, Spring 1974.

e. Reback, Gary L. "Fetal experimentation: moral, legal, and medical implications." *Stanford Law Review* 26 (5):1191–1207, May 1974.

f. Office of the Secretary, Department of Health, Education, and Welfare. "Protection of human subjects: proposed policy." *Federal Register* 39 (165):30648–30657, 23 August 1974.

g. Ramsey, Paul. *The Ethics of Fetal Research.* New Haven: Yale University Press, 1975.

46. Jonas, Hans. "Philosophical reflections on experimenting with human subjects." *Daedalus* 98 (2):219–247, Spring 1969. Ramsey, Paul. "Consent as a canon of loyalty with special reference to children in medical investigation." *In his The Patient as Person: Explorations in Medical Ethics.* New Haven: Yale University Press, 1970, p. 1–58.

47. McCormick, Richard A. "Proxy consent in the experimentation situation." *Perspectives in Biology and Medicine* 18 (1):2–20, Autumn 1974.

48. Louisell, David. "Abortion, the practice of medicine and the due process of law." *UCLA Law Review* 16 (2):233ff., February 1969. Note. "The law and the unborn child: the legal and logical inconsistencies." *Notre Dame Lawyer* 46:349ff., Winter 1971.

RICHARD WASSERSTROM

Ethical Issues Involved in Experimentation on the Non-Viable Human Fetus

THE STATUS OF THE FETUS

I do not believe that the question of the morality of experimentation on living, non-viable fetuses can be sensibly considered without some attention being paid at the outset to the question of what kind of an entity a human fetus is. Although some of the relevant arguments do not depend, even implicitly, upon an answer to this question, the great majority of them do. That this is so can be seen, I think from the fact that the question of experimentation is a very different one if the fetus is thought to be fundamentally like a piece of human tissue or organ, e.g., an appendix, than if the fetus is thought to be fundamentally like a fully developed, adult human being with normal capacities and abilities.

There are four different views that tend to be held concerning the status of the human fetus. They are: (a) that the fetus is in most if not all morally relevant respects like a fully developed, adult human being. At least two major arguments can be given in support of this position. The first is a theological argument which fixes conception as the time at which the entity acquires a soul. And since possession of a soul is what matters morally and what distinguishes human beings from other entities, the fetus is properly regarded as like all other persons. The second argument focuses upon the similarities between a developing fetus and a newly born infant. In briefest form, the argument goes as follows. It is clear that we regard a newly born infant as like an adult in all morally relevant respects. Infants as well as adults are regarded as persons who are entitled to the same sorts of

protection, respect, etc. But there are no significant differences between newly born infants and fetuses which are quite fully developed and about to be born. What is more, there is no point in the developmental life of the fetus which can be singled out as the morally significant point at which to distinguish a fetus not yet at that point from one which has developed beyond it and hence is now to be regarded as a person. Therefore, fetuses are properly regarded from the moment of conception as having the same basic status as an infant. And since infants are properly regarded as having the same basic status as adults, fetuses should also be so regarded.

Now, of course, on this view abortion, whether before or after viability, raises enormous moral problems, since it is morally comparable to infanticide and homicide, generally. And the morality of abortion *per se* is beyond the scope of the present inquiry. This view is nonetheless directly relevant, even on the assumption that abortion prior to viability is morally permissible. For on this view, for instance, experimentation ex utero [outside the uterus] upon a non-viable living fetus is to be seen as analogous to experimentation upon, say an adult human being who is in a coma and who will die within the next few hours. Thus, on this view, the moral problems of experimentation ex utero would be thought to be similar to those of experimentation upon adults whose deaths were imminent and who were themselves unconscious.

(b) That the fetus is in most if not all morally relevant respects like a piece of tissue or a discrete human organ, e.g., a bunch of hair or a kidney. The argument in support of this view focuses upon all of the ways in which fetuses are different from typical adults with typical abilities. In particular, the absence of an ability

Reprinted from National Commission for the Protection of Human Subjects of Biomedical and Behavioral Research, *Research on the Fetus: Appendix* (Washington, D.C.: U.S. Department of Health, Education, and Welfare, 1975).

to communicate, to act autonomously (morally, as well as physically), to be aware of one's own existence, and/or to experience sensations of pain and pleasure would singly and collectively be taken to be sufficient grounds for regarding the fetus as more like an organ growing within the woman's body than like any other kind of entity. It should be noted, too, that for our purposes this view includes all those positions which regard the status of the fetus as changing from something like a human organ to something else only at or after the moment of viability has been reached. For this inquiry is concerned only with experimentation upon non-viable fetuses.

On this view there are, I think, virtually no arguments against experimentation ex utero and only a few arguments against experimentation in utero. Whatever, for example, can properly be done to a severed human organ which still has certain life capacities—e.g., it is capable of being transplanted into another human, or it still maintains some of its organ function—can properly be done to the non-viable fetus ex utero in those few hours before its life functions have ceased.

(c) That the fetus is in most if not all morally relevant respects like an animal, such as a dog or a monkey. The fetus is, on this view, clearly not a person, nor is it just a collection of tissue or an organ. It is an entity which is at most entitled only to the same kind of respect that many (but not necessarily all) persons think is due to the "higher" animals. It is wrong to inflict needless cruelty on animals—perhaps because they do suffer or perhaps because of what this reveals about the character of the human imposing the cruelty. And fetuses are, basically in the same class.

On this view, too, there are comparatively few worries about experimentation ex utero on non-viable fetuses. At most, the worries are of the same sort that apply to experimentation upon living animals. For the most part, it is proper to regard them as objects to be controlled, altered, killed, or otherwise used for the benefit of humans—subject only to concerns relating to the infliction of needless and perhaps intentional pain and suffering upon the entities being experimented upon, and (in the

case of those higher animals we most identify with) to prohibitions upon their consumption as food.

(d) That the fetus is in a distinctive, relatively unique moral category, in which its status is close to but not identical with that of a typical adult. On this view the status of the fetus is both different from and superior to that of the "higher" animals. It is, perhaps, closest to the status of the newly born infant in a culture in which infanticide is regarded as a very different activity from murder or to the status of the insane, the mentally defective or slaves—again in cultures which see them as less than persons but as clearly superior to animals. The case for regarding fetuses as belonging to a special, discrete class of entities rests, I think, largely on the fetus' potential to become in the usual case a fully developed adult human being. Conceding that the fetus is significantly different from an adult in respect to such things as its present capacity to act autonomously, to experience self-consciousness, and perhaps even to experience pain, this view emphasizes the distinctiveness of the human fetus as the entity capable in the ordinary course of events of becoming a fully developed person. This view sees the value of human life in the things of genuine value or worth that persons are capable of producing, creating, enjoying, and being, e.g., works of art, interpersonal relations of love, trust and benevolence, and scientific and humanistic inquiries and reflections. Correspondingly, it sees the distinctive value of the fetus as being alone the kind of entity that can some day produce, create, enjoy and be these things of genuine value and worth.

It is, I think, especially important to notice the implications of this view for the morality of experimentation upon non-viable fetuses ex utero. For it is the non-viability of the fetus that goes, I believe, a long way toward making experimentation a substantially less troublesome act than it would otherwise be. That is to say, it is evident, I think, that on this view abortion is a morally worrisome act because it involves the destruction of an entity that possesses the potential to produce and be things of the highest value. However, if an abortion has been performed and if the fetus is still non-viable, then experimentation upon the fetus in no way affects the fetus' ability, or lack thereof, ever to realize any of its existing potential. On this view especially, abortion, not experimentation upon the non-viable fetus, is the fundamental, morally problematic activity.

SPECIFIC ISSUES RELATING TO EXPERIMENTATION EX UTERO

I propose now. . . to turn to an examination of what seem to me to be the specific issues that arise in thinking about the morality of experimentation upon non-viable, living, human fetuses ex utero. The examination will be divided into four parts: (a) an enumeration and analysis of the arguments against experimentation; (b) an enumeration and analysis of the arguments in favor of experimentation; (c) an enumeration and discussion of some specific problems that arise in respect to the question of consent; and (d) a statement of my own view about the permissibility of experimentation.

THE MAJOR ARGUMENTS AGAINST EXPERIMENTATION UPON NON-VIABLE, LIVING, HUMAN FETUSES EX UTERO

The arguments can be divided in a rough fashion into two groups: those that, on the one hand, oppose experimentation because of the possible, deleterious consequences that are thought to follow from the legitimization of such a practice; and those that, on the other hand, oppose experimentation because of some feature of the situation that is seen to be itself wrong or improper. I begin with the former collection of arguments—those that concentrate upon the possible, deleterious consequences.

Possible, deleterious consequences of permitting a practice of fetal experimentation. One general argument here is that if such a practice is permitted and well publicized, then individuals and, in some related sense, the society will become less sensitive to values and claims which are entitled to the greatest respect. Thus, one specific version of this general line of attack is the argument that individuals

will become less sensitive than they ought to be to the value of human life. Another specific claim is that individuals will become less sensitive than they ought to be to the rights and needs of persons who are, for one reason or other, incapable of looking after themselves, e.g., infants, the aged, and the seriously ill or retarded. Still a third, related worry is that individuals will become less sensitive than they ought to be to the claims of those persons whose deaths are reasonably thought to be certain and imminent, e.g., persons in the last stages of terminal illnesses. And a fourth, consequential concern is that individuals will become less sensitive than they ought to be to the rights of persons not to be the unwilling subjects of experimentation.

I think one thing that is of interest about all four of these arguments is that they can retain some if not all of their force irrespective of what is thought in fact to be the correct view about the kind of entity a fetus is. That is to say, consider the claim that permitting fetal research may lead individuals to become less sensitive than they ought to be to the rights and needs of persons who are, for one reason or another, incapable of looking after themselves. Even someone who is convinced that a fetus is basically like a human organ might nonetheless legitimately worry about the inferences that individuals would mistakenly draw from the permissibility of a practice of fetal research. As long as it is reasonable to believe that persons, in any significant number, might mistakenly suppose that the principle which justified fetal experimentation was a principle which justified experimentation upon any entity that was incapable of keeping itself alive without substantial human assistance, this is a deleterious consequence of a practice of fetal experimentation which would have to be taken into account. Of course, the more one thinks that a fetus is like other persons in most significant respects, the more one is also apt to think that individuals generally may confuse the case of the fetus with the case of those other entities whose claims to morally more sensitive treatment are nonetheless distinguishable.

A rather different consequential argument goes like this. Once it becomes permissible for experiments to be done on living, non-viable fetuses, such fetuses will come to be regarded as extremely useful in medical research. The increased demand for fetuses within the scientific community will lead to the creation of a variety of subtle as well as obvious incentives for persons both to have abortions and to have them in such a way that the fetus can be a useful object of experimentation. And this is undesirable for several reasons. To begin with, unless it is the case that abortion is a morally unproblematic action, it is wrong to develop a social practice which will encourage persons to have abortions. In addition, the fact that fetuses are useful objects of experimentation might lead members of the scientific and medical community unconsciously to distort or alter their views of when persons should have abortions. Doctors might in this way take into account non-medical reasons for advising patients to have abortions. And, finally, there is always the danger that the pressures and inducements would operate unequally throughout the society—persons from a low socioeconomic status would be the ones who were more likely to be attracted by the incentives and subjected to the pressures.

Still a third argument, which may or may not be consequentialist, points to the fact that many individuals will experience revulsion and will be in psychic turmoil when they learn of fetuses being treated in this way, i.e., as objects of experimentation. The revulsion and turmoil are comparable, although less universal, . . . [to] that encountered at the thought of such things as cannibalism, and the desecration of graves. If a large number of persons respond this way, then one argument against experimentation is that it will substantially impair social peace and harmony. Because they care so strongly, they will be led to act antagonistically toward the source of their discomfort. In addition, even if the numbers are not large, the severe quality of their reactions may justify prohibition simply on the ground that the gains of experimentation do not overbalance the pain and discomfort experienced by those who are so affected.

Arguments for the Intrinsic or Direct Wrongness of Fetal Experimentation. I can identify approximately a half-dozen arguments that in some direct, non-consequential way call into question the morality of fetal experimentation upon non-viable, living fetuses. More so than in the case of the consequential arguments, the force of these arguments often depends upon the status that it is thought ought properly be accorded the fetus.

The first two arguments relate to the principle involved in fetal experimentation. One such argument is this: to permit fetal experimentation is at least to commit oneself to the principle that it is permissible to perform comparable experiments upon any living person, provided only that we have good reason to believe that the person will die very soon, i.e., within a few hours, anyway. But since it is surely wrong to experiment on persons just because they will die anyway within a few hours, experimentation on non-viable, living fetuses lacks a coherent principle of support.

The other argument is similar: to permit fetal experimentation is to commit oneself to the principle that it is permissible to perform comparable experiments on all living persons, provided only that they are no longer conscious and will not regain their consciousness before they die. But since it is surely wrong to experiment on all such persons, experimentation on non-viable living fetuses lacks a coherent principle of support.

In both cases it is, I think, clear that the force of the argument depends upon the claim that fetuses are sufficiently like other human persons so that there are no plausible, reasonably persuasive grounds upon which to distinguish the way in which the fetus is treated from the way in which other persons, e.g., the terminally ill or the unconscious, could also properly be treated. The argument appeals both to a claim that it would be wrong to treat other persons in this way and to a claim that the case of fetal experimentation cannot be readily or convincingly distinguished.

A third argument concerns the concept of viability. It is this. The concept of viability is anything but a precise one, even within medical science. It is fundamentally the idea that the fewer the number of weeks of gestation the less likely it is that any medical means presently exists by which the fetus could be kept alive until it could function without artificial support. The problem is not just one of imaginary, theoretical possibilities. Given the present state of medical technology there will at best be a range within which it is relatively likely or unlikely that the fetus could be kept alive, i.e., is viable. This means that it is not the case that all fetuses classified as non-viable for purposes of experimentation would necessarily have died no matter what steps had been taken to try to maintain their lives. Now it is clear that once a fetus is viable it is wrong to experiment upon it in ways that are potentially harmful to it. But if this is so, then in some significant number of cases comparable experiments will be performed on fetuses classified ''non-viable'' but perhaps really viable.

The plausibility of this argument depends both upon the claim that deleterious experimentation upon viable fetuses would be wrong and upon the claim that a significant number of moderately developed fetuses determined to be non-viable might in fact have proved to have been viable, if they had not been the subjects of experimentation.

A fourth argument is this: We believe that fetal experiments which directly terminate either respiration or heartbeat are wrong; see, e.g., DHEW, ''Protection of Human Subjects: Policies and Procedures.'' But there is no real difference between that and engaging in experiments in which the risk of terminating respiration or heartbeat is substantially increased. Hence, if the former is wrong, the latter must be too.

I think this argument is surely correct in its insistence upon the absence of any convincing way to distinguish experiments which directly terminate either respiration or heartbeat from those that increase the risk of termination significantly. What remains the open question, however, is whether there is any good moral reason to regard as improper experiments which directly terminate the respiration or heartbeat of a non-viable fetus.

The fifth argument concerns the general question of the relationship between means and ends in morality. Let it be conceded, so this argument goes, that good ends, e.g., the prevention of premature births, are sought to be achieved through this kind of fetal experimentation. Nonetheless, if the means used to achieve that end are morally unacceptable, it is wrong to seek that end in this way. Hence the pursuit of a good end cannot justify experimentation on non-viable fetuses.

This argument leaves two questions unanswered. To begin with, the argument assumes rather than explains the immorality of this kind of experimentation on non-viable fetuses. Unless independent grounds are offered to establish the impropriety of such experiments, the argument is at best hypothetical: if such grounds exist, they cannot be overridden by the worth of the end that is sought. In addition, the argument assumes both the possibility of separating clearly means from ends and the wrongness of using bad means to achieve a good end. Neither assumption seems to me to be unproblematic, and both would require discussion and analysis of a sort which lies beyond the scope of this inquiry.

The remaining argument relates especially to those experiments which prolong the life of the non-viable fetus, but also to some experiments which do not. The argument is that all experiments which cause the fetus more pain than it would otherwise experience are bad just in virtue of this fact. I do think that it always counts against the doing of an action that it increases the amount of pain in the world, and it always counts substantially against the doing of an action that it increases the amount of pain experienced by human beings. Thus, this argument would, I think, be a relevant argument if it were the case that it was reasonable to think that the non-viable fetus had the present capacity to experience pain, even in the sense, say, that we think animals like dogs and horses do. And the argument would be an especially important one if it were the case that it was reasonable to think that the non-viable fetus possessed the present capacity to experience pain in roughly the same sense or way in which fully developed persons do.

As has already been indicated, some of the arguments depend quite directly upon what view is held concerning the status of the fetus, and others do not. More specifically, if the non-viable fetus is properly regarded as basically a human organ or piece of tissue, little if anything more than scientific curiosity is needed to justify experimentation. In the same way, if the non-viable fetus is properly regarded as basically like a higher animal, e.g., a monkey, genuine scientific curiosity coupled with the avoidance of unnecessary suffering, if any, is all that is required.

The chief argument that applies, even if the non-viable fetus enjoys some other, more significant status, consists in a threefold claim. First, things of great usefulness vis-à-vis the preservation and improvement of human lives can be learned from these experiments. Second, things of great usefulness vis-à-vis the preservation and improvement of human lives can only be learned from these experiments. And third, to describe the fetus as non-viable is to concede that no matter what is done, all signs of life will disappear from the fetus within a very short period of time, i.e., not more than four or five hours. Thus, it is claimed, the conjunction of utility, need and inevitability combine to establish the legitimacy of this kind of experimentation, irrespective of the status of the fetus.

One important objection that this argument must confront is this: if experimentation is justifiable under these conditions, then it is also justifiable in the case of a person who is unconscious, and who will die soon without regaining consciousness, e.g., because he or she is in the last stages of a terminal illness. But because it is wrong to experiment on adults who are in this state, it cannot consistently be maintained that it is right to experiment on the fetus.

At least two responses are possible. First, it might be argued that fetuses are just in a different class from adults. To be sure, there may not be anything intrinsically wrong with experimenting on an adult in the circumstances just described. However, to permit experiment-ation would be an unwise exception to the doctrine of the sanctity of human life. Because fetuses are perceived to be different entities from fully developed persons, to permit experimentation on them is not to create the same kind of dangerous exception.

Second, it might be argued that the two cases are distinguishable in that there is no analogue to the concept of non-viability in the case of the adult. That is to say, medical science cannot identify with confidence those cases in which an individual will die soon without regaining consciousness, in the same way in which it can identify with confidence those fetuses that are not yet viable.

There is one other argument in favor of experimentation that is worth noting. It is that if there is no good, moral reason to prohibit experimentation, then a decision to prohibit it encourages the practice of making social decisions on non-rational if not irrational grounds. And this is a generally unwise thing to do. That is to say, it might be maintained that experimentation should be prohibited just because it seems wrong or offensive even though no one can give a plausible account of why it ought to be so regarded. This argument is an answer to that way of proceeding. It is an argument for the importance of restricting scientific inquiry only if there are good reasons and not, for example, irrational or superstitious objections to the investigations.

THE ISSUE OF CONSENT

There is a general problem of consent that arises: namely, that the fetus will not have consented to anything. The question is whether that should make a difference. It might be argued, of course, that an experiment is always improper unless the subject of the experiment agrees or consents to being a subject. Since the fetus did not consent to being a subject, any experimentation upon the fetus is improper. The difficulty with this position is that there is no obvious way to decide whether the principle should apply to entities who are not capable of consenting, and if so, to which kinds of entities. It will depend upon the view that is taken of the status of the fetus, and the possible answers will parallel those discussed above in the first part of the paper. If the fetus is a person, then consent will be required (but so, *a fortiori,* should consent have been required for the abortion). . . . I conclude, therefore, that no new general problem is raised by the absence of the consent of the fetus to being the subject of experimentation.

There is, however, a related issue that is worth mentioning. It is possible, I think, to hold a variety of views about the status of the fetus and still believe that the mother, or perhaps both parents, have a legitimate claim to have their consent secured before any fetal experimentation occurs. The justification cannot, of course, be that to require the consent of the parents will protect the fetus from harm. This is because, having elected to terminate the pregnancy, the parents are already in a non-traditional, atypical relationship vis-à-vis the offspring. So it cannot be that the consent of the parents should be required as a means of protecting the fetus, or looking after its interests. Still, the parents may have sensibilities, attitudes, etc. that are deserving of respect—sensibilities, etc. that correspond to those of living persons toward a deceased relative. It is not exactly that they "own" the deceased, but that they do have a legitimate claim to decide how the body of the deceased shall be dealt with. In the same way, I think, parents of an aborted fetus could still quite often see themselves as being in a similar relationship to the fetus, such that they would feel themselves injured in serious ways were the fetus to become the subject of experimentation without their agreement. For this reason, I believe that the consent of the mother (in the case of an unmarried woman) or of both parents to any experimentation should be required before the abortion occurs, and that the nature of the proposed experiments should be explained carefully and fully to them.

RECOMMENDATIONS CONCERNING
EXPERIMENTATION EX UTERO

My own view is that the fetus enjoys the kind of unique moral status described in. . . (d)

above. Hence, abortion on demand seems to me to be a very troublesome moral issue. If the morality of the abortion is not in question, however, then I somewhat uncertainly conclude that experimentation ex utero may be permissible provided the following conditions are satisfied:

1. The consent of the mother (if unmarried) or of both parents should be procured before the abortion, and the experiments clearly described to those whose consent is required.

2. It should be determined by a body independent of those proposing the experiments that the experiments can reasonably be expected to yield important information or knowledge concerning the prevention of harm or the treatment of illness in other human beings. That same body should also determine that the desired information or knowledge is not reasonably obtainable in other ways.

3. Those medical persons who counsel a woman concerning abortion and secure the requisite consent should not be the same persons—or affiliated directly with those persons—who will be involved in the experimentation.

4. No experiments should be permitted on an aborted fetus which might in fact be viable, given the state of present medical ability.

SPECIFIC ISSUES RELATING TO
EXPERIMENTATION IN UTERO

The cases that seem to me to be problematic are those in which there is a reasonable risk that the experiment will be harmful to the fetus and in which the experiments are not undertaken in order to benefit the particular fetus. Much of what has been said about experimentation ex utero applies to these cases as well. In addition, however, there are several new arguments that are relevant only in these cases.

The most significant one against experimentation in utero is that the fetus' non-viability has not yet been established in the same way in which it has been in the case of experimentation ex utero. That is to say, in the latter case, the abortion has already occured and ex hypothesis the fetus cannot survive no matter what is done. In the former case, however, the abortion has yet to take place, and until it does there is always the genuine possibility that the mother may change her mind and decide not to have the abortion at all.

Because this is so, the possibility of intervening injury resulting from the experimentation creates the following dilemma. On the one hand, if the mother changes her mind and decides not to have the abortion, the chances have thereby been increased that she will give birth to a child who is unnecessarily injured. It seems unfair to the child, the society, and the parents to bring into the world a child with defects or disabilities that could have been prevented.

On the other hand, if the mother is required to proceed with the abortion because the experiments have been undertaken, the state is regarding the original consent to the abortion as irrevocable and it is, in essence, requiring her to submit to the abortion against her will.

There is, in addition, a related matter. The fact that potentially damaging experiments have been performed on the fetus will itself constitute an added inducement to the mother to go through with the abortion and not change her mind. That is to say, experimentation itself makes abortion more likely because the belief that the fetus has been injured will make the mother less likely to change her mind. If abortion is viewed as the kind of serious act that ought not be "artificially" encouraged, then the intervening experimentation may be objected to as just such an "artificial" inducement or encouragement to stay with the original decision to have the abortion.

For the above (and other) reasons I think it important that the decision to have an abortion be kept easily revocable, up until the time of the abortion. And for this reason I do not think that any experiments in utero should be permitted, where those experiments involve a substantial risk of injury to the fetus.

WILLARD GAYLIN AND MARC LAPPÉ

Fetal Politics: The Debate on Experimenting with the Unborn

. . .Our purpose here is not to describe the wide range of research that might be morally acceptable to a reasonable majority of people. It is, rather, to establish a minimal, plausible case for fetal experimentation.

To begin with, we will consider experimentation only on the living fetus. To allow the dead products of abortion a privilege and dignity beyond those of the dead body is irrational and offensive; as long as we permit autopsy and exploitation of parts of the human body, we should permit evaluation and use of the products of abortion.

Reprinted by permission of the authors from *Atlantic Monthly*, May 1975, pp. 66–71. Copyright © 1975 Willard Gaylin and Marc Lappé.

In establishing a minimal case, we should eliminate all research which could just as well be done on laboratory animals as on the fetus. The fetus must never be regarded as a convenient or inexpensive laboratory animal. We would draw an arbitrary line between *in utero* and *ex utero* research. Recognizing that a whole set of new considerations and new moral dilemmas are created when we extend the life of a fetus outside of the womb for purposes of experimentation, we would not consider this research. And we would distinguish our case from research done on the expendable or replenishable by-products of conception, notably those cells shed into the amniotic fluid or the fluid itself, recognizing that contingent upon adequate demonstration of the safety of obtaining these materials through "amniocentesis," this research raises special problems other than violating the integrity of the fetus.

The most justifiable experiment would seem to us to be that which is closest to the therapeutic model. Of course, in the case of abortion the fetus cannot be "helped" by being experimented upon since it is doomed to death anyhow, but perhaps its death can be ennobled because it serves those more fortunate. If the doomed fetus could be used to supply the information that would permit those same parents, or similar parents, a greater opportunity for a healthy wanted child, we would have a persuasive argument for experimentation. The classic example would involve a disease lethal or damaging to the gestating child and a vaccine or drug that would prevent the disease in an expectant mother. The vaccine has been proved harmless or the drug efficacious to adults, though its effect on the developing fetus is unknown, i.e., it may be harmless or therapeutic or it may be more destructive than the disease.

The development of the rubella vaccination against German measles is a prototypic example. Exposure to German measles causes serious abnormalities in 20 to 40 percent of exposed fetuses. To protect the developing fetus against infection, mothers must be immunized, but for many years no one knew whether the rubella vaccine would harm the fetus itself. Pre-abortion studies were virtually the only way to determine quickly the safety of rubella vaccine. The alternatives would be to give the vaccine to an exposed expectant mother who wanted her child, running the risk of seriously damaging or killing the child; not to give her the vaccine, allowing her the option of carrying to term a possibly congenitally defective child; to abort what might be a healthy fetus to avoid the roughly one-out-of-three odds of having a child with some defect. (We now bypass these dilemmas by vaccinating pre-adolescent girls or a maximal portion of the population of grade-schoolers.)

The alternative, to do research on fetuses, seems clearly the most humane solution. Since we know we are going to destroy, dismember, and discard the fetus in a procedure known as abortion, it seems a small indignity to expose it to the rubella vaccine just prior to that termination, and in the process determine whether or not there is an effect on the unborn child. At best the vaccine would not affect the child, and if the woman were to change her mind, the pregnancy would have been protected; at worst, the fetus would have been exposed to an attenuated form of a virus which otherwise causes abnormalities in one case out of three.

This minimal sort of research, which begins while the woman is still pregnant and ends with an assay of her aborted fetus, is precisely the research expressly prohibited by the new federal regulations, despite the knowledge that the testing of new vaccines or potential therapies for genetic diseases which might prevent congenital abnormalities or fetal death *requires* such study.

Consider the recent occurrences. In a joint study to determine the safety of the rubella vaccine, a research team headed by Dr. Antti Vaheri at the University of Helsinki, including workers at Case Western Reserve University and the National Institutes of Health, gave one form of rubella vaccine to thirty-five pregnant women some eleven to thirty days before abortion. In the United States, all that was done was to conduct a test for presence of the virus in the aborted fetus, yet the NIH contacted the U.S. researchers and "reached an agreement" with them to suspend further work.

In 1972, when smallpox broke out over a large area of Yugoslavia, the large-scale vaccination program there was hampered by a nagging uncertainty over whether a possible risk to an unborn child would exist if the vaccine virus were given to pregnant women. Because of this concern, women who were pregnant—and therefore, their fetuses—were denied protection from the ravages of smallpox which, since 1932, has been known to be capable of causing fetal death. More important, women who were vaccinated unknowingly while in the very early stages of pregnancy had to be urged to abort because of the unknown risks of the vaccine to their fetuses. As a result, many more fetal deaths were probably caused by our lack of knowledge than by the epidemic itself. If Yugoslavia or other countries had been encouraged, or permitted, to expose a small number of pregnant women already committed to abortion, we might have learned if the vaccine virus crossed the placenta, and much fetal death could have been avoided.

An appalling range of viral infection (chicken pox, mumps, measles, hepatitis, etc.) is associated with an increased risk of fetal disability or death, especially during the first trimester, and there is increasing need for research leading to the protection of the fetus from these agents.

One lesser known but serious condition during pregnancy is that caused by the cytolomegalovirus. This infection is estimated to cause between 1000 and 3000 cases of mental retardation in this country annually. As long as the vaccine research is not permitted, we will be encouraging abortion in all cases of exposure to this virus, since most parents will not want to run the risk of having a mentally retarded or seriously damaged child.

We find ourselves, therefore, in a peculiar position. The total destruction of one or two *normal* fetuses to protect against the possible birth of one *abnormal* fetus, under current law in the United States, is not legally objectionable. We allow and sometimes encourage just such a practice in the case of a male fetus at risk for hemophilia. Here, abortion of the *normal* male, virtually indistinguishable from its affected brother, is sanctioned to ensure that half the time, a hemophilic fetus is eliminated. Yet to do research which might save both infants on a fetus that is about to be destroyed is, if we accept the current status quo, morally objectionable. We will, in addition, have to permit the birth of many seriously crippled children when exposure to the virus or presence of genetic disease has not been detected, or the parent is morally opposed to abortion.

At some point it becomes unethical *not* to do fetal experimentation. We believe that point has been reached when the research has as its objective the saving of the lives (or the reduction of defects) of other, wanted fetuses. Certainly the cost of not doing studies which could provide a means to protect the developing fetus against a viral or bacterial infection which may be fatal or crippling is greater than the costs here incurred. The medical ethic "do no harm" would, of course, be violated—but we already violated that principle when we accepted the concept of abortion. The ultimate harm of destroying the fetus trivializes that which precedes it. Yet abortion is legal, and we are in the ridiculous position of having legalized abortion while prosecuting researchers. Four doctors are currently under indictment in Boston for having performed an experiment to determine if antibiotics to combat fetal syphilis could breach the placenta in therapeutic concentrations. The charge: "illegal dissection," as defined by an 1814 Massachusetts grave-robbing statute.

In an ideal world, no experimentation on any human beings, or on any living things, would be permitted. We do not live in a perfect world, and any experimentation on living creatures probably desensitizes us to a certain extent. As those creatures approach personhood, the restrictions on the experimentation become more urgent and more necessary. But "not doing" is a form of doing, as we have shown. Not permitting a treatment is permitting a disease. The distinctions between passive and active harm are increasingly difficult to determine. If we do not do research on unwanted fetuses, we will do it on wanted fetuses, and indeed on children. Every new utilization of a drug, operative procedure, vaccine, or antibiotic on a human patient is an experiment and involves an act of faith. Any laboratory animal differs in reaction from a human being in significant ways. The first person on whom any new procedure is used is therefore an experimental animal, and often subject to fatality. Since we did not test the thalidomides on unwanted fetuses, we tested them unwittingly on wanted ones.

"No experimentation" is not an option. Society demands the alleviation of diseases and deformities of children. We will continue to experiment. We have the choice only of which experimental population. At worst, fetal research degrades abortion by making it a vehicle for ends of no relevance to the specific life it takes; at best, however, it endows the process of abortion with human values it will not otherwise have.

In all of this we must never reduce even the unwanted fetus to the level of an experimental animal. We must recognize the nobility of that which it might have been: we must honor its potential. But we must not err in the opposite direction. We must not guard the "rights" of the about-to-be-destroyed fetus at the expense of the safety and health of the wanted, about-to-be-born child.

Experimentation with Prisoners

FRANK J. AYD, JR.

Drug Studies in Prisoner Volunteers

The use of prisoners as volunteer medical research subjects has been and is controversial. This is attested to by the statements made during the Congressional hearings, and by the Food and Drug Administration, the National Institutes of Health, and the Pharmaceutical Industry, after publication in the *New York Times* on July 28, 1969, of a lengthy, in-depth report on prisoner-participants in drug investigations and biomedical research.[1] Some say that, in any circumstance, the use of inmate volunteers is unethical and should be prohibited.[2] They cite some abuses and agree with Starzl[3] at the University of Colorado who stopped using prisoners as research subjects because "there is every reason to believe that this practice, however equitably handled in a local situation, would inevitably lead to abuse if accepted as a reasonable precedent and broadly applied."

The objectors to the use of prisoners as experimental subjects argue that these men and women are exploited, albeit for a good cause. The experiments usually are not for the volunteer's benefit. They possibly may advance scientific knowledge and aid others. Hence, the dissenters dispute the right of the prisoner to volunteer and question the motives for his willingness to be a "guinea pig." They doubt if informed consent can be obtained from incarcerated people who are paid to take a possibly toxic drug or to have a painful biopsy, contending that payment is coercion. They admit that prisoners who serve as research subjects seldom receive any reduction in sentences or favoritism regarding parole. Nevertheless, they believe that prisoners are further coerced into volunteering by their desire to exchange the monotony, oppressiveness, and often inhumane prison living conditions for the prestige and ego-satisfaction garnered from participation in potentially fruitful research and the admittedly better living conditions in a special research unit.

Despite all the misgivings that have been voiced and the objections that have been raised, the simple truth is that ethical studies

Reprinted with permission of the author and the publisher from *Southern Medical Journal*, Vol. 65, No. 4 (April 1972), pp. 440–44.

using prisoner volunteers for medical research have been done in the past and will be in the future. Furthermore, while there have been unethical experiments involving prisoners, it can be asserted forthrightly that they have been infrequent indeed. These exceptional abuses do not preclude ethical drug studies in prisoners but they do make it mandatory that investigators determine with as much certitude as possible: (1) the criteria necessary for assuring that the study is ethical, and (2) the safeguards that will minimize the risk of a study being unethical. To do this, consideration must be given to: (1) the clinical investigator, (2) the experimental subject, and (3) the purpose, design and conduct of the trial.

THE CLINICAL INVESTIGATOR

Beecher[4] has stated correctly, "A study is ethical or not at its inception." This being so, it is obvious that only the clinical investigator can assure that a trial is ethical. It is the clinical investigator who conceives the study, who is the architect of the protocol or at least its scientific and ethical judge, who is the selector of the participants, who is responsible for indoctrinating volunteers and for procuring their informed consent, who is the conductor or supervisor of the project, who must decide whether a trial is to continue or be terminated when side effects or complications arise, and who is the evaluator of the results of the trial.

Clearly a clinical investigator not only must be qualified by training and experience to execute a drug study, but he must be a man whose personal and professional ethical codes and whose moral integrity are impeccable. He also must be a conscientious, compassionate, and responsible scientist who unhesitatingly places the rights and welfare of his subjects over his desire to conduct and complete a drug study. Such a man will familiarize himself thoroughly with all available data on the investigational drug. He will refrain from extorting consent from volunteers who trust him implicitly. On the contrary, such an investigator will scrupulously provide the prospective subject with all the facts needed to make a prudent decision, so the volunteer can give or withhold informed consent. He acknowledges that his desire to make an important scientific discovery or a significant contribution to medical science through his research may unwittingly impel him to disregard the welfare and rights of his subjects. Consequently, such an investigator would submit willingly a complete protocol of the proposed drug study, prior to its initiation, for review by peers competent to evaluate its scientific and ethical merits or flaws. He also would have the protocol inspected and judged by anyone else: for example, prison officials, who have the right and duty to know fully what is proposed and how it will be performed, so that the study may be approved or disapproved. He will not object to but welcome monitoring by others qualified to do so from the inception to the conclusion of the study. He would do these things because he is not reluctant to have his conscience or his scientific expertise reinforced and to have the opinion of capable peers provide any corrective necessary.

EXPERIMENTAL SUBJECTS

Usually when a notice asking for volunteers to be experimental subjects is brought to the attention of prison inmates, more prisoners offer themselves than are needed for the research project. Since this happens even before the prisoners are given a detailed explanation of the nature of the study and the possible inconveniences, discomforts, and risks involved, it is important to know who volunteers and why.

Among the most often cited reasons for a prisoner's willingness to be an experimental subject are:

(1) Financial reward. I believe that a prisoner has the right to payment for serving as a research subject, just as nonprisoner volunteers are paid. However, I concur completely with Freund[5] who suggested that "the amount paid should not be so large as to constitute undue influence—that is, so large as to obscure an appreciation of the risk and weaken the will to self-preservation. We ought not be put in the business of buying lives."

(2) Hope for a reduction of sentence. This is no longer valid since prisoners who serve as

medical research subjects rarely receive any reduction in sentences or favoritism regarding parole.

(3) Direct or indirect seeking of medical or psychiatric help through professional advice, or a drug.

(4) To escape a lonely, tedious existence.

(5) To have something to do and talk about.

(6) To participate in what is looked upon as a stimulating, exciting adventure.

(7) A desire to prove to himself and to others that he can do something good and admirable.

(8) To command and receive respect and accolades from others. An experimental subject is no longer a nonentity in prison.

(9) Some form of psychopathology. For instance, many prisoners are "risk-takers" guided by the attitude "What have I got to lose?" They volunteer to be research subjects to gratify self-destructive urges.

(10) The absence of obligations to others.

(11) Simple curiosity.

These motives for offering to be a research subject by prisoners, with the exception of the hope for a reduction of sentence, are identical to those listed for nonprisoner volunteers by Lasagna and von Felsinger,[6] Pollin and Perlin,[7] and others.[8]

A prisoner who offers to participate in medical research has several reasons for his decision that to him seem realistic and valid. These motives create for him a psychologic set that impels him to volunteer and at times to mask or deny anything that would make him ineligible. This psychologic set of the prisoner volunteer poses a challenge to an investigator. He must be fully cognizant of its existence and be appreciative of the barrier it may be to securing informed consent. He must realize that he must take a very comprehensive history and do a very thorough work-up of the volunteer to be certain the prisoner is not deliberately hiding or denying any physical or mental condition that would make him an unsuitable research subject. Since a significant number of presumed "normal" volunteers for research projects may have various types and severity of psychopathology, a clinical investigator should look out for these individuals, not necessarily to exclude them from the study, but to be able to assess more accurately the drug responses they may have.

INFORMED CONSENT

There is no doubt that after a volunteer has been carefully screened to ascertain his suitability for inclusion in a drug trial, the major tasks of the investigator are the avoidance of even subtle coercion and the obtaining of informed consent. Precisely what the latter means and how it can be secured is the subject of much disagreement. Nevertheless, just as a prisoner has the right to volunteer, so too does he have the right to refuse. It is for this reason that a clinical investigator is legally and morally obliged to obtain informed consent. To enable an investigator to do this, the Food and Drug Administration, on August 30, 1966, set down the following guidelines for subject consent in regard to investigational new drug use in man:

"Consent" or "informed consent" means that the person involved has legal capacity to give consent, is so situated as to be able to exercise free power of choice, and is provided with a fair explanation of all material information concerning the administration of the investigational drug, or his possible use as a control, as to enable him to make an understanding decision as to his willingness to receive said investigational drug. This latter element requires that before the acceptance of an affirmative decision by such person the investigator should make known to him the nature, duration and purpose of the administration of said investigational drug; the method and means by which it is to be administered; all inconveniences and hazards reasonably to be expected, including the fact, where applicable, that the person may be used as a control; the existence of alternative forms of therapy, if any; and the effects upon his health or person that may possibly come from the administration of the investigational drug. Said patient's consent shall be obtained in writing by the investigator.

An investigator should be guided by the principle of doing what is just for an experimental subject. As pointed out by Angela Holder[9] in an excellent three-part report on informed consent, there are no definite standards that are imposed by law other than the obligation to refrain from misrepresentation. A prospective research subject has a right to know what is likely to happen but the courts agree that what and how much he is to be told is a matter of medical judgment. As long as the investigator attempts to be fair to all concerned and bears in mind that standards of due care require reasonable explanations, no court expects more of him. He is not required to explain in detail all imaginable risks when such explanation would be harmful, unnecessary, or unreasonable.

Any investigator capable of designing and conducting a first-class drug study should have the ingenuity necessary to obtain valid informed consent from a potential subject who is not psychotic or mentally incompetent. This may be difficult at times, but seldom is it impossible. I believe that fulfillment of the following steps should enable an investigator to decide if he has obtained informed consent:

(1) There should be a frank dialogue between investigator and volunteer, during which the investigator, in as simple terms and as concisely as possible, discusses the purposes and design of the study, the known or presumed indications for the drug and the animal and human data, if any, that support this, the dose(s) of the drug to be administered, the likely side effects, all tests to be done before, during, and at the end of the trial, and what kind of physical or mental symptoms or diseases definitely may make a participant at high risk. The volunteer should be encouraged to ask as many questions as he wishes. He should be told bluntly that it is fine to have implicit faith in the investigator but that he must not let this be overriding in his decision to participate in a research project.

(2) After the initial verbal indoctrination, the investigator should give the prospective subject a typewritten account of the same information about the proposed drug trial. This, too, should be brief and to the point. The volunteer should be urged to study this carefully and to write down any questions that occur to him. When he has reached his decision, he should request another interview with the investigator.

(3) During the second interview with the potential subject, the investigator repeats the information provided in the first verbal indoctrination and in the written communication and answers any questions asked. If the investigator is satisfied that the volunteer understands reasonably well what he is volunteering for and the possible inconveniences and hazards and is willing to sign the necessary consent form, he can assume that the consent is valid and informed. If the investigator is uncertain about the volunteer's comprehension of the proposed study, he should give him a questionnaire covering all the basic information given to him. The volunteer's replies to the questionnaire should suffice to determine if he understands and is capable of giving informed consent. The use of a questionnaire may seem troublesome but it can be worth the bother, since some individuals are poor verbal communicators and much better revealers of their comprehension, retention of information and ability to utilize information when they communicate in writing.

That investigators should use succinct explanations phrased in very simple language, when informing a prospective volunteer about a proposed drug trial has been documented very well by Epstein and Lasagna.[10] In a mock experimental situation set up to evaluate how well potential subjects comprehended the experiment and to what extent they were prepared to participate, volunteers were given 3 forms (short, medium, and long) providing information about the projected drug trial. The information contained in the 3 forms was similar in regard to its main points, differing primarily in the degree of descriptive material and hence in length. Epstein and Lasagna found that those who read the short form of the protocol in which the pertinent information was included without detailed elaboration retained significantly more of the important facts than did those shown either the intermediate or long protocol forms. Thus, they demonstrated persuasively that comprehension, maximum retention of information, and ability to utilize information intelligently is best when the presentation of data is brief and to the point.

PURPOSE, DESIGN, AND CONDUCT OF A TRIAL

Since drug studies involving prisoners usually are done for the benefit of others, it is imperative that the purpose, design and execution of the trial be such that it will provide not only scientifically valid and useful data but that it will adequately safeguard the prisoner's rights and welfare. Hence, to ensure that a proposed drug trial is ethical not only in purpose and design but in actual conduct, the investigator is obliged to have an adequately trained staff, to be sure that at all times there is ample interest in the prisoner as a person, and that there is never any lack of necessary medical supervision. The chief deficiencies in drug testing programs in prisons that have led to their criticism and halting, because they were deemed unethical, have been the lack of a qualified staff, insufficient concern for the prisoners' welfare, including inadequate safeguards for their health, improper medical supervision, and the inferior quality of the results obtained. To obviate some of these faults, it has been suggested that a Prison Experimental Review Committee be set up to advise prison boards on health risks to prisoners involved in drug testing programs.[11] In addition, because investigators may unwittingly lower their standards during a drug trial, there should be an independent watchdog body that monitors a drug study throughout for the protection and welfare of prisoner-participants.

EPILOGUE

There is no ethical problem associated with drug studies in prisoners that cannot be overcome by the assiduous efforts of a responsible clinical investigator, especially when he seeks and accepts the counsel and guidance of qualified peers. I agree completely with Hodges and Bean[12] that "the use of prison volunteers for medical research is justified and highly desirable for the investigator, for the subjects, and for society. It not only permits the conduct of human investigation under ideal circumstances, but it enables the participants to feel that they are serving a useful function as indeed they are." Furthermore, it should be stressed that, contrary to the surmise of those who consider prisoners as most unlikely to be reliable adherents to the protocol, the fact is they usually are most cooperative when a subject in a drug study. It is true that some deviate and do not disclose this for selfish reasons, just as nonprisoner volunteers sometimes do. The majority, however, do not deviate from the protocol, even when there is ample opportunity to do so. In fact, they not only comply as individuals but, because of their interest in the successful conclusion of a trial, they often police each other. Most prisoners enjoy being a member of a group doing something for the benefit of others. As McDonald[13] has pointed out, they develop a genuine esprit de corps. This can and has led to a marked improvement in behavior, independent of drug effects, as Stoffer and associates[14] have noted. The experience of these investigators derived from a drug study involving ex-addict female prisoners led them to conclude that even poorly behaved prisoners, with personality abnormalities, may make good subjects for clinical research and that many problems for the investigator can be avoided by choosing the appropriate design. Finally, I think it can be said that, more often than not, participation in a research project can and does benefit prisoners. This probably is their most important reward for being partners in medical research.

NOTES

1. Rugaber, W.: "Prison drug and plasma project leave fatal trail." *New York Times,* June 28, 1969, pp. 1, 20–21.

2. Pappworth, M. H.: *Human Guinea Pigs.* Boston, Beacon Press, 1967.

3. Starzl, T. E.: "Ethical problems in organ transplantation: clinician's point of view. In "Changing Mores of Biomedical Research." *Ann Intern Med* (Suppl 7) 67:35, 1967.

4. Beecher, H. K.: *Research and the Individual: Human Studies.* Boston, Little, Brown and Company, 1970.

5. Freund, P. A.: "Some reflections on consent." Conference on ethical aspects of experimentation on human subjects. *Daedalus* 98:314, 1969.

6. Lasagna, L., von Felsinger, J. M.: "The volunteer subject in research." *Science* 129:359–361, 1954.

7. Pollin, W., Perlin, S.: "Psychiatric evaluation of 'normal control' volunteers." *Amer J Psychiat* 115:129–133, 1958.

8. Beecher, H. K.: *Research and the Individual: Human Studies.* Boston, Little, Brown and Company, 1970.

9. Holder, A. R.: "Informed consent." *JAMA* 214:1181; 1383; 1661, 1970.

10. Epstein, L. C., Lasagna, L.: "Obtaining informed consent." *Arch Intern Med* (Chicago) 123:682–688, 1969.

11. Investigative Committee Report, Medical Association of the State of Alabama, May 30, 1969.

12. Hodges, R. E., Bean, W. B.: "The use of prisoners for medical research." *JAMA* 202:513–515, 1967.

13. McDonald, J. C.: "Why prisoners volunteer to be experimental subjects." *JAMA* 202:511–512, 1967.

14. Stoffer, S. S., Sapira, J. D., Meketon, B. F.: "Behavior in ex-addict female prisoners participating in a research study." *Compr Psychiat* 10:224–232, 1969.

ALEXANDER M. CAPRON

Medical Research in Prisons: Should a Moratorium Be Called?

A dozen years ago the late Edmond Cahn suggested the limits of human experimentation "require more attention and respect than lawyers, ethicists or experimental scientists have been giving them." In the past few years this concern has begun to be met as many scientific and lay bodies have cast a critical eye over experimental practice and consequences. I do not share the view of those scientists who have expressed alarm and dismay over this growing scrutiny. The objective of the biomedical scientists as well as of the "meddlesome intruders" is essentially the same—to reduce human suffering. This goal requires not only the advancement of knowledge through experimentation, but also adequate protection of human subjects.

It would be naive, however, to suggest that even full adherence to this laudable goal will mean that human research will be without costs. Yet it is precisely for this reason that I believe that the organs of government must play an active role in formulating policy for human experimentation and reviewing its consequences. Researchers defend their work by pointing to the benefits they may turn up "for

Reprinted with permission of the author and the Institute of Society, Ethics, and the Life Sciences from *Hastings Center Report*, Vol. 3, No. 3 (June 1973), pp. 4–6.

society," but it is doubtful that even with review by professional colleagues, they have the proper capability or authority to weigh all the societal benefits against the costs or consequences involved in their research. Thus, it is not only appropriate but very necessary that the United States Congress take part in answering a fundamental question: "When may a society, actively or by acquiescence, expose some of its members to harm in order to seek benefits for them, for others, or for society as a whole?"

Nowhere is that question more starkly posed than in the area of research with prisoners, on which I have been asked to comment. The special urgency of this issue arises from three factors: (1) the subjects involved are "captives" of the state and are only available for research at the state's sufferance; (2) their peculiar position not only renders their "consent" to participation questionable but also may lead to subtle, and often unintended, abuse by experimenters; and (3) the research is carried on in a context which lacks the peer influences and controls which characterize most other research settings.

My comments on the need for a thorough rethinking of prison research fall into two parts—first a broad question about the entire enterprise based on present practices, and second, a number of particular suggestions.

MORATORIUM ON PRISON RESEARCH

A quick survey of the recent literature pertaining to research on prisoners reveals such experiments as: (1) repeated bilateral testicular biopsies and injections of radioactive thymidine, conducted with Oregon inmates to study the rate of spermatogenesis: (2) drug testing and plasmapheresis programs in half-a-dozen institutions which left what was described as a "trail" of infection, illness and at least six deaths apparently resulting from the program; (3) research on the "aversive" conditioning effects of a drug (Anectine) which creates muscle paralysis and a sensation of suffocation (like drowning) with sixty-four "extreme acting-out criminal offenders" at the California Medical Facility. Five participants were signed up by the institution's Special Treatment Board "against their will" and another 18 indicated that "they involuntarily signed the treatment contract [in] that they felt some implied pressure to do so in the doctor's request"; (4) the use of Colorado prisoners as organ donors, a practice since halted; (5) the artificial creation of typhoid fever and other infections, in experiments conducted with Federal funds by investigators from the United States Army and the University of Maryland; (6) research, some of it sponsored by the Pentagon, on treatment for artificially induced fungi and bacteria, including Staphylococcus aureus, Candida albicans and Pseudomonas, which could cause serious—even fatal—infections; and (7) the experimental induction of scurvy in eleven prisoners in Iowa, two of whom escaped before they had developed such clinical signs as: swollen bleeding gums, perifollicular hemorrhages and congested follicles, joint swelling and pain, conjunctival hemorrhages, and bilateral femoral neuropathy. This list could be almost endlessly supplemented from medical literature as well as the popular press.

But the whole story is not told by concentrating only on the highly risky or painful studies. Just as troublesome is the huge volume of mundane and scientifically insignificant experimentation being done. In considering the combined weight of both types of current research I have reached the conclusion that a prompt and complete moratorium should be called on prison research. In other words, no new projects should be approved and wherever possible existing studies should be suspended or transferred to a non-prison setting.

I make such a far-reaching proposal because it seems the only sure way to accomplish two very important goals.

First: A moratorium is the only way to really shake up conventional, lockstep thinking on the use of prisoners as "guinea pigs." Only if we go back to the beginning and ask ourselves "Is this really necessary? Is this the best way?" will we get a true perspective.

Second: A moratorium would provide a real incentive for reevaluating the conditions, if any, under which prisoner research seems justified. At the same time, a cessation of research would provide a background of calm, rather than crisis in which to reach judgments and to formulate legislative and regulatory safeguards. Past attempts to frame guidelines or regulations have largely been responses to tragedies, or following revelations of abuses.

Objections can certainly be raised to a moratorium on prison research. It will become more difficult and expensive to conduct many studies, and some important work might be interfered with. The penal system will also be temporarily deprived of whatever financial and social benefits research programs provide.

The denial to prisoners of the opportunity to participate in research may also smack of "paternalism," but I believe that is inaccurate. I do not know whether most prisoners would support or oppose the moratorium, but I do not believe that is the prime question. The real concern is that we do what is right for society—which includes not only the avoidance of exploitation and harm to prisoners but also a proper regard for the direct and indirect costs to the state.

In many countries, including Great Britain, medical research gets along without using prisoners. That was the position taken in the World Medical Association's *Draft Code of Ethics on Human Experimentation* (1961), although that was watered down in the WMA's *Declaration of Helsinki* as adopted (1964) to refer to subjects being "in such a mental, physical, and legal state as to be able to exercise fully his power to consent."

PROBLEMS NEEDING RESOLUTION

I'd like now to comment on five specific points as examples of problems which should be resolved during a moratorium.

TYPE OF RESEARCH

Perhaps the first question which a moratorium would provoke would be whether a distinction should be drawn between studies employing prisoners as "normal volunteers" and those which are experimental forms of "treatment," based on a general penological objective or a specific psychiatric or behavioral goal for the individual prisoner. Though there would seem to be more justification (in terms of special need) for allowing the latter to resume, it would appear that such research involves some of the most troublesome types of interventions imaginable, not only in terms of psychosurgery but also in many studies on psychotropic and behavior-modifying drugs. Moreover, any analogy to the distinction between "subjects" and "patient-subjects" raises the question of who is really the "patient" (in terms of expected benefits) in such situations—the prisoner, the institution or society? Even more than in non-therapeutic drug research, the role of "patient-subject" seems to emphasize the forced options with which prisoners have to deal.

COMMITTEE REVIEW

Just as a few years ago an ideal of the clinical investigator ("intelligent, informed, conscientious, compassionate, responsible") was held out as the talisman of safe and proper human research, so it seems today that review by a committee of peers and intelligent laymen is conjured up as the magical protection. Yet the one is as certain to fail as the other—because medical education is not adequate to produce "ideal" investigators and because the regulatory bodies seem unwilling to devote the necessary ingenuity and energy to coming up with a really viable and productive committee mechanism.

First, there is much evidence that existing regulations are not well enforced. A second problem concerns what is expected of the committees. Can they do a good job without a substantial investment of time? It is also necessary to ask what function we expect the laymembers of such committees to serve. I am dubious of their ability to import "community values" into committee decision-making on an *ad hoc* basis, but I am even more skeptical of the creation of a new group of specialists in this type of work. Long-term membership in a committee would seem to me a sure-fire formula for unimaginative, routine and bureaucratic handling of the proposals.

Lay or "community" thought and values *are* very much needed in the context of formulating exact standards. On an individual case basis such input is needed to improve "informed consent" forms. This could well come by means of a "patient-subject" or "consumer" viewpoint (as expressed by prisoners). In addition to committee review, this would give prospective application the "reasonable man" standard for judging informed consent in each case, just as the recent cases in California [*Cobbs v. Grant*, 104 Cal. Rptr. 505 (1972)] and the District of Columbia [*Canterbury v. Spence*, 464 F.2d 772 (D.C. Cir. 1972)] now require its after-the-fact application according to the new standard for jury evaluations of informed consent adopted in those cases.

A final improvement in review committee procedures (which like the foregoing seems applicable outside the range of penal institutions) deserves special mention. If review committees are to progress and make "better" judgments, they need to learn from more than their own limited, local experience. Yet DHEW has done nothing, so far as I know, to develop communication among the committees. They could probably best undertake this by supporting the periodic publication of a "Clinical Investigations Reporter" established on an independent basis in a university (perhaps through joint law and medical school sponsorship). Through the resolution of "difficult cases" at the local level and on up the line, such a reporter would permit the committees to work together to develop a "common law" indicating the limits of permissibility on various parameters.

KINDS OF INSTITUTIONS

It may be that certain categories of institutions are inappropriate places for human research, either because of their condition or their population (pretrial detainees v. convicts). No limits of this sort have yet been explored.

CONSENT

Doubts about the validity of prisoner consent lie behind much of the current concern about research. Without rehashing all the old issues, I would like to mention two. First, it is necessary to make sure that information is clearly and accurately conveyed by someone who is knowledgeable enough to elaborate and answer prisoners' questions. Is it appropriate, as is now the practice in many cases, for the investigator to leave obtaining of consent to a (non-medical) subordinate?

What level of compensation is appropriate? Drawing the line between exploitation (too little paid) and undue influence (too much paid) is plainly a very hard task. Would it be useful to place restrictions on the use or destination of funds? The question of payment also raises the issue of prisoners working as lab assistants and clinical technicians, a continuing practice at many institutions which may be responsible for some gross scientific errors.

INDEMNIFICATION

Many experiments still contain exculpatory language on negligent injuries in their consent form. DHEW guidelines now prohibit this practice. We also need to consider a program of insurance for the subjects of research to cover all consequences of their participation, including those arising unforeseeably and without negligence; if we were committed to this policy we could devise ways to overcome the difficulties in distinguishing sequelae related to research from those that are unrelated.

SUGGESTED READINGS FOR CHAPTER 10

Books and Articles

Campbell, A. G. M. "Infants, Children, and Informed Consent." *British Medical Journal* 3 (August 3, 1974), 334–338.

Curran, William J., and Beecher, Henry K. "Experimentation in Children." *Journal of the American Medical Association* 210 (October 6, 1969), 77–83.

Hodges, Robert E., and Bean, William B. "The Use of Prisoners for Medical Research." *Journal of the American Medical Association* 202 (November 6, 1967), 177–179.

Ingelfinger, F. J. "Ethics of Experiments on Children." *New England Journal of Medicine* 288 (April 12, 1973), 791–792.

Jonsen, Albert R., *et al. Biomedical Experimentation on Prisoners*. San Francisco: Health Policy Program, University of California School of Medicine, 1975.

Lowe, Charles U.; Alexander, Duane; and Mishkin, Barbara. "Nontherapeutic Research on Children: An Ethical Dilemma." *Journal of Pediatrics* 84 (April, 1974), 468–472.

Marston, Robert Q. "Research on Minors, Prisoners, and the Mentally Ill." *New England Journal of Medicine* 288 (January 18, 1973), 158–159.

Mitford, Jessica. "Experiments Behind Bars." *Atlantic Monthly* 76 (January, 1973), 64–73.

Ramsey, Paul. *The Ethics of Fetal Research*. New Haven: Yale University Press, 1975.

Ramsey, Paul. "The Enforcement of Morals: Nontherapeutic Research on Children." *Hastings Center Report* 6 (August, 1976), 21–30.

Regan, Tom, and Singer, Peter. *Animal Rights and Human Obligations*. Englewood Cliffs, N.J.: Prentice-Hall, 1976.

Scarf, Maggie. "The Fetus As Guinea Pig." *New York Times Magazine*, October 19, 1975, pp. 13ff.

U.S., Department of Health, Education, and Welfare. "Protection of Human Subjects: Proposed

Policy." *Federal Register* 39 (August 23, 1974), 30648–30657.

U.S., National Commission for the Protection of Human Subjects. *Research on the Fetus: Report and Recommendations* and *Appendix*. Washington, D.C.: U.S. Department of Health, Education, and Welfare, 1975.

U.S., National Commission for the Protection of Human Subjects. *Research Involving Prisoners: Report and Recommendations* and *Appendix*. Washington, D.C.: U.S. Department of Health, Education, and Welfare, 1977.

Walters, LeRoy. "Ethical Issues in Experimentation on the Human Fetus." *Journal of Religious Ethics* 2 (Spring, 1974), 33–54.

Bibliographies

Sollitto, Sharmon and Veatch, Robert M., comps. *Bibliography of Society, Ethics and the Life Sciences*. Hastings-on-Hudson: Institute of Society, Ethics and the Life Sciences. Updated periodically. See under "Experimentation and Consent."

Walters, LeRoy, ed. *Bibliography of Bioethics*. Vols. 1- . Detroit: Gale Research Co. Issued annually. See under "Aborted Fetuses," "Children," "Fetuses," "Human Experimentation," and "Prisoners."

Part VI

BIOMEDICAL AND BEHAVIORAL TECHNOLOGIES

11.
Behavior Control

The term "behavior control" is a general label used to refer to biomedical, psychological, and social means of manipulating human actions, whether of an individual person or a group. It is defined by Perry London as "the ability to get someone to do one's bidding."[1] This definition seems to imply that behavior control is present only if one's behavior is being manipulated *by another party* and is a *coercive* manipulation. But biomedical and psychological controls might be used voluntarily by an individual to control his own behavior, as when one takes tranquilizers in order to reduce anxiety. Hence London's definition must be altered, though it is controversial how far and in which respects it should be augmented.

There is nothing very new about the idea that techniques can be used to control human behavior. Political authorities in many states have long known about pressure tactics used to control political dissidents. Even powerful drugs and brain surgery are not recent in origin. Relatively new, however, are several sophisticated applications of older control methods, as well as some novel techniques developed by modern science and psychology. The implications of these modern developments are currently being assessed in order to discover their efficacy as treatments, the precision with which predictions can be made using such techniques, and the conditions under which they are and are not ethically acceptable. Some of these techniques have aroused considerable public interest. Examples are the use of new tranquilizing and energizing drugs, psychotherapies, and programs of behavioral modification. Other techniques have received less extensive use, perhaps because of their relative unavailability. Examples include surgical operations on the brain in order to alter mental states or overt behavior (psychosurgery) and electrical stimulation of the brain (ESB).

The technologies of behavior control and the precision with which these technologies can be applied are likely to increase at a stunning pace. These technologies can be used as therapies for the treatment of illnesses; but they can also be used to manipulate, distort, and even destroy persons. In this chapter several of these techniques are studied in the attempt to discover the conditions, if any, under which these diverse techniques are ethically permissible.

MAJOR EMPIRICAL, CONCEPTUAL, AND ETHICAL CONTROVERSIES

Several problems recur no matter which form of behavior control is under consideration. Some problems are purely conceptual (What is behavior control? What is psychosurgery?, etc.), others largely empirical, and some distinctly ethical. Indeed, there seem to be three major types of problems, one of which is empirical, one conceptual, and one ethical.

1. *The empirical problem of adequate evidence.* Several problems of scientific evidence have arisen which are not specifically ethical in character, yet the answers to which heavily influence ethical judgments. For example, it is claimed by some experts that we know so little about the brain and the physiological effects of powerful drugs that we ought not to allow psychosurgery and various drug therapies until we have obtained controlled experimental evidence which supplies such information. It is claimed that we do not adequately understand what side-effects might occur, whether the results are irreversible, and which among the available therapies are most likely to be successful in permanently eliminating the undesired behavior. Other experts flatly disagree, arguing that the evidence is as good as that used in ordinary medical practice for the treatment of most diseases. This is not a matter which can be decided by non-medical laymen, including ethicists; but resolution of these disputes over empirical matters is nonetheless of decisive ethical relevance.

2. *The conceptual problem of distinguishing disease and deviancy.* The problem of the nature of disease was discussed in Chapter 3, but it reappears here in an especially interesting manner. The question is this: if behavior control therapies are medical treatments, as is usually claimed by those who employ them, then what is the disease being treated? Diagnoses of illness are often made on the basis of overt behavior—e.g., *violent* behavior. But is this behavior diseased or is it simply a behavioral manifestation of which we highly disapprove? Are we treating people for a disease, or are we punishing them? How in general is the distinction to be drawn between deviant behavior of which we disapprove but which is not diseased and behavior which is deviant because of a disease? The separation of the two is especially difficult if the diagnosis itself is made exclusively on the basis of observed behavior. They are less difficult to separate if, as some claim, definite structural abnormalities can be detected by (for example) x-rays and exploratory surgery. (These problems emerge with special vigor in the debates below between Mark and Chorover and between Szasz and Chodoff.)

3. *The ethical problem of informed consent.* The importance of this issue—which is treated in detail in Chapters 4 and 10—is re-emphasized in discussions of behavior control. Must one obtain voluntary informed consent in order to employ behavior control therapies? Ordinarily one would think so, but when persons have been involuntarily institutionalized in hospitals and prisons, must their informed consent still always be obtained? Is this necessary not only for major procedures such as psychosurgery but also for presumably milder forms of therapy, such as drugs and psychotherapy? And, finally, if the person is in a coercive environment such as a prison or hospital, under what conditions, if any, is it meaningful to say that consent is informed and voluntarily given? The issue of informed consent may be the most widely discussed of all those which arise—perhaps, as Bedau suggests in his article, because of the Nuremberg Code (see Chapter 9) and the Kaimowitz case (discussed in this chapter by Mason).

Though clearly difficult, it is ideal to resolve the relevant empirical and conceptual issues before approaching the ethical ones. And, as we shall now see, it is advisable to make basic decisions on ethical matters before consideration of legal issues.

THE LEGAL CONTROL OF BEHAVIOR CONTROL

The ethical justifiability of laws which restrict and/or permit the technologies of behavior control is itself a central and controversial issue. Ideally laws exist to protect people, most obviously from physical abuse, but from psychic and emotional abuse as well. Since the technologies of behavior control easily lend themselves to substantial physical and mental abuse, laws which safeguard individual and societal rights and liberties are obviously desirable. But the law has two sides. By ensuring liberty to one set of persons, it may unduly restrict the liberty of others. The acceptability of such limitation depends upon its justifiability, and when an adequate justification is not forthcoming, the law can itself become an instrument of oppression. Many, and perhaps the majority, of ethical problems of behavior control derive from asking the question, "Which uses of control technologies should be banned outright, which should be legally restricted though not prohibited, and which should be legally unrestrained?"

In attempting to answer this question, a distinction should be made between *coercive uses* and *voluntary uses* of behavior control technologies. Consider voluntary uses first. Sometimes patients freely submit to therapeutic uses of these technologies, as when they visit a psychiatrist or enroll in a behavior modification program in order to lose weight. If laws sharply restrict access to these techniques, they limit the freedom of both patients and practitioners. It is widely believed, however, that some behavior control technologies are so inherently dangerous that they should not be permitted, regardless of the desires of patients and practitioners. But should such voluntary uses of these techniques therefore be banned, and if so on what grounds? Clearly at bottom this question is a moral and not a legal one, for it asks what the law *ought* to be rather than what it *is*.

Coercive uses of behavior control technologies are perhaps less prevalent than voluntary uses, but they are by no means rare. Persons are involuntarily committed to institutions for mental treatment as a matter of common practice. Drug therapies and psychotherapy are forced on many of these persons. Potentially, all behavior control technologies could be similarly used by the state. States may be well- or ill–intentioned in this coercive use of behavior control techniques, but the same ethical question arises in either case: under what conditions, if any, is the state justified in the coercive use of these technologies in order to control the behavior of individual persons?

Ethically acceptable answers to the above questions must provide principled justifications of state intervention. To deny access to behavior control technologies is one way of limiting liberty, while the forced use of these therapies is undoubtedly an intervention, though some would deny that it limits liberty. In any event, the question of a principled justification of state intervention remains.[2] In this chapter almost all of the articles turn their attention to this problem, but problems of legal control are treated in detail by Shapiro and Mason, while Bedau and Beauchamp pay special attention to problems of voluntariness and coercion.

T. L. B.

NOTES

1. *Behavior Control* (New York: Harper & Row, 1969), p. 4.
2. The final article in Chapter 1, by Joel Feinberg, briefly outlines the most frequently proposed grounds for such coercion, and it might prove useful to refer to that essay when attempting to evaluate the claims made by various authors in this chapter.

MICHAEL H. SHAPIRO

Legislating the Control of Behavior Control

Psychotropic (mind-altering) drugs,[1] electrical stimulation of the brain (ESB) by implantation of electrodes,[2] psychosurgery,[3] and organic conditioning techniques are now available for extensive use by the state in controlling criminal, sick or otherwise aberrant or unwanted behavior. While these methods of control ("organic therapies")[4] have already brought substantial improvements in the treatment of mental illness, they portend substantial danger for personal freedom. Some of these therapies have already been used on various occasions in clearly objectionable ways and for clearly objectionable purposes.[5] Consider, for example, the experiments in aversive conditioning[6] with the drug Anectine performed at the California Medical Facility at Vacaville and the Atascadero State Mental Hospital. These chilling exercises, carried out on unwilling as well as "consenting" inmates,[7] were described by the "therapists" at Vacaville as:

an attempt to evaluate the effectiveness of an aversive treatment program utilizing Succinylcholine (anectine) as a means of suppressing such hazardous behavior [e.g., repeated assaults, attempted suicide]. The drug . . . was selected for use as a means of providing an extremely negative experience for association with the behavior in question. Succinylcholine, when injected intramuscularly, results in complete muscular paralysis including temporary respiratory arrest. Onset of effects is rapid and the reaction can be controlled by amount injected. It avoids many of the strenuous features which characterize other chemical aversion procedures . . . , allows for more precise control temporally, and is almost free of side effects. It was hypothesized that

Reprinted with permission of the publisher from *Southern California Law Review*, Vol. 47, No. 2 (February, 1974), pp. 240, 243–55, 260–65, 272f, 276f.

the association of such a frightening consequence (respiratory arrest, muscular paralysis) with certain behavioral acts would be effective in suppressing these acts. . . .

How severe is the anectine experience from the point of view of the patient? Sixteen likened it to dying. Three of these compared it to actual experiences in the past in which they had almost drowned. The majority described it as a terrible, scary, experience.[8]

Such gross assaults upon personal autonomy should dispatch any notions that officialdom in general or the medical profession in particular can safely be left to their own devices in determining the nature of and occasions for intervention in human mentation[9] for purposes of achieving mind/behavior control.

Psychosurgery is another—rather more drastic—organic therapy which has recently been performed on prisoners in California. Three inmates of Vacaville underwent a procedure known as stereotactic surgery, which destroys selected areas of brain tissue—in these cases, portions of their amygdalas. Psychosurgery, in any of its forms, is an irreversible procedure which may result in substantial, permanent and perhaps severely dysfunctional effects on mentation. While it has, from time to time, received favorable scientific reviews, its "therapeutic" value is seriously in doubt.

Projected applications of behavior control technologies are reflected in detailed proposals for making the release of prisoners and mental patients contingent upon their acceptance of implantation of electrodes both for direct control of behavior and for monitoring, or upon their agreement to use psychotropic drugs in prescribed ways. We are thus faced with the prospect of having significant numbers of people who, although appearing to be "free" (they are, after all, not behind bars or in padded cells), are subject either to the control of remote, external monitors who can alter psyches electronically, or to the influence of powerful psychoactive agents which constantly regulate mental functioning.

There is clear evidence that these and other organic behavior control techniques have been endorsed and recommended for use on prisoners and mental patients. Witness the specific recommendation of California's Director of Corrections that psychosurgery be used on violent prisoners;[10] the increasing pressures for the use of organic therapies and conditioning techniques, and the proposals for extensive neurobiological screening and preventive treatment.

These current and projected developments rather strongly suggest that legislatures and courts should bring under their aegis the problem of controlling the use of behavior control technologies. Such regulation ought to insure that rigorous restraints are placed on any state efforts toward mental "demolition" masquerading as "therapy." To do so without jeopardizing the plainly admirable goals of curing or arresting severe mental illness—and thereby achieving some measure of benefit to the victim/patient/prisoner, and some measure of public protection and benefit—is the critical legislative task to which this Article is addressed.

A PRECIS OF THE PROPOSED ALTERNATIVE STATUTES

During the 1973-74 session of the California Legislature, Assemblyman Alan Sieroty introduced legislation (Assembly Bill (AB) 2296) to control the use of organic therapies in California prisons. A more comprehensive draft statute (referred to hereafter as "Statute I") is contained in Appendix I [in original text]. The salient features of AB 2296 are these. (1) It records the proposition that protection of the integrity of thought and mentation is a fundamental constitutional right.[11] (2) It provides that informed consent is a necessary condition for the administration of organic therapies

upon those having the capacity for such consent, except for electroconvulsive therapy (ECT) in certain emergencies.[12] This entails that the state cannot impose organic therapy upon anyone who, even if suffering from mental disturbance, retains his capacity to decide whether to submit to therapy, and refuses it. Under this "per se" rule, his refusal simply ends the matter. (3) It provides that psychosurgery, electrical stimulation of the brain, and other organic therapies (as those terms are delimited in AB 2296)[13] require judicial authorization in every instance[14] (except for specified uses of ECT[15]). The purpose of the judicial proceeding is to determine whether informed consent has in fact been obtained, and to assess the medical soundness and propriety of the proposed therapy. (4) It provides that if a prisoner lacks the capacity for informed consent, neither psychosurgery nor ESB may be employed.[16] (We thus have another per se rule.[17]) (5) It sets forth stringent procedures for determining when organic therapy (other than psychosurgery or ESB) may be administered to those lacking the capacity for informed consent.[18] (6) It explicates the central concepts of "organic therapy" and "informed consent," and specifies the criteria and procedures required for determining the existence or lack of capacity for informed consent, and the procedures for securing such consent.[19]

Statute I goes beyond AB 2296 by including within the definition of "organic therapy" the use of all the several kinds of psychotropic drugs, and by extending coverage of the statute's provisions to persons involuntarily confined in mental hospitals. While Statute I requires that a person with the capacity for informed consent must give such consent as a precondition for administration of these drugs, when this consent is given prior judicial authorization is not required because chemotherapy, in general, is less intrusive than psychosurgery or certain other organic therapies. Furthermore, Statute I permits the use of drug therapy upon persons lacking the capacity for informed consent, in accordance with stringent provisions which govern the determination that such capacity is lacking and which require that the proposed chemotherapy be medically sound.

This Article will review the purposes and rationales of various critical sections of the alternative statutes, and will attempt to limn some of the major legal and moral issues at stake in deciding whether and how to use the behavior control technologies described here.

The principal goals of AB 2296 and Statute I are (1) to provide a buffer against the power of the state to control behavior, and (2) to do so without simultaneously ruining the possibility of restoring disturbed inmates to functionality and freedom. Too stringent restrictions or prohibitions on the use of organic therapies can plunge us into a Catch-22-like dilemma: "You may use any therapy you wish, as long as it doesn't work; if it works, it is forbidden." The conflicting aims of freedom from madness and freedom from state incursions upon personal autonomy are substantially accommodated by the requirement of informed consent. Prisoners who competently reject organic therapies will be free of them; those who give their informed consent may venture such therapies; and those who lack the capacity for informed consent are guaranteed an informed adjudication which is intended to restrain the arbitrary or improper exercise of the state's power.

The power to coercively apply organic therapies is as awesome and dangerous a power as any state may possess (planet-destroying capabilities aside). As already suggested, however, these therapies represent the most effective (and intrusive) medical advances we have had in treating mental illness. The statutes thus have to balance freedom from coercive therapy against freedom from the debilitation of mental illness: the effect of organic treatment foregone may be as destructive of human liberty and potential in an individual case as the effect of enforced treatment in another. If the state predicates the use of organic therapy upon the securing of informed consent, and also provides for stringent procedures regulating the use of such therapy upon those lacking the capacity for such consent, it will have taken a major step toward reconciling both freedoms.

THE CONSTITUTIONAL PROTECTION OF MENTATION

A. THE PRESUMPTIVE IMMORALITY OF SUBSTITUTION OF JUDGMENT: A COROLLARY OF THE VALUE OF PERSONAL AUTONOMY

The statutes reflect three major propositions. The first is a moral thesis: it is prima facie (presumptively) immoral for the state to effect substantial changes in a person's mentation[20] against his will. That is, mind control is prima facie wrong and must be justified on moral grounds adequate to overcome the presumption of immorality. This proposition is simply an instance of the general moral principle of personal autonomy that forcing individuals to do what they do not wish to do, or preventing them from doing what they wish to do, is prima facie wrong.[21] Such coercion—whether considered mind control or behavior control—seems aptly described by the expression "substitution of judgment."

The second proposition is that this moral presumption against enforced substitution of judgment is embodied in and informs certain constitutional provisions.

The third proposition, derivable in part from the second, is that the Constitution, through both its protection of communication under the first amendment and its protection of privacy, protects freedom of mentation[22] as a fundamental right which cannot be abridged except by demonstrating that the abridgment is necessary to further a compelling state interest. The conclusion that the state's action is "necessary" implies the corollary that there is no alternative method for furthering that interest which would be a less onerous burden upon the fundamental right.

Given the preceding theses, specific and stringent statutory prescripts should trammel the power of the state to employ organic therapies coercively, however benevolent the intentions of the state may be—and they may be insufferably benevolent. Since organic therapies may be able to substantially reconstruct one's psyche and to effect behavior control with considerable precision (and increasingly so as research continues), unchecked state power to confine and "treat" would be a massive danger to personal freedom.

. . .

The appropriate inquiry, then, concerns the extent to which a therapeutic regimen affects or intrudes upon mentation. Psychosurgery, for example, may severely affect mentation by permanent destruction of selected areas of the brain. A conditioning or learning program seeking to induce mental and behavioral changes, however, may affect mentation by the use of relatively mild reward or punishment stimuli, and thus would seem to involve a lesser intrusion or assault upon mentation. Since therapies vary in the degree to which we are inclined to view them as intrusive or non-intrusive, we must address some obvious questions: do therapies such as token economies, psychotherapy, moral suasion, or organic behavior modification programs like the Anectine conditioning program fall outside the scope of the first amendment because (unlike, e.g., psychosurgery or ESB) their effects on mentation are in some sense less intrusive? How do we identify among the infinitude of stimuli or conditions which have *some* effect on mentation those which should be deemed so assaultive of our mental autonomy, individuality, or personhood, that the state should be heavily burdened with justifying their use in altering mentation? A legal theory which characterized ordinary instructional methods in public schools, or the psychic effects of confinement *simpliciter,* as raising a threshold first amendment issue would hardly be satisfactory, even though the long run mentational effects may be substantial. Simply walking past a person's field of vision effects a change in his sensorium; but under ordinary circumstances we would not regard this as an instance of coercive mind control. In short, not every effort to change behavior by changing attitudes, emotions, or mentation generally constitutes coercive mind control.

Criteria of Intrusiveness. The limiting principles needed in determining whether a given mode of alteration of mentation raises a threshold first amendment claim seem, at least as a matter of ordinary intuition, to involve notions of the "intrusiveness" of its effects on mentation.

The concept of intrusiveness of a therapy or program in turn seems to involve the following criteria (which, while in the main conceptually distinct, are in fact interdependent):[23] (i) the extent to which the effects of the therapy upon mentation are reversible; (ii) the extent to which the resulting psychic state is "foreign," "abnormal" or "unnatural" for the person in question, rather than simply a restoration of his prior psychic state (this is closely related to the "magnitude" or "intensity" of the change); (iii) the rapidity with which the effects occur; (iv) the scope of the change in the total "ecology" of the mind's functions; (v) the extent to which one can resist *acting* in ways impelled by the psychic effects of the therapy; and (vi) the duration of the change. For present purposes, it is immaterial whether the change effects a constriction or amplification of a person's mental functioning, or whether the effects are "good" or "bad."

These criteria of intrusiveness require some elaboration. There are a number of senses of "irreversible." Effects of a therapy may simply endure or dissipate over time, and in this sense the notion of irreversibility refers simply to a lengthy duration of effect. Effects may also be reversible simply by withdrawing the psychotropic agent—e.g., deactivation or removal of an implanted electrode. But such reversibility may be entirely at the option of the therapist. If the patient cannot eliminate the psychotropic agent, or is prevented from doing so, the effects of the agent are appropriately described as "irreversible." Some therapies may be substantially immune from efforts of will to countermand their psychic effects. The effects of ESB, for example, are extremely difficult and perhaps in many cases impossible to erase by the unaided mental efforts of the patient, and for this reason may be considered irreversible. The effects of a given therapy may nevertheless be counteracted in certain ways. One drug may be neutralized by another, or perhaps by an effort of self-control ("I *will* stay awake!"), and its effects would thus be reversible in this sense. But if such "chasers" are unavailable, and "will power" is unavailing, then the effects are again properly described as "irreversible" during the period of effectiveness of the drug, which may be substantial. Finally, the therapy's effects may substantially dilute the patient's very desire to ward off its effects. Electrical stimulation of a pleasure center in the brain might well generate a preference for stasis in the new psychic condition.

The rather protean concept of irreversibility may thus, depending upon the circumstances, refer to extended duration of effect; to the fact that the patient alone cannot eliminate the psychotropic agent; to the fact that the effects of a given psychotropic agent may be immune from "will power," and may thus hold for a substantial time unless neutralized by some means unavailable to the patient; or to the fact that the therapy may erase any desire to avoid the effects of that therapy. Psychosurgery may produce effects irreversible in several of these senses. Although some of its effects may dissipate or be compensated for through the use of drugs, other effects seem to be permanent. Since the procedure destroys brain tissue which cannot regenerate, neither patient nor therapist has an option to "withdraw" the psychotropic agent. The "bleaching of the personality" or "blunting of emotions" effected by psychosurgery may in any event destroy the desire to alter one's newly-acquired psyche.

A second index of the instrusiveness of a mind-altering technique is the "unnatural" or "foreign" quality of its effects for the person in question, at least under normal circumstances. Consider, for example, the effects of ESB in producing word aphasia, or an orgasmic feeling without the customary erotic stimuli. The exhortations of a psychotherapist, however, do not generally produce highly abnormal states of mind, and since the subject ordinarily has an opportunity to accept or reject the suggestions or hortatory efforts of his mentors, it is rather an overstatement to talk of intrusive or coerced changes in mentation.

. . .

The Intrinsic Value of Mentation. Much of the preceding discussion was based on the the-

sis that mentation is *instrumentally* valuable in generating communication, and that this instrumental value would be impaired by attempts to excise certain kinds of mentation ("disordered," "solitary") from first amendment protection. There is, however, another consideration, which is that mentation is *intrinsically* valuable,[24] and therefore all mentation should be presumptively protected by the first amendment.[25] If so, the posited first amendment protection of mentation does not depend entirely on the protection of communication.

While we may accept the empiricist thesis that there can be little or no mentation without prior imprinting of the *tabula rasa* of our minds (a process substantially certain to involve human communication), solitary thought, thought only indirectly related to specific communications—indeed, mentation and mental activity generally—are, it is suggested, intended targets of the first amendment's protection. An historical analysis will not be ventured at this point, but the contention here is that the first amendment was intended to protect *thought*—whether or not such thought was likely to be instrumental in generating communication or action. In *Stanley v. Georgia* the Supreme Court said:

Our whole constitutional heritage rebels at the thought of giving government the power to control men's minds. . . . We are not certain that this argument [regulation is necessary to protect the "individual's mind from the effects of obscenity"] amounts to anything more than the assertion that the State has the right to control the moral content of a person's thoughts. . . . Whatever the power of the state to control public dissemination of ideas inimical to the public morality it cannot constitutionally premise legislation on the desirability of controlling a person's private thoughts.[26]

. . .

It appears that *Kaimowitz v. Department of Mental Health*[27] adopted the foregoing analysis of privacy as one of its rules of decision, relying both upon the first amendment's protection of privacy and upon inferences drawn from other constitutional provisions:

There is no privacy more deserving of constitutional protection than that of one's mind. . . .

Intrusion into one's intellect, when one is involuntarily detained and subject to the control of institutional authorities, is an intrusion into one's constitutionally protected right of privacy. If one is not protected in his thoughts, behavior, personality and identity, then the right of privacy becomes meaningless. [*Citing* Note, *Conditioning and Other Technologies Used to "Treat?" "Rehabilitate?" "Demolish?" Prisoners and Mental Patients*, 45 S. CAL. L. REV. 616, 663 (1972).]

. . .In the hierarchy of values, it is more important to protect one's mental processes than to protect even the privacy of the marital bed.[28]

PERSONAL AUTONOMY AND THE COERCIVE USE OF ORGANIC THERAPY AS A MEANS OF FURTHERING COMPELLING STATE INTERESTS

The conclusion of the preceding discussion was that there is a fundamental right against coercive governmental interference with mentation through the use of organic therapies. The existence of that right was inferred from the first amendment's protection of communication, its recognition of the instrumental and intrinsic values of mentation and personal autonomy, and also from the Constitution's general protection of privacy. Claims based upon fundamental constitutional rights are, however, defeasible. If the state can establish that a proposed course of action is necessary to further or achieve a compelling state interest, then it has constitutionally justified its resulting encroachment upon the fundamental right. This condition for defeasibility implies that the state must show that there are no alternative means of furthering that compelling interest which would place a less onerous burden upon the fundamental right.

How, in principle, can a state establish a compelling interest justifying the use of organic therapy as the least onerous means of furthering that interest? The state, no doubt, would cite as compelling interests the public safety; the restoration of a person to functionality, for the benefit of himself, his family, and society; and the costs of confinement, supervision or various modalities of treatment. The state would no doubt also claim that its techniques for freeing one from the burdens of

madness represented that means of effecting this liberation which trenched least upon the fundamental right of freedom of mentation. In short, the state would claim a right to compel treatment on both "social cost" and "paternalistic" grounds. . . .

NOTES

1. *Psychotropic* mens "mind-altering" or "affecting the psyche."

2. *Electrical stimulation of the brain* is described and explained in J. DELGADO. PHYSICAL CONTROL OF THE MIND: TOWARD A PSYCHOCIVILIZED SOCIETY 257 (1969) [hereinafter cited as PHYSICAL CONTROL]: "[M]ovements, sensations, emotions, desires, ideas, and a variety of psychological phenomena may be induced, inhibited, or modified by electrical stimulation of specific areas of the brain." Drugs are sometimes applied directly to selected brain areas through "micro-implants" or micro-pipettes.

3. Defining *psychosurgery* poses some difficulties. An accurate lexical definition might be this: surgery on the brain principally for purposes of altering or controlling mentation and behavior, whether or not such mentation and behavior is associated with "mental disorder," or with "diseased" portions of the brain. *See* the definitions in Kaimowitz v. Department of Mental Health, Civil No. 73-19434-AW (Wayne County, Mich., Cir. Ct., July 10, 1973), at 9–11.

4. *Organic Therapy* is defined in A.B. 2296, § 2670.5(c), and Statute I, § 2 (c). The expression refers to procedures which affect or alter through electrochemical or surgical means a person's thought patterns, sensations, feelings, perceptions, and mentation . . . or mental activity generally; or to *conditioning* techniques using the effects of electrical or chemical intervention into mental functioning as part of the conditioning program.

5. *See In re* Owens, No. 70J 21520 (Cook County, Ill., Cir. Ct., County Dep't, Juv. Div., July 9, 1971). There, Thorazine was used on juveniles without careful medical review, without investigation of less intrusive means for controlling conduct, and perhaps for purely punitive purposes. The court found that Thorazine, a phenothiazine antipsychotic drug (a "major tranquilizer") (W. CUTTING, HANDBOOK OF PHARMACOLOGY 677 (4th ed. 1969) [hereinafter cited as CUTTING]) was "used as a behavior control device for episodes of aggressive, assaultive, and destructive behavior." The court ordered that no intramuscular injection of Thorazine or other tranquilizer be administered "except as part of a treatment for medical or emotional illness or disorder." It also ordered that no such drug therapy could be given unless there had been a prior attempt to control the juvenile in other ways, and unless an attempt had been made to administer the drug orally with his consent. Presumably, if all these conditions were met the drug could be forcibly administered intramuscularly.

6. On the particular meanings of "aversion therapy," "operant" and "classical" conditioning, see American

Psychiatric Ass'n, *A Psychiatric Glossary,* 13–14, 22–23 (3d ed. 1969).

7. Mattocks & Jew, Assessment of an Aversive Treatment Program with Extreme Acting-Out Patients in a Psychiatric Facility for Criminal Offenders 5 (unpublished manuscript prepared for Dep't of Corrections, on file with the University of Southern California Law Library, undated).

8. *Id.* at 3, 15. In many cases, the drug was administered without the inmate's consent.

9. *Mentation* refers to cognition, understanding, perception, emotion—loosely, any mental functioning or activity. (This does not, for present purposes, include the regulation of the body's autonomic functions for which the brain is principally responsible). *See* Longo, *supra* note 3 [in original text], at 179; *Webster's New Third International Dictionary* (1966).

10. Letter from R. Procunier, Director of the Dep't of Corrections, to Robert L. Lawson, Executive Officer, California Council on Criminal Justice, Sept. 8, 1971, in *Rough Times* 204 (J. Agel ed. 1973). The letter indicates that it is a "letter of intent" proposing neurosurgical treatment of violent inmates, and proposes that "surgical and diagnostic procedures would be performed to locate centers in the brain which may have been previously damaged and which could serve as the focus for episodes of violent behavior. If these areas were located and it was verified that they were indeed the source of aggressive behavior, neurosurgery would be performed, directed at the previously found cerebral foci."

11. A.B. 2296, § 2670. The parallel section in Statute I is section 1.

12. A.B. 2296, §§ 2670(c), 2671; Statute I, §§ 2(c), 3.

13. The definitions of these terms differ in the two statutes.

14. A. B. 2296, § 2670.5(a)(1); Statute I, § 2(a)(1).

15. A.B. 2296, § 2671; Statute I, § 3.

16. A.B. 2296, § 2670.5(b); Statute I, § 2(b).

17. Unless otherwise specified, references herein to the "per se" rule designate the prohibition against treatment over the objection of persons having the capacity for informed consent.

18. A.B. 2296, §§ 2675–79; Statute I, §§ 8–12.

19. A.B. 2296, §§ 2672–73; Statute I, §§ 4–5.

20. "Mentation" is defined in note 9 *supra.* The changes may be in mood, cognition, perception—indeed, in the entire complex of mental functions and patterns which make up "personality" or "character" traits, and personal identity itself. *See generally* the sources cited in note 7 *supra* [in the original text].

21. *Cf.* H. L. A. Hart, *Law, Liberty and Morality,* 21–22 (1963): "[Restrictions on Liberty] may be thought of as calling for justification for several quite distinct reasons. The unimpeded exercise by individuals of free choice may be held a value in itself with which it is *prima facie* wrong to interfere; or it may be thought valuable because it enables individuals to experiment—even with living—and to discover things valuable both to themselves and to others."

22. The first amendment argument developed in the text at notes 51–54 *infra* [in the original text] was applied in Kaimowitz v. Department of Mental Health, Civil No. 73–19434-AW (Wayne County, Mich., Cir. Ct., July 10, 1973) excerpted at 42 U.S.L.W. 2063 (July 31, 1973).

23. These criteria appear to form a set, no member of which is necessary, and no member of which may be sufficient alone to justify the conclusion that the therapy is "intrusive." It is a familiar feature of general terms that their applicability may rest upon the presence of a "quorum" of factors in such a set. This combination of factors (frequently unspecifiable in advance) would then arguably justify the use of the general term.

24. In contrast to instrumental goods, some things are considered intrinsic goods " . . . because we value these things . . . not for what they lead to but for what they are." J. HOSPERS, HUMAN CONDUCT 105 (1961).

25. Justice Brandeis, concurring in Whitney v. California, 274 U.S. 357 (1927), stated: "Those who won our independence believed that the final end of the State was to make men free to develop their faculties; and that in its government the deliberative forces should prevail over the arbitrary. They valued liberty both as an end and as a means."

26. *Id.* at 565–66.

27. Civil No. 73–19434-AW (Wayne County, Mich., Cir. Ct., July 10, 1973).

28. *Id.* at 38–39.

HUGO ADAM BEDAU

Physical Interventions to Alter Behavior in a Punitive Environment: Some Moral Reflections on New Technology

I

There is, I suppose, a wide variety of techniques of social control that can be gathered together under the heading of physical intervention techniques. The term is chosen so as to be as inclusive as possible and yet to suggest an analogy to the medical notion of physical intervention for therapeutic purposes, since the role of medical research and medical administration in the development and the use of these techniques is a prominent feature of many of them. In order to be as specific as possible at the outset, I use the term "physical intervention techniques" to mean one or more of the following four sorts or sets of techniques:

(1) Psychosurgery (or neurosurgery). By this term I mean such methods as stereotaxic surgery, involving electrodes, radiation, or ultrasonic waves, to destroy deeply embedded brain tissue (Chorover, 1974). It was techniques of this sort that made the project at Boston City Hospital by Dr. Vernon Mark and his associates a matter of recent public (and even national) controversy (Haas, 1973).

(2) Drug (or chemo) therapy. By this term I mean such methods as the subcutaneous injection of apomorphine or other emetics, the use of anectine and prolixin to make the subject docile, not to say helpless, as well as the use of psychotropic drugs and drug-induced convulsive shock (Neville, 1974).

(3) Aversion therapy. By this term I mean such methods as the use of electric shock techniques to condition child molesters against further criminal conduct (Knight, 1974). Both aversion therapy and chemotherapy were

These excerpts from "Physical Interventions to Alter Behavior in a Punitive Environment: Some Moral Reflections on New Technology," by Hugo A. Bedau are reprinted from *American Behavioral Scientist*, Vol. 18, No. 5 (May/June 1975), pp. 657–678, by permission of the publisher, Sage Publications, Inc.

brought to public attention in the last few years through Stanley Kubrick's film of Anthony Burgess's novel *A Clockwork Orange* (Ricks, 1972).

(4) Sensory deprivation. By this term I mean such relatively crude and traditional methods as isolation and removal of the subject from all contact with the social environment and severe restrictions on his physical environment, as used, for instance in the initial phase of the now-defunct federally financed START program (Chicago Peoples Law Office, 1973; Oelsner, 1974a, 1974b).

On the other hand, I exclude various other relatively novel techniques, such as psychotechnology and sociotechnology, of the sort used by Synanon and Esalen, because like psychiatric techniques generally, these methods essentially depend on discursive cognitive intercourse between the subject and the controller. However corrupt these methods may become, either intentionally or through negligence and incompetence, they are still aided by methods of moral education of the sort on which Socrates and other moral teachers have relied. There are, no doubt, borderline cases between my extremes of physical intervention on the one side and cognitive discourse on the other (e.g., posthypnotic suggestion), but they need not trouble us here. It is enough for purposes of the present discussion to have a small set of clear cases under the former category, and I believe that the techniques mentioned above are just that.

Throughout this discussion, I shall consider these methods only in the context of criminology and penology. Thus, I exclude any consideration of their use as therapy in mental institutions or in private medical practice. I also exclude any consideration of them as *experimental research methods* in laboratories not linked to punitive-custodial institutions and not used on a clientele provided by the workings of the criminal justice system. For similar reasons, there is no more than a partial overlap between my subject and the large topic of the morality of operant conditioning and behavioral modification (Goodall, 1972; Russell, 1974). My notion of physical intervention techniques obviously extends beyond these purely behavioristic methods, while the use of those methods is by no means confined to punitive-custodial settings. Finally, I shall concentrate on the application of these techniques to violent and dangerous offenders, or at least, persons incarcerated because of violence and harm to others. It is, after all, usually the violent offender who poses the greatest challenge to safe custody and release and against whom repressive violence is usually judged to be least in need of explanation.

Given the variety of physical intervention techniques, the circumstances of their imposition, their consequences, and of our knowledge about them, it may seem well nigh impossible to offer any but the most platitudinous moral generalizations about them here. Platitudinous or profound, any such moral generalizations will depend on prior factual generalizations about these methods. What might such generalizations be? I suggest the following half dozen:

(1) These methods can be used without either the informed consent or the voluntary co-operation of the subject. Some of them can be used with the subject in irons, or sedated, or otherwise immobile; to a certain extent, each can be used only with subjects in some form of custody and control. They are often experienced as unpleasant and judged by the subject to be undesirable, and this reluctance can be overcome without recourse to methods which rely only on persuasion and cognitive exchange between the subject and the controller.

(2) Although administered by physicians or under medical supervision, these methods are not used in a truly therapeutic manner, because they are not used to cure any identifiable illness or disease or to rectify any clinical abnor-

mality. Since their use does not depend on prior medical diagnosis of physically based abnormality or sickness, their use need not cease as a consequence of subsequent medical diagnosis, either.

(3) These methods are used with the intention or purpose of altering the subject's behavior by affecting the internal physical states of the subject's body, nervous system, or brain. They characteristically work either directly via physical alteration of the body (e.g., neurosurgery) or indirectly via physical stimuli (e.g., sensory deprivation). Altering the subject's conscious cognitive states, therefore, is not really an intervening variable in the sequence which begins with these physical interventions and ends with his altered behavior.

(4) These methods are used to extinguish undesired behavior and to induce desired behaviors, where the behaviors in question are not necessarily identified and chosen by the subject, or by the subject in consultation with the controller. Insofar as either set of behaviors can be identified precisely at all, they can be chosen for the subject by the controller acting alone. To that extent, at least, the value system of the controller can arbitrarily supersede that of the subject.

(5) These methods are used with the intention to produce irreversible effects. The decay rate of the methods of operant conditioning is considerable, given the generally uncontrolled social environment in which the subject lives after his custody terminates. In theory, however, all these techniques would be as irreversible as are the surgical ones, if only it were known how to make them so.

(6) These methods can be used rationally only when certain empirical assumptions are accepted by the controllers. Chief among these are: the assumption that harmfulness to others and criminality generally are sociobehavioral effects or expressions of a person's inner physiological states; the assumption that further harmfulness or criminality can be prevented by altering those internal states; the assumption that crime (or at least aggressive and assaultive crimes against the person and against property) is an expression of some physiologically based

defect or excess, an abnormality; and the assumption that the controllers know what is better behavior for the subject (in at least some types of situation) than he does.

Among these six factual generalizations, the one most likely to provoke moral qualms is the fifth, because of the obvious way in which the autonomy, dignity, and self-respect of the subject of these techniques is denied by the controller from the onset of his use of such techniques. Some observers have been inclined to say that the purpose of physical intervention techniques is to make the subject better, to improve him in his own eyes, or at least to make him less unhappy with his surroundings and with himself. It is doubtful whether any of these techniques, in any significant sense of the terms "improve" and "better," can be said to improve the subject or to make him a better person. Such achievements seem in the nature of the case to be too much in a person's own hands for them to be the outcome of such involuntary methods as those here under review. Furthermore, these techniques may well destroy the very capacities needed by a person to make himself, or to become through maturation and experience, better than he now is; nor are these incapacities likely to be superseded by new and better capacities as the result of the use of such physical interventions. On the other hand, that these methods can make a person less unhappy with himself and less dangerous to others may well be true, and I will not dispute it. Still, these consequences, where they do occur, are at best only a by-product of the primary effects. For the chief purpose of these methods seems to be, first and foremost, to make the subject more tractable, less excitable, more manageable, for the sake of the custodial personnel charged with handling him on an immediate day-to-day basis, for the sake of other inmates with whom he must circulate while in custody, and finally for the sake of public safety after his release. It has been said by some doctors closely associated with the use of these techniques that they will transform a person into a "model citizen" (Haas, 1973: 6), "a responsible, well-adjusted citizen" (Chorover, 1974: 59). One is inclined to doubt

whether Locke, Rousseau, Kant, Jefferson, and Mill would have agreed that these techniques can have such results. Their ideal of citizenship was not the docile, receptive, unprotesting person that these methods are known typically to create.

II

Before turning directly to the questions of morality raised by these techniques of physical intervention, I think that it is important to notice that there are some significant questions of morality raised by the punitive setting in which these techniques are typically used. This can easily be seen by considering the morally different climates of four different punitive environments. To see how these environments look from the moral point of view, suppose that you have been convicted of a crime and have been sentenced to prison. You are given four punitive options among which you must choose. On option 1, your sentence is for a *fixed* term of years, so that your release is contingent only on the expiration of sentence and the passage of time. . . . On the next alternative, option 2, your sentence is for an indeterminate period, with expiration and release contingent on your satisfaction of certain *specific objective conditions.* . . . In contrast to this, your next alternative, option 3, provides that your sentence is for an indeterminate period, as in 2, only now your release is contingent on satisfying certain *subjective criteria.* Moreover, the judgment whether you satisfy them is not in your hands, or the hands of your peers (inside or outside of prison), or in the hands of an impartial tribunal, as in 2. It is entirely in the hands of your custodians. . . . The final alternative, option 4, would also give you an *indeterminate* sentence with release theoretically possible. But you are never informed of what the conditions or criteria are for your release. This is because *there are none;* the entire system is Kafkaesque from the moment you enter until (if ever) you leave.

We need not pause to consider whether actual imprisonment approximates more or less closely one rather than another of these four options, nor need we worry about the many possible variations within each option that we can conceive. What does matter is that we can see, from a moral point of view, that there are some important differences in terms of which it would be rational to rank options. On option 4, it would appear that the frustration, the powerlessness, the loss of dignity and significant freedom for the convict are the greatest.

. . .

As ideal types of imprisonment go, options 1 and 2 have advantages from the prisoner's point of view that are missing from options 3 and 4. Now it is crucial to realize that the prisoner's point of view is substantially that of the moral point of view itself. After all, his point of view is not merely one among others; his situation is surely the one that is designed to be the worst off among all those involved in the structure of punitive institutions. Its definitive character for the moral point of view is conclusive. I conclude, therefore, that there is ground for considerable doubt that the prison environment necessary to make sense of the use of physical intervention techniques is morally optimum; and if it is not morally optimum, then it is not morally acceptable at all.

III

It is now time to look more closely at the specific areas of moral concern that the new technology of physical intervention raises. Again, the way to identify what these problems are from the moral point of view is to see them from the perspective of the convict. In order to give this some bite, it is desirable to see how one would respond to these techniques if they were about to be imposed on oneself. Let us begin, therefore, with this consideration uppermost. Perhaps it will be sufficient if I merely list eight sets of problems in the form of questions, and add some brief explanatory comment on each as I go along.

(1) The problem of personal integrity. Does the convict have an inviolable, indefeasible,

absolute right to be himself, whatever and whoever he is, the product of whatever heredity and environment is his lot, even if he is deviant or dangerous to himself and others? To answer in the affirmative may entail that the convict will have to take the consequences that society imposes on persons who are dangerous to others. The use of physical intervention techniques, which would change the convict's physical nature in order to change his behavior, tends to imply that there is no such right. Or, if it is conceded by advocates of these techniques that convicts do have such a right, then it is argued that this right is outweighed by other considerations, either for the individual's own future good or for society's safety, or both. The trouble with such criticisms of the right of personal integrity, as many philosophers have shown (Morris, 1970; Dworkin, 1971), is that they do not take seriously the idea of such a right.

(2) The problem of immunity versus forfeiture of rights. What rights to the privacy and inviolability of body and mind should a person lose once he has been committed to a penal institution, in virtue of his status as a convicted dangerous offender? Is a person immune, morally speaking, from any harms or risks of of harm to himself at the hands of others, except when he waives his immunity? Or does the convict necessarily forfeit the right to personal privacy and psychophysical inviolability, as he obviously has forfeited the right of personal liberty? If he does forfeit them, what rights, exactly, are forfeited and on what grounds? For instance, does the convict also forfeit a right to treatment, i.e., to the preferred treatment from among those available to him?

(3) The problem of second-order or procedural rights. If the basic or first-order rights of the prisoner are not held to be inviolate, in virtue of his status as a convicted dangerous offender, then what rights does the convict have to the procedural protection of the suspension, waiver, or forfeiture of these basic rights? For instance, even if he has no right to refuse modes of physical intervention on his body and nervous system that the authorities judge to be appropriate for him, does he nevertheless have the right to informed notice, to

counsel, and to appeal, concerning the occasions, the extent, and the administration of these techniques?

(4) The problem of rights and goods. How should the convict resolve the conflict between his right (if he has a right) to be left alone, even inside prison, to serve his time free of quasi-therapeutic physical interventions, and his desire (if he has such a desire) to be free from the misery that his aggressive or other impulses cause him (never mind the misery they cause others), and thus freer to seek his own good in his own way? It appears he must waive his rights to be left as he is, if he is to obtain any of these goods by the route of the new technology of physical intervention.

(5) The problem of informed voluntary consent. With what right do custodial authorities use on prisoners any physical substance, stimuli, or technique of manipulation, without first obtaining the consent of the prisoner? How can this consent be construed to be informed unless the prisoner has had explained to him the nature of the physical intervention, the risks, and the probable consequences for him? When the circumstances of release from confinement approximate not the models 1 or 2 discussed earlier (recall section II above), but model 3 if not 4, is it even possible for a person to give his voluntary consent to such a regimen of treatment? Of all the moral problems posed by the new techniques of physical intervention, this is the one that has received the greatest publicity because of the Nuremberg Code and the recent Kaimowitz case (Boston University Law Review, 1974), and I shall return to it below (see section IV).

(6) The problem of paternalism versus authoritarianism. What are the limits on the use of coercion—on the kinds of coercion and on the actions coercively prevented or elicited—that one person may use on another in the name of the latter's own good? Is it true, as John Stuart Mill asserted over a century ago, that "the sole end for which mankind are warranted, individually or collectively, in interfering with the liberty of action of any of their members is self-protection. . . . His own good [that is, the good of the person whose conduct is coercively restrained] . . . is not sufficient warrant" (Mill, 1859:205)? How much illegitimate authoritarianism is bred on the margins of legitimate paternalism within the framework of total coercive institutions such as prisons? The fact that the intention of those who use the new techniques of physical intervention on convicts may be therapeutic does not alter either the authoritarian or paternalistic character of their use. Their use is necessarily authoritarian insofar as it is not contingent on the informed voluntary consent of the subject; it is necessarily not therapeutic unless it is used to alleviate a diagnosed illness (or abnormality) or its symptoms; it is necessarily paternalistic insofar as they are used not to protect society from the offender, but to make the offender better off or happier. Thus, it is entirely possible for these techniques to be simultaneously therapeutic, paternalistic, and authoritarian (contra Kittrie, 1971:3).

(7) The problem of deceptive labeling. Do we have the right to produce a condition or state in the subject in the name of treatment or institutional management that we would not have the right to produce in him in the name of punishment? When does enforced treatment, especially where it involves irreversible neurological and physical effects in the subject, become punitive control under a false therapeutic label? This problem arose recently in the controversial federal START program, as can be seen from these remarks taken from a radical prisoner publication:

The definition of the type of prisoner who will be the subject of START's programmatic behavioral conditioning is somewhat revealing:

> He is assaultive, and maliciously schemes to demonstrate his own physical prowess, usually pressuring the weaker more passive element of the population. Feelings of guilt are non-existent as he can easily rationalize maladaptive behavior, always projecting adversity onto others. He is usually verbal to discretely mask deceitful intent which makes him manipulative. He is egotistical to the utmost extreme, viewing himself as indestructable. He threatens the rehabilitation of a less sophisticated offender continually indoctrinating the latter that crime does pay.

It seems apparent that the description was designed to fit the politically aware prisoner who is well respected as a leader by fellow convicts and who understands and explains prisons in relation to their socio-economic and racial setting. The definition can be applied to any prisoner who resists prison fascism in any way [Chicago Peoples Law Office, 1972:6].

How is it possible that a person who is truly "assaultive," who is "always projecting adversity onto others," who is "manipulative" and "egotistical to the utmost extreme"—the criteria ostensibly used by the authorities to determine the convicts who should enter in the START program—could also be, in the language of the radical critics, "well respected as a leader by fellow convicts," or, for that matter, be "any prisoner who resists prison fascism in any way"? Critics of the START program who would condemn it in this way appear to be talking about a totally different set of criteria from those formulated by the START spokesmen; nor is it seriously conceivable that although the two sets of criteria are totally independent of each other, as their wording surely establishes, they are still substantially coextensive because in application they identify one and the same group of convicts. Nevertheless, the most influential and respected recent treatise on crime and punishment favors programs very much like START for a clientele of prisoners "whom nobody else wants, those whom other institutions reject because they are too disruptive, too turbulent, too unpromising" (Morris and Hawkins, 1970: 198). While these words may not perfectly describe the "new breed" of prisoner (Sykes, 1974), it may seem, understandably, to the spokesmen for radical prison reform that the leaders of this new breed will be among those headed for "special segregation units" and the new technology of physical intervention, because they will be judged "too disruptive, too turbulent, too unpromising" to be left among the general convict population. After all, this seems to have been just the kind of judgment made by the authorities on George Jackson while he was at Soledad Prison in California. So the radical critics of START and other such programs may be right after all.

(8) *The problem of blaming the victim.* In a society replete with social injustices of every sort, why should those who resort to self-help, violence, and victimization of others by direct personal encounter in order to have their way in the world be subjected not only to stigmatization and loss of personal liberty through criminal conviction, but also be subjected to the abuses of personal integrity and autonomy that the new technology of physical intervention necessarily encourages? Is it so clear that what we know about the etiology of criminal violence shows that allocation of social resources to the new technology is a good investment? Or would it be better to suspend altogether the development of such techniques and to devote the money and energy thereby available to the analysis and alleviation of social injustice?

Are any of these moral problems novel and peculiar to the situation in which we find ourselves because of the development of new techniques of physical intervention? Or are all of these problems familiar to us because they are essentially continuous with other techniques that have been with us since the earliest period of systematic imprisonment as a mode of punishment? (One should beware the inference that because the techniques under discussion are new, therefore the moral problems they pose must be new. That would be like arguing from the novelty of electronic surveillance techniques, or the novelty of death by radiation poisoning, to the conclusion that these techniques must pose different moral problems than wire-tapping or handguns.) My suspicion is that these new techniques are historically continuous, at least to some extent, with the mentality manifest in older and cruder methods, in particular with hanging the murderer, maiming the thief, castrating the rapist, sterilizing the defective, and lobotomizing the violent. Like these older techniques, the justification for the new ones straddles the ground between incapacitating the offender and visiting retribution of him for the harm he has caused others. Perhaps the chief differences between the older and the newer methods are two. One is that the newer methods are not always irreversible, whereas all of the older ones were. The other is that the newer methods are designed to leave the convict more or less able to conduct his affairs without further strict confinement, whereas the older methods were far more incapacitating. While these two differences are by no means negligible, it is also true that if we appraise these older techniques by reference to the check list set out earlier of basic characteristics that more or less define the newer techniques (see Section I), the continuity between the two sets of methods is rather striking. To the degree that this continuity is undeniable and dominates the discontinuities, like the two mentioned above, then the classic moral objections directed against the older techniques will apply to the newer ones, too.

IV

Given moral qualms of the sort reviewed above, what is their consequence for the policy questions surrounding the use of these new techniques? There are fundamentally only three policy alternatives, and we can reduce them to two very rapidly. One extreme policy position is, of course, that (1) there should be an unlimited and unregulated use of physical intervention techniques on violent or dangerous offenders. I take it, however, that no one seriously defends this alternative. However inconclusive one may find the moral doubts raised in the previous discussion, they presumably suffice to rule position 1 out. Even if they do not, there is little or no chance as things now stand that anyone will obtain the legal power to implement position 1. The important lower court decision in the Kaimowitz case, rendered in July 1973, seems likely to set the trend of the law in this regard, despite somewhat contrary earlier rulings in other cases (Rothman, 1973). It is true that the entire ethos of our society lies in the direction leading to position 1, for we live in an experimental culture. Our curiosity about ourselves and how our environment and even our heredity can be altered so as to treat our behavior as a dependent variable knows few moral bounds. Confronting modern experimental behavioral and medical science with the

chronic problem of violent crime can hardly result in anything but a readiness to try methods of physical intervention, with at most grudging concessions to the legal procedural rights of the offender as the sole buffer against irresponsible use and experimentation with such techniques. Nevertheless, the specter of Nazi-type experimentation looms whenever safeguards are removed. Consequently there is little likelihood that the initial policy alternative under discussion here will ever be openly defended and adopted.

That leaves us with a choice between two other policy alternatives. One is (2) a limited and regulated use of techniques of physical intervention, with the limits and controls drawn to reflect a judicious response to the moral problems we have examined. The other alternative is (3) the absolute prohibition of the use of any techniques of physical intervention on the convict, no matter what the scientific judgment may be of the violence and dangerousness to which the offender is prone and of safety and effectiveness of the intervention techniques. For myself, I am doubtful whether to defend position 2 or 3. My inclination is to defend position 2, but as I am unsure where to draw the necessary lines and of how to respond to all the difficulties raised earlier, my inclination in favor of this alternative fluctuates. In the remainder of these remarks, I can do little more than try to show how at least some of the difficulties from the moral point of view can be met, or partially met. To that extent I will argue against alternative 3 and thus help us back into the middle ground offered by alternative 2.

The absolute prohibition of physical intervention on the mind and body of a convict is a natural extension of the absolute prohibitions of corporal and capital punishments, which I along with many other moralists have long favored (Bedau, 1964, 1967). Yet it is clear that these new techniques are not intended to be used in a purely incapacitative, retributive, socially defensive way. They have elements of rehabilitation and therapy that are undeniable. So it is not going to be possible to condemn them on the same grounds that suffice to reject the older and cruder methods of bodily incapacitation. Nor is it possible to condemn all use of these methods by appeal to the kind of reasoning stemming from the Kantian tradition in moral philosophy, with its emphasis on "the dignity of the person," whether in the fairly simple form in which some appeal to these ideas (Kittrie, 1971: 393) or in the quite sophisticated form stemming from the theory of distributive justice developed by Rawls (1971). If we take the Kantian philosophy in its simpler, traditional form, then it would require us to base all our punishments in part on the principle that society has a "right of retaliation" against offenders, whereas most theorists of crime and punishment now find such a notion noxious. If we take this philosophy in its latest and most subtle form, we may well discover new and plausible grounds for abandoning a number of traditional methods of dealing with juvenile offenders (Kohlberg, 1974) and with adult prisoners generally (Morris, 1974: 81–83). Nevertheless, the idea of judging the rationality of modes of punitive treatment from the point of view of a person in "the original position" (roughly, in a hypothetical "state of nature") will not suffice to rule out in their entirety the use of physical interventions that hold out the hope of helping a convict who cannot be helped as much by any less severe technique. Since it would be rational for a person to choose to have such interventions visited on him, much as it would be rational for a dying patient to risk experimental surgery to save his life, the use of such techniques on dangerous and violent offenders in a punitive environment cannot be wholly ruled out. If the moral point of view can be systematically represented by the rationalistic moral reasoning that Rawls (1971) has developed, then the moral point of view will not entail alternative 3.

In this light it is useful to reconsider the role to be played by informed voluntary consent in the present context. Perhaps the strongest and simplest argument for something like alternative 3 is the following:

(i) No one may be subjected to physical intervention techniques unless he has granted his informed voluntary consent.

(ii) No one in prison can give his informed voluntary consent to the use of such methods.

∴ (iii) No one in prison may be subjected to these techniques.

In the wake of Kaimowitz, there seems to be considerable readiness to accept premise ii. The reasoning seems to be that premise ii follows because (a) incarceration is itself a constraint on the exercise of free choice and voluntary consent, and (b) a prisoner grants his consent to undergo these techniques against the background of a system of custody and release essentially based on the subjective models discussed earlier (section II above). This argument seems to me reasonably strong, though it is only empirical, not a priori. That is, it is not claimed to be logically impossible for a prisoner to consent voluntarily to anything at all, or to anything proposed to him by his jailers with effects they cannot fully control, that he cannot fully understand, and that involve physical intervention with his body. All that is insisted is that in the typical case, informed voluntary consent cannot be reliably given by persons under prison discipline to quasi-therapeutic methods of physical intervention. Such a stronger, a priori argument to establish premise ii is tempting, but it would be incorrect, in my opinion. Anyway, the empirical argument of (a) and (b) is strong enough; and I, for one, am willing to accept premise ii as at least establishing a presumption against the possibility of informed voluntary consent by prisoners which the law must respect.

But what about premise i? It is a very strong premise indeed, so strong that it is conspicuously missing from the "therapeutic bill of rights" proposed by Kittrie (1971: 400–404), and it is implicitly denied by Morris and Hawkins (1970: 197–200). Theorists of crime and punishment are not about to accept premise i because it would bar any possible judgment of the authorities that in the absence of physical interventions the offender will continue to be a real danger to society, including prison society (other inmates and the custodial staff). Thus, the judgment by the offender's custodians that he is dangerous and a threat to the well-being of others remains the trump card against any ace from the side of the offender. Such a judgment of dangerousness can be sufficient to justify physical intervention in those cases where it is also judged that the intervention is the least repressive, least destructive method to inflict on the offender that is also sufficient to reduce or eliminate his dangerousness. The right of the authorities in custody over an offender to make such a judgment of dangerousness and to act on it, with consequences of a far-reaching sort, would be defended (if anyone bothered to defend it) along the following lines. First, no one has the right to be the final judge of whether he is a menace to others; no one has veto rights over the judgment of others that he is a menace to them. Second, the offender, by virtue of his conviction of a serious criminal offense involving violence to the person, has already been proved dangerous to others. Prima facie, there is now a burden of proof on him to show why he should not be regarded as someone ready and willing to be dangerous in the future. Third, if he gives evidence while in custody that he is still dangerous, then it is reasonable to consider the methods sufficient to reduce or eliminate the likelihood of his further violence against others, and to use on him the least repressive, least brutal method sufficient to that end. If this reasoning is accepted, premise i of our original argument must be rejected, and we are well on our way to the discussion of the remaining alternative from among our original three, to wit, the limits and conditions under which the new techniques of physical intervention may properly be used.

Thus, the rejection of premise i in our argument earlier prevents us from drawing the conclusion that no prisoner may be involuntarily subjected to physical interventions designed to make him less dangerous to others. While this does not dispose of that conclusion (nothing short of proving it to be self-contradictory would do this), it does tend to direct us toward policy alternative 2 by requiring us to back away from alternative 3. If this analysis is correct, and my reasoning so far is in the right direction, then the chief task on which morality, law, and social science need to be brought to bear concerns exactly where, at present, and on what grounds the new techniques of physical intervention may be employed. If it is wrong to prohibit their use under any conditions, as I am inclined to think it is, then it remains to be shown precisely where the line must be drawn to divide permissible use of such interventions from impermissible use.

REFERENCES

BEDAU, H. A. (1967) "A social philosopher looks at the death penalty." *Amer. J. of Psychiatry* 123 (May): 1361–1370.

——— [ed.] (1964) *The Death Penalty in America.* New York: Doubleday Anchor.

Boston University Law Review (1974) "Kaimowitz v. Department of Mental Health: a right to be free from experimental psychosurgery?" 54 (March): 301–339.

Chicago Peoples Law Office (1973) "Check out your mind: behavior modification experimentation and control in prison and a national proposal to fight it." (unpublished memorandum)

CHOROVER, S. L. (1974) "The pacification of the brain." *Psychology Today* 7 (May): 59–69.

DWORKIN, R. M. (1971) "Taking rights seriously," pp. 168–194 in E. V. Rostow (ed.) *Is Law Dead?* New York: Simon & Schuster.

GOODALL, K. (1972) "Shapers at work." *Psychology Today* 5 (November): 53–63, 132–138.

HAAS, F. (1973) "The making of a human vegetable." *Outlook on Criminal Justice in the Commonwealth* (Mid-December): 1, 6.

KITTRIE, N. N. (1971) *The Right to Be Different: Deviance and Enforced Therapy.* Baltimore: Johns Hopkins Univ. Press.

KNIGHT, M. (1974) "Child molesters try 'shock' cure." *New York Times* (May 21): 43.

KOHLBERG, L. (1974) Position paper. Conference on Moral Development and Juvenile Justice, October. (unpublished)

MILL, J. S. (1859) "On liberty," pp. 126–250 in M. Warnock (ed.) *John Sturat Mill: On Liberty, Utilitarianism, Essay on Bentham.* Cleveland: World Publishing.

MORRIS, H. (1970) "Persons and punishment," pp. 111–134 in A. I. Melden (ed.) *Human Rights.* Belmont, Calif.: Wadsworth.

MORRIS, H. (1970) "Persons and punishment," pp. 111–134 in A. I. Melden (ed.) *Human Rights.* Belmont, Calif.: Wadsworth.

MORRIS, N. (1974) *The Future of Imprisonment.* Chicago: Univ. of Chicago Press.

—— and G. HAWKINS (1970) *The Honest Politician's Guide to Crime Control.* Chicago: Univ. of Chicago Press.

OELSNER, L. (1974a) "U. S. ends project on jail inmates." *New York Times* (February 7): 12.

—— (1974b) "U. S. bars crime fund use on behavior modification." *New York Times* (February 15): 54.

RAWLS, J. (1971) *A Theory of Justice.* Cambridge: Harvard Univ. Press.

RICKS, C. (1972) "Horror show." *New York Review* (April 6): 28–31.

ROTHMAN, D. (1973) "Decarcerating prisoners and patients." *Civil Liberties Review* 1 (Fall): 8–30.

RUSSELL, E. W. (1974) "The power of behavior control: a critique of behavior modification methods." *J. of Clinical Psychology Monograph Supplement* 43 (April): 1–30.

SYKES, G. M. (1974) "The new breed of prisoner." *New York Times* (April 21): IV, 5.

TOM L. BEAUCHAMP

Paternalism and Bio-behavioral Control

Recently ethical and legal philosophers have shown a revival of interest in whether paternalistic reasons are ever good reasons for the limitation of individual liberties in the form of coercive laws. A special target has been John Stuart Mill, whose searching criticisms of paternalism in *On Liberty* are now widely regarded as too sweeping and insufficiently guarded. Against these recent trends in philosophy I argue in this paper that: (1) Mill's critique of paternalism is in all essentials sustainable; (2) Even his most sympathetic critics (especially Dworkin, Feinberg and Hart) have not demonstrated that paternalism is justified; (3) Paternalistic reasons for bio-behavioral control are both common and dangerous, yet are, like all forms of paternalism, irrelevant to the justification of coercive limitation of liberty.

Reprinted from *The Monist,* Vol. 60, No. 1 (January 1977) with the permission of the author and the publisher.

I use the term "bio-behavioral control" to cover the following set of technological capacities:

A. Information control
  1. Psychotherapy
  2. Behavioral engineering
B. Bio-psychological control
  1. Electrical stimulation of the brain (ESB) and psychosurgery
  2. Psychotropic drugs
C. Bio-medical control
  1. Life-sustaining and reproductive controls
  2. Genetic engineering

. . .

I shall first briefly survey a few selected examples of paternalistic justifications for coercive bio-behavioral interventions. I then pass on to general philosophical concerns about the nature and merit of paternalism, including a defense of Mill against his critics.

Recent technology indicates that we are now capable of biologically and behaviorally controlling the course of human development in ways previously unavailable. Once we began to learn the physical and environmental processes which control human development an area rife with possibilities for human engineering emerged. Recently, inheritable alterations in human cells have been produced by means such as the initiation of viral infection. Various drug therapies, surgical procedures, and behavior-modification techniques continue to produce impressive results. These control capabilities presage that both "favorable" and "unfavorable" alterations may be required by the state, or at least introduced on a massive scale. Some on the vanguard of these developments contend that we can and should engineer the production of children, "improve" as a whole the human stock we breed, and introduce more rigorous social controls through bio-behavioral techniques. They offer a wide range of justifications for their envisioned alterations. It would be foolish to attempt here to assess the full complement of justifications for coercive bio-behavioral intervention which have been offered, and I wish to emphasize that I restrict my arguments exclusively to available paternalistic justifications. (Since the authors cited attempt to provide the strongest possible case for their positions, they sometimes offer a mixed set of justifications which are not *purely* paternalistic.)

INVOLUNTARY COMMITMENT AND THERAPY ON GROUNDS OF INSANITY

Involuntary commitment to therapeutic environments is common. The justification offered for both commitment and forced therapy is often overtly paternalistic. Sometimes language as vague as the "patient's need for treatment" is used, and at other times "dangerous to self" and in "need of custody" suffice by law as criteria of commitment. Forced bio-behavioral therapeutic techniques are legally permitted after the patient has been committed. The first and most crucial coercive act requiring justification, however, is the commitment

itself. A typical problem case is that of Mrs. Catherine Lake, who suffered from arteriosclerosis causing temporary confusion and mild loss of memory, interspersed with times of mental alertness and rationality. All parties agreed that Mrs. Lake never harmed anyone or presented any threat of danger, yet she was committed to a mental institution because she often seemed in a confused and defenseless state. At her trial, while apparently fully rational, she testified that she knew the risk of living outside the hospital and preferred to take that risk rather than be in the hospital environment. The Court of Appeals denied her petition, arguing that she is "mentally ill," "is a danger to herself . . . and is not competent to care for herself." The legal justification cited by the Court was a statute which "provides for involuntary hospitalization of a person who is 'mentally ill and, because of that illness, is likely to injure himself' . . . ."[1] Such reasoning is widespread today, despite forceful arguments by psychiatrists that the harmless "mentally sick" are often competent to make rational judgments.

EUGENIC STERILIZATION

Eugenic sterilization laws are still in effect in over half the states in the U. S. The retarded have been a special target, since they along with criminals, epileptics, alcoholics, and other vulnerable groups have been alleged to have genetically rooted mental and physical disabilities. Since the retarded are often childlike and unaware of their responsibilities, the rearing of children is frequently a heavy burden. For such reasons it has been considered in their own best interest that they be sterilized, even if they do not agree or fail to comprehend the decision.[2] Irvin B. Hill, writing about the sterilization of mentally deficient persons in prison, argues as follows:

A mentally deficient person is not a suitable parent for either a normal or a subnormal child, and children would be an added burden to an already handicapped individual, who does well to support himself. It would be unfair to the state, *to the individual,* and particularly *to his potential children,* to permit his release without the *protection* of sterilization. . . .

> . . . It has been the policy of the State of Oregon to sterilize mentally deficient persons before releasing them from its institution and . . . this program has been of benefit from economic, social, *and eugenic* standpoints. . . . It *assists the individual* in his transition to a non-institutional life; and it relieves the state of the financial burden. . . . [3]

While not a pure paternalistic justification for eugenic control, it is partially paternalistic and is the kind of reasoning which, once canonized into law, can easily become purely paternalistic in coercive environments. Free and informed consent is unlikely in the context of penal institutions, especially when one is dealing with mentally deficient persons. They can be bribed with offers of freedom and intimidated by threats that their confinement will be extended. Although we now know both that most retarded persons are born from parents of normal intelligence and that the retarded often have children of normal intelligence, prison and other custodial environments continue to give rise to the sort of paternalistically motivated interventions suggested by Hill.

PSYCHOSURGERY

Psychosurgery is an intentional surgical intervention on a person's brain which can easily alter such capacities as memory, emotion, speech, and reasoning. It has been condemned by some as destructive of human autonomy, and praised by others as restorative of human autonomy. Dr. Orlando J. Andy, a practitioner, is one supporter, partially on paternalistic grounds:

> [Psychosurgery] should be performed on patients who are *a detriment to themselves* and to society. It should be *used for custodial purposes* when a patient requires constant attention. . . .
> It should be used in the adolescent and pediatric age group *in order to allow the developing brain to mature* with as *normal* a reaction to its environment as possible. . . .
> *The patient must have confidence and trust* in the physician or physician's recommendation. The final decision, however, to have an operation should be left to the patient and relatives. I do not operate without their support, consent, and request. [4]

It is again questionable whether the notion of consent can be meaningfully applied. The consent of relatives must often be solely relied upon, and it is easily obtainable—for the relatives' selfish or paternalistic reasons. [5] Psychotropic and other powerful drugs are often used without consent, and sometimes consent is not even requested for psychosurgery, as in a recent British case where a magistrate ordered involuntary psychosurgery for a compulsive gambler and psychopath charged with larceny and misrepresentation. [6] It is interesting to note that throughout his testimony Dr. Andy appeals to the idea that psychosurgery is in the best interests of the patient, will result in a wider range of freedom, removes extreme risks otherwise present, and removes otherwise irreversible health deficiencies. As we shall see, these are precisely the sort of justifying reasons advanced by the supporters of paternalism.

BEHAVIORAL ENGINEERING

Some behavioral psychologists notoriously employ paternalistic justifications for modifying children's behavior, as do proponents of amphetamines for hyperkinetic children. But some utopian ideals, as instanced by Skinner, are far more broadly paternalistic:

> The literature of freedom has encouraged escape from or attack upon all controllers. . . . What is overlooked is control which does not have aversive consequences at any time. . . . The technology has been most successful . . . in child care, schools, and the management of retardates and institutionalized psychotics. . . .
> The problem is to design a world which will be liked not by people as they now are but by those who live in it. "I wouldn't like it" is the complaint of the individualist who puts forth his own susceptibilities to reinforcement as established values. . . . A better world will be liked by those who live in it because it has been designed with an eye to what is, or can be, most reinforcing. . . . [7]

This forward-looking paternalism justifies coercive controls on grounds that the designer provides positive benefits in every individual's own best interest. Skinner repeatedly observes that such techniques will become more and more attractive as social problems such as overpopulation increase. He is probably right.

In these four examples I have been emphasizing only the active side of potential paternalistic coercion, but the distinction between actively *requiring* a person to do *x* and passively *not allowing* a person to do *x* is worthy of notice. For example, a state might for paternalistic reasons require that violent rioters undergo psychosurgery, yet not allow epileptics to have the same operation. This could result in a two-sided paternalism: rioters should have the operation because it's better for them than prison confinement, but it's too dangerous for epileptics because of possible side-effects. Such passive coercion is likely to be the most subtle, least noticed, and most widely prevalent form of paternalism. Yet the laws spawned may be highly controversial. It is not difficult to find such paternalistic laws against euthanasia with patient consent, the use of drugs not productive of socially harmful behavior, and psychosurgery with patient consent. Examples of this form of paternalism are found in Peter Breggin's polemic against psychosurgery (also by implication euthanasia) and in Vernon Mark's discussion of coercive psychotherapeutic intervention:

We can recognize the individual's right to harm or kill himself, but we can never permit *someone else* to harm him *or to help him* toward his self-maiming or suicide.[8]

Thomas Szasz . . . states that therapists should not interfere with a patient's "free will," if he wants to kill himself. The medical model is far more humane, for it views self-destructive tendencies, especially in drug-intoxicated or temporarily disturbed patients, as symptoms of disease that require some form of intervention.[9]

. . .

THE NATURE AND TYPES OF PATERNALISM

Paternalistically motivated laws are thought to be justified because they work to prevent persons from harming themselves. This justification for limiting individual liberty presumably supplements more widely accepted justifications such as the prevention of harm by others and the maintenance of public order. Whether paternalistic reasons are *good* reasons will occupy us momentarily, but first some agreement must be reached concerning proper use of the word "paternalism." If one operates with a definition as loose as H. L. A.

Hart's—"the protection of people against themselves"[10]—misunderstandings readily follow. Legislation intended to help citizens protect themselves from inadvertent acts, such as mutilating their hands in garbage disposals, would on this definition seem paternalistic. Gerald Dworkin has provided a better definition, which I accept with only two innocuous modifications (in brackets): Paternalism is "the [coercive] interference with a person's liberty of action justified by [protective or beneficent] reasons referring exclusively to the welfare, good, happiness, needs, interests or values of the person being coerced."[11]

Joel Feinberg has quite properly distinguished two types of paternalism:[12]

1. *Legal paternalism*—the justification of state coercion to protect individuals from self-inflicted harm.

2. *Extreme paternalism*—the justification of state coercion to benefit individual persons.

Skinner is an example of the second type, our other figures of the first.

Feinberg also considers the possibility that there are two kinds of paternalism, strong and weak, a distinction which presumably cuts across the above categories. He explains the weak form as follows (113 [50]):

The state has the right to prevent self-regarding harmful conduct only when it is substantially non-voluntary or when temporary intervention is necessary to establish whether it is voluntary or not.

The class of nonvoluntary cases includes cases where there is consent but not adequately informed consent. The strong form holds that the state has the right to coercively protect or benefit a person even when his contrary choices are informed and voluntary. The problem with this distinction, as Feinberg himself argues, is that "weak paternalism" is not paternalism in any interesting sense, because it is not a liberty limiting principle *independent* of the "harm to others" principle (113, 124). For this reason I restrict use of the term "paternalism" to strong paternalism. However, it is important to see that the "temporary intervention" mentioned above is both coercive and justified on what might deceptively appear to be paternalistic grounds. Mill believed that a person ignorant of a potential danger which might befall him could justifiably be restrained, so long as the coercion was temporary and only for the purpose of rendering the person informed, in which case he would be free to choose whatever course he wished. Mill regarded this—correctly, I think—as temporary but justified coercion which is not "real infringement" of liberty:

If either a public officer or anyone else saw a person attempting to cross a bridge which had been ascertained to be unsafe, and there were no time to warn him of his danger, they might seize him and turn him back, without any real infringement of his liberty; for liberty consists in doing what one desires, and he does not desire to fall into the river.[13]

It is not a question of protecting a man *against himself* or of interfering with his *liberty of action*. He is not *acting* at all in regard to this danger. He needs protection from something which is precisely *not himself,* not his intended action, not in any remote sense of his own making. While I am here embellishing Mill, this seems to me clearly the direction of his argument. Mill goes on to say that once the man has been fully informed and understands the dangers of the bridge, then he should be free to traverse it, if he wishes. I shall be arguing in support of Mill's conclusions, and I shall call this justification of *temporary* intervention "Mill's proviso."

. . .

Dworkin, Feinberg, and Hart have had the good sense to examine the proper or justified limits of Mill's principles. Hart suggests that because there has been a general decline in the belief that individuals always or even frequently know their own interest best or are capable of free, informed consent, we no longer accept Mill's protests against paternalism, and in fact accept at least legal paternalism as a "perfectly coherent policy" (H, 32f). Supposedly it is for paternalistic reasons that we think a person should not be allowed to sell himself into slavery, barter himself to a doctor for dangerous experiments, or take morphine purely for the sake of pleasure.

. . .

I shall not, unfortunately, have space to explore the individual arguments of these philosophers. Instead I treat them as a collective unit. But I believe there is something approximating a consensus among Dworkin and Hart that there are conditions which justify paternalistic interventions, even though individually they may be neither necessary nor sufficient conditions for justified coercion. Their views can be concisely combined and systematically ordered as follows:

The Principle of Paternalism justifies liberty-limiting legislation and other coercive interferences. The Principle states that: S justifiably coerces P by intervention I if (but not only if):

Justifying Aim Condition
1. By performing I, S is protecting P against himself,

Restricting Conditions
2. Reasonable grounds indicate that P either
   (a) does not know his own best interest, though this is knowable by S (cf. H, 32), *OR*
   (b) does know his own best interest, yet is insufficiently motivated to pursue it unless legally required to do so (cf. D, 77f),
3. I achieves a wider range of freedom for P,
4. I avoids an extreme, manifestly unreasonable risk to P,
5. I avoids serious evils which P might cause himself through decisions which are far-reaching, potentially dangerous and irreversible, and where no *rational* alternative is more highly valued by P (cf. D, 78–80),[14]

Weighting Condition[15]
6. The general presumption against coercion is outweighed by the significance of the above conditions, which also must outweigh other principles (e.g., confidentiality, privacy) that restrict intervention. . . .

In addition to these conditions Hart and Feinberg distinguish voluntary and involuntary assumptions of a risk and stress the importance of the degree of voluntariness (F, 110 f [48]). Factors which constrain free choice such as inadequate reflection, transitory desires, inner psychological compulsions, family pressures, etc. are seen as factors "which diminish the significance to be attached to an apparently free choice or to consent" (H, 33). I shall have more to say about the role of voluntariness momentarily.

Dworkin and Hart proceed by citing practices most would agree are justified and sometimes spring from paternalistic motives. It is then assumed that if the conditions justifying these (paternalistically motivated) practices can be listed, they are independent of the harm principle, and paternalism has been justified. Accordingly, no Mill-supportive example can dent or falsify such an analysis, because it has already been assumed (not, I think, *argued*) that instances of *justified paternalism* have been given. Now *if* the methodology and the assumptions just mentioned are admitted, I do not believe this thesis can be gainsaid.

· · ·

Dworkin, Feinberg, and Hart [present] troublesome cases [which] center on situations where persons are (a) ignorant and (b) less than fully voluntary in acting. All ignorance cases can be handled, I believe, by Mill's proviso. Once someone is adequately informed (assuming this is possible and assuming the person is able to act on the information), the decision should rest with the agent. Cases of involuntary acts or less than fully voluntary acts are more troublesome only because there are degrees of voluntariness. Fully involuntary acts are not especially difficult, however, nor did they seem so to Mill. Feinberg has this point just right:

Neither should we expect anti-paternalistic individualism to deny protection to a person from his own nonvoluntary choices, for insofar as the choices are not voluntary they are just as alien to him as the choices of someone else (F, 112 [48]).

Such harmful "actions" involve harms caused by conditions either unknown to the relevant persons or beyond their control, and *for this reason* are subject to coercive intervention. . . .

Still, what are we to say about those actions which are partially voluntary and partially involuntary—e.g., those performed under behavior control devices such as subliminal advertising, and drug therapy, or in circumstances involving alcoholic stimulation, mob-inspired enthusiasm, retardation, and neurotic compulsion? I see no reason why all these cases should not be treated like ignorance cases. We may (assuming objectivity and knowledge on our part) justifiably protect a man from harm which might result directly from his drunkenness or retardation. To the extent one protects him from causes beyond his knowledge and control, to that extent (subject perhaps to further specific qualifications) one justifiably intervenes. If a potentially injurable person genuinely has "cloudy judgment" or is being deceived through ignorance, his choices are substantially nonvoluntary. And if he can be injured *because* of these conditions, we may justifiably restrain his action. But once informed of the dangers of his action, if and when a context can be provided where voluntary choice is meaningfully possible, he cannot justifiably be further restrained. Mrs. Lake provided us earlier with an excellent anti-paternalistic example where coercion is *not* justified. Severely retarded persons provide a useful example where coercion *is* justified. Those with minimal or no language skills are not capable of voluntary choice. It is sometimes contended, however, that they must be protected against themselves by involuntary sterilization, in order that they not enter into sexual relations. This piece of paternalism has matters reversed. Such persons seldom have sexual relations unless exploited by others. Any coercion should be aimed at protecting them from exploitation and should be justified by the harm principle. There are less intrusive means to the end of protection than sterilization. Also, if such persons can be taught language skills and acquire a meaningful measure of free choice, our obligations to them are altered, and coercion would no longer be justified. The case is similar with non-rational behavior control techniques, which typically are used to alter the "choices" a man makes, without his understanding or consenting to the alterations. To the extent such actions truly are controlled, it is meaningless to say they are chosen, though no doubt the degree of control and voluntariness rest on a multi-level continuum.

. . .

THE JUSTIFICATION OF JUSTIFYING PRINCIPLES

Reasonable and informed persons differ concerning those actions which should and should not be coercively restrained; they also differ over the acceptability of those justifying principles invoked as grounds for such interventions. They can disagree vigorously over the proper interpretation of cases such as those I have advanced. Nowhere do they disagree more than in the area of cases which some take to be *hard cases* in test of the sufficiency of a particular principle to justify interference (as, say, suicide and slavery are hard cases for the harm principle) or (2) *hard core cases* favoring the sufficiency of a principle (as, say, the mentally ill needing treatment are considered by some hard core cases for paternalistic principles). One man's clinching paradigm may be the butt of another's attack. In such cases we often say that two disputants cannot bring their moral intuitions into harmony. So in the present dispute over paternalism, it might be argued, I am simply unable to bring my Mill-aligned intuitions into accord with those of Dworkin and Hart; yet there are cases . . . which have an attractive moral sway in the direction of paternalism. Cases of suicide, slavery, treatment of the retarded, and drug controls [are examples]. . . . The question must now be raised whether anything further can be said to adjudicate our differences.

First, a couple of methodological points are in order. I would agree that the systematic use of examples has its limits and may yield inconclusive results. I share the scepticism of those contemporary philosophers who believe that reliance upon intuition and upon quasi-legal notions such as the "outweighing" of one right or principle by another may ultimately fail to resolve important issues. Also, I am prepared to agree that ethical argument by analysis of examples is not purely descriptive of our common ethical beliefs, and hence is not simply a matter of systematically bringing general intuitions into harmony. Often such argument is *revisionary* of our ethical beliefs. Examples shock intuition and alter belief. In the end disagreements such as, say, mine with Dworkin, may largely reduce to arguments concerning why moral beliefs ought to be readjusted. To argue, then, that paternalism is never justified may well be a way of arguing that we ought to regard it as never justified. I accept the view that moral philosophy should be in the business of providing such arguments.

Why, then, ought paternalism to be judged unacceptable? The dominant reason is that paternalistic principles are too broad and hence justify too much. Robert Harris has correctly pointed out that Hart's description of paternalism would in principle "justify the imposition of a Spartan-like regimen requiring rigorous physical exercise and abstention from smoking, drinking, and hazardous pastimes."[16] The more thoughtful restrictions on paternalism proposed by Dworkin and Feinberg would disallow this sort of extreme, but still leave unacceptable latitude, especially in contexts where bio-behavioral controls are most likely to be abused. Prison environments and therapeutic agencies have thrived on the use of paternalistic justifications. Paternalism potentially gives prison wardens, psychosurgeons, and state officials a good reason for coercively using most any means in order to achieve ends they believe in the subject's best interest. It is demonstrable that allowing this latitude of judgment is dangerous and acutely uncontrollable. This is as true of Feinberg, Hart, and Dworkin's hard core cases in favor of paternalism as it is elsewhere.

Paternalists, then, leave us with unresolved problems concerning the scope of the principle. Suppose, for example, that a man risks his life for the advance of medicine by submitting to an unreasonably risky experiment, an act which most would think not in his own interest. Are we to commend him or coercively restrain him? Paternalism strongly suggests that it would be permissible to coercively restrain such a person. Yet if that is so, then the state is permitted to restrain coercively its morally heroic citizens, not to mention its martyrs, if they act—as such people frequently do—in a manner "harmful" to themselves. I do not see how paternalism can be patched up by adding further conditions about the actions of heroes and martyrs. It would increasingly come to bear the marks of an ad hoc and gratuitous principle which is not genuinely independent of the harm principle.

It is universally acknowledged that the harm principle justifiably permits coercive interventions. No other justifying principle occupies such a non-controversial status. Perhaps this will and ought to change. But before we agree to supplementary liberty limiting principles, it would seem the better part of caution to be as certain as possible that the harm principle will not suffice and that the evils the supplementary principles enable us to prevent are greater than the evils they inadvertently permit.

NOTES

1. The relevant court documents are found in Jay Katz, Joseph Goldstein, and Alan M. Dershowits, *Psychoanalysis, Psychiatry, and Law* (New York: The Free Press, 1967), pp. 552–54, 710–13.

2. The history of such justifications in American Society can be found in Kenneth M. Ludmerer, *Genetics and American Society* (Baltimore: The Johns Hopkins University Press, 1972) and in Mark H. Haller, *Eugenics* (New Brunswick, New Jersey: Rutgers University Press, 1963).

3. Irvin B. Hill, "Sterilizations in Oregon," *American Journal of Mental Deficiency*, Vol. 54 (1950), p. 403. Italics added.

4. Testimony before U. S. Senate Subcommittee of the Committee on Labor and Public Welfare, on "Quality of Health Care—Human Experimentation," Friday, February 23, 1973 (Washington, D. C., Government Printing Office), pp. 351 f. Italics added.

5. This claim is vigorously argued by Peter Breggin, "The Second Wave," *Mental Hygiene* (March, 1973), p. 393. It is more soberly argued by Vernon H. Mark and Robert Neville in "Brain Surgery in Aggressive Epileptics," *Journal of the American Medical Association* 226, No. 7 (November 12, 1973), p. 771.

6. Cf. Nicholas Kittrie, *The Right to be Different: Deviance and Enforced Therapy* (Baltimore: The Johns Hopkins Press, 1971), p. 354. This book is a useful resource for legal invocations of *parens patriae* powers. On the use of both Drugs and Psychosurgery, see Michael H. Shapiro, "Legislating the Control of Behavior Control: Autonomy and the Coercive Use of Organic Therapies," 47 *Southern California Law Review* (1974), pp. 237–356. [Reprinted as the first article in this chapter]

7. *Beyond Freedom and Dignity* (New York: Bantam Books, 1971), pp. 38, 142, 156.

8. Peter Breggin, "The Second Wave," p. 393. (Second italics added.)

9. Vernon Mark, "A Psychosurgeon's Case for Psychosurgery," *Psychology Today*, Vol. 8, No. 2 (July, 1974), p. 84.

10. H. L. A. Hart, *Law, Liberty, and Morality* (Stanford: Stanford University Press, 1963), p. 31. Hereafter abbreviated *H*.

11. Gerald Dworkin, "Paternalism," *The Monist*, Vol. 56 (January, 1972), p. 65. Hereafter abbreviated *D*.

12. "Legal Paternalism," *The Canadian Journal of Philosophy*, Vol. I (1971), pp. 105–24. This paper is reworked in *Social Philosophy* (Englewood Cliffs: Prentice-Hall, 1973). Hereafter both are abbreviated *F*, with references to the latter in brackets. The distinction mentioned above is best made in *Social Philosophy*, p. 33, and in his "'Harmless Immoralities' and Offensive Nuisances," *Issues in Law and Morality*, ed. N. S. Care and T. K. Trelogan (Cleveland: Case Western Reserve University Press, 1973), pp. 83 f.

13. Mill, *On Liberty* (Indianapolis: Liberal Arts Press, 1956), p. 117. Feinberg deals with this example (112 [49]), but I am unsure whether he believes Mill's conclusion [is] correct.

14. Cf. the similar condition justifying paternalism given by R. S. Downie, *Roles and Values* (London: Methuen and Company, 1971), p. 108.

15. My formulation of the Weighting Condition is indebted to Michael D. Bayles, "Comments: Offensive Conduct and the Law, " in *Issues in Law and Morality (op. cit.)*, pp. 112 f.

16. "Private Consensual Adult Behavior: The Requirement of Harm to Others in the Enforcement of Morality," 14 *UCLA Law Review* (1967), p. 585n.

VERNON H. MARK

The Case for Psychosurgery

INTRODUCTION

The continuing controversy surrounding psychosurgery is responsible not only for greater public awareness of the procedure but also for the publication of misinformation that has hindered rational discourse and policy planning relating to its use. An informed discussion of psychosurgery must proceed from at least a general familiarity with the medical data. It is therefore the purpose of this article to provide a brief summary of the research in this area and to correct the more significant distortions regarding psychosurgical practice that have surfaced in the course of the anti-psychosurgery campaign. . . .

A SURVEY OF THE MEDICAL FINDINGS

CLASSICAL PSYCHOSURGERY

In its classical sense, psychosurgery includes operations on the frontal lobes or their connections in the brain to relieve the symptoms of intractable depression, agitation, compulsion, delusion, hallucination and ideas of reference in patients with no known brain disease. Such surgery is performed only when psychiatric treatment, drug therapy, electroconvulsive treatment and other forms of environmental therapy have failed to relieve the patient's symptoms.

Frontal lobe surgery was initiated by the clinical trials of Moniz,[1] a Nobel Laureate. Although it is most effective in treating agitation and depression, the operation of radical frontal lobotomy was widely performed in the

United States for the relief of symptoms in agitated schizophrenic patients. Many of these patients were institutionalized, and controlled studies, such as those of the United States Veterans Administration,[2] showed that the condition of the operated patients improved in terms of their ability to leave mental institutions and carry on integrated lives in non-institutional settings. However, some of these patients paid the unacceptably high price of severe emotional blunting and intellectual deterioration for their treatment. Thus, with the advent of powerful ataractic drugs—Thorazine, Stelazine and Haldoperidol, for example—capable of achieving the same therapeutic goals without surgery, the performance of radical frontal lobe surgery in the United States ceased.

More restricted forms of frontal lobe surgery were developed in this country by Foltz and White[3] and by Thomas Ballantine.[4] However, these studies were developed more fully in Great Britain where the more limited popularity and use of psychosurgery made it less susceptible to replacement by drug therapy. Cairns and his associates at Oxford University began to modify frontal lobe operations so that small portions of the frontal lobe were ablated to produce specific relief of symptoms.[5] They initiated the operation of cingulotomy in which the destructive lesion is restricted to a small bundle of fibers called the cingulum. Fortunately, critical British psychiatrists evaluated an extensive series of patients prior to surgery and followed them for several years afterward. A review of their published studies indicates that restricted forms of frontal surgery may be therapeutic when other methods of treatment have proved ineffective.[6]

Reprinted with permission of the publisher from *Boston University Law Review*, Vol. 54, No. 2 (March 1974), pp. 217–230.

Psychosurgery has expanded beyond its classical meaning to include any neurosurgical operation that affects human behavior, even if the patients being treated have obvious brain disease. The most controversial patients within this expanded definition are those who have epilepsy and psychiatric symptoms, often including abnormally aggressive behavior.[7]

Although the brain responds to the environment as an integrated unit, an individual's brain mechanisms are limited by their ontogenetic and phylogenetic development. It is therefore a specialized portion of the brain, the limbic system, that more directly governs "fight or flight" behavior, sexuality, appetite and emotional tone. As broadly defined, the limbic system or limbic brain includes the medial-frontal lobes and orbital surfaces, the cingulum, amygdala, hippocampus, hypothalamus and portions of the thalamus, mid-brain and mid-line commissures.[8]

The limbic brain may be damaged by head injury, infections such as virus encephalitis and rabies, brain tumors, hemorrhage, infarcts, poisons, and lack of oxygen such as may occur in febrile convulsions. One of the more common diseases afflicting the limbic brain, however, is focal epilepsy.[9] Such epilepsy may be associated with behavioral abnormalities, and the focus may originate from the inner or medial-anterior portion of the temporal lobe. A typical attack of temporal lobe epilepsy which includes such foci produces the following symptoms: hallucinations of taste or smell associated with momentary lapses in consciousness, lip-smacking, head and eye turning, mental confusion, inappropriate speech, repetitive inappropriate movements and, at times, major motor seizures.

Episodes of violence appear to be occasionally related to this variety of epilepsy. Currie and his colleagues, for example, have shown that abnormal aggressivity, sometimes motivated by unreasoning and overwhelming fear, may occur either preceding or during the seizure itself or in the stage of post-ictal confusion.[10] Much more frequently, however, episodes of catastrophic rage occur between seizures. Walker, who has demonstrated that implanted electrodes may detect frequent seizures deep within the brain that are undetectable from the surface of the brain or head, believes that these repeated deep seizures bear an important relationship to the inter-ictal rage characteristic of epileptic patients with limbic foci.[11]

If anti-convulsant and ataractic drugs and psychiatric treatment fail to relieve the symptoms associated with temporal lobe epilepsy, surgical treatment involving the removal of the anterior portion of the temporal lobe is usually administered. Specifically, such surgery includes the complete removal of amygdala, hippocampus in its anterior third and surface structures on the lateral portion of the lobe. However, in an attempt to achieve the same kind of therapy with less destruction of brain tissue, stereotactic methods have been developed. Tiny electrodes implanted into the amygdala may now be used for recording, stimulating and destroying restricted portions of tissue with heat.[12] The preservation of as much brain tissue as possible is, of course, always to be desired, but sterotactic methods are particularly useful for patients who have epileptic foci in both temporal lobes, because the bilateral, complete removal of anterior temporal lobes would severely limit recent memory and intellectual functioning. Indeed, this complication occasionally occurs when both temporal lobes are damaged before surgery is accomplished.

Because the clinical signs of temporal lobe epilepsy are not as dramatic as those of major motor seizures and the surface confirmation of a temporal lobe attack is difficult, critics of this kind of surgery argue that the diagnosis of the disorder is indefinite and dependent upon the vagaries of a brain wave recording. Recent studies prove, however, that most patients with temporal lobe epilepsy have definite structural changes in the brain which can be seen on special x-rays called pneumoencephalograms[13] or in the specimens of temporal lobes removed when temporal lobectomy is performed. Falconer has reported that 25–50 percent of the temporal lobe epileptic patients surveyed in various series displayed abnormal aggressivity. About 80 percent of temporal lobe segments removed at surgery contained gross or microscopic abnormalities situated in the anterior and medial portions. About 50 percent of these patients had a scar called mesial sclerosis in the anterior temporal region, 10 percent had infarcts, atrophy or other gross lesions, and approximately 20 percent had small brain tumors called hamartomas.[14]

Studies by Walker and Blumer[15] and by Falconer[16] demonstrate that temporal lobe surgery may relieve epileptic patients of their seizures, abnormal aggressivity and other psychiatric symptoms. In the words of one who has reviewed this data, "this careful but uncontrolled series would hardly lend support to an indiscriminate use of brain surgery for management of disordered behavior, [but] it lends equally little support to those who would forbid any surgery of this type under all circumstances."[17]

Cooper and Gilman have achieved similar results without removing brain tissue.[18] Through the implantation of stimulating electrodes on top of the cerebellum, or small brain, they have stopped epileptic seizures by electrical stimulation. In one patient in particular, in whom epileptic seizures were associated with catastrophic rage and destructive violence, cerebellar stimulation completely reversed both these symptoms and the seizures themselves. Seizures and violence recurred when the stimulation was no longer administered, but the symptoms disappeared once again when it was resumed.

PSYCHOSURGERY AND STRUCTURAL BRAIN DAMAGE

Catastrophic rage may develop in association with rabies, head injury, hydrocephalus and large brain tumors. Although such tumors usually grow so rapidly and are so disabling that aggressivity is not a major complaint, some patients do have this symptom.

Three Case Histories. Patient *A*,[19] brought to the hospital after trying to decapitate his wife with a meat cleaver, was in an agitated, aggressive state and had to be restrained from tearing at people with his nails and teeth. A distinctive personality change had occurred five months prior to his admission to the hospital. He had become slovenly in his habits, filthy in his body care, insulting to his wife and fellow workers, and he complained of weakness in one arm and of headaches. An examination revealed that his optic nerve heads were swollen with increased intracranial pressure. In addition, a mass lesion in the right frontal area of the brain impinged upon the base of the frontal lobe and pressed internal connections from the anterior temporal lobe. Part of this mass, it was discovered through surgery, consisted of swollen dead brain tissue which has been destroyed by a tumor the size of a small tangerine. After the removal of this tumor—a variety known as meningioma—the patient did not threaten the life of his wife for another 20 years, during which time he worked for 17 years at one job. The recurrence of his condition has prompted a repeat neurological examination at the present time.

Damage to the limbic brain is frequently caused by head injury. Occasionally, such injury results in the swelling of spaces inside the head, the ventricles. This condition, called hydrocephalus, is usually accompanied by increased placidity and even torpor, but hyper-aggressivity and attack behavior may also appear.

Patient *B*[20] was hit by an automobile and sustained a head injury. In a convalescent home, unusual symptoms of mental disturbance and aggressive behavior began to appear. His language patterns changed abruptly and he became hostile, repeatedly attacking nurses by tackling them to the ground and then proceeding to bite them. Studies of his brain indicated a remarkable dilation of his ventricles. Surgery known as the ventriculo-atrial shunt was performed in which spinal fluid is shunted into the right heart through a valve. By reducing the excess fluid in his ventricles, the operation successfully reversed the patient's symptoms, including his abnormal aggressivity.

Head injuries that do not result in hydrocephalus may also be related to abnormal aggressivity. Patient C^{21} suffered a severe head injury when the bicycle he was riding collided with a truck. Upon his admission to the emergency room, the patient began to terrorize nurses, doctors and attendants. His wild and agitated state lasted for 36 hours, and, during periods of apparent lucidity, he denied having any memory of the collision or his wild behavior. Initial arteriograms were normal but were followed by a typical temporal lobe epileptic attack ushered in by a feeling of floating and brief unconsciousness. These symptoms were subsequently followed by a series of major motor seizures and seizures involving one arm and leg with rapidly advancing paralysis and coma. It was then discovered, through a repeat arteriogram and surgery, that the patient's brain had a huge swollen hemisphere with blood over the surface and pockets of blood in the depths of the temporal and parietal lobes. An extensive, external decompression saved the patient's life and promoted the recovery of some function in the previously paralyzed arm and leg. Moreover, his emotional behavior is now normal.

The Role of the Environment. The relationship between brain abnormalities and abnormal behavior does not necessarily negate the role of social and cultural factors in the course of diagnosis or treatment. All human behavior is the result of interaction between the brain and the environment and must therefore be analyzed on an individual basis. It is our assumption that an individual with a damaged brain, particularly if the injury is in the limbic system, is less able to respond appropriately to environmental stress than the individual with a normal brain. The relevance of environmental considerations as opposed to physiological factors must be evaluated in each case. Thus, one patient who, during an epileptic seizure, put a knife into the heart of a stranger who brushed against her had a relatively small environmental component influencing her behavior. On the other hand, however, a patient who had a violent quarrel with his family directly preceding an epileptic seizure and who smashed a wall in the post-ictal phase probably had an important environmental component provoking his violence.

THE ANTI-PSYCHOSURGERY CAMPAIGN

In 1967, Dr. William Sweet, Dr. Frank Ervin and I wrote a letter to the *Journal of the American Medical Association* about the possible role of brain dysfunction in individuals who killed or maimed others in urban riots.[22] For several years, this preliminary statement was, like most letters to the editor, largely ignored. Subsequently, it was superseded by more complete statements in a book[23] and an article.[24] The anti-psychosurgery campaign initiated in 1972,[25] however, suddenly invested the letter with false significance. These critics have claimed that this letter and our other writings advocated psychosurgery for urban rioters by linking the riots to brain disease and by treating biological factors at the expense of socio-cultural conditions.[26] A reading of the letter reveals, however, that the use of psychosurgery on urban rioters was not discussed, but rather that the possible role of brain disease in individual violence was presented. Moreover, the letter explicitly recognized the severe social problems of urban centers. Similarly, the critics have generally ignored our suggestion in 1970 that the investigation of the causes of violence include consideration of police and National Guard activity.[27]

Pervading the criticism of neurological treatment for personal violence is concern that it is directed primarily against the poor and the underprivileged and that it has marked overtones of racism. It has been charged, for example, that the Neuro-Research Foundation which supported some of our work has moved from the "middle- and upper-class" Massachusetts General Hospital to the Boston City Hospital, a "beleaguered public institution [that] caters primarily to black and lower class patients. . . ."[28]

During the last decade, Dr. William Sweet and I have operated on 13 patients with epilepsy affecting the limbic system and associated with abnormal aggressivity. Eleven of these patients were operated on at Massachusetts General Hospital and two of them—both nonresidents of Boston—were operated on at

Boston City Hospital. The Neuro-Research Foundation did not move to Boston City Hospital. With the assistance of the National Institutes of Health, it has supported research at both of these Boston hospitals. Although the physical facilities at Boston City Hospital were significantly improved with help from the Foundation, these facilities are used for all neurological patients and not solely for patients with behavior disorders. Finally, it is important to note that to date no psychosurgery of the classical form has been performed at Boston City Hospital, although such procedures properly continue to be performed in Boston's private hospitals.

More distressing and misleading, however, is the charge of racism.[29] A theory that some violence is caused by brain disease in no way implies that it is characteristic of blacks. Indeed, it is the theory that personal violence is caused exclusively by social conditions that may direct our attention to the black ghettos. Thus, our theory of violence does not have any racially suspect political implications.

In addition, it is our experience that there is no special correlation between violence and race. The physician in the emergency room and the clinic witnesses the results of violence in both upper class and lower class homes. Although ghetto violence may be reported more often and may be more visible due to its spilling out of overcrowded homes into the streets, from the physician's perspective the color of violence is claret, not black or white.

The victims of unreported violence are just as severely injured as the ghetto victims of blunt instruments or knives. MacDonald, for example, has shown that some automobile drivers are intent upon committing suicide or murder.[30] McFarland indicates that over half of all fatal automobile accidents are related to alcoholism,[31] and there is evidence that the limbic brain is affected preferentially by alcohol.[32] Indeed, alcoholic intoxication may affect the brain as severely as brain tumors, infections and injuries. The difference in incapacitation is one of duration rather than severity.

The disproportionate prevalence of violence in the ghetto becomes more apparent than real in light of such widespread automobile violence and the domestic violence that is more often revealed in the divorce court than in the police court. Thus, a biological model of violence cannot concentrate on one race, ethnic group or other social segment of the population. Conversely, once the violence is identified as related to environment, it may then be associated with such groups through the application of a subculture theory.

There is, however, a danger of de facto racism that should not be minimized. Certain institutions in which blacks are disproportionately represented may present their inmates as candidates for psychiatric neurosurgery for custodial or punitive motives. This form of racism should be combatted through the limitation of psychiatric neurosurgery to cases where brain pathological disorders are well defined. In addition, the safeguards of requiring informed consent and regulating institutional action should receive adequate attention. Under present conditions, it would seem that the performance of psychosurgery on convicted felons should be prohibited.

THE RELATIVE BENEFITS OF PSYCHOSURGERY AND OTHER FORMS OF PSYCHIATRIC TREATMENT

To fully appreciate the cost-benefit ratio of psychosurgery, it must be compared with the results obtained by nonsurgical forms of treatment. Environmental manipulation, psychoanalysis, behavior therapy and other forms of psychotherapy may be successful in relieving the symptoms of certain patients, but it has been recently reported that no valid statistical data indicate that any particular form of psychotherapy is more effective in treating seriously ill mental patients than any other form of treatment or even chance alone.[33] Furthermore, recent studies of the effectiveness of psychotherapy are said to be characterized by serious methodological flaws invalidating their conclusions.[34]

Any discussion of the hazards of psychosurgery should also take note of the significant hazards associated with psychotherapy. Yalom and Lieberman, for example, have studied encounter group casualties.[35] Of 209 university undergraduates who entered 18 encounter groups which met for a total of 30 hours each, 39 did not complete the schedule and were considered dropouts. Sixteen of the remaining test group subjects were judged to be casualties. In other words, they experienced significant, negative effects that endured for many months. Another patient in the series committed suicide.

Drug therapy with neuroleptic agents—Thorazine, Stelazine and Haldol, for example—has proved to be more effective than inert substances or conventional sedatives.[36] Over 250 million people have taken these drugs since their introduction in the 1950s.[37] Although a single dose of any antipsychotic drug is seldom dangerous, the administration of these agents over a period of weeks or months may cause a number of side effects and complications. A syndrome resembling Parkinson's disease is common and some of the drugs may occasionally produce a fatal leukopenia.

An unusual syndrome known as tardive dyskinesia has been observed in patients receiving these agents over a long period of time. It consists of slow, rythmical movements in the region of the mouth with protrusion of the tongue, smacking of the lips, blowing of the cheeks, side-to-side movements of the chin and other bizarre muscular activities. This condition becomes dangerous when breathing or motor coordination are impaired. There is no known treatment for this condition, and it continues even after drug therapy is discontinued. Although definitive studies on the intellectual and emotional effects of the syndrome have not been conducted, pathological studies indicate that structural changes in the brain do occur.[38] The dilemma faced by psychopharmacologists has been recently articulated as follows: "Because of the lack of adequate substitutes for the neuroleptic drugs in the treatment of psychosis, tardive dyskinesia has been accepted as an undesirable but occasionally unavoidable price to be paid for the benefits of prolonged neuroleptic therapy." [39]

. . .

V. CONCLUSION

Although the arguments of the . . . anti-psychosurgeons may be countered on several grounds, the responsibility of neurosurgeons to properly diagnose and treat their patients is not, by this critique, diminished. It is clear, however, that the function of the neurosurgeon requires reference not only to medical consideration, but to legal, ethical, social and political ones as well. Thus, it is particularly appropriate for the physician and surgeon in charge of the patient to make their decisions in conjunction with a multidisciplinary committee composed of independent persons skilled in the relevant scientific and nonscientific disciplines. This symposium is a welcome first step in the development of such multidisciplinary committees as a responsible method of resolving the dilemmas raised by psychosurgery in particular and by modern medicine in general.

NOTES

1. Moniz, "Les Premieres Tentatives Opératoires dans le Traitement de Certaines Psychoses", 91 *L'Encephale* 1 (1936).

2. *Hearings on Psychosurgery Before the Subcomm. on Health of the Comm. on Labor and Public Welfare Meeting Jointly with the Subcomm. on Health and Hospitals of the Comm. on Veterans' Affairs*, 93d Cong., 1st Sess. (1973) (remarks of D. Johnson & M. Musser).

3. Foltz & White, "Pain 'Relief' by Frontal Cingulotomy," 19 *J. Neurosurg*. 89 (1962).

4. Ballantine, Cassidy, Flanagan & Marino, "Stereotaxic Anterior Cingulotomy for Neuro-psychiatric Illness and Intractable Pain," 26 *J. Neurosurg*. 488 (1967).

5. Whitty, Duffield, Tow & Cairns, "Anterior Cingulectomy in the Treatment of Mental Disease," 1 *Lancet* 475 (1952).

6. Sweet, "Treatment of Medically Intractable Mental Disease by Limited Frontal Leucotomy—Justifiable?," 289 *New Eng. J. Med*. 1117 (1973).

7. *See, e.g.,* Mark & Sweet, "The Role of Limbic Brain Dysfunction in Aggression," *Research Publications of the Association for Research in Nervous & Mental Disease*, Vol. 52, Ch. 8 (to be published in 1974).

8. For a more extensive discussion of the limbic system see V. Mark & F. Ervin, *Violence and the Brain*, 13–24 (1970).

9. "Epilepsy itself is not a disease. It is a symptom of brain dysfunction and electrical disorganization within the brain. This disorganization is manifested inside the brain as

a very noticeable electrical discharge marked by an increase in both amplitude and frequency of the brain waves." *Id.* at 60.

10. Currie, Heathfield, Henson & Scott, "Clinical Course and Prognosis of Temporal Lobe Epilepsy." 94 *Brain* 173 (1971).

11. Walker, "Man and His Temporal Lobes," 1 *Surg. Neurol.* 69 (1973).

12. For an extensive discussion of stereotactic surgery see V. Mark & F. Ervin, *supra* note 8, at 69–87.

13. *See id.* at 112–24 (especially Fig. 28).

14. Falconer & Taylor, "Surgical Treatment of Drug-Resistant Epilepsy Due to Mesial Temporal Sclerosis," 19 *Arch. Neurol.* 353, 356 (1968).

15. Walker & Blumer, "Long-Term Effects of Temporal Lobe Lesions on Sexual Behavior and Aggressivity," in *The Neurobiology of Violence* (W. Fields & W. Sweet, eds.)

16. Falconer, "Reversibility by Temporal-Lobe Resection of the Behavioral Abnormalities of Temporal-Lobe Epilepsy." 289 *New Eng. J. Med.* 451 (1973).

17. Geschwind, "Effects of Temporal-Lobe Surgery on Behavior," 289 *New Eng. J. Med.* 480, 481 (1973).

18. Address By I. Cooper & S. Gilman, "The Effect of Chronic Cerebellar Stimulation upon Muscular Hypertonus and Epilepsy in Man." The American Neurological Association, Montreal, June 12, 1973.

19. V. Mark & F. Ervin, *supra* note 8, at 58–59.

20. Crowell, Tew & Mark, "Aggressive Dementia Associated with Normal Pressure Hydrocephalus," 23 *Neurology* 461 (1973).

21. This case has not been published in the medical literature.

22. Mark, Sweet & Ervin, "Role of Brain Disease in Riots and Urban Violence," 201 *J.A.M.A.* 895 (1967). Because of this letter's significance to the anti-psychosurgeons, it has been reprinted in full: "*To the Editor:* —That poverty, unemployment, slum housing, and inadequate education underlie the nation's urban riots is well known, but the obviousness of these causes may have blinded us to the more subtle role of other possible factors, including brain dysfunction in the rioters who engaged in arson, sniping, and physical assault.

"The urgent needs of underprivileged urban centers for jobs, education and better housing should not be minimized, but to believe that these factors are solely responsible for the present urban riots is to overlook some of the newer medical evidence about the personal aspects of violent behaviors.

"It is important to realize that only a small number of the millions of slum dwellers have taken part in the riots, and that only a sub-fraction of these rioters have indulged in arson, sniping, and assault. Yet, if slum conditions alone determined and initiated riots, why are the vast majority of slum dwellers able to resist the temptations of unrestrained violence? Is there something peculiar about the violent slum dweller that differentiates him from his peaceful neighbor?

"There is evidence from several sources, recently collated by the Neuro-Research Foundation, that brain dysfunction related to a focal lesion plays a significant role in the violent and assaultive behavior of thoroughly studied patients. Individuals with electroencephalographic abnormalities in the temporal region have been found to have a much greater frequency of behavioral abnormalities (such as poor impulse control, assaultiveness and psychosis) than is present in people with a normal brain wave pattern.

"On the other hand, French and South African reports disclosed that persons arrested for murder had six to nine times the frequency of abnormal brain waves as occur in the population at large. Delinquent psychopaths tested in a medical center for federal prisoners in the United States had an almost equally high frequency of abnormal brain wave patterns. Stafford-Clark and Taylor divided 64 English prisoners accused of murder into five categories. They found only one of 11 prisoners guilty of killing in self-defense, or in the commission of another crime, with an abnormal brain wave. Four out of 16 murderers with a clear homicidal motive had electroencephalographic abnormalities, but an abnormal pattern was present in 11 of 15 prisoners who did not have a motive for committing murder. It would be of more than passing interest to find what percentage of the attempted and completed murders committed during the recent wave of riots were done without a motive.

"Finally, it is an unjustified distortion to conclude that the urban rioter has a monopoly on violence. It pervades every social, ethnic, and racial stratum of our society. The real lesson of the urban rioting is that, besides the need to study the social fabric that creates the riot atmosphere, we need intensive research and clinical studies of the *individuals* committing the violence. The goal of such studies would be to pinpoint, diagnose, and treat those people with low violence thresholds before they contribute to further tragedies."

Id. (footnotes omitted).

New evidence on the urban riots was reviewed, and the authors' emphasis on the violence of *individuals* received elaboration in September 1970: "One of the outstanding features of the widespread urban riots that have recently swept through the United States is the relatively small amount of personal violence committed compared to the large number of people taking part in the riot. In the Watts community of 330,000 people, there were about 10,000 rioters; 37 people were killed, and 118 were wounded by gun fire. Many of these people were killed by police and National Guard troops and some were killed when they were unwittingly left behind in burning buildings. It is our opinion that the riot atmosphere represents a powerful environmental influence on all those people taking part in the riot. The fact that so few people were killed or injured in these riots makes us believe that unusually strong control mechanisms were operating both in the individual rioters and in the police and National Guard troops who sought to keep the riot under control. It would be particularly interesting under these circumstances to examine in detail those individuals who did cause serious injury or death—be they rioters or members of the police and National Guard."
V. Mark & F. Ervin, *supra* note 8, at 151–52.

23. V. Mark & F. Ervin, *supra* note 8.

24. Mark & Neville, "Brain Surgery in Aggressive Epileptics: Social and Ethical Implications," 226 *J.A.M.A.* 765 (1973).

25. *See* Breggin, "The Return of Lobotomy and Psychosurgery," *reprinted in* 118 *Cong. Rec.* E1602 (daily ed. Feb. 24, 1972).

26. *See, e.g., Breggin,* "New Information in the Debate over Psychosurgery," reprinted in 118 *Cong. Rec.* E3380 (daily ed. Mar. 30, 1972): Chorover, "Big Brother and Psychotechnology," *Psychology Today,* Oct. 1973, at 43, 47–48.

27. *See* note 22 *supra.*

28. Chorover, *supra* note 26, at 48.

26. *See, e.g.,* Progressive Labor Party, Smash "Scientific" Racism (unpublished leaflet on file at Boston University Law Review); Breggin, Letter to the Editor on *Psychosurgery,* 226 *J.A.M.A.* 1121 (1973). The following response to this charge has appeared in somewhat different form in Mark & Neville, *supra* note 24, at 768–69; and in Mark, 227 *J.A.M.A.* 943 (1974).

30.MacDonald, "Suicide and Homicide by Automobile," 121 *Am. J. Psychiat,* 366 (1964).

31. McFarland, Ryan & Dingman, "Etiology of Motor-Vehicle Accidents," 278 *New Eng. J. Med.* 1383, 1384 (1968).

32 Lee, "Effect of Alcohol Injections on Blood-Brain Barrier," 23 *Q. J. Studies on Alcohol* 4 (1962).

33. Grinker, "Emerging Concepts of Mental Illness and Models of Treatment: The Medical Point of View," 125 *Am. J. Psychiat.* 865, 866 (1969).

34. Dyrud & Holzman, "The Psychotherapy of Schizophrenia: Does It Work?," 130 *Am. J. Psychiat.* 670 (1973).

35. Yalom & Lieberman, "A Study of Encounter Group Casualties," 25 *Arch. Gen. Psychiat.* 16 (1971).

36. Crane, "Clinical Psychopharmacology in Its 20th Year," 181 *Science* 124 (1973).

37. *Id.* at 124.

38. Christensen, Moller & Faurbye, "Neuropathological Investigation of 28 Brains from Patients with Dyskinesia," 46 *Acta Psychiat. Scand.* 14 (1970).

39. American College of Neuropsychopharmacology—FDA Task Force, Neurological Syndromes Associated with Antipsychotic Drug Use: A Special Report, 28 *Arch. Gen. Psychiat.* 463, 465 (Schiele et al. eds. 1973).

STEPHAN L. CHOROVER

Psychosurgery: A Neuropsychological Perspective

INTRODUCTION

We are still far from understanding how our brains give rise to the varied phenomena of our subjective experience. But despite our relative ignorance, we biologists and behavioral scientists stand today in a position comparable to that occupied by our colleagues in nuclear physics almost 30 years ago. In 1945, developments in that field led to the atomic bomb and ushered in a new world of ethical and social problems. During the past few decades, developments in the biobehavioral sciences have spawned a wide-ranging psychotechnology, a varied arsenal of tools and techniques for predicting and modifying human social behavior. The continued development and deployment of this psychotechnology has also engendered serious ethical and social problems that can no longer be ignored.

Reprinted with permission of the publisher from *Boston University Law Review,* Vol. 54, No. 2 (March 1974), pp. 231, 239–48.

Psychosurgery is among the more controversial forms of psychotechnology. Also known as "psychiatric neurosurgery," "mental surgery," "functional neurosurgery" and "sedative neurosurgery," psychosurgery may be defined as brain surgery that has as its primary purpose the alteration of thoughts, social behavior patterns, personality characteristics, emotional reactions, or some similar aspects of subjective experience in human beings.[1]. . .

PSYCHOSURGERY FOR VIOLENCE

It has long been popularly believed that there is a close association between epilepsy and violence. The phrase "a fit of anger" nicely epitomizes this view. Over the years, a large number of clinical studies have dealt with this question. After reviewing the available literature and assessing the clinical experience of neurologists who have cared for many patients with seizure disorders, a recent study sponsored by the National Institute of Neurological Diseases and Stroke concluded that "violence and aggressive acts do occur in patients with temporal lobe epilepsy but such are rare, perhaps no more frequent than in the general population.''[2]

Two of the best known cases of this kind are "Thomas R." and "Julia S." Their pseudonyms have entered the vocabulary of psychosurgery, their cases have been fictionalized in a best-selling novel,[3] and they continue to arouse public interest as purported successes of Drs. Vernon H. Mark and Frank R. Ervin, the authors of the controversial *Violence and the Brain*. Bearing in mind that the existence of a causal connection between epilepsy and violence remains an open question in the view of most neurologists, let us consider each of these cases in turn.

THE CASE OF THOMAS R.

The Presentation by Mark and Ervin. Thomas is introduced to Mark and Ervin's readers in the following passages:[4]

He was a brilliant [*sic*] 34-year-old engineer with several important patents to his credit. Despite his muscular physique it was difficult to believe he was capable of an act of violence when he was not enraged, for his manner was quiet and reserved, and he was both courteous and sympathetic.

Despite a history of physical illness, Thomas managed to educate himself as an engineer.

He was an extremely talented, inventive man, but his behavior at times was unpredictable and even frankly psychotic. He was seen and treated by psychiatrists over a period of 7 years with no effect on his destructive outbursts of violence.

Thomas's chief problem was his violent rage; this was sometimes directed at his co-workers and friends, but it was mostly expressed toward his wife and children. He was very paranoid, and harbored grudges which eventually produced an explosion of anger. He often felt that people were gratuitously insulting to him. . . .

For example, during a conversation with his wife,

he would seize upon some innocuous remark and interpret it as an insult. At first, he would try to ignore what she had said, but could not help brooding; and the more he thought about it, the surer he felt that his wife no longer loved him and was "carrying on with a neighbor." Eventually he would

reproach his wife for these faults, and she would hotly deny them. Her denials were enough to set him off into a frenzy of violence.

Thomas was referred to Mark and Ervin by a psychiatrist who they say had concluded that "prolonged psychiatric treatment did not improve his behavior and . . . that his spells of staring, automatisms and rage represented an unusual form of temporal lobe seizure."[5] An electroencephalographic examination revealed electrical brain activity considered by them to be indicative of epilepsy, and additional tests suggested the presence of other brain abnormalities. After experimenting with a wide range of pharmacological agents, none of which proved therapeutic, they decided to proceed with stereotaxic surgery. Arrays of electrodes were implanted in both temporal lobes with their ends reaching the nucleus amygdala. The "optimal site for destructive lesions"[6] was sought through repeated stimulation and recording. Stimulation in one portion of the amygdala "produced a complaint of pain, and a feeling of 'I am losing control'," two reactions that marked the onset of Thomas' periods of violence. However, stimulation of a portion of the amygdala just four millimeters to the side produced the opposite reactions of detachment, "hyperrelaxation" and a "feeling like Demerol."[7]

Mark and Ervin's account of how they obtained Thomas' consent to their proposed surgery is revealing both in terms of what is said and what is left unsaid. They viewed Thomas as keenly aware of personal insults and highly sensitive to threats, and found that "the suggestion that the medial portion of his temporal lobe was to be destroyed . . . would provoke wild, disordered thinking."[8] At this point in their discussion, they acknowledge in a footnote the physician's "extraordinary responsibility" of safeguarding the rights of the patient and of securing his free and informed consent.[9] But, they continue, "[u]nder the effects of lateral amygdala stimulation, [Thomas] showed bland acquiescence to the suggestion" that psychosurgery be performed.[10]

However, 12 hours later, when this effect had worn off, Thomas turned wild and unmanageable. The idea of anyone's making a destructive lesion in his brain enraged him. He absolutely refused any further therapy, and it took many weeks of patient explanation before he accepted the idea of bilateral lesions [*sic*] being made in his medial amygdala.[11]

Since Mark and Ervin considered Thomas' rage inappropriate and were, by their own account, able to blunt it by lateral amygdala stimulation, it is perhaps not surprising to learn that Thomas finally "accepted the idea." Directly following this quoted passage, we are informed of the success of the procedure in these brief sentences: "Four years have passed since the operation, during which time Thomas has not had a single episode of rage. He continues, however, to have an occasional epileptic seizure with periods of confusion and disordered thinking."[12]

The reader, recalling Mark and Ervin's original assertion that Thomas' "chief problem was his violent rage"[13] and that he exhibited some preoperative seizures and confused or disordered thinking, may reasonably conclude from this account that bilateral amygdalectomy has not only improved Thomas' condition, but has also effected a specific and total cure of his chief complaint. The rage is allegedly gone, the other preoperative symptoms remain essentially unchanged, and no postoperative side effects are mentioned. In light of the devastating effects of bilateral amygdalectomy on the social behavior of nonhuman primates, the apparently successful outcome of Thomas' case seems remarkable indeed. The implied absence of any adverse social reactions appears especially unexpected. Is it sufficient, however, to rely on mere implications? Highly relevant information is not provided by the published case histories. Prior to his operation, Thomas was married and supported his family through his work as an engineer. It would seem that a full account of the effects of his psychosurgery should include, for example, information concerning his marriage and his employment.

Contradictory Reports. At the request of Thomas' family an independent follow-up of Thomas' case has been performed by Dr. Peter R. Breggin, a psychiatrist and well-known critic of psychosurgery.[14] Dr. Breggin interviewed the patient and his family, reviewed the hospital charts made before and after surgery and discussed the case with several well-informed individuals.

According to Dr. Breggin, Thomas was continuously employed through December 1965. During that year he began to have serious marital problems which prompted visits to his wife's psychiatrist. Breggin conducted a telephone interview with this psychiatrist during which he was told that Thomas' wife was indeed afraid of him, but that no actual harm was done to her.[15] Moreover, writes Breggin:

[the] psychiatrist remembers that Thomas was depressed, but not sufficiently depressed to warrant electroshock or drugs. His memory is entirely consistent with the hospital records which report no hallucinations, delusions, paranoid ideas or signs of difficulty with thinking. In the charts, his most serious psychiatric diagnosis is "personality pattern disturbance," [a classification] reserved for mild problems with no psychotic symptomatology.[16]

Finally, certain hospital charts state that "[h]e has never been in any trouble at work or otherwise for aggressive behavior."[17] In short, Dr. Breggin's account stands in sharp contrast to the published assertions of Drs. Mark and Ervin. Indeed, Breggin claims that the only incidence of violence mentioned in Thomas' hospital files were those provoked by Mark and Ervin themselves.

Thomas was treated by Mark and Ervin from October 1966 until his release from Massachusetts General Hospital on August 27, 1967. He subsequently returned with his mother to the west coast, unable to rejoin his wife and children because his wife had, during his treatment, filed for divorce. Eventually, she married the man about whom Thomas had allegedly been paranoid.[18] Shortly after the operation, it became apparent that Thomas was socially confused and unable to cope with the complexities of normal life. He was soon admitted to a west coast Veterans Administration hospital where he was placed on a locked ward and given heavy doses of medication. Breggin's account suggests that Thomas' new physicians did not have access to his medical records from Massachusetts General Hospital. Indeed, they regarded his comments concerning Mark and Ervin's procedures as evidence of his delusional state of mind.[19] After six months of confinement, he was discharged with a diagnosis of "schizophrenic reaction, paranoid type."[20] At present, Breggin claims, Thomas is totally unable to work, is incapable of caring for himself and must periodically be rehospitalized as assaultive and psychotic.

Dr. Breggin is not the only available source of information about Thomas' postoperative history. His follow-up study has recently been supplemented by a complaint filed in behalf of the patient[21] and is generally consistent with information the author has obtained from other sources.[22] In August 1972, Dr. Ernst Rodin, a Detroit neurosurgeon, visited Dr. Mark's project in Boston. Rodin, at that time a co-author of a proposal to perform psychosurgery on involuntarily incarcerated individuals,[23] made the visit "to obtain the most up-to-date information on the results of surgery for aggressive behavior in human beings. . . ."[24] Hoping that this inquiry would strengthen his proposal, Rodin was all the more disturbed by the disparities he discovered between the published accounts and the information available at first hand. Specifically, Dr. Ira Sherwin, a neurologist involved with the project, told Rodin that "he was not aware of any genuinely successful cases"[25] and that Thomas R. "will never be able to function in Society."[26]

THE CASE OF JULIA S.

The Presentation by Mark and Ervin. Julia S., another one of Mark and Ervin's celebrated patients, is the daughter of a well-to-do physician. She is described as being "an attractive, pleasant, cherubic blonde who looked much younger than her age of 21."[27] Starting with an attack of encephalitis before the age of two, she had a long history of brain disease. Her epileptic seizures began at about the age of 10, some being grand-mal convulsions, but most appearing to be petit-mal, or psycho-motor, seizures characterized by "brief lapses of consciousness, staring, lip smacking, and chewing."[28] Between seizures, Julia's behavior was marked by "severe temper tantrums followed by extreme remorse."[29] She also experienced "racing spells," which began with terrifying feelings of panic and ended in her rapidly running aimlessly about the streets. At least 12 people are said to have been assaulted by her, and when she was 18, she seriously injured other women in two separate stabbing incidents.[30]

Because Julia failed to respond to extensive psychotherapy, drugs and electroshock, Mark and Ervin concluded that her case "clearly illustrates the point that violent behavior caused by brain dysfunction cannot be modified except by treating the dysfunction itself."[31] Accordingly, they explored Julia's brain, producing rage reactions with the aid of amygdala electrodes and a telemetry device called a "stimoceiver." Finally, lesions were made in the "appropriate areas." *Violence and the Brain,* which was published two years after Julia's operation, contains the following evaluation by Mark and Ervin:

It is still too early to assess the results of the procedure, but she had only two mild rage episodes in the first postoperative year and none in the second. Since she had generalized brain disease and multiple areas of epileptic activity, it is not surprising that epileptic seizures have not been eliminated, or that her psychotic episodes have continued at the postoperative level.[32]

Contradictory Reports. The author is aware of no independent and detailed follow-up studies that may have been made of Julia's case. However, a former member of the project staff, a professional person who was particularly concerned about Julia and in a position permitting almost constant observation of her, recalls that Mark and Ervin's treatments made Julia more despondent and brought an end to her guitar playing and to her desire to engage in intellectual discussion.[33]

PSYCHOSURGERY AND DEVIANCE CONTROL

Results obtained in both animals and human beings raise serious doubts about the purported merits of psychosurgery. The continued performance of the procedure when its scientific foundations remain dubious and its therapeutic value has yet to be established may justifiably be considered questionable or even irresponsible. What is more ominous, however, is the increasing promotion and practice of psychosurgery as a technique of deviance control. The development of psychosurgery is another example of the time-honored practice of reducing complex social problems to the status of personal infirmities.[34] The authors of *Violence and the Brain* are among those who have advanced the view that social deviance and interpersonal violence in our society may be attributable to some kind of "brain dysfunction." It follows from this view that amygdalectomy may be an appropriate treatment for individuals whose brain dysfunction results in "a low threshold for impulsive violence."[35]

Other psychosurgeons have also advocated their medical procedures as an approach to social policy planning in the area of deviance control. At the Second International Conference of Psychosurgery in 1970, for example, Dr. M. Hunter Brown, a California psychosurgeon, urged his colleagues "to initiate pilot programs for precise rehabilitation of the prisoner-patient who is often young and intelligent, yet incapable of controlling various forms of violence."[36] Jessica Mitford has recently noted, however, that the increasing popularity of behavior alteration programs among penologists is in part due to their interest in suppressing those prisoners who interpret prison life in socioeconomic or racial terms.[37] These suggested uses for psychosurgery clearly involve more than medical considerations.

Foreign psychosurgeons, it would seem, have been at least as devoted to deviance control as their American counterparts. During 1972, a group of German neurosurgeons performed stereotaxic psychosurgery involving the destruction of a portion of the hypothalamus upon "22 male patients, 20 of them being sexual deviants, one suffering from neurotic 'pseudo homosexuality' and one from intractable addiction to alcohol and drugs."[38] According to their report, "15 of the sexual deviants obtained a good result which was in most cases excellent with complete harmonization of sexual and social behavior."[39] In only one case were poor results acknowledged, and no cases of serious side effects were reported. In an earlier report, however, these same researchers found that their first three patients suffered a postoperative "incapacity to indulge in erotic fantasies and stimulating visions."[40] This obliteration of the patients' fantasy lives inexplicably failed to qualify as an untoward side effect in the more recent description of the same operations.

Psychosurgery explicitly aimed at taming hyperactive children has been performed in India, Thailand, Japan and the United States. In a summary of 115 patients,[41] including 39 children under the age of 11, one team recently claimed that the destruction of the cingulate gyrus, amygdala and regions of the hypothalamus "proved to be useful in the management of patients who previously could not be managed by other means."[42] An American psychosurgeon who favors the selective destruction of the thalamus in such cases has claimed to have obtained "good" or "fair" results in a majority of operations.[43] It is impossible to assess his findings in an objective fashion because of his characteristically unilluminating case reports, of which the following is typical:

A seven-year-old mentally retarded child had sudden attacks of screaming, yelling, running and beating his head against the wall. The walls were actually indented by the blows.

Following thalamotomy three years ago, the patient did not display the wild, aggressive and screaming behavior. The improved behavior was an enjoyment for both the child and the parents.[44]

CONCLUSION

Because the weight of the available evidence indicates that limbic system psychosurgery produces a marked deterioration in behavior, serious impairments of judgment and other disastrous social adjustment effects, and because psychosurgeons have failed to provide balanced accounts of their cases, it would appear prudent for the medical profession and the relevant regulatory agencies of state and federal government to act promptly along the following lines. First, there should be an explicit recognition that psychosurgery is a highly experimental procedure and not a proven therapeutic one as is so often alleged by its contemporary proponents. Second, psychosurgery should not be performed upon children, prisoners, involuntarily held or committed mental patients, or those deemed to be mentally retarded. Third, a registry and assessment mechanism should be established to collect and disseminate information on present and past practices in psychosurgery. One function of such an agency might be the systematic psychological assessment of surviving psychosurgery patients and post-mortem examinations of their brain tissue when they die. Fourth, there should be a temporary moratorium on all further psychosurgical operations until the risks can be weighed against the benefits descovered by a systematic and impartial review of the field.[45] Finally, basic research on brain mechanisms and behavior should be supported and extended. Carefully pursued and properly interpreted, such research offers the only reliable course of action for increasing our understanding of human brain function and its relation to behavior. A better understanding of this kind, coupled with broader public education in the brain sciences, should ultimately provide the best possible defense against the simplistic theories upon which much of contemporary psychosurgery has been built.

It would be a mistake, however, to view psychosurgery in a social vacuum. Although it has unique characteristics, psychosurgery is, in terms of social policy, merely one of a large number of psychotechnological means that are continually being advanced to deal with troublesome individuals or groups. The relevant "target populations" are vaguely defined as "aggressive," "assaultive," "volatile," "acting-out," "disruptive," "incorrigible," "uncooperative," or "dangerous." The possibility that such behavior may be justifiable is generally ignored as are the social consequences of discouraging diversity. Indeed,

the physical and chemical control of disruptive behavior has been suggested in every futuristic model of technological fascism. Insofar as the causes of social conflict actually lie in the domain of social affairs, psychotechnological treatment of deviants should be regarded as a perversion of medicine and a distinct threat to individual liberty. The time has come to examine the entire spectrum of psychotechnology and to question the prevalent ideologies of behavioral prediction, modification and control. We must try, most of all, to assess the impact and social consequences of psychotechnology in the broad contexts of politics and public policy. For to deny the power and political appeal of repressive psychotechnology is to expedite its encroachment, and to refrain from combatting it is to surrender not only our constitutional freedom, but also our human dignity.

NOTES

1. This is essentially the definition given by Dr. Bertram S. Brown, Director of the National Institute of Mental Health. *See Hearings on S. 974, S. 878 and S.J. Res. 71 Before the Subcomm. on Health of the Senate Comm. on Labor and Public Welfare,* 93d Cong., 1st Sess., pt. 2, at 339 (1973).

2. Goldstein, "Brain Research and Violent Behavior," 30 *Arch. Neurol.* 1, 28 (1974).

3. *See* M. Crichton, *The Terminal Man* (1972). Thomas appears to be the model for Harry Benson, the title character in Crichton's novel. Ellis, the fictional neurosurgeon in the book, expresses with some literary license Mark and Ervin's view that psychomotor epilepsy and other brain damage are major factors in contemporary social violence and that psychosurgery offers a rational approach to the prevention of such violence. In this connection, it is of interest to note that Crichton has added a postscript to the paperback edition of the book which reveals: "In the face of considerable controversy among clinical neuroscientists, I am persuaded that the understanding of the relationship between organic brain damage and violent behavior is not so clear as I thought at the time I wrote the book." *Id.* at 282 (1973 ed.).

4. Mark & Ervin, *Violence and the Brain,* 93–94 (1970).

5. Mark & Ervin, "Is There a Need to Evaluate the Individuals Producing Human Violence?,"*Psychiat. Opinion,* Aug. 1968, at 32, 33.

6. *Id.* at 33.

7. Mark & Ervin 96.

8. Mark & Ervin, *supra* note 5, at 34.

9. *Id.*

10. *Id.*

11. Mark & Ervin 96–97.

12. *Id.* at 97.

13. *Id.* at 93.

14. Breggin, "An Independent Followup of a Person Operated upon for Violence and Epilepsy" by Drs. Vernon Mark, Frank Ervin and William Sweet of the Neuro-Research Foundation of Boston, *Rough Times,* Nov.-Dec. 1973, at 8, col. 1.

15. *Id.* at 8, col. 3.

16. *Id.*

17. *Id.*

18. *Id.* at 9, col. 2. For a description of this aspect of his "paranoia" see Mark & Ervin 93–94.

19. Thomas' discharge summary from the Veterans Administration Hospital reads: "Patient stated that . . . Massachusetts General Hospital were [*sic*] controlling him by creating lesions in his brain tissue some time before. Stated that they can control him, control his moods and control his actions, they can turn him up or turn him down." Breggin, *supra* note 22, at 9, col. 2. *See also* Memorandum, note 14 *infra,* at 4.

20. Breggin, *supra* note 14, at 9, col. 3.

21. Kille v. Mark, Civil No. 681998 (Super. Ct., Suffolk County, Mass., filed Dec. 3, 1973).

22. Hunt, "The Politics of Psychosurgery," Part I, *Real Paper* (Boston), May 30, 1973, at 1, col. 1, *reprinted in Rough Times,* Sept.-Oct. 1973, at 2, col. 1; Hunt, "The Politics of Psychosurgery," Part II, *Real Paper* (Boston), June 13, 1973, at 8, col. 1, *reprinted in Rough Times,* Nov.-Dec. 1973, at 6, col. 1; Trotter, Violent Brains (unpublished manuscript written for Ralph Nader's Center for Responsive Law, Washington, D. C.); Memorandum from Dr. Ernst Rodin to Dr. J. S. Gottlieb, Aug. 9, 1972, submitted as Exhibit AC-4 in Kaimowitz v. Department of Mental Health, Civil No. 73-19434-AW (Cir. Ct., Wayne County, Mich., July 10, 1973).

23. This proposed research was ultimately blocked in Kaimowitz v. Department of Mental Health, Civil No. 73-19434-AW (Cir. Ct., Wayne County, Mich., July 10, 1973), discussed elsewhere in this symposium. *See* comment, *"Kaimowitz v. Department of Mental Health:* A Right to Be Free from Experimental Psychosurgery?", 54 B.U.L. Rev. 301 (1974). [Reprinted —see next article in this chapter.]

24. Memorandum, *supra* note 22, at 1.

25. *Id.* at 4.

26. *Id.*

27. Mark & Ervin 97.

28. *Id.*

29. *Id.*

30. *Id.* at 97–98.

31. *Id.* at 98.

32. *Id.* at 107–08. As late as 1972, the authors were similarly uninformative: "It is still too early to assess the results of the procedure, but the frequency of both the rage attacks and epileptic seizures have been markedly decreased since operation." Mark, Ervin & Sweet, "Deep Temporal Lobe Stimulation in Man," in *The Neurobiology of the Amygdala, supra* note 23, [in original text] at 485, 494. *See also* Trotter, *supra* note 22, at 12 [in original text].

33. The author is in possession of an extensive record of personal observations made by this member of the project staff, who wishes to remain anonymous.

34. *See* Chorover, "Big Brother and Psychotechnology," *Psychology Today,* Oct. 1973, at 43, 45.

35. Mark & Ervin 2.

36. E. Valenstein, *Brain Control: A Critical Examination of Brain Stimulation and Psychosurgery,* 255 (1973).

37. *See* Mitford, "The Torture Cure," *Harper's,* Aug. 1973, at 16. *See also* J. Mitford, *Kind and Usual Punishment* (1973).

38. Müller, Roeder & Orthner, "Further Results of Stereotaxis in the Human Hypothalamus in Sexual Deviations, First Use of This Operation in Addiction to Drugs," 16 *Neurochirurgia* 113 (1973).

39. *Id.*

40. Roeder & Miller, "Zur Stereotaktischen Heilung der Pädophilin Homosexualität," 94 *Deutsch. Med. Wochnschr.* 409 (1969).

41. Balasubramaniam, Kanaka, Ramanugam & Ramanurthi, "Surgical Treatment of Hyperkinetic and Behavior Disorder," 54 *Int'l. Surgery* 18 (1970).

42. *Id.* at 22.

43. *Hearings, supra* note 1, at 353 (testimony of Dr. Orlando J. Andy).

44. *Id.* at 348. *See also* Andy, "Neurosurgical Treatment of Abnormal Behavior," 252 *Am. J. Med. Sci.* 232, 236–37 (1966), *reprinted in Hearings, supra* note 1, at 417, 421–22.

45. *See* S.J. Res. 86, 93d Cong., 1st Sess. (1973). This resolution, introduced by Senator Beall, calls for a two-year moratorium during which the Secretary of Health, Education and Welfare would compile and analyze the available data.

JOHN R. MASON

Kaimowitz v. Department of Mental Health:*
A Right to Be Free From Experimental Psychosurgery

INTRODUCTION

Kaimowitz v. Department of Mental Health,[1] a recent decision by Michigan's Wayne County Circuit Court, represents the first judicial response to an issue that is certain to produce future litigation and public controversy:[2] the legal and medical dilemma of psychosurgical intervention into the human brain. Psychosurgery can be provisionally defined as a related set of neurological operations, all of which seek to alter behavior through the destruction of tiny patches of brain tissue despite the absence of a clinically established disease. It is accepted neurosurgical practice to use electroradial or ultrasonic techniques on brain tumors or to ameliorate disorders such as Parkinson's disease by surgical operations on the brain.[3] These operations, however, are not psychosurgical because they are performed on diseased tissue or on a recognized clinical syndrome.

In contrast, psychosurgery destroys abnormal tissue, or even normal tissue, in order to prevent some specified behavior. The medical community is uncertain whether such procedures eradicate any clinically verifiable "disease"; that they modify human behavior is indubitable. The most controversial use of psychosurgery is the destruction of brain cells believed by some scientists to be sources of aggression in certain "uncontrollable" persons.

THE CASE OF JOHN DOE

In early 1972, John Doe, a 36-year-old mental patient at Michigan's Ionia State Hospital, was invited by the director of the Department of Mental Health to participate in a state-funded experiment. The experiment's goal was to test the comparative efficacy of two methods of reducing aggression in chronically violent wards of the state. One method involved the administration of cyproterone acetate, a drug which renders the recipient impotent as well as docile; the other method entailed psychosurgical destruction of areas of the brain which evidenced abnormal electrical discharge during periods of aggression which, by hypothesis, the subject could not control.[4]

John Doe, who had been civilly committed to the Department's care as a sexual psychopath at age 18, agreed to participate in the psychosurgery treatment group. On the strength of his signed consent Doe's parents also gave their written permission for the experiment to commence. The next step in the experimental design would have been implantation of 10 monitoring electrodes into the patient's brain. This research program came to an abrupt halt, however, when Michigan Legal Services attorney Gabe Kaimowitz brought suit to block the experiment.

Kaimowitz asked that the state be enjoined from performing psychosurgery on John Doe or on any other similarly situated person, but the patient himself resented this outside intervention and continued to manifest willingness to receive experimental treatment.[5] The court then appointed independent counsel to represent Doe's interests.[6] A habeas corpus petition was brought on his behalf alleging that the Michigan criminal psychopath statute,[7] under which Doe had been committed, was unconstitutional. On March 23, 1973, the Wayne County Circuit Court granted Doe his freedom holding that the psychopath statute could not withstand challenge under the equal protection clause.

Although John Doe was technically free and

*Civil No. 73–19434-AW (Circuit Court, Wayne County, Mich., July 10, 1973).

Reprinted with permission of the publisher from *Boston University Law Review*, Vol. 54, No. 2 (March 1974), pp. 30l–3, 319–27, 335–39.

the state had moved to withdraw funds for the experiment, the court reasoned that additional questions raised by Kaimowitz were not moot because he represented the class of Michigan mental patients potentially subject to psychosurgical experimentation.[8] Throughout spring 1973 the court listened to extensive argument and complex expert testimony about the brain. The court also took notice of Doe's considered decision not to go ahead with the experiment, a reversal of the position he had maintained previously. The court then issued the following rulings: first, patients involuntarily committed in state institutions are legally incapable of giving competent, voluntary, knowledgeable consent to experimental psychosurgical operations which will irreversibly destroy brain tissue;[9] second, the first amendment freedoms of speech and expression presuppose a right to generate ideas which could be destroyed or impaired by psychosurgery;[10] third, the constitutional right to privacy would be frustrated by unwarranted medical intrusion into a patient's brain.[11]

The Wayne County Circuit Court expressly refused to rule on the concomitant question whether the proposed psychosurgery amounted to a violation of the eighth amendment ban on cruel and unusual punishment "because of the many other legal and constitutional reasons for holding that the involuntarily detained mental patient may not give an informed and valid consent to experimental psychosurgery."[12] Also, it appears from the opinion that the court did not consider its rulings on the first amendment and the right of privacy issues to be essential to its holding on the issue of informed consent. However, the constitutional arguments advanced by the court are at least strong dicta meriting analytic attention from those concerned with the case's wider implications. *Kaimowitz* is probably the most important opinion yet published regarding the law's attempt to cope with man's recently augmented power to control behavior. . . .

THE *KAIMOWITZ* CONSENT STANDARD: ITS LEGAL SIGNIFICANCE AND EFFECT ON BRAIN RESEARCH

The court's discussion of the three elements that comprise informed consent focuses on the predicament of individuals who have been committed by the state to institutional care. Feeling that these persons are peculiarly vulnerable to pressures which might impair their judgment, *Kaimowitz* holds that they can neither freely choose experimental psychosurgery nor expect real benefit from the operation. In examining the reasoning of the Wayne County Circuit Court, it is important to probe the internal coherence of its consent standard in order to assess the cogency of the opinion's logic and the breadth of the court's holding. It is equally important to examine the opinion in the context of the concept of a "right to treatment" and the evident need for further research on the brain. An opinion so sensitive to the rights of involuntarily committed mental patients should be approached with their long-term welfare in mind.

The court is correct in noting that mental patients commonly are not given opportunities to make decisions, and undoubtedly this operates to diminish their sense of personal dignity and reduce their competence to reflect on the risks accompanying experimental treatment. John Doe, for example, was dependent on institutional authorities for the privilege to walk on the hospital grounds, have picnics with his family, or even to have a lamp in his room. Although rules like these may have justification in certain circumstances, it is clear that Doe's 18-year dependence on the institution was a factor in inducing his original decision to agree to the operation. Indeed, Doe did not finally revoke his consent until his freedom had been granted during the trial's initial phase. While litigation proceeded for purposes of the declaratory judgment, he elected to remain at Ionia State Hospital for a short time in order to gain composure before returning to the community. During this interim Doe read *Violence and the Brain*. His subsequent testimony was that this period of reading and reflection had allowed him time to "stop and reconsider an awful lot."[13]

It is questionable whether an institution falling below the treatment standards delineated in *Wyatt* could be considered a milieu capable of nurturing competent consent to experimental psychosurgery.[14] In large, warehouse-like wards furnishing merely custodial care, it is unlikely that patients have received enough therapy or decision-making experience to enable them to make a momentous decision—whether to undergo a dangerous experimental treatment—with requisite competence. Competency cannot be fostered in an environment where patients are neglected or dehumanized. Moreover, if no treatment plan is provided and carried out for an individual, his sanity, which is certainly a necessary condition of competent choice, will never be restored. Since many underequipped state hospitals must allocate a large portion of staff time to control rather than to therapy, the "violent" mental patient often becomes stigmatized and cut off from whatever meager treatment the institution can offer him.[15]

It should not be imagined, however, that if all state hospitals were brought up to the standards prescribed in *Wyatt* that this alone would dispose of *Kaimowitz'* concern about the competency of an involuntarily committed person's consent to experimental psychosurgery. Competency is an attribute an individual could possess regardless of the general quality of care in the institution in which he is confined. In custodial institutions which fall below *Wyatt* standards, there is often a small group of patients who have decision-making capabilities that can be effectively exercised, usually because these persons are institutionally misplaced or have benefitted from special staff attention. Conversely, even in a hospital vastly exceeding *Wyatt* standards, which offered every patient intensive therapy, there might still be persons who, because of a focal brain disorder, were "uncontrollably" violent and unresponsive to less drastic treatment, yet nonetheless able to make the decision to receive psychosurgery. Such cases would be rare, but for these persons psychosurgery might be a genuine option.

Since competency is a question which ultimately turns on the psychological capacity of an individual patient, it seems that the *Kai-*

mowitz court intended that judicial review of this component of its consent standard would be carried out on a case-by-case basis. The opinion notes, for example, that at some future time an involuntarily detained mental patient could consent to a *demonstrably therapeutic* amygdalotomy.[16] This suggestion would be absurd if it were supposed that competency was a trait which could never be established in any member of the entire mental patient population. A judge or a review committee could undertake the determination of whether a patient was capable of consenting to therapeutic psychosurgery. While the consent of a mental patient should be strictly scrutinized for competency, a person's competency to consent ought not to be conclusively presumed lacking simply *because* he is involuntarily committed.

Kaimowitz' view of consent's second component—voluntariness—however, is that voluntary consent is not practicable in a situation of *inherent* inequality between doctors and administrators and the patients in their care. The results of such a holding are far-reaching. First, since the consent of an *involuntarily* committed person to surgery might always be tainted by a tacit desire to obtain release, apparently no manifestation of consent, however emotionally compelling, could pass this standard of review. This prohibitive notion of voluntariness seems to undermine the case-by-case review of patient consent implied in the court's standard for competency. Second, the danger that consent to experimental psychosurgery might be procured by promising the inmate his liberty seems just as great a threat in a prison as it does in a mental hospital. This problem would be especially acute in "progressive" penal institutions where many of the inmates are confined under an indeterminate sentence which can be shortened for "cooperation" or "good behavior." *Kaimowitz* can be expected to spawn a series of cases challenging any future plans for amygdalotomies on prisoners.[17] Third, while the court is aware of psychosurgery's therapeutic potential and obviously considers some form of research vital to the development of this new treatment, perilous *experimental* research is a precondition of any *verifiably therapeutic* amygdalotomy which could be developed in the future. It may be possible that, given the court's absolute ban on experimentation on the involuntarily committed, no research subjects will be available. Thus, it is important to examine which, if any, avenues of research are left open by the opinion.

As a practical matter, virtually all psychosurgical research has been stopped as a result of the case.[18] If a doctor in a jurisdiction following *Kaimowitz* wanted to perform an experimental amygdalotomy for violence, he would have to find a subject in the class of persons who are "uncontrollably" aggressive, desirous of an operation, and free from the pressures imposed on free choice by institutional control. Barring an influx of violent patients into the offices of private psychosurgeons, however, membership in such a class is probably small or nonexistent. Thus, it is unlikely that significant, controlled studies of the procedure can be generated in this manner.

In deciding to halt experimental psychosurgery in institutions, the *Kaimowitz* court seems to have been most influenced by the irreversible effects of brain surgery, and by the poor risk-benefit ratio such an operation offers to patients.[19] But the court expressly disclaimed any "desire to impede medical progress" and suggested that "[o]ther avenues of research must be utilized and developed."[20] Morever, the opinion indicates elsewhere that consent will be less closely scrutinized as the risk-benefit ratio becomes more favorable.

Informed consent is a requirement of variable demands. Being certain that a patient has consented adequately to an operation, for example, is much more important when doctors are going to undertake an experimental, dangerous, and intrusive procedure than, for example, when they are going to remove an appendix.[21]

This suggests that experimental brain exploration could be undertaken on involuntarily committed persons if the purpose were therapeutic, the results unlikely to be irreversible, and the risk of collateral side-effects small. Under such circumstances presumably the court would regard the voluntariness of consent as less difficult to establish.

Even if the opinion *is* interpreted in some such fashion, the court appears to be de-

manding a temporary, but total, ban on psychosurgery generally when it claims that valid consent must be "knowledgeable." The court's view is that it is our "lack of knowledge about the subject [of experimental brain surgery]" which makes consent impossible at the present time.[22] This implies that a patient cannot consent to an operation on the brain which involves unknown hazards—even if the subject has been warned that such hazards may exist and that they are grave. Read in isolation from the rest of the opinion this would mean that the court held, as a matter of public policy, that individuals may not assume the risk of such an operation.

By taking the position that the brain is so inherently beyond our present knowledge that knowledgeable consent to experimental psychosurgery is impossible, *Kaimowitz* appears to pose additional difficulties for future research. It is possible that animal studies cannot fully replicate the functioning of the human brain for experimental purposes. Consequently, even if these studies are supplemented with nonintrusive studies with human subjects, it may be difficult to obtain the data necessary to determine whether amygdalotomies on human beings can ever be therapeutic. And if, as the court appears to imply, the reason amygdalotomies cannot presently be performed is because of our limited grasp of the brain and its functioning, it would appear impossible for *anyone*—involuntarily committed mental patient or ordinary citizen—to validly consent to such a procedure at the present time.

On this reading of the case, even the small class of "uncontrollably" violent persons who reside outside institutions and are willing to undergo an amygdalotomy could not give valid consent. Such a holding could have been reached by finding experimental psychosurgery to be a modern equivalent of the common law crime of mayhem. But mayhem has traditionally been confined to a class of actions which result in *certain* damage to the body.[23] In contrast, while an amygdalotomy does involve great risks, it is the very *uncertainty* of the operation's outcome which persuaded the *Kaimowitz* court to ban the procedure for the involuntarily committed.

However, even if amygdalotomies are so dangerous that knowledgeable consent to them should be prohibited as a matter of policy, it does not necessarily follow that psychosurgical operations with more favorable risk-benefit ratios are also illegal. Cingulotomy and "orbital undercutting," procedures which are typically performed on patients who have not been institutionalized, could also be performed on competently consenting institutionalized persons —provided that the therapeutic accuracy of such operations is substantially that reported by their practitioners. Research employing electrical stimulation of the brain (ESB) should also remain viable after *Kaimowitz* since it involves only minimal risk of irreversible brain damage. Despite the fact that these avenues of research remain open, it appears that researchers have concluded that psychosurgery of any kind will be illegal per se if courts in their jurisdictions follow *Kaimowitz*. While this result would be just if all psychosurgery were as risky as the experiment narrowly escaped by John Doe, it would be a mistake to think that *Kaimowitz,* even if adopted by other jurisdictions, would foreclose judicial approval of safer psychosurgical methods.

An interpretation of the opinion as implying a total ban on all psychosurgery can be avoided by reading the case as proscribing merely a specific operation—amygdalotomy—and applying only to a unique class—the involuntarily committed. Although the court refers repeatedly to "psychosurgery," rather than limiting its discussion specifically to amygdalotomies, it is clear that the procedure under consideration is the sort of amygdalotomy proposed for John Doe. Such an operation is rightly termed "experimental" by the court, and it would be distinguishable from any provably therapeutic surgical technique. The court itself explicitly acknowledged the possibility that a therapeutic form of amygdalotomy might be developed in the future, and that "it [could be] possible, with appropriate review mechanisms, that involuntarily detained mental patients could consent to such an operation."[24] Similarly, throughout the opinion the *Kaimowitz* court speaks of the situation of "involuntarily confined mental patients." For example, the court refers only in passing to experimentation on prisoners,[25] however analogous their situation is to that of mental patients.

Additional support for the interpretation that the court's holding concerns only mental patients can be found in the following language:

[I]nvoluntarily detained mental patients cannot give informed and adequate consent to experimental psychosurgical procedures on the brain.

The three basic elements of informed consent— competency, knowledge, and voluntariness—*cannot be ascertained with a degree of reliability* warranting resort to use of such an invasive procedure.[26]

This rationale resembles the position taken by the American Orthopsychiatric Association in its amicus brief that the substantial doubts surrounding each component of consent, when considered in cumulation, must result in a per se rule against finding adequate consent in any specific instance.[27] And since "competency" and "voluntariness" were only at issue in *Kaimowitz* because of the fact of involuntary commitment, the court appears to be referring only to the class of mental patients of which John Doe was a member.

If this is indeed the court's view, then the internal logic of its holding is difficult to comprehend. If no one can presently give valid consent to any amygdalotomy "knowledgeably," as parts of the opinion suggest, it is unnecessary to create a special per se rule for involuntarily committed mental patients. And if the court's holding is limited to such mental patients, "voluntariness" alone would be a criterion of consent which could not be met in any case. Thus, there is no need to cumulate doubts to reach the opinion's result.

Also, in the event that animal studies and nonintrusive research on human subjects someday are completed without resulting in the development of a therapeutic amygdalotomy, a per se rule would shut off competent involuntarily committed persons from access to an operation they might legitimately desire.

Under *Wyatt,* which furnishes only *procedural* safeguards for experimental research, consent to such an operation could be given if proper review took place. If *Kaimowitz* is followed, however, its determination of *public policy* would preclude a court from approving the consent of an involuntarily committed person to experimental psychosurgery even if consent had been found competent and voluntary by an acceptable review committee.[28] Therefore, it is possible that experimental psychosurgery might someday be unavailable only to the small class of institutionalized persons who truly desire the operation. Ironically, then, the *Kaimowitz* per se rule may be creating a situation in which a "right" to be free from treatment could be used to deny the privilege to make personal medical decisions which the court was at pains to secure in John Doe's particular case.[29] . . .

Kaimowitz can furnish general guidance on the issue of informed consent to psychosurgery, but the precise holding of the case should be limited to experimental, irreversible psychosurgery on "uncontrollably" aggressive, involuntarily committed persons. It is vital that such persons be protected from the jeopardy which confronted John Doe, but it would be tragic if his case became a precedent which could be misinterpreted in such a way as to stifle the development of research on the brain or to deny mental patients access to safer electronic therapies which are just becoming available.

. . .

Neurosurgeons may feel that the danger that creative research will be thwarted is greatly increased by the *Kaimowitz* decision and by the provision for community participation in the review of medical experiments envisioned by the new DHEW guidelines. Legal commentators sympathetic to the "right to treatment" concept have also expressed reservations about the competence of courts, in particular, to assess the value of proposed treatment plans for specific individuals.[30] But if *Kaimowitz,* as this Comment has suggested, proscribes only irreversible operations on violent, involuntarily committed mental patients, then it is possible to allow experimentation on the brain using ESB and ICSS [intercranial self-stimulation] to continue. By using these less drastic experimental methods, researchers may develop enough data to permit psychosurgery to become an effective therapy of last resort for a delimited class of focal brain disorders.

There is an additional advantage to permitting research to proceed in this manner. If experimentation does indicate that some verifiable clinical syndrome correlates with "uncontrollable" aggression, then psychosurgery will be viewed as an operation aimed at a brain dysfunction comparable to epilepsy[31]—not as a "laundered lobotomy" or a tool of repression. If no such "dyscontrol syndrome" is discovered, then this verdict will have been reached by scientific inquiry unhampered by judicial fiat. Dr. Mark has recently stated his belief that psychosurgery should be closely confined within the parameters of the medical model: "It is one thing to advocate neurosurgical procedures for certain kinds of violent behavior caused by organic brain disease or dysfunction. It is quite another to advocate them as general methods of behavior control."[32] On the other hand, he acknowledges that "we have not developed significant tests . . . to establish what the functional norms are with respect to the limbic brain,"[33] a concession that makes it difficult to distinguish between which operations are performed on "organic brain disease or dysfunction" and those which are merely aimed at "behavior control." *Kaimowitz* does not foreclose scientific discovery of such norms, if such norms exist, and, if they were made explicit by the psychosurgeons, then it would also be possible to determine with greater clarity what they mean by brain pathology which results in violence.

Surely, however, the court was right to set a limit on the "right to treatment" where dangerous experimentation is proposed. It is inappropriate to allow research to proceed when scientists themselves have not even articulated criteria which would define the existence of a violence syndrome. The *Kaimowitz* opinion does proscribe irreversible psychosurgical operations of the type proposed for John Doe. Read correctly, that proscription should neither forestall scientific inquiry nor deny available therapies to those who cannot be treated by other means.

CONCLUSION

Courts are not the only legal institutions presently concerned with psychosurgery. In Oregon the state legislature has passed a statute mandating review of all psychosurgical proposals by a medical committee. In Massachusetts the Commissioner of Mental Health has announced his intention of appoint a task force on the technique, and State Senator Chester Atkins has introduced legislation that would regulate psychosurgery throughout the Commonwealth. On the federal level there are the proposed DHEW guidelines to protect experimental subjects, and the United States Congress is currently considering several proposals that would ban, suspend, or regulate experimental psychosurgery.

A statutory response to this subject can be of only the most general kind. As research on brain functioning progresses, science may be able to offer a more precise treatment with less risk of damaging side-effects than it can furnish today. The concept of *experimental* psychosurgery may contract as ESB or ICSS tests enable surgery or implanted pacemakers to become effective therapies of last resort for consenting patients who cannot be helped by less drastic treatment methods. Whatever the effect of future legislation or administrative action, *Kaimowitz* will remain the most adventurous attempt yet made by the judiciary to respond to new medical techniques that augment both the power to cure and the power to control. Interpreted properly, the opinion exhibits a practical accommodation between scientific research, therapeutic needs and individual rights within the framework of the common law.

NOTES

1. Civil No. 73–1944-AW (Cir. Ct., Wayne County, Mich., July 10, 1973) (all citations are to slip opinion), *summarized at* 42 U.S.L.W. 2063 (July 31, 1973).

2. *E.g.,* Kille v. Mark, No. 681998 (Super. Ct., Suffolk County, Mass., filed Dec. 3, 1973) (suit for negligence brought by patient operated on for violent rage).

3. Kaimowitz v. Department of Mental Health, slip op. at 10–11. *But see* Chorover, "Psychosurgery: A Neuropsychological Perspective," 54 *B.U.L. Rev.* 231 (1974). [Reprinted—see preceding article.]

4. The study's research design is described more fully in J. Gottlieb & E. Rodin, "Proposal for the Study of the Treatment of Uncontrollable Aggression at the Lafayette Clinic," *reprinted in* Kaimowitz v. Department of Mental Health, slip op., appendix.

5. Attorney Kaimowitz entered the proceedings on his own motion, premising the suit on his standing as a Michigan taxpayer. Interview with Francis A. Allen, Attorney for Intervenor-Plaintiff, in Boston, Feb. 4, 1974.

6. *Id.*

7. Mich. Comp. Laws §§ 780.501 *et seq.* (1948) (Criminal Sexual Psychopathic Persons Act), *repealed,* Pub. Act 143 (1968).

8. The Department of Mental Health was unsuccessful in its ensuing effort to obtain an Order of Superintending Control for a Stay of Proceedings. On March 26, 1973, the court of appeals denied the stay. Kaimowitz v. Department of Mental Health, slip op. at 7 n.8.

9. *Id.* at 31–32.

10. *Id.* at 35–36.

11. *Id.* at 38–39.

12. *Id.* at 39.

13. N.Y. Times, Apr. 5, 1973, at 26, col 1.

14. Three years prior to *Kaimowitz* the Wayne County Circuit Court had itself found conditions at Ionia State Hospital to be substandard and in violation of a statutory and constitutional "right to treatment."

15. Restraint of aggressive patients in crowded state hospitals is often accomplished by large doses of pacifying drugs. Administration of these substances temporarily stupifies the patient. Because of the disruption he has caused, an aggressive patient is less likely to receive staff attention in the future. Although moderate chemical restraints frequently may benefit certain individuals, their very power is an invitation to abuse when conditions call for a quick response to patient violence and less restrictive alternatives are unavailable to the staff.

16. Kaimowitz v. Department of Mental Health, slip op. at 40.

17. *See* Mark, "Brain Surgery in Aggressive Epileptics," *Hastings Center Report,* Feb. 1973, at 1. "Prison inmates suffering from epilepsy should receive only medical treatment; surgical therapy should not be carried out, because of the difficulty in obtaining truly informed consent." *Id.* at 5 n.1. This position apparently would preclude amygdalotomies even on prisoners suffering from temporal lobe epilepsy.

18. N.Y. *Times,* Mar. 18, 1973, § 4, at 14, col 1.

19. Kaimowitz v. Department of Mental Health, slip op. at 13.

20. *Id.* at 15.

21. *Id.* at 22.

22. *Id*. at 27.

23. *E.g.,* State v. Bass, 255 N.C. 42, 120 S.E.2d 580 (1961) (severed fingers).

24. Kaimowitz v. Department of Mental Health, slip op. at 40.

25. *Id*. at 3l–32 nn.24–25.

26. Kaimowitz v. Department of Mental Health, slip op. at 3l–32 (emphasis added) (footnote omitted).

27. Brief for American Orthopsychiatric Ass'n as Amicus Curiae at 60: "[T]he legal adequacy of all three elements of consent . . . is 'suspect' and, as a matter of law, these suspicious [*sic*] when taken in combination should render the consent of *any* mental patient invalid within the framework of tort law."

28. Kaimowitz v. Department of Mental Health, slip op. at 40 n.27, indicates that the court considered the DHEW guidelines in force at that time to be adequate review mechanisms in the event medical knowledge develops to the point where amygdalotomies are demonstrably therapeutic. A fortiori the stronger guidelines recently proposed by the Department would be acceptable.

29. The *Kaimowitz* court, slip op. at 18 n.18, quoted with approval, the language of Justice Cardozo in Schloendorff v. Society of New York Hosps., 211 N.Y. 125, 129, 105 N.E. 92, 93 (1914): "Every human being of adult years or sound mind has a right to determine what shall be done with his own body. . . ."

See Kaimowitz v. Department of Mental Health, *su-* *pra* at l2–13 (emphasis added), where the court stated that "[a]ny experimentation on the human brain, especially when it involves an intrusive, irreversible procedure in a none [*sic*] life-threatening situation, should be undertaken with extreme caution, *and then only when* answers cannot be obtained from animal experimentation and from nonintrusive human experimentation." This language can be read to suggest that the court would permit an involuntarily committed mental patient to consent to an experimental amygdalotomy if less dangerous avenues of research have been exhausted at some date in the future, but the court nowhere develops a discussion of this possibility.

30. *See, e.g.,* Reisner, "Psychiatric Hospitalization and the Constitution: Some Observations on Emerging Trends," 1973 *U. Ill. L.F.* 9.

31. For a discussion of epilepsy see Wilder, "The Clinical Neurophsyiology of Epilepsy: A Survey of Current Research," *NINDB Monograph No. 8* (NIH 1968).

32. Mark & Neville, "Brain Surgery in Aggressive Epileptics: Social and Ethical Implications," 226 *J.A.M.A.* 769 (1973).

33. Mark & Southgate, "Violence and Brain Disease," Clinical Pathological Conference, 216 *J.A.M.A.* 1025, 1033 (1971).

Involuntary Commitment

THOMAS S. SZASZ

Involuntary Mental Hospitalization: A Crime Against Humanity

I

For some time now I have maintained that commitment—that is, the detention of persons in mental institutions against their will—is a form of imprisonment;[1] that such deprivation of liberty is contrary to the moral principles embodied in the Declaration of Independence and the Constitution of the United States;[2] and

that it is a crass violation of contemporary concepts of fundamental human rights.[3] The practice of "sane" men incarcerating their "insane" fellow men in "mental hospitals" can be compared to that of white men enslaving black men. In short, I consider commitment a crime against humanity.

Existing social institutions and practices, especially if honored by prolonged usage, are generally experienced and accepted as good and valuable. For thousands of years slavery was considered a "natural" social arrangement for the securing of human labor; it was sanctioned by public opinion, religious dogma, church, and state;[4] it was abolished a mere one hundred years ago in the United States; and it is still a prevalent social practice in some parts of the world, notably in Africa.[5] Since its origin, approximately three centuries ago, commitment of the insane has enjoyed equally widespread support; physicians, lawyers, and the laity have asserted, as if with a single voice, the therapeutic desirability and social necessity of institutional psychiatry. My claim that commitment is a crime against humanity may thus be countered—as indeed it has been—by maintaining, first, that the practice is beneficial for the mentally ill, and second, that it is necessary for the protection of the mentally healthy members of society.

Illustrative of the first argument is Slovenko's assertion that "Reliance solely on voluntary hospital admission procedures ignores the fact that some persons may desire care and custody but cannot communicate their desire directly."[6] Imprisonment in mental hospitals is here portrayed—by a professor of law!—as a service provided to persons by the state because they "desire" it but do not know how to ask for it. Felix defends involuntary mental hospitalization by asserting simply, "We *do* [his italics] deal with illnesses of the mind."[7]

Illustrative of the second argument is Guttmacher's characterization of my book *Law, Liberty, and Psychiatry* as ". . . a pernicious book . . . certain to produce intolerable and unwarranted anxiety in the families of psychiatric patients."[8] This is an admission of the fact that the families of "psychiatric patients" frequently resort to the use of force in order to control their "loved ones," and that when attention is directed to this practice it creates embarrassment and guilt. On the other hand, Felix simply defines the psychiatrist's duty as the protection of society: "Tomorrow's psychiatrist will be, as is his counterpart today, one of the gatekeepers of his community."[9]

These conventional explanations of the nature and uses of commitment are, however, but culturally accepted justifications for certain quasi-medical forms of social control, exercised especially against individuals and groups whose behavior does not violate criminal laws but threatens established social values.

II

What is the evidence that commitment does not serve the purpose of helping or treating people whose behavior deviates from or threatens prevailing social norms or moral standards; and who, because they inconvenience their families, neighbors, or superiors, may be incriminated as "mentally ill"?

1. *The medical evidence.* Mental illness is a metaphor. If by "disease" we mean a disorder of the physiochemical machinery of the human body, then we can assert that what we call functional mental diseases are not diseases at all.[10] Persons said to be suffering from such disorders are socially deviant or inept, or in conflict with individuals, groups, or institutions. Since they do not suffer from disease, it is impossible to "treat" them for any sickness.

Although the term "mentally ill" is usually applied to persons who do not suffer from bodily disease, it is sometimes applied also to persons who do (for example, to individuals intoxicated with alcohol or other drugs, or to elderly people suffering from degenerative disease of the brain). However, when patients with demonstrable diseases of the brain are involuntarily hospitalized, the primary purpose is to exercise social control over their behavior,[11] treatment of the disease is, at best, a secondary consideration. Frequently, therapy is non-existent, and custodial care is dubbed "treatment."

In short, the commitment of persons suffering from "functional psychoses" serves moral and social, rather than medical and therapeutic, purposes. Hence, even if, as a result of future research, certain conditions now believed to be "functional" mental illnesses were to be shown to be "organic," my argument against involuntary mental hospitalization would remain unaffected.

2. *The moral evidence.* In free societies, the relationship between physician and patient is predicated on the legal presumption that the

individual "owns" his body and his personality.[12] The physician can examine and treat a patient only with his consent; the latter is free to reject treatment (for example, an operation for cancer).[13] After death, "ownership" of the person's body is transferred to his heirs; the physician must obtain permission from the patient's relatives for a postmortem examination. John Stuart Mill explicitly affirmed that ". . . each person is the proper guardian of his own health, whether bodily, or mental and spiritual."[14] Commitment is incompatible with this moral principle.

3. *The historical evidence.* Commitment practices flourished long before there were any mental or psychiatric "treatments" of "mental diseases." Indeed, madness or mental illness was not always a necessary condition for commitment. For example, in the seventeenth century, "children of artisans and other poor inhabitants of Paris up to the age of 25, . . . girls who were debauched or in evident danger of being debauched, . . ." and other "misérables" of the community, such as epileptics, people with venereal diseases, and poor people with chronic diseases of all sorts, were all considered fit subjects for confinement in the Hôpital Général.[15] And, in 1860, when Mrs. Packard was incarcerated for disagreeing with her minister-husband,[16] the commitment laws of the State of Illinois explicitly proclaimed that ". . . married women . . . may be entered or detained in the hospital at the request of the husband of the woman or the guardian . . . , without the evidence of insanity required in other cases."[17] It is surely no coincidence that this piece of legislation was enacted and enforced at about the same time that Mill published his essay *The Subjection of Women*.[18]

4. *The literary evidence.* Involuntary mental hospitalization plays a significant part in numerous short stories and novels from many countries. In none that I have encountered is commitment portrayed as helpful to the hospitalized person; instead, it is always depicted as an arrangement serving interests antagonistic to those of the so-called patient.[19]

III

The claim that commitment of the "mentally ill" is necessary for the protection of the "mentally healthy" is more difficult to refute, not because it is valid, but because the danger that "mental patients" supposedly pose is of such an extremely vague nature.

1. *The medical evidence.* The same reasoning applies as earlier: If "mental illness" is not a disease, there is no medical justification for protection from disease. Hence, the analogy between mental illness and contagious disease falls to the ground: The justification for isolating or otherwise constraining patients with tuberculosis or typhoid fever cannot be extended to patients with "mental illness."

Moreover, because the accepted contemporary psychiatric view of mental illness fails to distinguish between illness as a biological condition and as a social role,[20] it is not only false, but also dangerously misleading, especially if used to justify social action. In this view, regardless of its "causes"—anatomical, genetic, chemical, psychological, or social—mental illness has "objective existence." A person either has or has not a mental illness; he is either mentally sick or mentally healthy. Even if a person is cast in the role of mental patient against his will, his "mental illness" exists "objectively"; and even if, as in the case of the Very Important Person, he is never treated as a mental patient, his "mental illness" still exists "objectively"—apart from the activities of the psychiatrist.[21]

The upshot is that the term "mental illness" is perfectly suited for mystification: It disregards the crucial question of whether the individual assumes the role of mental patient voluntarily, and hence wishes to engage in some sort of interaction with a psychiatrist; or whether he is cast in that role against his will, and hence is opposed to such a relationship. This obscurity is then usually employed strategically, either by the subject himself to advance *his* interests, or by the subject's adversaries to advance *their* interests.

In contrast to this view, I maintain, first, that the involuntarily hospitalized mental patient is, by definition, the occupant of an ascribed role; and, second, that the "mental disease" of such a person—unless the use of this term is restricted to demonstrable lesions or malfunctions of the brain—is always the product of interaction between psychiatrist and patient.

2. *The moral evidence.* The crucial ingredient in involuntary mental hospitalization is coercion. Since coercion is the exercise of power, it is always a moral and political act. Accordingly, regardless of its medical justification, commitment is primarily a moral and political phenomenon—just as, regardless of its anthropological and economic justifications, slavery was primarily a moral and political phenomenon.

Although psychiatric methods of coercion are indisputably useful for those who employ them, they are clearly not indispensable for dealing with the problems that so-called mental patients pose for those about them. If an individual threatens others by virtue of his beliefs or actions, he could be dealt with by methods other than "medical": if his conduct is ethically offensive, moral sanctions against him might be appropriate; if forbidden by law, legal sanctions might be appropriate. In my opinion, both informal, moral sanctions, such as social ostracism or divorce, and formal, judicial sanctions, such as fine and imprisonment, are more dignified and less injurious to the human spirit than the quasi-medical psychiatric sanction of involuntary mental hospitalization.[22]

3. *The historical evidence.* To be sure, confinement of so-called mentally ill persons does protect the community from certain problems. If it didn't, the arrangement would not have come into being and would not have persisted. However, the question we ought to ask is not *whether* commitment protects the community from "dangerous mental patients," but rather from precisely *what danger* it protects and by *what means?* In what way were prostitutes or vagrants dangerous in seventeenth century Paris? Or married women in nineteenth century Illinois?

It is significant, moreover, that there is hardly a prominent person who, during the past fifty years or so, has not been diagnosed by a psychiatrist as suffering from some type of "mental illness." Barry Goldwater was called

a "paranoid schizophrenic";[23] Whittaker Chambers, a "psychopathic personality";[24] Woodrow Wilson, a "neurotic" frequently "very close to psychosis";[25] and Jesus, "a born degenerate" with a "fixed delusional system," and a "paranoid" with a "clinical picture [so typical] that it is hardly conceivable that people can even question the accuracy of the diagnosis."[26] The list is endless.

Sometimes, psychiatrists declare the same person sane *and* insane, depending on the political dictates of their superiors and the social demand of the moment. Before his trial and execution, Adolph Eichmann was examined by several psychiatrists, all of whom declared him to be normal; after he was put to death, "medical evidence" of his insanity was released and widely circulated.

According to Hannah Arendt, "Half a dozen psychiatrists had certified him [Eichmann] as 'normal.' " One psychiatrist asserted, ". . . his whole psychological outlook, his attitude toward his wife and children, mother and father, sisters and friends, was 'not only normal but most desirable.' . . ." And the minister who regularly visited him in prison declared that Eichmann was "a man with very positive ideas."[27] After Eichmann was executed, Gideon Hausner, the Attorney General of Israel, who had prosecuted him, disclosed in an article in *The Saturday Evening Post* that psychiatrists diagnosed Eichmann as " 'a man obsessed with a dangerous and insatiable urge to kill,' 'a perverted, sadistic personality.' "[28]

Whether or not men like those mentioned above are considered "dangerous" depends on the observer's religious beliefs, political convictions, and social situation. Furthermore, the "dangerousness" of such persons—whatever we may think of them—is not analogous to that of a person with tuberculosis or typhoid fever; nor would rendering such a person "non-dangerous" be comparable to rendering a patient with a contagious disease non-infectious.

In short, I hold—and I submit that the historical evidence bears me out—that people are committed to mental hospitals neither because they are "dangerous," nor because they are "mentally ill," but rather because they are society's scapegoats, whose persecution is justified by psychiatric propaganda and rhetoric.[29]

4. *The literary evidence.* No one contests that involuntary mental hospitalization of the so-called dangerously insane "protects" the community. Disagreement centers on the nature of the threat facing society, and on the methods and legitimacy of the protection it employs. In this connection, we may recall that slavery, too, "protected" the community: it freed the slaveowners from manual labor. Commitment likewise shields the non-hospitalized members of society: first, from having to accommodate themselves to the annoying or idiosyncratic demands of certain members of the community who have not violated any criminal statutes; and, second, from having to prosecute, try, convict, and punish members of the community who have broken the law but who either might not be convicted in court, or, if they would be, might not be restrained as effectively or as long in prison as in a mental hospital. The literary evidence cited earlier fully supports this interpretation of the function of involuntary mental hospitalization.

IV

I have suggested that commitment constitutes a social arrangement whereby one part of society secures certain advantages for itself at the expense of another part. To do so, the oppressors must possess an ideology to justify their aims and actions; and they must be able to enlist the police power of the state to impose their will on the oppressed members. What makes such an arrangement a "crime against humanity"? It may be argued that the use of state power is legitimate when law-abiding citizens punish lawbreakers. What is the difference between this use of state power and its use in commitment?

In the first place, the difference between committing the "insane" and imprisoning the "criminal" is the same as that between the rule of man and the rule of law:[30] whereas the "insane" are subjected to the coercive controls of the state because persons more powerful than they have labeled them as "psychotic," "criminals" are subjected to such controls because

they have violated legal rules applicable equally to all.

The second difference between these two proceedings lies in their professed aims. The principal purpose of imprisoning criminals is to protect the liberties of the law-abiding members of society.[31] Since the individual subject to commitment is not considered a threat to liberty in the same way as the accused criminal is (if he were, he would be prosecuted), his removal from society cannot be justified on the same grounds. Justification for commitment must thus rest on its therapeutic promise and potential: it will help restore the "patient" to "mental health." But if this can be accomplished only at the cost of robbing the individual of liberty, "involuntary mental hospitalization" becomes only a verbal camouflage for what is, in effect, punishment. This "therapeutic" punishment differs, however, from traditional judicial punishment, in that the accused criminal enjoys a rich panoply of constitutional protections against false accusation and oppressive prosecution, whereas the accused mental patient is deprived of these protections.[32]

. . .

V

A basic assumption of American slavery was that the Negro was racially inferior to the Caucasian. "There is no malice toward the Negro in Ulrich Phillips' work," wrote Stanley Elkins about the author's book *American Negro Slavery,* a work sympathetic with the Southern position. "Phillips was deeply fond of the Negroes as a people; it was just that he could not take them seriously as men and women; they were children."[33]

Similarly, the basic assumption of institutional psychiatry is that the mentally ill person is psychologically and socially inferior to the mentally healthy. He is like a child: he does not know what is in his best interests and therefore needs others to control and protect him.[34] Psychiatrists often care deeply for their involuntary patients, whom they consider—in contrast with the merely "neurotic" persons—

"psychotic," which is to say, "very sick." Hence, such patients must be cared for as the "irresponsible children" they are considered to be.

The perspective of paternalism has played an exceedingly important part in justifying both slavery and involuntary mental hospitalization. Aristotle defined slavery as "an essentially domestic relationship"; in so doing, wrote Davis, he "endowed it with the sanction of paternal authority, and helped to establish a precedent that would govern discussions of political philosophers as late as the eighteenth century."[35] The relationship between psychiatrists and mental patients has been and continues to be viewed in the same way. "If a man brings his daughter to me from California," declares Braceland, "because she is in manifest danger of falling into vice or in some way disgracing herself, he doesn't expect me to let her loose in my hometown for that same thing to happen."[36] Indeed, almost any article or book dealing with the "care" of involuntary mental patients may be cited to illustrate the contention that physicians fall back on paternalism to justify their coercive control over the unco-operative patient. "Certain cases" [not individuals!]—writes Solomon in an article on suicide—". . . must be considered irresponsible, not only with respect to violent impulses, but also in all medical matters." In this class, which he labels "The Irresponsible," he places "Children," "The Mentally Retarded," "The Psychotic," and "The Severely or Terminally Ill." Solomon's conclusion is that "Repugnant though it may be, he [the physician] may have to act against the patient's wishes in order to protect the patient's life and that of others."[37] The fact that, as in the case of slavery, the physician needs the police power of the state to maintain his relationship with his involuntary patient does not alter this self-serving image of institutional psychiatry.

Paternalism is the crucial explanation for the stubborn contradiction and conflict about whether the practices employed by slaveholders and institutional psychiatrists are "therapeutic" or "noxious." Masters and psychiatrists profess their benevolence; their slaves and involuntary patients protest against their malevolence. As Seymour Halleck puts it: ". . . the psychiatrist experiences himself as a helping person, but his patient may see him as a jailer. Both views are partially correct."[38] Not so. Both views are completely correct. Each is a proposition about a different subject: the former, about the psychiatrist's self-image; the latter, about the involuntary mental patient's image of his captor.

NOTES

1. Szasz, T. S.: "Commitment of the mentally ill: Treatment or social restraint?" *J. Nerv. & Ment. Dis.* 125:293–307 (Apr.–June) 1957.

2. Szasz, T. S.: *Law, Liberty, and Psychiatry: An Inquiry into the Social Uses of Mental Health Practices* (New York: Macmillan, 1963), pp. 149–90.

3. Ibid., pp. 223–55.

4. Davis, D. B.: *The Problem of Slavery in Western Culture* (Ithaca, N. Y.: Cornell University Press, 1966).

5. See Cohen, R.: "Slavery in Africa." *Trans-Action* 4:44–56 (Jan.–Feb.), 1967; Tobin, R. L.: "Slavery still plagues the earth." *Saturday Review*, May 6, 1967, pp. 24–25.

6. Slovenko, R.: "The psychiatric patient, liberty, and the law." *Amer. J. Psychiatry*, 121:534–39 (Dec.), 1964, p. 536.

7. Felix, R. H.: "The image of the psychiatrist: Past, present, and future." *Amer. J. Psychiatry*, 121:318–22 (Oct.), 1964, p. 320.

8. Guttmacher, M. S.: "Critique of views of Thomas Szasz on legal psychiatry." *AMA Arch. Gen. Psychiatry*, 10:238–45 (March), 1964, p. 244.

9. Felix, op. cit., p. 231.

10. See szasz, T. S.: "The myth of mental illness." This volume [original source] pp. 12–24; *The Myth of Mental Illness: Foundations of a Theory of Personal Conduct* (New York: Hoeber-Harper, 1961); "Mental illness is a myth." *The New York Times Magazine*, June 12, 1966, pp. 30 and 90–92.

11. See, for example, Noyes, A. P.: *Modern Clinical Psychiatry*, 4th ed. (Philadelphia: Saunders, 1956), p. 278.

12. Szasz, T. S.: "The ethics of birth control; or, who owns your body?" *The Humanist*, 20:332–36 (Nov.–Dec.) 1960.

13. Hirsch, B. D.: "Informed consent to treatment," in Averbach, A. and Belli, M. M., eds., *Tort and Medical Yearbook* (Indianapolis: Bobbs-Merrill, 1961), Vol. I, pp. 631–38.

14. Mill, J. S.: *On Liberty* [1859] (Chicago: Regnery, 1955), p. 18.

15. Rosen, G.: "Social attitudes to irrationality and madness in 17th and 18th century Europe." *J. Hist. Med. & Allied Sciences*, 18:220–40 (1963), p. 223.

16. Packard, E. W. P.: *Modern Persecution, or Insane Asylums Unveiled*, 2 Vols. (Hartford: Case, Lockwood, and Brainard, 1873).

17. Illinois Statute Book, Sessions Laws 15, Section 10, 1851. Quoted in Packard, E. P. W.: *The Prisoner's Hidden Life* (Chicago: published by the author, 1868), p. 37.

18. Mill, J. S.: *The Subjection of Women* [1869] (London: Dent, 1965).

19. See, for example, Chekhov, A. P.: *Ward No. 6*, [1892], in *Seven Short Novels by Chekhov* (New York: Bantam Books, 1963), pp. 106–57; De Assis, M.: *The Psychiatrist* [1881–82], in De Assis, M., *The Psychiatrist and Other Stories* (Berkeley and Los Angeles: University of California Press, 1963), pp. 1–45; London, J.: *The Iron Heel* [1907] (New York: Sagamore Press, 1957); Porter, K. A.: *Noon Wine* [1937], in Porter, K. A., *Pale Horse, Pale Rider: Three Short Novels* (New York: Signet, 1965), pp. 62–112; Kesey, K.: *One Flew Over the Cuckoo's Nest (New York: Viking, 1962);* Tarsis, V.: *Ward 7: An Autobiographical Novel* (London and Glasgow: Collins and Harvill, 1965).

20. See Szasz, T. S.: "Alcoholism: A socio-ethical perspective." *Western Medicine,* 7:15–21 (Dec.) 1966.

21. See, for example, Rogow, A. A.: *James Forrestal: A Study of Personality, Politics, and Policy* (New York: Macmillan, 1964); for a detailed criticism of this view, see Szasz, T. S.: "Psychiatric classification as a strategy of personal constraint." This volume [original source] pp. 190–217.

22. Szasz, T. S.: *Psychiatric Justice* (New York: Macmillan, 1965).

23. "The Unconscious of a Conservative: A Special Issue on the Mind of Barry Goldwater." *Fact,* Sept.–Oct. 1964.

24. Zeligs, M. A.: *Friendship and Fratricide: An Analysis of Whittaker Chambers and Alger Hiss* (New York: Viking, 1967).

25. Freud, S. and Bullitt, W. C.: *Thomas Woodrow Wilson: A Psychological Study* (Boston: Houghton Mifflin, 1967).

26. Quoted in Schweitzer, A.: *The Psychiatric Study of Jesus* [1913] transl. by Charles R. Joy (Boston: Beacon Press, 1956), pp. 37, 40–41.

27. Arendt, H.: *Eichmann in Jerusalem: A Report on the Banality of Evil* (New York: Viking, 1963), p. 22.

28. Ibid., pp. 22–23.

29. For a full articulation and documentation of this thesis, see Szasz, T. S.: *The Manufacture of Madness: A Comparative Study of the Inquisition and the Mental Health Movement* (New York: Harper & Row, 1970).

30. Hayek, F. A.: *The Constitution of Liberty* (Chicago: University of Chicago Press, 1960), especially pp. 162–92.

31. Mabbott, J. D.: "Punishment" [1939], in Olafson, F. A., ed., *Justice and Social Policy: A Collection of Essays* (Englewood Cliffs, N.J.: Prentice-Hall, 1961), pp. 39–54.

32. For documentation, see Szasz, T. S.: *Law, Liberty, and Psychiatry: An Inquiry into the Social Uses of Mental Health Practices* (New York: Macmillan, 1963); *Psychiatric Justice* (New York: Macmillan, 1965).

33. Elkins, S. M.: *Slavery: A Problem in American Institutional and Intellectual Life* [1959] (New York: Universal Library, 1963), p. 10.

34. See, for example, Linn, L.: *A Handbook of Hospital Psychiatry* (New York: International Universities Press, 1955), pp. 420–22; Braceland, F. J.: Statement, in *Constitutional Rights of the Mentally Ill* (Washington, D. C.: U. S. Government Printing Office, 1961), pp. 63–74; Rankin, R. S. and Dallmayr, W. B.: "Rights of Patients in Mental Hospitals," in *Constitutional Rights of the Mentally Ill, supra,* pp. 329–70.

35. Davis, op. cit., p. 69.

36. Braceland, op. cit., p. 71.

37. Solomon, P.: "The burden of responsibility in suicide." *JAMA,* 199:321–24 (Jan. 30), 1967.

38. Halleck, S. L.: *Psychiatry and the Dilemmas of Crime* (New York: Harper & Row, 1967), p. 230.

PAUL CHODOFF

The Case for Involuntary Hospitalization of the Mentally Ill

I will begin this paper with a series of vignettes designed to illustrate graphically the question that is my focus: under what conditions, if any, does society have the right to apply coercion to an individual to hospitalize him against his will, by reason of mental illness?

Case 1. A woman in her mid 50s, with no previous overt behavioral difficulties, comes to believe that she is worthless and insignificant. She is completely preoccupied with her guilt and is increasingly unavailable for the ordinary

Reprinted with permission of the author and the publisher from *American Journal of Psychiatry,* Vol. 133, No. 5 (May 1976), pp. 496–501. Copyright 1976, the American Psychiatric Association.

demands of life. She eats very little because of her conviction that the food should go to others whose need is greater than hers, and her physical condition progressively deteriorates. Although she will talk to others about herself, she insists that she is not sick, only bad. She refuses medication, and when hospitalization is suggested she also refuses that on the grounds that she would be taking up space that otherwise could be occupied by those who merit treatment more than she.

Case 2. For the past 6 years the behavior of a 42-year-old woman has been disturbed for periods of 3 months or longer. After recovery from her most recent episode she has been at home, functioning at a borderline level. A month ago she again started to withdraw from her environment. She pays increasingly less attention to her bodily needs, talks very little, and does not respond to questions or attention from those about her. She lapses into a mute state and lies in her bed in a totally passive fashion. She does not respond to other people, does not eat, and does not void. When her arm is raised from the bed it remains for several minutes in the position in which it is left. Her medical history and a physical examination reveal no evidence of primary physical illness.

Case 3. A man with a history of alcoholism has been on a binge for several weeks. He remains at home doing little else than drinking. He eats very little. He becomes tremulous and misinterprets spots on the wall as animals about to attack him, and he complains of "creeping" sensations in his body, which he attributes to infestation by insects. He does not seek help voluntarily, insists there is nothing wrong with him, and despite his wife's entreaties he continues to drink.

Case 4. Passersby and station personnel observe that a young woman has been spending several days at Union Station in Washington, D.C. Her behavior appears strange to others. She is finally befriended by a newspaper reporter who becomes aware that her perception of her situation is profoundly unrealistic and that she is, in fact, delusional. He persuades her to accompany him to St. Elizabeths Hos-

pital, where she is examined by a psychiatrist who recommends admission. She refuses hospitalization and the psychiatrist allows her to leave. She returns to Union Station. A few days later she is found dead, murdered, on one of the surrounding streets.

Case 5. A government attorney in his late 30s begins to display pressured speech and hyperactivity. He is too busy to sleep and eats very little. He talks rapidly, becomes irritable when interrupted, and makes phone calls all over the country in furtherance of his political ambitions, which are to begin a campaign for the Presidency of the United States. He makes many purchases, some very expensive, thus running through a great deal of money. He is rude and tactless to his friends, who are offended by his behavior, and his job is in jeopardy. In spite of his wife's pleas he insists that he does not have the time to seek or accept treatment, and he refuses hospitalization. This is not the first such disturbance for this individual; in fact, very similar episodes have been occurring at roughly 2-year intervals since he was 18 years old.

Case 6. Passersby in a campus area observe two young women standing together, staring at each other, for over an hour. Their behavior attracts attention, and eventually the police take the pair to a nearby precinct station for questioning. They refuse to answer questions and sit mutely, staring into space. The police request some type of psychiatric examination but are informed by the city attorney's office that state law (Michigan) allows persons to be held for observation only if they appear obviously dangerous to themselves or others. In this case, since the women do not seem homicidal or suicidal, they do not qualify for observation and are released.

Less than 30 hours later the two women are found on the floor of their campus apartment, screaming and writhing in pain with their clothes ablaze from a self-made pyre. One woman recovers; the other dies. There is no conclusive evidence that drugs were involved (1).

Most, if not all, people would agree that the behavior described in these vignettes deviates significantly from even elastic definitions of normality. However, it is clear that there would not be a similar consensus on how to react to this kind of behavior and that there is a considerable and increasing ferment about what attitude the organized elements of our society should take toward such individuals. Everyone has a stake in this important issue, but the debate about it takes place principally among psychiatrists, lawyers, the courts, and law enforcement agencies.

Points of view about the question of involuntary hospitalization fall into the following three principal groups: the "abolitionists," medical model psychiatrists, and civil liberties lawyers.

THE ABOLITIONISTS

Those holding this position would assert that in none of the cases I have described should involuntary hospitalization be a viable option because, quite simply, it should never be resorted to under any circumstances. As Szasz (2) has put it, "we should value liberty more highly than mental health no matter how defined" and "no one should be deprived of his freedom for the sake of his mental health." Ennis (3) has said that the goal "is nothing less than the abolition of involuntary hospitalization."

Prominent among the abolitionists are the "anti-psychiatrists," who, somewhat surprisingly, count in their ranks a number of well-known psychiatrists. For them mental illness simply does not exist in the field of psychiatry (4). They reject entirely the medical model of mental illness and insist that acceptance of it relies on a fiction accepted jointly by the state and by psychiatrists as a device for exerting social control over annoying or unconventional people. The anti-psychiatrists hold that these people ought to be afforded the dignity of being held responsible for their behavior and required to accept its consequences. In addition, some members of this group believe that the phenomena of "mental illness" often represent essentially a tortured protest against the insanities of an irrational society (5). They maintain that society should not be encouraged in its oppressive course by affixing a pejorative label to its victims.

Among the abolitionists are some civil liberties lawyers who both assert their passionate support of the magisterial importance of individual liberty and react with repugnance and impatience to what they see as the abuses of psychiatric practice in this field—the commitment of some individuals for flimsy and possibly self-serving reasons and their inhuman warehousing in penal institutions wrongly called "hospitals."

The abolitionists do not oppose psychiatric treatment when it is conducted with the agreement of those being treated. I have no doubt that they would try to gain the consent of the individuals described earlier to undergo treatment, including hospitalization. The psychiatrists in this group would be very likely to confine their treatment methods to psychotherapeutic efforts to influence the aberrant behavior. They would be unlikely to use drugs and would certainly eschew such somatic therapies as ECT*. If efforts to enlist voluntary compliance with treatment failed, the abolitionists would not employ any means of coercion. Instead, they would step aside and allow social, legal, and community sanctions to take their course. If a human being should be jailed or a human life lost as a result of this attitude, they would accept it as a necessary evil to be tolerated in order to avoid the greater evil of unjustified loss of liberty for others (6).

THE MEDICAL MODEL PSYCHIATRISTS

I use this admittedly awkward and not entirely accurate label to designate the position of a substantial number of psychiatrists. They believe that mental illness is a meaningful concept and that under certain conditions its existence justifies the state's exercise, under the doctrine of parens patriae, of its right and obligation to arrange for the hospitalization of the sick individual even though coercion is involved and he is deprived of his liberty. I believe that these psychiatrists would recommend involuntary hospitalization for all six of the patients described earlier.

*Electroconvulsive therapy.—Ed.

THE MEDICAL MODEL

There was a time, before they were considered to be ill, when individuals who displayed the kind of behavior I described earlier were put in "ships of fools" to wander the seas or were left to the mercies, sometimes tender but often savage, of uncomprehending communities that regarded them as either possessed or bad. During the Enlightenment and the early nineteenth century, however, these individuals gradually came to be regarded as sick people to be included under the humane and caring umbrella of the Judeo-Christian attitude toward illness. This attitude, which may have reached its height during the era of moral treatment in the early nineteenth century, has had unexpected and ambiguous consequences. It became overextended and partially perverted, and these excesses led to the reaction that is so strong a current in today's attitude toward mental illness.

However, reaction itself can go too far, and I believe that this is already happening. Witness the disastrous consequences of the precipitate dehospitalization that is occurring all over the country. To remove the protective mantle of illness from these disturbed people is to expose them, their families, and their communities to consequences that are certainly maladaptive and possibly irreparable. Are we really acting in accordance with their best interests when we allow them to "die with their rights on" (1) or when we condemn them to a "preservation of liberty which is actually so destructive as to constitute another form of imprisonment" (7)? Will they not suffer "if [a] liberty they cannot enjoy is made superior to a health that must sometimes be forced on them" (8)?

Many of those who reject the medical model out of hand as inapplicable to so-called "mental illness" have tended to oversimplify its meaning and have, in fact, equated it almost entirely with organic disease. It is necessary to recognize that it is a complex concept and that there is a lack of agreement about its meaning. Sophisticated definitions of the medical model do not require only the demonstration of unequivocal organic pathology. A broader formulation, put forward by sociologists and deriving largely from Talcott Parsons' description of the sick role (9), extends the domain of illness to encompass certain forms of social deviance as well as biological disorders. According to this definition, the medical model is characterized not only by organicity but also by being negatively valued by society, by "nonvoluntariness," thus exempting its exemplars from blame, and by the understanding that physicians are the technically competent experts to deal with its effects (10).

Except for the question of organic disease, the patients I described earlier conform well to this broader conception of the medical model. They are all suffering both emotionally and physically, they are incapable by an effort of will of stopping or changing their destructive behavior, and those around them consider them to be in an undesirable sick state and to require medical attention.

Categorizing the behavior of these patients as involuntary may be criticized as evidence of an intolerably paternalistic and antitherapeutic attitude that fosters the very failure to take responsibility for their lives and behavior that the therapist should uncover rather than encourage. However, it must also be acknowledged that these severely ill people are not capable at a conscious level of deciding what is best for themselves and that in order to help them examine their behavior and motivation, it is necessary that they be alive and available for treatment. Their verbal message that they will not accept treatment may at the same time be conveying other more covert messages—that they are desperate and want help even though they cannot ask for it (11).

Although organic pathology may not be the only determinant of the medical model, it is of course an important one and it should not be avoided in any discussion of mental illness. There would be no question that the previously described patient with delirium tremens is suffering from a toxic form of brain disease. There are a significant number of other patients who require involuntary hospitalization because of organic brain syndrome due to various causes. Among those who are not overtly organically ill, most of the candidates for involuntary hospitalization suffer from schizophrenia or one of the major affective disorders. A growing and increasingly impressive body of evidence points to the presence of an important genetic-biological factor in these conditions; thus, many of them qualify on these grounds as illnesses.

Despite the revisionist efforts of the anti-psychiatrists, mental illness *does* exist. It does not by any means include all of the people being treated by psychiatrists (or by nonpsychiatrist physicians), but it does encompass those few desperately sick people for whom involuntary commitment must be considered. In the words of a recent article, "The problem is that mental illness is not a myth. It is not some palpable falsehood propagated among the populace by power-mad psychiatrists, but a cruel and bitter reality that has been with the human race since antiquity" (12, p. 1483).

CRITERIA FOR INVOLUNTARY HOSPITALIZATION

Procedures for involuntary hospitalization should be instituted for individuals who require care and treatment because of diagnosable mental illness that produces symptoms, including marked impairment in judgment, that disrupt their intrapsychic and interpersonal functioning. All three of these criteria must be met before involuntary hospitalization can be instituted.

1. Mental illness. This concept has already been discussed, but it should be repeated that only a belief in the existence of illness justifies involuntary commitment. It is a fundamental assumption that makes aberrant behavior a medical matter and its care the concern of physicians.

2. Disruption of functioning. This involves combinations of serious and often obvious disturbances that are both intrapsychic (for example, the suffering of severe depression) and interpersonal (for example, withdrawal from others because of depression). It does not include minor peccadilloes or eccentricities. Furthermore, the behavior in question must represent symptoms of the mental illness from which the patient is suffering. Among these symptoms are actions that are imminently or potentially dangerous in a physical sense to self

or others, as well as other manifestations of mental illness such as those in the cases I have described. This is not to ignore dangerousness as a criterion for commitment but rather to put it in its proper place as one of a number of symptoms of the illness. A further manifestation of the illness, and indeed, the one that makes involuntary rather than voluntary hospitalization necessary, is impairment of the patient's judgment to such a degree that he is unable to consider his condition and make decisions about it in his own interests.

3. Need for care and treatment. The goal of physicians is to treat and cure their patients; however, sometimes they can only ameliorate the suffering of their patients and sometimes all they can offer is care. It is not possible to predict whether someone will respond to treatment; nevertheless, the need for treatment and the availability of facilities to carry it out constitute essential preconditions that must be met to justify requiring anyone to give up his freedom. If mental hospital patients have a right to treatment, then psychiatrists have a right to ask for treatability as a front-door as well as a back-door criterion for commitment (7). All of the six individuals I described earlier could have been treated with a reasonable expectation of returning to a more normal state of functioning.

I believe that the objections to this formulation can be summarized as follows.

1. The whole structure founders for those who maintain that mental illness is a fiction.

2. These criteria are also untenable to those who hold liberty to be such a supreme value that the presence of mental illness per se does not constitute justification for depriving an individual of his freedom; only when such illness is manifested by clearly dangerous behavior may commitment be considered. For reasons to be discussed later, I agree with those psychiatrists (13, 14) who do not believe that dangerousness should be elevated to primacy above other manifestations of mental illness as a sine qua non for involuntary hospitalization.

3. The medical model criteria are "soft" and subjective and depend on the fallible judgment of psychiatrists. This is a valid objection.

There is no reliable blood test for schizophrenia and no method for injecting grey cells into psychiatrists. A relatively small number of cases will always fall within a grey area that will be difficult to judge. In those extreme cases in which the question of commitment arises, competent and ethical psychiatrists should be able to use these criteria without doing violence to individual liberties and with the expectation of good results. Furthermore, the possible "fuzziness" of some aspects of the medical model approach is certainly no greater than that of the supposedly "objective" criteria for dangerousness, and there is little reason to believe that lawyers and judges are any less fallible than psychiatrists.

4. Commitment procedures in the hands of psychiatrists are subject to intolerable abuses. Here, as Peszke said, "It is imperative that we differentiate between the principle of the process of civil commitment and the practice itself" (13, p. 825). Abuses can contaminate both the medical and the dangerousness approaches, and I believe that the abuses stemming from the abolitionist view of no commitment at all are even greater. Measures to abate abuses of the medical approach include judicial review and the abandonment of indeterminate commitment. In the course of commitment proceedings and thereafter, patients should have access to competent and compassionate legal counsel. However, this latter safeguard may itself be subject to abuse if the legal counsel acts solely in the adversary tradition and undertakes to carry out the patient's wishes even when they may be destructive.

COMMENT

The criteria and procedures outlined will apply most appropriately to initial episodes and recurrent attacks of mental illness. To put it simply, it is necessary to find a way to satisfy legal and humanitarian considerations and yet allow psychiatrists access to initially or acutely ill patients in order to do the best they can for them. However, there are some involuntary patients who have received adequate and active treatment but have not responded satis-

factorily. An irreducible minimum of such cases, principally among those with brain disorders and process schizophrenia, will not improve sufficiently to be able to adapt to even a tolerant society.

The decision of what to do at this point is not an easy one, and it should certainly not be in the hands of psychiatrists alone. With some justification they can state that they have been given the thankless job of caring, often with inadequate facilities, for badly damaged people and that they are now being subjected to criticism for keeping these patients locked up. No one really knows what to do with these patients. It may be that when treatment has failed they exchange their sick role for what has been called the impaired role (15), which implies a permanent negative evaluation of them coupled with a somewhat less benign societal attitude. At this point, perhaps a case can be made for giving greater importance to the criteria for dangerousness and releasing such patients if they do not pose a threat to others. However, I do not believe that the release into the community of these severely malfunctioning individuals will serve their interests even though it may satisfy formal notions of right and wrong.

It should be emphasized that the number of individuals for whom involuntary commitment must be considered is small (although, under the influence of current pressures, it may be smaller than it should be). Even severe mental illness can often be handled by securing the cooperation of the patient, and certainly one of the favorable efforts. However, the distinction between voluntary and involuntary hospitalization is sometimes more formal than meaningful. How "voluntary" are the actions of an individual who is being buffeted by the threats, entreaties, and tears of his family?

I believe, however, that we are at a point (at least in some jurisdictions) where, having rebounded from an era in which involuntary commitment was too easy and employed too often, we are now entering one in which it is becoming very difficult to commit anyone, even in urgent cases. Faced with the moral obloquy that has come to pervade the atmosphere in which the decision to involuntarily hospitalize is considered, some psychiatrists, especially younger ones, have become, as Stone (16) put it, "soft as grapes" when faced with the prospect of committing anyone under any circumstances.

THE CIVIL LIBERTIES LAWYERS

I use this admittedly inexact label to designate those members of the legal profession who do not in principle reject the necessity for involuntary hospitalization but who do reject or wish to diminish the importance of medical model criteria in the hands of psychiatrists. Accordingly, the civil liberties lawyers, in dealing with the problem of involuntary hospitalization, have enlisted themselves under the standard of dangerousness, which they hold to be more objective and capable of being dealt with in a sounder evidentiary manner than the medical model criteria. For them the question is not whether mental illness, even of disabling degree, is present, but only whether it has resulted in the probability of behavior dangerous to others or to self. Thus they would scrutinize the cases previously described for evidence of such dangerousness and would make the decision about involuntary hospitalization accordingly. They would probably feel that commitment is not indicated in most of these cases, since they were selected as illustrative of severe mental illness in which outstanding evidence of physical dangerousness was not present.

The dangerousness standard is being used increasingly not only to supplement criteria for mental illness but, in fact, to replace them entirely. The recent Supreme Court decision in *O'Connor v. Donaldson* (17) is certainly a long step in this direction. In addition, "dangerousness" is increasingly being understood to refer to the probability that the individual will inflict harm on himself or others in a specific physical manner rather than in other ways. This tendency has perhaps been carried to its ultimate in the *Lessard v. Schmidt* case (18) in Wisconsin, which restricted suitability for commitment to the "extreme likelihood that if the person is not confined, he will do immediate harm to himself or others." (This decision was set aside by the U.S. Supreme Court in 1974.) In a recent Washington, D.C., Superior Court case (19) the instructions to the jury stated that

the government must prove that the defendant was likely to cause "substantial physical harm to himself or others in the reasonably foreseeable future."

For the following reasons, the dangerousness standard is an inappropriate and dangerous indicator to use in judging the conditions under which someone should be involuntarily hospitalized. Dangerousness is being taken out of its proper context as one among other symptoms of the presence of severe mental illness that should be the determining factor.

1. To concentrate on dangerousness (especially to others) as the sole criterion for involuntary hospitalization deprives many mentally ill persons of the protection and treatment that they urgently require. A psychiatrist under the constraints of the dangerousness rule, faced with an out-of-control manic individual whose frantic behavior the psychiatrist truly believes to be a disguised call for help, would have to say, "Sorry, I would like to help you but I can't because you haven't threatened anybody and you are not suicidal." Since psychiatrists are admittedly not very good at accurately predicting dangerousness to others, the evidentiary standards for commitment will be very stringent. This will result in mental hospitals becoming prisons for a small population of volatile, highly assaultive, and untreatable patients (14).

2. The attempt to differentiate rigidly (especially in regard to danger to self) between physical and other kinds of self-destructive behavior is artificial, unrealistic, and unworkable. It will tend to confront psychiatrists who want to help their patients with the same kind of dilemma they were faced with when justification for therapeutic abortion on psychiatric grounds depended on evidence of suicidal intent. The advocates of the dangerousness standard seem to be more comfortable with and pay more attention to the factor of dangerousness to others even though it is a much less frequent and much less significant consequence of mental illness than is danger to self.

3. The emphasis on dangerousness (again, especially to others) is a real obstacle to the right-to-treatment movement since it prevents the hospitalization and therefore the treatment of the population most amenable to various kinds of therapy.

4. Emphasis on the criterion of dangerousness to others moves involuntary commitment from a civil to a criminal procedure, thus, as Stone (14) put it, imposing the procedures of one terrible system on another. Involuntary commitment on these grounds becomes a form of preventive detention and makes the psychiatrist a kind of glorified policeman.

5 Emphasis on dangerousness rather than mental disability and helplessness will hasten the process of deinstitutionalization. Recent reports (20, 21) have shown that these patients are not being rehabilitated and reintegrated into the community, but rather, that the burden of custodialism has been shifted from the hospital to the community.

6 As previously mentioned, emphasis on the dangerousness criterion may be a tactic of some of the abolitionists among the civil liberties lawyers (22) to end involuntary hospitalization by reducing it to an unworkable absurdity.

DISCUSSION

It is obvious that it is good to be at liberty and that it is good to be free from the consequences of disabling and dehumanizing illness. Sometimes these two values are incompatible, and in the heat of the passions that are often aroused by opposing views of right and wrong, the partisans of each view may tend to minimize the importance of the other. Both sides can present their horror stories—the psychiatrists, their dead victims of the failure of the involuntary hospitalization process, and the lawyers, their Donaldsons. There is a real danger that instead of acknowledging the difficulty of the problem, the two camps will become polarized, with a consequent rush toward extreme and untenable solutions rather than working toward reasonable ones.

The path taken by those whom I have labeled the abolitionists is an example of the barren results that ensue when an absolute solution is imposed on a complex problem. There are human beings who will suffer greatly if the abolitionists succeed in elevating an abstract principle into an unbreakable law with no exceptions. I find myself oppressed and repelled by their position, which seems to stem from an ideological rigidity which ignores that element of the contingent immanent in the structure of human existence. It is devoid of compassion.

The positions of those who espouse the medical model and the dangerousness approaches to commitment are, one hopes, not completely irreconcilable. To some extent these differences are a result of the vantage points from which lawyers and psychiatrists view mental illness and commitment. The lawyers see and are concerned with the failures and abuses of the process. Furthermore, as a result of their training, they tend to apply principles to classes of people rather than to take each instance as unique. The psychiatrists, on the other hand, are required to deal practically with the singular needs of individuals. They approach the problem from a clinical rather than a deductive stance. As physicians, they want to be in a position to take care of and to help suffering people whom they regard as sick patients. They sometimes become impatient with the rules that prevent them from doing this.

I believe we are now witnessing a pendular swing in which the rights of the mentally ill to be treated and protected are being set aside in the rush to give them their freedom at whatever cost. But is freedom defined only by the absence of external constraints? Internal physiological or psychological processes can contribute to a throttling of the spirit that is as painful as any applied from the outside. The "wild" manic individual without his lithium, the panicky hallucinator without his injection of fluphenazine hydrochloride and the understanding support of a concerned staff, the sodden alcoholic—are they free? Sometimes, as Woody Guthrie said, "Freedom means no place to go."

Today the civil liberties lawyers are in the ascendancy and the psychiatrists on the defensive to a degree that is harmful to individual needs and the public welfare. Redress and a more balanced position will not come from further extension of the dangerousness doctrine. I favor a return to the use of medical criteria by psychiatrists—psychiatrists, however, who have been chastened by the buffeting they have received and are quite willing to go along with even strict legal safeguards as long as they are constructive and not tyrannical.

REFERENCES

1. Treffert, D. A.: "The practical limits of patients' rights." *Psychiatric Annals* 5(4):91–96, 1971.

2. Szasz T.: *Law, Liberty and Psychiatry*, New York, Macmillan Co., 1963.

3. Ennis, B.: *Prisoners of Psychiatry*, New York, Harcourt Brace Jovanovich, 1972.

4. Szasz, T.: *The Myth of Mental Illness*, New York, Harper & Row, 1961.

5. Laing, R.: *The Politics of Experience*, New York, Ballantine Books, 1967.

6. Ennis, B.: "Ennis on 'Donaldson'." *Psychiatric News*, Dec 3, 1975, pp 4, 19, 37.

7. Peele, R., Chodoff, P., Taub, N.: "Involuntary hospitalization and treatability. Observations from the DC experience." *Catholic University Law Review* 23:744–753, 1974.

8. Michels, R.: "The Right to Refuse Psychotropic Drugs." *Hastings Center Report*, Hastings-on-Hudson, NY, 1973.

9. Parsons, T.: *The Social System*. New York, Free Press, 1951.

10. Veatch, R. M.: "The medical model: its nature and problems." *Hastings Center Studies* 1(3):59–76, 1973.

11. Katz, J.: "The right to treatment—an enchanting legal fiction?" *University of Chicago Law Review* 36:755–783, 1969.

12. Moore, M. S.: "Some myths about mental illness." *Arch Gen Psychiatry* 32:1483–1497, 1975.

13. Peszke, M. A.: "Is dangerousness an issue for physicians in emergency commitment?" *Am J Psychiatry* 132:825–828, 1975.

14. Stone, A. A.: "Comment on Peszke, M. A.: Is dangerousness an issue for physicians in emergency commitment?" Ibid. 829–831.

15. Siegler, M., Osmond, H.: *Models of Madness, Models of Medicine*. New York, Macmillan Co., 1974.

16. Stone, A.: Lecture for course on The Law, Litigation, and Mental Health Services. Adelphi, Md, Mental Health Study Center, September 1974.

17. O'Connor v Donaldson, 43 USLW 4929 (1975).

18. Lessard v Schmidt, 349 F Supp 1078, 1092 (ED Wis 1972).

19. In re Johnnie Hargrove, Washington, DC., Superior Court Mental Health number 506–75, 1975.

20. Rachlin, S., Pam, A., Milton, J.: "Civil liberties versus involuntary hospitalization." *Am J Psychiatry* 132:189–191, 1975.

21. Kirk, S. A., Therrien, M. E.: "Community mental health myths and the fate of former hospitalized patients." *Psychiatry* 38:209–217, 1975.

22. Dershowitz, A. A.: "Dangerousness as a criterion for confinement." *Bulletin of the American Academy of Psychiatry and the Law* 2:172–179, 1974.

SUGGESTED READINGS
FOR CHAPTER FOR CHAPTER 11

Books and Articles

Ayd, Frank J., ed. *Medical, Moral and Legal Issues in Mental Health Care*. Baltimore:Williams & Wilkins, 1974.

Dworkin, Gerald. "Autonomy and Behavior Control." *Hastings Center Report* 6 (February, 1976), 23–28.

Katz, Jay, *et al.*, eds. *Psychoanalysis, Psychiatry and Law*. New York: Free Press, 1967.

London, Perry. *Behavior Control*. New York: Harper & Row, 1971.

Mark, Vernon and Ervin, Frank. *Violence and the Brain*. New York: Harper & Row, 1970.

Michigan, Circuit Court for Wayne County. *Kaimowitz v. Department of Mental Health*. Civil No. 73–19434–AW (July 10, 1973).

Murphy, Jeffrie G. "Total Institutions and the Possibility of Consent to Organic Therapies." *Human Rights* 5 (Fall, 1975), 25–45.

"New Technologies and Strategies for Social Control: Ethical and Practical Limits." *American Behavioral Scientist* 18 (May/June, 1975). Special issue.

Rosenhan, D. L. "On Being Sane in Insane Places." *Science* 179 (January, 1973), 250–58.

"Symposium: Psychosurgery." *Boston University Law Review* 54 (March, 1974). Special issue.

Szasz, Thomas. *Ideology and Insanity*. New York: Doubleday Anchor, 1970.

Szasz, Thomas. *The Myth of Mental Illness*. New York: Hoeber, 1961.

U.S., National Commission for the Protection of Human Subjects. *Psychosurgery: Report and Recommendations* and *Appendix*. Washington, D.C.: U.S. Department of Health, Education, and Welfare, 1977.

Valenstein, Eliot S. *Brain Control: A Critical Examination of Brain Stimulation and Psychosurgery*. New York: Wiley, 1973.

"Viewpoints on Behavioral Issues in Closed Institutions." *Arizona Law Review* 17 (No. 1, 1975). Special issue.

Wexler, David B. "Mental Health Law and the Movement Toward Voluntary Treatment." *California Law Review* 62 (May, 1974), 671–92.

Bibliographies

Sollitto, Sharmon, and Veatch, Robert M., comps. *Bibliography of Society, Ethics and the Life Sciences*. Hastings-on-Hudson, N.Y.: Institute of Society, Ethics and the Life Sciences. Updated periodically. See under "Behavior Control."

Walters, LeRoy, ed. *Bibliography of Bioethics*. Vols. 1- . Detroit: Gale Research Co. Issued annually. See under "Behavior Control," "Electrical Stimulation of the Brain," "Electroconvulsive Therapy," "Involuntary Commitment," "Operant Conditioning," and "Psychosurgery."

12.
Genetic Intervention and Reproductive Technologies

The preceding chapter focused on techniques for controlling human behavior. In this final chapter we shall examine the medical and social applications of several recent developments in genetics and related fields.

GENETIC TESTING AND GENETIC SCREENING

Genetic Testing of Adults, Children and Newborns. Many of the basic laws of heredity were first discovered in the nineteenth century by the Austrian biologist and monk, Gregor Mendel. During the twentieth century geneticists and physicians have become increasingly aware of the significant hereditary component in many human diseases. In the early 1970s more than 1,600 genetically-related disorders had been identified. By the mid-1970s this number had grown to approximately 2,300.[1]

In some cases, genetic testing (by means of biochemical studies or chromosomal analysis) assists in the treatment of a patient's disorder. For example, such testing is currently employed to detect phenylketonuria (PKU) in newborn infants. If diagnosed early, this genetically-based "inborn error of metabolism" can be controlled by means of a special diet, and the brain damage which may otherwise result from the disease can be limited. On the other hand, some genetic conditions can be diagnosed for which neither a cure nor preventive measures are available. Huntington's chorea is a late developing, genetically-caused disease which strikes its victims at age 35 to 45 and produces rapid mental and physical deterioration and death within five years. Although diagnosis of Huntington's chorea is possible after the onset of the disease, no effective treatment can at present be offered to chorea victims.

Medicine's ability to diagnose an increasing number of hereditary disorders can be viewed as merely an extension to a new sphere of its general diagnostic capabilities. However, the fact that hereditary disorders are genetically transmitted from one generation to the next makes it possible for medicine to go a step beyond the *diagnosis* of disease in an individual to *predictions* concerning the genetic characteristics of the individual's offspring. For example, genetic testing can detect the "carriers" of approximately 50 recessive conditions—disorders, that is, in which persons who have one normal gene and one variant gene at the same location on paired chromosomes generally do not suffer any ill effects. If two carriers of the same recessive trait reproduce, however, there is a one-in-four chance that their offspring will inherit the variant gene from both parents and will thus be afflicted with the disease. One example of a recessive disorder detectable through genetic testing is Tay-Sachs disease. This disease, which is most common in Jewish persons of eastern European heritage, leads to the gradual debilitation and death of afflicted infants before the age of five. By the application of Mendel's laws of heredity, one can predict that, on average, two Tay-Sachs carriers who produce four children will have a family in which one child is afflicted with Tay-Sachs disease, two children carry the recessive trait for Tay-Sachs disease, and one child is completely free of the gene for Tay-Sachs disease.

Prenatal Diagnosis. In the late 1960s new techniques were developed which allow genetic testing to be extended to the fetus *in utero*. During the middle trimester of pregnancy, a pregnant woman can request a procedure called amniocentesis, in which a sample of amniotic fluid is removed from the sac which surrounds the fetus. This fluid is then subjected to laboratory analysis. By the mid-1970s approximately fifty genetic or chromosomal disorders, such as Down's syndrome, could be detected by this method. If the diagnosis reveals that a fetus is afflicted with such a disorder, the parents are then faced with the decision whether to have the fetus aborted.

In addition to amniocentesis, other methods for the prenatal detection of genetic disease are being developed. One new device, the fetoscope, has been used experimentally to visualize various parts of the fetus. With the aid of the fetoscope physicians may one day be able to detect anatomical abnormalities in the developing fetus. Techniques for drawing samples of fetal blood from the placenta have also been tested. These techniques may make possible the detection of fetuses afflicted with blood disorders, such as sickle-cell disease.

There are close links between the issue of prenatal genetic diagnosis and several questions discussed in earlier chapters of this book. One's ethical evaluation of prenatal diagnosis and selective abortion will depend in part upon one's view of fetal status and one's analysis of ethical issues in abortion (Chapter 5). A clear parallel also exists between the selective abortion of genetically defective fetuses and the practice of allowing genetically handicapped newborn infants to die (Chapter 7); indeed, the practice of selective abortion is likely to affect the attitudes of parents and health professionals toward genetically afflicted newborns.[2]

The technical aspects of prenatal diagnosis are discussed in the introductory essay by Theodore Friedmann. The second essay in the chapter, by Daniel Callahan, provides a philosophical perspective on genetic disease. Callahan suggests that the concept of genetic "defect," "abnormality," or "disease" may presuppose a value-laden model of the perfect human being. (His discussion at this point parallels the general debate concerning the concepts of health and disease, as illustrated in Chapter 3.) Callahan's essay also warns that the intensification of efforts to detect and conquer genetic disease may lead to a narrow utilitarian calculus which would, "quite literally, put a price on everyone's head." In his view, the campaign to alleviate or eradicate genetic disorders should be coupled with respect for the self-determination of prospective parents and with a concern to provide improved medical care to genetically-afflicted persons.

Programs of Genetic Screening. Genetic screening involves no *medical* procedures other than the genetic testing techniques described above; screening simply applies the techniques of genetic testing to large numbers of persons. Two types of genetic screening programs can be envisioned, voluntary and involuntary programs. If one combines the voluntary-involuntary distinction with the varieties of genetic testing previously enumerated, the categories shown in Figure 1 emerge.

Some genetic screening programs of the 1960s and 1970s have been voluntary and have sought to discover already-born individuals suffering from a particular disease, for example, phenylketonuria (PKU). They thus correspond to category 1 below. In 1963, however, Massachusetts began a program of mandatory testing for PKU in all newborns (category 5). Since 1963 most other states in the United States have instituted similar programs of mandatory PKU screening.[3] A qualitatively new stage in genetic screening was reached in the late 1960s, when programs were

FIGURE 1: GENETIC SCREENING PROGRAMS

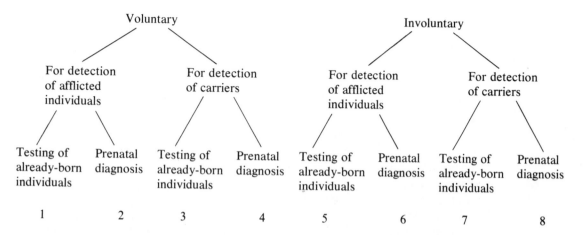

initiated which sought to detect *carriers* of specific recessive traits rather than *sufferers* from particular genetic diseases. In the case of Tay-Sachs disease all carrier-screening programs were voluntary (category 3); however, several states passed laws which required the establishment of programs to screen for carriers of sickle-cell trait (category 7).[4] In addition, voluntary programs of screening have been established for pregnant women 35 years of age and older who desire prenatal diagnosis for the detection of fetuses afflicted with chromosomal abnormalities (category 2). No screening programs corresponding to categories 4, 6, and 8 have been instituted.

In the excerpt from *The Ethics of Genetic Control* published in this chapter, Joseph Fletcher advocates the use of a straightforward utilitarian calculus in decisions concerning programs of genetic screening. In his view, to allow a foreseen and preventable harm is equivalent to causing the harm in question. (This point is reminiscent of debates concerning killing and letting die in Chapter 7.) Consequently, Fletcher regards an emphasis on reproductive rights and the right to privacy as both egocentric and eugenically disastrous.

In contrast, the report of the Hastings Center Research Group emphasizes the rights and interests of individuals and families. The report rejects as illegitimate the use of genetic screening programs for the attainment of eugenic goals. It also opposes all involuntary programs of genetic screening, arguing that "there is currently no public health justification for mandatory screening." The right of individual privacy and the possible impact of genetic screening programs on particular individuals and social groups are accorded highest priority in the position statement of the Research Group.

Contrasting factual and normative assumptions seem to underlie these two divergent approaches to genetic screening. Descriptively, Fletcher—perhaps drawing upon the views of the late H. J. Muller[5]—presupposes that laissez-faire reproduction will further pollute the already-deteriorating human gene pool. In contrast, the report of the Hastings Center Research Group implicitly denies that such a "clear and present" genetic danger exists.[6]

Prescriptively, the two essays reflect different viewpoints on the obligations of present persons to members of future generations. In a manner reminiscent of Jonas' approach to human experimentation (Chapter 9), the Research Group rejects mandatory screening as an illegitimate means to the end of eugenic progress. By implication, the group denies that the present generation has a moral obligation to bequeath an optimal gene pool to its near or distant descendants. Fletcher, however, advocates compulsory genetic screening as a way of fulfilling obligations to both future and present generations.

IN VITRO FERTILIZATION, CLONING, AND GENETIC INTERVENTION

The issues treated in the first section of this chapter, genetic testing and genetic screening, are matters of immediate concern for health professionals, public policy-makers, and citizens in general. In contrast, the second and final section of the present chapter focuses on several potential *future* applications of research in genetics, reproductive biology, and molecular biology. (The essay by Bernard Davis provides a succinct overview of projected trends in genetic research.)

In Vitro Fertilization. Since 1932, when Aldous Huxley published *Brave New World.* the idea of uniting human sperm and ova in the laboratory has been a significant theme in the literature of science fiction. In the 1970s, fiction is on the verge of being translated into fact. In vitro fertilization—literally, fertilization "in glass"—has been successfully accomplished in several species of animals. It seems likely that successful test-tube fertilization and embryo transfer in humans will be achieved by 1980, if not before. Indeed, during 1976 the British embryologist R. G. Edwards and his colleague Patrick Steptoe announced that, following in vitro fertilization, an embryo was transferred to a woman where it implanted; however, since implantation occured in one of the woman's Fallopian tubes, rather than in the uterus as intended, the pregnancy had to be terminated after thirteen weeks.[7]

James Watson's essay reviews the scientific steps which have led toward in vitro fertilization in humans and surveys several pro and con arguments. Proponents of in vitro fertilization note that many women who are infertile because of blocked Fallopian tubes, or oviducts, could be enabled to bear children with the aid of this technique. Without denying the potential benefits of in vitro fertilization in the alleviation of infertility, opponents of the technique argue that its use separates reproduction from the sexual relationship and may lead to the widespread employment of surrogate mothers. According to Watson, it is not yet clear whether advocates or opponents of in vitro fertilization will succeed in having their views prevail in the political process.

Cloning. The English verb "clone" is derived from the Greek work Klōn (twig or slip) and refers to a method by which offspring are produced asexually. Unlike sexual reproduction, which combines genetic material from two parents, asexual reproduction, or cloning, results in offspring which are genetically identical to a single parent. For example, if one were to cut a branch from a tree, place the branch in water until roots sprouted, then plant the branch, one would have created a clone of the tree from which the branch had been cut. The clone would contain exactly the same genes as the parent tree.

Watson describes how a clonal frog was produced in Oxford in the 1960s. In this case the nucleus of a maternal egg was removed and the nucleus of an adult cell inserted in its place. By this method a frog embryo was produced which was genetically identical to the adult "donor" frog. In fact, the cloned frog was in many ways the identical twin of the parent frog. Watson reports that similar experiments have been performed with mice and predicts that by 1990, or perhaps 2120, a clonal human being will also be produced.

Watson's essay remains primarily descriptive, depicting cloning experiments as a logical extension of Edwards' research on in vitro fertilization. In contrast, Davis ventures to speculate on some of the potential benefits and hazards of human cloning. While both authors agree that if the cloning of human beings becomes feasible some limits will need to be set, Watson urges that careful consideration be given to the development of an international public policy on human cloning *before* this powerful new technology is in fact developed.

Genetic Intervention. As noted above, the human race is afflicted by approximately 2,300 identifiable genetic or chromosomal disorders. Genetic testing reveals the presence of some of these disorders; however, only in few cases are satisfactory dietary or medical treatments available for detectable disorders. (Selective abortion following prenatal diagnosis eliminates, rather than cures, the genetically-defective fetus.)

One response to this rather bleak situation is the attempt to develop therapies which correct such abnormalities at the genetic level. Davis describes two approaches to the repair of genetic material, one of which would be used in the nonreproductive cells, the other of which would seek to eliminate genetic defects in sperm and ova prior to reproduction. Robert Sinsheimer's essay describes a newly developed method for combining genetic material from diverse species. The ability of molecular biologists to produce recombinant DNA molecules will contribute substantially to our understanding of genetic defects and may one day provide a mechanism for the repair of defective human genes.

The notion of "repair" presupposes a conception of health and disease, and it is but a short step from the elimination of genetic defects to the enhancement of human genetic capabilities. The essays of Davis and Sinsheimer present an interesting contrast in their fundamental approach to genetic intervention in humans. Davis expresses confidence that the benefits of scientific advance will outweigh the costs and argues that attempts by society to limit the progress of science will ultimately be detrimental. Sinsheimer, however, presents a more cautious perspective. In his view, the enthusiastic use of new genetic capabilities in large-scale programs of genetic engineering could introduce "a sudden major discontinuity in the human gene pool" and thus destroy the delicate balance between biological evolution and human culture.

L. W.

NOTES

1. Victor A. McKusick, *Mendelian Inheritance in Man* (4th ed.; Baltimore: Johns Hopkins University Press, 1975), p. xii.

2. John Fletcher, "Attitudes toward Defective Newborns," *Hastings Center Studies* 2 (January, 1974), 21–32.

3. Tabitha M. Powledge, "Genetic Screening as a Political and Social Development," in Daniel Bergsma, ed., *Ethical, Social and Legal Dimensions of Screening for Human Genetic Disease* (Miami: Symposia Specialists, 1974), pp. 30–32.

4. *Ibid.*, pp. 33–34.

5. "The Guidance of Human Evolution," *Perspectives in Biology and Medicine* 3 (Autumn, 1959), 1–43.

6. On this point see Marc Lappé, "Moral Obligations and the Fallacies of Genetic Control," *Theological Studies* 33 (September, 1972), 411–427.

7. P. C. Steptoe and R. G. Edwards, "Reimplantation of a Human Embryo with Subsequent Tubal Pregnancy," *Lancet* 1 (April 24, 1976), 880–882.

THEODORE FRIEDMANN

Prenatal Diagnosis of Genetic Disease

More than 1,600 human diseases caused by defects in the content or the expression of the genetic information in DNA have been identified. Some of these diseases are very rare; others, such as cystic fibrosis and sickle-cell anemia, are relatively common and are responsible for much illness and death. It has been estimated that more than 25 percent of the hospitalizations of children are for illnesses with a major genetic component. Thanks to new techniques of biochemistry and cell biology, we are learning a great deal about the biochemical mechanisms that lead from a genetic defect to clinical disease. Particularly important has been the discovery that cells from patients can be grown and studied in tissue culture in artificial nutrient media, and that these cells often continue to express the abnormal function of a mutant gene. As a result genetic manipulative techniques are being developed through which man may acquire the ability to control aspects of his own evolution, to eliminate disease and even to improve his genetic makeup. Another application of these techniques is prenatal genetic diagnosis.

The ability to establish the diagnosis of genetic disease prior to birth came through studies of the fluid that bathes the developing fetus within the amniotic cavity: a sac surrounding the fetus that is lined by two layers of cells (the chorion and the amnion) and is filled with fluid derived mainly from fetal urine and fetal respiratory secretions. Suspended in the fluid are viable cells shed from the fetal skin and respiratory tract, and perhaps from the fetally derived lining of the cavity itself. Amniocentesis, the

removal of fluid from the amniotic cavity by needle puncture, became useful and important in the early 1960's for the detection of unborn infants who ran the risk of Rh incompatibility. When an Rh-negative mother carries an Rh-positive fetus, the mother may become sensitized to the "foreign" red blood cells from the fetus, and the antibodies that develop may in later pregnancies cross the placenta, cleave to the fetus's red blood cells and cause the destruction of red cells, severe anemia, brain damage and even death. . . . Obstetricians discovered that they could estimate the degree of blood destruction by measuring the concentration of hemoglobin breakdown products in the amniotic fluid.

During amniocentesis for Rh disease it became clear that much useful information could be obtained by examining cells in the amniotic fluid. In 1949 Murray Barr of Canada had discovered that nerve cells from female cats were distinguishable from those of the male by the presence in the female cells of a darkly staining piece of chromosomal material on the nuclear membrane. These "Barr bodies" were then found to characterize female cells in many other mammals, including human females. Mary Lyon of England subsequently found that early in mammalian embryogenesis one of the two X chromosomes in female cells (male cells have only one X chromosome and a Y chromosome) randomly becomes condensed and inactive. In the unusual instances where cells have more than two X chromosomes all except one are condensed. In male cells condensation does not take place. The altered physical properties of these condensed chromosomes give rise to their staining characteristics.

From *Scientific American*, Vol. 255, No. 5 (November 1971), pp. 34–42. Reprinted with permission. Copyright © 1971 by Scientific American, Inc.

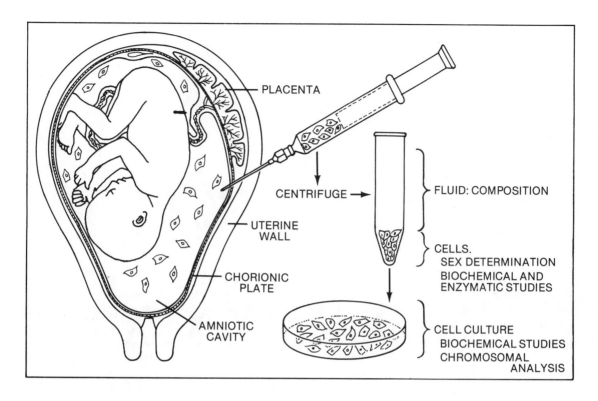

SAMPLE OF FLUID surrounding the fetus is taken by inserting a sterile needle into the amniotic cavity and withdrawing a small amount of fluid. The process is called amniocentesis. The fluid, derived mostly from fetal urine and secretions, contains fetal cells *(not drawn to scale)*. Care must be taken not to puncture the placenta or the fetus. The sample is centrifuged to separate cells and fluid. A variety of tests can be made. Optimum time for the amniotic tap for genetic diagnosis is about the 16th week of gestation.

Since amniotic-fluid cells are mostly fetal in origin, investigators turned to them as an unprecedentedly valuable material for detecting the kinds of genetic disease that are caused by mutations on the X chromosome and that therefore affect only males. The best-known of the "X-linked" diseases is the bleeding disorder hemophilia. In this disease a deficiency of one of the protein factors required for clotting results in prolonged and intractable bleeding, particularly at sites of traumatic injury.

An ovum from a female carrier of hemophilia will have either a normal X chromosome or a defective one. After fertilization half of all the resulting males will receive as their only X chromosome the one carrying the mutant gene.

Since there is no normal copy of the gene from the father such males will express the defect fully. (The father must pass his Y chromosome in order for the fetus to be male.) The other males will be normal, since they have by chance received the normal X chromosome from the mother. Therefore detection of a female fetus *in utero* by the presence of Barr bodies in a pregnancy in which there is a risk of hemophilia rules out the possibility of disease, although 50 percent of the females will be carriers. A male fetus, however, may be either affected or normal.

Predictions can also be made on the genetic constitution of the fetus in the case of diseases associated with an abnormal number of chromosomes or arrangement of chromosomes. In

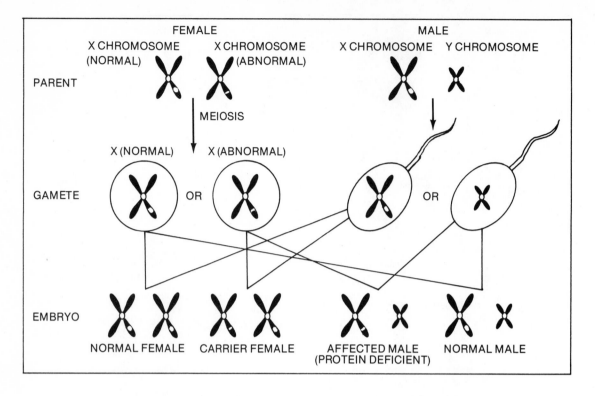

HEMOPHILIA is transmitted by mothers who have a defective gene for a clotting protein in one of their X chromosomes. Female offspring do not develop the disease because they receive at least one X chromosome that is not defective, but half of them like their mother will be carriers. A male offspring has a 50 percent chance of getting the defective gene and being afflicted with the disease.

1959 the French geneticist Jérôme Lejeune discovered that patients with mongolism (now usually called Down's syndrome) have no mutant or defective gene but rather carry an extra chromosome that in itself is probably normal. We now know that most cases of Down's syndrome are caused by a defect in the separation of chromosomes, called nondisjunction, in the developing egg resulting in the formation of ova with two No. 21 chromosomes instead of the usual one.

When such an egg is fertilized by a normal sperm, the result is an embryo carrying three normal No. 21 chromosomes. This "trisomy" of chromosome No. 21 causes Down's syndrome. An important feature of this kind of Down's syndrome is its increased incidence

with advanced maternal age. A pregnant woman 40 years old is more than 10 times as likely to have an affected infant as one 25 years old. The disease is the single most common chromosomal aberration found in live-born infants.

In a rarer type of Down's syndrome the extra chromosome No. 21 is translocated onto another chromosome. A healthy carrier mother has only 45 chromosomes instead of the usual 46, but the total amount of genetic information is normal. During the formation of the ovum, however, segregation of chromosomes can give rise to an ovum carrying the translocated No. 21 plus the free No. 21. Fertilization of such an ovum leads to an embryo with an apparently normal chromosome num-

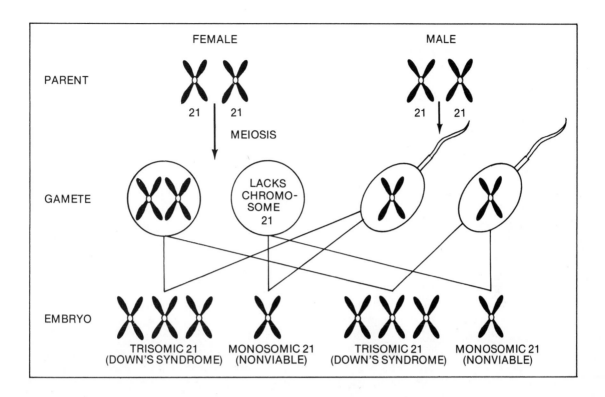

DOWN'S SYNDROME, or Mongolism, results when chromosomes fail to separate (nondisjunction) during meiosis, giving rise to some ova with two No. 21 chromosomes. When the ovum with the extra chromosome is fertilized, the embryo develops abnormally.

ber, but with an extra chromosome No. 21. The abnormalities in this kind of Down's syndrome are similar to those in the nondisjunction type.

Parallel with developments in cell biology have been advances in our knowledge of the flow of genetic information from DNA through RNA to protein. The precise biochemical defects involved in several hundred human disorders have been discovered, and this is due largely to the realization that tissue-culture cells from patients often continue to show the biochemical defect characteristic of a given disease. Such culture methods have most often used skin cells, but recently geneticists have learned that amniotic-fluid cells can also be cultured and used diagnostically.

· · ·

Some 40 genetic diseases can now be di-

agnosed prenatally by tests on the amniotic fluid and its cells. Several referral centers, including the one at the University of California at San Diego, have facilities for performing all or almost all of these tests. It is likely that other methods of prenatal diagnosis will eventually become available, such as studying changes in the enzyme patterns in the mother's blood or even detecting fetal cells in the mother's circulation. Meanwhile the increased availability (and probable automation) of assay procedures, including chromosome analysis, will lead to widespread prenatal diagnosis through amniocentesis in the next few years. This fact compels us to reflect on several important questions.

The most obvious question concerns the safety of the procedure itself. For prenatal diagnostic purposes the optimum time to perform amniocentesis seems to be around the 16th week of gestation. By that time enough amniotic fluid has accumulated for a sample to be easily obtained by needle puncture. The fetus is small and not likely to be traumatized, and sufficient time is still available to grow amniotic cells, perform the diagnostic procedures and proceed with a therapeutic abortion if that is desired. In the hands of the relatively small number of experienced individuals now performing amniocentesis the procedure does not seem to present much danger of traumatic injury to the mother or the fetus. The fetal parts can be manipulated away from the site of the needle puncture, and the placenta can be located by ultrasonic methods. One may expect traumatic complications to increase temporarily as less experienced physicians with insufficient specialized training begin to perform amniocentesis. Since any diagnostic procedure with a small but irreducible rate of complications is justifiably used only if the conditions being searched for lead to disease or damage much more frequently than the diagnostic procedure itself, it is important that these questions of safety be answered.

A more vexing problem concerns the possibility of developmental damage to the fetus through interference with the fetal environment, perhaps as a consequence of removal of fluid and its metabolites or through changes in pressure within the uterus. To detect this kind of damage would require a long-term developmental and intellectual evaluation of infants who had experienced amniocentesis. The National Institute of Child Health and Human Development is now undertaking such studies through a newly organized Amniocentesis Registry, which will collect and evaluate long-term effects of the procedure on fetus and mother. Preliminary claims for the safety of amniocentesis have already been made, but since experience with the procedure is still limited, we must be prepared for the possibility that some untoward effects on the fetus will become evident as the number of amniotic taps increases.

If we assume that the procedure will prove to be relatively safe, we can ask how and for what purpose we want to use such methods of prenatal genetic diagnosis. Some have suggested that prenatal genetic screening through amniocentesis may become a routine part of prenatal care—similar to tests on the mother for syphilis, diabetes and high blood pressure—as an effort to detect most fetal diseases and malformations before birth. This possibility seems remote. The problem of creating facilities to evaluate the three million births per year in the U.S. are of course immense, and many local and regional centers would have to be established. More important is the probability that there is almost certain to be a risk inherent in amniocentesis greater than the probability of detecting an abnormal fetus in an unselected population. This objection will obviously need to be modified if less hazardous methods of obtaining fetal genetic information are developed.

The most obvious purpose of such procedures is to reduce or eliminate the occurrence of genetic diseases that impose a devastating emotional burden on parents and often cause suffering and death in affected children. At present the only genetic diseases that might be detected *in utero* are those in which tissue-culture cells in the laboratory express the genetic abnormality of the disease, or those in which biochemical abnormalities are present in urine and other excretions and might therefore appear in the amniotic fluid. So far most developmental abnormalities, such as congenital heart disease, cannot be detected before birth.

Among the 1,600 genetic diseases that now are recognized, there will almost certainly be many that will not be expressed in the cells or the fluid obtained by amniocentesis. It is believed that all cells in the body, regardless of their function in differentiated tissues, carry the same genetic information. Any individual cell is therefore theoretically capable of performing functions of all other kinds of cells in that organism. We also know, however, that only some kinds of cells can conduct specialized functions such as the making of hemoglobin. If methods could not be found to activate or uncover the genes for hemoglobin in the skin or amniotic-fluid cells of patients with genetic forms of anemia, it might not be possible to detect these diseases in the uterus.

One factor that hinders the development of effective programs for the prevention of genetic diseases is the difficulty of identifying the pregnancies that are at risk. One of the clearest current indications for amniocentesis is advanced maternal age, since that is associated with the greatly increased risk of Down's syndrome. It has been estimated that if all pregnancies in women 35 years of age or older were evaluated by *in utero* detection methods, the rate of occurrence of this disease would be reduced to half the present level if selective abortion were practiced. Such age criteria, however, do not apply in many genetic disorders.

The other common indication for amniocentesis is a pregnancy in a woman who has previously borne a child with a genetic disease; this is called retrospective detection. If the disease is a dominant one such as Huntington's chorea, the risk of disease to the fetus is 50 percent. Monitoring subsequent pregnancies could readily detect all cases except those due to new mutations. Selective abortion on affected fetuses could virtually eliminate the disease. Unfortunately screening methods for Huntington's chorea and other dominant diseases are not available. If the disease is a recessive one, the potential effect of retrospective detection and selective abortion is much less impressive. We can expect to find only a small number of new cases, since the initial cases are all missed and subsequent pregnancies carry only a 25 percent probability of producing an affected child. If we assume a reproductive goal of two normal children per family, the number of new cases detected would at best be only 34 percent of the total. The effect of such programs on individual families known to have a history of genetic abnormality can nonetheless be great.

If prenatal diagnosis and selective abortion were coupled with extensive screening programs to find heterozygous carriers*, profound reductions might be achieved in the incidence of some recessive diseases. If the screening program could detect each family in which both parents were carriers, the monitoring of all pregnancies in only those families would result

*Individuals who possess a specific recessive gene but are not themselves afflicted with a genetic disease.—Ed.

in the detection of virtually all new cases of a recessive disease, and selective abortion for affected fetuses could be practiced. It is possible that with such a regime only cases caused by mutations would occur. Programs of this kind would necessarily be elaborate and expensive, but geneticists have already undertaken programs to detect and prevent new cases of Tay-Sachs disease. Since the frequency of the gene for Tay-Sachs disease among Ashkenazy Jews is 10 times that of the general population, marriages among Jews are being screened by blood tests of both partners. In families where both husband and wife are found to be carriers it is planned to monitor all pregnancies and to offer abortions in cases where the fetus is found to be affected.

Cost-benefit analyses have shown that detection programs for Tay-Sachs disease and Down's syndrome alone would result in very large savings for individual families and for society as a whole if affected fetuses were aborted instead of being born and ultimately institutionalized at state expense. Four thousand infants with Down's syndrome are born each year in the U.S., and lifetime institutional care for each one costs approximately $250,000. Such analyses, however, seldom define what they consider the benefit. Is it only black figures in the ledger instead of red? Economic considerations are undeniably important, but it seems a dangerous precedent to justify screening and selective abortion programs solely on the basis of comparing their cost with the economic burden to families and to society. One could argue cogently that we should be more willing to spend money for the elimination of disease even if it proves to be uneconomical.

Recently some geneticists, notably Arno G. Motulsky of the University of Washington School of Medicine and James V. Neel of the University of Michigan, have become concerned with the possibility that large-scale genetic manipulations such as prenatal detection and abortion might lead to detrimental changes in the quality and the diversity of the human gene pool. Such changes might be the inadvertent result of programs to eliminate disease or the deliberate consequence of eugenic programs to eliminate certain undesirable genes from the population.

Motulsky and Neel have recently shown that programs of prenatal detection and selective abortion might bring about unexpected increases in the frequency of genes for some diseases. As an illustration let us assume that in the future each family will have two normal children and will compensate for fetuses lost through abortion. Under these conditions the prevention of natural gene loss through death or nonreproducibility of the affected homozygotes* could lead to an increase over many generations of 50 percent in the gene frequency. For cystic fibrosis this means that over 50 generations the frequency of carriers in a population would increase from its present 5 percent to a new equilibrium level of 7.5 percent. Motulsky considers that, in view of the long time required, the change is minimal and probably of no real concern, particularly when it is compared with the effect on gene frequencies of a program of premarital counseling and the prevention of mating between heterozygous carriers. If any selective advantage exists for the heterozygote and persists in the future, as seems to be the case with sickle-cell anemia and cystic fibrosis, the frequency of carriers might rise over many generations to a startling level of 50 percent. Every second person would be a carrier.

Another startling effect could occur in X-linked diseases such as hemophilia, where no distinction can yet be made between affected and normal males *in utero*. If abortion of all male fetuses in carrier mothers were to become widespread, the result could be a 50 percent increase in the gene frequency *with each generation*.

The directed elimination of genes by selective abortion after prenatal detection is certainly feasible and, as Motulsky shows, is probably not deleterious in most instances. The gene responsible for a dominant disease such as Huntington's chorea could be virtually

*Individuals afflicted with a recessive genetic disease. —Ed.

eliminated with a modest detection and abortion program, although that is not yet possible since biochemical tests for this disease and other dominant diseases are not available. It is unlikely that the loss of such a gene would in any way be injurious to the species. The elimination of genes for recessive diseases, however, would require not only much more elaborate screening programs for large segments of the population but also the abortion of all unaffected heterozygous fetuses. It is difficult to see how this could ever be justified.

Geneticists realize that genetic diversity is important for ensuring the adaptability, and therefore the survival, of a species in the face of continually changing evolutionary selective pressures. Presumably the human species is no exception. This is not to say that our present gene pool is an optimum one, and it is certain that the evolution of our gene pool is continuing even now. Although one might argue that some changes can be made in our gene pool that are evolutionarily neutral or even advantageous, we must question our ability to use this capacity to even partially direct our genetic future with sufficient wisdom and foresight.

Until now prenatal diagnosis combined with selective abortion has been applied mostly in cases where there has been little or no doubt about the inevitability of disease with a demonstrated genetic abnormality. We are now, however, beginning to understand more about the role of normal genetic variation in man, and about the existence of aberrations that are not so closely associated with disease. Several recent clinical situations have emphasized the uncertainties in the relationship between the existence of a genetic abnormality and the development of clinical disease. A chromosomal abnormality, the XYY syndrome, has recently been described in which some men have an extra Y chromosome. Clinical studies have suggested that such men are statistically more likely to develop aggressive antisocial behavior than normal XY males. Some of the affected men are criminals but most are not, and most important of all we have no firm evidence that it is the extra chromosome that is directly responsible for the suspected tendency toward criminal behavior.

In another instance a normal parent carrying a translocation of material from a No. 3 chromosome to another chromosome has given birth to a child with apparently the identical chromosomal abnormality but with severe mental retardation. The detection in fetal cells of this kind of translocation would therefore not have helped in determining if the fetus were destined to be severely retarded or of normal intelligence. These findings illustrate the fact that in some cases our knowledge of the mechanism by which a defective gene leads to the development of human clinical disease is inadequate. We may also recall that some genes may confer a selective advantage on heterozygous carriers. Heterozygotes for sickle-cell anemia are less susceptible to infection with malaria. It is probable that other genes that are detrimental under some conditions are of value to the species. Knowledge of such challenges to our diagnostic and prognostic accuracy may make it increasingly difficult to provide information on which prospective parents can make informed and intelligent decisions.

Some fear that in a society where abortion is becoming acceptable, increasingly arbitrary standards may be applied in the making of decisions on the fitness or desirability of a given fetus. In present circumstances it is not difficult to imagine the emergence of pressures to set standards for desirability in genetically determined human characteristics. At the moment it is not at all clear how these standards might be arrived at, and whose standards they might be. Neel has pointed out that condemning many of today's infants to famine and inadequate development does not display greater respect for the quality of human life than is found in primitive societies that practice infanticide with undesired or defective newborn infants. Others have questioned the moral justification for making these life-death decisions. Through recent upheavals in our social, legal and religious institutions we are now faced with the dilemma of assigning to the fetus certain rights. In several instances damages have been awarded on behalf of fetuses in criminal and tort suits. At the same time abortion laws have been liberalized to the point of suggesting that early fetuses do not have the right to life if the mother wants to abort a pregnancy. Prenatal genetic diagnosis seemed at first no different from most other new diagnostic methods. Now we see that we are faced with problems of assigning values to individuals with given genetic characteristics and designing programs directed against them. Until now most of these characteristics have been associated with severe clinical disease. Now we are not always certain what the existence of genetic anomalies will mean to the health of an individual. These uncertainties could result in an accentuation of the conflict in our society between personal choice and governmental control, which could possibly come in the form of selected programs of compulsory screening and mandatory abortion for some conditions that are deemed socially intolerable. The obviously dangerous extensions of such a practice would impinge so drastically on our individual liberties as to make them unacceptable and morally unjustifiable.

Intriguing developments in our legal concepts of the unborn child seem imminent, since there are certain to be legal tests of the liability of parents and others for offspring born with genetically determined handicaps that are predictable. Such "wrongful life" suits have already been brought on behalf of illegitimate infants and some infants born with severe developmental defects due to prenatal infection with syphilis and German measles. Similar suits involving genetic diseases will soon test the concept that we—as parents, physicians and human beings—have obligations to the unborn to protect them from the likelihood of genetically determined defects. One may hope that advances in other social institutions will at the same time help us to resolve our individual and societal attitudes toward life, born and unborn.

DANIEL CALLAHAN

The Meaning and Significance of Genetic Disease: Philosophical Perspectives

I want to raise here the question of why we are concerned with genetic disease and how we might appropriately look upon it. I will leave to others a treatment of the various ethical problems which the detection and treatment of genetic disease pose. Instead, I will focus my attention on the kind of human, social and cultural perspectives brought to bear on genetic disease, and the way in which they tend to establish the framework within which ethical issues are discerned and handled. This is important not only because these perspectives are interesting in themselves, but also because I am convinced that ethical systems, codes, and insights spring ultimately from assessments of the meaning and significance of human existence. All of us, I believe, have certain images of life, certain fundamental stances toward reality, certain sets of assumptions about the nature of things. Taken together, they help to determine the way questions are framed, priorities of interest established, emotional commitments made, fears, hopes and anxieties aroused. The first question I want to pose concerning genetic disease is this: What image of human existence is pertinent as a framework for determining our response to the reality of genetic disease?

When I was about seven I was approached one day on a playground by a very odd-looking boy of perhaps twelve or thirteen, stumbling, misshapen and with a rather silly, though friendly smile on his face. My reaction was a mixture of horror, fear, and curiosity. I wanted to stare at him and study him, but at the same time I wanted to run home as fast as I could. I resolved the dilemma at first by moving carefully backwards as he kept coming toward me,

Reprinted with permission of the publisher from Bruce Hilton, *et al.* eds., *Ethical Issues in Human Genetics: Genetic Counseling and the Use of Genetic Knowledge* (New York: Plenum Publishing Corp., 1973), pp. 83–90.

trying to keep him at a safe distance. But he kept coming and, eventually, I did run home, certain that if I did not he would "get me." He represented an alien, utterly inexplicable phenomenon.

No one, of course, had told me about Down's syndrome, and no one did for many years after. My parents said vaguely that he was "sick" and that "he wouldn't hurt me," but little more. That he was the child of a close neighbor, usually hidden, was something I had to deduce for myself. All the adults in the neighborhood, it seems, knew about him, but all tacitly engaged in a highly successful conspiracy to say nothing about the matter—indeed, to evade all pointed questions asked by innocent children. Eventually, the mongoloid I had encountered simply disappeared, no doubt into some institution.

I mention this incident because it seems to me to sum up one pervasive, almost instinctual human reaction to genetic disease. The defective human being has historically seemed a mysterious, awesome, terrifying creature—almost a separate, subhuman species—to be shunned altogether, explained away by means of elaborate religious mythologies, or given a special meaning, either as an omen of good or of evil. Of course, we now know more about genetic disease. We have some notion of why these hitherto strange creatures issue forth from the womb as defectives, and we think we have some ways of coping with what we are now able to classify as an abnormality.

But it would be a mistake to think that the old sense of mystery, awe, and terror does not live on. Surely the pervasive parental fear of bearing a defective child is not just because of the troubles of raising such a child, though that is a most serious matter. The fear seems much deeper than that, as if a defective child would represent a supreme undoing of the parents' image of themselves and reality. I am reminded of the conviction of many philosophers of antiquity that there is an irrational, irreducible surd element in the universe, which constantly breaks through our visions and structures of ordered rationality. Genetic disease, long before it was labeled as that, was a case in point. One might in the instance of a hunting accident be able to discern a causal logic; the accident, however unacceptable, at least made sense. Genetic disease made no sense whatever; a defective child just arrived, out of some primeval darkness. A terror before the darkness still endures.

Yet, unlike our ancestors, we are no longer willing to be cowed. We are beginning to fight back, and the steps being taken follow a familiar script. We try to understand the mystery, by turning it into a problem rather than a mystery; then, with our cool-headed, rational explanation in hand we set ourselves to doing something about it—we label it a "disease" and then we try to "conquer" it. The change in our image of reality is evident here. Our ancestors had no choice but to be terrorized, and thus in compensation to find some symbolic means by which the philosophical absurdity of the defective existence could be understood and lived with. For our part, we act—fast, hard, and with all the technical means at our disposal.

The results are becoming evident. We are beginning to understand genetic disease, to know how to diagnose its presence, and, in some cases, how to cure it. Increasingly, it is becoming possible for those who do not want to bear defective children not to bear them. Since no one wants to bear such a child, just as they do not want to contract cancer or coronary disease, we are all that much the better off.

Yet at the level of broad philosophical perspective, I believe we should anticipate some problems. The conquest of genetic disease proceeds from the optimistic assumption that physical reality can be understood and that its aberrations can be minimized or eliminated. Nature can be brought to heel. That has been the assumption of the medical sciences generally, and its successes have served as the best possible arguments against those who still believe there is a surd element in reality. Unfortunately, though, the fact of the matter is that we have just begun the conquest of genetic disease; it may be decades or centuries before the last defective child is born into the world. If a heuristic optimism is a necessity in order that the struggle against the disease is to go forward, this ought not to blind us to the fact that there is far more of what we do not know than of what we do, and far more genetic diseases that we have not conquered than we have.

In the meantime, during a great transition period which has no discernible end point, what ought to be the philosophical significance we attribute to genetic disease and genetically defective human beings? What ought our image of the world be and what place ought genetic disease to have within it? Let me point to some items on the present cultural horizon which seem to me to bespeak some dilemmas which need to be considered.

First, we still speak much of freedom of parental choice in the use of genetic information. And it is still common for genetic counselors to reassure parents that a defective fetus or child is "not their fault." Yet it is possible to detect tendencies which could eventually rob people of their choice and "blame" them for the defective children they bring into the world. If there is something of a paradox here at first sight, it soon disappears. For the corollary to giving people freedom of choice is to make them responsible for the choices they make. It is then only a very short step to begin distinguishing between responsible and irresponsible choices; social pressure begins to put in an appearance. Thus, while in principle the parents of a fetus with a detected case of Down's syndrome are still left free to decide whether to carry it to term, it is not difficult to discern an undercurrent in counseling literature and discussion that would classify such a decision as irresponsible. This is amplified in a subtle way. Abortion is said to be "medically indicated" in such cases, as if what is essentially an ethical decision has now become nothing but medical.

I am not concerned here with whether the

decision in this or similar circumstances is irresponsible, or whether an abortion ought to be performed. I only want to point out that if and when we begin holding parents responsible for the children they bring into the world, and blaming them for what we take to be irresponsible choices, we may then have a result worse than that which flowed from the superstition of our ancestors. We will then share with our ancestors the view that a defective child is a curse but then, unlike them, provide no comfort whatever other than the ascetic reward of praise or blame for socially acceptable behavior in the face of the curse. In a word, it is simply not clear to me that in this circumstance an image of the world which, based on fierce rationality, would hold every person responsible for every jot and title of his or her behavior is altogether preferable to one which, while it could give them no choice, did not judge them either. And, of course, if we begin blaming those who make what we term "irresponsible" choices, then the freedom of choice now extolled in genetic counseling would become a mockery.

Second, while it has no doubt always been the case that parents of defective children have had to count the financial costs, the introduction of modern cost-accounting and cost-benefit analysis into the genetic equation adds a distinctively different element. We can now, quite literally, put a price on everyone's head, working out the long-term financial costs to individuals and societies of caring for a defective child.

But let us observe a curiosity. It was counted a great advance of the modern mind when a bookkeeping God, with his minutely maintained ledger of good and bad deeds, was noisily rejected. Yet here we are, beginning to keep our own books, and using them increasingly as a determinant in deciding whether or not defectives should be allowed the privilege of birth, and their parents the privilege of parenthood. Moreover, we seem to have forgotten the reason why the bookkeeping God was rejected—because it seemed eminently unjust, insensitive, and outrageous that a scorecard be kept on human lives. Indeed, we are even worse than that old God; for at least in his ledger everything was supposedly recorded. But our cost-benefit analysis totes up one item only—what the financial liability of the defective will be, what he will cost us in terms of taxes, institutional facilities, the time of medical personnel, and so on. Needless to say, this kind of reckoning is prone to be weak in comparing the costs of the defective against the cost of other patently foolish public and private expenditures which are accepted with barely a word of protest. What is society spending on cosmetics this year? Nor does this kind of reckoning have much to say about ways of reconstructing the social and political order to make possible a more humane treatment of those considered a social liability—the poor, the aged, the unfit. No, for the kind of cost-benefit analysis which seems to be emerging in genetic calculations goes only in the cost direction; it is seemingly assumed that the benefits to a society which decided simply to bear the costs of humane care are either nonexistent or simply too intangible to be worth much bother.

Third, behind the human horror at genetic defectiveness lurks, one must suppose, an image of the perfect human being. The very language of "defect," "abnormality," "disease," and "risk" presupposes such an image, a kind of prototype of perfection. In the past there seemed little which could be done to realize the prototype; it was contemplated as a platonic form, well out of reach. Eventually, a kind of wisdom developed. Since it appeared clear that, even if there is a perfect human being to be conceived or imagined, the price of pursuing and imposing it is very high in terms of the ways it can change our response to actually existing human beings. Human diversity began to be appreciated and justified. In fact, behind modern society's at least verbal commitment to civil rights, to justice for all, lies a rejection of images of individual perfection and uniformity. A similar pattern has been manifest in even the purely scientific sphere, with a rejection in biology and zoology of monotypical modes of analysis and classification (which stressed a fixed, static concept of type) in favor of a populationist approach (which makes

Yet because of the advances in the detection and cure of genetic disease—the ghost of the perfect human being, once sensibly laid to rest, is putting in his appearance again. And I believe we are beginning to see evidence of what this means: a heightened anxiety on the part of prospective parents about bearing a defective child, increased social pressure against those who would bear a child deviating from the norm of perfection, and, at what I hope is not the leading edge but a fringe only, hints that the sensible society of the future will of course deny parents the right to bring into the world any child who could not measure up, who would be a burden upon society.

There have surely been abuses and a good deal of plain silliness in recent rejections of purported ethical absolutes and ethical objectivity, of fixed codes, of rigid notions of the "human" and the "non-human," of the worthy and the unworthy, of static notions of perfection and imperfection. But on the whole, this rejection has helped to soften life, to provide a defense against the totalitarian reformer, to widen our appreciation of the value of human differences, variations and dissimilarities, to lead us to construct visions of political and social orders which can encompass and profit from variety. An image of man based on a pluralistic rather than a monistic conception of reality has been hard-won. It would be a supreme irony if, in the name of even greater progress, there was reintroduced the old monistic, monotypical kind of thinking, this time, as before, in the name of value, good order, and a mythical notion of perfection.

Fourth, every image of the world and reality carries with it a correlative view of the nature of human community. It is not for nothing that political reformers and revolutionaries (think only of Karl Marx) have felt that the condition for a change in ethical and political thinking is, first of all, a change in metaphysical thinking. An egalitarian social structure can, only with difficulty and patch-work logic, be built upon a metaphysic of fixed hierarchical realities. Participatory democracy has nothing going for it in a society which secretly believes that some

people are inherently lower than others and thus not fit to govern themselves.

It would be a mistake to say that past human societies adapted happily and well to the reality of genetic disease and defect. Yet there did develop the humane response that society as a whole should share the burden of caring for the defective, that the parents or family should not be left with sole responsibility for the care and survival of the defective. Moreover, in laws against infanticide, child neglect and abuse, there was reflected a belief that society has an obligation toward children, an obligation which holds good regardless of their physical or mental condition. We can see in these historical developments a concept of community and society which tried to respond to human diversity, even that diversity represented by the grossly abnormal. So, too, it was perceived that any effective recognition of diversity—which means a recognition of actual inequalities of individual assets and liabilities in society—required a joint sharing of responsibility by all for all, so that those least equipped by nature or nurture to function would not be inevitable losers.

This cultural development represented a great milestone in human history, even if our society and most others have hardly succeeded in living up to the obligations which it entailed. We created public institutions for defectives, only too often to treat them like animals once we gave them the benefit of admission to those institutions. Nonetheless, the introduction of the very notion of common and public responsibility represented a triumph of great magnitude. A triumph, I am sorry to say, which would all be for nothing if we accept the idea that defectives and their parents have no right to burden the rest of us with their troubles, or that it is naive to find a social solution for a problem which can be done away with by a scientific solution.

I would not want to be misunderstood here. Nothing I have said should be construed as an objection to the further development and refinement of genetic knowledge and the art of genetic counseling. On the contrary, the suffering brought on by genetic disease warrants nothing less than a full-scale social, scientific and economic effort to eliminate, cure or alleviate these afflictions. My concern, rather, is with the spirit in which such an effort is undertaken, with the kind of philosophical perspective which should lie behind it, and with the social context in which it is carried out.

Genetic disease will not be done away with overnight, if ever. At the simplest level, there is at least a requirement that people's hopes not be raised too high too precipitately; that will just set the stage for even more suffering. More important though is the question of how we are to continue living in the company of genetic disease, even as vigorous steps are taken to minimize its impact. As Professor Crow has emphasized, the reality of genetic disease is that it is a recurrent disease brought about by the continued reintroduction of defective genes by mutation. The overarching dilemma I have tried to sketch comes to this: How can we manage both to live humanely with genetic disease and yet to conquer it at the same time? Both goals seem imperative and yet the logic of each is different. We cure disease by ceasing to romanticize it, by gathering our powers to attack it, by making it an enemy to be conquered. We learn to live with a disease, however, in a very different way; by trying to accept and cherish those who manifest the disease, by shaping social structures and institutions which will soften the individual suffering brought on by the disease, by refusing to make the bearer of the disease our economic, social, or political enemy.

Our communal task, I believe, is to find a way of combining both logics. That will not be easy, if only because most people find it easier to cope with one idea than with two at the same time. It will mean, for instance, simultaneously working to improve the societal treatment and respect accorded those born with defects, and working to extend our genetic knowledge and applying it to genetic counseling. It will mean taking the idea of free choice seriously, allowing parents to make their own choice without penalizing them socially for the choices they

make, or condemning them for those choices which will increase the financial costs to society. Part of the very meaning of human community, I would contend, entails a willingness of society to bear the social costs of individual freedom.

It will mean some care in the way we use language. As physical organisms we stand "at risk" of genetic disease, as do our children and our descendants; as cultural beings, however, we stand "at risk" also in another sense, of seeing our values, our better instincts, and our humanity diseased and crippled. If odds are to be calculated, then let both sets of risks be included in our general equation. Moreover, if the "risk" of genetic disease is to be calculated, and better calculated, let it be remembered that no set of mathematical statistics can, by themselves, "indicate" what we ought to do in response to the realities they delineate. That requires the introduction of ethical premises, and those premises, in turn, require some coherent notion of what the human good is. When we speak of the good of "the patient," let it not be the case, in the first place, that we use the term "patient" only for those we think desirable to treat (using some clinical term for the rest—fetus, conceptus, neonate); or, in the second place, that the decision if and how to treat a patient not be made a matter of how we, as individuals or community, happen to feel about the intrinsic worth of that patient. Beyond that, particular care is needed when we speak of someone or some group's "good." It is not all that easy to know what is good for the individual, for the family and for society, though one might gather otherwise in light of the many confident statements made on the subject. As a descriptive term indicating deviation from a statistical mean, the word "abnormal" can be very helpful, as a philosophical term, indicating some mandatory level of social and genetic fitness— a prototype of human perfection—it can be very hazardous.

To conquer a disease is to reflect a view of the world. It is also to create a partially new world and a new view of human possibilities. How we go about dealing with genetic disease —the kinds of counseling techniques developed, the professional consensuses which emerge, the attitudes developed toward carriers of defects and toward the children many of them will bear, the kinds of choices which emerge and the positions taken on the nature of those choices—will both reflect one world and bring another into being. That is a heavy burden to bear and we had better be aware of it.

JOSEPH FLETCHER

The Ethics of Genetic Control

COSTS AND BENEFITS

The essence of tragedy is the conflict of one good with another. The conflict of good with evil is only melodrama. We often have to calculate the relative desirability of things. We pay for what we get, always. Choosing high quality fetuses and rejecting low quality ones is not tragedy; sad, but not agonizing.

A heavier trial of the spirit and a real test of responsible judgment, if we want to exert serious control, would be a problem like deciding whether to induce abortion when only one of a pair of nonidentical twins has an untreatable metabolic disorder. It would mean losing a good baby to prevent a bad one. But even here compassionate control should not hesitate: the good one is still only potential, and pregnancy could—at least ordinarily—be restarted. It is far more callous not to prevent the fate of a foreseeably diseased baby than it is disappointing to postpone a good one for a matter of only months.

To be responsible, to take control and reject low quality life, only seems cruel or callous to the morally superficial. Actually, it is practical compassion. Robert Louis Stevenson was shocked at first when he found the Polynesians practicing "infanticide," Their ignorance of contraception and obstetrics meant they had to resort to "abortion at birth" when a newborn turned out to be defective, or when the small atolls they lived on simply could not yield food and shelter for any more people. It was loving concern for *actual* children in their radically finite world which led them to abortion and population control; a matter of costs and benefits.

Stevenson said, somewhat bemused, that never had he seen people anywhere who loved their children as much as those coral reef dwellers did. Of course. The world's finiteness is harder to hide on a Pacific coral reef.

Not to control, and not to weigh one thing against another, would be subhuman. A mature ethics is social, not egocentric. Call it what you will—mathematical morality, ethical arithmetic, moral calculus—we are obliged in conscience to think of benefits relative to costs.

Trying to be responsible we have to calculate. We issue drivers' licenses, for example, even though the cars of some will become lethal weapons; it is the price we pay for motor transport. If we could tell which applicants for a license will be killers we would not license them. It used to be that we had no way of knowing which couples were carrying a common gene defect or which pregnancies were positive for it. But now we *can* know; we have lost that excuse for taking genetic risks. To go right ahead with coital reproduction in many couples' cases is like walking down a line of children blindfolded and deliberately maiming every fourth child. It is cruel and insane to deprive normal but disadvantaged children of the care we could give them with the $1,500,000,000 we spend in public costs for preventable retardates.

Ethics is not loftily independent of economics and utilitarian or distributive justice. Economics deals with preferences among competing choices, and utility aims at spreading expectable benefits. What we need morally is a telescope, not just a microscope.

.   .   .

RIGHTS AND REGULATION

All alleged human rights cease to be right, become unjust, when their exercise would victimize innocent third parties and bystanders. All rights are "imperfect," not absolute or uncontingent. We might say this particularly of the so-called "right to privacy" as it bears on propagating at will and inordinately. The social welfare and protection of third parties has a prior claim. The "right" to reproduce, like all others, is—morally weighed—really only a privilege.

A worrisome side to the practice of control is whether it should ever be imposed or must always be voluntary. If people could be relied upon to be compassionate we would have no reason to even consider mandatory controls. But there are too many who do not control their lives out of moral concern; they are self-centered about what they do or neglect to do, even though they may be "cagey" about it. Large families and a pious disregard of genetic counseling, like refusing to undergo vaccinations until it is made a matter of police enforcement, show how the common welfare often has to be safeguarded by compulsory control or what Garrett Hardin calls "mutual coercion mutually agreed upon."[1]

Coercion is a dirty word to liberals, but all social controls—e.g., the government's tax powers—are really what the majority agree upon, however reluctantly, out of enlightened self-interest and a *quid pro quo* willingness to give up something to get something better. It

might be protection from overpopulation, for instance. Ideally it is better to do the moral thing freely, but sometimes it is more compassionate to force it to be done than to sacrifice the well-being of the many to the ego-centric "rights" of the few. This obviously is the ethics of a sane society. Compulsory controls on reproduction would not, of course, fit present interpretations of due process in the fifth and fourteenth amendments to the Constitution.[2] Here, as in so many other ways, the law lags behind the ethics of modern medicine and public health knowledge.

SCREENING

A good illustration of the tension between rights and regulation takes shape in trying to control hereditary disease. Each of us carries from five to ten genetic faults. If they match up in sexual roulette, tragedy results. How can we avoid or curtail the danger? Denmark prohibits marriages of certain couples unless they are sterilized. But if this method of control and prevention is used, or any other, how do we find out *who* are the ones who should not marry or, if they do, should not have babies by the natural or coital mode? Screening by one means or another is the obvious way to fulfill our obligation to potential children, as well as to the community which has to suffer when defectives are born.

The law in most countries is far behind our emerging medical information. People are not required to make their bad genes known to their mates nor are physicians required to reveal the facts. A man with polycystic kidney disease is not required to let it be known—even though it is highly immoral (unjust) to keep knowledge of such a hereditary disaster (renal failure in middle age) from his children and those they marry. Medical genetics will continue to isolate more and more such diseases, so that as our ability to prevent disease and tragedy increases so does the moral guilt of secrecy, indifference to the consequences for others, and fatalistic inaction.

Conquering infectious diseases reduces the cause of the trouble, but to conquer genetic diseases *increases* the cause or source of the trouble. This dysgenic effect is the first big-scale moral dilemma for medicine—truly a dilemma. Infections come from the environment around us but genetic faults come from within us, and therefore any line of genetic sufferers allowed to propagate will spread their disease through more and more carriers. As we cut down on the infectious diseases we are threatened with a relative rise in deaths and debility due to genetic disorders. We are now approaching a situation in which genetic causes account for as many *or more* deaths than "disease" in the popular sense.

Our moral obligation to undergo voluntary screening, if it is indicated, is too obvious to underline. The squeeze here, ethically, is that the social good often requires *mass* screening. When it is voluntary it is "nicer," as we see in the popular acceptance of tests for cervical cancer. But let it be compulsory if need be, for the common good—Hardin's "mutual coercion mutually agreed upon." Francis Crick has said that "if we can get across to people the idea that their children are not entirely their own business and that it is not a private matter, it would be an enormous step forward."[3] The biophysicist Leroy Augenstein estimated in 1972 that a total of 6 per cent of births or one out of seventeen, are defective. Of these, he said, forty thousand to fifty thousand children every year "are so defective that they don't know that they are human beings."[4] His figures are more impressive than his formulation, however; if an individual cannot "know" he is a human being he is not a human being.

Parents of adopted children and donors of AID are much more carefully screened and selected than "natural" parents—which is logically ridiculous even though we can understand how it came about. A socially conscientious system would be a national registry; blood and skin tests done routinely at birth and fed into a computer-gene scanner would pick up all anomalies, and they would be printed out on data cards and filed; then when marriage licenses are applied for, the cards would be read in comparison machines to find incompatibilities and homozygous conditions.

The objection is, predictably, that it would "violate" a "right"—the right to privacy. It is even said, in a brazen attack on reason itself, that we have a "right to *not* know." Which is more important, the alleged "privacy" or the good of the couple as well as of their progeny and society? (The couple could unite anyway, of course, but on the condition Denmark makes—that sterilization is done for one or both of them. And they could even still have children by medical and donor assistance, bypassing their own faulty fertility.)

Screening is no more an invasion of privacy than "contact tracing" in the treatment of venereal disease, or income tax and public health records, or compulsory flouridation of the water, or the age-old codes of consanguinity (which were only based on nonsense). A good education for those who balk would be a week's stay in the wards of a state institution for the "retarded"—a term used to cover a host of terrible distortions of humanity. Just let them *see* the nature and extent of it; that would convince them.

NOTES

1. *Exploring New Ethics for Survival*. New York: The Viking Press, 1972, pp. 260–62.

2. F. Grad, "Legislative Responses to the New Biology: Limits and Possibilities," U.C.L.A. *Law Review*, 15 (February 1968), 486.

3. Quoted by A. Rosenfeld, *The Second Genesis: The Coming Control of Life*. Englewood Cliffs, N.J.: Prentice-Hall, 1969, p. 161.

4. "Birth Defects," *Humanistic Perspectives in Medical Ethics*, ed., M. Visscher. London: Pemberton Publishing Co., 1972, p. 207.

Ethical and Social Issues in Screening for Genetic Disease

. . . A number of large-scale genetic screening programs for sickle-cell trait and sickle-cell anemia, and at least one for the carrier state in Tay-Sachs disease, have been initiated. Further proliferation of genetic screening programs for these and other genetic diseases seems likely, and in some cases participation in these programs may be made compulsory by statute.* Since screening programs acquire genetic information from large numbers of normal and asymptomatic (e.g., carrier state) individuals and families, often after only brief medical contact, their operation generally falls outside the usual patient-initiated doctor-patient relation. As a result, traditional applications of ethical guidelines for confidentiality and individual physician responsibility are uncertain in mass screening programs. Thus, we believe it important that attempts be made now to clarify some ethical, social and legal questions concerning the establishment and operation of such programs. Although we recognize that there are deep divisions regarding the morality of abortion and that certain views would question prenatal diagnosis so far as it involves abortion, we shall not discuss these issues here. In what follows, we have considered the goals that genetic screening programs may serve and have described some principles that we believe are essential to their proper operation.

GOALS SERVED BY SCREENING

It is crucial that screening programs be structured on the basis of one or more clearly

A report from the Research Group on Ethical, Social and Legal Issues in Genetic Counseling and Genetic Engineering of the Institute of Society, Ethics and the Life Sciences. Reprinted with permission from the *New England Journal of Medicine,* Vol. 286 (May 25, 1972), pp. 1129–1132.

*Massachusetts approved an act (Chapter 491 of Acts and Resolves, 1971) on July 1, 1971, "requiring the testing of blood for sickle trait or anemia as a prerequisite to school attendance."

identified goals and that such goals be formulated well before screening actually begins. We believe it will prove costly in scientific and human terms to omit or defer a careful evaluation of program objectives. Although there are three distinguishable categories of goals that screening programs may serve, we believe the most important goals are those that either contribute to improving the health of persons who suffer from genetic disorders, or allow carriers for a given variant gene to make informed choices regarding reproduction, or move toward alleviating the anxieties of families and communities faced with the prospect of serious genetic disease. The following are representative statements of goals that have been used to justify screening programs.

THE PROVISION OF BENEFITS TO INDIVIDUALS AND FAMILIES

Such benefits may arise from enabling couples found by screening to be at risk for transmitting a genetic disease to take genetic information into account in making responsible decisions about having or not having children. This usually is done by providing genetic counseling services and informing couples about the nature of existing alternatives and potential therapies (e.g., sickle-cell screening). Another advantage consists in detecting asymptomatic persons at birth when amelioration of the sequelae of a genetic disease is already possible —e.g., screening for phenylketonuria (PKU). Still another is providing means for couples, found at risk by screening, to have children free from a severe and untreatable genetic disease (e.g., Tay-Sachs screening).

ACQUISITION OF KNOWLEDGE ABOUT GENETIC DISEASE

Laboratory research and theoretical studies have had a major role in helping to understand fundamental aspects of human genetic diseases. In addition, however, some large-scale screening programs may be needed to determine frequencies of rare diseases and to establish new correlations between genes or groups of genes and disease. In some such screening programs, no therapy may be immediately available for the pathologic condition, although the information derived from them may lead to therapeutic benefits in the future. Research programs aimed primarily at the acquisition of genetic knowledge per se are important. Yet we believe their value is enhanced when they also contribute information that is useful for counseling individuals or for public-health purposes.

REDUCTION OF THE FREQUENCY OF APPARENTLY DELETERIOUS GENES

Although little is known about the possible beneficial (or detrimental) effects of most deleterious recessive genes in the heterozygous state, the reduction of their frequency would be one way to decrease the occurrence of suffering caused by their homozygous manifestations. Nevertheless, as a goal of screening programs, the means required to approach this objective appear to be both practically and morally unacceptable. Virtually everyone carries a small number of deleterious or lethal recessive genes, and to reduce the frequency of a particular recessive gene to near the level maintained by recurrent mutation, most or all persons heterozygous for that gene would have either to refrain from procreation entirely or to monitor all their offspring in utero and abort not only affected homozygote fetuses but also the larger number of heterozygote carriers for the gene.[1-3] However, substantial reduction in the frequency of a recessive disease is possible by prenatal screening and selective abortion, or by counseling persons with the same trait to refrain from marriage or childbearing.[3] Nevertheless, these means of reducing the suffering concomitant to recessive disease raise moral questions of their own.

PRINCIPLES FOR THE DESIGN AND OPERATION OF SCREENING PROGRAMS

ATTAINABLE PURPOSE

Before a program is undertaken, planners should have ascertained through pilot projects and other studies that the program's purposes are attainable. Articulating attainable purposes is necessary if the program is to avoid promising (or seeming to promise) results or benefits that it cannot deliver. It is also desirable to update program design and objectives continually in the light of the program experience and new medical developments. Consideration might also be given to incorporating additional purposes—for example, sickle-cell screening programs might profitably enlarge their scope to include other hemoglobinopathies[4] as well as general screening for anemia.[5]

COMMUNITY PARTICIPATION

From the outset program planners should involve the communities affected by screening in formulating program design and objectives, in administering the actual operation of the program, and in reviewing results. This involvement may include the lay, religious and medical communities as in the Baltimore Tay-Sachs program.[6] Considerable effort should be expended to make program objectives clear to the public, and to encourage participation. Recent articles describing detection programs for Tay-Sachs-disease heterozygotes[6] and for persons with sickle-cell trait or disease[7] have stressed the educational aspect of program design as the crucial component of successful operation. The principal value of community participation is to afford individuals knowledge of the availability and self-determination in the choice of this type of medical service. Educated community involvement is also a means of reducing the potential risk that those identified as genetically variant will be stigmatized or ostracized socially.

EQUAL ACCESS

Information about screening and screening facilities should be open and available to all. To make testing most useful for certain conditions, priority should be given to informing certain well defined populations in which the condition occurs with definitely greater frequency, such as hemoglobin S in blacks and deficient hexosaminidase A (Tay-Sachs disease) among Ashkenazi Jews.

ADEQUATE TESTING PROCEDURES

To avoid the problems that occurred initially in PKU screening,[8] testing procedures should be accurate, should provide maximal information, and should be subject to minimum misinterpretation. For detection of autosomal recessive conditions* like sickle-cell anemia, for example, the test used should accurately distinguish between those carrying the trait and those homozygous for the variant gene.[4,9]

ABSENCE OF COMPULSION

As a general principle, we strongly urge that no screening program have policies that would in any way impose constraints on childbearing by individuals of any specific genetic constitution, or would stigmatize couples who, with full knowledge of the genetic risks, still desire children of their own. It is unjustifiable to promulgate standards for normalcy based on genetic constitution. Consequently, genetic screening programs should be conducted on a voluntary basis. Although vaccination against contagious diseases and premarital blood tests are sometimes made mandatory to protect the public health, there is currently no public-health justification for mandatory screening for the prevention of genetic disease. The conditions being tested for in screening programs are neither "contagious" nor, for the most part, susceptible to treatment at present.[10]

INFORMED CONSENT

Screening should be conducted only with the informed consent of those tested or of the parents or legal representatives of minors. We seriously question the rationale of screening preschool minors or preadolescents for sickle-cell disease or trait since there is a substantial danger of stigmatization and little medical value in detecting the carrier state at this age. However, in the light of recent information that sickle-cell crises can potentially be mitigated,[10] a beneficial alternative would be newborn screening that could identify the SS homozygote in early life, and thereby anticipate the

*Recessive conditions not linked to the sex chromosomes.—Ed.

problems and complications associated with sickle-cell disease and provide early counseling to the parents.

In addition to obtaining signed consent documents, it is the program director's obligation to assure that knowledgeable consent is obtained from all those screened, to design and implement informational procedures, and to review the consent procedure for its effectiveness. The guidelines available from the Department of Health, Education, and Welfare[11] provide a useful model for formulating such consent procedures.

PROTECTION OF SUBJECTS

Since genetic screening is generally undertaken with relatively untried testing procedures[9] and is vitally concerned with the acquisition of new knowledge, it ought properly to be considered a form of "human experimentation." Although most screening entails only minimum physical hazard for the participants, there is a risk of possible psychologic or social injury, and screening programs should consequently be conducted according to the guidelines set forth by HEW for the protection of research subjects.[11]

ACCESS TO INFORMATION

A screening program should fully and clearly disclose to the community and all persons being screened its policies for informing those screened of the results of the tests performed on them. As a general rule all unambiguous diagnostic results should be made available to the person, his legal representative, or a physician authorized by him. Where full disclosure is not practiced, the burden of justifying nondisclosure lies with those who would withhold information. If an adequate educational program has been offered on the meaning of diagnostic criteria and subjects participate in the screening voluntarily, it may generally be assumed that they are emotionally prepared to accept the information derived from the testing.

PROVISION OF COUNSELING

Well trained genetic counselors should be readily available to provide adequate assistance (including repeated counseling sessions if necessary) for persons identified as heterozygotes or more rarely homozygotes by the screening program. As a general rule, counseling should be nondirective, with an emphasis on informing the client and not making decisions for him.[12] The need for defining appropriate qualifications for genetic counselors in the context of screening programs and for providing adequate numbers of trained counselors remains an urgent one. It is the ongoing responsibility of the program directors to evaluate the effectiveness of their program by follow-up surveys of their counseling services. This may include steps (taken with the prior understanding and approval of the subjects screened) to determine how well the information about genetic status has been understood and how it has affected the participants' lives.

UNDERSTANDABLE RELATION TO THERAPY

As part of the educational process that precedes the actual testing program, the nature and cost of available therapies or maintenance programs for affected offspring, combined with an understandable description of their possible benefits and risks, should be given to all persons to be screened. We believe this is one of the items of information that subjects need in deciding whether or not to participate in the program. In addition, acceptance of research therapy should not be a precondition for participation in screening, nor should acceptance of screening be construed as tacit acceptance of such therapy. Both those doing the testing and those doing the counseling ought to keep abreast of existing and imminent developments in diagnosis and therapy[10,13–15] so that the goals of the program and information offered to those being screened will be consistent with the therapeutic options available.

PROTECTION OF RIGHT OF PRIVACY

Well formulated procedures should be set up in advance of actual screening to protect the rights of privacy of individuals and their families. We note that the majority of states do not have statutes that recognize the confidentiality of public-health information or are even minimally adequate to protect individual privacy.[16] Researchers therefore have a particularly strong obligation to protect screening information. Consequently, we favor policies of informing only the person to be screened or, with his permission, a designated physician or medical facility, of having records kept in code, of prohibiting storage of noncoded information in data banks where telephone computer access is possible and of limiting private and public access only to anonymous data to be used for statistical purposes.

CONCLUSIONS

Even if the above guidelines are followed, some risk will remain that the information derived from genetic screening will be misused. Such misuse or misinterpretation must be seen as one of the principal potentially deleterious consequences of screening programs. Several medical researchers have recently cautioned their colleagues of the potential for misinterpretation of the clinical meaning of sickle "trait" and "disease."[5] We are concerned about the dangers of societal misinterpretation of similar conditions and the possibility of widespread and undesirable labeling of individuals on a genetic basis. For instance, the lay public may incorrectly conclude that persons with sickle trait are seriously handicapped in their ability to function effectively in society. Moreover, protecting the confidentiality of test results will not shield all such subjects from a felt sense of stigmatization nor from personal anxieties stemming from their own misinterpretation of their carrier status. Extreme caution should therefore be exercised before steps that lend themselves to stigmatization are taken—for example, stigmatization can arise from recommending restrictions on young children's physical activities under normal conditions because of sickle-cell trait, or from denying life-insurance coverage to adult trait carriers, neither of which are currently medically indicated. In view of such collateral risks of screening, it is essential that each program's periodic review include careful consideration of the social and psychologic ramifications of its operation.

REFERENCES

1. Crow, J. F.: *Population perspective, Ethical Issues in Genetic Counseling and the Use of Genetic Knowledge.* Edited by P. Condliffe, D. Callahan, B. Hilton, et. al. New York, Plenum Press, 1973.

2. Morton, N. E.: "Population genetics and disease control." *Soc. Biol.* 18: 243–251, 1971.

3. Motulsky, A. G., Frazier G. R., Felsenstein, J.: "Public health and long-term genetic implications of intrauterine diagnosis and selective abortion", *Intrauterine Diagnosis* (Birth Defects Original Article Series Vol. 7, No. 5). Edited by D. Bergsma. New York, The National Foundation, 1971, pp. 22–32.

4. Barnes, M. G., Komarmy L., Novack, A. H.: "A comprehensive screening program for hemoglobinopathies." *JAMA* 219:701–705, 1972.

5. Beutler, E., Boggs, D. R., Heller, P., et. al.: "Hazards of indiscriminate screening for sickling." *N. Engl. J. Med.* 285:1485–1486, 1971.

6. Kaback, M. M., Zieger, R. S.: "The John F. Kennedy Institute Tay Sachs program: practical and ethical issues in an adult genetic screening program", *Ethical Issues in Genetic Counseling and the Use of Genetic Knowledge.* Edited by P. Condliffe, D. Callahan, B. Hilton, et. al. New York, Plenum Press, 1973.

7. Nalbandian, R. M., Nichols, B. M., Heustis, A. E., et. al.: "An automated mass screening program for sickle cell disease." *JAMA* 218:1680–1682, 1971.

8. Bessman, P. S., Swazey, J. P.: "PKU: a study of biomedical legislation", *Human Aspects of Biomedical Innovation.* Edited by E. Mendelsohn, J. P. Swazey, I. Traviss. Cambridge, Harvard University Press, 1971, pp. 49–76.

9. Nalbandian, R. M., Henry, R. L., Lusher, J. M., et. al.: "Sickledex test for hemoglobin S.: a critique." *JAMA* 218:1679–1680, 1971.

10. May, A., Bellingham, A. J., Huehns, E. R.: "Effect of cyanate on sickling". *Lancet* 1:658–661, 1972.

11. *The Institutional Guide To DHEW Policy on Protection of Human Subjects, Grants Administration Manual,* Chapter 1–40. (DHEW Publication No [NIH] 72–102). Washington, D. C., Division of Research Grants, Department of Health, Education, and Welfare, 1971.

12. Sorenson, J. R.: *Social Aspects of Applied Human Genetics* (Social Science Frontiers No. 3). New York, Russell Sage Foundation, 1971.

13. McCurdy, P. R., Mahmood, L.: "Intravenous urea treatment of the painful crisis of sickle-cell disease: a preliminary report." *N. Engl. J. Med.* 285:992–994, 1971.

14. Gillette, P. N., Manning, J. M., Cerami, A.: "Increased survival of sickle-cell erythrocytes after treatment *in vitro* with sodium cyanate." *Proc. Natl. Acad. Sci. U. S. A.* 68:2791–2793, 1971.

15. Hollenberg, M. D., Kaback, M. M., Kazazian, H. H., Jr.: "Adult hemoglobin, synthesis by reticulocytes from the human fetus at midtrimester." *Science* 174:698–702, 1971.

16. Schwitzgebel, R. B.: "Confidentiality of research information in public health studies." *Harv. Leg. Comment* 6:187–197, 1969.

In Vitro Fertilization, Cloning, and Genetic Intervention

BERNARD D. DAVIS

Prospects for Genetic Intervention in Man

Extrapolating from the spectacular successes of molecular genetics, a number of essays and symposia (*1*) have considered the feasibility of various forms of genetic intervention (*2*) in man. Some of these statements, and many articles in the popular press, have tended toward exuberant, Promethean predictions of unlimited control and have led the public to expect the blueprinting of human personalities. Most geneticists, however, have had more restrained second thoughts.

Nevertheless, recent alarms about this problem have caused wide public concern, and understandably so. With nuclear energy threat-

Reprinted with permission of the author and the publisher from *Science,* Vol. 170 (December 18, 1970), pp. 1279–1283. Copyright 1970 by the American Association for the Advancement of Science.

ening global catastrophe and with so many other technological advances visibly damaging the quality of life, who would wish to have scientists tampering with man's inner nature? Indeed, fear of such manipulation may arouse even more anxiety than fear of death. The mass media have accordingly welcomed sensational pronouncements about the dangers.

While such dangers clearly exist, it also seems clear that some scientists have dramatized them (3) in order to help persuade the public of the need for radical changes in our form of government (4). But however laudable the desire to improve our social structure, and however urgent the need to improve our protection against harmful uses of science and technology, exaggeration of the dangers from genetics will inevitably contribute to an already distorted public view, which increasingly blames science for our problems and ignores its contributions to our welfare. Indeed, irresponsible hyperbole on the genetic issue has already influenced the funding of research (5). It therefore seems important to try to assess objectively the prospects for modifying the pattern of genes of a human being by various means. But let us first note two genetic principles that must be taken into account.

RELEVANT GENETIC PRINCIPLES

Polygenic traits and behavioral genetics. The recognition of a gene, in classical genetics, depends on following the distribution of two alternative forms (alleles) from parents to progeny. In the early years of genetics, after the rediscovery of Mendel's laws in 1900, this analysis was possible only for those genes that exerted an all-or-none control over a corresponding monogenic trait—for example, flower color, eye color, or a hereditary disease such as hemophilia. The study of such genes has continued to dominate genetics. However, monogenic traits constitute a small, special class. Most traits are polygenic: that is, they depend on multiple genes, and so they vary continuously rather than in an all-or-none manner. Moreover, each gene itself is polymorphic— that is, it is capable of existing, as a result of mutation, in a variety of different forms (alleles); and though the protein products of these alleles differ only slightly in structure, they often differ markedly in activity.

For our purpose it is especially pertinent that the most interesting human traits—relating to intelligence, temperament, and physical structure—are highly polygenic. Indeed, man undoubtedly has hundreds of thousands of genes for polygenic traits, compared with a few hundred recognizable through their control over monogenic traits. However, the study of polygenic inheritance is still primitive; and the difference from monogenic inheritance has received little public attention. Education on the distinction between monogenic and polygenic inheritance is clearly important if the public is to distinguish between realistic and wild projections for future developments in genetic intervention in man.

Interaction of heredity and environment. The study of polygenic inheritance is difficult in part because it requires statistical analysis of the consequences of reassortment, among the progeny, of many interacting genes. In addition, even a full set of relevant genes does not fixedly determine the corresponding trait. Rather, most genes contribute to determining a *range of potential* for a given trait in an individual, while his past and present environments determine his phenotype (that is, his actual state) within that range. At a molecular level the explanation is now clear: the structure of a gene determines the structure of a corresponding protein, while the interaction of the gene with subtle regulatory mechanisms, which respond to stimuli from the environment, determines the amount of the protein made. Hence, the ancient formulation of the question of heredity versus environment (nature versus nurture) in qualitative terms has presented a false dichotomy, which has led only to sterile arguments.

POSSIBILITIES IN GENETIC MANIPULATION

Somatic cell alteration. Bacterial genes can already be isolated (6) and synthesized (7); and while the isolation of human genes still appears to be a formidable task, it may also be accomplished quite soon. We would then be able to synthesize and to modify human genes in the test tube. However, the incorporation of externally supplied genes into human cells is another matter. For while small blocs of genes can be introduced in bacteria, either as naked DNA (transformation) or as part of a nonlethal virus (transduction), we have no basis for estimating how hard it will be to overcome the obstacles to applying these methods to human cells. And if it does become possible to incorporate a desired gene into some cells, in the intact body, incorporation into all the cells that could profit thereby may well remain difficult. It thus seems possible that diseases depending on deficiency of an extracellular product, such as insulin, may be curable long before the bulk of hereditary diseases, where an externally supplied gene can benefit only those defective cells that have incorporated it and can then make the missing cell component.

Such a one-shot cure of a hereditary disease, if possible, would clearly be a major improvement over the current practice of continually supplying a missing gene product, such as insulin. (It could be argued that improving the soma in this way, without altering the germ cells, would help perpetuate hereditary defectives; but so does conventional medical therapy.) The danger of undesired side effects, of course, would have to be evaluated, and the day-to-day medical use of such material would have to be regulated: but these problems do not seem to differ significantly from those encountered with any novel therapeutic agent.

Germ cell alteration. Germ cells may prove more amenable than somatic cells to the introduction of DNA, since they could be exposed in the test tube and therefore in a more uniform and controllable manner. Another conceivable approach might be that of *directed mutagenesis:* the use of agents that would bring about a specific desired alteration in the DNA, such as reversal of a mutation that had made a gene defective. So far, however, efforts to find such directive agents have not been successful: all known mutagenic agents cause virtually random mutations, of which the vast majority

are harmful rather than helpful. Indeed, before a mutagen could be directed to a particular site it would probably have to be attached first to a molecule that could selectively recognize a particular stretch of DNA (8); hence a highly selective mutagen would have to be at least as complex as the material required for selective genetic recombination.

If predictable genetic alteration of germ cells should become possible it would be even more useful than somatic cure of monogenic diseases, for it could allow an individual with a defective gene to generate his own progeny without condemning them to inherit that gene. Moreover, there would be a long-term evolutionary advantage, since not only the immediate product of the correction but also subsequent generations would be free of the disease.

Genetic modification of behavior. In contrast to the cure of specific monogenic diseases, improvement of the highly polygenic behavioral traits would almost certainly require the replacement, in germ cells, of a large but specific complement of DNA. Since I find such replacement, in a controlled manner, very hard to imagine, I suspect that such modifications will remain indefinitely in the realm of science fiction, like the currently popular extrapolation from the transplantation of a kidney or a heart, with a few tubular connections, to that of a brain, with hundreds of thousands of specific neural connections. However, this consideration would not apply to the possibility of impairing cerebral function by genetic transfer, since certain monogenic diseases are known to cause such impairment.

Copying by asexual reproduction (cloning). We now know that all the differentiated somatic cells of an animal (those from muscle, skin, and the like) contain, in their nuclei, the same complete set of genes. Every somatic cell thus contains all the genetic information required for copying the whole organism. In different cells different subsets of genes are active, while the remainder are inactive. Accordingly, if it should become possible to reverse the regulatory mechanism responsible for this differentiation any cell could be used to start an embryo. The individual could then be developed in the uterus of a foster mother, or eventually in a glorified test tube, and would be an exact genetic copy of its single parent. Such asexual reproduction could thus be used to produce individuals of strictly predictable genetic endowment; and there would be no theoretical limit to the size of the resulting clone (that is, the set of identical individuals derivable from a single parent and from successive generations of copies).

Though differentiation is completely reversible in the cells of plants (as in the transfer of cuttings), it is ordinarily quite irreversible in the cells of higher animals. This stability, however, depends on the interaction of the nucleus with the surrounding cytoplasm; and it is now possible to transfer a nucleus, by microsurgery or cell fusion, into the cytoplasm of a different kind of cell. Indeed, in frogs differentiation has been completely reversed in this way: when the nucleus of an egg cell is replaced by a nucleus from an intestinal cell embryonic development of the hybrid cell can produce a genetic replica of the donor of the nucleus (9). This result will probably also be accomplished, and perhaps quite soon, with cells from mammals. Indeed, there is considerable economic incentive to achieve this goal, since the copying of champion livestock could substantially increase food production.

Another type of cloning can already be accomplished in mammals: when the relatively undifferentiated cells of an early mouse embryo are gently separated each can be used to start a new embryo (10). A large set of identical twins can thus be produced. However, they would be copies of an embryo of undetermined genetic structure, rather than of an already known adult. This procedure therefore does not seem tempting in man, unless the production of identical twins (or of greater multiplets) should develop special social values, such as those suggested by Aldous Huxley in *Brave New World*.

Predetermination of sex. Though no one has yet succeeded in directly controlling sex by separating XX and XY sperm cells, this technical problem should be soluble. Moreover, in principle it is already possible to achieve the same objective indirectly by aborting embryos of the undesired sex: for the sex of the embryo can be diagnosed by tapping the amniotic fluid (amniocentesis) and examining the cells released into that fluid by the embryo.

Wide use of either method might cause a marked imbalance in the sex ratio in the population, which could lead to changes in our present family structure (and might even be welcomed in a world suffering from overpopulation). Alternatively, new social or legal pressures might be developed to avert a threatened imbalance (11). But though there would obviously be novel social problems, I do not think they would strain our powers of social adaptation nearly as much as some urgent present problems.

Selective reproduction. A discussion of the prospects for molecular and cellular intervention in human heredity, would be incomplete without noting that any society wishing to direct the evolution of its gene pool already has available an alternative approach: selective breeding. This application of classical, transmission genetics has been used empirically since Neolithic times, not only in animal husbandry, but also, in various ways (for example, polygamy, *droit de seigneur,* caste system), in certain human cultures. Declaring a moratorium on genetic research, in order to forestall possible future control of our gene pool, would therefore be locking the barn after the horse was stolen.

Having reviewed various technical possibilities, I would now like to comment on the dangers that might be presented by their fulfillment and to compare these with the consequences of efforts to prevent this development.

EVALUATION OF THE DANGERS

Gene transfer. I have presented the view that if we eventually develop the ability to incorporate genes into human germ cells, and thus to repair monogenic defects, we would still be far from specifying highly polygenic behavioral traits. And with somatic cells such an influence seems altogether excluded. For though genes undoubtedly direct in considerable detail the pattern of development of the brain, with its network of connections of 10 billion or more nerve cells, the introduction of new DNA following this development clearly could not redirect the already formed network; neither could we expect it to modify the effect of learning on brain function.

To be sure, since we as yet have little firm knowledge of behavioral genetics we cannot exclude the possibility that a few key genes might play an especially large role in determining various intellectual or artistic potentials or emotional patterns. But even if it should turn out to be technically possible to tailor the psyche significantly by the exchange of a small number of genes in germ cells, it seems extremely improbable that this procedure would be put to practical use. For it will always be much easier, as Lederberg (12) has emphasized, to obtain almost any desired genetic pattern by copying from the enormous store already displayed in nature's catalog.

While the improvement of cerebral function by polygenic transfer thus seems extremely unlikely, one cannot so readily exclude the technical possibility of impairing this function by transfer of a monogenic defect. And having seen genocide in Germany and massive defoliation in Vietnam, we can hardly assume that a high level of civilization provides a guarantee against such an evil use of science. However, several considerations argue against the likelihood that such a future technical possibility would be converted into reality. The most important is that monogenic diseases, involving hormonal imbalance or enzymatic deficiencies, produce gross behavioral defects, whose usefulness to a tyrant is hard to imagine. Moreover, even if gene transfer is achieved in cooperating individuals, an enormous social effort would still be required to extend it, for political or military purposes, to mass populations. Finally, in contrast to the development of nuclear energy, which arose as an extension of already accepted military practices, the potential medical value of gene transfer is much more evident than its military value; hence a

"genetic bomb" could hardly be sprung on the public as a secret weapon. Accordingly, we are under no moral obligation to sacrifice genetic advances now in order to forestall such remote dangers: if and when gene transfer in man becomes a reality there would still be time to assert the cultural and medical traditions that would promote its beneficial use and oppose its abuse.

This last obstacle would be eliminated if it should prove possible to develop a virus that could be used to infect a population secretly with specific genes, and it is the prospect of this ultimate horror that seems to cause most concern. However, for reasons that I have presented above the technical possibility of producing useful modifications of personality by infections of germ cells seems extremely remote, and the possibility of doing so by infecting somatic cells in an already developed individual seems altogether excluded. These fears thus do not seem realistic enough to help guide present policy. Nevertheless, the problem cannot be entirely ignored; in a country that has recently been embarrassed by its accumulation of rockets containing nerve gas even the remote possibility of handing viral toys to Dr. Strangelove will require vigilance.

Genetic copies. If the cloning of mammals becomes technically feasible its extension to man will undoubtedly be very tempting, on the grounds that enrichment for proved talent by this means might enormously enhance our culture, while the risk of harm seemed small. Since society may be faced with the need to make decisions in this area quite soon, I would like to offer a few comments in the hope of encouraging public discussion.

On the one hand, in fields such as mathematics or music, where major achievements are restricted to a few especially gifted people, an increase in their number might be enormously beneficial—either as a continuous supply from one generation to another or as an expanded supply within a generation. On the other hand, a succession of identical geniuses might exert an excessively conservative influence, depriving society of the richness that comes from our inexhaustible supply of new combinations of genes. Or genius might fail to flower, if its drive depended heavily on parental influence or on cultural climate. And in the literary, social, and political areas the cultural climate surely plays so large a role that there may be little basis for expecting outstanding achievement to be continued by a scion. The world might thus be quite disappointed by the contributions of another Tolstoy, Churchill, or Martin Luther King, or even another Newton or Mozart. Moreover, though experience with monozygotic twins is somewhat reassuring, persons produced by copying might suffer from a novel kind of "identity crisis."

Though our system of values clearly places us under moral obligation to do everything possible to cure disease, there is no comparable basis for using cloning to advance culture. The responsibility for initiating such a radical departure in human reproduction would be grave, and surely many will feel that we should not do so. But I suspect that it would be impossible to enforce any such prohibition completely: the potential gain seems too large, and the procedure would require the cooperation of only a very small group of people. Hence whatever the initial social consensus, I suspect that a stable attitude would not emerge until after some early tests, whether legal or illegal, had demonstrated the magnitude of the problems and of the gains.

A much greater threat, I believe, would be the use of cloning for the large-scale amplification of a few selected individuals. Who would wish to send a child to a school with a large set of identical twins as his classmates? Moreover, the success of a species depends not only on its adaptation to its present environment but also on its possession of sufficient genetic variety to include some individuals who could survive in any future environment. Hence if cloning were extended to the point of markedly homogenizing the population, it could create an evolutionary danger. However, we have already lived for a long time with a similar possibility: any male can provide a virtually limitless supply of germ cells, which can be used in artificial insemination; yet genetic homogenization by this means has not

become the slightest threat. Since cloning is unlikely to become nearly so easy it is difficult to see a rational basis for the fear that its technical possibility would increase the threat.

Implications for genetic research. Though the dangers from genetics seem to me very small compared with the immense potential benefits, they do exist; its applications could conceivably be used unwisely and even malevolently. But such potential abuses cannot be prevented by curtailing genetic research. For one thing, we already have on hand a powerful tool (selective breeding) that could be used to influence the human gene pool, and this technique could be used as wisely or unwisely as any future additional techniques. Moreover, since the greatest fear is that some tyrant might use genetic tools to regulate behavior, and especially to depress human potential, it is important to note that we already have on hand pharmacological, surgical, nutritional, and psychological methods that could generate parallel problems much sooner. Clearly, we shall have to struggle, in a crowded and unsettled world, to prevent such a horrifying misuse of science and to preserve and promote the ideal of universal human dignity. If we succeed in developing suitable controls we can expect to apply them to any later developments in genetics. If we fail—as we may—limitations on the progress of genetics will not help.

If, in panic, our society should curtail fundamental genetic research, we would pay a huge price. We would slow our current progress in recognizing defective genes and preventing their spread; and we would block the possibility of learning to repair genetic defects. The sacrifice would be even greater in the field of cancer; for we are on the threshold of a revolutionary improvement in the control of these malignant hereditary changes in somatic cells, and this achievement will depend on the same fundamental research that also contributes toward the possibilities of cloning and of gene transfer in man. Finally, it is hardly necessary to note the long and continuing record of nonmedical benefits from genetics, including increased production and improved quality of livestock and crops, steadier production based on resistance to infections, vastly increased yields in antibiotic and other industrial fermentations, and, far from least, the pride that mankind can feel in one of its most imaginative and creative cultural achievements: understanding of some of the most fundamental aspects of our own physical nature and that of the living world around us.

While specific curtailment of genetic research thus seems impossible to justify, we should also consider briefly the broader proposal (see, for example, 8) that we may have to limit the rate of progress of science in general, if we wish to prevent new powers from developing faster than an inadequate institutional framework can be adjusted to handle them. While one can hardly deny that this argument may be valid in the abstract, its application to our present situation seems to me dangerous. No basis is yet in sight for calculating an optimal rate of scientific advance. Moreover, only recently have we become generally aware of the need to assess and control the true social and environmental costs of various uses of technology. Recognition of a problem is the first step toward its solution, and now that we have taken this step it would seem reasonable to assume, until proved otherwise, that further scientific advance can contribute to the solutions faster than it will expand the problems.

. . .

REFERENCES AND NOTES

1. P. B. Medawar, *The Future of Man* (Basic Books, New York, 1960); Symposium on "Evolution and Man's Progress," *Daedalus* (Summer, 1961); G. Wolstenholme, Ed., *Man and His Future* (Little, Brown, Boston, 1963); J. Lederberg, *Nature* 198, 428 (1963); J. S. Huxley, *Essays of a Humanist* (Harper and Row, New York, 1964); T. M. Sonneborn, Ed., *The Control of Human Heredity and Evolution* (Macmillan, New York, 1965); R. D. Hotchkiss, *J. Hered.* 56, 197 (1965); J. D. Roslansky, Ed., *Genetics and the Future of Man* (Appleton-Century-Crofts, New York, 1966); N. H. Horowitz, *Perspect. Biol. Med.* 9, 349 (1966).

2. The term *"genetic engineering"* seemed at first to be a convenient designation for applied molecular and cellular genetics. However, I agree with J. Lederberg [*The New York Times*, Letters to the editor, 26 September (1970)] that the overtones of this phrase are undesirable.

3. Editorials, *Nature* 224, 834, 1241 (1969); J. Shapiro, L. Eron, J. Beckwith, *ibid.*, p. 1337.

4. J. Beckwith, *Bacteriol. Rev.* 34, 222 (1970).

5. P. Handler, *Fed. Proc.* 29, 1089 (1970).

6. J. Shapiro, L. MacHattie, L. Eron, G. Ihler, K. Ippen, J. Beckwith, *Nature* 224, 768 (1969).

7. K. L. Agarwal, and 12 others, *ibid.* 227, 27 (1970).

8. S. E. Luria, in *The Control of Human Heredity and Evolution*, T. M. Sonneborn, Ed. (Macmillan, New York, 1965), p. 1.

9. R. Briggs and T. J. King, in *The Cell*, J. Brachet and A. E. Mirsky, Eds. (Academic Press, New York, 1959), vol. 1; J. B. Gurdon and H. R. Woodward, *Biol. Rev.* 43, 244 (1968).

10. B. Mintz, *J. Exp. Zool.* 157, 85, 273 (1964).

11. A. Etzioni, *Science* 161, 1107 (1968).

12. J. Lederberg, *Amer. Natur.* 100, 519 (1966).

JAMES D. WATSON

The Future of Asexual Reproduction

Several years ago a most remarkable frog grew up in Oxford. Its origin did not lie in the union of a haploid sperm cell with a haploid egg, the fertilization process which ordinarily gives each higher animal a mixture of paternal and maternal genes. Instead this frog arose from an enucleated egg, into which had been inserted a diploid nucleus from the intestinal cell of an adult frog. Microsurgical removal of the maternal nucleus from this egg had denuded it of any genetic material.

But by subsequently gaining a diploid nucleus (as opposed to the haploid form found in a sperm) the egg acquired the chromosome number normally present in a fertilized egg. As such it could be activated to divide, thereby setting into motion the successive embryological states which culminate in an adult frog.

The genetic origin of this frog was thus very different from that of all previous frogs, one half of whose chromosomes came from the male parent through the sperm, the other half from the female parent which produced the egg. Normal fertilization processes, by combining genetic material from two different parents, always generate progeny uniquely different from either parent.

CLONAL REPRODUCTION OF FROGS

In contrast, the Oxford frog derived *all* its genetic material from the individual whose intestinal cell was used as the nuclear donor. The genetic complement of all its diploid somatic cells (as opposed to its haploid sex cells) was thus identical to that in the donor frog. So, in effect, it was an identical twin of the donor frog born some months before. Furthermore, since every adult frog contains millions of cells capable of being used as nuclear sources, the original donor could have served as the genetic

Reprinted with permission of the author from *Intellectual Digest*, Vol. 2, No. 2 (1971), pp. 115–125.

parent of thousands of progeny identical to itself.

This type of reproduction is generally referred to as a *clonal* reproduction. (A *clone* is the aggregate of the asexually produced progeny of a single cell; for example, all the descendants of a single bacteria present as a colony upon a Petri dish.) The genetic identicalness of all members of a clone arises from the fact that the normal process of cell division (called mitosis) produces two daughter cells with identical chromosomal complements. The nuclei of the cells found in the frog's intestine are thus identical to those which could be found, say, in its liver or brain.

CELL DIFFERENTIATION

In contrast, the cell division process called meiosis, which generates the sex cells, reduces the chromosome number by half. Only one of each pair of homologous chromosomes enters a sperm or egg. Moreover, a completely random event determines whether the given chromosome is of male or female origin.

So no two eggs (or sperm) arising in a given individual are ever genetically equivalent. No two sexually produced frogs, having the same two parents, thus will be identical unless they arise by the rare splitting of an already divided fertilized egg into two separate daughter cells, each of which goes on to develop into a complete embryo. (This is the process by which identical human twins are produced.) In contrast, all the members of a clone produced by mitosis will be identical, except for the occasional mutant cell resulting from rarely occurring somatic gene mutations.

The existence of the first clonal frog, the result of the work of the English zoologist John Gurdon, was a very important scientific event. He settled the long-controversial biological dilemma of whether the process of cell differentiation in frogs was primarily a cytoplasmic or a nuclear event. During embryological development, the progeny cells which result from the cell divisions commencing after fertilization become changed (differentiated) into a variety of morphologically and functionally different cell types. For example, muscle cells, nerve cells, and skin cells of a single individual all have a common ancestor in one fertilized egg.

Most differentiated animal cells, when isolated from contact with other cells, continue to divide and maintain their specific differentiated state. This fact posed the question of the nature of the factors which maintain the specific form of a given differentiated cell. In particular, does differentiation occur through irreversible changes in the nucleus which somehow alter its chromosomal makeup, perhaps by the mutation of specific genes?

Gurdon's clonal frog cleanly settled this point by showing that a nucleus taken from a highly differentiated cell still retains its capacity for directing the development of a completely normal frog. Differentiation thus does not involve gene mutations. Instead, it must be based upon complicated interactions between the nucleus and cytoplasm, interactions which effectively command certain genes to produce the specific gene products needed for a given differentiated state.

THE MORAL ISSUE

But as soon as one such specialized nucleus is removed from its given cytoplasmic environment, for example by microsurgical introduction into a new cytoplasmic environment, the instructions which its genes receive are no longer the same and a new set of genes will go into action. In particular, when the nucleus of a differentiated frog cell is placed inside an enucleated unfertilized egg, it quickly sets in motion the successive steps of embryological development leading first to the tadpole stage and finally to an adult frog.

The question of course arises, will this same basic principle hold for the large majority of differentiated cells? Now I suspect most biologists will guess yes. In general, very fundamental phenomena, of which differentiation is one, do not have a different molecular basis from one organism to another. Moreover, it is already clear that differentiation in several plant species does not involve irreversible nuclear changes. Now it is routinely possible to produce mature plants starting from highly specialized somatic cells of diploid chromosome number. For example, mature carrot plants can be produced from single callus cells that are placed in proper nutritional environments. Thus it is highly likely that the embryological development of most higher animals, including man, involves the creation of countless numbers of somatic nuclei each capable of serving as the complete genetic material for a new organism. This means that, theoretically, all forms of higher animal life may in effect be capable of clonal reproduction.

If true, this situation could have very startling consequences as to the nature of human life, a fact soon appreciated by many magazine editors, one of whom commissioned a cover with multiple copies of Ringo Starr, another of whom gave us overblown multiple likenesses of the current sex goddess Raquel Welch. It takes little imagination to perceive that different people will have highly different fantasies; perhaps with some imagining the existence of countless people with the features of Picasso or Frank Sinatra or Walt Frazier or Doris Day. And would monarchs like the Shah of Iran, knowing they might never be able to have a normal male heir, consider the possibility of having a son whose genetic constitution would be identical to their own?

Clearly even more bizarre possibilities can be thought of, and so we might have expected that many biologists, particularly those whose work impinges upon these possibilities, would seriously ponder their implications, and begin a dialogue which would educate the world's citizens and offer suggestions which our legislative bodies might consider in framing national science policies. On the whole, however, this is not at all what has happened. Though a number of scientific papers devoted to the problem of genetic engineering have casually mentioned that clonal reproduction may someday be with us (the discussion to which I am party) they have been so vague and devoid of meaningful time estimates as to be virtually soporific.

Does this effective silence imply a conspiracy to keep the general public unaware of a potential threat to their basic ways of life? Could it be motivated by fear that the general reaction will be a further damning of all science, thereby decreasing even more the limited money available for pure research? Or does it merely tell us that most scientists do live such an ivory-tower existence that they are capable of thinking rationally only about pure science, dismissing more practical matters as subjects for the lawyers, students, clergy, and politicians to face up to in a real way?

One or both of these possibilities may explain why the occasional scientist has not taken cloning before the public. The main reason, however, I suspect, is that the prospect to most biologists looks too remote and chancy—not worthy of immediate attention when other matters, like nuclear weapon overproliferation and pesticide and auto-exhaust pollutions, present society with immediate threats to its orderly continuation. Though scientists as a group are the most future-oriented of all professions (some investment bankers would probably disagree) there are few of us who concentrate on events unlikely to become reality within the next decade or two.

CLONING OF MAMMALS

Behind the general belief that the development of techniques for cloning any mammal, including man, lies far in the future, are fundamental differences between the embryological development of mammals and of amphibians like the frog. These differences reflect the very different environments in which amphibian and mammalian embryos develop. All the frog's embryological development, even in the beginning fertilization stages, occurs in vitro, outside the body of the female parent, generally in the nutrient-poor environment of freshwater lakes and ponds. Thus all the food supply necessary for growth to a developmental stage capable of independent feeding, in the case of a frog to the tadpole stage, must initially be present within the unfertilized egg. As a result,

amphibian eggs are not only always relatively large but all their developmental stages are capable of relatively easy experimental investigation.

In great contrast are the eggs of placental, bearing mammals. Their eggs are relatively small, since they have to contain only the nourishment necessary to reach approximately the 64-cell stage. At this point the tiny embryo implants itself on the wall of the uterus, a placenta forms, and all the food molecules necessary for subsequent embryonic growth come from the female parent.

Not only does the small size of such mammalian eggs make experimentation very difficult, but even more important, all the stages of development normally occur within the ovary, oviduct, or uterus. Moreover, there seems to be no real prospect that any mammal can ever be raised totally in vitro. Thus detailed knowledge about the exact steps in the embryogeny of any mammal is much, much less complete than that of amphibians, all of whose development normally occurs in vitro.

The cloning of any mammal thus will be far from a routine task. In particular, the techniques of micromanipulation used to insert nuclei into frog's eggs cannot now be applied to eggs in the mammalian size range. They are likely to be irreversibly damaged by the introduction of a nucleus whose diameter is only some two or three times less than that of the egg itself. And if somehow a trick were ever found to successfully insert a diploid nucleus, the equally challenging task of finding conditions for the in-vitro growth of the modified egg through to the adult stage would still lie ahead. Thus the clonal production of human beings has seemed to most geneticists an event so unlikely as to not be worth the stirring up of public attention.

This assessment would be correct if the pace of research on human reproductive biology were to continue at the current rate. With a few exceptions, work on the early developmental processes in man has not been seriously pushed either here in the United States or elsewhere. As a result, there exists a scientific lacuna so serious that it deeply disturbs those people who realistically worry about over-population problems. They believe that more basic biological knowledge about human reproductive processes would be very helpful in slowing down the fearful rise in the number of human beings.

Consequently, there is already much "population" money available to induce more people to move into the field of reproductive biology, hopefully to learn in great detail the step-by-step processes by which a human egg is ovulated, fertilized, and cleaved, and moves down the oviduct to implant on the uterine wall.

A key ingredient to obtaining this information is the development of methods by which the early embryological stages of mammals can be studied in vitro. For as long as study is restricted to work on intact animals, experimental work, as distinguished from observational analysis, will be virtually impossible.

NUCLEAR INSERTION

Most importantly, though unknown even to most biologists, the beginnings of first-rate research on the in-vitro cultivation of mammalian eggs has already occurred. Techniques are in fact available for the isolation of mouse eggs, their fertilization in vitro, and subsequent cultivation under test-tube conditions which permit growth to the 64-cell stage. At this point the embryonic body (called a blastocyst) can be surgically implanted back into the uterus of a living mouse, where it can eventually develop to the stage at which normal birth occurs.

This means that most of the techniques that will be needed to produce a clonal mouse are already available. The only serious obstacles remaining are the development of methods for the removal of the haploid maternal nucleus and the subsequent addition of a diploid adult nucleus. Now there are hints that the enucleation problem will not be serious. For some years it has been known that addition of the mitotic poison colchicine to preovulatory mice leads to abnormal meiotic divisions, which frequently produce nucleus-free eggs. Moreover,

very recent work suggests that colchicine in vitro acts similarly. When it is added to unfertilized eggs which have been surgically removed from a living mouse, healthy enucleated eggs are produced.

And furthermore, it looks as if the nuclear insertion process may not be nearly as tricky as it was first thought. This change of opinion comes from the development of very simple methods for the fusing of two cells to yield a single cell containing the genetic compounds of both donor cells. Though the existence of rare examples of cell fusion was first clearly demonstrated in Paris by Barski in 1962, not until 1966 did Henry Harris and John Watkins, working in the pathology department of Oxford University, develop a routine method for easily fusing almost any two desired cells. Their contribution was the introduction of Sendai virus (a close relative of the common flu viruses) killed by ultraviolet light.

In some way not yet understood, adsorption of large numbers of Sendai particles so modifies cell surfaces that when two treated cells touch each other, portions of the opposing cell surfaces effectively dissolve, thereby creating one much larger cell containing two nuclei. Subsequently these nuclei often coalesce, yielding a single nucleus containing all the chromosomes present in both original nuclei.

During the past three years, Christopher Graham, also at Oxford, has been using Sendai virus to fuse mouse eggs with diploid adult mouse cells. The resulting cells still retain the essential features of an egg, because even the relatively small mouse eggs are much larger than most diploid adult cells. While the fused eggs can divide several times, they so far have not yet developed into blastocysts, the stage necessary for successful implantation into the mouse uterus. Conceivably this limitation results from the need to remove the zona pellucida (a normal protective covering) for the Sendai virus fusing trick.

EXPERIMENTING WITH HUMAN EGGS

Conditions must thus be found either to fuse eggs which retain the zona pellucida or which permit unprotected denuded eggs to develop normally to blastocysts. A reasonable guess is that Graham will succeed, if not this year, most likely within this coming decade. The clonal mammal then will no longer be science fiction.

A likely consequence will be the initiation of similar experiments with a variety of other mammals; first, with easily obtainable laboratory varieties of hamsters, rats, and rabbits, and soon afterwards with economically important domestic animals such as cattle, sheep, and pigs. Though introduction of such methods into animal husbandry might seem at first like economic madness, many veterinarians may suspect otherwise, knowing well the very large prices currently paid for prize animals. Moreover, such research would certainly liven up many agricultural schools, since some of their faculty would jump at something more exciting than the now very routine breeding programs inspired by Mendelian genetics.

So we must expect that, unless somehow strongly discouraged, veterinarians throughout the world someday will attempt the cloning of uniquely valuable domestic animals. One can certainly imagine wealthy racehorse owners wondering whether with a better jockey their prize three-year-old would have been unbeatable. While Nijinsky eventually lost his last two races, might a clonal derivative win every time?

At first consideration, it would seem likely that cloning of many domestic species would have to occur before serious thought would be given to the development of clinical procedures which would make human cloning more than a theoretical possibility. This way of thinking presupposes that the primary purpose for such methodological development need be cloning itself. If this in fact were the objective, the normal and legal objections that would undoubtedly crop up most certainly would effectively prevent the legal granting of the medical facilities needed for extensive in-vitro experiments with human eggs.

If, however, the stated objective is to probe the human reproductive process so that better contraceptive methods can be obtained, the reaction of the general public will be much harder to predict. Though many people will look with horror at any test-tube work with

human eggs, others will breathe more easily if something is being done to prevent the world from being crushed by overpopulation. Until several years ago, this latter group was numerically relatively small and without favor in virtually any political circle. Today, however, taboos which would have seemed unbreakable just a decade ago are rapidly being overturned —witness the recent action of the United States Congress in overwhelmingly passing legislation to promote family planning. Even more significant was the action of New York state in making abortions the legal right of any women who desire them.

It thus seems virtually inevitable that for one reason or another the number of people studying all aspects of human embryogeny will greatly increase. Not only will the amount of classical observational analysis increase, but even more important, direct experimentation with human eggs most likely will soon be the main preoccupation of a number of intelligent, highly qualified biologists.

Already there exists one such individual, R. G. Edwards, an English reproductive biologist now working in the physiology department of Cambridge University. Originally trained as an embryologist and with some ten years experience in growing mouse embryos in vitro, he focuses his attention on the test-tube growth of human eggs. His original source of material was immature eggs (oocytes) obtained from ovarian tissue that had been surgically excised for reasons completely incidental to his work. From this tissue, Edwards removed the eggs from their surrounding follicles. As such, they were not yet capable of fertilization, since most eggs within human ovaries are present in the dictyotene, a stage just at the beginning of the two meiotic divisions which generate haploid eggs.

But by placing dictyotene-phase eggs in a culture medium similar to that previously worked out for the in-vitro maturation of mouse eggs, the remaining steps of meiosis occur, and some 36 hours later bring the eggs to metaphase II, the stage where normal ovulation occurs. Then when human sperm are added, fertilization occurs, yielding a diploid nucleus capable of dividing several times. However, no fertilized in-vitro matured egg has ever yet developed up to the blastocyst stage. Some factor not yet understood must go wrong during the in-vitro meiosis.

To circumvent this difficulty. Edwards, together with his clinical colleague, P. C. Steptoe of Oldham General Hospital, has devised a simple surgical method for the removal of healthy human eggs after they have completed much of meiosis, but before the ovulation step which releases free eggs from their follicles into the oviduct. Called laparoscopy, it is a relatively minor operation which, while requiring general anesthesia, generally only requires a 24-hour hospital stay.

HELP FOR INFERTILE WOMEN

Prior to the operation, a regimen of hormone treatment (gonadotrophins) is given to induce follicle maturation and egg development through the early stages of meiosis. Laparoscopy is then performed, some four hours before ovulation would normally occur. The ovaries so exposed usually contain highly enlarged follicles with thinning walls, through which the desired oocytes can be carefully removed. These procedures have now reached the state where healthy eggs can be obtained from over half the follicles examined.

Such preovulating oocytes are very suitable for subsequent embryological investigations. Fertilization rapidly ensues after the addition of human sperm, and in contrast to those eggs which had undergone meiotic divisions in vitro, these in-vivo matured eggs generally begin normal cleavage divisions. Already many embryos have developed to the eight-cell stage, while a few have become blastocysts, the stage where successful implantation into a human uterus should not be too difficult to achieve. In fact, Edwards and Steptoe hope to accomplish implantation and subsequent growth into a normal baby within this coming year.

The question naturally arises: why should any woman willingly submit to such operations? There is clearly some danger involved

every time Steptoe operates. Nonetheless, he and Edwards believe that the risks involved are more than counterbalanced by the fact that their research may develop methods which make their patients able to bear children. All their patients, though having normal menstrual cycles, are infertile, conceivably because many have blocked oviducts which prevent passage of their eggs into the uterus. If so, in-vitro growth of their eggs up to the blastocyst stage may circumvent their infertility, thereby allowing normal childbirth. Moreover, since the sex of a blastocyst is easily determined by chromosomal analysis, such women would be able to decide whether to give birth to a boy or a girl.

SELECTIVE CLONING

Clearly, if Edwards and Steptoe succeed, their success will be followed up in many other places. The number of such infertile women, while small on a relative percentage basis, is likely to be large on an absolute basis. Within the United States there could conceivably be 100,000 or so women who would like a similar chance to have their own babies.

At the same time we must anticipate strong, if not hysterical, reactions from many quarters. The certainty that the ready availability of this medical technique will open up the possibility of hiring out unrelated women to carry a given baby to term is bound to outrage many people. For there is absolutely no reason why the blastocyst need be implanted in the same woman from whom the preovulatory eggs were obtained. So many women with anatomical complications which prohibit successful childbearing would be strongly tempted to find a suitable surrogate. And it is easy to imagine that many women who just don't want the discomforts of pregnancy would also seek this very different form of motherhood.

Some very hard decisions may soon be upon us. The vague potential for abhorrent misuse should not necessarily weigh more strongly than the unhappiness which thousands of married couples feel when they are unable to have their own children. Different societies are likely to view the matter differently, and it would be surprising if all were to come to the same conclusion. We must, therefore, assume that techniques for the in-vitro manipulation of human eggs are likely to be general medical practice, capable of routine performance in many major nations, within some ten to twenty years.

The situation would then be ripe for extensive efforts, either legal or illegal, at human cloning. No reason, of course, dictates that such experiments need occur. Most of the medical people capable of such experimentation would probably stay totally clear of any step which in any way looked as if its real purpose was to clone. But it would be shortsighted to believe that everyone will instinctively recoil from such purposes. Some people may quite sincerely believe that the world desperately needs many copies of the really exceptional people if we are to fight our way out of the ever-increasing computer-mediated complexity that so frequently makes our individual brains inadequate.

Moreover, given the widespread development of safe clinical procedures for handling human eggs, cloning experiments would not be prohibitively expensive. They need not be restricted to the superpowers—medium-sized, if not minor, countries all now possess the resources needed for eventual success. Furthermore, there need not exist the coercion of a totalitarian state to provide the surrogate mothers. There are already such widespread divergences as to the sacredness of the act of human reproduction that the boring meaninglessness of the lives of many women would be sufficient cause for their willingness to participate in such experimentation, be it legal or illegal. Thus, if the matter proceeds in its current nondirected fashion, a human being—born of clonal reproduction—most likely will appear on the earth within the next twenty to fifty years, and conceivably even sooner, if some nation actively promotes the venture.

THE ASEXUALLY PRODUCED CHILD

The reaction of most people to the arrival of this asexually produced child will, I suspect, be one of despair. The nature of the bond between parents and their children, not to mention ev-

eryone's values about their individual uniqueness, could be changed beyond recognition if such children became a common occurrence.

Many people, particularly those with strong religious backgrounds, already believe we should *now* deemphasize all forms of research which could lead to circumvention of the normal sexual reproductive processes. If this step were taken, experiments on cell fusion might no longer be supported by federal funds or tax-exempt organizations. Prohibition of such research would most certainly put off the day when diploid nuclei will satisfactorily be inserted into enucleated human eggs. It would be even more effective to take steps quickly to make illegal, or to reaffirm the illegality of, any experimental work with human embryos.

Neither of these prohibitions, however, is likely to be made. In the first place, the cell-fusion technique now offers one of the best avenues for understanding the genetic basis of cancer. Today all over the world cancer cells are being fused with normal cells to pinpoint those specific chromosomes responsible for given forms of cancer.

In addition, fusion techniques are the basis of many genetic efforts to unravel the biochemistry of diseases such as cystic fibrosis or multiple sclerosis. Any attempts to stop such work by using the argument that cloning represents a greater threat than a disease like cancer is likely to be considered irresponsible by virtually anyone able to understand the matter.

Though more people would initially go along with a prohibition against work on human embryos, many may have a change of heart when they ponder the problem which the population explosion poses. The current projections are so horrendous that responsible people are likely to consider the need for more basic embryological facts much more relevant to our self-interest than the not-very-immediate threat of a few clonal men existing some decades ahead. And the potentially militant lobby of infertile couples who see test-tube conception as their only route to the joys of raising children of their own making would carry even more weight. So, scientists like Edwards are likely to get a go-ahead if, almost perversely, the immediate consequences of research supported by "population money" will be the production of even more babies.

Complicating any possible effort at effective legislative guidance is the multiplicity of places where work like Edwards' could occur, thereby making it most unlikely that such manipulations would have the same legal (or illegal) status throughout the world. We must assume that if Edwards and Steptoe produce a really workable method for restoring fertility, large numbers of women will search out those places where it is legal (or possible), just as now they search out places where abortions can easily be obtained.

Thus, all nations formulating policies to handle the implications of in-vitro human embryo experimentation must realize that the problem is essentially an international one. Even if one or more countries stop such research, such action could effectively be neutralized by the response of a neighboring country.

This most disconcerting impotence holds even for the United States. If our congressional representatives, upon learning where the matter now stands, decided they wanted none of it and passed very strict laws against human embryo experimentation, their action would not seriously set back the current scientific and medical momentum which brings us close to the possibility of surrogate mothers, if not of human clonal reproduction. This is because the relevant experiments are being done not in the United States but largely in England. This is partly a matter of chance, but also a consequence of the advanced state of English cell biology. In certain areas it is far more adventurous and imaginative than its American counterpart. There is no American university with the strength in experimental embryology that Oxford possesses.

We must not assume, however, that the important decisions today lie only before the British government. Very soon we must anticipate that a number of biologists and clinicians of other countries, sensing the potential excitement, will move into this area. So even if the current English effort were stifled, similar experimentation could soon begin elsewhere. Thus it appears to me most desirable that as many people as possible be informed about the new ways of human reproduction and their potential consequences, both good and bad.

This is a matter far too important to be left solely in the hands of the scientific and medical communities. The belief that surrogate mothers and clonal babies are inevitable because science always moves forward, an attitude expressed to me recently by a scientific colleague, represents a form of laissez-faire nonsense dismally reminiscent of the creed that American business, if left to itself, will solve everybody's problems.

Just as the success of a corporate body in making money need not advance the human condition, neither does every scientific advance automatically make our lives more "meaningful." No doubt the person whose experimental skill eventually brought forth a clonal baby would be given wide notoriety. But the child, growing up in the knowledge that the world wants another Picasso, would view his creator in a different light.

FOR THE FUTURE

Thus I would hope that over the next decade far-reaching discussion will occur, at the informal as well as the formal legislative level, about the many problems which are bound to arise if test-tube conception becomes a common occurrence. On some matters a sufficient international consciousness might develop to make possible some form of international agreement before the cat is totally out of the bag. A blanket declaration of the worldwide illegality of human cloning might be one result of a serious effort to ask the world in which directions it wishes to move.

Admittedly, the vast effort needed for even the most limited international arrangement will deter those who believe the matter is now of only marginal importance, and that in effect it might be a red herring designed to take our minds off our callous attitudes toward war, poverty, and racial prejudice. But if we do not think about the matter now, the possibility of our having a free choice will one day suddenly be gone.

ROBERT SINSHEIMER

Troubled Dawn for Genetic Engineering

The essence of engineering is design and, thus, the essence of genetic engineering, as distinct from applied genetics, is the introduction of human design into the formulation of new genes and new genetic combinations. These methods thus supplement the older methods which rely upon the intelligent selection and perpetuation of those chance genetic combinations which arise in the natural breeding process.

The possibility of genetic engineering derives from major advances in DNA technology —in the means of synthesising, analysing, transposing and generally manipulating the basic genetic substance of life. Three major advances have all neatly combined to permit this striking accomplishment: these are, 1, the discovery of means for the cleavage of DNA at highly specific sites; 2, the development of simple and generally applicable methods for the joining of DNA molecules; and 3, the discovery of effective techniques for the introduction of DNA into previously refractory organisms.

The art of DNA cleavage and degradation languished in a crude and unsatisfactory state until the discovery and more recent application of enzymes known as restriction endonucleases. These enzymes protect the host cells against invasion by foreign genomes by specifically severing the intruding DNA strands. For the purposes of genetic engineering, restriction enzymes provide a reservoir of means to cleave DNA molecules reproducibly at a limited number of sites by recognising specific tracts of DNA ranging for four to eight nucleotides in length. These sites may be deliberately varied by the choice of the restriction enzyme.

This article first appeared in *New Scientist, London, The Weekly Review of Science and Technology,* Vol. 68 (October 16, 1975). Reprinted with permission.

The enzymes cut both strands of the DNA double helix, and the break may be at the same base pair or staggered by several bases (Figure 1). In the latter case the two fragments of DNA are each left with a terminal unpaired strand—a so-called cohesive or "sticky" end. This is particularly valuable in joining together two pieces of DNA end to end.

The number of susceptible tracts in a DNA obviously depends on the particular DNA and the particular enzyme. In some important instances there is only one such tract. For instance, the restriction enzyme coded by the *E. coli* drug resistance transfer factor I—Eco RI —cleaves the DNA of the simian virus 40 at only one site. Similarly it cleaves the circular DNA of the plasmid PSC 101 at only one site, The DNA of bacteriophage lambda is, however, severed at five sites. It is possible to produce mutants of lambda with progressively fewer sites, until lambda strains are now available with just one or two sites.

For some purposes more numerous cleavage sites are useful. In a number of laboratories, including my own, the ϕX virus RF can be cut at up to 13 sites using selected restriction enzymes. Because these enzymes yield overlapping fragments, a physical map of the DNA can be formed and correlated with the viral genetic map.

Restriction enzymes thus permit us to obtain specific fragments of DNA. For genetic engineering one would like to be able to rejoin such fragments in arbitrary ways. Two general methods have been developed to achieve this both of which depend on the "sticky end" principle in which complementary single strand ends combine (Figures 1 and 2). Restriction enzymes which inflict staggered cuts automatically produce "sticky ends" in the DNA chain severed. Alternatively, a combination of enzymic and chemical manipulation can create a "sticky end".

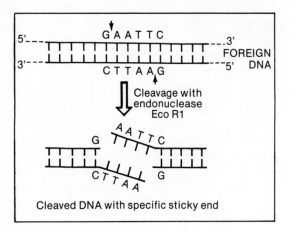

Figure 1. Endonucleases can cleave double stranded DNA at one point, or staggered as shown in the diagram. The staggered cut produces sticky ends which can join with sections of DNA severed by the same enzyme.

MODIFIED PLASMIDS IN E. COLI

By these means, then, any arbitrarily selected piece of DNA from any source can be inserted into the DNA of an appropriately chosen plasmid or virus. The new combination must then, for most purposes, be reintroduced into an appropriate host cell. This was achieved just a few years ago when Stanley Cohen, at Stanford, discovered that plasmid DNA could be reintroduced, albeit with low efficiency, into appropriately treated *E. coli* cells and that these could then subsequently grow and propagate the plasmid. Foreign genes can therefore be introduced into *E. coli* plasmids which can be propagated indefinitely in ordinary bacterial cultures. As one instance, the ribosomal RNA genes of *Xenopus laevis* (the African clawed toad) have been introduced into an *E. coli* plasmid and propagated for over 100 cell generations. And these genes are transcribed in their new host (Figure 2).

A similar result can, in principle, be achieved with the bacteriophage lambda. A

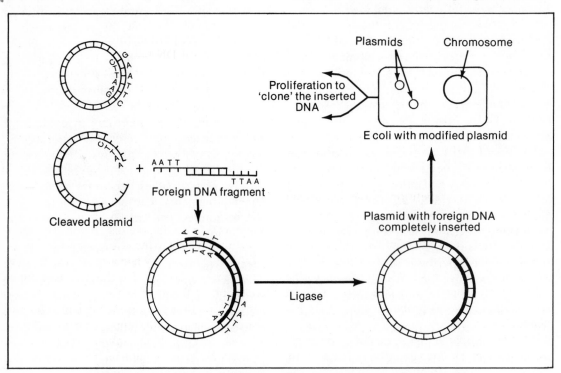

Figure 2. Cloning a gene: a nick is made in the circular DNA of a plasmid; the required DNA sequence, excised with the same restriction enzyme, is inserted into the gap; the DNA chains are repaired by a ligase enzyme; the plasmids are reintroduced into *E. coli;* when the coli culture multiplies, the plasmids, and the foreign genes with them, are multiplied (cloned) too.

foreign gene can be inserted into lambda DNA; spheroplasts or treated cells infected with this DNA will yield virus which can then be used to infect normal cells. By clever manipulation a recombinant DNA can be obtained which can subsequently be integrated into the host chromosome and propagated thereafter with the host.

To what purposes may these novel genetic combinations be put? One can conceive of a variety of benign purposes. Unfortunately one can also conceive of malign purposes, and of major, if unintended, hazards.

The first purposes that come to mind are of a purely scientific character. The structure and organisation of the eukaryotic (higher organism) genome is currently being studied intensively. This research has been grossly impeded by the complexity of these genomes and the lack of means to isolate particular portions in adequate quantities for experimental analysis. The insertion of fragments of eukaryotic DNA into plasmids, followed by cloning (cellular multiplication), permits one to grow cultures of any size containing just one particular fragment. At present the choice of fragments to be inserted cannot in general be precisely defined, although some prior selection can be introduced. However, ingenious methods are being devised to permit subsequent selection of those bacterial clones carrying fragments of particular interest.

Clones of bacteria bearing, say, histone genes, ribosomal RNA genes, genes from individual bands of *Drosophila* DNA, DNA of a certain degree of repetition in the sea urchin genome, and so forth, are currently being investigated. There are numerous questions to ask and numerous matters of interest concerning the transcription and translation of such genes in the bacterial host: for instance, the rates at which they may mutate, and the use of such cloned genes as probes of the eukaryotic genome.

It is very probable that in time the appropriate genes can be introduced into bacteria to convert them into biochemical factories for producing complex substances of medical importance: for example, insulin (for which a shortage seems imminent), growth hormone, specific antibodies, and clotting factor VIII

which is defective in hemophiliacs. Even if these specific genes cannot be isolated from the appropriate organisms, the chances of synthesising them from scratch are now significant.

Other more grandiose applications of microbial genetic engineering can be envisaged. The transfer of genes for nitrogen fixation into presently inept species might have very significant agricultural applications. Appropriate design might permit appreciable modifications of the normal bacterial flora of the human mouth with a significant impact upon the incidence of dental caries. Even major industrial processes might be carried out by appropriately planned microorganisms.

However, we must remember that we are creating here novel, self-propagating organisms. And with that reminder, another darker side appears on this scene of brilliant scientific enterprise. For instance, for scientific purposes there is great interest in the insertion of particular regions of viral DNA into plasmids —particularly, portions of oncogenic (cancer-inducing) viral DNA—so as to be able to obtain such portions and their gene products in quantity and subsequently to study the effects of these substances on their normal host cells. Abruptly we come to the potential hazard of research in this field, in fact the specific hazard which inspired the widely known "moratorium" proposed last year by a committee of the US National Academy, chaired by Paul Berg.

This moratorium and its related issues deserve very considerable discussion. Briefly, it became apparent to the scientists involved—at almost the last hour when all of the techniques were really at hand—that they were about to create novel forms of self-propagating organisms—derivatives of strains known to be normal components of the human intestinal flora—with almost completely unknown potential for biological havoc. Could an *Escherichia coli* strain carrying all or part of an oncogenic virus become resident in the human intestine? Could it thereby become a possible source of malignancy? Could such a strain spread throughout a human population? What would be the consequence if even an insulin-secreting strain became an intestinal resident? Not to mention the more malign or just plain stupid scenarios such as those which depict the insertion of the gene for botulinus toxin into *Escherichia coli.*

UNKNOWN PROBABILITIES

Unfortunately the answers to these questions in terms of probabilities that some of these strains could persist in the intestines, the probabilities that the modified plasmids might be transferred to other strains, better adapted to intestinal life, the probabilities that the genome of an oncogenic virus could escape, could be taken up, could transform a host cell, are all largely unknown.

Following the call for a moratorium a conference was held at Asilomar at the end of last February to assess these problems. While it proved possible to rank various types of proposed experiments with respect to potential hazard, for the reasons already stated it proved impossible to establish, on any secure basis, the absolute magnitude of hazard. Various distinguished scientists differed very widely, but sincerely, in their estimates. Historical experience indicated that simple reliance upon the physical containment of these new organisms could not be completely effective.

In the end a broad, but not universal, consensus was reached which recommended that the seemingly more dangerous experiments be deferred until means of "biological containment" could be developed to supplement physical containment. By biological containment is meant the crippling of all vehicles— cells or viruses—intended to carry the recombinant genomes through the insertion of a variety of genetic defects so as to reduce very greatly the likelihood that the organisms could survive outside of a protective, carefully supplemented laboratory culture.

This seems a sensible and responsible compromise. However, several of the less prominent aspects of the Asilomar conference also deserve much thought. The lens of Asilomar was focused sharply upon the potential biological and medical hazard of this new research,

but other issues drifted in and out of the field of discussion. There was, for instance, no specific consideration of the wisdom of diverting appreciable research funds and talent to this field, in lieu of others. An indirect discussion of this question was perhaps implicit in the description of the significance and scientific potential of research in this field presented by those who were impatient of any delay.

Indeed the eagerness of the researchers to get on with the work in this field was most evident. To a scientist this was exhilarating. Obviously these new techniques open many previously closed doorways leading to the potential resolution of long-standing and important problems. I think also there is a certain romance in this joining together of DNA molecules that diverged billions of years ago and have pursued separate paths through all of these millenia. Personally I feel confident one could easily justify this new research direction. But a sociologist of science might see other under-currents in this impetuous eagerness, and the bright scientific promise should not blind us to the realities of other concerns.

Nor was there any sustained discussion at Asilomar of ancillary issues such as the absolute right of free inquiry claimed quite vigorously by some of the participants. Here, I think, we have come to recognise that there are limits to the practice of any human activity. To impose any limit upon freedom of inquiry is especially bitter for the scientist whose life is one of inquiry; but science has become too potent. It is no longer enough to wave the flag of Galileo.

Rights are not found in nature. Rights are conferred within a human society and for each there is expected a corresponding responsibility. Inevitably at some boundaries different rights come into conflict and the exercise of a right should not destroy the society that conferred it. We recognise this in other fields. Freedom of the press is a right but it is subject to restraints, such as libel and obscenity and, perhaps more dubiously, national security. The right to experiment on human beings is obviously constrained. Similarly, would we wish to claim the right of individual scientists to be free to create novel self-perpetuating organisms likely to spread about the planet in an uncontrollable manner for better or worse? I think not.

This does not mean we cannot advance our science or that we must doubt its ultimate beneficence. It simply means that we must be able to look at what we do in a mature way.

There was, at Asilomar, no explicit consideration of the potential broader social or ethical implications of initiating this line of research—of its role, as a possible prelude to longer-range, broader-scale genetic engineering of the flora and fauna of the planet, including, ultimately, man. It is not yet clear how these techniques may be applied to higher organisms but we should not underestimate scientific ingenuity. Indeed the oncogenic viruses may provide a key; and mitochondria may serve as analogues for plasmids.

CONTROLLED EVOLUTION?

How far will we want to develop genetic engineering? Do we want to assume the basic responsibility for life on this planet—to develop new living forms for our own purpose? Shall we take into our own hands our own future evolution? These are profound issues which involve science but also transcend science. They deserve our most serious and continuing thought. I can here mention only a very few of the more salient considerations.

Clearly the advent of genetic engineering, even merely in the microbial world, brings new responsibilities to accompany the new potentials. It is always thus when we introduce the element of human design. The distant, yet much discussed application of genetic engineering to mankind would place this equation at the centre of all future human history. It would in the end make human design responsible for human nature. It is a responsibility to give pause, especially if one recognises that the prerequisite for responsibility is the ability to forecast, to make reliable estimates of the consequence.

Can we really forecast the consequence for mankind, for human society, of any major change in the human gene pool? The more I have reflected on this the more I have come to doubt it. I do not refer here to the alleviation of individual genetic defects—or, if you will, to the occasional introduction of a genetic clone —but more broadly to the genetic redefinition of man. Our social structures have evolved so as to be more or less well adapted to the array of talents and personalities emergent by chance from the existing gene pool and developed through our cultural agencies. In our social endeavours we have, biologically, remained cradled in that web of evolutionary nature which bore us and which has undoubtedly provided a most valuable safety net as we have in our fumbling way created and tried our varied cultural forms.

To introduce a sudden major discontinuity in the human gene pool might well create a major mismatch between our social order and our individual capacities. Even a minor perturbation such as a marked change in the sex ratio from its present near equality could shake our social structures—or consider the impact of a major change in the human life span. Can we really predict the results of such a perturbation? And if we cannot foresee the consequence, do we go ahead?

It is difficult for a scientist to conceive that there are certain matters best left unknown, at least for a time. But science is the major organ of inquiry for a society—and perhaps a society, like an organism, must follow a developmental programme in which the genetic information is revealed in an orderly sequence.

The dawn of genetic engineering is troubled. In part this is the spirit of the time—the very idea of progress through science is in question. People seriously wonder if through our cleverness we may not blunder into worse dilemmas than we seek to solve. They are concerned not only for the vagrant lethal virus or the escaped mutant deadly microbe, but also for the awful potential that we might inadvertently so arm the anarchic in our society as to shatter its bonds or conversely so arm the tyrannical in our society as to forever imprison liberty.

It is grievous that the elan of science must be tempered, that the glowing conviction that knowledge is good and that man can with knowledge lift himself out of hapless impotence must now be shaded with doubt and caution. But in this we join a long tradition. The fetters that are part of the human condition are not so easily struck.

We confront again, the enduring paradox of emergence. We are each a unit, each alone. Yet, bonded together, we are so much more. As individuals men will have always to accept their genetic constraints, but as a species we can transcend our inheritance and mould it to our purpose—if we can trust ourselves with such powers. As geneticists we can continue to evolve possibilities and take the long view.

SUGGESTED READINGS FOR CHAPTER 12

Books and Articles

Bergsma, Daniel, ed. *Ethical, Social, and Legal Dimensions of Screening for Human Genetic Disease*. Birth Defects: Original Article Series, Vol. 10, No. 6. Miami: Symposium Specialists, 1974.

Cohen, Stanley N. "Recombinant DNA: Fact and Fiction." *Science* 195 (February 18, 1977), 654–657.

Edwards, Robert G., and Sharpe, David J. "Social Values and Research in Human Embryology." *Nature* 231 (May 14, 1971), 87–91.

Fletcher, John. "The Brink: The Parent-Child Bond in the Genetic Revolution." *Theological Studies* 33 (September, 1972), 457–485.

Fletcher, Joseph. *The Ethics of Genetic Control: Ending Reproductive Roulette*. Garden City, N. Y.: Doubleday Anchor, 1974.

Friedmann, Theodore, and Roblin, Richard O. "Gene Therapy for Human Genetic Disease?" *Science* 175 (March 3, 1972), 949–955.

Golding, Martin. "Ethical Issues in Biological Engineering." *UCLA Law Review* 15 (February, 1968), 443–479.

Hilton, Bruce, *et al.*, eds. *Ethical Issues in Human Genetics: Genetic Counseling and the Use of Genetic Knowledge*. New York: Plenum Press, 1973.

Humber, James M., and Almeder, Robert E., eds. *Biomedical Ethics and the Law*. New York: Plenum Press, 1976. Part IV.

Kass, Leon R. "Making Babies: The New Biology and the 'Old' Morality." *Public Interest*, No. 26 (Winter, 1972), 18–56.

Lappé, Marc. "Moral Obligations and the Fallacies of Genetic Control." *Theological Studies* 33 (September, 1972), 411–427.

Lappé, Marc, and Morison, Robert S., eds. "Ethical and Scientific Issues Posed by Human Uses of Molecular Genetics." *Annals of the New York Academy of Sciences* 265 (January 23, 1976), 1–208.

Milunsky, Aubrey, and Annas, George J., eds. *Genetics and the Law*. New York: Plenum Press, 1976.

Muller, H. J. "The Guidance of Human Evolution." *Perspectives in Biology and Medicine* 3 (Autumn, 1959), 1–43.

National Research Council, Committee for the Study of Inborn Errors of Metabolism. *Genetic Screening: Programs, Principles, and Research*. Washington, D. C.: National Academy of Sciences, 1975.

Ramsey, Paul. *Fabricated Man: The Ethics of Genetic Control*. New Haven: Yale University Press, 1970.

Veatch, Robert M. "Ethical Issues in Genetics." In Steinberg, Arthur G., and Bearn, Alexander G., eds. *Progress in Medical Genetics*, Volume 10. New York: Grune and Stratton, 1974. Pp. 223–264.

Walters, LeRoy. "Technology Assessment and Genetics." *Theological Studies* 33 (December, 1972), 666–683.

Waltz, Jon R. and Thigpen, Carol R. "Genetic Screening and Counseling: The Legal and Ethical Issues." *Northwestern University Law Review* 68 (September/October, 1973), 696–768.

Bibliographies

Sollitto, Sharmon, and Veatch, Robert M., comps. *Bibliography of Society, Ethics and the Life Sciences*. Hastings-on-Hudson, N.Y.: Institute of Society, Ethics and the Life Sciences. Updated periodically. See under "Genetics, Fertilization, and Birth."

Walters, LeRoy, ed. *Bibliography of Bioethics*. Vols. 1- . Detroit: Gale Research Company. Issued annually. See under "Cloning," "DNA Therapy," "Genetic Counseling," "Genetic Intervention," "Genetic Screening," "In Vitro Fertilization," and "Recombinant DNA Molecule Research."

THE LETTERS OF
MICHELANGELO

Volume Two

1537 - 1563

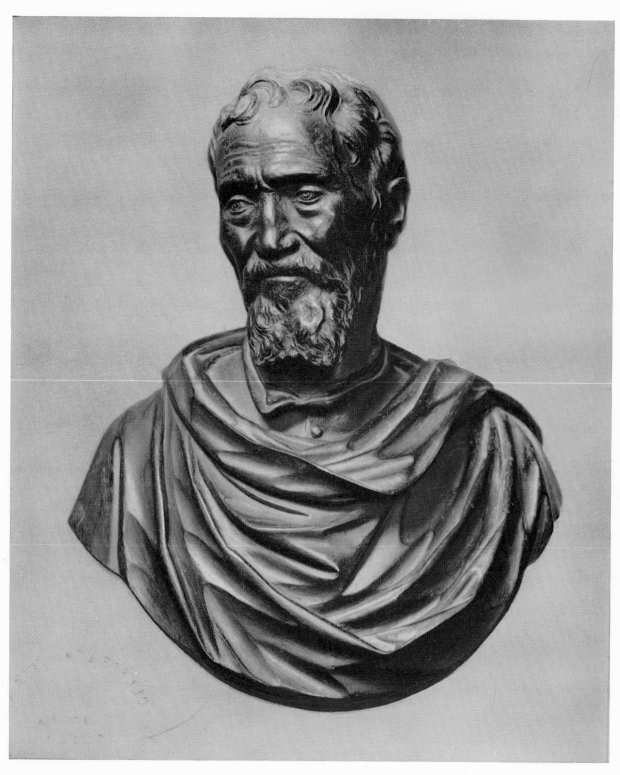

Michelangelo

Giovanni da Bologna
Casa Buonarroti, Florence

THE LETTERS OF
MICHELANGELO

Translated from the original Tuscan
Edited & Annotated

in Two Volumes

by

E. H. RAMSDEN

Volume Two
1537-1563

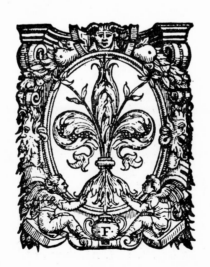

STANFORD UNIVERSITY PRESS
1963

Stanford University Press
Stanford, California
1963

Designed by Margot Eates
Printed in Great Britain by W. & J. Mackay & Company Ltd, Chatham

Process and line blocks by The Bryant Engraving Company Ltd (Wace Group)
Basingwerk Parchment and Matt Art Papers by Grosvenor, Chater & Company Ltd
Bound in the United States of America

Contents of Volume II

Continued overleaf

Contents of Volume II

List of Plates

ix

List of Plates

List of Plates

THE INTRODUCTION

The Introduction

hen Michelangelo reached Rome on September 23rd 1534 Clement VII was already *in extremis*; two days later he was dead.[1] Now, for the first time for eighteen years, Michelangelo, being released from the service of the Medici, found himself at liberty to complete the Tomb of Julius in fulfilment of his obligation to the della Rovere heirs. But his anticipated freedom was not to be enjoyed. For no less than thirty years the new Pope, Paul III, who, before his elevation on October 13th had been recognized as perhaps the most learned, astute and distinguished of all the members of the Sacred College, had apparently cherished a desire to command Michelangelo's services[2] and now that he was in a position to do so, he was not to be denied.

According to a communication from the Venetian envoy in Rome to the Imperial ambassador in Venice,[3] as early as the beginning of 1534, Pope Clement had so far prevailed upon Michelangelo that he had undertaken to execute the enormous fresco for the altar wall of the Sistine Chapel. The subject then proposed was said to be *The Resurrection*, a theme in some respects more suitable for that position than *The Last Judgment*, which is more commonly reserved for the liturgical west end of a church.

That there could be any valid reason for the abandonment of this great project owing to the death of his predecessor was not a notion that the resolute Farnese Pope was prepared for a moment to entertain, however importunately Michelangelo might plead his prior engagement to the Duke of Urbino. But Michelangelo remained obdurate and even thought of leaving Rome to continue the Tomb elsewhere. Finally, however, Paul III, attended by eight of the cardinals, went to visit him in his house in the Macel de' Corvi.[4] Here, while they were all admiring the marbles and the cartoons, the Cardinal of Mantua, Ercole Gonzaga, suddenly exclaimed that the figure of Moses alone would suffice to do honour to the Tomb of Julius. Then the Pope, being still unable to induce Michelangelo to enter his service, himself undertook to arrange matters with the Duke, and in such a way, that at last Michelangelo found himself with no option but to yield. On September 1st 1535[5] he was formally appointed a member of the Pope's household, with a place at his table and, what was perhaps even more relevant, with a salary of twelve hundred *scudi* a year.[6]

It is true that in consequence he was no longer his own master, any more than he had been for the past thirty years or was to be for the rest of his life; it is true that he had virtually to abandon his first love, sculpture, and to cleave unto his second, painting; it is true that he had to bear the burden of the Tomb for another ten years, yet even so,

xv

life in Rome was not without its compensations, since of all places upon earth that was where he most ardently desired to be.

In 1532, probably in December, he had been introduced to Tommaso de' Cavalieri, a young Roman nobleman of great personal distinction, by whose appearance and manners he had been instantly captivated. There is no doubt whatever that Michelangelo loved him passionately and that he was completely carried away.

From the evident embarrassment of his second letter, (and particularly of the draft,[7]) it is obvious that he had made no concealment of his feelings in the first. This frank avowal not only of admiration but also of love, from a man of Michelangelo's eminence, might be more difficult to understand, were it not for what is known of his peculiar susceptibility, in the first place, and of Cavalieri's peculiar quality, in the second: in virtue of which much that to grosser minds might be suspect in such a relationship is seen to be blameless. And that the relationship was open to misinterpretation no-one was more aware than Michelangelo himself, who in one of the numerous sonnets he addressed to Cavalieri, spoke of 'the vulgar, vain, malignant horde', men who, being incapable of conceiving the sublimer aspirations of the soul even – *un casto amor* – were prompt to attribute to others the baser inclinations of which they are conscious within themselves.[8]

A confession, upon which it would be difficult to place too much emphasis, is recorded by an intimate friend of his, Donato Giannotti, in his famous *Dialoghi*, and is certainly authentic. The occasion was a day in Rome devoted to two conversations, in which Michelangelo was the principal speaker, and in which Luigi del Riccio, Antonio Petroneo and Giannotti himself also took part. At noon they proposed to go their several ways and to meet again later, whereupon del Riccio invited them all to dine at his house, but this Michelangelo declined to do, not, however, because he did not care for the society of his friends, but because, paradoxically, he cared for it too much. This, no less than the extent to which he exemplified the Greek maxim, γνῶθι σεαυτὸν, is amply borne out by what follows. In justification of his refusal of del Riccio's invitation, he said this of himself, 'I am a man more inclined than anyone who ever lived to care for people. Whenever I see anyone possessed of some gift which shows him to be more apt in the performance or expression of anything than others, I become, perforce, enamoured of him and am constrained to abandon myself to him in such a way that I am no longer my own, but wholly his.'[9] Seeing then, as he went on to explain, that his three companions were all gentlemen of parts, he would be reft from himself and lost and confounded for days, if, without respite, he were to give himself up entirely to them, and to others whom he might meet at del Riccio's house. It was therefore imperative for him to withdraw for a short space in order that he might, as it were, return to himself. The same thought is re-echoed in certain of his madrigals in which, being unable any longer to endure the exquisite agony of *l'estremo ardore* by which he was consumed, he cried unto the god of Love to restore him to himself that he might die – *Deh rendim' a me stresso, acciò ch' i'mora.*[10]

In other words, being conscious of the hypersensitivity of his nature, he knew it to be essential for the preservation of his equilibrium, both as an artist and as a man, to maintain a certain measure of isolation, and this, not because he was a misanthrope and a recluse, as everyone has always contended, but because he was exactly the reverse, being all too prone to love not wisely but too well.

Understandably, the appeal for Michelangelo was always primarily and in a heightened degree through the eyes:

> *Passa per gli occhi al core in un momento*
> *Qualunque obbietto di beltà lor sia.*[11]

So that he easily became intoxicated, not only with the physical beauty of human beings:

> *Che cosa è questa, amore,*
> *Ch' al cor entra per gli occhi;*[12]

but to an even more impelling extent with the spiritual beauty of the soul, as it is communicated through the eyes. The theme is, indeed, recurrent in his poetry – *Sol d'uno sguardo fui prigione e preda*,[13] or again, *Tu c' hai negli occhi tutto 'l paradiso*.[14] One remembers, too, the words he used in a letter to Cavalieri, written in August 1533 – 'Imagine, if the eye were also playing its part, the state in which I should find myself.'[15]

Even without confirmation of the fact that Tommaso de' Cavalieri pre-eminently fulfilled the classic conception of καλὸς κἀγαθός we should be justified, from this remark alone, in believing him to have been a man of singular quality. Happily, however, confirmation of this belief is not wanting. On the occasion of his second discourse to the Florentine Academy in the spring of 1547,[16] Benedetto Varchi described him as being a young Roman of great nobility, in whom, 'besides his incomparable beauty', he perceived, as he said, 'such graceful manners, so excellent an endowment and so charming a demeanour that he indeed deserved, and still deserves, the more to be loved the better he is known.'[17]

If this was the impression made upon Varchi by the impact of a unique personality, how much greater must that impact have been upon a man of Michelangelo's particular sensibility. It is therefore small wonder that, at a time when he was unusually lonely, disappointed, frustrated and bereft, he should have been 'the first to move' in initiating the friendship and should almost at once have become, as he confessed in one of his sonnets to Cavalieri, 'the captive of an arméd cavalier':

> *Maraviglia non è se, nud' e solo,*
> *Resto prigion d'un Cavalier armato.*[18]

One cannot too much regret that no draft of Michelangelo's first letter has been preserved, though something of its contents may perhaps be gauged from the tone, not so much of the second letter, as of the draft which it superseded, in which the extent to which he had become enamoured is manifest. What Cavalieri's feelings must have been on receiving such a letter from the greatest artist in Europe are difficult to imagine, but the letter he wrote in reply was in all respects becoming.[19]

> I have received your letter which was as gratifying to me as it was unexpected. I say unexpected, because I do not deem myself worthy that a man of your eminence should deign to write to me.
>
> As to what Pierantonio said to you in praise of me and of those works of mine which you yourself have seen and on account of which you pretend to show me no little affection, I say in reply to you that they were insufficient to cause a man of such excellence as yourself and without a second, let alone a peer on earth, to write to a youth – a mere babe and therefore as ignorant as can be. At the same time, I do not wish to infer that you are a liar. I think, nay rather, I am certain that the cause of the affection you bear me is this – that being a man supreme in art yourself – or rather the epitome of art itself – you are constrained to love those who are the followers and lovers of art, among whom, according to my capacity, I yield to few.
>
> I promise you truly that the love I bear you in exchange is equal or perhaps greater than I ever bore any man, neither have I ever desired any friendship more than I do yours. And if not in other things, at least in this I possess excellent judgment and of this you would have proof if fortune, who opposes me only in this, had not willed that now, when I should be able to enjoy your company, I should be slightly indisposed. Unless she begins to torment me anew, I certainly hope to be cured within a few days and to come and visit you and to fulfil my obligations, if that would please you.
>
> In the meantime, I shall spend at least two hours a day enjoying the contemplation of your two drawings which Pierantonio has brought me, the which the more I study them the more do they delight me, and I shall assuage the worst of my indisposition thinking of the expectation which the said Pierantonio has given me of being able to see other things of yours.
>
> That I may not be tedious, I will not write at greater length. Only I would remind you, should you have occasion to do so, to avail yourself of my services.
>
> And to you do I continuously commend me.
>
> > Your most affectionate servant
> > Tommao Cavalieri

The whole tone of the letter bespeaks the enchantment of the character. His scepticism about Michelangelo's alleged reason for writing is charmingly conveyed, while the simple and graceful manner of his acceptance of the honour done him could hardly be surpassed. From then on the friendship developed in a fashion that is perhaps unique. Cavalieri was certainly in no doubt as to his good fortune; this is made clear in a letter of Bartolomeo Angiolini's to Michelangelo, written on September 6th 1533. 'Your Messer Tommao,' he wrote, 'is very grateful in the recognition that he has been so favoured by God as to have acquired such a friendship with a man as endowed as you are, and he was the more grateful when I told him that you would soon be returning, which he desires more than anything else.' In another letter Angiolini wrote, saying, 'as far as I can see he has no less affection for you than you have for him', and in yet another, 'From what he says, he shows himself to have no other desire in the world except your return, because he says when he is with you he is happy, because he possesses everything he desires in this world. So much so that if you are consumed with a desire to return, he burns with the desire that you should.'[20]

The correspondence on both sides leaves us in no doubt that the feeling they entertained for each other was intense, but it is equally certain that the relationship, ardent though it was, always remained Platonic, a fact which no reputable biographer has ever disputed. To maintain that Michelangelo had no passionate longings of a physical kind would, however, be to deny the evidence of the poems, such, for instance as the sonnet, *S' i' avessi creduto al primo sguardo*,[21] but, equally, to imagine that he ever contemplated their indulgence or failed to sublimate them would be to disregard the evidence of others, as, for example, *Non vider gli occhi miei cosa mortale*,[22] or another of equal significance, *Ben può talor col casto e buon desio*.[23] Thus, for all the fascination which, as a personality, Cavalieri possessed for Michelangelo, especially it would seem in certain mannerisms, as in the particular way in which he opened and closed his eyes, if one may judge from the lines:

> *Perc' al superchio ardore,*
> *Che toglie e rende poi*
> *Il chiudere e l'aprir degli occhi tuoi*,[24]

the friendship was for him essentially an inspiration. To this, likewise, the poems bear witness, notably perhaps *Veggio co' bei vostri occhi un dolce lume*, and *Io mi son caro assai più ch'io non soglio*;[25] which are instinct with the strange exhilaration of a sublimated passion, which could not but be beyond the comprehension of the Aretinos of this world, who chose, and still choose, to interpret what lies beyond their own experience in terms of their own littleness. Had Michelangelo's association with Cavalieri been on a lower level it would scarcely have endured for the rest of his life. Whenever he had need of him, Cavalieri was always at hand and was always sent for immediately when anything went wrong.[26] Yet even so Michelangelo could still take umbrage with the dearest of all his friends, as happened over some misunderstanding which occurred in the autumn of 1561, when Cavalieri, obviously hurt and perplexed by his manner, wrote to him in these terms:[27]

Molto Mag^(co) S^(or) mio

For some days past I have been under the impression that you have some grievance against me, I know not what, but yesterday I was convinced of it when I called at your house. Not being able to imagine the reason I wanted to write you this letter, so that, if you are so disposed, you can enlighten me, for I am more than certain that I have never injured you, but you too easily give credence to those whom perhaps you ought least to believe and someone has perhaps told you some lie, lest I might one day discover to you the many rascalities that are committed in your name, which do you little honour. If you want to know what they are you shall, but I cannot, nor, being able, would I force them upon you. But I assure you, if you do not want me for a friend you can say so, but you will never prevent me from being a friend to you and always seeking to serve you. Only yesterday I came to show you a letter from the Duke of Florence and to spare you trouble, as I have always done up till now, and you may be certain that you have no better friend than I. I do not want to enlarge upon this, but if it now appears to you otherwise, I hope within a little while, if you wish, that you will enlighten me, for I know that you know that I have always been a friend to you without any self-interest whatever. Now I would not say more, that I may not appear to justify myself over anything, which is not the case, for I cannot imagine in any way what you have against me. But I beg and adjure you by the love you bear towards God that you will tell me, so that I may be able to undeceive you. And having nothing else to say, I commend me to you. From my house on the 15th day of November 1561.

Your servant
Tommao de' Cavalieri

This is the last of Cavalieri's letters that have survived, but from the devotion implicit in it throughout, which is as marked as the veneration shown in his first letter of almost thirty years before, there can be no question but that the slight estrangement between them was of short duration and that he never ceased to serve, to solace and sustain him. Confirmation of this fact is found in Diomede Leoni's letter of February 15th 1564 to Lionardo, written three days before Michelangelo's death in which, having advised him not to press himself unduly on the roads in the bad weather, he ended by saying, 'you may feel at ease when you remember that Messer Tommaso Cavalieri, Messer Daniele and I are here to render every possible assistance.'[28]

This proneness to take offence characterized Michelangelo throughout his life and was the cause of much unhappiness both to himself and to others. It arose, of course, from his inordinate sensitivity, on the one hand, and from his natural diffidence, on the other. For just as it is obvious from the remark about Cardinal Riario he made in his first letter from Rome,[29] 'he seemed pleased to see me', that he was conscious of the least nuance in the attitude of people towards him, so he always remained *pusilanimo a richiedere*[30] when it came to seeking concessions for himself.

Being easily hurt, he either flared up, as he did with Luigi del Riccio over the engraving, and said more perhaps than he intended, or withdrew, as he did with Cavalieri over some imagined grievance, and said nothing. Which of the two was the more disconcerting for his friends it would be hard to say. On the whole the latter would appear to have been the more difficult to cope with, if one may judge from a letter of Francesco da Sangallo's, written in all probability towards the end of 1524, when Michelangelo had been so dissatisfied with his carving of part of the frieze of masks in the Medici Chapel that he had only authorized the payment of part of the sum due to him.[31] In this letter Sangallo spoke of his distress at the sour looks and angry countenance with which Michelangelo had confronted him on several occasions during the past weeks, without explaining his reasons or giving him an opportunity to vindicate himself, which clearly shows that it was Michelangelo's silence and failure to reveal the cause of his displeasure that Sangallo found particularly hard to bear. But so greatly did he value his esteem that he was not prepared to let the matter go by default and having reminded him of their long friendship he begged to be allowed to see him and to receive an explanation, assuring him that he would forego the friendship of everyone he knew rather than lose his, having always looked upon him as a father as he always would.[32] In face of such an appeal it is difficult to suppose that Michelangelo did not relent, just as it is difficult, in spite of Vasari's insistence on the point, to believe that he never forgave Sebastiano del Piombo for his temerity in having the altar wall of the Sistine Chapel prepared for oil instead of for fresco without consulting him[33] – a foolish move on Sebastiano's part, no doubt, and one which could not fail to have aroused Michelangelo's ire at the time. But one cannot be convinced that they remained estranged, in view of the fact that they had been intimately associated for many years, that Sebastiano was recognized to be the best company in the world (an attraction which Michelangelo always found hard to resist) and that after Sebastiano's death in the summer of 1547 he did not fail to support the claims of Guglielmo della Porta to the office of *piombatore* – a sculptor whom Sebastiano had introduced to him in 1537.[34]

So undue an emphasis has, however, been placed upon this propensity of his to quarrel that it has even been pretended that the loss of his friends mentioned in one of his letters written in 1556[35] was due not to death, which is clearly stated, but to the churlishness of his behaviour towards them – a misreading unworthy of mention except to show the lengths to which would-be recondite criticism can sometimes be carried.[36] Being, as has already been remarked, abnormally sensitive, it cannot be denied that he was always quick to take offence and apt at times to imagine insults where none were intended, but he was not quarrelsome in a provocative sense. Courteous himself, as his letters testify, he expected a like courtesy from others and was not to be insulted with impunity, even by Popes. Also, because he moved in a world beset by intrigues, of which, by reason of his eminence, he himself became a focus (as the terms of Cavalieri's letter quoted above make plain), he inevitably grew more suspicious as he grew older, particularly as the bitterness of his personal experience was not such as to render him otherwise.

But standing in need of kindness and consideration himself, he was no less ready to extend the same kindness and consideration to others. After Maestro Bernardino's failure to cast the statue of Julius II at the first attempt, he not only made every allowance for him, but on Maestro Bernardino's return to Florence sought to protect him from any subsequent recriminations, as we know from his letter to Buonarroto, in which he said, 'Maestro Bernardino left here yesterday. If he should say anything to you, be nice to him – and leave it at that'[37] – an injunction that argues a professional respect for a colleague which makes it hard to credit the story that he publicly taunted Leonardo da Vinci with his failure to cast the Sforza horse.[38]

A respect for the feelings of other people also prevailed with him even when he had been exasperated beyond measure. For while he might inveigh against the 'dunghill of a boy', whom he dismissed from his service in 1513, he was nevertheless careful not to offend the boy's parents. 'If you speak to the lad's father,' he wrote in a postscript to the same letter,[39] 'tell him kindly about the affair; say that he is a good lad, but too refined and not suited to my service.' In other words, though not slow to wrath in the everyday things of life, nor willing to suffer fools gladly, his wrath soon abated, his bark, as the saying is, being ever worse than his bite. Similarly, when hardly able to contain himself over the quarrels which arose between Maestro Giovanni and Urbino about the work they had contracted to do for the frame for the Tomb of Julius, he enlisted the help of Luigi del Riccio, in order that the affair might be settled in a manner not only satisfactory to himself, but fair to both of them. With an appealing bluntness he confessed, however, that, if they came to blows and anything were to happen to either of them, though he would be sorry about Maestro Giovanni, he would be much more sorry about Urbino, because he had brought him up.[40]

Thus, despite a pardonable loss of patience (and contrary to the findings of the irresponsible and purblind) he was characterized not only by an innate courtesy, but also by a surpassing largeness of heart. Never was he asked to do anyone a kindness that he did not endeavour to do it if it lay within his power, whether this involved the order for a dagger to please Aldobrandini, the entertainment of Lorenzo Strozzi to gratify Buonarroto, an enquiry after the health of a Spanish painter to allay the fears of his relatives, the purchase of a seal to oblige Tanagli, or a letter of recommendation to assist Sebastiano – whatever it might be, no-one appealed to him in vain.[41] And when he was unable to do what was asked of him, he hastened to say so, that his friends and acquaintances might not depend on him fruitlessly.[42] If Guicciardini wanted him to redeem a farm, he did so; if Francesca asked alms to enable a wretched girl (with no alternative open to her) to enter a convent, he supplied it; if Fattucci desired a sight of his sonnets or those by Vittoria Colonna, he sent them; if Cornelia made a request for cloth, he procured it; if Vasari was in need of his intervention, he intervened.[43] And although when Lionardo wished to purchase a property against his uncle's better judgment, Michelangelo might pretend that he would have to find the money himself, he afterwards forwarded the necessary amount, just the same.[44]

And what of his attitude towards his subordinates and of theirs towards him? Even in the early days he assured his father that he had always done more for them than he need have done, and he repeated the same thing some seventeen years later in a letter to Piero Gondi.[45] Yet even so, this made neither for peace nor popularity, since on his own showing his workmen found him 'in some way strange and obsessed'.[46] This was largely because they were unused to a master who was at once a genius and a perfectionist, who, being above corruption himself, expected not only an honest, but a good day's work as well and was not disposed to tolerate anything less. 'We are hard put to it with a hundred eyes to keep one of them at work',[47] he wrote in 1526 and nothing in his experience ever convinced him that constant supervision was not necessary. But a stern and uncompromising refusal to countenance the deception and graft inseparable, then as now, from the furtherance of any great enterprise was no more calculated to commend him to the *soprastanti* of the Basilica in Rome than it had been to endear him to the *Operai* at the Duomo in Florence. The principle that 'promises, gratuities and presents corrupt justice'[48] was against the tradition and came not within their purview, but the consciousness of inferiority engendered by the knowledge that it did not, served only to increase their animosity towards him.

If, therefore, he was hated, as Romain Rolland was at such pains to insist,[49] it was in this context, and in this context only, in which his vigilance and rectitude were as much despised by his rivals and professional colleagues as they were resented by those immediately or remotely under his authority.[50] When it came to a more personal relationship, however, the case was different. Then his kindly and at times almost paternal attitude towards those who worked for him became apparent. Who but Michelangelo, when burdened with cares, at eighty years of age, and at the height of his fame, would have taken the trouble to remit to Florence a mere couple of *scudi* on behalf of one of his labourers at the Basilica, and would have been so concerned to see that the man's mother should receive the money?[51] Again, in the case of his father's old servant, Mona Margherita, his kindness and consideration were unfailing,[52] while she, for her part, was apparently devoted to him, since in his letter to Michelangelo of January 4th 1533 Stefano Lunetti, who was ill, wrote to him saying, 'Mona Margherita comes to see me every week. She says it seems to her like a thousand years awaiting your return';[53] and though perhaps not exactly on a par, the attitude of the wife of the bailiff who had acted as caretaker during his absence from Rome seems to have been similar, if we may credit Sebastiano del Piombo's amused reference to her in August 1532, when he said, 'the bailiff's wife is in love with you; she has made an offer of the beds, the furniture and everything she possesses down to the hens. I have not liked to accept anything without your permission, but as she will be your neighbour, she may be useful to you.'[54]

From this remark of Sebastiano's we see at once that Michelangelo's style of living was not pretentious; but it would be a mistake to suppose that he always meant precisely the same thing by the statement, 'I live poorly', which is recurrent in the letters, or precisely what we should mean by a use of the term *poveramente* to-day. In his early years in Rome, when his family was nothing but a liability and he had no-one to depend upon but himself, he certainly knew the meaning of privation, so much so at times that his father felt constrained to warn him that to live frugally was one thing, to live penuriously another.[55] We know, too, that he lived in appalling conditions in Bologna while working on the bronze Pope, not, however, by choice, but of necessity. Though not quite so bad, conditions do not appear to have been appreciably different during the four years in which he was engaged on the Sistine vault, since, when Buonarroto asked him to entertain Lorenzo Strozzi when he was passing through Rome, he received this reply: 'I do not think you realize how I am living here. However, I must forgive you for that' – a comment from which we may draw the conclusion that it had never occurred to Buonarroto that his brother's circumstances would not be such as to permit him to entertain Lorenzo, at least adequately, on this occasion.[56] But Michelangelo was right. His brother could not have realized how great was the pressure under which he laboured nor how inadequate were the rewards, because, for some reason impossible to ascertain, the artist (like the scholar) seems to be expected to work infinitely harder than anyone else for infinitely less, as if, forsooth, it were all delight and that delight sufficient to physic all pains. But alas it is not, as Michelangelo knew to his cost, for at this time he was scarcely able to provide for his own necessities. Only those lacking altogether in imagination would expect his letters to his family to be filled, under these circumstances, with sensitive observations on his art (about which they cared little and of which they would soon have grown heartily sick) rather than with the day to day problems of living, which impinged upon him no less than upon everyone else. The visions of the painter are perpetuated in the vault; the cares of the man in his letters.

With his return to Rome at the beginning of 1513 the most precarious years of his career were over. Then it was that he took up residence in the Macel de' Corvi, in the house purchased for him by the della Rovere for the purpose of executing the Julius Tomb. This property is thus described in the Contract of 1516: 'A house of several storeys, with reception rooms, bedrooms, grounds, a vegetable garden, wells and other buildings.'[57] Included among the latter were two *casette*, or cottages, one of which was occupied at the time of Michelangelo's death by his assistant, Pierluigi Gaeta. This we learn from the agreement of May 1st 1564, whereby Daniele da Volterra rented the house from Lionardo, except for the rooms in the tower, which Lionardo retained for his own occasional use when he was in Rome.[58] So that, although by Renaissance standards the house was not palatial, the property as a whole was not inconsiderable, as may be judged both from the description and from the price which the Buonarroti obtained for it when they sold it to a certain Stefano Lunghi in 1605 for three thousand eight hundred *scudi*, a sum substantially higher than the amount which Michelangelo knew he would have to pay for the imposing house he had wished to buy for his nephew in Florence.

Here, then, Michelangelo settled down with his assistants, apprentices and at least one servant, since a Bolognese *fante* is specifically mentioned,[59] intending, as he informed his father, to live 'simply' (not as heretofore 'poorly') in his own house.[60] It is true that many years later, when he employed both men and women servants, he told Lionardo that he lived 'poorly' but that he paid well,[61] by which, however, he clearly did not mean 'poorly' in the poverty-stricken sense in which he had formerly used the term, but rather, it would seem, 'poorly' in comparison with the great households of the cardinals and prelates with whom he habitually associated at that period of his life. Nor in such a context could he have thought of his mode of life as other than 'poor', when one considers that according to the census of 1526/27 the *bocchi* in the household of Niccolò Ridolfi had numbered one hundred and eighty and that this was a modest retinue in comparison with that of Alessandro Farnese, the future Pope, whose household comprised no fewer than three hundred and six mouths in all.[62] But because Michelangelo lived 'simply' in a way adapted to the requirements of his profession, this does not mean that he lived in a state of squalid disorder, as some have imagined. Indeed, from such indications as we possess, we should be justified in reaching a different conclusion. In the same way, a great deal that has been said concerning his attitude to dress and his way of living generally may be discounted, being as it is, not only without foundation, but such balderdash as to be palpably untrue.

Much of the misunderstanding that has arisen in this connection may be traced to the passage in which Condivi, when discussing Michelangelo's appearance and habits, says this of him; 'Many a time when he was more robust, he had slept in his clothes with his slippers on',[63] a statement which, while undoubtedly true, requires some qualification. How often when living in impossible conditions in Bologna, may he not have flung himself down just as he was, worn out with fatigue and anxiety, during his prodigious labours on the bronze Pope; how often, too, after a long hard day in the mountains, when his strength and patience had been taxed to the uttermost, may he not have been glad to sleep as best he could with the added protection of his clothes when it was cold. But to suppose that he did so either by habit or from choice would be as ridiculous as to suppose that he slept four in a bed by preference and not of necessity.[64] No doubt stories of his early days lost nothing in the telling when he afterwards recalled them for the benefit of artists of a younger generation, some of whom failed to realize that Michelangelo could not always be taken seriously, being given, as he was, to nothing if not to exaggeration, of which a notable example is provided by the postscript to his letter to Giovansimone of 1509 and another by one of his letters to Lodovico, written about three years later;[65] neither of which is wanting in picturesque embellishment. Did he really slough his skin like a snake when he removed the dogskin slippers which, as an old man, he wore 'for months together' beneath his hose?[66] It seems highly unlikely from every point of view. Was he, in fact, unable to read letters or to look at drawings except with his head thrown back for months after the completion of the Sistine vault, because of the injury caused to his sight?[67] If this was so, it certainly seems strange that there is no mention of such a disability in the letters which he was writing normally throughout the period in question. Did he really 'feel no fatigue'[68] during the four long years during which he toiled on the vault – *non sendo in loco bon* – standing and lying in every conceivable position in the effort to accomplish his task? Certainly this was not the case, if we are to believe the evidence of his own letters and of the bitter, though amusing, verses on the subject, which he addressed to his friend, Giovanni da Pistoia.[69] During periods such as these, when he was immersed in work of a peculiarly difficult and intensive kind, it must be obvious that he would have had neither the time, the occasion, nor the energy to concern himself with matters of dress, but to suppose on that account that he was habitually indifferent to appearances would be to ignore the probabilities and such evidence as we have at our command.

No-one as proud as Michelangelo of what he believed to be the noble descent of his family, no-one as anxious to re-establish its fortunes and to maintain its honour, and no-one as insistent as he that his relations should do him credit, is likely under normal circumstances to have been negligent about his own appearance. In 1540 he had sent a not very tactful message to his brother Gismondo, whose habit of 'trudging after oxen' caused him much annoyance, in these words: 'Tell him', he wrote to Lionardo, 'that he does us little honour in making a peasant of himself',[70] and when a year later Lionardo wished to visit Rome, Michelangelo wrote to him saying, 'You must wait until next Lent . . . when I will send you money to equip yourself that you may not come here like a nobody.'[71] Being a true Florentine and having a brother in the wool-trade, besides, he was himself an excellent judge of cloth, and always insisted upon the best both for himself and for other people.[72] He was particular about the fit of his own clothes and had procured a length of satin for a doublet for himself of so superior a quality that he deemed it suitable to present to Arcadelt in acknowledgment of his services.[73] His fury when Lionardo sent him a present of shirts 'so coarse', as he said, 'that there's not a peasant in Rome who would not be ashamed to wear them',[74] leaves us, moreover, in no doubt as to the quality of the linen he wore, of which he possessed an ample supply, according to the inventory of his effects taken after his death.[75] Though somewhat worn, like the garments of most old men, the clothes then remaining in his wardrobe were handsome rather than otherwise, as one would expect from the description of the Cordovan leather boots made to his own design which he habitually wore, and from the style of the black damask doublets in which he was invariably depicted in the portraits and in the engravings with which we are familiar. This type of garment he seems generally to have worn during the later years of his life and it was in a doublet such as this, with spurred boots upon his feet and a velvet cap of antique cut upon his head, that he was finally interred.[76]

So much then for this 'irritable old recluse' and his mode of life in the squalor and isolation of the 'hovel' in the Macel de' Corvi of which we sometimes hear tell[77] – the 'hovel' which, together with its contents, he estimated to be worth several thousands of *scudi* and in which, for all his pride, he seems, strangely enough, not to have been ashamed to receive the envoy of the Duke of Florence![78]

The first twelve years of Michelangelo's permanent residence in Rome were, beyond question, the richest years of his life, both intellectually and spiritually, and, since the days of his youth, also the happiest. These were the years of his most intimate and profound relationships and the least troubled of the last thirty troubled years of his life in Rome. While remaining as always deeply attached to his Messer Tommao, and while enjoying the devoted support, first of Bartolomeo Angiolini, and afterwards of Luigi del Riccio, he now entered upon a new experience – a close friendship with a woman, but of a rare and special kind.

At the time of his first meeting with Vittoria Colonna in 1536 she had been a widow for eleven years, seven of which she is traditionally held to have spent in mourning for her husband, Ferrante d'Avalos, Marchese di Pescara, of whom, however, she had seen very little during their sixteen years of married life, as after the first three which they spent in Ischia together he had been continually at the wars. The last occasion on which she saw him was in 1522, three years before his death, and then only briefly. She had, nevertheless, been grief-stricken at her loss and had found such consolation as might be hers in writing innumerable poems to his memory. All the same, the notion that it was because she was still unable to assuage her sorrow after seven years that she at last 'disposed herself to the raising of her mind above earthly affairs and fixed them on divine ones, convinced that this was the only means of freeing the soul from those affections whence come most of this world's bitterness'[79] would seem to lack verisimilitude. In all probability it would be truer to say that her bereavement, followed so soon after by the sack of Rome, which had shattered the City and appalled the whole of Europe, had disposed her, on her return to Rome, to seek a less ceremonious and less lonely way of life than that to which she had been accustomed. This could then best be found in monasteries where, attended by her own servants and without taking the veil, she could take some part in the conventual life, for which she would appear to have had a natural aptitude. Thus it was that she became increasingly absorbed in the religious controversies of the day which formed the principal preoccupation of the society in which she moved. She knew and corresponded with all the leading churchmen and humanists of the age, amongst whom she was held in the highest repute, while she herself held sufficiently liberal views to have become almost dangerously involved with Fra Bernardino Ochino, to whom, prior to his apostasy, she had even gone to the length of signing herself, 'Your Reverence's most obedient daughter and disciple'. Happily, however, she drew back in time. For she had been so far implicated that one of the questions on which Pietro Carnesecchi was closely pressed, during his trial before the Inquisition many years later, was the degree to which he had been influenced by her views.[80] It was not, however, until she placed herself under the spiritual guidance of Cardinal Pole (who in the eyes of the fanatical Caraffa Pope did not escape suspicion of heresy himself) that she finally found, at least in some measure, that tranquility of soul for which she yearned.

What it was that originally attracted Vittoria Colonna and Michelangelo to each other can only be surmised. By conventional standards she was not beautiful, despite the fact that at the time of her marriage 'the chroniclers had agreed that nowhere could be found a more beautiful, virtuous and gifted couple', but in this connection we cannot lose sight of the fact that all brides are beautiful and all bridegrooms virtuous – at least for the time being, and it had not yet been said of the Marchese that 'there was not to be found in his day anyone more deeply dyed in perfidy or more courageous in arms'.[81] As to the Marchesa, had she been beautiful, Ariosto could not have failed to mention it in his lines in praise of her, which are devoted, however, entirely to the virtues of the mind, in which she was certainly not wanting. But if not beautiful, her quality, as portrayed by Francisco d'Ollanda particularly in the first of his three Dialogues (and there seems no reason to doubt his veracity), is unmistakable. In every sense of the term, a great lady, she was characterized at once by that dignity of bearing and that ease of manner by which the aristocrat is pre-eminently distinguished. And not only so, for though contemplative by nature, she possessed a lightness of touch and a social grace which Ollanda, for his part, found entirely delightful. Nor was he less impressed by her insight where Michelangelo was concerned and by the skill with which she induced him to do as she desired for the benefit and pleasure of herself and the rest of the company. But in any case, as Ollanda put it, 'the Marchesa was bound to conquer, nor do I see who could defend himself against her'. As for Michelangelo, he was powerless to resist her and perhaps in his heart of hearts he had no real wish to do so.

Once again, by reason of the burning ardour of his nature, he had caught fire. Potentially romantic, the feeling he entertained for her was intense and the level of their communion something that he had never before experienced. To him she appeared beautiful perhaps above all in virtue of that transcendent 'beauty of the inward soul', communicated through the eyes, the eyes by which he was always and so strangely haunted – *Che gli occhi senza 'l cor non han virtute*.[82] And in this connection the rather pathetic lines in which he lamented his own ugliness – *Mentre i begli occhi giri* – (which Frey seems justified in associating with Vittoria Colonna) may also be quoted:

> *Ben par che 'l ciel s'adiri,*
> *Che 'n si begli occhi io me veggia si brutto,*
> *E ne' miei brutti ti veggia si bella.*

It is from lines such as these, taken in conjunction with some of the other poems he addressed to her, especially *Se'l troppo indugio ha più grazia e ventura*,[83] one of the most moving of the sonnets, that the extent to which his feeling amounted once again to a sublimated passion can best be gauged. For her the friendship was on rather a different plane, though the tenderness of her regard for him and her appreciation of his qualities matched his own for her. In the Portuguese Dialogues she is recorded as having said to him, 'In Rome those who know you esteem you more than your works; those who do not know you esteem the least part of you, even the work of your hands.'[84]

Of his own vulnerability no-one was more aware than Michelangelo himself, who, in one of the sonnets, *Al cor di zolfo, alla carne di stoppa*, written at about this time or according to Frey, a little earlier, so aptly describes the state of his mind at this time that it may not be out of place to quote it in full in Symonds's translation, which is sufficiently felicitious to render the spirit of the original:

> A heart of flaming sulphur, flesh of tow,
>> Bones of dry wood, a soul without a guide
>> To curb the fiery will, the ruffling pride
>> Of fierce desires that from the passions flow;
> A sightless mind that weak and lame doth go
>> Mid snares and pitfalls scattered far and wide:
>> What wonder if the first chance brand applied
>> To fuel massed like this should make it glow?
> Add beauteous art, which, brought with us from heaven,
>> Will conquer nature; – so divine a power
>> Belongs to him who strives with every nerve.
> If I was made for art, from childhood given
>> A prey for burning beauty to devour,
>> I blame the mistress I was born to serve.[85]

'A soul without a guide' – *Alma senza guida* – this apparently was what he felt himself to be in a world of changing beliefs, and declining faith, a state of bewilderment not unknown to Vittoria Colonna herself, who had expressed a comparable sentiment in one of her own sonnets:

> . . . . *ed in me ancora*
> *Ragion vuol che nel mal cresca la fede.*[86]

All things considered, it is unlikely that Michelangelo was either as perplexed in mind or as intellectually troubled by the conflict of religious opinions as she had been before she was able to say with confidence, as she did in 1541 in a letter to her kinswoman, the beautiful Giulia Gonzaga, who was also involved with the *spirituali*, 'I owe the health of both my soul and my body to Cardinal Pole; the former was endangered by superstition, the latter by misrule.'[87] Over the crucial question of the doctrine of justification he wisely advised her 'to believe that she could only be saved by faith, but to act as if she could only be saved by works',[88] than which a more judicious compromise could hardly be found. For Michelangelo the case was different. To begin with, he had less time to devote to scholastic considerations, and if he was troubled at all by matters of dogma it was only superficially so. Rather was he oppressed by a sense of his own sins and shortcomings – *Carico d'anni e di peccati pieno*[89] – and by doubts as to the sufficiency of his own faith – faith which he once described as the gift of gifts – *Il don de' doni*[90] – in which, even at a much later date, he felt himself to be deficient. Perhaps it was that his faith was of a different order from that which was vaunted in his day, since it had nothing in common with the ecstasies of the converted. One cannot imagine that he would have had any more use for the tears and tremblings of the saints than he had for the sanctity of the master-weaver's wife,[91] or that he would ever have vied with any cardinal for the privilege of holding the basin for the vomiting of St. Philip Neri.[92]

Though naturally prone at times to waver – *Ora in sul destra, ora in sul manco piede*[93] – he was in fact sustained throughout his life by a profound yet simple trust in God, and during a long and arduous pilgrimage may fairly be said to have fulfilled the ancient Hebrew ideal of the God-fearing man; 'He hath showed thee, O man, what is good; and what doth the Lord require of thee, but to do justly and to love mercy and to walk humbly with thy God.'[94] Nor, beyond the inevitable change of vision from the 'dreams of youth' to the reflections of old age, is there anything to show that he ever became intrinsically different from what he had always been; for it is noticeable that in many respects he never changed. There is, for example, no appreciable difference between the tone and style of his first extant letters and his last, except that he prefaced the first three with a religious invocation, which he never afterwards used; while only in a letter to Buonarroto written in 1517 did he conclude, for some unaccountable reason, with the words *Cristo vi guardi*.[95] In none of his other letters did he make use of any of the customary formulae – *Dio di male vi guardi* – *Cristo sano vi conservi* – *Iddio vi prosperi* – still less of the abbreviation, *Iddio etc.* – which would suggest that there was nothing either perfunctory, sanctimonious, or superstitious in his approach.

In general, however, Michelangelo observed the conventions of his period, conforming outwardly to the forms of worship prescribed by the Church and accepting inwardly the basic principles of his creed with the simplicity of a child. There is no question but that the hope of heaven was very real to him and that he found immense comfort in the expectation of paradise. This thought was, after all, the main solace to him for the death, first of his brother and then of his father:

> *E se 'l pensier, nel quale i' mi profondo,*
> *Non fussi che 'l ben morto in ciel si ridi*
> *Del timor del morire in questo mondo:*
>
> *Cresciere' 'l duol: ma' dolorosi stridi*
> *Temprati son d' una credenza ferma,*
> *Che 'l ben vissuto, a morte me' s' annidi.*[96]

But if he believed like a child, like a child he also stood in need of reassurance and encouragement, guidance and consolation. And this, in large measure, Vittoria Colonna was able to give him, with something perhaps of a mother's tenderness, a type of affection he had never known, but which may not have come any more amiss to him, old though he was, than it came to Reginald Pole, when his own mother died upon the scaffold.[97] But it was not only in the role of a human comforter that she meant so much to him; it was also in that of a spiritual mentor in whom he reposed a confidence as implicit as that which Dante reposed in Beatrice – *quella donna ch' a Dio mi meneva*.[98] He might, indeed, have used the very words of the poet himself, had he not sung for her so many songs of his own, in none of which is the dual role in which he conceived her, as being at once both the end, and the means of its attainment, more beautifully expressed than in this, one of the most famous of his madrigals:

> *A l' alta tuo lucente diadema*
> *Per la strada erta e lunga*
> *Non è, donna, chi giunga,*
> *S' umiltà non v' aggiugni e cortesia:*
> *Il montar cresce, e 'l mie valore scema;*
> *E la lena mi manca a mezza via.*
> *Che tuo beltà pur sia*
> *Superna, al cor par che diletto renda,*
> *Che d' ogni rara altezza è giotto e vago:*
> *Po' per gioir della tuo leggiadria,*
> *Bramo pur che discenda*
> *Là dov' aggiungo: e 'n tal pensier m' appago,*
> *Se 'l tuo sdegnio presago,*
> *Per basso amare e alto odiar tuo stato,*
> *A te stessa perdona il mie peccato.*[99]

Yet greatly though he loved her, being, as Condivi records, 'enamoured of her divine spirit', she, for her part, loved him tenderly in return, and 'often came to Rome from Viterbo and other places, whither she went for her pleasure and to pass the summer, for no other reason but to see him'. From among many whom he thought to be *più nobil genti* she singled him out and invariably treated him with an esteem becoming both to his age and to his eminence. On one occasion she addressed him as *Unico maestro Michelangelo et mio singularissimo amico* and on another she sent him this letter with a copy of her poems:

Magnifico Messer Michelangelo,

So great is the fame conferred upon you by your art that you might perhaps never have believed that either through time or through any other cause it would prove to be subject to death, unless that divine light had entered your heart, which has shown to you that earthly glory, however long it may endure, has nevertheless its own second death. Therefore, beholding in your sculpture the beneficence of the

One Who has made you a supreme master, you will recognize that by my writings which are, as it were, already dead, I give thanks to the Lord only because by writing I used to offend Him less than I now do by idleness. And I beg you to accept this my attempt as an earnest of future works. At your command.[100]

This gift, and the almost apologetic note which accompanied it, Michelangelo acknowledged with extraordinary grace in the following sonnet, which reveals, in some ways better than almost anything else, the essential charm of their relationship:

> *Felice spirto, che con zelo ardente,*
>   *Vecchio alla morte, in vita il mio cor tieni,*
>   *E fra mill' altri tuo' diletti e beni*
>   *Me sol saluti fra più nobil gente;*
> *Come mi fusti agli occhi, or alla mente,*
>   *Per l'altru' fiate, a consolar mi vieni:*
>   *Onde la speme il duol par che raffreni,*
>   *Che non men che 'l disio l' anima sente.*
> *Dunche trovando in te chi per me parla,*
>   *Grazia di te per me fra tante cure,*
>   *Tal grazia ne ringrazia chi ti scrive.*
> *Che sconcia e grand' usur saria a farla,*
>   *Donandoti turpissime pitture*
>   *Per riaver persone belle e vive.*[101]

Thus it is that the truth of Michelangelo's last recorded words concerning her is borne in upon us – 'The Marchesa di Pescara was devoted to me', he wrote, 'and I no less to her.'[102] Nor, we may surmise, would the Marchesa herself have complained had she foreseen that ultimately it would be 'his name that has carried hers across the ages'.

On March 20th 1546 Michelangelo received the supreme honour of Roman citizenship.[103] But he always remained a Florentine at heart and only towards the end of his life, when the unprecedented amiabilities of the Duke finally reconciled him to the new régime, did he cease to lament the feuds and factions which had in the end deprived the city of her republican liberties. The nostalgia which he still felt for his native Tuscany – *Toscana nostra* – some ten years or more after his final departure is briefly indicated by Donato Giannotti in the first of his *Dialoghi*,[104] which affords a pleasant insight into the ease and intimacy of the relationship which existed between some of the Florentines in Rome, whether *fuorusciti* or not. It also shows the readiness with which Michelangelo gave of himself to his friends when he was at leisure and in a mood to do so.

'Well met', he exclaimed with pleasure when one morning he and Giannotti encountered Luigi del Riccio and Antonio Petroneo, as they were walking towards St. John Lateran, 'this is a fortunate chance to have met you here.' And then, in answer to Antonio's remark that he and del Riccio would be more than happy if Michelangelo and Giannotti would join them in their walk, he replied, with that touch of irony for which he was famous, 'If to-day your happiness consists in having us for company, you have come by it; because we are ready to join you.' After further amusing interchanges, as they went along, the conversation turned upon Dante and the length of time he had spent in the exploration of Hell and Purgatory, a conversation in which for once, and contrary to his usual practice, Michelangelo took the lead. The discussion continued until about midday when the friends parted with the intention of meeting again after vespers outside the house of Francesco Priscianese, the printer. Giannotti and Antonio were late, having been detained by their patron, Cardinal Ridolfi, who would have kept Giannotti even longer had he not learnt that he had an appointment with Michelangelo, whereupon, as Giannotti remarked to his companions, as they approached, 'he released me at once without another word, so great is his pleasure in gratifying such a man over anything, however small it may be.'

While Michelangelo and del Riccio had been waiting for the others, Priscianese had taken them round and shown them the printing presses, in which Michelangelo displayed great interest and on taking leave of him to continue their walk in the direction of the Porta del Popolo, Michelangelo turned to him saying, 'Messer Francesco, all I can say is that you may always rest assured that I am not only willing but anxious to be of service to you.'

In the dissertation which followed Giannotti took no part until the end, and then he entered into an animated, not to say a heated, discussion with Michelangelo as to whether Dante was justified in consigning Brutus and Cassius to the jaws of Lucifer,[105] Giannotti, the republican *par excellence*, maintaining that he was not; Michelangelo, the *dantista*, maintaining that he was. To the amusement of the others they persisted in their arguments for some time, each stoutly contending for his own view, until at last, still unconvinced, Giannotti gave up, saying that he would see Michelangelo home and that if he were cross with him, he would make his peace on the way. But before they separated del Riccio asked Michelangelo to recite the sonnet he had recently composed in praise of Dante, *Quella benigna stella che co' suoi*,[106] which Michelangelo consented to do, though averring that it was unworthy of their ears.

After del Riccio's death Giannotti became the closest of Michelangelo's Florentine contemporaries (or virtual contemporaries) in Rome, despite his frequent absences, first in the suite of Cardinal Ridolfi and after his death in that of the French Cardinal, François de Tournon. But that was not yet, and in the meantime Michelangelo and del Riccio maintained a day to day relationship of the most intimate and delightful kind. All that we know of del Riccio's character leaves us with the impression of a man with a genius for friendship. Generous, noble, kind and considerate, in a way seldom encountered, he and Michelangelo shared not only the minor pleasures of life, involving an endless exchange of small courtesies and communications, 'part banter, part affection', such as are savoured by all who understand the true meaning of friendship, but also the major anxieties and griefs from which few are exempt. And in nothing is this more evident than in the way in which Michelangelo endeavoured to solace and to cheer del Riccio when he suddenly found himself bereft by the death of his young kinsman, Cecchino de' Bracci, the apple of his eye and the idol of the Florentine circle in Rome.

According to Symonds,[107] del Riccio and Michelangelo 'were drawn together by a common love of poetry and by the charm of *[this]* rarely gifted youth'. Although the emphasis is wrong as regards Cecchino, there can be no doubt that del Riccio possessed what Michelangelo called 'the spirit of poetry' and that it was mainly to divert him after Cecchino's death that he undertook to send him fifteen or sixteen[108] *polizini* (perhaps one for each year of the boy's age). To say of these epigrams that 'they rate low among his poems, having too much of scholastic trifling and too little of the accent of strong feeling in them,' is to postulate an intention that never existed. Much of this verse Michelangelo himself valued, as we know, at 'one sturgeon's egg' and no more, and to imagine otherwise is to misunderstand the nature of the whole proceeding. Whenever del Riccio sent him some delicacy, as he frequently did, he composed a quatrain in return, to which from time to time he would add a note such as, 'I did not mean to send you this, because it is very stupid, but the trout and truffles would prevail even with heaven'; and on another occasion, 'Nonsense! the fount is dry – you must wait till it rains. You are in too much of a hurry', from all of which it is obvious that Michelangelo was not himself emotionally involved, regretful though he was, like Giannotti and others, at the premature death of a youth to whom they were all attached, but who was as dear to the childless del Riccio as a son.[109]

To one of these quatrains Michelangelo added two lines in jest, which were afterwards omitted by del Riccio in the fair copy in the Magliabechiano Codex and by Guasti in his edition of the *Rime*, but were included by Frey in his edition of the *Dichtungen*.[110] The quatrain in question is as follows:

> *La carne terra, qui l' ossa mie prive*
> *De' lor begli occhi e del leggiandro aspetto,*
> *Fan fede a quel ch' i' fu grazia e diletto*
> *In che carcer quaggiù l' anima vive.*

lines which in English may be rendered:

> My flesh become dust and my bones which here repose,
> Deprived of the beautiful eyes and the fair countenance,
> Attest to him to whom I was an object of affection and delight
> In what a prison-house the spirit dwelt below.

The parody of the last two lines which Michelangelo added ran thus:

> *Fan fede a quel ch' i' fu grazia nel letto*
> *Che abbracciava, e'n che l' anima vive.*

To anyone who looks at these two lines with attention, it instantly becomes clear that Michelangelo, with his typically Renaissance penchant for a pun, happened to observe the ease with which a salacious twist could be given to the lines merely by substituting the words *nel letto* for *diletto*, and *che abbracciava* for *che carcer*, so that they would then read, 'Attest to him to whom I was an object of affection in bed in what an embrace the spirit dwelt below.' To these lines – a mere *jeu d'esprit* on Michelangelo's part, which he could not resist sending once he had thought of it – he added a note saying, 'Learn these last two lines, which are a moral lesson, and this I'm sending you as a reckoning for the fifteen *polizini*.' It is a pity he wrote them, because it has lead to the assumption that he intended them to be taken as a covert rebuke to del Riccio, an assumption that could only be made by those unfamiliar with his sardonic sense of humour. Yet more pompous rot has been talked about these two lines than can well be believed. Thus from America we have the following – 'I must now call [*sic*] the reader's attention to Quatrain No. 19. The two-line variant, which follows it, shows clearly that Michelangelo knew something else about Luigi del Riccio's admiration for the lad. But he too had once asked Luigi to inform him whether "our idol" [*Cecchino*], of whom he had dreamed, would encourage him or threaten him.'[111] This in all conscience is foolish enough, but what of this? '. . . there is strong reason to suppose that the artist entered into homosexual relations with the fifteen-year-old Cecchino Bracci, at whose death he composed fifty poems of an admiring nature, but revealing no nobility of feeling. Indeed, the ribald verses of LXXIII, 19, with their salacious footnote to Luigi del Riccio, which editors also pass under [*sic*] silence, compromise both the artist and his friend del Riccio.'[112] To this there is but one retort, albeit of the ungodly, – Tush ! and again, Tush !

Yet notwithstanding the inherent absurdity of the idea that both men were implicated, it might be as well to examine the circumstances a little more closely, lest some measure of special pleading might here seem to be involved.

As to del Riccio, it can only be said that from all we know of his character and despite the unpredictability of human nature where sex is concerned, nothing in the world would seem more unlikely than that he would either himself have corrupted the boy, whose guardian he was, or have allowed anyone else to do so. While as to Michelangelo, it has already been shown that, whether or not he ever had physical relations with men of his own age, he was most certainly not a paederast.[113] But apart from that, does it seem feasible, at a period when he was much concerned for the welfare of his soul, when he had long since come to think of himself as being *si presso a morte, e si lontan da Dio*,[114] and when he was in close spiritual communion with Vittoria Colonna, to whom, as she wrote, he had spoken of Christ with such a fervent and humble heart, that at the age of nearly sixty-nine, a man such as Michelangelo, should at the same time be indulging in an illicit relationship with a boy not yet sixteen years of age? And if it does not, what is the explanation of the parody, if a serious answer must be found for a piece of verbal ingenuity of no consequence? In all probability, it referred back to something that had been previously discussed. Ever since the uncovering of *The Last Judgment* three years before, when the Theatines had been the first to object to the nudities,[115] Michelangelo had been open to accusations of impudicity and perhaps worse, and it may be that some base insinuation in the vein of Aretino had recently been made, and that in the distorted lines he was only indicating to del Riccio how fatally easy it was to falsify anything, if one had a mind to do so. But, most pertinently of all, had there been any truth in the innuendo, the variant would never have been added.

In speaking of del Riccio's omission of the two lines quoted above, Frey says that he did rightly, as likewise did Michelangelo the Younger, but he contends that in Guasti's case this procedure is incomprehensible because 'he should have known Michelangelo better'. For, as he goes on to say, 'cynicisms of this kind are nothing more than casual observations and provide no basis for judging the poet, his eroticism, or the relationship between del Riccio and Cecchino. At most the addition of the two lines shows that in Michelangelo's case the composition of these epitaphs was nothing more than an occasional stylistic exercise.'[116]

Throughout the last years of Michelangelo's work on the Tomb of Julius II del Riccio was a constant support to him in every possible way. Like the long Petition to Paul III, the letter to Cardinal Farnese[117] is almost certainly in his hand. He it was who formulated the letters to the bank, who interpreted documents, who intervened in quarrels between Michelangelo's assistants, and performed any such services of which he stood in need. He it was who tried to improve Lionardo's relations with his uncle, who cared for Michelangelo in his own apartments on two occasions when he was ill, and who gave every proof of what he conceived to be the nature of friendship. To this conception he made allusion in an answering madrigal to one of Michelangelo's, in which the latter acknowledged his indebtedness to del Riccio for his kindness on one of the aforementioned occasions:

> *Non debbe esser molesta*
> *Alcuna cortesia*
> *Fra li amici, et antica opinione*
> *Del mondo è stata questa:*
> *Ch' ogni cosa sia*
> *Fra lor comune; et entrar già in prigione*
> *L' uno a morir per l' altro; e di ragione,*
> *Roba, vita et onor fra lor si dona,*
> *Dunque fra noi nascier non può quistione;*
> *Poi che a nulla amicizia non perdona.*[118]

On neither side, therefore, was there the least doubt as to what Michelangelo recognized to be 'the true friendship that exists between us'; for which reason the misunderstanding that arose over the engraving[119] must have come as an extraordinary shock to each of them in turn: to Michelangelo, who thought, though he could scarcely credit it, that del Riccio had insulted and intended to dupe him; to del Riccio who could hardly believe it possible that Michelangelo could imagine such a thing or could so far misinterpret his intentions. There are grounds for thinking, moreover, that of the two it was del Riccio who was finally the more hurt and the more offended and that Michelangelo had to exercise a good deal of tact before a complete reconciliation was effected.

Although Bartolomeo Angiolini may have known him almost, if not quite as well, no-one among Michelangelo's many friends knew him more intimately or understood him better than Luigi del Riccio. For just as Giovanni Maria della Porta had observed the expediency of getting the Duke of Urbino to write Michelangelo a line in his own hand about the ratification of the Contract of 1532, since, as he said, 'I am told that with the knowledge of Your Lordship's good-will this man would show himself to be amenable and would work miracles',[120] so del Riccio, while never making the mistake of taking his objections too seriously, always remained mindful of the fact that though he might be cajoled he could never be coerced. This was why he was able to persuade Michelangelo to accede to the Pope's wishes, even when initially he had been least inclined to do so, an ability of which the papal entourage was well aware.

Towards Paul III himself, for whom he had a considerable liking and respect, Michelangelo behaved, apparently, with the same frankness and ease of manner that he had used towards Julius II and Clement VII. Being born, as he said of himself, with a dislike of ceremony and dissimulation, he declined to gratify the Pope by standing about all day like a courtier, when he was not needed, believing, as he told Ollanda, that he served His Holiness better by working for him in his own house. 'Sometimes, I may tell you,' he added, 'my important duties have given me so much licence, that when I am talking to the Pope I put this old felt hat nonchalantly on my head and talk to him very frankly, but he does not put me to death on that account.' On the contrary, one may imagine that like his predecessors Pope Paul found such an approach, which never transgressed the boundary of good manners, exceedingly refreshing, even more so perhaps than the *trebbiano* and the fruit which Michelangelo was accustomed to present to him from time to time. But if one thing is more certain than another, it is that he valued Michelangelo's services almost beyond price and was prepared to accommodate him in every way possible. Evidence of this is afforded by the pains that were taken by Cardinal Farnese not only to protect his interests over the Po Ferry, but also to ease his mind over the Tomb.[121] There is, however, another item of considerable interest in connection with Michelangelo's relations with Pope Pagolo, and that is a note from Jacopo Melighini intimating the Pope's desire to see the Pauline frescoes and to talk to him *if it were not inconvenient*, as His Holiness was alone and *asked him to say at what time he could come*. This note was sent round to Michelangelo on the feast of San Lorenzo, August 10th, but the year remains conjectural.[122] The terms in which it is couched are, however, so accommodating and so far from being in the nature of a command, that one is tempted to wonder whether something more than a desire to enjoy Michelangelo's company did not lie behind it. Was the note not perhaps written in 1546, and had not the Pope learnt of the death of his architect, Antonio da Sangallo? And if so, was he not minded to sound Michelangelo as to a possible successor to Sangallo at St. Peter's? The question as far as Michelangelo was concerned was an ominous one, but whether or not the interview in question took place immediately after Sangallo's death or later on, by the August of 1546 Michelangelo was about to enter upon one of the two most desolate periods of his life.

Little did he think when, on the morning of his discourse on Dante, he proposed the contemplation of death as a man's best defence against the sunderings of the world and as the most effective means of restoring him to himself,[123] that it would not be the light of his own lantern that would be the first to be quenched; for, as he remarked to Vasari a few years later, 'I am so old that Death has frequently plucked me by the mantle to take me away with him.'[124] Instead, however, he it was who was left to face the darkness which descended upon him, as one by one the lanterns in the hands of those, for the most part, younger than himself fell to the ground. To his intense grief and consternation Luigi del Riccio died in the autumn of 1546, leaving him bereft not only of the most intimate of all his friends, but of the man upon whom he was most dependent for help and advice in his many concerns, public and private alike. Nor does it seem that he ever found anyone to take del Riccio's place in anything like the same way, though later on Francesco Bandini appears to have acted to some extent for him in business matters and to have become a close friend as well.

Almost it might seem as if to try him to the uttermost, as gold in the furnace is tried, scarcely had he become accustomed to the void left by the death of Luigi del Riccio, when he was overwhelmed by another and no less devastating grief – the loss of Vittoria Colonna, who died some four months later, on February 25th 1547. She had been ill for some time, perhaps with a recurrence of the malady from which she had suffered while at Viterbo in 1543, when Girolamo Fracastoro, the celebrated Veronese physician to the Council of Trent, had been consulted. Yet even so, nothing could mitigate the shock of her passing. And, when he afterwards went to see her to take his final leave, to his lasting regret 'he did not kiss her on the brow or on the cheek, as he did kiss her hand.'[125] For some time after this he remained sorrowfully at home in a state of utter desolation that can better be imagined than described, but which is indicated in the last paragraph of a letter to his old friend Fattucci, written towards the end of March, in which he said, 'Having been very unhappy lately, I have been at home and in going through some of my things a great number of the trifles *[meaning his poems]* which I formerly used to send you came to hand, from among which I'm sending you four. . . . You will say rightly that I am old and distracted, but I assure you that only distractions prevent one from being beside oneself with grief.'[126]

Though aroused somewhat from his lethargy by the receipt of a manuscript copy of Varchi's *Due Lezioni* delivered to the Florentine Academy, which undoubtedly afforded him enormous pleasure and gratification, the undercurrent of his emotions is nevertheless discernible in the letters of acknowledgment which he wrote in reply to Luca Martini and to Benedetto Varchi himself. To the one he described himself as being 'not only an old man, but almost numbered among the dead', while to the other he expressed himself in even more moving terms when he said, 'I am an old man and death has robbed me of the dreams of youth – may those who do not know what old age means bear it with what patience they may when they reach it, because it cannot be imagined beforehand.'[127]

He was now seventy-two years of age and of these years he had spent forty-two in the service of four out of five successive Popes. But what in terms of professional satisfaction and personal fulfilment had this service meant to him? In the case of one private and two public commissions he had been obliged to default; the finished cartoon for *The Battle of Cascina* had been destroyed; the bronze figure of Julius II, which he had wrought at such pains and without profit to himself, had been cast down. By a superhuman effort he had completed the Sistine vault. and had been cheated of half his reward. He had been forced to undertake the façade of San Lorenzo and had lost three of the best years of his life in the marble quarries at Pietra Santa, at the end of which the contract, to his intense mortification, had been cancelled. He had begun work on the New Sacristy, the Laurentian Library and the Medici Tombs, and had been obliged to abandon them before they were little more than half finished. Of two lesser commissions that he had been able to fulfil, one had proved a failure and the other had disappeared. In the case of the first, *The Risen Christ*, in order, as it were, to make amends, but against the advice of his friend Lionardo the saddler, he had, with immense generosity, presented Metello Vari with another but unfinished figure of Christ, which Vari had seen and desired to possess.[128] In the case of the second, the *Leda*, its loss was not only to be regretted on artistic grounds, but because it was this that had proved to be a contributary cause of the premature death of his assistant, Antonio Mini.[129] Then, on his return to Rome, Michelangelo had been obliged, contrary to his own inclinations, to undertake the painting of *The Last Judgment* and of the two frescoes in the Pauline Chapel. Last of all, there had been the fiasco of the Tomb of Julius, the whole bitterness of which is summed up in his outcry to Cardinal Farnese – 'It is borne in upon me that I lost the whole of my youth chained to this Tomb'.[130] And not only so. Even when he was ostensibly quit of it in 1545, the matter was not at an end; for unbelievable though it may seem, the issues involved were still under discussion as late as 1553. In fact, Michelangelo, knowing the monument to be as little creditable to himself as it was unworthy of the Duke, became so perturbed by the things alleged against him that

Annibale Caro, secretary to Cardinal Farnese, with whom he had recently become friendly, moved by compassion for an old man, finally felt impelled to plead Michelangelo's cause with the Duke. In a letter addressed to the Duke's secretary, Antonio Gallo, Caro, while making no attempt to exonerate Michelangelo entirely, asked 'such remission and pardon as the great are wont to offer to men of genius such as Michelangelo', since thereby the Duke might be a means of prolonging the life of so singular a man, for, as Caro assured him, 'Michelangelo is in such a fret at being in disgrace with His Excellency that this alone might be the occasion of shortening his days'.[131] Whether or not the Duke acceded to Caro's request and granted Michelangelo the consolation of which he stood in need is not known. The last reference to the affair is contained in another letter of Caro's, dated November 17th, in which he wrote thanking Gallo for his willingness to submit the case to the Duke and assuring him of Michelangelo's continuing gratitude for his good offices towards him.

In face of all this it is hardly surprising that Michelangelo, in speaking of fate and fortune in the lottery of life, should have come to think of himself as being darkly dowered, or, as he himself expressed it, *Et a me consegnaro il tempo bruno*.[132]

But no patrons were ever satisfied. Always, before he had been able to complete one commission, he was required to undertake another, and until the day of his death he was to know no respite. It was thus, precisely at a time when he had but recently been freed from the encumbrance of the Tomb; when he was still labouring on the second Pauline fresco, a task in his own view unsuited to an old man; when he was broken in spirit by the death of the two friends on whom, apart from Cavalieri and for different reasons, he had most relied, that he was compelled, wholly against his will, to undertake another task, yet more onerous than all the rest – the rebuilding of the Basilica of St. Peter. It was not, however, until two years later, on October 11th 1549, by a brief of Paul III, that supreme powers were granted to him as architect of the fabric, in succession to Antonio da Sangallo. A month later the great Farnese Pope was dead.

At the beginning of 1550, probably on Sunday, February 16th, Michelangelo again wrote to his old friend Fattucci, to whom he had written in such heartbroken terms two years before, when, in desperate need of sympathy, he had ended by saying, 'Reply to me about something, I beg of you.'[133] This time, having referred to the election of the new Pope, Julius III, he continued in these words: 'As regards my own affairs, I should be grateful, and you would be doing me the greatest kindness, if you would let me know, truthfully and without scruple, how Lionardo's affairs are going, because he is young and I am anxious about him, and more so because he is alone and without guidance.'[134]

Here spoke the true Michelangelo, whose kindly interest and genuine concern for his nephew's welfare remained constant, despite the apparent harshness of some of his letters to the boy, with whom he had by now been in correspondence for nearly ten years. Unfortunately for himself, Lionardo seems to have been lacking in just those assets most needed to recommend him to his illustrious uncle. He was not good looking; he was wanting in tact and humour; he did not write a fair italic hand. The first short-coming, though no doubt regrettable in Michelangelo's eyes, could not be held against him; the second was more serious; but the third was unforgivable, because it betrayed a lack of consideration for others, which Michelangelo rightly regarded, and tacitly assumed by his own conduct, to be the foundation of good manners. 'If you had to write to the biggest ass in the world, I believe you'd write with more care', he exclaimed angrily in a letter of 1546.[135] And, seeing that he never ceased to hear about the illegibility of his letters, one would have thought that in sheer self-defence, Lionardo would have learnt to write, if not a beautiful hand like Michelangelo's own, at least one that his uncle could read without being 'thrown into a fever' every time he received a letter. There is, moreover, no question but that he would have done himself an incalculable service had he had the nous to do so. 'I am certain', wrote del Riccio in 1545,[136] 'that if you fall in with him and are conciliatory over little things, you will have whatever you want.' But Lionardo was not heedful of good advice and continually managed to get across his uncle in various ways. Whether owing to his own error of judgment or to Fattucci's, he certainly made an initial mistake in not going to Rome when he was expected, on the completion of *The Last Judgment*, which everyone else was flocking to see. Michelangelo was neither flattered by this, nor pleased by the boy's mercenary choice of the additional fifty *scudi* promised him, if he did not come,[137] and it may fairly be said that it was at this time that he gained the impression that, like the rest of the family, Lionardo was less attached to him himself than to his much coveted wealth. Nor, is there any reason to suppose that he was wrong,[138] if we may judge from Lionardo's subsequent behaviour when his uncle was ill. Like his father, Lionardo owed everything that he possessed to Michelangelo, who, being given rather amusingly to telling members of his family what they should or should not have said on any given occasion,[139] always had a proper appreciation of the right attitude to be adopted. It was not that he required fulsome thanks, but he did require a little kindly courtesy in recognition of what he had done and of the hardships he had endured in order that his family might not have to endure any.[140] And in comparison with what he had suffered, it may well have seemed to him that he was justified when he said to Lionardo in his letter of February 6th 1546, 'You have all lived on me for forty years now, and not so much as a kind word have I ever had from you.'[141]

It is noticeable, however, that the relations between them improved considerably after Lionardo's marriage, about which there was so much ado. But while he must have grown heartily tired of Michelangelo's repetitive advice to him about choosing a bride, Lionardo can never have been in any doubt that it was his happiness and well-being, and nothing else, that Michelangelo really had at heart. This emerges over and over again; yet anxious though he was that Lionardo should marry, he was not prepared to urge it upon him against the young man's own inclinations, or if he had any scruples in the matter, which Michelangelo came to think might be the case, partly because the negotiations were so long drawn out and partly because he had no great confidence in the fruitfulness of the Buonarroti.[142] After all, of his four brothers only Buonarroto had married, while, as to his own attitude to marriage, there are grounds for thinking that more may be revealed in what he said to his nephew in his letter of June 24th 1552 than in the famous excuse recorded by Vasari, that in his art he already had a wife too many and that his works were his children[143] – a reply calculated to reveal less than nothing, true though it may have been up to a point. 'If, however, you do not feel physically capable of marriage', he wrote, 'it is better to contrive to keep oneself alive than to commit suicide in order to beget others'[144] – a shrewd piece of advice certainly (though, as it turned out, he need not have been apprehensive), but it is permissible to wonder whether it may not be considerably more than that.

Had Michelangelo been of a less ardent and impulsive temperament and less prone to be carried away by his response to people who appealed to him, this evasive answer about his failure to marry might seem more convincing. But as it is, there are certain aspects of the matter which must give us pause. His obvious pleasure in children, as shown both in the way in which he portrayed them and in his remarks to Cornelia Colonelli about caring for his namesake, the little Michelangelo d'Amadore;[145] his extraordinary tenderness, as exemplified particularly in numerous of his early works, as well as other indications of his potential aptitude for marriage, have already been discussed,[146] and seeing that he was, as he said of himself, *Al desir pronto, alla vaghezza troppa,*[147] it is difficult to imagine that at some time or other in the days of his youth he would not have committed himself irrevocably to a beautiful face and a sympathetic heart, if it had not been for some kind of inhibition (apart from the claims of his art) such as that which emerges in the three stanzas of one of the longer poems, *Io crederrei, se tu fussi di sasso.*[148] In these verses, which exist only in an unpolished and fragmentary state, he speaks of his passion for a woman who had only to look at him to make him glow, who had only to smile at him or greet him in the street to inflame him, but to whom, if she spoke to him or asked anything of him, he was unable to reply or to make any response whatever, so that in an instant his desire failed and his hopes had, perforce, to yield to his inhibition. Hence, as he continued:

> *I' sento in me non so che grand' amore*
> *Che quasi arrivere' 'nsino alle stelle:*
> *E quando alcuna volta il vo' trar fore,*
> *Non ho buco si grande nella pelle,*
> *Che nol faccia a uscirne assa' minore*
> *Parere, e le mie cose assai men belle:*
> *C' amore o forza, el dirne è grazia sola;*
> *E men ne dice chi più alto vola.*

– in other words, although the intensity of his emotion was such that it could, he felt, almost outsoar the stars, he was unable by any means within his power to give it expression.

In his commentary on these verses Carl Frey had this to say: 'Michelangelo's personal experience and poetic imagination appear to be inextricably interwoven. . . . These poetic creations are of a particularly intimate nature and were not meant for other eyes; they were written only for the artist himself.'[149] The fragmentary condition in which these stanzas exist, the choice of simile and the complete frankness of statement confirm this, but Frey is surely wrong when he says that 'the poet was guided entirely by his powerful imagination and the incidents he portrays are exaggerated'. For it must be borne in mind that much which to the average understanding may seem to be exaggerated was not so in Michelangelo's case. Where a lesser imagination had envisaged 'the twelve Apostles in the lunettes and the usual ornamentations to fill the remaining area',[150] Michelangelo had envisaged all the splendours of the Sistine vault. His reactions to the vicissitudes of life, whether he was in a mood of elation or of despondence, can accordingly only be assessed, and must of necessity be interpreted, in terms of his enormous creative capacity. When impassioned, he was indeed impassioned; when frustrated, he was indeed frustrated; when cheerful, cheerful, and when downcast, downcast; the scale of his response being, in fact, commensurate with the scale of his genius.

To men of lesser ability such reactions must necessarily have seemed excessive and it was probably this more than anything else that led to the notion that Michelangelo was 'strange and obsessed', the *pazzia* of which he was commonly accused (which cannot, incidentally, be translated as 'madness') being nothing more than an undue obsession with the particular object with which he happened to be preoccupied. Thus, in the quarrels already referred to between Messer Giovanni and Urbino over the Tomb, he asked del Riccio to intervene in what to anyone else in his position would have been a mere matter of routine, simply because, as he put it, 'to make this statement in front of those fellows completely exhausts me and I have no breath left to speak'.[151] If then, over a matter such as this – and there are many analogous examples of this tendency that could be cited from the letters – he easily became overwrought, how much more vulnerable must he have been when it came to affairs of the heart which touched him more nearly.

Nevertheless, to argue inductively on a subject such as the foregoing and to attempt to draw conclusions of some importance from premises that may appear at first sight to be slender in the extreme, would be hazardous were it not manifest that there were some situations, of a particularly personal kind, in which for Michelangelo as a poet the venting of his pent-up emotions in the form of verse amounted to nothing short of a necessity, since not otherwise would he have been able to contain himself. By their very nature the stanzas discussed above cannot therefore be lightly dismissed as being applicable to one isolated experience. Rather would they appear, when read in conjunction with the view expressed in his letter to Lionardo, when considered in the light of the Buonarroti's sexual deficiency, and when related to certain aspects of his own work and personality, which have already been examined,[152] to provide confirmatory evidence of a psycho-somatic condition to which, at least at times, he appears to have been subject. There is, accordingly, a strong presumption that what we have here is a personal confession of a peculiarly intimate kind, a form of apology undertaken subconsciously to relieve what might otherwise have developed into a trauma. Or, to put it differently, his impotence was in proportion to his passion, and he knew it – *E men ne dice chi più alto vola.*

If this were indeed the case, nothing would be more natural than that he should seek, as it were, to exorcise his feelings of frustration by giving vent to them, just as he had done in other situations and was to do again. When his fury against Giovanni da Pistoia knew no bounds, he poured forth a flood of invective that spared Giovanni nothing;[153] when faced with the physical manifestations of the stone during the crisis of his disorder, he left nothing unsaid,[154] not because he revelled in it, but precisely because he did not, for only by the use of a means of catharsis of a more or less violent kind was he able in any degree to control his revulsion. But as in the case of the *stanze* – *Io crederri se tu fussi di sasso* – here again we cannot suppose that the *capitolo* – *I' sto rinchiuso come la midolla* – (which exists only in the Giannotti *codicetto*) was written for eyes other than his own, even allowing for the fact that, like Dante, Michelangelo was not bred in a mawkish tradition.

Although at this time Michelangelo could find no words bitter enough in which to describe his condition, through the ministrations of his physician, Realdo Colombo, he made a reasonably good recovery and was able to assure Lionardo that in other respects he was much as he had been at thirty years of age, 'but', he added, 'I am . . . in need of God's help. So tell Francesca to pray for me and tell her that if she knew the state I have been in, she would see that she is not without companions in affliction.'[155] Poor Francesca, she was at this time only about thirty years of age herself, yet Michelangelo already thought of her as a companion in affliction, not because of any peculiar misfortune of her own, but because such was the intolerable fate of the women of her day; who, when scarcely more than children, were either given in marriage to men not of their own choice, or immured in convents not of their own volition. There were a few exceptions, among whom Sofonisba Anguisciola may be numbered, the child of enlightened parents, to whom Michelangelo showed great kindness and offered every encouragement during her two years in Rome, prior to her appointment as court painter to Queen Isabella of Spain in 1559.[156] Otherwise, it was only the ladies of the great houses, like Vittoria Colonna and Giulia Gonzaga, women of birth and culture, who had, besides, the inestimable good fortune to be childless, who enjoyed any measure of independence or could be said, in any appreciable sense, to have lived or savoured life at all.

Though not substantially different from that of her contemporaries, Francesca's lot was perhaps rather better than most. From Michelangelo's obvious liking and respect for him, it may be deduced that her husband, Michele Guicciardini, was more considerate than many, and he does not seem to have been frequently absent from home. Yet even so, and although after the death of the fourth child born to her, she mercifully had no more, there is frequent mention in the letters of the fact that she was ailing and ill-content, a matter of much concern to Michelangelo, who often wrote to her and sent her messages in an attempt to comfort and encourage her. Like Lionardo and Guicciardini, she too wanted to go to Rome and made one abortive attempt to do so, but unfortunately at a moment when Michelangelo was himself too harassed to receive her.[157] So that although it was she and not her brother to whom Michelangelo was really attached, and she and not her brother who dearly loved him in return, she never saw him again after he left Florence in 1534 and was, moreover, beside herself with grief when rumours of his death reached Florence in January 1546.[158]

The pitiable plight of these hapless girls bartered in the marriage market or consigned to the cloister is amply exemplified both in Michelangelo's charitable efforts to give alms where there was most need and, in Sir Thomas Browne's words, particularly 'where want [*was*] silently clamorous'; and in the quest for a bride for Lionardo, which was diligently pursued in accordance with the age old precepts formulated by Paolo di Ser Pace da Certaldo – 'When thou takest a wife, have a care that she is born of a good father and mother . . . and take great heed that the wife thou choosest is not born of a family where there is sickness or consumption or scrofula or madness or scurvy or gout.'[159]

In his final choice Lionardo was certainly fortunate and his wife, Cassandra Ridolfi, perhaps happier, though hardly less wearied, than most, with the almost yearly arrival of another child which, not unnaturally, seldom survived. Michelangelo's pleasure in this marriage was altogether charming; his satisfaction in having spoken to her kinsman, Lorenzo Ridolfi, about it and in having, in his own words, 'said all the correct things better than I thought I could';[160] his desire to mark the fact that 'she is the wife of a nephew of mine' by giving her some token of the relationship, perhaps in the form of a fine necklace of valuable pearls which 'I'm told . . . would be appropriate', but above all in his gratification in Lionardo's contentment and in the success of the marriage, as expressed in one of his letters written nearly a year later, in which he said, 'you write me of your continued happiness with Cassandra. We must thank [*God*] for it, and all the more so because this is something sufficiently rare. Thank her and commend me to her and if anything here would please her, let me know.'[161] Clearly, he was enormously relieved that Lionardo was no longer alone and without companionship and was only too anxious to show his gratitude to Cassandra in any way that Lionardo might suggest. It is only a pity that he himself was unable to witness 'the beginnings of another Buonnarroto'[162] which, perhaps for more reasons than one, afforded him such singular pleasure and satisfaction.

With the close of the long conclave following the death of Paul III, in the course of which Cardinal Niccolò Ridolfi, who had been known to be *papabile*, died unexpectedly, and the Cardinal of England, Reginald Pole, who would otherwise have received the tiara, refused election by homage, the three loneliest and most profoundly unhappy years that Michelangelo had ever known came to an end.

Holding office, as he did, by virtue of a papal brief, and being, as he was, a member of the papal household, the outcome of this, as of the three ensuing conclaves, was a matter of some moment to him, since with every change of pontificate his own position was liable to be affected. By great good fortune, in Julius III, who was elected on February 8th 1550, he acquired a patron who could not have been more favourably disposed towards him. While the new Pope's admiration for his genius was no less than that evinced by Paul III, his consideration for his infirmity was greater. 'Having respect for his age, he understands well and appreciates his greatness,' wrote Condivi, 'but wishes not to burden him with more than he is willing to do.'[163] At the same time, Julius always consulted him and sought his advice over the many architectural projects he initiated, for some of which Michelangelo supplied both designs and models. But he was so much given to changing his mind over everything he undertook that Michelangelo once remarked to a friend that he 'had a mind like a weather-cock on a bell-tower, turned about by every wind'. All the same, as far as Michelangelo was concerned, he remained unmoved, despite the pressure brought to bear upon him by the Sangallo faction and others who sought to contrive his downfall. Hence, instead of revoking the authority granted by the brief of 1549, Julius confirmed it and spared no pains to protect him against the attacks of the malevolent who never ceased to harass him in every possible way; indeed, as Vasari records, 'he thought so much of Michelangelo that he always sided with him against the cardinals'.[164] The sincerity of his regard and his disinterested appreciation of Michelangelo's qualities is still further attested by Condivi, who, however partisan some may consider him to have been, cannot, during the pontificate in which he was writing and in a work dedicated to Julius III himself, have made such a statement as the following, had it been unfounded: 'As I heard from the Most Reverend Monsignor di Forli [*Tantecose*], his chamberlain, the Pope has often said that (if it were possible) he would willingly take of his own years and of his own blood to add to the life of Michelangelo, that the world might not so soon be deprived of such a man. I also, having access to His Holiness, heard this from his own lips with my own ears, and more also.'[165] It is noteworthy, moreover, that to Ascanio Condivi himself (who recorded the advice in the dedication of his *Vita di Michelangelo Buonarroti*) Julius could propose nothing better than that he should strive to imitate the virtues of Michelangelo.

Such gestures of confidence and amiability, gratifying though they might be, were, however, of less immediate benefit to Michelangelo, once he had been assured of his position, than Giorgio Vasari's arrival in Rome shortly afterwards, in obedience to the command he had received from Julius prior to his self-predicted elevation.

The companionship of the younger man, who had always been attentive to him, and who now spent some part of every day in his company and consulted him about all the new commissions with which he had been entrusted, gave him a new interest in life and his spirits noticeably revived. This Michelangelo realized himself when he wrote, 'seeing that you revive the dead, I am not surprised that you should prolong the life of the living, or rather half-living, long since hastening towards the grave'.[166] Among other things, during this Jubilee year they visited the seven churches, the Pope, in deference to Michelangelo's age, having given them both permission to ride instead of going on foot, thereby granting them a double indulgence. Between churches, according to Vasari, they pleasantly beguiled the time with 'many fine and useful discussions on the arts and crafts.' It is obvious also that Michelangelo was much more himself, and ever ready to indulge his sardonic sense of humour, as he did one day when they were crossing the Ponte Santa Maria, the rebuilding of which, through the intrigues of underlings, had been taken out of his hands and given to Nanni di Baccio Bigio, who had removed a great quantity of the travertine he had put in to strengthen the foundations. 'Giorgio,' he said, 'this bridge shakes; let us ride carefully, lest it should give way while we are on it.' Nor, as it befell, was he much mistaken; five years later, when the Tiber flooded it collapsed altogether, and though rebuilt has ever since been known as the Ponte Rotto – a tribute to Nanni's prowess, which is corroborated by the account of his efforts at Ancona, where, in attempting to clear the port at small cost, he was said to have done more damage in one day than the sea in ten years.[167]

Although Vasari did not continue for any length of time in the Pope's service, he and Michelangelo remained constantly in touch, the very pleasing relationship which existed between them being clearly reflected in their correspondence. But no matter whether he was in Rome or in Florence, Vasari always proved a solicitous and understanding friend, on whom Michelangelo could rely, especially over the troubles he had constantly to face and the molestation he had perpetually to endure through the intrigues of his persecutors at the Basilica. The knowledge of Vasari's influence with the Duke of Florence and of the Duke's generous and affable disposition towards himself must have been a considerable moral support to him, particularly during the brief pontificate of Marcellus II, whose election in April 1553 cannot but have caused him great consternation, in view of the new pontiff's known readiness to comfort his enemies, of which, as Cardinal Cervini, he had given ample proof during his tenure of office as Prefect of the fabric of St. Peter's. But Michelangelo's consternation was short lived, for scarcely had he reached a decision to leave Rome and to return to Florence when, to his relief and to the relief of the Curia, Marcellus died.

To have had to leave Rome at eighty years of age to take up his abode even in his native city, which he had left so long before that it was almost as if he had never been there, would, in any case, have imposed so severe a strain upon him that it is questionable whether he would have survived. But to have had to do so with the knowledge that he was abandoning his work on the fabric at a stage when the work was advanced and there was money to spend on it, and with the conviction that the eight years he had spent on it would be wasted, must have rendered his demise a certainty. By this time, and in spite of all that he had suffered and would, as he must have known, continue to suffer, he was wholly dedicated to the task which had been imposed upon him against his will and in face of every argument he could advance in support of his plea to be spared so great a burden. 'Many people believe, as I do myself,' he wrote in a letter to Lionardo, two years later, 'that I was put there by God', and for this reason he was unwilling to abandon it, unless he was obliged, because to do so would, he felt, bring disgrace upon him throughout Christendom and would, besides, lay a grievous sin upon his soul.[168] He was therefore grateful to be able to continue his service, with the same powers as before, under Paul IV, who succeeded Marcellus II on May 23rd 1555.

But even this did not mean that he was at the end of the troubles and vexations by which he was continually beset. In August of the same year his faithful Urbino became seriously ill, so that he was not only deprived of his services, of which he stood almost hourly in need, but had the anxiety and distress of his indisposition to bear as well. Then in November, when he could not longer conceal the certainty of its tragic outcome, even from himself, he received the announcement of the death of his brother Gismondo.[169] Though they had never been very close to each other and though Michelangelo had been hurt by his silence when Giovansimone died seven years before, his decease at such a moment cannot but have increased the wretchedness and intensified the poignancy of a situation that was already acute, as Urbino's condition gradually grew worse.

The simple dignity of the terms in which Michelangelo conveyed the news to Lionardo, when the end came, was equalled only by the ineffable pain of the communication. 'I must tell you that last night, the third of December, at nine o'clock, Francesco, called Urbino, passed from this life to my intense grief, leaving me so stricken and troubled that it would have been more easeful to die with him, because of the love I bore him.'[170] Of the many sorrows he had known this was in some respects the most unbearable of all. Old and defenceless, he was so stupefied by the shock that for some weeks he lost all count of time, the extent to which he remained inconsolable being emphasized in his letter to Vasari written about two months later, in which the same heart-broken cry he had uttered in his letter to Lionardo was heard again. After speaking of the exemplary death Urbino had died, he went on to refer to his own forlorn predicament; 'I have had him twenty-six years and found him entirely loyal and devoted; and now, when I had made him rich and expected him to be a stay and support to me in my old age, he has vanished from me and nothing is left to me but the hope of seeing him again in Paradise.'[171] Well therefore might Varchi speak in his funeral oration of the miseries, the tribulation, the anguish and the torments of human life and of the bitter tears which Michelangelo shed over the death of his faithful and devoted servant.[172]

Something of the same sentiment is expressed in the sonnet, *Per croce e grazia e per diverse pene* which he addressed a little later to Lodovico Beccadelli, a close friend, who had recently taken up his appointment as archbishop of Ragusa.[173] Beccadelli was very homesick and during his absence kept up an intermittent correspondence with Michelangelo, whom he always remembered in his prayers and with whom he was happy to resume his friendship when he returned to Rome. In the sonnet in question Michelangelo spoke feelingly of his loss – *E piango e parlo del mio morto Urbino* – who might, he says, have otherwise gone with him across the sea and over the mountains to visit Beccadelli, but who now drew him by a different road to the place of his habitation, where he was waiting to receive him.

In the meantime Michelangelo was left to go on alone, bearing as best he could the many burdens by which he was encumbered – the thought of which had caused Urbino more anguish than the thought of death itself.

Though very different in character from those of his predecessors whom Michelangelo had served, Paul IV was no less anxious than they to avail himself of the services of a man who was now so famous as to have become a legend in his own time, as we learn from a letter of Piero Vettori to his friend Vincenzo Borghini, dated January 4th 1557. In it he gave him an account of certain gentlemen from Germany who, being on a visit to Rome, had so keen a desire just to *see* Michelangelo, that he had given them an introduction, as a result of which Michelangelo had been pleased to satisfy their curiosity and had kindly received them at his house.[174] Evidently, as Ollanda had remarked twenty years before, 'a man not as surly as people imagine'.[175]

Nowhere is the extent to which Michelangelo was sought after, even by this bigoted and ferocious pontiff, more vividly confirmed than in a despatch from the Florentine ambassador, Bongianni Gianfigliazzi, dated September 28th 1558, in which he reported a conversation he had recently had with Francesco Bandini. It reads in part as follows:

> On Sunday evening Bandini came to see me and told me that that morning he had been to the Minerva to hear Mass with Michelangelo Buonarroti, who had told him that His Holiness required his attendance every day, that he had had long discussions with the Pope, though he spent most of the time listening, [*Paul IV being a vociferous talker*] and that he had informed His Holiness that he was now an old man and that he [*the Pope*] had other architects and capable men about him much superior to himself and that he could obtain designs from them. He also said that His Holiness had made so many proposals that he was amazed. . . . On being asked what these designs were, he replied, 'It suffices that they are *cose grande, grandissime*.' Being pressed still further, he replied, '*Cose da . . .*' but had stopped short, saying, 'It is not seemly that I should discuss a pope. . . .'[176]

But the Caraffa Pope had missed his opportunity; not because Michelangelo was no longer capable of providing him with any designs he required, which was very far from being the case, but because little more of his pontificate remained to him. The first years, during which he had availed himself of Michelangelo's services on the fortifications of the City, had been spent in an ill-advised conflict with Spain, as a result of which the work on St. Peter's had been brought almost to a standstill and Michelangelo himself had taken refuge in Spoleto for fear that Rome might again be sacked. And in this connection it is worthy of remark that almost the first thing that the Pope had done, once the scare was over, had been to send a special messenger to Spoleto to command Michelangelo's return.[177] He was presumably anxious that the work on the Basilica should be resumed with as little delay as possible.

It was during the months immediately following this resumption of work on the building that the mistake was made over the vaulting of the *Cappella del Re,* which Michelangelo found so humiliating and his rivals so heartening. But though more acute, the anguish of mind he had to endure on this occasion was not substantially different from that to which by this time he must have become inured. From the outset the opposition he had had to meet at the Basilica had been formidable, nor indeed, in one sense, was it lessened by the brief of 1549 which granted him supreme powers. Never in the whole history of art can an artist have received a greater tribute to his genius as an architect or to his character as a man. No limits were set either to his freedom or to his authority, and in the unswerving confidence that the powers granted him would never be abused, the mandate granted by Paul III was renewed by three Popes in succession. The veneration accorded him by the potentates whom he served was equalled, however, only by the animosities of his inferiors who sought to supplant him. He had, in addition, to contend with the venality of his underlings, who resented the stand he took from the outset against all the forms of graft to which they were accustomed. But in the eyes, whether of his masters, his rivals, or his subordinates, his own probity was always beyond question. By the incalculable wisdom of his decision to refuse all emoluments over and above his annual salary, as supreme sculptor, painter and architect to the Vatican, he secured his exemption from any and every charge of self-seeking and from any and every suspicion of partiality, no matter what course he chose to pursue in respect of 'demolitions and constructions of whatever kind'.[178]

Thus, in the words of Pastor, 'the self-denial and the determination with which, in spite of all opposition, he remained true to his great purpose gives a truly tragic consecration to his closing years'.[179] And in some of the simple statements in his own letters this is borne out. 'I am an old man,' he wrote in the concluding paragraph of his letter of December 2nd 1558 to Lionardo, 'and here I am bearing great burdens, which seems not to be recognized; and I do so for the love of God, in Whom is all my hope.'[180] Yet notwithstanding the renewed offers of the Duke to receive him, that he might end his days in peace, he continued to bear them, though touched to the core by the Duke's concern. This is confirmed by Giovan Francesco Lottini's letter to Cosimo I of July 7th 1557, in which he said:

Michelangelo Buonarroti is, in fact, so old that though he still wishes to do so, he is unable to stir very far and now seldom or rarely goes to St. Peter's, besides which the model *[i.e. of the cupola]* will take months and months to complete and he is obliged and anxious to complete it. When I made him Your Excellency's offer, he was moved to tears and one could see that he was desirous of serving You if he had the power, but, in fact, he cannot do so, as besides the stone, he has other troublesome disorders.[181]

But though deprived of his services, except in regard to the designs for San Giovanni de' Fiorentini, which Michelangelo prepared for him, the Duke was not finally deprived of making his acquaintance, which he did in the autumn of 1560, when he paid a state visit to the Pope of his choice, Pius IV, who had been elected on Christmas Day of the previous year. According to Vasari's account of the visit, 'Immediately on the arrival of Duke Cosimo and the Duchess, Eleanora, Michelangelo went to see them and did so several times during their stay in Rome.' Vasari makes no mention, however, of the Duke's visit to Michelangelo which is specifically noted by Varchi.[182] Probably both versions are correct, but in either case, nothing in his career became the Duke more (and he was a proud man) than the veneration he showed on this occasion for an artist whose services he could no longer hope to command, but whom he recognized to be, beyond doubt, the first of the Florentines. And as in life, so in death he was prepared to do him honour, for as he said in his letter to the Academicians four years later, when the obsequies were under discussion, 'such is the affection we bear to the rare genius of Michelangelo Buonarroti'.[183]

The time, however, was not yet. But during the four years, or rather less, that still remained to him, Michelangelo was not to be spared any of the vexations which by this time must have become only too familiar, though he had now acquired a new assistant, Pierluigi Gaeta, who lived in his house and on whom he could rely with some confidence, while he had in addition become greatly attached to Daniele Ricciarelli and to Tiberio Calcagni, whom he saw constantly, and who could always be called upon in case of need. Such need arose in August 1561, when he had a seizure after working for several hours in the heat on the designs for the Porta Pia. On this occasion Tommaso de' Cavalieri and Francesco Bandini were also summoned by Antonio Francese, a servant whom he had for a number of years. At first it was thought that he was dying, but in a few days he had completely recovered and seemed extremely well.[184] He made no mention of this seizure to Lionardo, at least as far as we know, and except for an attack of colic in the winter of 1562, he seems, though frail, to have remained in tolerably good health for the rest of his life, so much so that in July 1562 Ricciarelli was able to assure Lionardo that, except for being a little weak in the legs, there was not much the matter with him.[185]

This was certainly just as well, in view of the fresh calumnies to which he was subjected shortly afterwards,[186] in countering which he displayed a vigour such as he was accustomed to display whenever his honour or good faith were impugned. But Pius IV, 'who not only loved him, but honoured him and held him dear'[187] was no more persuaded to believe the accusations against him now than he had been three years before, when Michelangelo tendered his resignation to Cardinal Carpi, who, though one of his best friends, nevertheless seems somehow to have been persuaded to believe that things were not going well at the Basilica, when in fact they could not have been going better.[188] After a full investigation the charges brought against him on this occasion in respect of the fabric also proved to be unfounded and for the last time Michelangelo's honour was vindicated.

The torments which he had endured for nearly seventeen years were now at an end. With Antonio Francese and his other servants to look after him; with Pierluigi Gaeta at his right hand; and with Francesco da Cortona to deputize for him at the Basilica, he was at last left to live the rest of his life in peace.[189] Five months more remained to him, during which time he was still able to carve. On Saturday, February 12th, he spent all day working on the *[Rondanini] Pietà* and would have done so again on the following day, had Antonio not reminded him that it was Sunday. Then on the Monday, the opening of Carnival week, he was taken ill, and the news spread rapidly through the City. He sent for Daniele Ricciarelli and as soon as he arrived told him quite simply that he was dying – *O Daniello, io sono spacciato; mi ti racomando, non mi abandonare*.[190] His most intimate friends, Tommaso de' Cavalieri, Diomede Leoni and Tiberio Calcagni gathered round him and he asked that Lionardo should be informed. He lingered for another four days and then at the *Ave Maria* on Friday evening, remembering the Passion of Christ and believing, as he had always believed, that 'if life pleases us we ought not to fear death which comes from the hand of the same Master',[191] he gave up his soul to God.

On the evening of the same day, February 18th 1564, Gherardo Fidelissimi, one of the doctors who had been in attendance, wrote to Cosimo I to inform him of the death of Michelangelo and to acquaint him with the desire he had expressed to be buried in Florence. He wrote at once, he said, knowing how high a regard the Duke had entertained for the rare endowments of the deceased, 'the greatest man that the world has ever known'.[192] These are words of supreme praise, which may seem the more inordinate when we consider that they were used by a subject in addressing his prince. But may we not echo the comment made in a similar connection, when it was said of Sir Thomas More, another of the superlatively great figures of the Renaissance, that he came ' "as near perfection as our nature will permit" . . . strange words these, yet can we say that they are an exaggeration?'[193]

If not as an artist, certainly as a man, Michelangelo himself would have been the first to disclaim any such pre-eminence.

> *Non è più bassa e vil cosa terrena*
> *Che quel che, senza te, me sento e sono;*[194]

he had written when, oppressed with a sense of his own imperfection, he had tried, almost hourly, to accustom himself to the thought of approaching death, or, as he had expressed it in another sonnet, in lines that are strangely moving in their indication of his persistent need of solace:

> *Nè pinger, nè scolpir fia più che quieti*
> *L' anima volta a quel Amore divino*
> *Che aperse, a prender noi, in croce le braccia.*[195]

These lines, which were written ten years before he died, show not only how long he had dwelt within the shadow of death, but also how deeply he was concerned with the contemplation of God, with the life of the soul and with man's paramount obligation to prepare himself for his passing from this world to the next. In the course of his funeral oration Benedetto Varchi placed some emphasis upon the value and, indeed, the necessity of this concern for the spiritual ends of human existence. 'Man's supreme felicity and ultimate beatitude consist', he said, 'in understanding, in loving and in serving God perfectly' and 'in his meditation on death Michelangelo attained his ultimate perfection, his ultimate felicity and his ultimate beatitude.'[196] 'Who was ever more religious?' he asked, 'Who ever lived a more godly life? Who ever died a more Christian death than Buonarroti?' And, in the qualified sense in which he posed the question, that is to say, in the sense that no-one who, having received the lively Oracles of God, had ever striven more valiantly to obey them, Varchi was probably not far wrong. For himself, however, Michelangelo made no claims. He merely said, 'Before men, I do not say before God, I count myself an honest man.'[197] Yet whether or not the claims made for him in this respect were too high, it cannot be doubted but that here, truly, was 'a holy and humble man of heart'.

It was, in any case, in this spirit and for the salvation of his soul that he devoted the last years of his life to that art which God had assigned to him,[198] and to the furtherance of a task which he knew he would not live to see completed. But if in this lay the ultimate frustration and the ultimate tragedy of a life devoted to creative ends, in this probably more than in anything else lay the ultimate triumph and the ultimate glory of a life devoted in no less a degree to the service of God. It is perhaps not for us to ask how it should be that all the suffering and all the toil he endured, in order that the Basilica might be brought to a stage at which it could not afterwards be altered or changed into another form should prove to have been in vain. Unlike Milton, we can only remain silent before an inscrutable providence, without presuming 'to justify the ways of God to men'.

But in this at least Michelangelo was blessed, if of so much else he was deprived, namely, in the multitude of his friendships. Esteemed by the learned and liked and respected by everyone in all walks of life, by women as well as by men, his close friends, as Varchi observed, were *copiosissimi*.[199] Wherever he went he was welcomed; 'If you want to give everyone pleasure, come to supper at the bank this evening,' wrote Luigi del Riccio,[200] while, if we may base our conclusions on Vasari's account of his own reception when he called on Michelangelo unexpectedly,[201] we see clearly that his affection for them was no less than theirs for him. But it was, more especially, for their desire to serve him that the attitude of his friends was notable, an attitude epitomized in a confession of one of his assistants, Giovanni da Reggio, who in October 1520 wrote to him from Rome saying, 'I am doing everything I can, because so great are my obligations towards you, that as long as I live I would place my life and everything I have in the world at your disposal – and after death also, if I were able.'[202]

But above all, Michelangelo evoked in men a protective instinct that is so marked as to be unaccountable, except on a psychological basis. And it is herein that the crux of his whole temperament lies. For only in the postulation of an essential ambivalence in his nature, or, in a manner of speaking, *un uomo in una donna, anzi uno dio,*[203] or vice versa, can the problem of the intersexuality of his art and the bisexuality of his loves be satisfactorily resolved. This hypothesis, that there existed in him a uniquely balanced sexual duality, would also account for much else, both in his art and in his experience alike; for a rare intermingling of tenderness and power in the first, and of passion and pain in the second. It would explain the extremes of feeling to which he was subject, a sublime capacity for exaltation on the one hand, and a terrifying capacity for suffering on the other. It would also explain some of the peculiar difficulties he encountered in the management of men, his tendency to be *pusilanimo a richiedere*, his need always to be escorted, his diffidence, his suspicion, his qualms and his vulnerability, all of which suggest a certain difficulty of adjustment in a world which takes little or no cognizance of any variation from the accepted norm. But in this connection it cannot be too strongly emphasized that no imputation of effeminacy is here involved. To speak of a subtle interfusion of the finer qualities of both sexes is not (as some may think) to detract from the character, but rather to give it an added grace which is not to be despised. For although the hypersensibility thus engendered inevitably acquainted him with an anguish of spirit unknown to the average man, it also enhanced his creative powers, and, as far as we are able to judge, endowed him, as a personality, with an unwonted charm and an undeniable magnetism.

Being thus possessed of a wider vision, a deeper insight, a more intuitive understanding, a greater compassion and a heightened response to life – *Dal bello a bel fur fatti gli occhi mei*[204] – he conceived of his art in the most sublime terms of which man is capable, even as a means of progression towards that divine beauty to which the soul aspires, passing 'from fair forms to fair pursuits, from fair pursuits to fair perceptions, until from fair perceptions it attains at last to the perception of that which is nothing but the perception of absolute beauty itself'.[205]

So much, then, for the artist, who became known in his own lifetime as the divine

Michelangelo. But what of the man? If it be true that life has meaning in proportion to its form and that, like a work of art, in order to satisfy the conception of greatness, it, too, must be 'serious, complete and of a certain magnitude',[206] can it finally be said that as a man Michelangelo satisfied this conception? In answer to this question, let Vittoria Colonna be the last to speak, as she turns to him, saying, 'In Rome those who know you esteem you more than your works; those who do not know you, esteem the least part of you, even the work of your hands.' To which Michelangelo replies, 'Perchance, Signora, you attribute to me more than I deserve. . . .'[207]

References to which the superior numbers in the text of the Introduction relate. Titles of works not included in the Bibliography are here given in full

1. *No. 434.*
2. *Condivi, L.*
3. *Pastor, X, p. 363.*
4. *Condivi, LI.*
5. *Gotti, II, p. 123.*
6. *Appendix 33.*
7. *No. 91 & Draft 4.*
8. *J. A. Symonds, The Sonnets of Michelangelo, London, 1904, p. 59.*
9. *Giannotti, Dialogi, p. 68 et seq.*
10. *Guasti, p. 52.*
11. *Ibid., p. 220.*
12. *Ibid., p. 50.*
13. *Ibid., p. 115.*
14. *Ibid., p. 186.*
15. *No. 193.*
16. *Appendix 37.*
17. *Guasti, p. cviii.*
18. *Ibid., p. 189.*
19. *Symonds, II, p. 400 et seq.*
20. *Ibid., II, p. 396.*
21. *Guasti, p. 211.*
22. *Ibid., p. 214.*
23. *Ibid., p. 225.*
24. *Ibid., p. 52.*
25. *Ibid., pp. 188, 177*
26. *Daelli, No. 23.*
27. *Symonds, II, p. 402.*
28. *Ibid., II, p. 319.*

29. *No. 1.*
30. *Gaye, II, p. 231.*
31. *Milanesi, p. 596.*
32. *Frey, Briefe, p. 338 et seq.*
33. *Vasari, V, p. 584.*
34. *Ibid., VII, p. 546.*
35. *No. 419.*
36. *Robert J. Clements, Michelangelo's Theory of Art, London, 1963, p. 385 et passim.*

37. No. 29.
38. Carl Frey, *Il Codice Magliabechiano,* Berlin, 1892, p. 115.
39. No. 90.
40. No. 214.
41. Nos. 9, 51, 71, 55, 145.
42. No. 71.
43. Nos. 206, 416, 357, 432, 348.
44. Nos. 352, 416.
45. Nos. 13, 161.
46. No. 161.
47. No. 177.
48. No. 315.
49. Rolland, p. 25 et seq. Cf. Vol. I, pp. xxvi, xxvii.
50. Nos. 128, 130.
51. Nos. 396, 397, 400.
52. Nos. 185, 200, 203, 204, 205.
53. Frey, *Briefe,* p. 337.
54. Milanesi, *Corr.,* p. 102.

55. Frey, *Briefe,* p. 1.
56. No. 51.
57. Milanesi, p. 651.
58. Gasparoni, p. 158 et seq.
59. No. 124.
60. No. 89. Cf. No. 82.
61. No. 350.
62. Lanciani, p. 56.
63. Condivi, LXVI.
64. No. 9.
65. Nos. 49, 90.
66. Condivi, LXVI & Vasari, VII, p. 285.
67. Vasari, VII, p. 178.
68. Ibid.
69. No. 51 & Guasti, p. 158.
70. No. 205.
71. No. 210.
72. Nos. 94, 384, 394, 432.
73. Nos. 150, 216.
74. No. 203.

75. Gotti, II, p. 149 et seq.
76. Gaye, III, p. 133.
77. Michele Saponaro, *Michelangelo,* trans. C. J. Richards, London, 1951, passim.
78. No. 402.

79. Lawley, p. 53 et seq.
80. Colonna, *Carteggio,* p. 331.
81. Lawley, pp. 7, 38.
82. Guasti, p. 57.
83. Ibid., pp. 116, 209.
84. F. de Holanda, *De La Pintura Antigua,* ed. M. Denis, Madrid 1921, p. 150.
85. Guasti, p. 176: Symonds, *Sonnets,* p. 20.
86. Colonna, *Rime,* p. 111.
87. Colonna, *Carteggio,* p. 238.
88. Schenk, p. 99.
89. Guasti, p. 238.
90. Ibid., p. 234.
91. No. 337.
92. Ponnelle & Bordet, p. 504.
93. Guasti, p. 30.
94. Micah, VI, 8.
95. Milanesi cxiii, here omitted, being fragmentary.
96. Guasti, p. 297.
97. Schenk, p. 93.
98. Dante, *Paradiso,* xviii, 4.
99. Guasti, p. 46.
100. Colonna, *Carteggio,* p. 322.
101. Guasti, p. 168.
102. No. 347.

103. Vasari, VII, p. 300.
104. Giannotti, *Dialogi,* p. 39.
105. Dante, *Inferno,* XXXIV, ll.64–69.
106. Giannotti, *Dialogi,* p. 98.
107. Symonds, II, pp. 71, 153
108. Guasti, pp. 10, 9, 15.
109. Appendix 30.

110. *Frey, Dicht., pp. 69, 383 (Note: Epigram No. 19 corresponds to No. 17 in Guasti's edition.)*
111. *Tusiani, p. 183*
112. *Clements, op. cit., p. 89.*
113. *Vol. I, p. xlvi–xlviii.*
114. *Guasti, p. 239.*
115. *Pastor, XII, p. 659.*
116. *Frey, Dicht., p. 383.*
117. *Nos. 219, 227.*
118. *Guasti, p. 28.*
119. *No. 244 & Appendix 27, pt. II.*
120. *Gotti, II, p. 79.*

121. *Appendixes 33, 31*
122. *Daelli, No. 8.*
123. *Giannotti, Dialogi, p. 69.*
124. *Vasari, VII, p. 282.*
125. *Condivi, LXIII.*
126. *No. 281.*
127. *Nos. 279, 280.*
128. *Frey, Briefe, pp. 184, 186, 188*
129. *Vol. I, p. xlvi.*
130. *No. 227.*
131. *Caro, II, p. 50, & Duppa, p. 149 et seq. (Note: Duppa's arguments against the date 1553 – August 20th – are inadmissible.)*
132. *Gausti, p. 202.*
133. *No. 281.*
134. *No. 343.*
135. *No. 269.*
136. *Steinmann, p. 53.*
137. *No. 213.*
138. *Appendix 34.*
139. *Nos. 92, 262, 278.*
140. *No. 185.*
141. *No. 262.*
142. *Nos. 427, 444, 461.*
143. *Vasari, VII, p. 281.*
144. *No. 371.*

145. *No. 431.*
146. *Vol. I, p. li.*
147. *Symonds, Sonnets, p. 20.*
148. *Guasti, p. 329, stanzas 11–13.*
149. *Frey, Dicht., p. 322.*
150. *No. 157.*
151. *No. 214.*
152. *Vol. I, p. li et seq.*
153. *Guasti, p. 160.*
154. *Ibid., p. 294*
155. *No. 323.*
156. *Vasari, VI, p. 498 et seq., & Papini, 573 et seq.*
157. *No. 214.*
158. *Gotti, I, p. 299 & Appendix 34.*
159. *Guido Biagi, Men and Manners in Old Florence, London, 1909, p. 68.*
160. *No. 379.*
161. *No. 386.*
162. *Nos. 388, 389.*

163. *Condivi, LVIII.*
164. *Vasari, VII, p. 233.*
165. *Condivi, LVIII.*
166. *No. 348.*
167. *Vasari, VII, pp. 288, 235, 266.*
168. *Nos. 435, 398.*
169. *No. 407.*
170. *No. 408.*
171. *No. 410.*
172. *Benedetto Varchi, Orazione di Messer B. V., Florence, 1564, pp. 42, 44.*
173. *Guasti, p. 235: Beccadelli, p. 15.*

174. *Steinmann, p. 32; Gaye, II, p. 418.*
175. *F. d' Olanda, I Dialoghi michelangioleschi, ed. E. M. Bessone Aureli, Rome, 1926, p. 155.*
176. *Steinmann & Wittkower, p. 425.*
177. *Appendix 43: No. 435.*

178. *Appendix 44, p. 308.*
179. *Pastor, XVI, p. 452.*
180. *No. 444.*
181. *Gaye, III, p. 14.*
182. *Vasari, VII, p. 200; Varchi, Orazione, p. 45.*
183. *Vasari, VII, p. 291.*
184. *Daelli, No. 23.*
185. *Ibid., No. 24.*
186. *Appendix 44.*
187. *Varchi, Orazione, p. 44.*
188. *No. 462.*
189. *Cf. No. 76.*
190. *Gotti, I, p. 357.*
191. *Vasari, VII, p. 278.*

192. *Gaye, III, p. 126.*
193. *'The Times', April 1st, 1935.*
194. *Guasti, p. 232.*
195. *Ibid., p. 230.*
196. *Varchi, Orazione, p. 61 et seq.*
197. *No. 227.*
198. *Cf. No. 212.*
199. *Varchi, Orazione, p. 43.*
200. *Steinmann, p. 34.*
201. *Appendix 39: Vasari, VIII, p. 330.*
202. *Frey, Briefe, p. 160.*
203. *Guasti, p. 94.*
204. *Ibid., p. 34.*
205. *Plato, Symposium, 211 C.*
206. *Vol. I, p. xxiv.*
207. *Holanda, De la Pintura Antigua, p. 150.*

Chronology : 1534-1564

This chronology is designed as a framework to the letters, in order that Michelangelo's main movements and the work on which he was principally engaged during successive periods may be co-ordinated with his correspondence. The works executed under contract, or to which specific dates may be assigned, are indicated in larger type; those that were executed pari passu or to which no specific dates may be assigned, are indicated in smaller type. The relative type sizes have, therefore, no relevance to the question of artistic merit.

For exhaustive chronologies the reader is referred to A. Venturi, IX, Pt. I, pp. 627–714, or to H. Thode, I, pp. 343–484.

	1534	ROME
		Election of Paul III (Alessandro Farnese) – *October 13th.*
	1535	ROME
		Expenses for preparatory work connected with the painting of *The Last Judgment* sanctioned by the *Camerario* – *April.*
TOMB OF JULIUS II		Brief appointing Michelangelo supreme sculptor, painter and architect to the Vatican at a salary of 1,200 *scudi* a year – *September 1st.*
THE LAST JUDGMENT *(cartoons)*		Brief granting him the reserves of the Po ferry at Piacenza – *September 1st.*
		Payments for the scaffolding for the execution of *The Last Judgment* – *December 7th.*
	1536	ROME
		Payments for further preparations of the altar wall of the Sistine Chapel – *January–April.*
		Michelangelo at work on *The Last Judgment* – *May.*
THE LAST JUDGMENT TOMB OF JULIUS II		Michelangelo introduced to Vittoria Colonna, Marchesa di Pescara.
		Motu proprio exempting Michelangelo from the legal penalties consequent upon his non-fulfilment of the Contract of 1532 for the Tomb of Julius II – *November 17th.*

THE LAST JUDGMENT
CAMPIDOGLIO
(designs)

1537 ROME

Visit of Paul III to the Sistine Chapel to view the partially completed fresco – *February 4th*.

Execution of a model for a salt for the Duke of Urbino – *July*.

Marriage of Michelangelo's niece, Francesca Buonarroti to Michele Guicciardini.

Anton Maria Piccolomini ceded his right to proceed against Michelangelo for the non-fulfilment of the contracts of 1501, 1504 to Paolo de' Panciatichi – *December 5th*.

1538 ROME

Registration of the brief of September 1st 1535 in the *Libri della Camera* – *May 9th*.

Death of Francesco Maria della Rovere, Duke of Urbino – *October 20th*.

Meetings at the church of San Silvestro di Monte Cavallo between Vittoria Colonna, Michelangelo, Francisco d'Ollanda and others – *October 13th, October 20th, November 3rd*.

1539 ROME

1540 ROME

Motu proprio exempting Michelangelo from observance of the statutes of the *Corporazione degli Scarpellini e Marmorai* of Rome – *February*.

Beginning of Michelangelo's correspondence with his nephew, Lionardo Buonarroti – *July*.

Payment made for lowering of the scaffolding in the Sistine Chapel – *December 15th*.

Death of Bartolomeo Angiolini – *December 28th*.

1541 ROME

Conflict between Paul III and Ascanio Colonna over the salt tax. Vittoria Colonna withdrew to the Monastery of San Paolo in Orvieto – *March*.

Vittoria Colonna returned to the Monastery of San Silvestro in Capite in Rome – *August*.

Vittoria Colonna took up residence in the Monastery of Santa Caterina in Viterbo – *October*.

THE LAST JUDGMENT

Completion of *The Last Judgment* – uncovered *October 31st.*

Negotiations with the Duke of Urbino over the Tomb of Julius II and the allocation of certain figures to other masters to enable Michelangelo to undertake the frescoes in the Pauline Chapel – *November.*

The Last Judgment uncovered to the public – *December 25th.*

1542　ROME

Michelangelo's Petition to Paul III in respect of the Tomb of Julius II – *July 20th.*

Fourth and last Contract with the heirs for the Tomb of Julius II – *August 20th.*

Payment to Michelangelo's assistant, Urbino, for the grinding of the colours for the fresco *The Conversion of St. Paul* – *November 16th.*

1543　ROME

Vittoria Colonna taken ill in Viterbo.

Motu proprio appointing Urbino conservator of the paintings in the Vatican chapels – *October 26th.*

1544　ROME

THE CONVERSION OF ST. PAUL
TOMB OF JULIUS II

Death of Cecchino de' Bracci – *January 8th.*

Michelangelo attended a conference on the fortifications of the *Borgo* – *February 25th.*

Vittoria Colonna returned to Rome and took up residence in the Monastery of Sant' Anna de' Funari – *June.*

Michelangelo taken seriously ill. Nursed by Luigi del Riccio in the Strozzi-Ulivieri palace – *July–August.*

Fire on the roof of the Sistine Chapel – *December 31st.*

1545　ROME

Completion of the Tomb of Julius II – *February.*

THE CONVERSION OF ST. PAUL

Paul III viewed the completed fresco of *The Conversion of St. Paul* – *July 12th.*

BASILICA OF ST. PETER
THE MARTYRDOM OF ST. PETER

Payment to Urbino for preparatory work in connection with the second fresco – *The Martyrdom of St. Peter* – *August.*

Council of Trent – opening session – *December.*

Luigi del Riccio returned to Rome from Lyons – *December.*

Michelangelo again taken ill and nursed by del Riccio in the Strozzi-Ulivieri palace – *December–January.*

BASILICA OF ST. PETER
THE MARTYRDOM OF ST. PETER

1546 ROME

Michelangelo returned to his own house in the Macel de' Corvi – *January 16th.*

Luigi del Riccio left for Venice on business – *March.*

CORNICE OF THE FARNESE PALACE

Michelangelo received the honour of Roman citizenship – *March 20th.*

Death of Antonio da Sangallo – *August 3rd.*

Death of Luigi del Riccio – *September/October.*

1547 ROME

Michelangelo appointed architect of St. Peter's in succession to Antonio da Sangallo – *January 1st.*

Death of Vittoria Colonna – *February 25th.*

Benedetto Varchi delivered two discourses, one on Michelangelo's sonnets, to the Florentine Academy – *March 6th, 13th.*

Death of Francis I of France – *March 31st.*

Last payment in respect of the Po ferry – *April.*

Death of Sebastiano del Piombo – *June.*

Request by Michelangelo for the measurement of the cupola and lantern of Santa Maria del Fiore, Florence – *July.*

BASILICA OF ST. PETER
THE MARTYRDOM OF ST. PETER

1548 ROME

Death of Michelangelo's brother, Giovan Simone – *January 9th.*

Michelangelo granted the revenues of the office of Civil Notary of the Romagna in lieu of those of the Po ferry – *October 2nd.*

1549 ROME

Michelangelo ill with a severe attack of the stone – *March.*

Brief conferring upon Michelangelo supreme powers as architect of St. Peter's – *October 11th.*

Paul III viewed the almost completed fresco of *The Martyrdom of St. Peter* – *October 13th.*

Death of Paul III – *November 10th.*

BASILICA OF ST. PETER
THE MARTYRDOM OF ST. PETER

1550   ROME

Publication of *Due Lezioni* by Benedetto Varchi – *January 12th.*

Election of Julius III (Gianmaria Ciocchi del Monte) – *February 8th.*

Completion of *The Martyrdom of St. Peter.*

Publication of *Le Vite* by Giorgio Vasari.

1551   ROME

Michelangelo confirmed in his office as architect of St. Peter's after defending himself before the Deputies in the presence of the Pope – *January.*

1552   ROME

Brief renewing the terms of Michelangelo's appointment as architect of St. Peter's – *January 23rd.*

Collation for the workmen at St. Peter's to celebrate the completion of the cornice at the base of the drum – *February 24th.*

BASILICA OF ST. PETER
SANTA MARIA DEL FIORE PIETÀ

1553   ROME

Marriage of Michelangelo's nephew Lionardo Buonarroti to Cassandra di Donato Ridolfi – *May 16th.*

Publication of *Vita di Michelangelo Buonarroti* by Ascanio Condivi – *July.*

1554   ROME

Birth of a son, Buonarroto, to Lionardo and Cassandra – *April.*

1555   ROME

Death of Julius III – *March 23rd.*

Election of Marcellus II (Marcello Cervini) – *April 9th.*

BASILICA OF ST. PETER

Michelangelo in correspondence with Vasari about his return to Florence.

Death of Marcellus II – *May 1st.*

Election of Paul IV (Gianpietro Caraffa) – *May 23rd.*

Michelangelo deprived of the revenues of the office of Civil Notary of the Romagna – *May.*

Death of Michelangelo's brother Sigismondo – *November 13th.*

Death of Francesco d'Amadore (Urbino) – *December 3rd.*

1556 ROME, SPOLETO

Abdication of the Spanish throne by Charles V in favour of his son Philip II – *January 16th.*

Rome being threatened by the Spaniards under the Duke of Alba and the work at St. Peter's being suspended Michelangelo took refuge at Spoleto – *September.*

Michelangelo arrived in Rome, having been recalled by special messenger – *October 31st.*

1557 ROME

Discovery of the error made in the vaulting of the Cappella del Re, St. Peter's – *April.*

Initiation of the model of the cupola of St. Peter's.

1558 ROME

Death of Charles V in retirement at Yuste – *September 21st.*

1559 ROME

Death of Henry II of France – *July 10th.*

Death of Paul IV – *August 18th.*

Michelangelo approached about plans for S. Giovanni dei Fiorentini in Rome – *October.*

Election of Pius IV (Gian Angelo de' Medici) – *December 25th.*

S. GIOVANNI DEI FIORENTINI
(designs)

1560 ROME

Michelangelo tendered his resignation to Cardinal Ridolfo da Carpi – *September 13th.*

S. MARIA DEGLI ANGELI
ALLE TERME DI DIOCLEZIANO
(designs)

PORTA PIA
(designs)

Cosimo, Duke of Florence and Eleanora of Toledo on state visit to Rome – *November.*

Completion of the model of the cupola of St. Peter's.

1561   ROME

Michelangelo had a seizure but quickly recovered – *August.*

Don Francesco, son of Cosimo I in Rome – *November.*

1562   ROME

The Duke of Florence refused to support Nanni di Baccio Bigio in his intrigues against Michelangelo – *April.*

BASILICA OF ST. PETER
RONDANINI PIETÀ

1563   ROME

Michelangelo elected second Academician (the Duke being the first) of the *Accademia del Disegno* in Florence – *January 31st.*

Intrigues of Nanni di Baccio Bigio against Michelangelo – *August/September.*

1564   ROME

Beginning of Michelangelo's last illness – *Monday, February 14th.*

Death of Michelangelo – *Friday, February 18th.*

Obsequies of the divine Michelangelo Buonarroti
in the church of San Lorenzo in Florence
(prior to entombment in Santa Croce)
July 14th
1564.

IX

LETTERS
199 - 212

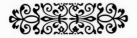

From Rome
1537 - 1542

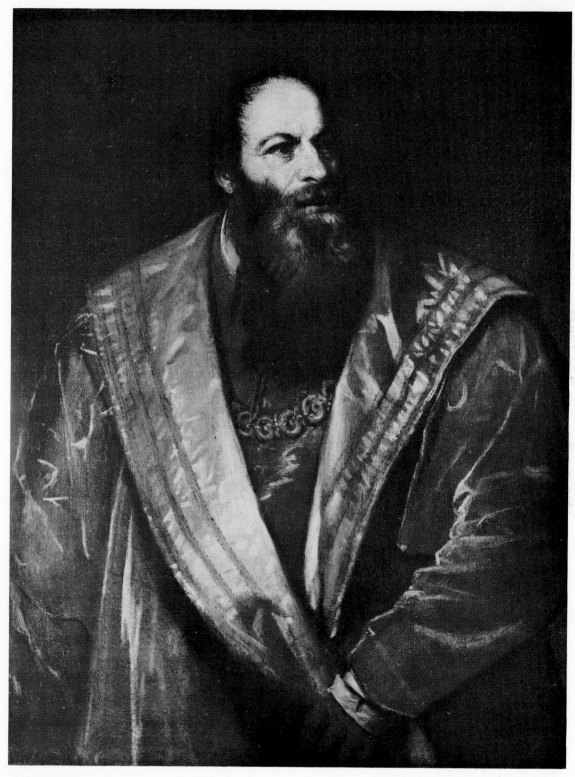

1. *Pietro Aretino*

Titian
Palazzo Pitti, Florence

IX. From Rome : 1537-1542

¶ [To the Magnificent Messer Pietro Aretino in Venice]

199

Published
Source
Mil. cdxxi
From Rome
September 1537

Magnificent Messer Pietro,[1] my lord and brother — The receipt of your letter has caused me at once both pleasure and regret. I was exceedingly pleased because it came from you, who are uniquely gifted among men, and yet I was also very regretful, because, having completed a large part of the composition, I cannot put your conception in hand, which is so perfect that, if the Day of Judgment were passed and you had seen it in person, your words could not have described it better.

Now as to your writing about me, I not only say in reply that I should welcome it, but I entreat you to do so, since kings and emperors deem it the highest honour to be mentioned by your pen.[2] In the meantime, should I have anything that might be to your taste, I offer it to you with all my heart.

In conclusion, do not, for the sake of seeing the painting I am doing, break your resolve not to come to Rome, because that would be too much. I commend me to you.[3]

MICHELANGELO BUONARROTI

1. Pietro Aretino (1492–1556), the 'Scourge of Princes', who, in his letter of September 15th 1537, which was couched in fulsome terms, had had the temerity to make gratuitous suggestions about the way in which 'The Last Judgment' should be treated. Because Michelangelo ignored this advice and failed to comply with his request for drawings, Aretino took his revenge, after the completion of the fresco, by sending him one of the most cruel and vindictive letters ever written (Gaye, II, p. 332 & Symonds, II, pp. 45 et seq.).

2. Aretino reverts to this phrase in the above-mentioned letter of November 1545.

3. This letter was published by Bernardino Pino in 1574 (I, p. 287). The original autograph is no longer extant.

¶ To Gismondo di Lodovico Buonarroti in Florence

200

Buonarroti
Archives
Mil. cxxxiv
From Rome
(1537)

Gismondo — I'm sending twenty ducats to Florence, at the rate of seven *lire* each; I've paid them over to Bartolomeo Angiolini here, to be made payable to you there through Bonifazio Fazzi. So, as soon as you get this, go and get them, and take ten for yourself, and give five of them to Mona Margherita; give the other five to Lionardo,[1] if he's behaving himself; if not, spend them on anything needed for the house;

acknowledge receipt, and give the letter to Bonifazio's bank, or to anyone else you like, and direct it to Bartolomeo Angiolini at the Customs.

MICHELANGELO IN ROME

1. *Lionardo di Buonarroto, Michelangelo's nephew.*

201 ¶ [TO THE SIGNORA VITTORIA COLONNA, MARCHESA DI PESCARA]

*Private
Collection
Mil. cdliv
From Rome
(Winter 1538/9)*

Before taking possession, Signora, of the things which Your Ladyship has several times wished to give me, I wanted, in order to receive them as little unworthily as possible, to execute something for you by my own hand. Then I came to realize that the grace of God cannot be bought, and that to keep you waiting is a grievous sin. I confess my fault and willingly accept the things in question. And when they are in my possession I shall think myself in paradise, not because they are in my house, but because I am in theirs; wherefore I shall be under an even greater obligation to Your Ladyship than I am, if that were possible.

The bearer of this will be Urbino, my assistant, whom Your Ladyship could inform when you wish me to come and see the head of Christ you promised to show me. I commend me to you.[1]

Your Ladyship's servant,

MICHELANGELO BUONARROTI

1. *This letter is written under the sonnet – 'Per esser manco almen, Signiora, indegnio' (Guasti, p. 169). See Appendix 26. The letter actually received by the Marchesa, which was formerly in the Archivio Silvestri, was unknown to both Milanesi and Guasti. It has recently been acquired through a London bookseller by a private collector. Milanesi's text was based on an autograph in the Casa Buonarroti and differs from Guasti's in omitting the words 'servitore di vostra Signoria', and both from the original in omitting the words 'di Cristo' after the word 'testa'.*

202 ¶ [TO THE SIGNORA VITTORIA COLONNA, MARCHESA DI PESCARA]

*Vatican Codex
Mil. cdlv
From Rome
(Spring 1539)*

Signora Marchesa — Seeing that I am in Rome, I do not think it was necessary to have left the Crucifix with Messer Tommao[1] and to have made him an intermediary between your ladyship and me, your servant, to the end that I might serve you; particularly as I had desired to perform more for you than for anyone on earth I ever knew.

But the great task[2] on which I have been and am engaged has prevented me from making this known to Your Ladyship. And because I know that you know that love requires no task-master, and that he who loves slumbers not – still less had he need of intermediaries. And although it may have seemed that I had forgotten, I was executing something I had not mentioned, in order to add something that was not expected. My plan has been spoilt.[3]

'*Mal fa chi tanta fè. . . .*'[4]

Your Ladyship's servant,

MICHELANGELO BUONARROTI IN ROME

1. *Cavalieri. See Appendix 26.*

2. *The painting of 'The Last Judgment'.*

3. *In the autograph the madrigal 'Ora in sul destro ora manco piede . . .' (Guasti, p. 30) is written at right-angles to the letter at the foot of the page, which is signed at the bottom, but upside down.*

4. *'Mal fa chi tanta fè si tosta oblia' (v. 5, l. 9) from Petrarch's canzone, 'S' i' 'l dissi mai, ch' i' vegna in odio a quella . . .' (Petrarch, p. 272).*

¶ TO LIONARDO BUONARROTI IN FLORENCE

203

British Museum Mil. cxxxvii From Rome July (10th/17th) 1540

Lionardo — I have received three shirts together with your letter, and am very surprised that you should have sent them to me, as they're so coarse that there's not a peasant in Rome who wouldn't be ashamed to wear them. Had they been finer, however, I shouldn't have wanted you to send them, because when I need any I'll send the money to buy them.

As to the farm at Pazzolatica,[1] in a fortnight or three weeks[2] I'll have seven hundred ducats paid to Bonifazio Fazi in Florence in order to redeem it but it must first be seen what security Michele will give for them, so that your sister could withdraw the dowery that was given her, should she happen to wish to do so, for any reason. So talk it over with Gismondo and let me have an answer; because unless I see that the seven hundred are properly secured, I shan't redeem it. I think that's all. Encourage Mona Margherita to keep up her spirits, and see that you treat her kindly in word and deed, and try to be a man of honour yourself – otherwise, I would have you understand that you'll inherit nothing of mine.

MICHELANGELO IN ROME

1. *On the marriage of his niece, Francesca, to Michele Guicciardini, Michelangelo had given her the farm at Pazzolatica as her dowery. Apparently Michele now wished to have the capital, and Michelangelo therefore agreed to redeem the farm for 700 ducats, provided he was satisfied that Michele would secure the money in such a way that it could revert to Francesca in case of need. After the trouble which the Buonarroti family had had over the dowery of Mona Cassandra (see Nos. 45–50), Michelangelo was very punctilious in the matter of doweries. See Appendix 41.*

2. *The letter is endorsed 'Assumption', i.e. August 15th, which evidently indicates the day on which payment was received. See No. 204.*

204

*Buonarroti
Archives
Mil. cxxxi
From Rome
August 7th
1540*

¶ [To Giovan Simone di Lodovico Buonarroti in Florence]

Giovan Simone — This morning, the seventh day of August 1540, I've paid to Bartolomeo Angiolini six hundred and fifty gold *scudi* in gold,[1] which he will remit to Florence to Bonifazio Fazzi for the redeeming of the farm at Pazzolatica. So when you've notified Michele and Bonifazio tells him that he has the seven hundred ducats to pay him at the rate of seven *lire* each, and as soon as he [*i.e. Michele*] gives a guarantee of receipt, you can at once take over the farm. So you and the priest[2] can go and talk to Bonifazio and he'll tell you what must be done.

Also, I wish you to understand that since I've been in Rome I've sent you about two thousand ducats, including these last, and I've always paid Bartolomeo Angiolini in advance the equivalent of all that I've sent; and since I'm not keeping a record of anything, and since we're mortal and a new generation is growing up, I should like it always to be clear for the benefit of whoever survives me, that the said money came from me. So, I should like you to talk it over with Bonifazio and if this is legal, get him to enter it in such a way that it will always be clear that it came from me. That's all I have to say about this.

Be considerate to Mona Margherita and tell her that, if these two farms are ploughed again, she will be able to keep a servant as I wrote her.

MICHELANGELO IN ROME

1. *For exchange purposes the scudo was worth more than the ducat.*

2. *i.e. Messer Giovan Francesco Fattucci, to whose spiritual care Michelangelo entrusted his brother's children, Francesca and Lionardo, when he left Florence finally in 1534.*

¶ To Lionardo di Buonarroto Simoni in Florence

*British
Museum
Mil. cxxxvi
From Rome
September 25th
1540*

205

Lionardo — I have a letter from Gismondo which says that he wants me to get my agents in Florence to give him nine bushels of grain. I don't know who my agents in Florence are, but I do know that I haven't given charge of my property to one more than to another. So tell Mona Margherita to give him what she can spare, and tell him from me that he does us little credit in making a peasant of himself. Also tell Mona Margherita not to give anything to anyone on my account, apart from members of the family, because I do not want anyone to go to her and pretend to be acting for me, and to cheat her over something, as Donato del Sera[1] did, since he had no authority from me and I didn't owe him a *scudo*. Therefore tell her this from me, and tell her to keep up her spirits. And try to be a man of honour yourself.

Michelangelo in Rome

1. *A relative of Michelangelo's on his mother's side.*

¶ To Lionardo di Buonarroto

*British
Museum
Mil. cxxxviii
From Rome
November 13th
1540*

206

Lionardo — Michele writes me that he wants me to appoint a proxy, to whom he may renounce the farm at Pazzolatica. I have made Giovansimone and Gismondo my proxies and he can renounce it to them. The power of attorney will be enclosed with this. So give it to them, that they may receive the said farm from Michele and the receipt for the money he has received.

The news of Mona Margherita's death has been a great grief to me – more so than if she had been my sister – for she was a good woman; and because she grew old in our service and because my father commended her to my care, God is my witness that I intended before long to make some provision for her. For this He has not pleased that she should tarry. Alas!

With regard to the management of the house, you'll have to take thought for it yourselves and not look to me, because I'm old and have great difficulty in managing for myself.[1] You have enough to enable you to keep a capable servant and to live like men of honour, if you are united in peace together; and for my part I'll help you as long as I live; if you are not, I'll wash my hands of it.

Also, I should like you to confer with the said Michele, to see how much of the money he spent on the house and on bulls at Pazzolatica remains outstanding, excluding the taxes which have been paid, as he wrote me.

Your[2] Michelangelo in Rome

1. *Michelangelo seems to have had a great deal of trouble with his servants, as witness the number of engagements and dismissals noted in the Ricordi.*

2. *In the autograph 'your' is crossed through, as he did not sign himself in this manner to his nephew.*

207

¶ To Lionardo di Buonarroto in Florence

British Museum Mil. cxxxix From Rome December 18th 1540

Lionardo — I've here paid fifty ducats, at seven *lire* each, to Bartolomeo *Angiolini*[1] to remit to the Fazzi in Florence. So get Ser Giovan Francesco to go to the bank with you, and first of all get the bank to repay him the money he paid on my behalf for the field I bought. And get the bank to state on what account I'm repaying him the said money, in order that it may always be clear that this has been done and that it has been repaid through a third party. And have the balance of the said money paid to Guicciardino in the same way – that is to say, have it stated on what account. The balance he requires for the settlement of the debt due to him I'll include when I happen to be sending more money, as it's not convenient now. I think that's all.

Michelangelo in Rome

1. *Angiolini died ten days later (Frey, Briefe, p. 283).*

208

¶ [To Messer Luigi del Riccio in Rome]

Buonarroti Archives Mil. cdxlii From Rome (March 1541)

Messer Luigi,[1] my dear Signor — I'm sending my assistant, Gabbriello,[2] to you in order that you may give him the money in question. He is trustworthy; you can safely give it to him. I think that's all. I've recovered and hope to live another few years, since Heaven has placed my health in the hands of Messer Baccio[3] and in the *trebbiano*[4] supplied by the Ulivieri.

Your servant

Michelangelo in the Macel dei Corvi

1. *Luigi del Riccio, head of the Strozzi-Ulivieri banking house in Rome. He took over the management of Michelangelo's affairs after Angiolini's death. See Appendix 27.*

2. *Scipione Gabbrielli.*

8

3. *A few months before he completed 'The Last Judgment' Michelangelo fell from the scaffolding and severely injured his leg. He was attended by the Florentine physician, Bartolomeo Rontini. This fall is referred to by Niccolò Martelli in his letter to Rontini of April 10th 1541 (Martelli, 10v).*

4. *A sweet white wine evidently supplied from the Ulivieri estates by Luigi del Riccio.*

¶ To Lionardo Buonarroti in Florence

209

Buonarroti Archives Mil. cxli From Rome (August) 1541

Lionardo — I learn from your letter that you want to come to Rome this September. I think Lent might be the time to come; therefore, as you've delayed so long, you can wait until then, and in the meantime I'll see how my affairs proceed, because they're not going as I wish.[1] Try to become a man of honour and bear in mind what your father left you and what you have now and thank God for it. I want you to go and see Michele Guicciardini and tell him that I learn from his letter that he is well, and how content he is with the three sons he has, which has given me great pleasure. And although Francesca isn't very well, as she writes me, tell her from me that in this world one can't be wholly fortunate, and that she must be patient. Commend me to her, and say I won't answer her further just now, because I cannot. And commend me to him.

MICHELANGELO BUONARROTI IN ROME

1. *He probably refers to the Pope's wish that, on the completion of 'The Last Judgment', he should proceed to the painting of the Pauline Chapel.*

¶ To Lionardo di Buonarroto Simoni in Florence

210

Buonarroti Archives Mil. cxlii From Rome August 20th 1541

Lionardo — You write me that you want to come to Rome with Guicciardino this September. I tell you that this is not convenient yet, because it would only add to my vexations, over and above my other troubles. I say the same as regards Michele, because I'm so busy[1] that I haven't time to pay attention to you, and every little thing extra is a great bother to me, not excepting even having to write this. You must wait until next Lent, when I'll send for you and will send you money to equip yourself, that you may not come here like a nobody. I also wrote to Michele and advised him likewise to wait until next Lent, so that I may entertain him, as I shall be free. But perhaps he has some business in Rome that makes it necessary for him to be here in September – I don't know. But if this is not the case, I again advise him not to come until next

Lent, because this September I shan't have time for more than a word with him, particularly as Urbino, my assistant, is going to Urbino this September, and leaving me here alone with so many vexations. To have to do the cooking for the two of you would be the last straw. Read this letter to Michele and ask him to wait until next Lent, as I've said. Learn to write, for you seem to me to go from bad to worse.

MICHELANGELO IN ROME

1. *i.e. on the final stages of 'The Last Judgment'. On the completion of the fresco the Chapel was formally reopened on October 31st 1541.*

211

¶ TO LIONARDO DI BUONARROTO SIMONI IN FLORENCE

Buonarroti Archives Mil. cxliii From Rome January 19th 1542

Although I've written to the priest,[1] I meant to write the same thing to you; then I hadn't time and also because writing is a bother to me. I'm enclosing with this the letter to the priest, which is open, from which you can see what I wanted to write to you; which is that I'm sending you fifty gold *scudi* in gold and instructions as to what you are to do with the money if you want to come to Rome, and likewise how you are to use them if I send you fifty more, supposing you don't want to come. The said fifty gold *scudi* in gold, which I'm sending you, I've sent this morning, the nineteenth day of January, by Urbino my assistant, to Bartolomeo Bettini, that is to say to the Cavalcanti and Giraldi; I'm enclosing the letter of exchange with this. Take it to the Salviati and they'll pay you the money. Make out the receipt correctly, that is to say, for the amount received from me in Rome.[2]

Read the priest's letter and then give it to him – or rather, give it to him first and he'll read it to you; and be guided by him as to coming or not coming. And if you decide to come let me know first, as I'll arrange with some honest muleteer here for you to come with him. And if you really want to come, don't let Michele know about it, because I can't put him up, as you'll see if you come.

The said Michele has written to me that he wants me to send him nine ducats and two thirds, which he says were still owing when I redeemed the farm at Pazzolatica. He asked me for them before, but the priest wrote and told me that when he did the accounts with him, he showed him that he wasn't owed them. So ask the priest to tell you, or to write and tell me, whether I have to send him the money or not.

MICHELANGELO IN ROME

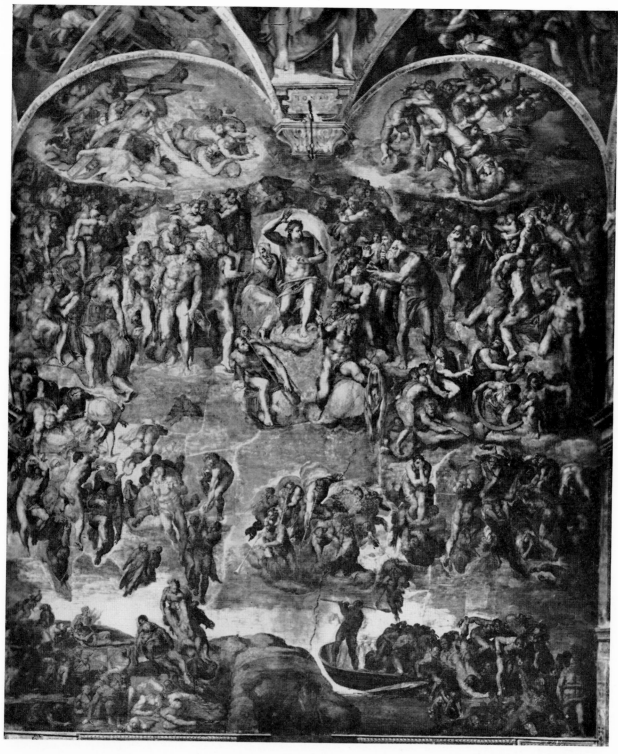

2. *The Last Judgment*

Michelangelo
Sistine Chapel, Rome

1.   *i.e. Ser Giovan Francesco Fattucci.*

2.   *The receipt was to be made out for the number of scudi paid into the bank in Rome, and not for the number of ducats drawn from the bank in Florence.*

212

¶ [To Messer Niccolò Martelli in Florence]

Biblioteca Nazionale, Florence Mil. cdxxii From Rome January 20th 1542

Messer Niccolò[1] — I have received your letter through Messer Vincenzo Perini,[2] with two sonnets and a madrigal.[3] The letter and the sonnet addressed to me are wonderful, so much so that anyone would be deserving of censure who found anything in them to censure.[4]

The truth is that you bestow so many praises upon me that, if paradise were within me, far fewer would suffice. I see that you imagined me to be the man that would to God I were. I am a poor fellow, and of little worth, plodding along in that art which God has assigned to me, in order to prolong my life as long as I can. And thus, such as I am, I am at your service and at the service of the whole Martelli house. Both for the letter and for the sonnets I thank you, but not as I should, because an equal height of courtesy is beyond me. I am ever yours. From Rome on the 20th day of January 1542.

MICHELANGELO BUONARROTI

1.   *Niccolò Martelli, a member of the Accademia Fiorentina (see Appendix 37), had written to Michelangelo on December 4th [1541] on the occasion of the uncovering of 'The Last Judgment'. In publishing his own letter, together with Michelangelo's reply, in 1546 (p. 9v) he supplied the year (evidently omitted in the original) and mistakenly supposed it to have been written in 1540 instead of 1541.*

2.   *Vincenzo Perini (afterwards Treasurer of the Romagna) had forwarded the letters and begged in return that he might see Michelangelo's answer. On March 28th 1542 Martelli accordingly sent him a copy of it, declining, however, to part with the original which he regarded as being among his most treasured possessions. Martelli likewise misdated this letter by one year (p. 9r).*

3.   *Frey, Dicht., pp. 265 et seq.*

4.   *This refers to Martelli's request that Michelangelo would censure anything he found deserving of censure in the poems he had sent – not as being in any way worthy of Michelangelo, but as a token of his affectionate regard.*

X

LETTERS
213 - 249

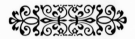

From Rome
1542 - 1545

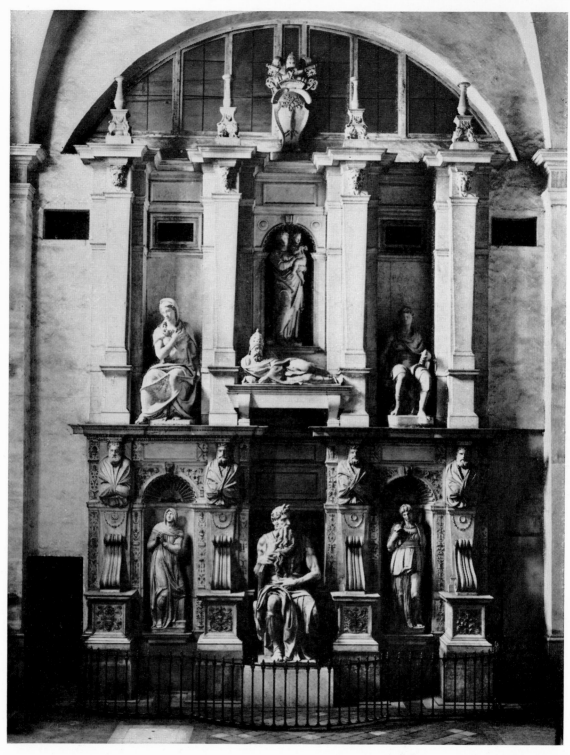

3. The Tomb of Julius II

Michelangelo
S. Pietro in Vincoli, Rome

X. From Rome : 1542-1545

¶ To Lionardo di Buonarroto

Buonarroti
Archives
Mil. cxliv
From Rome
February 4th
1542

213

Lionardo — You write me that you don't think you'll come,[1] and that you'll use the fifty *scudi*, supposing that I send the other fifty, to invest in the shop. I'd send them shortly, but first I want the agreement of Giovan Simone and of Gismondo, because I want them to be present when the money is invested in the shop, and I want things properly arranged by them and with their agreement, as I wrote you, because they are my brothers. So I'm writing to them about it. Get them to reply to me as to their agreement, and I will not fail to do as I've said.

I wrote and told you that Guicciardini had asked me for nine *scudi*, or rather ducats, and two thirds which he said were still owing when I redeemed the farm at Pazzolatica, and I told you to let me know whether he was owed them or not. You haven't replied to me. So ask Messer Giovan Francesco to tell you whether in fact I owe them to him, and write and tell me so that I may send them to him. I think that's all.

On the 4th day of February 1542.

MICHELANGELO IN ROME

---

1. *i.e. to Rome. This would seem to have been a major error of judgment either on Lionardo's part or on Fattucci's. It was probably this decision which led Michelangelo to think that Lionardo cared only for his money.*

¶ To Messer Luigi del Riccio in Rome

Buonarroti
Archives
Mil. cdxxxii
From Rome
May 1542

214

Messer Luigi, my dear Signor — As you have dealt with this disagreement which has arisen between Urbino and Maestro Giovanni, and as you are not involved in it, you can give a fair ruling about it. As you are aware, I gave them the work in order to do each of them a good turn. Now, because the one is too grasping and the other no less unreasonable, this difficulty has arisen between them, which might lead to a serious quarrel resulting in blows or death. Should such a thing happen to either of them, I should be sorry about Messer Giovanni, but much more so about Urbino, because I've brought him up. Therefore, if the terms of the partnership[1] permit, I think they should both be dismissed and that the work should revert unconditionally to me, so that their stupidity may not be my ruin, and I can get on with it. Although I have been advised to divide the said work, and to allot one part to the one and one to the other, I cannot do this, and to give it ....[2] to either one of them alone would be to wrong the one to whom I did not give it. It therefore seems to me that there is no other course but to leave the work in my hands, so that I can get on with it.

As to the money, that is the hundred *scudi* I paid, and as to the work they have done, let them arrange it between themselves in such a way that I may not be the loser. I beg you to get them to agree as best you can, because this would be an act of charity.

And since one of them may perhaps wish to prove that the little that has been done he has done entirely himself and, in addition to the money he has already received, is owed much more – should this be the case, I too can prove that I have lost a month of my time on the said work, owing to their bestial ineptitude, and have held up the work for the Pope, which means a loss to me of more than two hundred *scudi*; so that I am owed much more by them than they by the work.

Messer Luigi, I have made this statement to you in writing, because to make it in front of these fellows by word of mouth completely exhausts me, so that I have no breath left to speak.

YOUR MICHELANGELO BUONARROTI IN THE MACELLO DE' POVERI[3]

1. *A contract, whereby Michelangelo allocated the completion of the architectural frame for the Tomb of Julius II to his assistant, Urbino (Francesco di Bernardino d'Amadore da Urbino) and to Maestro Giovanni de' Marchesi da Saltri jointly, had been drawn up on May 16th 1542. But as the two could not agree, it had to be cancelled. Another was drawn up on June 1st of the same year (Milanesi, pp. 710, 712). See Appendix 28.*

2. *There is a tear in the MS. at this point.*

3. *Michelangelo here alters 'Ravens' Lane' to 'Poor Men's Lane'.*

215   ¶ [TO MESSER LUIGI DEL RICCIO IN ROME]

Buonarroti Archives Mil. cdxxiii From Rome (May 1542)

I sent this[1] to Florence some time ago. I'm now sending it to you, as I have revised it to suit the occasion more nearly, so that you may, if you like it, consign it to the flame, that is to say, to the one that consumes me. Also, I would ask another favour of you – that is, would you resolve a certain doubt in which I was left last night, because, when in a dream I greeted our idol[2] he seemed to me both to smile and to threaten me. Not knowing which of the two to hold by, I beg you to find out from him, and when we meet on Sunday to resolve it for me.

Yours, with infinite obligation and always.

[Unsigned]

If you like it, have it written out properly and give it to those chords which hold men captive without distinction and remember me to Messer Donato.[3]

1. *A madrigal or sonnet. For the interpretation of this letter see Appendix 29.*

2. *Francesco (Cecchino) de' Bracci. See Appendix 30.*

3. *Donato Giannotti (1492–1573). A Florentine man of letters and an ardent republican. On the fall of the Republic, he joined the 'fuorusciti' and lived both in Venice and in Rome, where, in the service of Cardinal Ridolfi, he became a leading member of the intellectual circle in which Michelangelo moved. Michelangelo figures in his 'Dialoghi' and it was at Donato's instigation that he executed the bust of Brutus for Cardinal Ridolfi (1501–1550).*

¶ [To Messer Luigi del Riccio in Rome]

216

*Buonarroti
Archives
Mil. cdxxix
From Rome
(May/June
1542)*

Messer Luigi — I think I should do something so as not to appear ungrateful to Arcadente.[1] So if you think of giving him some token, I'll return you whatever you give him. I have a piece of satin for a doublet at home, which Messer Girolamo[2] got for me. If you approve, I'll send it to you to give him. Tell Urbino or one of the others what you think. I'll settle with you for everything.

Your Michelangelo

1. *Jacques Arcadelt (c.1505–c.1567), the eminent Flemish composer, who became a member of the Julian Choir in 1539 and of the Sistine Choir in 1540. See Appendix 29.*

2. *Perhaps Girolamo Ubaldini, the merchant banker.*

¶ To Messer Luigi del Riccio at the Bank

217

*Buonarroti
Archives
Mil. cdxxviii
From Rome
(May/June
1542)*

Messer Luigi, my dear Signor — Arcadente's air[1] is considered to be a beautiful thing, and as, according to what he says, he understands that it has given no less pleasure to me than to you who commissioned it, I do not wish to appear ungrateful to him in a matter like this. I therefore beg you to think of some present to make him, either of silks[2] or money, and to let me know, and I'll do as you say without any hesitation. That's all I have to tell you. I commend me to you, and to Messer Donato, and to heaven and earth.

YOUR MICHELANGELO once again

1. *This letter is written under the madrigal 'Spargendo il senso il troppo ardor cocente' (Guasti, p. 82). See Appendix 29.*

2. *A typical gift of the period. Cf. Landucci, p. 314.*

218

Buonarroti Archives Mil. cdxxxi From Rome July 1542

¶ [TO MESSER LUIGI DEL RICCIO IN ROME]

Messer Luigi, my dear Signor — I'm sending you by Urbino, my assistant, twenty *scudi* for you to give to Maestro Giovanni[1] for the work of which you are cognizant, and as Urbino is also drawing a profit from the said work, I must give another twenty to him, which will make forty; so that I shall have already spent a hundred and forty *scudi*. And of the said work, not sixty *scudi*'s worth has been done. Maestro Giovanni will have had seventy-five *scudi*, of which thirty is profit. Since the company was formed, Urbino has spent the balance of the hundred I paid out at the beginning on the marbles and on daily wages (Maestro Giovanni having received fifty-five); but for two months Urbino has not had anything, when he should have the same profit as Maestro Giovanni, that is to say, thirty ducats as profit on the work. But I'll content him with twenty.

Since the decision was made and given in writing about the amount of the aforesaid work that has been done, I have assessed it myself, and I find that not a tenth part of it has been done. But I was very glad that the men who assessed it estimated a seventh[2] in Maestro Giovanni's favour, so he cannot complain. But there is nothing that can be done about it. And if anyone has cause to complain, it is I more than anyone else, because I have lost two months of my time over it by troubling myself with ......[3] but I'm more upset over the Pope's anger than over the two hundred *scudi*.

I presume too much on your kindness. God grant I may be able to repay you.

Maestro Giovanni must release the marbles which remain on the Campidoglio. I am not letting him remove those for which he has already been paid, as this was one of the causes of the differences which arose between them. And he must give a discharge for everything else in the same way.

YOUR MICHELANGELO : ROME

1. *See Note 1, No. 214.*

2. *On July 8th 1542, three men, Maestro Giuliano, Maestro Bernardino da Marco, and Andrea Bevel-acqua, scarpellino, had been called in to assess the amount that had been done on the frame for the Tomb of Julius, and had adjudged it to be one-seventh, as against Michelangelo's own estimate of one-tenth (Milanesi, p. 714, and Gaye, II, pp. 291 et seq.).*

3. *There is a tear in the MS. at this point.*

¶ PETITION TO POPE PAUL III

Biblioteca Nazionale Florence Mil. cdxxxiii From Rome July 20th 1542

219

Messer Michelangelo Buonarroti, having undertaken a long time ago to execute the Tomb of Pope Julius in Santo Piero in Vincola, in accordance with certain terms and conditions, as by a contract drawn up by Messer Bartolomeo Cappello, under date, the 18th day of April 1532 appears: and being afterwards required and constrained by His Holiness Our Lord, Pope Paul the Third, to execute the painting of his new chapel, and being unable to attend to that and to the finishing of the Tomb, he came, through the mediation of His Holiness, to a new agreement with the Illustrious Lord Duke of Urbino, to whom the charge of the aforesaid Tomb has fallen, as from one of the Duke's letters, dated the 6th day of March 1542 is evident; whereby of six statues that are to be built into the said Tomb, the said Messer Michelangelo might allocate three to a good and approved master to finish and to build into the said work; and the other three, in-cluding the Moses, he had himself to finish with his own hand, and, similarly, he was obliged to have the architectural frame completed, that is to say, the rest of the orna-ment of the said Tomb, in the style of the first part that had been completed. Whence, in order to give effect to the said agreement, the aforesaid Messer Michelangelo allocated the finishing of the said three statues, which were well advanced – that is, one of Our Lady with the Child in her arms, standing, and one Prophet and one Sibyl, seated, to Raffaello da Montelupo, a Florentine, recognized as being among the best masters of the present time, for four hundred *scudi*, as by the written agreement between them ap-pears; and the rest of the architectural frame and ornament of the Tomb, with the ex-ception of the crowning pediment,[1] he allocated in like manner to Maestro Giovanni de' Marchesi and to Francesco da Urbino, *scarpellini* and stone carvers, for seven hundred *scudi*, as by the written undertaking between them appears. It remained to him to finish the three statues by his own hand, that is, the Moses and two Captives; the which three statues are almost finished. But because the said two Captives were executed when the work was designed to be much larger, and was to include many other statues, which work was afterwards in the above-mentioned contract curtailed and reduced; for this reason they are unsuited to the present design, nor would they by any means be appro-priate for it. Therefore, the said Messer Michelangelo, in order not to fail to honour

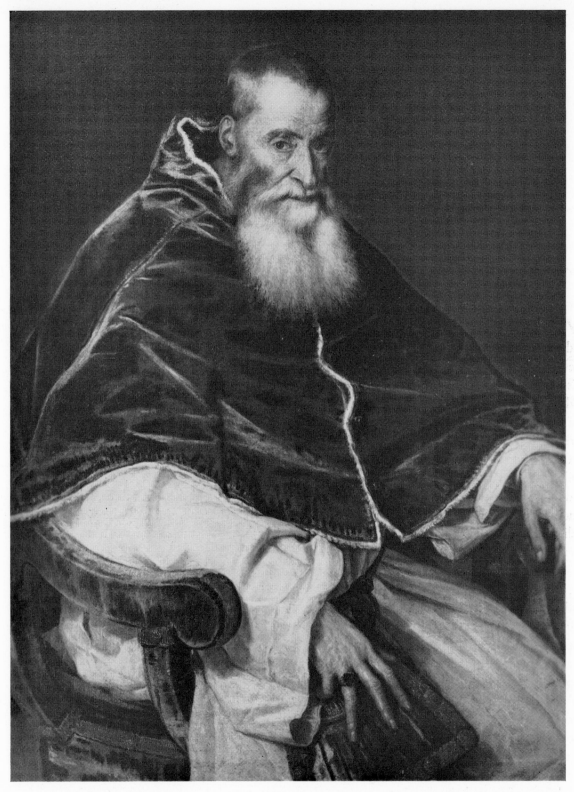

4. *Pope Paul III*　　　　　　　　　　　　　　　　　　　　　　　*Titian*
Museo Nazionale, Naples

his obligation, began the other statues to go in the same zone as the Moses, the Contemplative Life and the Active, which are well enough advanced to be easily finished by other masters. But the said Messer Michelangelo, being again required by His said Holiness, Our Lord Pope Paul the Third, and urged to begin work on his chapel and to carry it to completion, as stated above, the which is a great task, which requires his personal attention complete and undistracted by any other concern, the said Michelangelo, being an old man, and desiring to serve His Holiness with all his powers; being also constrained and compelled by him in the matter, and being unable to do so, unless he is first released entirely from this work of Pope Julius, which keeps him in a state of physical and mental suspense, petitions His Holiness, since he is resolved that he should work for him, to negotiate with the the Illustrious Lord Duke of Urbino for his complete release from the said Tomb, cancelling and annulling every obligation between them, on the following unequivocal terms. First, the said Michelangelo requests permission to be allowed to allocate the other two statues that remain to be finished to the said Raffaello da Montelupo, or to whomsoever else His Excellency pleases, for a fair price to be determined, which he thinks will be about 200 *scudi*; and the Moses he wishes to deliver, finished by himself. And further, he is willing to deposit the full sum of money that is to go into the finishing of the said work – notwithstanding the inconvenience it will be to him, and much though he has contributed towards the said work – that is, the balance that remains outstanding of the amount he has not yet paid to Raffaello da Montelupo to finish the three statues allocated, as above, which is about 300 *scudi*, and the balance outstanding, which he has not yet paid for the working of the architectural frame and ornament, which is about 500 *scudi*; and the 200 *scudi*, or whatever will be needed to finish the last two statues, besides a hundred ducats, which are to go to the finishing of the crowning pediment of the said Tomb; which in all amounts to between 1,100 and 1,200 *scudi*, or whatever shall be necessary, which he will deposit in Rome in a suitable bank, in the name of the aforesaid Illustrious Lord Duke, in his own name, and in that of the work, with the express condition that the sum is to be used to finish the said work, and for nothing else, nor is to be touched or removed for any other purpose. And he is agreeable, besides this, as far as he is able, to superintend the said work on the statues and ornamentation, so that it may be finished with that diligence which is required. And in this way His Excellency will be assured that the work will be finished and will know where the money is to be found to effect it, and will be able, through his agents, to press for the continuance of the work, and to have it brought to completion. This is much to be desired, because Michelangelo is very old and is fully occupied on work which he will with difficulty have time to finish, let alone to do anything else. And Messer Michelangelo shall remain entirely free and shall be able to work for and to fulfil the wishes of His Holiness, whom he hereby petitions to cause a letter to be written to His Excellency, requesting him to give the requisite order here, and to send a mandate empowering his release from every contract and obligation existing between them.[2]

1. *i.e. 'frontispezio'. It is difficult to interpret this word, unless we suppose that Michelangelo intended to surmount the work with a central pediment. Had this been carried out it would, to some extent, have mitigated the weakness of the upper zone and have given meaning to the flanking candelabra.*

2. *This petition, which is in the handwriting of Luigi del Riccio, is endorsed with a note 'Copy of a document given by Messer Michelangelo Buonarroti to Messer Piergiovanni, Master of the Robes to Our Lord, on the 20th day of July, 1542 . See Appendix 28.*

220

Buonarroti Archives Mil. cdxxiv From Rome (July/August) 1542

❡ To Messer Luigi del Riccio, dearest friend

Messer Luigi — I am sending you a bag of documents,[1] so that you may see which is the one to be sent to Cortese.[2] Please tell Urbino which is the right one, so that he may have it copied out and may wait and pay for it, and afterwards take it to the said Cortese. But if you cannot attend to it to-day, Urbino can bring the said documents back to me, and I'll send them back to you another time, when it is convenient.

Also, I beg you to send me my draft[3] and Perino's, or rather Pierino's,[4] and also that sonnet I sent you, so that I may revise it and look it over carefully, as you bid me.

Your Michelangelo

1. *Documents relating to the Tomb of Julius II.*

2. *Messer Jacopo Cortese, a public notary or member of the Romana Curia Causarum. He had been one of the procurators at the drawing up of the Contract of April 1532 and was to be one of the witnesses to the new Contract of August 1542 (Milanesi, pp. 703, 716).*

3. *i.e. a draft of a sonnet or madrigal.*

4. *Probably Perino del Vaga, alias Piero Buonaccorsi. See Vol. I, Appendix 20.*

221

Buonarroti Archives Mil. cdxxv From Rome (August) 1542

❡ [To Messer Luigi del Riccio in Rome]

Messer Luigi, my dear Signor — I am earnestly begging a very great favour of you. It is that you would look at a document that Cortese has drawn up for me, as I do not understand it, and, as Urbino will explain to you, I cannot come to see you. In order not to seem ungrateful to him, please would you thank him and commend me to him, and for yourself, forgive me my too great temerity.

Your Michelangelo

¶ To Messer Luigi del Riccio, dearest friend

*Buonarroti
Archives
Mil. cdxxx
From Rome
August 30th
1542*

Messer Luigi — A poor man with no-one to serve him is guilty of these lapses.[1] Yesterday[2] I could neither come nor could I reply to your letter, because my crowd came home late.

I therefore make my apologies to you personally, and beg you to make my apologies to Messer Salvestro[3] and to commend me to Cecchino.

[Unsigned]

1. *In his letter of August 29th Luigi had asked him to dinner, saying, 'If you want to give everyone pleasure come to supper at the bank this evening' (Frey, Dicht., p. 530).*

2. *August 29th was the Feast of the Decollation of St. John the Baptist and a general holiday. Michelangelo had presumably given Urbino and the rest of his household the day off and therefore had no one to send in the morning or to attend him at night.*

3. *Messer Salvestro da Montaguto, one of his bankers.*

¶ [To Messer Luigi del Riccio in Rome]

*Buonarroti
Archives
Mil. cdxxvii
From Rome
(August/
September
1542)*

Messer Luigi — You, who have the spirit of poetry – please would you shorten and revise one of these madrigals, whichever seems to you the least lamentable, as I have to give it to a friend of ours.[1]

Your Michelangelo

1. *This note is appended to the madrigal 'Non è senza periglio', the other one being that beginning 'Sotto duo belle ciglia' (Guasti, pp. 129, 130).*

¶ To Messer Luigi del Riccio, my dear Signor and faithful friend

*Buonarroti
Archives
Mil. cdxxvi
From Rome
(September)
1542*

Messer Luigi, my dear Signor — Love has ratified the contract I made between him and myself:[1] but as to the other ratification,[2] of which you are cognizant, so far I don't know anyone who thinks me worthy of it. So I commend me to you, to Messer Donato, and to the third,[3] first or last as you please.

Your Michelangelo Buonarroti, full of troubles, Rome

Old things, fit for the fire, not to be seen by anyone.[4]

1. *This note accompanies two madrigals, 'Ben sarà 'l fiero ardore' and 'Perch' all' superchio ardore,' (Guasti, pp. 51, 52, Dicht, p. 419). It is to these that the first line of the letter refers.*

2. *The ratification of the last contract for the Tomb of Julius II. See Appendix 28.*

3. *Cecchino de' Bracci.*

4. *This refers to the madrigals which he evidently considered a poor effort.*

225 ¶ To Monsignor .... Datary

*Buonarroti
Archives
Mil. cdxxxviii
From Rome
October 17th
1542*

Reverend and magnificient Lord Datary[1] — Of the regular salary of 50 *scudi* a month, which Our Lord grants me, I am owed payment for eight months, that is to say from February until now, which amounts at the end of this month to four hundred Italian gold *scudi* in gold. Would you be kind enough to pay them to Salvestro da Montaguto and Company for me, and to continue to make them a regular payment month by month, for which a receipt will be given. I should be glad if the payment might be made promptly. I commend myself to your reverend and magnificent Lordship, and I pray God He may grant you your desires.

From my house in the Macello de' Corvi on the 17th day of October 1542.

At Your Lordship's command,

MICHELANGELO BUONARROTI

1. *The office of Datary was held at this time by Niccolò Ardinghelli (1503–1547), a Florentine. The letter is a copy in Luigi del Riccio's hand.*

226 ¶ To Messer Luigi del Riccio

*British
Museum
Mil. cdxxxiv
From Rome
October/
November 1542*

Messer Luigi, dear friend — Messer Pier Giovanni[1] is continually urging me to start painting.[2] I don't think I can for another four to six days as yet, because, as anyone can see, the *arricciato*[3] isn't dry enough for me to begin.

But there is another thing that worries me more than the *arricciato* and prevents me not only from painting, but from living life at all; namely that the ratification[4] hasn't come. I realize that I'm being put off, so much so that I'm completely desperate. I've bled myself white to the amount of one thousand four hundred *scudi*, of which I would have availed myself for the work of seven years, during which time I could have done two tombs, let alone one. This I did in order to be able to live in peace and to give my mind entirely to the service of the Pope. Now I find myself without the money and with

Messer Lugi amico caro · io so molto sollecitato damesser preu giouanni alcomin
ciare adipignere · e come siguo uedete · aora p quattro o sei di no credo pote
re · p che larricciato no esecho i modo che si possa comiciare lma ce unal
tra cosa che mi da piu noia che lauricciato · e che no che dipignere vio
mi lascia uiuere comesta e laretisficagione che no niene e conosco ch me
date parose · i modo che io sono ingra dispetatione · io mi so canato delcu
ore mille quattro ceto scudi che marebbon seruito sette anni allauorare
che arei fatto dua sepulture no che una equesto o fatto p potere stare
i pace e seruire slpapa co tucto il cuore ora mi truo no mato i danari
e co piu guerra e afanni che mai · quello che o fatto circa i detti danari
lo fatto col conseno delduca e col contratto della liberatione eora che
io glo sborsati no me laretisficatione · i modo ch si puo molto be uedete
che significa questa cosa senza scriuerlo · basta che p la fede di treta
sei anni e p essersi donato uolotariamete austui io no merito altro la
pictura e lascultura lafatica e lafede mai uo uinato e una tuttauia di
male i peggio · meglio mera ne primi anni che io mi fussi messo afare
zolfanegh che no sarei intata passio me · io scriuo questo auostra s
o dir come o mo che mi uuol bene e che amarregiata questa cosa esame
iluero lo faro i te deue alpapa accio che esappi che io no posso uiue
re no che di pignere e se o dato speraza di comiciare lo dato co la
speraza della deta uestisficagioni che e gia n mese ch ci auea aessere
no uoglio piu stare sotto questo peso ne essere ogni di uitupato p giutator
da chi ma tosto canita e lo uove lamorte o slpapa solo me ne posso
canare

Yostro michelagnolo buo
naruoti

more worries and troubles than ever. What I did with regard to the said money, I did on the assumption of having the Duke's agreement and of being released from the contract. And now that I've disbursed the money, the ratification hasn't come, so that it's obvious what this means, without my telling you. Let it suffice that this is all I deserve in return for thirty-six years of fair dealing and ungrudging devotion to others. Painting and sculpture, hard work and fair dealing have been my ruin and things go continually from bad to worse. It would have been better had I been put to making matches[5] in my youth, than to be in such a fret!

I'm telling you this, because, as one who is kindly disposed towards me and has dealt with the matter and knows the truth, you can apprise the Pope of it, so that he may know that I am unable to live life at all, much less to paint. And if I have given an expectation of starting work, I've given it in the expectation of receiving the ratification, which should have been here a month ago. I will not bear this burden any longer, nor be insulted as a cheat by those who have deprived me of life and honour. Only death or the Pope can release me.

Your Michelangelo Buonarroti

1. *Pier Giovanni Alliotti (d.c.1562), Master of the Robes to Paul III. He was created Bishop of Forli (his birthplace) in 1551. He concerned himself with everything at the Vatican from the purchase of cloth for the Pope's robes to taking delivery of Michelangelo's colours. He was known to Michelangelo as 'Tantecose', because he complained that he had so many things ('tante cose') to attend to.*

2. *The frescoes in the Pauline Chapel, which he began in November 1542.*

3. *'Arricciato', the layer of plaster applied to a wall to be painted in fresco, beneath the final layer, 'intonaco', which is applied as required during the course of the painting.*

4. *See Appendix 28.*

5. *According to Dr. W. T. O'Dea, this is the earliest post-classical reference known concerning sulphur matches, 'zolfanelli'. Their manufacture was extremely simple (O'Dea, p. 234).*

227 ¶ To Monsignore ....

Biblioteca
Nazionale
Florence
Mil. cdxxxv
From Rome
October/
November
1542

Monsignore[1] — Your Lordship sends to tell me that I should paint and not worry about anything else. I reply that one paints with the head and not with the hands, and if one cannot concentrate, one brings disgrace upon oneself. Therefore, until my affair is settled, I can do no good work. The ratification of the last contract hasn't come, and on the strength of the other – the one drawn up in Clement's presence[2] – I am stoned every day, as if I had crucified Christ. I maintain that the said contract did not indicate that it was read over in Pope Clement's presence, as did the copy I afterwards had of it.

And this was because, when Clement had sent me to Florence that same day, Gianmaria of Modena, the ambassador,[3] got together with the notary and made him extend its scope to suit himself. So that when I returned and had access to it I found included in the contract a thousand ducats[4] more than had been specified; I found the house in which I'm living included and several other snags designed to ruin me, which Clement would not have tolerated. And Frate Sebastiano can bear witness to the fact that he wanted me to inform the Pope of this and to get the notary hanged. But I did not want to, because I remained under no obligation to carry out something which I could not have carried out had I been left free. I swear that I am not aware of having had the said money, which the contract states and which Gianmaria said that he found I had had.

But let us assume that I have had it – since I have acknowledged receipt and cannot repudiate the contract – and other moneys, if others be alleged, and let everything be put together, and then consider what I did for Pope Julius at Bologna, at Florence, at Rome, in bronze, in marble and in painting, and all the time I spent in his service, which was the whole time he was Pope – and then consider what I merit. On the basis of the salary paid me by Pope Pagolo,[5] I maintain, with a clear conscience, that the heirs of Pope Julius owe me five thousand *scudi*. I maintain, moreover, that such was the reward I received for my pains from Pope Julius – fool that I was not to know how to manage my affairs – that were it not for what I have received from Pope Pagolo, I should be dying of hunger to-day. But according to these ambassadors, it seems that I have enriched myself and robbed the sanctuary. They are making a great outcry, and I ought to be able to find a way of putting them to silence but I'm no good at it. Gianmaria, the ambassador at the time of the old Duke,[6] when the above-mentioned contract was drawn up in Clement's presence, told me when I returned from Florence and began working on the Tomb of Julius, that if I wanted to do the Duke a great favour, I should go with God, as he couldn't be bothered about the Tomb, though he took it very ill that I should serve Pope Pagolo. Then it was that I realized why he had had the house included in the contract – in order that I might be got to go away, and that they, on the strength of the contract, might rush in and take possession. So it is obvious what they are aiming at, and they are bringing disgrace on our opponents, their masters. This ambassador[7] who has recently arrived, enquired first of all what I had in Florence, because he wanted to see what stage the Tomb had reached. It is borne in upon me that I lost the whole of my youth, chained to this Tomb, contending, as far as I was able, against the demands of Pope Leo and Clement. An excessive honesty, which went unrecognized, has been my ruin. Such was my fate. I see many people, with an income of two or three thousand *scudi*, lying in bed, while I contrive, with the utmost exertion, to bring myself to poverty.

But to return to the painting. It is not in my power to refuse Pope Pagolo anything. I shall paint ill-content, and shall produce things that are ill-contenting. I have told Your Lordship this, because, if the opportunity occurs, you will be better able to acquaint

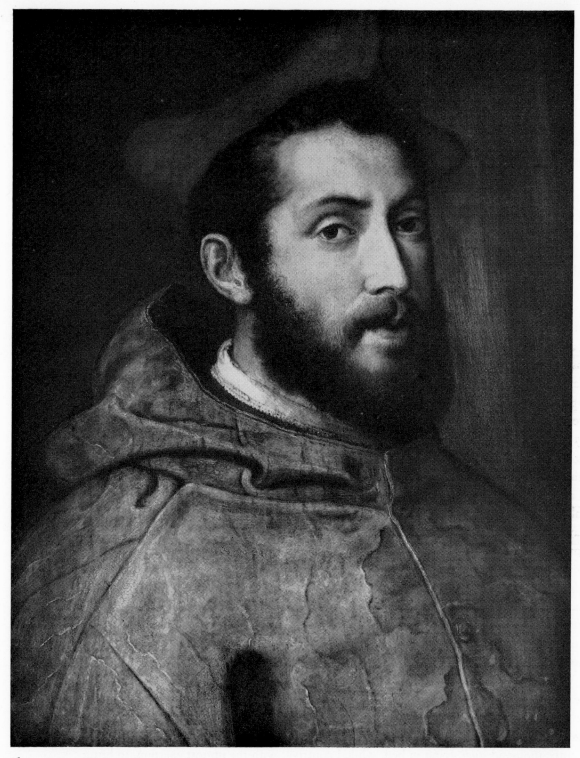

6. *Cardinal Alessandro Farnese*

Titian
Palazzo Corsini, Rome

the Pope with the truth. Also, I should be glad that the Pope should understand, in order that he may know the grounds on which this campaign is waged against me.

May those understand who can.

Your Lordship's servant,

MICHELANGELO

Several things that ought also to be said occur to me – that is, that this ambassador says that I lent Pope Julius's money at interest, and grew rich on it, as if Pope Julius had paid me eight thousand ducats in advance. The money that I had for the Tomb was intended for the expenses incurred for the said Tomb at that time; it will be seen to approximate to the sum that should be stated in the contract drawn up in the time of Clement; since, in the first year of Julius when he commissioned the Tomb, I was in Carrara for eight months, quarrying marbles, which I transported to the Piazza of St. Peter's, where I had the workshop behind Santa Caterina. Afterwards, Pope Julius decided not to have the Tomb done in his lifetime, and set me to painting. Then he kept me in Bologna for two years, to do the bronze Pope, which was destroyed. Then I returned to Rome and remained in his service until his death, always keeping open house, continuing to live, without an allowance and without a salary, on the money for the Tomb, because I had no other income.

Then, after the death of Julius, Aginensis wanted to proceed with the said Tomb, but on a larger scale. I therefore moved the marbles to the Macello de' Corvi and had that part executed which is now built in in Santo Pietro in Vincola, and executed the figures which I have in my house.

At this time, Pope Leo, who did not want me to execute the said Tomb, pretended that he wished to execute the façade of San Lorenzo in Florence and asked Aginensis for my services. He had therefore perforce to give me leave, with the proviso that I should do the said Tomb of Julius in Florence. While I was in Florence for the said façade of San Lorenzo, as I hadn't marbles there for the Tomb of Julius, I returned to Carrara and stayed there thirteen months, and transported all the marbles for the said Tomb to Florence, and built a workshop in which to execute them, and began working. At this time Aginensis sent Messer Francesco Palavicini, who is to-day the Bishop of Aleria, to urge me on, and he saw the workshop and all the said marbles and the figures blocked out for the said Tomb, which are still there to-day. Seeing this, that is to say that I was working for the said Tomb, Medici, who afterwards became Pope Clement, who was living in Florence, did not permit me to proceed, and I continued to be impeded in this way until Medici became Clement. Then in his presence the last contract up to now for the said Tomb was afterwards drawn up, in which it was stated that I had received the eight thousand ducats, which they say I lent at interest. But I want to confess a wrong-doing to Your Lordship – that is, that while I was at Carrara, when I stayed there thirteen months for the said Tomb, being in need of money, I spent a thousand *scudi* on marbles for the said work, which Pope Leo had sent me for the façade of San Lorenzo, or rather to keep me occupied, and I made him excuses, pretending there were difficulties. This I did for the love I bore the said work, for which I am repaid by being called a thief and a usurer by ignorant people who, at that time, weren't even born.

I am giving Your Lordship this account because I'm glad to have the opportunity of justifying myself in your eyes and in those of the Pope, to whom people have spoken ill of me, against whom Messer Piergiovanni says he has had to defend me, according to what he writes me; and also in order that Your Lordship may say a word in my defence, if you have the opportunity of doing so, because I'm telling the truth. Before men – I do not say before God – I count myself to be an honest man, because I've never cheated anyone; and also because in defending myself against these miscreants I am bound sometimes to become obsessed, as you see.

I beg Your Lordship to read this account when you have time and to do me this service, remembering that there are still witnesses to a great many of the things stated. Again, if the Pope were to see it I should be glad, and if the whole world were to see it, because I'm telling the truth, and there is much more I could say, and I'm not a thieving usurer, but a Florentine citizen of noble family, the son of an honest man, and not from Cagli.[8]

Since writing, a message has been sent me on behalf of Urbino's ambassador, to the effect that if I want the ratification, I should examine my conscience. My answer is that he has fashioned a Michelangelo of his own, made of the same stuff as himself.

But to proceed with the matter of the Tomb of Pope Julius, I repeat that after he changed his mind, as I've said, that is about doing it in his lifetime, several barges arrived at the Ripa with the marbles I had ordered at Carrara some time before, and as I was in need of money to pay the dues (not being able to get it from the Pope, as he had thought better about the undertaking) Baldassare Balducci, that is to say the bank of Messer Jacopo Gallo, lent me a hundred and fifty, or rather two hundred ducats, in order to pay the dues on the aforesaid marbles. And as at that time the *scarpellini* who had been engaged to do the said Tomb – some of whom are still alive – had come from Florence, and as I had equipped the house behind Santa Caterina, which Julius had given me, with beds and other furniture for the men who were to do the architectural frame and other things for the said Tomb, I found myself much embarrassed without money. And because I had urged the Pope as far as I could to proceed with it, one morning when I went to talk to him about it, he had me turned out by a groom. And when a Bishop of Lucca,[9] who witnessed this, said to the groom, 'Do you not know who this is?' the groom said to me, 'Pardon me, sir, these were my orders.' I went home, and wrote to the Pope, saying, 'Most Blessed Father – I was turned out of the Palace this morning by order of Your Holiness. I must therefore inform You that from now onwards, if You want me, You must seek me elsewhere than in Rome'. And I sent this letter to Messer Agostino, a steward, to give to the Pope. And at home I called a certain Cosimo, a carpenter in my service, who was making furniture for the house, and a *scarpellino* who was then in my service and is alive to-day, and said to them, 'Go and get a Jew and sell the contents of the house, and then return to Florence'. And I myself went and took a post horse and set out for Florence. The Pope, having received my letter, sent five horsemen after me; they caught me up at Poggibonsi at about ten o'clock at night and gave me a letter from the Pope, which said, 'Immediately on receipt of this, return to Rome, upon pain of Our displeasure'. The said horsemen asked me to reply, in order to show that they had found me. I made answer to the Pope that whenever he discharged his obligations towards me, I would return; otherwise he could never hope to get me back. And while I was in Florence Julius sent three briefs to the Signoria. When the last one arrived the Signoria sent for me and said, 'We do not propose to go to war with Pope Julius over you. You must go, and if you will return to him, we will give you a letter of such authority that if he does you any harm, it will be done to this Signoria.' Thus ordered, I returned to the Pope. It would take a long time to relate what followed. It suffices that this affair caused me a loss of one thousand ducats, because as soon as I had left Rome there was a great row, to the shame of the Pope, and nearly all the marbles I had in the Piazza of St. Peter's were stolen from me, and particularly the small pieces, so that I afterwards had to replace them. Thus I declare and affirm that the heirs of Pope Julius owe me five thousand ducats by way of indemnity. And those who have robbed me of my youth, my honour and my possessions, call me a thief! And again, as I've said before, Urbino's ambassador sends to tell me to examine my conscience first, and then I'll get a sight of the ratification from the Duke.[10] He did not say this before he made me deposit 1,400 ducats! In respect of these things of which I write I can only be mistaken as to the dates between then and now; everything else is true, and truer than I can say.

I beg Your Lordship, for the love of God and of the truth, to read all this when you have time, so that when the opportunity occurs you may be able to defend me to the Pope against those who speak ill of me without any knowledge of anything, and on false grounds have put it into the Duke's head that I am an arrant rascal. All the discords that arose between Pope Julius and me were owing to the envy of Bramante and Raphael of Urbino; and this is the reason why he did not proceed with the Tomb in his lifetime, in order to ruin me. And Raphael had good reason to be envious, since what he knew of art he learnt from me.

1. *For the identification of the cardinal addressed, Alessandro Farnese, see Appendix 31. This letter is a copy, perhaps in Luigi del Riccio's hand.*

2. *The contract was drawn up on April 29th 1532.*

3. *Giovanmaria della Porta da Modena, ambassador of Francesco Maria della Rovere, Duke of Urbino.*

4. *This would appear to have been a very irregular proceeding. According to Condivi, the alteration was not made when the contract was drawn up, but when it was engrossed. The contract published by Milanesi (p. 702) is a copy made by Luigi del Riccio, not of the original, but of the copy received by Michelangelo, as the sum received is given as 8,000 gold ducats of the Camera, and the house in*

the Macel de' Corvi is also included. Unfortunately no trace of the contract in dispute, which was drawn up by Bartolomeo Cappello, notary to the Apostolic Camera, can now be found either in the Archivio Segreto Vaticano or in the Archivio di Stato di Roma, though diligent search has been made for it. This would be explained if Condivi's statement is correct.

5. *i.e. Paul III.*

6. *Francesco Maria della Rovere. He died in 1538.*

7. *Girolamo Tiranno.*

8. *Cagli, a small township near Urbino. The precise significance of the phrase has now been lost, but it is evidently an expression of contempt equivalent to the modern Florentine phrase, 'Non vengo da Mugello'.*

9. *Cardinal Galleoto Franciotti (d. 1508) a nephew of Julius II, a young churchman of high repute.*

10. *Guidobaldo della Rovere. In 1547 he married Vittoria Farnese, granddaughter of Paul III.*

---

228   ¶ [To Messer Luigi del Riccio in Rome]

Buonarroti Archives Mil. cdxxxvi From Rome November 1542

Messer Luigi — I believe you may have an opportunity of finding out at the Palace what stage my affair has reached concerning the ratification, of which you are cognizant. I therefore beg you to do so if you can, because it would be the greatest kindness and because, as I wrote and told you before, I am unable to live life at all, much less to paint. And I think that, as an emissary[1] has been sent from the Duke without it, it may be a long affair and something may be put into the Pope's head to delay it. So if you can, I beg you to let me have some information.

Your Michelangelo

1. *Girolamo Genga (1476–1551), a painter in the service of the Duke of Urbino, who in 1531 had offered to act as an intermediary between the Duke and Michelangelo (Milanesi, Corr., p. 42: Vasari, 'Pros. Cron.', p. 388: and Appendix 28). He reached Rome in the middle of November.*

---

229   ¶ [To Messer Luigi del Riccio in Rome]

Buonarroti Archives Mil. cdxxxvii From Rome November 1542

Messer Luigi, dear friend — As I see the ratification isn't coming, I've made up my mind to stay at home and finish the three figures,[1] as I agreed with the Duke. It will suit me much better than dragging myself to the Palace every day. And those who choose to be cross must be cross. It is enough for me that I have acted in such a way that the Pope can't complain about me. The ratification was no benefit whatever to me, but to His Holiness, who wanted me to paint. It suffices that I am not prepared to run between the Pope and the Duke, and if the former, seeing that I have abandoned his painting, sends for the ambassador, it might perhaps be as well to acquaint the latter with my decision, so that he may know what to reply, should you think this advisable. It is to this end I'm writing to you about it.

YOUR MICHELANGELO

1. *This was what he was finally obliged to do in order to obtain the ratification. See No. 248.*

¶ TO GISMONDO DI LODOVICO BUONARROTI SIMONI IN FLORENCE

230

Gismondo — I'm sending you fifty gold *scudi* in gold, which I've paid to-day, the sixteenth day of December, here in Rome to the bank of Messer Salvestro da Montaguto, to have paid to you there in Florence. So go to the bank of the Capponi, and they'll be paid to you. Put them to your own use, and when you give the receipt, say – for the amount which Michelangelo has paid in Rome at the bank of Messer Salvestro da Montaguto – as is stated, and advise me of the receipt.

On the sixteenth day of December 1542.

MICHELANGELO BUONARROTI IN ROME

*Buonarroti
Archives
Mil. cxxxv
From Rome
December 16th
1542*

¶ TO LIONARDO DI BUONARROTO SIMONI IN FLORENCE

231

Lionardo — I learn from your letter and from the priest's where you handed in the contract to be forwarded to me; it didn't arrive here, and I'm certain about it, because Bettino[1] would have sent it direct to me at home. So I assume that it was retained at the bank there, where you handed it in. If you want me to get it, give it to Francesco d'Antonio Salvetti to direct to Luigi del Riccio[2] here, and it will be given to me at once and I'll ratify it. I think that's all.

I'm not writing to the priest because I haven't time. Commend me to him and thank him for his pains and the trouble he takes for us. And when you write to me, do not put 'Michelangelo Simoni' nor 'sculptor' on the outside. It is sufficient to say 'Michelangelo Buonarroti', as that's how I'm known here, and inform the priest of this likewise.

On the fourteenth day of April 1543.

MICHELANGELO BUONARROTI IN ROME

*Buonarroti
Archives
Mil. cxlvii
From Rome
April 14th
1543*

1. *Bartolomeo Bettini (d. 1551) of the Cavalcanti bank in Rome.*

2. *Endorsed in Luigi del Riccio's hand 'Messer Francesco Salvetti; give it into his own hand and get an answer to it'. Francesco Salvetti was a relative of del Riccio's and at one time there was some thought that he might enter into a partnership with Lionardo (Steinmann, pp. 53 et seq.).*

232

*Buonarroti
Archives
Mil. cxlv
From Rome
April (28th)
1543*

¶ To Lionardo di Buonarroto Simoni in Florence

Lionardo — I received the contract on Saturday evening, and the ratification will be enclosed with this. It wasn't executed before, because the contract hadn't come before, having been held up by the people to whom you gave it to forward to me. I have nothing else to tell you, nor have I time to write, nor have I yet read the letters. Thank the priest on my behalf, because he has put himself to a lot of trouble for us, and has done us a great service, and particularly to you people in Florence.

MICHELANGELO BUONARROTI IN ROME

233

*British
Museum
Mil. cxlvi
From Rome
(May 12th)
1543*

¶ To Lionardo di Buonarroto Simoni in Florence

Lionardo — I have had a search made at all the banks in Rome, and haven't found that any contract, except the last, for which I sent the ratification, has arrived here. We therefore think that it has been retained in Florence. If no letters or things of importance were enclosed, there is no need to think any more about it; if there were, we must put up with it. You wrote me that you have received the ratification and given it to the priest. I'm glad about this, since I don't think it's turned out badly; indeed, it's my belief that it has turned out well. I think that's all. Commend me to him, that is to Messer Giovan Francesco, and thank him on my behalf. I'm glad that you have spoken to Bettini;[1] commend me to him also, and thank him when you meet him.

MICHELANGELO IN ROME

1. *i.e. Bartolomeo Bettini was presumably on a visit to Florence.*

¶ [To Messer Luigi del Riccio]

234

*Buonarroti
Archives
Mil. cdxliv
From Rome
February 1544*

I should be ashamed, being so much in your company, not sometimes to speak in Latin,[1] albeit incorrectly.

Donato's sonnet[2] seems to me as fine as anything written in our time. But, having poor taste, I am no more able to judge of cloth newly-spun, although of the Romagna, than of worn brocades, which make even a tailor's dummy appear fine.

Write to him,[3] tell him this, give him this, and commend me to him.

[Unsigned]

1. *This note appears under the madrigal, 'S'è ver, com' è, che dopo il corpo viva,' (Guasti, p. 26), into which Michelangelo had introduced a Latin phrase.*

2. *The madrigal was written on the death of Cecchino de' Bracci, Luigi del Riccio's young kinsman, who died on January 8th 1544. It was written in answer to a sonnet by Donato Giannotti on the same subject, 'Messer Luigi mio di noi che sia', which bore the note, 'Magnificent Messer Luigi – since I wrote to you, I have produced a sonnet; I'm sending it to you, such as it is. Show it to Michelangelo as to a critic' (Frey, Dicht., p. 269). The date of Giannotti's note was January 30th 1544. It reached Rome on February 7th.*

3. *i.e. Donato Giannotti.*

¶ To Messer Luigi del Riccio

235

*Buonarroti
Archives
Mil. cdxlvii
From Rome
(February)
1544*

Our dead friend speaks, saying, 'If Heaven took every beauty from all other men on earth to make me alone beautiful, as it did, and if by divine decree on the Day of Judgment I had to return as I was when alive, it follows from this that the beauty, which Heaven gave me, cannot be restored to those from whom it was taken, but that I must be eternally more beautiful than others, and they ugly.' But this is the reverse of the conceit you suggested to me yesterday – one is fanciful and the other true.[1]

[Unsigned]

1. *This note accompanies one of the forty-eight epigrams and epitaphs (No. 8, Guasti, p. 7) which Michelangelo wrote for Luigi del Riccio on the death of Cecchino de' Bracci.*

236   ¶ [To the Castellan of the Castel Sant' Angelo in Rome]

*Buonarroti
Archives
Mil. cdxl
From Rome
February 26th
1544*

Monsignore the Castellan[1] — With reference to the model[2] under discussion yesterday, I didn't speak the whole of my mind, as I was requested to do by your lordship, because I thought it would give too much offence to those for whom I have a great regard – namely Captain Giovan Francesco,[3] from whom I differ over certain matters. For it seems to me that the bastions which have been begun can with reason, and must of necessity, be retained and continued. If this is not done, I am afraid we may be worse off, because with so many opinions and such diverse models I think they have greatly confused the Pope and so wearied him that if he came to no decision about anything, he might fail either to follow this course or to adopt some other, which would be disastrous and would do little credit to His Holiness. Therefore, as I've said, I think we should go on, I do not say with every single thing that has been begun, but only with the stretch of the Monte,[4] improving certain things, on the advice of the said Captain Giovan Francesco, without damaging what has been done, in order to take the opportunity of getting rid of the existing superintendence,[5] if it is as it is said to be, and of installing the said Captain Giovan Francesco, whom I regard as being altogether able and upright. If this were done, for the honour of the Pope I would place myself at his disposal, as I have been asked to do several times, not as a colleague, but altogether as a subordinate.

From the Spinegli to the Castello I should not do more than make a ditch, because if it were properly repaired, the corridor[6] is sufficient.

On the XXVI day of February 1544.[7]

Your Lordship's servant,

Michelangelo Buonarroti

---

1.   *Tiberio Crispi (1498–1566). He was connected (illegitimately) with the Farnese family and he received his cardinal's hat (at the instance, it is said, of the Pope's daughter Constanza) at the Consistory of December 19th 1544. Condivi mentions him as being among Michelangelo's friends, Michelangelo 'finding in him, besides his many excellent qualities, a rare and excellent judgment'.*

2.   *A model of the fortifications of the Borgo, anciently the citadel of the Papacy. See Appendix 32.*

3.   *Captain Giovan Francesco Montemellino da Perugia, a military engineer, sometime Captain of the Guard at the Castel Sant' Angelo.*

4.   *i.e. Monte Mario.*

5.   *i.e. that of Antonio Sangallo. The reference is deliberately oblique.*

6.   *i.e. the covered way, which then connected the Vatican with the Castel Sant' Angelo.*

7.   *This letter is a copy in Luigi del Riccio's hand.*

¶ To Lionardo di Buonarroto Simoni in Florence

237

Lionardo — I learn from your letter that the marbles[1] have been valued at one hundred and seventy *scudi*. As to what is to be done with the money when it is paid to you, I think, if my brothers agree, that it should be invested for you in a shop, wherever they think suitable, and that you should draw the licit interest[2] on it; but that you should not be able to lay it out in any other way without their permission. I also think that you should try to sell the workshop where the said marbles are, and should invest the money you get for it on the same conditions as that derived from the marbles. Later I'll be able to add more money to it, depending on how you behave yourself, as it doesn't seem to me you've yet learnt to write.

I've replied to Messer Giovan Francesco about the head of the Duke,[3] that I cannot attend to it there; it is true that I cannot, owing to the anxieties I have, but even more owing to old age, because I cannot see my way clear.

As to buying Luigi Gerardi's farm, about which you had a letter written to me, I don't think it a good thing to have another in Florence besides the one I've got, because to have more property there is only to have more anxiety, if I were unable to work. It therefore seems to me better to buy something somewhere else, from which I myself could enjoy the benefit in my old age, because the income the Pope allows me could be withdrawn, if I were unable to work. I've already had to make a stand for it twice. So answer the priest as to the said farm, about which he wrote me. I have nothing else to say to you. Try to do your best.[4]

Michelangelo in Rome

Buonarroti Archives Mil. cxlviii From Rome March 29th 1544

1. *The marbles left in the workshop in the Via Mozza.*

2. *i.e. interest not falling under the ban of the Church as being usurious.*

3. *A head of Cosimo de' Medici, Duke of Florence.*

4. *The letter is endorsed in Luigi del Riccio's hand, 'Messer Francesco Salvetti: deliver into his own hand and send the answer'.*

¶ [To Lionardo di Buonarroto Simoni]

238

Lionardo — I have been ill[1] and you have come in place of Ser Giovan Francesco, to kill me off and to see if I've left anything. Isn't all that you've had from me in Florence enough for you? You cannot deny you're like your father, who turned me out of my own house in Florence. I'd have you know that I've made my will in such a way that you need think no more about what I've got in Rome. So go with God, and

Buonarroti Archives Mil. cxlix From Rome July 11th 1544

don't come near me any more and never write to me again, and do as the priest tells you.[2]

MICHELANGELO

1. *Michelangelo was dangerously ill in the summer of 1544 and was nursed by Luigi del Riccio in his apartments in the Strozzi Palace. On July 21st del Riccio wrote to Roberto Strozzi in Lyons, saying that Michelangelo had been free of fever for several days, but was still very weak (Gaye, II, p. 296). The above letter, which was probably handed to Lionardo when he called to see his uncle, was therefore written while Michelangelo was still in a state of high fever. For the justification of Michelangelo's attitude on this occasion, and again when he was ill in 1546, see Appendix 34.*

2. *The letter is endorsed in Lionardo's hand, '1544. Received on the 11th day of July in Rome'.*

239

Buonarroti Archives Mil. cdxlviii From Rome (July/August 1544)

¶ [TO MESSER LUIGI DEL RICCIO]

I'm making you a return for the melons[1] with a draft,[2] but not the design as yet; but I'll certainly do it, as I can design a better one.[3] Commend me to Baccio[4] and tell him that if I had those concoctions here which he gave me there with you,[5] I should be another Gratian.[6] And thank him on my behalf.

[Unsigned]

1. *This note was written in reply to a letter from Luigi del Riccio, who had sent him a present of two melons from Lunghezza and a flask of Greek wine from San Gimignano saying, 'enjoy them for my sake' (Steinmann, p. 39).*

2. *The lines on Cecchino de' Bracci beginning 'Dal ciel fu la beltà mie diva e 'ntera' (Guasti, p. 13).*

3. *A drawing for a carving of Cecchino's head for which del Riccio had bought the marble on June 3rd. Michelangelo disliked the designs which del Riccio had previously sent him and had undertaken to do a better one.*

4. *Presumably Bartolomeo Rontini, his physician.*

5. *i.e. when he was nursed in the Strozzi-Ulivieri Palace.*

6. *The Emperor Gratian (359–383), who was noted for his gluttony and indolence.*

¶ To Messer Luigi del Riccio, friend, or rather, honoured patron, in Rome

240

*Buonarroti
Archives
Mil. cdxxxix
From Rome
(August 1544)*

My dear Messer Luigi — Because I know that you are as much an adept at formalities as I am a stranger to them, and because I have received from Monsignor Todi[1] a present which Urbino will tell you about, which I am sharing with you, I beg you, believing you to be a friend of his lordship's, to thank him in my name, when you conveniently can, with that formality which is as easy to you as it is difficult to me, and to make me your debtor for a few trifles.[2]

YOUR MICHELANGELO BUONARROTI

1. *Federigo Cesi, Bishop of Todi (1500–1565). He was a Clerk of the Camera and received his cardinal's hat at the Consistory of December 1544. He was a notable collector of antiquities, among which there were several pieces greatly admired by Michelangelo.*

2. *At this period trout, ravioli, caviar, melons, and other delicacies were constantly exchanged between friends. Gifts such as these Michelangelo frequently acknowledged in verses which he referred to as 'berlingozzi' pastries or as we might say, trifles. See Guasti, p. 19.*

¶ Lionardo di Buonarroto Simoni in Florence

241

*Buonarroti
Archives
Mil. cl
From Rome
December 6th
1544*

Lionardo — I do not want, however,[1] to fail you in that which I thought of doing some time ago, that is, to help you, if I learn that you are behaving yourself properly. So enclosed with this will be a letter addressed to Giovan Simone and Gismondo, in which I'm writing to tell them what I'm thinking of doing for you. But I do not propose to act without their advice. So give it to them, and tell them to answer me.

MICHELANGELO BUONARROTI IN ROME

1. *The use of the word 'however' is sufficiently amusing in the context if this characteristic letter is, as it appears to be, the first communication Lionardo received from his uncle after a lapse of five months. Cf. No. 238.*

242

Buonarroti
Archives
Mil. cxxxii
From Rome
December 6th
1544

¶ To Giovan Simone and Gismondo

Some time ago I thought of investing, little by little, up to a thousand *scudi* in the wool trade for Lionardo, if he's behaving himself properly, on this condition that he cannot withdraw it or use it for anything else without your permission. And to begin with I'm sending two hundred *scudi*, which I will shortly make payable there, if you tell me in reply that I should do so. And if you think I should do this, you must be careful that it's not invested in a risky concern, because I didn't find the money by the wayside. Tell me in reply what you think I should do. You are better able to judge than I am and to observe Lionardo's behaviour and whether he's fit to look after it.

Michelangelo Buonarroti in Rome

243

Buonarroti
Archives
Mil. cli
From Rome
December 27th
1544

¶ To Lionardo di Buonarroto Simoni in Florence

Lionardo — I have paid two hundred gold *scudi* in gold into the Covoni bank here, which will be paid to you there, to use as I wrote you in my last letter. So go to the Capponi with Gismondo or with Giovan Simone, and the money will be paid to you, that is, you will be paid two hundred gold *scudi* in gold, which I have paid in here. My proposal is that Giovan Simone and Gismondo should invest them for you in their name in the wool trade, if you think this would be safe; and that my name is on no account to be mentioned in connection with it; with this proviso, that the interest is to be yours, and that none of the said money can be laid out, removed or used for any other purpose, unless you are all three agreed, that is, Giovan Simone, Gismondo and you. And when you invest the money in the shop I wish you to ask Michele Guicciardini to be present with Giovan Simone and Gismondo, so that no mistake may be made as to the proper drawing up of the documents, because I think he understands these things and will gladly see to it on my behalf. And then get Giovan Simone and Gismondo to write acknowledging receipt of the said money and telling me how you have arranged matters, and commend me to Michele. And if neither Giovan Simone nor Gismondo can go with you to collect the said money, it will be given to you on your own to take to them, so that it may be used as stated above.

And when you make out the receipt for the said money at the Capponi's, make it out for the amount the Covoni received 'from Michelangelo in Rome'.

The letter of exchange from the Covoni for the Capponi will be enclosed with this, on which the said money will be paid to you.

Send me a copy of the transaction with the firm with which you invest the said money.

In Rome on the twenty-seventh day of December fifteen hundred and forty-four – style of the Incarnation.[1]

MICHELANGELO BUONARROTI IN ROME

1. *As the transaction was being arranged in Florence, Michelangelo here adopts the Florentine method of reckoning. In Rome the year was reckoned indifferently from December 25th or January 1st, in Florence from March 25th.*

¶ [TO MESSER LUIGI DEL RICCIO]

244

Messer Luigi — You seem to think that I shall reply to you as you wish me to, when it may well be the contrary. You give me what I refused, and you refuse me what I asked of you. Nor do you err unknowingly, since you sent it to me by Ercole, being ashamed to give it to me yourself.

It is still within the power of one who delivered me from death to insult me; but now I do not know which is the heavier to bear – this insult or death. I therefore beg and entreat you by the true friendship which exists between us to have that plate which I do not like destroyed, and to have the impressions that have been printed burnt; and if you are doing a traffic in me, do not allow others to do so, too. But if you shatter me utterly, I shall do exactly the same, not with you, but with your things.[1]

MICHELANGELO BUONARROTI

Not a painter, or a sculptor, or an architect,
but what you will; but not a drunkard, as I
told you when I was with you.[2]

*Buonarroti
Archives
Mil. cdlx
From Rome
(January 1545)*

1. *For the interpretation of this letter, see Appendix 27, Part II.*

2. *There is an inferior version of Plate 7 which may well be an impression from the plate to which Michelangelo understandably objected. The engraving here reproduced was evidently acceptable, as it was issued in 1545 and again in 1546, with an amended date.*

41

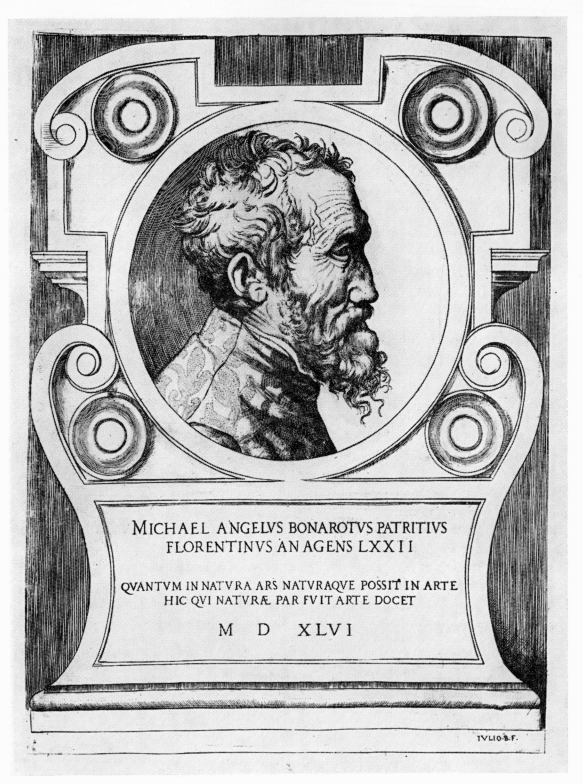

MICHAEL ANGELVS BONAROTVS PATRITIVS
FLORENTINVS AN AGENS LXXII

QVANTVM IN NATVRA ARS NATVRAQVE POSSIT IN ARTE
HIC QVI NATVRÆ PAR FVIT ARTE DOCET

M   D   XLVI

IVLIO·B·F·

7. *Michelangelo Buonarroti*   *Giulio Bonasone*

¶ To Lionardo di Buonarroto Simoni in Florence

245

*Buonarroti
Archives
Mil. clii
From Rome
January (10th)
1545*

Lionardo — I have had the receipt for the two hundred *scudi* from you and from Giovan Simone. As to investing it in one place rather than in another, I have no advice to give you, nor can I, because I'm not there and don't know anything about it. Francesco Salvetti, a relative of Luigi del Riccio's here, has written to say that your employers are very sound and honest men; however, do whatever you think will not result in a loss.

I think that's all. Commend me to Guicciardino.

MICHELANGELO IN ROME

¶ To Messer Luigi del Riccio

246

*Buonarroti
Archives
Mil. cdliii
From Rome
(January 1545)*

Messer Luigi — You are aware that the fire has exposed part of the Chapel.[1] I therefore think that it should be covered over again as it was, as soon as possible, if only roughly, until the spring, because the rain is not only spoiling the paintings, but is also cracking the walls. And because the walls are in process of settling in the normal way, the rain would not be at all good for them. I'm writing this in order that the Pope may not be put to some great expense to the advantage rather of other people than of the Chapel. So please would you make this clear, either when speaking to the Pope, or through Messer Aurelio,[2] to whom I also beg you to commend me.

YOUR MICHELANGELO

1. *A fire damaged part of the roof of the Sistine Chapel (not the Pauline Chapel, as stated by Milanesi) on the night of December 31st 1544. Payments were made for certain repairs in January 1545 (Archivio Camerale; Parte I^ – Serie: Fabbriche – Registro No. 1513, carta VI^ – State Archives, Rome).*

2. *Messer Aurelio Silvestri, a chamberlain to Paul III.*

¶ [To Messer Salvestro da Montaguto and Company in Rome]

247

*British
Museum
Mil. cdxliii
From Rome
January 25th
1545*

Magnificent Messer Salvestro and Company of Rome *per l'adrieto e per loro*[1] Antonio Covoni and Company — Will you be pleased to pay to Raffaello da Montelupo, sculptor, fifty *scudi* in silver, at ten julians per *scudo*, which is the only balance he can claim[2] for doing the three marble statues, and putting them in place at Santo Pietro in Vincola in the Tomb of Pope Julius; that is, for Our Lady with the Child in her arms, a Sibyl and a Prophet. For these, according to the agreement, he should be owed one

Mag.ci messer salvestro da monte onto e compagni di roma y la driet.
e ploro antonio consori e compagni sarete contenti pagare al
raffaello da monte lupo scultore scudi cinquanta di moneta
a gulii dieci y scudo che sono y ogni resto di quello potessi
a domadare y factura delle tre statue di marmo facte e messe
a sato pietro in cola nella sepultura di papa iulio cioe
y una nostra dona col puto in braccio e una sibilla e un profeta
delle quali se codo le convetioni resterebbe avere scudi ceto
sessanta ma y che y essere stato malato e no naver possuto
e aver fatto lavorare a altri stamo convenuti da chordo da vii
questi scudi cinquata y ogni resto che di cosi piglierete la
ricevuta y ne doghi a coto degli scudi ceto sessanta che mi
restano in deposito y detto coto Da roma alli vii di vi
di genaro 1545 — a Nativitate

Yo sero mi ch... la mio lo buo nano ti di ma propin

Vista per me Hier.o Tir.o oro Du
cale d'Urbino et approuata in quāt
li detti cinquanta scudi gli siano
debiti secondo il tenor del contratto
fatto co detto my Raphaello y mano
del Cappello, et no altriment ne
per altro modo dah cum di Sop
alli 27. di Gen.o 1545

Il med.o Hier.o Titano

hundred and seventy *scudi*; but because he has been ill and unable to do them, and has had to have the work done by others, we have agreed to pay him only this balance of fifty *scudi*. Will you obtain a receipt for this, and deduct the sum from the hundred and seventy *scudi* that remain to you in the said account. From Rome, on the twenty-fifth day of January, 1545, style of the Nativity.

YOUR MICHELANGELO BUONARROTI in his own hand

Seen and approved by me,
Hieronimo Tiranno, envoy
to the Duke of Urbino,
in respect of the said
fifty *scudi*, which are
owed according to the
terms of the contract
made with the said Messer
Raffaello, drawn by Cappello,[3]
for this purpose and no other.
Given as above, on the 27th day
of January 1545.

THE SAME HIERONIMO TIRANNO

1. *The meaning of the words in italics remains obscure.*

2. *As will be seen from No. 248, Raffaello da Montelupo was subsequently paid in full.*

3. *Bartolomeo Cappello, 'notarius rogatus'.*

¶ [TO MESSER SALVESTRO MONTAGUTO AND COMPANY IN ROME]

248

Magnificent Messer Salvestro and Company of Rome *per l'adrieto* — As is known to you, when I, being in the service of Our Lord, Pope Paul the Third, and being occupied in painting his new Chapel and unable to complete the Tomb of Pope Julius the Second in Santo Pietro in Vincola, and His Holiness, Our Lord, aforesaid, having intervened, a contract was drawn up by agreement with the Magnificent Hieronimo Tiranno, envoy of the Illustrious Lord Duke of Urbino, which contract his Excellency afterwards ratified, I deposited with you further sums of money, in order to finish the said work, of which, Raffaello da Montelupo was owed 445 *scudi*[1] at ten julians per *scudo*, being the balance of 550 *scudi* at the same rate. This was for finishing five marble statues,

*Biblioteca
Nazionale
Florence
Mil. cdxlv
From Rome
February 3rd
1545*

begun and blocked out by me and commissioned by the aforesaid ambassador of the Duke of Urbino – that is, Our Lady with the Child in her arms, a Sibyl, a Prophet, an Active Life and a Contemplative Life, as appears in full in the contract drawn up by Messer Bartolomeo Cappello, notary to the Camera, under date twenty-first [*sic*] of August 1542. Of these five statues, Our Lord having at my entreaty and in order to gratify me granted me a little time, I finished two myself, that is the Contemplative Life and the Active, for the same price for which the said Raffaello was to do them, and out of the same money he would have had. And afterwards the said Raffaello finished the other three and built them into the said Tomb, as may be seen. Therefore, will you pay him, at his convenience, one hundred and seventy *scudi* in silver, at ten julians per *scudo*, which remain to you in hand of the said sum, and obtain from him a final receipt, and one drawn, furthermore, by the said notary, by which he declares himself satisfied and fully paid for the said work, and post them to the account of the said sum which remains to you in hand. *Et bene valete.*

From Rome, on the 3rd day of February, 1545, style of the Nativity.[2]

YOUR MICHELANGELO BUONARROTI IN ROME

1. *According to the agreement made with him on February 27th 1542 (Milanesi, p. 709) Raffaello da Montelupo was to receive 400 scudi for completing the three statues, Our Lady, a Sibyl and a Prophet. Later, a further agreement was made for finishing the Active Life and the Contemplative Life for 150 scudi. When the last agreement for the Tomb was drawn on August 20th 1542, he had already received 105 scudi, leaving a balance of 445. In 1543 (Gaye, II, p. 304) he received 125 scudi, leaving a balance of the 400 due to him for the three statues, of 170 scudi.*

2. *This letter, which is a copy in Luigi del Riccio's hand, was obviously drafted by him, on the basis of Michelangelo's draft (No. 7).*

249

¶ [TO MESSER LUIGI DEL RICCIO IN ROME]

Buonarroti Archives Mil. cdli From Rome (February) 1545

Messer Luigi, dear friend—When I come to your house please would you treat me as I treat you when you come to mine. You let me come and be a nuisance to you, without telling me, so that I remain a presumptuous buffalo even in the eyes of the servants.

I think I shall be giving orders on Thursday to move the figures to San Pietro in Vincola, as I told you before, and as I want to pay for the moving of them out of the money for the said figures, which remains to you in hand, I think I'll make out an order for the said money for the ambassador to sign, so that nothing can ever be said, either to you or to me.[1] So would you please make out a draft of the said order, as you think it ought to be.

I did not recognize the son[2] of Messer Bindo Altoviti yesterday morning, and if you wanted to bring him here, you could have said so openly, because I hold myself at the service of Messer Bindo and all his family.

[Unsigned]

1. *This letter brings to an end the Tragedy of the Tomb – 'si ponga silenzio perpetua a questo negocio di sepultura per conto di detto messer Michelagnolo' (Milanesi, p. 716).*

2. *Giovanbattista (d. 1590), the second son of the Florentine banker, Bindo d'Antonio Altoviti (1491– 1557). The Altoviti were prominent among the 'fuorusciti', but, owing to their wealth and influence, were not declared rebels until they lent support to the Sienese in the war with Florence in 1554/55.*

XI

LETTERS
250 - 273

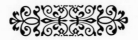

From Rome
1545 - 1546

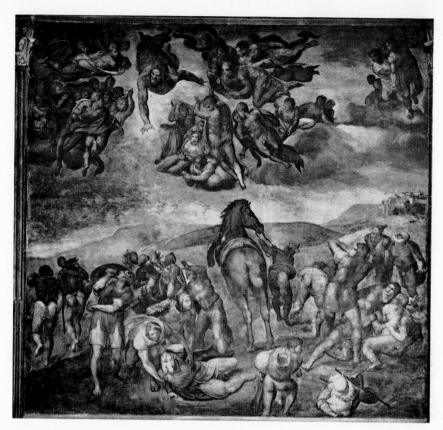

a. The Conversion of St. Paul

9. *The Frescoes of the Pauline Chapel*
Michelangelo
The Vatican, Rome

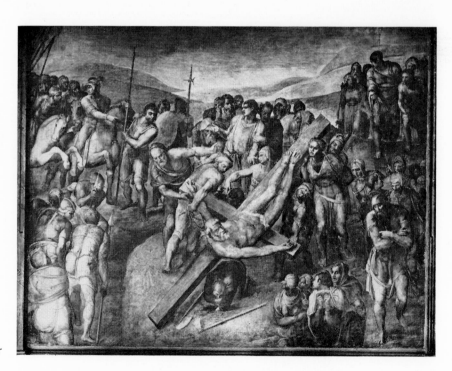

b. The Martyrdom of St. Peter

XI. From Rome : 1545-1546

250

¶ [To Messer Luigi del Riccio in Rome]

Messer Luigi — Please would you send me back the last madrigal which you don't understand, so that I may revise it, because that importunate beggar for drafts – that is Urbino – was in such a hurry he didn't let me look it over.[1]

About our spending the day together tomorrow, I make you my apologies, because the weather is bad and I have business at home. The day we were going to spend tomorrow, we'll spend later on, this coming Lent,[2] at Lunghezza[3] with a fat tench.

[Unsigned]

*Buonarroti
Archives
Mil. cdxlix
From Rome
(February 14th
1545)*

1. *This note is written under the madrigal 'Nella memoria delle cose belle' (Guasti, p. 42).*

2. *In 1545 Ash Wednesday fell on February 18th.*

3. *Lunghezza, the Strozzi villa on the road to Tivoli, which they used to visit together.*

¶ To Lionardo di Buonarroto Simoni in Florence

251

Lionardo — I learn from your letters that you have not yet found anywhere to invest the money I sent you, since, according to what you write me, those who have the means to trade for themselves don't want other people's money. It is therefore a sign that those who accept other people's money haven't the means of trading on their own account, so that it's risky. So I am pleased that you are proceeding slowly about placing it anywhere, so as not to squander it, because it would be your loss. Little by little, when I can, I'll send you up to a thousand ducats, as I wrote you. Afterwards I must think of my own needs in life, because I'm an old man and cannot any longer endure fatigue. I want to give up the ferry the Pope granted me,[1] because it is too much of a nuisance and I have good reason for not wanting to hold it. So I must make an income here, in order to be able to manage better than I'm doing. So learn to keep what you've got, because I cannot do any more for you.

I learn that Michele has had a son and that he and Francesca are well. I'm very pleased about it. I believe he now has four children. God grant they may be a comfort

*Buonarroti
Archives
Mil. cliii
From Rome
February 14th
1545*

to him. Commend me to him, and thank him on my behalf for the trouble he takes in your interest, for it is in mine no less. I'm very grateful to him for this. I'm not answering his letter, because I didn't altogether understand it, and also because I think this will do just as well. Therefore read it to him.[2]

MICHELANGELO BUONARROTI IN ROME

1. *The ferry – Il Porto del Po at Piacenza. See Appendix 33.*

2. *Endorsed in Luigi del Riccio's hand 'Lionardo del Riccio, have it delivered into his own hand'.*

252　　　¶ TO MESSER LUIGI DEL RICCIO IN ROME

Buonarroti Archives Mil. cdxlvi From Rome March 13th (1545)

To-day, the thirteenth day of March, I have received a hundred *scudi* from Melighino[1] for my salary for last January and February.

Messer Luigi — I have never received money from Melighino for which I haven't given a receipt. Therefore, if I've made a mistake, it can be seen from the receipts I've given in my own hand.

YOUR MICHELANGELO BUONARROTI

1. *Jacopo Melighini da Ferrara (d. 1549), an accountant at St. Peter's and co-architect with Michelangelo to Paul III (Vasari, V, p. 471).*

253　　　¶ TO LIONARDO DI BUONARROTO SIMONI IN FLORENCE

Buonarroti Archives Mil. cliv From Rome April (4th) 1545

Lionardo — I learn from your letter that you still haven't done anything; I assure you there's no need to hurry nor to make a great ado about it with your friends either, because one comes across few who are honest.

I thought of sending the same amount of money again within two months, but I don't like your keeping it in the house, because it's risky. However, I'll do as you all write and tell me; but as I'm not there, and cannot judge what can best be done with it these days, I leave it to you. If you think you can do something safer and more profitable with it, do as you think. I'll endeavour to send you all that I've promised within a year. That's all I have to say. Commend me to Michele and to Francesca.

MICHELANGELO IN ROME

¶ To Lionardo di Buonarroto Simoni in Florence

254

*Buonarroti
Archives
Mil. clv
From Rome
May 9th 1545*

Lionardo — I don't think it is possible to deposit money at interest anywhere without its being usurious, unless there is as much chance of loss as of gain. When I wrote and told you that if you wanted to do something else with the money I sent you that you thought would be safer, I meant buying something, like that land belonging to Niccolò della Buca, or anything else you thought suitable, and not depositing it in a bank at all, because they're all fraudulent.

I also wrote that I had the same amount of money available and told you all to write and tell me whether you wanted me to send it now or not, as you haven't yet discovered a way of using it, so answer me, and I'll act accordingly.

You wrote and told me of the office you've been given. I reply that you are a young man and have seen very little. I would remind you that in Florence it is better to retire than to advance.

Tell Giovan Simone that the new commentary on Dante by a Lucchese[1] hasn't been very well received by people who know anything, so there's no need to pay any attention to it. There's no other new one that I'm aware of.

Commend me to Michele Guicciardini and tell him that I'm well, but have many worries – so many that I haven't time to eat. So make my apologies to him, if I don't answer him. You can read this to him which will be the same thing. And tell Francesca to pray to God for me.

Also, if anyone writes to you on my account, I warn you not to rely on it, unless there is a line in my own hand.

[Unsigned]

1. *Alessandro Vellutello, whose commentary was first published in Venice by Marcolini in 1544.*

¶ To Lionardo di Buonarroto Simoni in Florence

255

*Buonarroti
Archives
Mil. clvi
From Rome
May 23rd 1545*

Lionardo — I have paid to-day, this twenty-third day of May, 1545, to the Covoni in Rome two hundred gold *scudi* in gold, to be paid to you there. So go to the Capponi, you and Giovan Simone or Gismondo, as you like, and they will be paid to you, that is, you will be paid two hundred gold *scudi* in gold, which I have paid in here. Make out the receipt accordingly and send me a copy.[1]

Michelangelo in Rome

1. *Endorsed in Luigi del Riccio's hand, 'Lionardo del Riccio, deliver safely'.*

256

¶ To Lionardo di Buonarroto Simoni in Florence

*Buonarroti
Archives
Mil. clviii
From Rome
July 4th 1545*

Lionardo — As to the *trebbiano*, I gave the receipt for forty-five flasks to the carter who brought it, and I wrote and told you not to send me anything unless I ask for it, and I do so again. As to coming to an arrangement about the money, it seems to me that Giovane Simone understands about it better than you do, because by going slowly one makes fewer mistakes. You have the wherewithal to live and are not being turned out, so you must be patient, and don't talk much about it, for fear of its being stolen. And when I can, I'll send you the rest up to the amount I promised.

Michelangelo in Rome

257

¶ [To Messer Luigi del Riccio]

*Buonarroti
Archives
Mil. cdlvi
From Rome
(Summer 1545)*

Messer Luigi — That friend, if it's that one you're talking about, might be welcome, if it suited him; but you and Messer Donato together have spoken so ill of him to me, that you've damped my ardour. So from now on be on your guard against introducing him. Tomorrow after dinner, I'll come to you and do whatever you command me.[1]

[Unsigned]

1. This note appears to refer to the appointment of someone to undertake the management of Michelangelo's affairs during Luigi del Riccio's absence from Rome, probably between July and December 1545.

258

¶ [To Messer Luigi del Riccio]

*Buonarroti
Archives
Mil. cdl
From Rome
(Autumn 1545)*

Messer Luigi — I commend me to you and to those you love, Messer Giuliano and Messer Roberto,[1] of whom you write me. I am at their service and if I do not do what is fitting, I'm fleeing my creditors, because I have a great debt[2] and little money.[3]

Your Michelangelo in that same Macel[4]

1. Giuliano di Pierfrancesco de' Medici (d. 1588) and Roberto Strozzi (d. 1566), his brother-in-law, who had married Maddalena de' Medici in 1539. They were resident in Lyons.

2. *Michelangelo refers to the hospitality he received at the Palazzo Strozzi-Ulivieri during his illness.*

3. *This note accompanies the madrigal 'Non sempre al mondo è si pregiato e caro' (Guasti, p. 27), which suggests an answer to criticism, perhaps to the invective contained in Pietro Aretino's letter of November 1545. The original, of which this is an autograph copy, was probably addressed to del Riccio in Lyons.*

4. *The signature is omitted by Milanesi, but is included by Guasti.*

¶ To Messer Luigi del Riccio, dear friend, in Lyons

259

Buonarroti Archives Mil. cdlvii From Rome (November) 1545

Messer Luigi, dear friend — All your friends, particularly Messer Donato and I, are very grieved about your illness, and more so as we are unable to help you in any way. But let us hope at least that it will prove to be slight – God grant it may be so.

In another letter I wrote and told you that if you were staying long, I thought of coming to see you, and this I repeat; because, having lost the ferry at Piacenza,[1] and being unable to remain in Rome without an income, I'm thinking of using up the little I have on hostelries, rather than staying cooped up like a beggar in Rome. I'm therefore inclined, unless anything else befalls, to go to St. James of Galicia[2] after Easter, and if you haven't returned, to start from wherever I hear you may be.

Urbino has spoken to Messer Aurelio[3] and will do so again, and from what he tells me, you will have the position you wanted for Cecchino's tomb,[4] and the said tomb is almost finished and will turn out a fine thing.[5]

Your Michelangelo Buonarroti in Rome

1. *Payments in respect of the Po ferry were suspended between August 1545 and February 1546. See Appendix 33.*

2. *The Shrine of Santiago de Compostela in Spain, one of the most famous places of pilgrimage in the Middle Ages.*

3. *Aurelio Silvestri, a chamberlain to Paul III.*

4. *In S. Maria in Aracoeli, where it may still be seen to-day.*

5. *Endorsed in del Riccio's hand '1545: from Messer Michelangelo Buonarroti, sent to and returned from Lyons on the 22nd day of December'.*

260

*Buonarroti
Archives
Mil. clx
From Rome
January 9th
1546*

¶ To his dearest Lionardo Buonarroti, as to a son, in Florence

Lionardo — I have to-day, this ninth day of January 1545,[1] paid to Messer Luigi del Riccio here in Rome six hundred gold *scudi* in gold, which he will make payable to you there in Florence, in order to complete the sum of a thousand *scudi* I promised you. So go to Piero di Gino Capponi[2] and they will be paid to you. Make out the receipt for them for the amount paid here, as stated.

And the said Messer Luigi will write below my intention towards you, because I'm not feeling well and can't write any more;[3] however, I have recovered and shall be all right, thank God – thus I pray, and do you do the same.

Besides the above-mentioned money, I have decided to provide Giovan Simone, Gismondo and you with three thousand *scudi* in gold, that is a thousand to each of you, but jointly, with this proviso that the money is invested in property or in something else that will bring you in an income, and that it remains in the family. So go and see about putting it into some good sound property, and when you find something that you think suitable let me know, so that I may provide the money. And this letter is common to all three of you. As I think that's all, I commend me to you. God etc. etc.[4]

In Rome on the aforesaid day.

I, Michelangelo Buonarroti in Rome

1. *N.S. 1546.*

2. *Piero di Gino Capponi (1508–1568). He was among the prominent citizens who later went on the embassy of obedience to Pius IV in 1559.*

3. *From here on the rest of the letter (except for the signature) is in the hand of Luigi del Riccio, who added what he imagined to be an acceptable address and conclusion to the letter. These additions could hardly have been less characteristic of the way in which Michelangelo was in the habit of addressing his nephew. For Luigi's covering letter to Lionardo, see Appendix 34.*

4. *del Riccio usually concluded his own letters to Lionardo 'God prosper you', 'God be with you', or 'God content you'.*

261

*Buonarroti
Archives
Mil. clxi
From Rome
January 16th
1546*

¶ To his dearest Lionardo Buonarroti, as to a son, in Florence

Dearest Lionardo — I wrote to you last Saturday, on the 9th, and remitted to you 600 *scudi* at Piero Capponi's, through Luigi del Riccio, as you will have seen. To this I'm awaiting a reply.

I also told you that I had decided to provide Giovansimone, Gismondo and you with three thousand *scudi*, as soon as you found a sound property in which to invest them, so that they may remain in the family; and I told you to go in search of something and to keep me informed daily.

I now hear from a great friend of mine here that the properties belonging to Francesco Corboli, who is living in Venice and went bankrupt some months ago, are being sold. And these, I am told, comprise an old house in Florence in the Santo Spirito quarter, and certain possessions situated at Monte Spertoli, including six yoke of oxen and a large house, or small mansion, suitable for an inn, which should go for an inclusive price or almost. So I want Giovansimone and you to find out all particulars and to enquire how much the *decima*[1] is, from what the income is derived in cash and in kind, what state the properties are in, and whether they are free from incumbrances, and what you think they are worth. Send me an answer about everything as soon as you can.[2]

As I am not feeling well,[3] Messer Luigi del Riccio has written to you in my place about certain properties that have been put in my way, as you will learn. So go into the matter carefully, and reply quickly.

MICHELANGELO BUONARROTI IN ROME

1. *The 'decima' was a 10 per cent tax on property which was imposed from time to time.*

2. *The letter, as witness the beginning, is written in Luigi del Riccio's hand up to this point. The rest was added by Michelangelo.*

3. *Although not fully recovered, Michelangelo returned to his own house on the day on which this letter was written (Frey, Dicht., p. 532). See Appendix 34.*

¶ To Lionardo di Buonarroto Simoni in Florence

262

Lionardo — You've been mighty quick in giving me information about the Corboli properties. I did not think you were back in Florence yet. Were you afraid, perhaps because it was put into your head, that I might change my mind? I tell you that I want to proceed slowly, because the money to pay for them I earned here with exertions[1] such as are unknown to those born clothed and shod like you.

As to your having come to Rome in such a rush, I don't know whether you would have come so quickly had I been starving and in want. It suffices that you throw away money you haven't earned, so great is your anxiety not to lose this inheritance.[2] And then you say that you were under an obligation to come, because of the love you bear me. Cupboard love! If you had loved me, you would now have written to me, saying, 'Michelangelo, spend the three thousand *scudi* there on yourself, because you have given us so much that it's enough for us. We care more for you than for your possessions'.[3]

You have all lived on me for forty years now, and not so much as a kind word have I ever had from you.

Buonarroti
Archives
Mil. clxii
From Rome
February 6th
1546

It is true that last year[4] you were so exhorted and admonished[5] that you were shamed into sending me a pack-load of *trebbiano*. Would that you hadn't sent even that!

I'm not writing you this because I don't want to buy; I do want to buy, in order to provide an income for myself, because I cannot work any more. But I want to proceed slowly in order not to buy a liability. So don't be in a hurry.

MICHELANGELO IN ROME

If anything should be said or demanded of you on my behalf, don't believe anyone, unless you have a line in my hand. The thousand ducats, or rather *scudi*, I sent you – if you will reflect on what can happen with shops, either through bad management or anything else, you will buy properties, because they are a sounder proposition. However, make up your own minds, and do what you think best.

1. *Cf. his words to Buonarroto, No. 81.*

2. *See Appendix 34.*

3. *Cf. his words to Lodovico, No. 50.*

4. *In June 1545.*

5. *By Luigi del Riccio. See Appendix 27, Part I.*

263　¶ TO LIONARDO DI BUONARROTO SIMONI IN FLORENCE

Buonarroti Archives Mil. clxiii From Rome February 13th 1546

Lionardo — About buying, or investing the money I've sent you in a shop, make up your own minds between you, and do what you believe to be best, because I'm not acquainted with the position.

As to the Corboli properties, I've had some information about them which doesn't please me, that is, that there is an *arbitrio*[1] of twenty-five *scudi*. If this were true, it would be the last straw, having bought them. I'm also told that some of their relations have some sort of claim on them.

I don't understand these things, so you must proceed slowly and keep your eyes open, and if it turns out to be a safe proposition you should be prepared to buy at a reasonable price, if they're good properties and particularly if they lie together within well-defined boundaries.

So look into it and let me know what you find out and what they are judged to be worth. That's all I have to say. Commend me to Guicciardino and to Francesca.

I need to provide myself with an income, because it would not be right to draw what I have had up till now from the Pope, if I were unable to work any more[2] and the said properties would form part of the said income. And for your sake I'd rather buy in Florence than elsewhere, either these properties or others.

MICHELANGELO BUONARROTI IN ROME

1. *The 'arbitrio' was 'an individual valuation, and the "decima" a general percentage of property' (Staley, p. 192).*
2. *Cf. Luigi del Riccio's correspondence, quoted in Appendix 33.*

¶ TO MESSER LUIGI DEL RICCIO IN ROME

264

Messer Luigi, dearest friend — I had decided, as you know, to take the Corboli properties at a reasonable price. I now draw back, the reason being that besides the *decima*, they are subject to an *arbitrio* of twenty-five *scudi*, which would be imposed on me twenty-five times a year.[1] I don't want, therefore, to keep you any longer in suspense; so look after your own interests in the matter as well as you can.[2] I commend me to you.

YOUR MICHELANGELO

Buonarroti Archives Mil. cdlviii From Rome (February/ March) 1546

1. *In saying that the 'arbitrio' would be imposed on him twenty-five times a year, Michelangelo infers that the authorities would assess him at an exorbitant rate.*
2. *Perhaps Luigi del Riccio, who came from the Santo Spirito Quarter in Florence, was considering the possibility of buying the Corboli property as an investment for himself, if Michelangelo decided to withdraw. Alternatively, he may have been negotiating the sale.*

¶ TO LIONARDO DI BUONARROTO SIMONI IN FLORENCE

265

Lionardo — You write me that you have found a means of forming a company with one of the magistrates and others, and that I might get some information about it. I'm not acquainted with, and have no means of getting information about a thing like this. But because to-day there are nothing but frauds, and one can trust nobody, I advise you to proceed slowly, particularly as you are not in want; and in proceeding slowly one discovers many things and particularly that anyone who opens a shop in a trade in which

Buonarroti Archives Mil. clxiv From Rome March 6th 1546

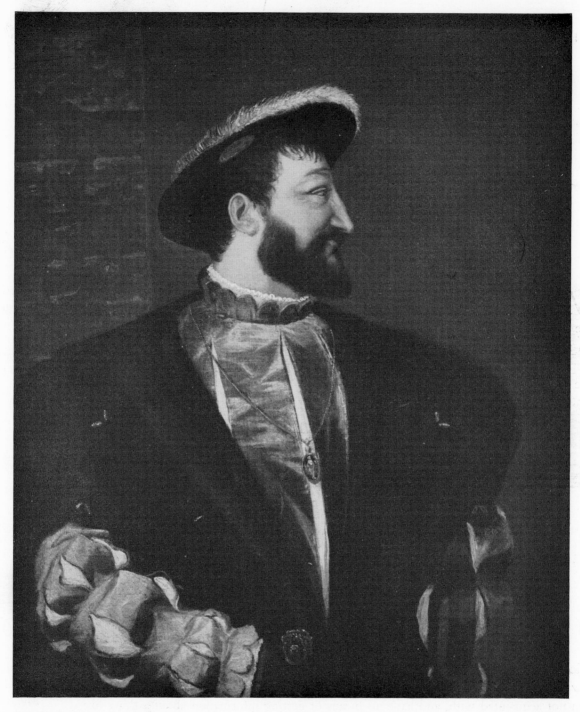

10. *Francis I, King of France*

Titian
Musée du Louvre, Paris

he is not experienced is soon ruined. And it's no use thinking one could make it good in these days.

As to the Corboli lands, I've had differing reports about them, and because, from my long experience, I'm suspicious, I've relinquished them, so that in my old age I may not be involved in some dispute, and you in others after I'm gone. So do no more about it.

MICHELANGELO BUONARROTI IN ROME

¶ TO THE MOST CHRISTIAN KING OF FRANCE

266

*Buonarroti
Archives
Mil. cdlix
From Rome
April 26th
1546*

Sacred Majesty[1] — I know not which is the greater, the favour or the wonder that Your Majesty should deign to write to a man like me, and still further to request of him examples of his work, which are in no way worthy of Your Majesty's name. But such as they are, be it known to Your Majesty that for a long time I have desired to serve You, but have been unable to do so, because even in Italy I have not had sufficient opportunities to devote myself to my art.

Now I am an old man and shall be engaged for some months on work for Pope Pagolo. But if, on its completion, a little of life remains to me, I will endeavour to put into effect the desire which, as I have said, I have had for a long time, that is to say to execute for Your Majesty a work in marble, in bronze and in painting. But if death baulks me in this desire of mine, I will not fail to fulfil it in the next life, where one no longer grows old, if it be possible to carve and to paint there.[2] And I pray God to grant Your Majesty a long and happy life. From Rome on the xxvi day of April mdxlvi.

Your Most Christian Majesty's

Most humble servant

MICHELANGELO BUONARROTI

1. *Francis I, King of France (1515–1547), had written to Michelangelo on February 8th 1546 expressing his desire to acquire something by his hand and asking besides for a cast of 'The Risen Christ' in Santa Maria sopra Minerva and of the 'Madonna delle Febbre' now in St. Peter's.*

2. *In this draft in the Casa Buonarroti the formal flourish with which the letter concludes is in the hand of Donato Giannotti. Luigi del Riccio was absent from Rome at this time and Giannotti in his stead was assisting Michelangelo in matters such as this.*

267

*Buonarroti
Archives
Mil. clxvi
From Rome
April 30th
1546*

❡ To Lionardo di Buonarroto Simoni in Florence

Lionardo — I've had the shirts. Later I learnt from another letter of yours about the income from a mill which is for sale, and lastly you wrote me about another property near Florence. The mill is not to my liking, because I've no confidence in an income based on water;[1] also, the one about which you now write to me seems to me too near Florence. If one could find something at a distance of eight or ten miles, it would seem to me more suitable; but there is no hurry. So don't make such an ado about it. I think that's all. When I don't answer you, bear in mind that I have other things to think about besides writing letters. Commend me to Guicciardino and to Francesca.

MICHELANGELO BUONARROTI IN ROME

1. *He had had, after all, some experience of 'an income based on water' – viz. the Po ferry.*

268

*Buonarroti
Archives
Mil. clxvii
From Rome
May 26th
1546*

❡ To Lionardo di Buonarroto Simoni in Florence

Lionardo — I've received the contract,[1] which seems to me all right, so thank Messer Giovan Francesco, because he has done me a great kindness, and beg him to thank Bernardo Bini[2] and commend me to him. I think that's all, because I wrote and told you in my last letter what you may do about the buying of something that seems to you suitable, provided that you have a sound title and that there are no grounds for litigation.

Enclosed with this will be one for Messer Giovan Francesco. Give it to him and commend me to him.

MICHELANGELO BUONARROTI IN ROME

1. *Probably the public quittance for the money he had received for the Tomb of Julius II (Condivi, lii).*

2. *Bernardo Bini, the banker through whom the payments for the Tomb of Julius II had been made to Michelangelo between 1513 and 1518 (Gotti, II, p. 52 et seq.).*

¶ To Lionardo di Buonarroto Simoni in Florence

269

*Buonarroti
Archives
Mil. clxviii
From Rome
June 5th
1546*

Lionardo — I have had a copy made of the draft of the power of attorney, without without *[sic]* alteration. I'm making you my attorney and sending it to you. Have it checked and if it's what you all want, it's good enough for me, because I've other things to think about[1] besides powers of attorney. And don't write to me any more; because every time I get a letter from you, I'm thrown into a fever, such a struggle do I have to read it. I do not know where you learnt to write. If you had to write to the biggest ass in the world, I believe you'd write with more care. So there's no need to add to my vexations, because I've enough of them already. It is up to you have the power of attorney checked and examined. And if you don't, it's your loss.

Michelangelo in Rome

1. *He was engaged at this time on the early stages of the work on the second fresco, 'The Crucifixion of St. Peter', in the Pauline Chapel (Tolnay, V., p. 143).*

¶ To Lionardo di Buonarroto Simoni in Florence

270

*Buonarroti
Archives
Mil. clxix
From Rome
September 4th
1546*

Lionardo — You've written me a long rigmarole about a trifle which only annoys me. About the money about the money *[sic]* of which you write, telling me how you have to spend it, decide between yourselves and spend it on what you most need. I don't think there's anything else, and I've no time for writing either.

Michelangelo in Rome

¶ To Lionardo di Buonarroto Simoni in Florence

271

*Buonarroti
Archives
Mil. clxx
From Rome
November 13th
1546*

Lionardo — I haven't written to you since you informed me about the business you've had about setting up the shop. I tell you there's no hurry and if you were to wait another year, I don't think there would be any harm at all, as you have enough to live on. I've recently been thinking that it might be a good thing to buy an imposing house in Florence for fifteen hundred *scudi* or thereabouts, or for more, if more be needed; because the one where you're living isn't large enough, as you must take a wife, and again it would be a good lodgment for this money, as I'm an old man. So look round and let me know.

I've recently received a letter from Francesca. I want you to go and tell her that I'll do all that she wrote and asked me to do, and that although I haven't written to her, I haven't on that account forgotten her or Michele either; but I'm too much occupied and haven't time for writing. Commend me to Michele and to her.

MICHELANGELO IN ROME

272

Buonarroti Archives Mil. clxxi From Rome December 4th 1546

¶ To Lionardo di Buonarroto Simoni in Florence

Lionardo — I've received sixteen *marzolini*[1] cheeses and paid the muleteer four julians. You should have received the letter I wrote you about buying an imposing house, and now, as I write, I've been brought a letter of yours, acknowledging its receipt, in which you tell me that you would go and see Michele and Francesca and would deliver the message. Commend me to them. About buying the house, I re-affirm the same, that is, that you should seek to buy an imposing house for fifteen hundred or two thousand *scudi*, if possible in our Quarter.[2] And as soon as you have found something suitable, I'll have the money paid to you there. I say this, because an imposing house in the city redounds much more to one's credit, because it is more in evidence than farm lands, since we are, after all, citizens descended from a very noble family.[3] I have always striven to resuscitate our house, but I have not had brothers worthy of this. So strive to do what I tell you and get Gismondo to return to live in Florence, so that it should no longer be said here, to my great shame, that I have a brother at Settignano who trudges after oxen. And when you've bought the house, other things can also be bought.

One day, when I've time, I'll tell you about our origins and whence and when we came to Florence, of which perhaps you are all in ignorance. It would therefore be wrong to abandon what God has given us.[4]

MICHELANGELO BUONARROTI IN ROME

1. *Marzolino, an excellently flavoured cheese made near Florence.*

2. *The Quarter of Santa Croce.*

3. *Michelangelo believed his family to be descended from the Counts of Canossa, a claim that has since been shown to be without foundation.*

4. *Endorsed in another hand 'Messer Giovanni Ulivieri – please have it delivered'.*

¶ To Lionardo di Buonarroto Simoni in Florence

Lionardo — You write me that you have heard of more houses to buy, among which you write me about the one that belonged to Zanobi Buondelmonte,[1] which seems to me more imposing than all the others. Therefore I think it would be as well to find out the lowest price, and if it is a sound proposition, take it. But do not rely upon Bernardo Basso. Pretend to believe him, but don't credit him in any way, because he is thoroughly dishonest. So be discreet, as one has to be, particularly when buying. The Via Ghibellina in our Quarter would please me well enough, but the cellars flood every winter; so think it over and be well advised, and when you and my brothers have come to a decision, let me know the price, and I'll have whatever is required paid in Florence.

About a month ago I had a letter from Messer Giovan Francesco with another enclosed, which hadn't anything in it; so make my apologies if I don't answer and commend me to him.

When you write, direct the letters to Bettino, that is, to the Cavalcanti, or to Girolamo Ubaldini. That's all. Commend me to Michele and to Francesca.

Michelangelo in Rome

Buonarroti Archives Mil. clix From Rome December 31st 1546

1. *Zanobi Buondelmonte (1491–1527) had played a prominent part in the Republican struggle against the Medici. He was eventually driven into exile, but in 1527, after the sack of Rome, he returned to Florence, where he died of the plague in the same year (Litta, VII, tav. xi).*

XII

LETTERS
274 - 341

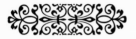

From Rome
1547 - 1549

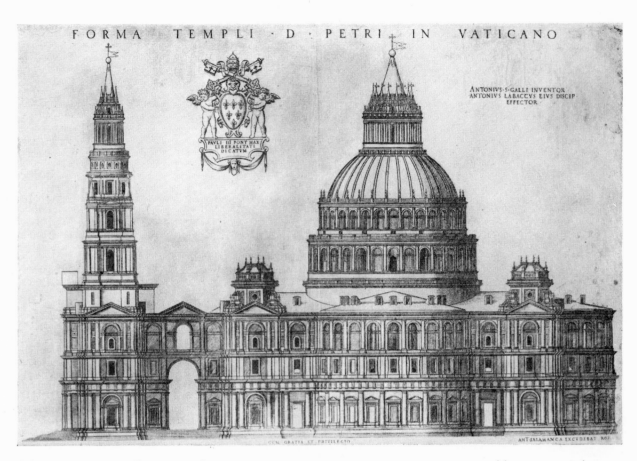

FORMA TEMPLI · D · PETRI · IN · VATICANO

ANTONIVS·S·GALLI INVENTOR
ANTONIVS LABACCVS EIVS DISCIP
EFFECTOR

PAVLI III PONT MAX
LIBERALITATI
DICATVM

CVM GRATIA ET PRIVILEGIO

ANT SALAMANCA EXCVDEBAT ROE

11. *Antonio Sangallo's Project for St. Peter's*   *Engraved by Antonio Salamanca*

XII. From Rome : 1547-1549

¶ [To Messer Bartolomeo Ferratini in Rome]

274

*Buonarroti
Archives
Mil. cdlxxiv
From Rome
(January 1547)*

Messer Bartolomeo,[1] dear friend — One cannot deny that Bramante was as skilled in architecture as anyone since the time of the ancients. He it was who laid down the first plan of St. Peter's,[2] not full of confusion, but clear, simple, luminous and detached in such a way that it in no wise impinged upon the Palace. It was held to be a beautiful design, and manifestly still is, so that anyone who has departed from Bramante's arrangement, as Sangallo has done, has departed from the true course; and that this is so can be seen by anyone who looks at his model with unprejudiced eyes.

He, with that outer ambulatory[3] of his, in the first place takes away all the light from Bramante's plan; and not only this, but does so when it has no light of its own, and so many dark lurking places above and below that they afford ample opportunity for innumerable rascalities, such as the hiding of exiles, the coining of base money, the raping of nuns and other rascalities, so that at night, when the said church closes, it would need twenty-five men to seek out those who remained hidden inside, whom it would be a job to find. Then, there would be this other drawback – that by surrounding the said composition of Bramante's with the addition shown in the model,[4] the Pauline Chapel, the Offices of the Piombo, the Ruota and many other buildings would have to be demolished; nor do I think that the Sistine Chapel would survive intact. As regards the part of the outer ambulatory that has been built, which they say cost a hundred thousand *scudi*, this is not true, because it could be done for sixteen thousand, and little would be lost if it were pulled down, because the dressed stones and the foundations could not come in more useful and the fabric would be two hundred thousand *scudi* to the good in cost and three hundred years in time. This is as I see it and without prejudice – because to gain my point would be greatly to my detriment. And if you are able to persuade the Pope of this, you will be doing me a favour, because I'm not feeling very well.

Your Michelangelo

If Sangallo's model is adhered to, it also follows that all that has been done in my time[5] may be pulled down, which would be a great loss.

1. *For the identification of the recipient of this letter see Appendix 36.*

2. *See Appendix 44.*

3. *The ambulatory to the south had already been built to door level.*

4. *The ambulatory to the north.*

5. *i.e. the buildings to the north of St. Peter's built during his lifetime.*

275

*Buonarroti
Archives
Mil. clxxiii
From Rome
January 22nd
1547*

¶ To Lionardo di Buonarroto Simoni in Florence

Lionardo — I learn from your letter that you've employed a go-between, or rather an agent, in the matter of the Buondelmonte's house, and that you hear that the price is 2,400 *scudi*. You wrote me to this effect in your other letter. It seems to me a large sum of money and I don't believe in these days, if they are looking for a sale, that they'll find ready cash like mine. So go and find out and let me know. And in the meantime you can look for something else, and, as I wrote and told you, something in our Quarter would please me; but I think the flooding of the cellars is a drawback. As to beginning to send the money to Florence, I want to send it by the usual route, as in the time of Messer Luigi, that is to say, to have it paid to you there by the Capponi, and to find out to whom I should pay it here. So if you can, find out from the said Capponi and let me know, because I will begin *[to send]* the money little by little for the said house.[1]

MICHELANGELO IN ROME

1. *Endorsed in another hand, 'Ser Ulivieri, deliver at once because it is from a friend and is important.'*

276

*Buonarroti
Archives
Mil. clxxiv
From Rome
February 11th
1547*

¶ To Lionardo di Buonarroto Simoni in Florence

Lionardo — I have to-day, this 11th day of February 1546,[1] taken five hundred gold *scudi* in gold to Messer Bindo Altoviti so that he may make them payable there to the same amount; and they will be paid to you accordingly by the Capponi. The bill of exchange will therefore be enclosed with this. You and Gismondo must go and fetch them; make out the receipt correctly, that is, for the amount I have paid here in cash, and send me a copy. And when you write to me, address the letter to Messer Girolamo Ubaldini. And if you keep the money in the house, let not the right hand know what the left hand doeth, because it's very risky. As to buying a house, don't concern yourself with anyone who does not wish to sell, because the money is of no less value than the houses; if not this one, then another.

MICHELANGELO BUONARROTI IN ROME

1. *N.S. 1547*

¶ TO LIONARDO DI BUONARROTO SIMONI IN FLORENCE

277

Buonarroti Archives Mil. clxxv From Rome March 5th 1547

Lionardo — I learn from your last letter that you've received the five hundred *scudi* which I sent you and the copy of the receipt,[1] and this morning, the fifth day of March 1546[2] I have taken to Messer Bindo Altoviti the other five hundred gold *scudi* in gold, that he may make them payable there by the Capponi in the same manner, either to you or to Gismondo, or to both of you. And enclosed with this will be the bill of exchange. So go and get them and make out the receipt correctly and send me a copy. And when you've bought the house I'll send you the balance, when you let me know. What I'm doing is only because you must take a wife and the house where you're living doesn't seem to me suitable. I'll leave you and my brothers to think about this, so let me know when and what you've decided, so that I can give you my opinion. I think it would be a good thing, because if one dies without an heir everything goes to the Hospital.[3] I think that's all. Commend me to the priest.

MICHELANGELO BUONARROTI IN ROME

1. *What he meant was, that he, not Lionardo, had had the receipt. Owing to the death of Vittoria Colonna, he was in a state of great distress at this time. Cf. No. 281.*

2. *N.S. 1547.*

3. *Presumably Santa Maria Nuova.*

¶ TO LIONARDO DI BUONARROTO SIMONI IN FLORENCE

278

British Museum Mil. clxxvi From Rome March 26th 1547

Lionardo —I've had the receipt for the *scudi* you received from the Capponi, for those which I here paid out to the Altoviti, but I'm astonished that Gismondo did not go with you, either for this last amount or for the first, because what I'm sending *[I'm sending]* no less for them than for you. But you write and thank me for the kindness I'm doing you, and you should have written, '*We* thank you for the kindness you're doing *us*'. I'm sending you this money on the same conditions as those which I wrote and told you about when I sent the money for investment in a shop – that is, that you might not do anything without the consent of my brothers. I wrote you about buying a house, because if you think of taking a wife, which seems to me essential, the house where you're living isn't large enough for the purpose; but if you can't find anything suitable, I think you could enlarge the one in the Via Ghibellina where you're living, that is, you could complete the roof-line round the corner into the other street, by buying the small house which is below, if that would be large enough. However, I think it would be better if you could manage to make a sound and imposing purchase, and I'll send you the balance.

As regards a wife, several people here have made suggestions to me, some of which please me, and some not. I expect they've also spoken to you about it. So if you've turned your mind to it, and if you have a fancy for one rather than another, let me know. And I'll give you my opinion. I think that's all.

MICHELANGELO BUONARROTI IN ROME

279

*Published
Source
Mil. cdlxiii
From Rome
(March) 1547*

¶ [TO MESSER LUCA MARTINI IN FLORENCE]

Magnificent Messer Luca[1] — Through Messer Bartolomeo Bettini I have received a letter of yours, together with a treatise – a commentary on a sonnet by my hand. The sonnet is indeed by me, but the commentary is from Heaven and is really admirable, I do not say in my judgment but in that of learned men and of Messer Donato Giannotti in particular, who can't put it down. He commends himself to you.

As regards the sonnet, I know it for what it's worth; but be that as it may, I cannot pretend that I do not feel a little vainglorious in being the subject of so fine and learned a commentary. And as I perceive from his words of praise that I appear to its author to be what I am not, I beg you to express my acknowledgments to him in terms befitting such devotion, affection and courtesy. I beg you to do this, because I feel myself to be of little worth and he who is well esteemed ought not to tempt fortune. It is better to remain silent than to fall from on high.

I am an old man and death has robbed me of the dreams of youth – may those who do not know what old age means bear it with what patience they may when they reach it, because it cannot be imagined beforehand.

Commend me, as I've said, to Varchi, as being enamoured of his gifts and at his service wherever I am.

Yours and at your service in all that lies in my power,

MICHELANGELO BUONARROTI IN ROME

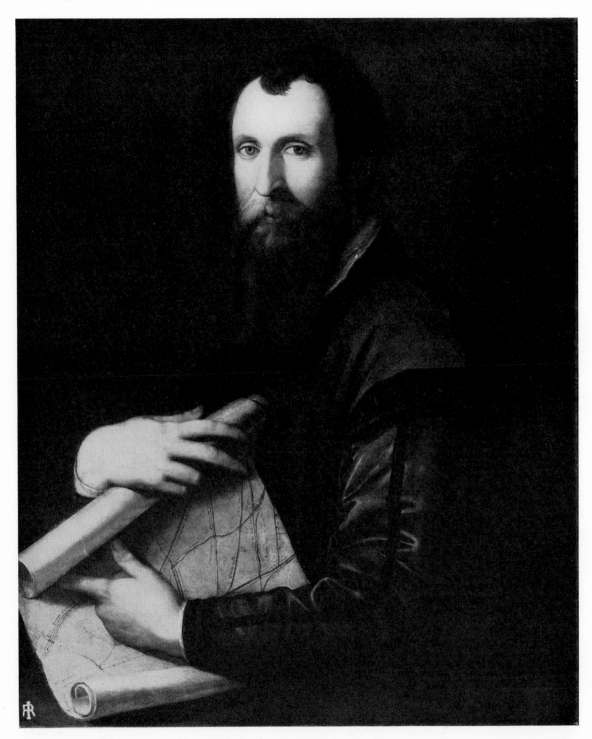

12. *Luca Martini*

Angelo Bronzino
Palazzo Pitti, Florence

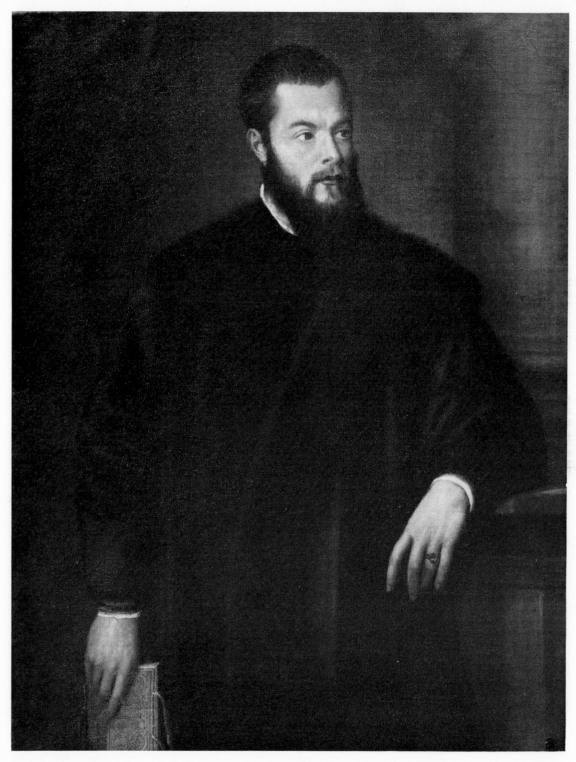

13. *Benedetto Varchi*

Titian
Kunsthistorisches Museum, Vienna

1. *Luca Martini, a member of the Accademia Fiorentina and a notable patron of the arts (see Appendix 37). He was much in the counsels of Duke Cosimo I and persuaded him to recall Benedetto Varchi from exile. He held office as Provveditore of the Mercato Nuovo, and later at Pisa where he was responsible for the draining of the marshes (Vasari, VI, pp. 125 et seq., and Vasari, VII, p. 600).*

¶ To Messer Benedetto Varchi

280

*Buonarroti
Archives
Mil. cdlxii
From Rome
(March) 1547*

Messer Benedetto[1] — So that it may indeed be evident that I have received your treatise, as I have, I will make some attempt to reply to the question asked of me, unlearned though I am.

I admit that it seems to me that painting may be held to be good in the degree in which it approximates to relief, and relief to be bad in the degree in which it approximates to painting. I used therefore to think that painting derived its light from sculpture and that between the two the difference was as that between the sun and the moon.

Now, since I have read the passage in your paper where you say that, philosophically speaking, things which have the same end are one and the same, I have altered my opinion and maintain that, if in face of greater difficulties, impediments and labours, greater judgment does not make for greater nobility, then painting and sculpture are one and the same, and being held to be so, no painter ought to think less of sculpture than of painting, and similarly no sculptor less of painting than of sculpture. By sculpture I mean that which is fashioned by the effort of cutting away, that which is fashioned by the method of building up being like unto painting. It suffices that as both, that is to say sculpture and painting, proceed from one and the same faculty of understanding, we may bring them to amicable terms and desist from such disputes, because they take up more time than the execution of the figures themselves. If he who wrote that painting is nobler than sculpture understood as little about the other things of which he writes – my maidservant could have expressed them better.

There are an infinite number of things, still unsaid, which could be said of kindred arts, but, as I've said, they would take up too much time, and I've little to spare, because I am not only an old man, but almost numbered among the dead. I therefore beg you to have me excused. I commend me to you and thank you to the best of my ability for the too great honour you do me, of which I am undeserving.

Your Michelangelo Buonarroti in Rome

1. *Benedetto Varchi (1502–1565), a Florentine scholar, critic, and historian, who published this letter, among others, in 1549 (N.S. 1550). The original is not extant. The copy in the Buonarroti Archives is endorsed by Michelangelo the Younger as follows, 'Given me by Cavaliere Pierantonio di Giulio de' Nobili'. For the circumstances in which the letter was written see Appendix 37.*

281

*British
Museum
Mil. cdlxv
From Rome
(March) 1547*

¶ To Giovan Francesco, priest in Santa Maria in Florence

Messer Giovan Francesco — As it is a long time since I've written to you and in order to prove to you by this that I'm still alive, and in order to learn from a letter of yours the same of you, I'm writing you these few lines.

I commend me to you and beg you to see that the enclosed letter reaches Messer Benedetto Varchi, the light and splendour of the Florentine Academy,[1] as I believe he's a great friend of yours. Give it to him and thank him on my behalf better than I am doing or can do myself.

Having been very unhappy lately,[2] I have been at home, and in going through some of my things a great number of these trifles, which I formerly used to send you, came to hand, from among which I'm sending you four, which I may perhaps have sent you before. You'll say rightly that I'm old and distracted, but I assure you that only distractions prevent one from being beside oneself with grief. So don't be surprised about it. Reply to me about something I beg of you. I remain always[3]

Your Michelangelo Buonarroti in Rome

1. *Cf. Draft 4, n. 3.*

2. *Vittoria Colonna had died in February and Luigi del Riccio four months previously.*

3. *See also Draft 9.*

282

*British
Museum
Mil. clxv
From Rome
April 29th
1547*

¶ To Lionardo di Buonarroto Simoni in Florence

Lionardo — The house in the Via de' Martegli doesn't please me, because it doesn't seem to me to be our kind of street. Take the one belonging to the Arte della Lana in the Via de' Servi, if it's suitable as to the rooms and other things, since it has a sound title. Let me know the amount by which you will be short and I'll have it paid to you at once. But take care that you're not cheated, and that a rumour of your wanting to buy a house may not cause a running up of the price. I think you should have a look at it, that is to say, you should first look at it very carefully and ascertain its value; and if you find that the price is unreasonable, leave it to those to whom it is acceptable, because the money wasn't found by the wayside. However, I'll send you the money needed, as I've said, and I give you free leave to take it or leave it, as you think best. I think that's all. Let me know what you've done.

On the twenty-ninth of April.

As regards buying, I'm not saying you must be particular as to ten *scudi*, but as to the honesty of the deal.

MICHELANGELO BUONARROTI IN ROME

¶ TO LIONARDO DI BUONARROTO SIMONI IN FLORENCE

283

British Museum Mil. clxxvii From Rome (May 14th) 1547

Lionardo — The bearer of this will be a *scarpellino* from Settignano, named Jacopo, who says he wants to sell certain lands near ours, a place called Fraschetta. So tell Gismondo about it and see what they're like. And if it would be a good thing to buy them, and if the title is sound, so that one's not buying a liability, let me know the price. And if it's not very much, I'll send you the money. As to buying the house, I don't suppose you've done anything more. About the other matter you must please yourself. All that matters to me is that you should let me know first. I think that's all.

MICHELANGELO IN ROME

¶ TO LIONARDO DI BUONARROTO SIMONI IN FLORENCE

284

British Museum Mil. clxxviii From Rome June 18th 1547

Lionardo — I understand about the Fraschetta farm from your letters. That's all there is to it. You need think no more about it. You write me that the house in the Via de' Servi was sold by auction and was not suitable in any case. And yet you seemed to like it at first, according to what you wrote me. But if it's sold it may be for the best. The one belonging to Giovanni Corsi,[1] about which you now write me is, I understand, the one at the corner of the Piazza di Santa Croce, opposite the Orlandini's house, which pleases me, if it pleases you. But I should be very doubtful about the title, if it's being sold. So if they're selling it, and we're thinking of buying it, you must keep your eyes wide open. And if it's for sale, let me know what they're asking for it. I know it's an old house, and I believe it's very badly arranged inside.

I've received a pack-load of *trebbiano*, less six flasks of the forty; three were broken, three of them were left with the Customs and I sent ten of them to the Pope. I hope to God it's good. I think that's all. Commend me to Guicciardino and to Francesca and to Messer Giovan Francesco.

MICHELANGELO IN ROME

1. *Giovanni di Bardo Corsi (1472–1547), a diplomat and philosopher. He played a leading part in public affairs (Mecatti, p. 172).*

285

*British
Museum
Mil. clxxxv
From Rome
July 30th 1547*

⁋ To Lionardo di Buonarroto Simoni in Florence

Lionardo — I learn from your last letter about the purchase of the house that Giovanni Corsi[1] is dead and that you do not know what the heirs will be doing about his house. You also wrote me that you think Zanobi Buondelmonte's will be for sale, which would be no less to my liking than the one belonging to the Corsi. But I think whichever of the two is available should be taken regardless of a hundred *scudi* or so, provided that the soundness of the title is thoroughly investigated, which I think should be done as soon as possible, because having, or wishing to take a wife, it would be better for you from every point of view to do so while I'm alive, rather than after my death.

In order to complete the transfer of the money, which I estimate will be needed to meet the price of either of the said houses, I will begin, perhaps next week, to send you a few *scudi*. And as, enclosed with yours, you sent me a begging letter, will you give the lady in question what you think suitable from the amount I shall be sending you. I think that's all. Commend me to Guicciardino and to Francesca. Commend me also to Messer Giovan Francesco and make my apologies, because if I do not discharge my obligations it is because I'm too harassed.

MICHELANGELO IN ROME

I want you to get, through Messer Giovan Francesco, the height of the cupola of Santa Maria del Fiore from where the lantern begins to the ground, and then the overall height of the lantern, and to send it to me. Also send me in the letter the measured length of a third of a Florentine *braccio*.[2]

1. *Giovanni Corsi had died on July 17th.*
2. *The first intimation of the building of the dome of St. Peter's.*

286

*British
Museum
Mil. clxxxvi
From Rome
August 6th
1547*

⁋ To Lionardo di Buonarroto Simoni in Florence

Lionardo — I'm sending five hundred and fifty gold *scudi* in gold, which I have just paid here to Messer Bartolomeo Bettini. You must go and get it from the Salviati, as instructed in the draft which will be enclosed with this. Make out the receipt correctly, that is, for the same amount as the said Bartolomeo has received in Rome. And send me a copy of it. I'm sending you the said five hundred *scudi* on account to add to the thousand I sent you for the purchase of the house. The balance that will still be needed for the said purchase I'll send you, when you let me know. From the fifty *scudi*, give four or six of them to that lady whose letter you sent me with your last one, if you think it suitable. As to the rest of the fifty, I'll tell you what I want you to do with them when you send me the receipt. On the sixth day of August 1547.

MICHELANGELO IN ROME

¶ TO LIONARDO DI BUONARROTO SIMONI IN FLORENCE

287

*British
Museum
Mil. clxxxvii
From Rome
September 3rd
1547*

Lionardo — I've had your letter with the receipt for the five hundred and fifty gold *scudi* in gold which I paid here to Bettino. You write me that you're going to present four[1] of them to that lady for the love of God, which pleases me. The balance of the fifty I also wish to be spent for the love of God, partly for the soul of Buonarroto, your father, and partly for mine. So look out for some impoverished fellow citizen with daughters to be married or placed in a convent,[2] and give it to him – but on the quiet – and take care not to be tricked and get a receipt for it and send it to me. *[I say on the quiet]* because in speaking of fellow citizens I know that when in need they are ashamed to go round begging. As regards taking a wife, I tell you I cannot present one lady to you rather than another, because it is so long since I was in Florence that I am unable to judge of the status of the citizens. So you must decide among yourselves and when you have found someone to your liking, I shall be very glad to have some information about it.

You sent me a brass rule, as if I were a builder or a carpenter and had to carry it around with me. I was ashamed to have it in the house and gave it away.

Francesca writes me that she is not well and that she has four children and is very troubled about not being well. I am very sorry about it; in other respects I do not think she lacks for anything. As regards troubles I think I have many more than she has and old age in addition, and I haven't time to entertain relatives. So on my behalf urge her to be patient and commend me to Guicciardino.

I advise you to spend the money I've sent you on something good, properties or otherwise, because it is very risky to keep it by you, particularly these days. So contrive to sleep with your eyes open.

MICHELANGELO BUONARROTI IN ROME

1. *When given the choice of making a donation of four or six scudi, Lionardo characteristically chose to give four. Cf. No. 290.*

2. *'Assai è manifesto quanto sia miglior la fortuna degli uomini che quella delle donne' (Dovizi, 'Calandria', Act II, Sc. 1).*

288

*British
Museum
Mil. clxxix
From Rome
September 24th
1547*

⁋ To Lionardo di Buonarroto Simoni in Florence

Lionardo — Late this evening I had a letter of yours, but I've little time for writing. As to the house belonging to the Corsi, you told me the last time you wrote to me about it that a rich neighbour was inclined to take it, but if he does not I make no doubt it's a risky thing. So keep your eyes open, so as not to buy a liability. Otherwise, if you like it, buy it at a reasonable price if you can get it. As to the donation, it is enough for me to know for certain that you've made it, and it is enough for me to have the Monastery's receipt, and you've no need to make any mention of me.

I was as grieved about Guicciardino's baby as if it had been my own son. Encourage them to bear it patiently and commend me to them. Commend me to Messer Giovan Francesco, thank him, and ask him to hold me excused if I don't discharge my obligations to him, because I am beset by too many worries and particularly now that I've lost the ferry[1] and am reduced to living on capital. God help us. I think that's all. Ask Messer Giovan Francesco to commend me to Bugiardino[2] if he's still alive.

MICHELANGELO BUONARROTI IN ROME

1. *See Appendix 33.*

2. *Giuliano Bugiardini, a painter and old associate of Michelangelo's. He died on February 17th 1554, at the age of 79. For the portrait of Michelangelo attributed to him see the frontispiece to Volume I.*

289

*British
Museum
Mil. clxxxi
From Rome
October 1st
1547*

⁋ To Lionardo di Buonarroto Simoni in Florence

Lionardo — From what I understand of your last letter about the house belonging to the Corsi, it seems to me that there is little to be said for it and much against it. It seems to me that one shouldn't take these old houses, unless they're very cheap, because when the repairs have to be undertaken one nearly always finds so much wrong with them that it would be better to build a new one altogether. Again, I don't like it, because it is unhealthy owing to the dampness of the ground floor. I think the cellar, about which you tell me nothing, may be worse, and according to what you write, only the title is sound. As to the price, you tell me it is one thousand six hundred florins. I don't know why florins,[1] but whatever they are, I think it would cost more than the purchase price to put it in order. Nevertheless, as it is in an imposing position, I do not say definitely that you shouldn't take it, particularly as the title is sound, as you write me. Therefore, consider it carefully, and whatever you do I'll always take to be for the best, because it is a risky thing to keep the money by one. I think that's all, except that if you decide to take it, have it properly surveyed and get it for the lowest price you can.

MICHELANGELO BUONARROTI IN ROME

1. *The florin had been largely superseded, first by the ducat and then by the scudo. See Appendix 3.*

¶ TO LIONARDO DI BUONARROTO SIMONI IN FLORENCE

290

British Museum Mil. clxxx From Rome October 15th 1547

Lionardo — You write me that the sale of the house belonging to the Corsi is being postponed, as repairs to the wall are needed, and that for the time being you're turning your attention to the shop and that you've found someone to form a partnership with you. It seems to me that if the facing of the outside wall of the said house were in good repair and the title were sound, we ought to take it, in order to find a lodgment for that money. And the inside can then be put to rights little by little. After the said house has been bought, you will have a sufficient balance to enable you to form a partnership in a shop – though it doesn't seem to me the time to cast the money to the winds. It is my experience that it is only in virtue of landed property that families establish themselves in Florence. So make up your mind to the best of your ability, for whatever you do, you'll be doing for yourselves.

As to the almsgiving, it seems to me that you're too lax. If you do not give of my money for the soul of your father, still less will you give of your own. Commend me to Messer Giovan Francesco and thank him, and tell him that as to providing you with a wife, I'm expecting a friend of mine,[1] who is absent from Rome, who wishes to put three or four proposals before me. I'll let you know about them and we'll see if there's anything in them for us.

MICHELANGELO BUONARROTI IN ROME

1. *Donato Giannotti, who, in the train of his patron, Cardinal Ridolfi, generally returned to Rome from Bagnaia, the Cardinal's summer residence, at about this time.*

291

*British
Museum
Mil. cxcv
From Rome
October 22nd
1547*

¶ To Lionardo di Buonarroto Simoni in Florence

Lionardo — I'm glad that you have informed me about the decree,[1] because if up till now I've been on my guard about talking to the exiles and associating with them, I'll be much more on my guard in future. As regards my being ill,[2] in the Strozzi's house, I do not consider that I stayed in their house, but in the apartment of Messer Luigi del Riccio, who was a very great friend of mine; nor, since Bartolomeo Angiolini died,[3] have I found anyone to look after my affairs who did so better or more devotedly than he. But since he died I no longer frequent the said house, to which all Rome can bear witness, and to the kind of life I lead, as I am always alone; I go about very little and talk to no-one, least of all to Florentines; but if I'm greeted in the street I cannot but respond with a kindly word and pass on – though, if I were informed as to which are the exiles, I would make no response at all. But, as I've said, from now on I'll be very much on my guard, particularly as I have so many other anxieties that life is a burden.

As regards setting up a shop, do whatever you think will turn out successfully, because it's not my profession and I cannot give you any good advice. I only say this to you, that if you waste the money you have you may never be able to recover it.

MICHELANGELO IN ROME

1. *See Appendix 38.*

2. *See Appendix 27. The Strozzi were among the leading 'fuorusciti'.*

3. *On December 28th 1540 (Frey, p. 283).*

292

*British
Museum
Mil. clxxxiv
From Rome
November 5th
1547*

¶ To Lionardo di Buonarroto Simoni in Florence

Lionardo — I've got the receipt for the donation, which I'm pleased about. As regards the house belonging to the Corsi, if there are neighbours who want it, let them take it and say that you don't want to stand in anyone's way; see what happens and wait to be approached.

Commend me to Messer Giovan Francesco and thank him on my behalf; because I'm much obliged to him. And tell him that that worthy man who replied to him that I did not concern myself with public affairs cannot but be a man of nice discrimination, because he spoke the truth. Would that my affairs in Rome gave me no more anxiety than those of State.

I cannot reply to you about the other house about which you write me, as I couldn't make the letter out. Never do I get a letter from you that I am not thrown into a fever before I manage to read it. I do not know where you learnt to write. No consideration!

MICHELANGELO IN ROME

¶ TO LIONARDO DI BUONARROTO SIMONI IN FLORENCE

293

British Museum Mil. clxxxii From Rome November 12th 1547

Lionardo — I wrote to you about taking a wife and informed you about three who had been mentioned to me here; one is the daughter of Alamanno de' Medici, another the daughter of Domenico Gugni, and the other the daughter of Cherubino Fortini.[1] I do not know any of these gentlemen, so can speak to you neither well nor ill of them, nor can I counsel you in favour of one lady rather than another. So if Michele Guicciardini would be prepared to go to a little trouble for us, he could make enquiries and advise us in the matter, and likewise if he is apprised of anything else. So beg him on my behalf to do this, and commend me to him.

As regards the purchase of the house – this seems to me essential before taking a wife, because I know the one where you're all living isn't big enough. So when you write to me about it, see that I am able to understand the letters, if you want me to answer you as to my opinion. Messer Giovan Francesco could also give good guidance about these matters, because he is old and experienced. Commend me to him. But above all, it is the guidance of God that we need, because it is a big decision. And I would remind you that between the wife and the husband there should be a difference of at least ten years, and have an eye to a sound constitution as well as to character. That's all I have to say.

MICHELANGELO IN ROME

1. *Apparently all three proposals had been put forward by Donato Giannotti, who was, however, particularly concerned in pressing the claims of the daughter of Alamanno di Bernardo de' Medici (1501–1572). In his letter of December 10th to the eminent humanist, Pietro Vettori (1499–1585) in Florence, Giannotti sent Alamanno a message, though in guarded terms, indicating that the match had been approved in principle, and on December 24th he wrote again saying, 'If you see Alamanno de' Medici, tell him that I have received his letter . . . and that when I have the opportunity I will not fail to do as he desires' (Giannotti, P.V., p. 125).*

294

*British
Museum
Mil. clxxxiii
From Rome
November 19th
1547*

❡ To Lionardo di Buonarroto Simoni in Florence

Lionardo — I've received fourteen *marzolini* cheeses, but I repeat what I've written you on other occasions – you should not send me anything unless I ask you to do so.

As regards the house belonging to the Corsi, I suspect that this parade of others being after it is being made in order to alarm you. The offer you have made seems to me all right, the said house being what it is inside. So wait a little and see.

As regards the other house which you say is near the Alberti's corner, it seems to me to be too expensive in view of its size and of its being unfinished. I repeat, however, that I cannot judge of things when I'm so far removed from them. And I make the same answer about setting up a shop; it's not my profession and I don't know enough to discuss it with you. It is up to you whether you make a success or a failure.

As regards the taking of a wife, I wrote to you about three who had been mentioned to me here. I'm not giving you advice about any of them, because I've no information about Florentine citizens. Guicciardino will be able to help you in matters like this. Commend me to him and to Francesca.

Michelangelo Buonarroti in Rome

295

*British
Museum
Mil. clxxii
From Rome
December 3rd
1547*

❡ To Lionardo di Buonarroto Simoni in Florence

Lionardo — About a year ago a book written by a Florentine chronicler came into my hands in which I found a Buonarroto Simoni, who was a member of the Signoria several times, about two hundred years ago, if I remember rightly. And then a Simone Buonarroti and then a Michele di Buonarroto Simoni and then a Francesco Buonarroti. I did not find Lionardo, the father of our father Lodovico, who was a member of the Signoria, because it did not come down as late as that. So I think you should sign yourself as 'Lionardo di Buonarroto Buonarroti Simoni'. There's nothing more to say in answer to your letter because I have not yet learnt anything about the girl or about the house that I can tell you.

Michelangelo in Rome

¶ To Lionardo di Buonarroto Simoni in Florence

296

Lionardo — I learn from your letter that a lawsuit is pending over certain lands at Settignano and that I must send you a power of attorney to enable you to defend it. The power of attorney will be enclosed with this, and I think I shall have to send you a book of contracts which I had made up in the correct form by Ser Giovanni da Romena,[1] which cost me eighteen ducats, in which the contract for the said lands cannot but be included. And together with the book I'll send some additional contracts and ratifications and other legal documents which represent my worldly possessions. So I want you to find a trustworthy carrier and to send him to me when he comes to Rome. And I'll give him a parcel of the said documents which will weigh about twenty pounds. And I want you to come to terms with him and not to be particular within half a *scudo* in order to ensure that he delivers them to you safely. And tell him that when he brings your letter acknowledging receipt I, too, will give him something.

As to the shop, Guicciardino writes me that you have invited him to enter into a partnership; but you write me that he invited you. Let it be as it may, provided that matters are made clear, because we aren't well off for friends and relatives and can't afford to quarrel. As to the name of the firm, I should certainly add that of 'Simone' and if it's too long, those who can't read it needn't.

[Unsigned]

British Museum Mil. clxxxviii From Rome December 17th 1547

1. *Giovanni da Romena was the notary who drew up the contract for the purchase of the properties which Michelangelo bought in June 1512. See No. 76, n. 1.*

¶ To Lionardo di Buonarroto Simoni in Florence

297

Lionardo — You write me that you have been applied to with reference to the Funds which are held as security for the farm I bought from Pier Tedaldi[1] because they want to buy part of the land comprised in the same title, and that you cannot consent to this without my permission. I give you permission to do whatever you think best, as I should do myself, if I were there. Last week I sent you the power of attorney you asked me for and I wrote and told you to find a trustworthy carrier and to send him to me with a letter from you, when he comes to Rome, because I want to give him a bundle of legal documents, which will weigh about twenty pounds, in which there will be a book of contracts, which I had made up by Ser Giovanni da Romena, with other contracts and legal documents of the utmost importance. Therefore agree a price with the carrier there and do not be particular within half a *scudo*, and pay him there, so that he

British Museum Mil. clxxxix From Rome December 24th 1547

may be the more certain to deliver it. I think that's all. On the twenty-fourth day of December 1547.

MICHELANGELO BUONARROTI IN ROME

1. *This was the farm at Rovezzano for the purchase of which Michelangelo entered into a complicated agreement in October 1519 (Milanesi, p. 581).*

298

British Museum Mil. cxc From Rome January 6th 1548

¶ To Lionardo di Buonarroto Simoni in Florence

Lionardo — A man who says he is the son of the carrier Lorenzo del Cione came to me to-day with your letter to collect the parcel of contracts which I wrote and told you I'd send you. I don't know him, but believing him to be the man you sent to collect them, I gave them to him, but with some misgiving, because they're very valuable. On its receipt you will write me through the same carrier and I'll give him something as I wrote you. I've put them in a box and wrapped it twice round in oiled cloth, and it is corded in such a way that water cannot damage it. That's all I have to say. On I know not what date, but to-day is Epiphany.[1]

In the book of contracts there is a letter from Count Alessandro da Canossa[2] which I recently came across at home. He once came to visit me in Rome as a relative. Take care of it.

MICHELANGELO BUONARROTI IN ROME

1. *He seems always to have been vague about the date of Epiphany. Cf. No. 39.*

2. *The letter was dated October 8th 1520. Michelangelo believed his family to be descended from Simone da Canossa, who was podestà of Florence in 1250. The Marchese Giuseppe Campori disproved this in his 'Catalogo degli Artisti italiani e stranieri negli Stati Estensi', Modena, 1855 (Milanesi, p. 216).*

299

British Museum Mil. cxci From Rome January 16th 1548

¶ To Lionardo di Buonarroto Simoni in Florence

Lionardo — The news of Giovansimone's death[1] reached me in your last letter. It has been a very great grief to me, because, old though I am, I had hoped to see him before he died and before I die myself. It has pleased God that it should be as it is, and we must be resigned. I should be glad to hear in detail how he died and whether he died having made confession and having received the Sacrament, together with all those things ordained by the Church; because if he received them and I knew of it, I should be less grieved.

As regards the legal documents and the book of contracts for which I wrote and told you to send the muleteer, I gave them to the man who came with your letter on the day of Epiphany, if I remember rightly, which was, I believe, ten days ago to-day.[2] I gave them to him in a large box wrapped in waxed cloth, corded and well packed. So see that you get it and advise me of its receipt, because it's very valuable. That's all I can say to you this time, because I was late in receiving the letter and I haven't time for writing.

Commend me to Guicciardino and to Francesca and to Messer Giovan Francesco.

MICHELANGELO BUONARROTI IN ROME

1. *Giovansimone died on January 9th 1548 and was buried in the family vault in Santa Croce.*

2. *There is a discrepancy between Michelangelo's dating and Lionardo's endorsement, which reads: '1547. From Rome. Received on the 26th Day of January from the 21st of the said month.' As Michelangelo's recollection as to the date would appear to be correct, we must suppose that the delivery of the letter was delayed and that Lionardo endorsed it accordingly. 1547 [O.S.].*

¶ TO LIONARDO DI BUONARROTO SIMONI IN FLORENCE

300

British Museum Mil. cxcii From Rome January 28th 1548

Lionardo — I learn from your letter that you have received the box with the book of contracts which arrived opportunely and were needed, as I thought. As to the house belonging to the Corsi, I think it would be as well to wait as long as possible and see what happens and not to be rushed.

As to the partnership there's no need to send me a copy of the deed, because I don't understand about it. If you succeed the success will be your own.

As regards the death of Giovansimone about which you write me, you pass it over very lightly, since you do not give me any more detailed information about anything nor about what he left. I would remind you that he was my brother, no matter what he was like, and that it cannot but be that I should be grieved and should wish that something should be done for the welfare of his soul, such as I did for the soul of your father. So take care not to be ungrateful for what has been done for you, who were without anything in the world. I'm astonished at Gismondo, who hasn't sent me a line about it, since it concerns him as much as it concerns me – and what concerns you is what we wish and nothing else.

MICHELANGELO IN ROME

301

British Museum Mil. cxciii From Rome February 4th 1548

¶ To Lionardo di Buonarroto Simoni in Florence

Lionardo — Since I last wrote to you I discovered a letter at home, in which you inform me about everything of Giovansimone's that was found. Afterwards I received another one informing me in detail about his death. As to what he left, you might have given me the information in your first letter, so that I should not have had to find it out from others, as I had to, before I heard about it from you, which made me exceedingly angry. As to his death, you write me that although he did not receive everything ordained by the Church, he died, nevertheless, in a state of perfect contrition, which, if this is the case, suffices for salvation. As to what he left, according to law Gismondo is the heir, as he did not make a will, and with this I enjoin you to do what you can for the good of his soul, and do not hesitate about money, because I won't fail you in what you do.

As regards the contracts and the legal documents which I sent you, take great care of them, because they may still be needed. As to the house belonging to the Corsi, I think you should abide by the offer you made, because if they want to sell it, if it's in the state you tell me it is in, I don't believe they'll get more for it in these days. I think that's all.

MICHELANGELO BUONARROTI IN ROME

302

British Museum Mil. cxciv From Rome February 18th 1548

¶ To Lionardo di Buonarroto Simoni in Florence

Lionardo — I wrote you that I had received a letter of yours, after all, about everything that Giovansimone has left and that according to law Gismondo is the heir to everything and that you should do what you can for the good of his soul and that I will not fail you.

For a choice of wives I told you of three who have been mentioned to me here. You've sent me no reply about this. It's up to you to marry or not to marry, or rather to choose one girl rather than another, provided she is of noble family and well brought up and rather without a dowery than with a large one, so that you may live in peace.

I think that's all. Thank Francesca and encourage her to be patient and commend me to Michele and to her.

MICHELANGELO BUONARROTI IN ROME

¶ To Lionardo di Buonarroto Simoni in Florence

303

Lionardo — I haven't replied to your last letter before, because I wasn't able to. As regards your taking a wife[1] you say you think it better to leave it for the summer. If you think so, I think so too.

As to going to Loreto as to going to Loreto[2] for your father's sake, if it was a vow, I think you should certainly fulfil it. If it is for the good of his soul you wish to do this, I would much rather give you the money you would spend on the journey to spend for him in alms in Florence, than to do anything else, because if you give the money to the priests, God knows what they do with it. Besides, it does not seem to me opportune to lose the time when you are setting up a shop. Therefore, if you wish to succeed, you must keep your nose to the grindstone and put aside youthful whims. I think that's all.

As regards the house belonging to the Corsi, I should like to know whether anyone ever spoke to you about it afterwards. Commend me to the priest, to Guicciardino and to Francesca.

On the 7th day of April 1548.

MICHELANGELO IN ROME

Buonarroti Archives Mil. cxcvi From Rome April 7th 1548

1. *On the same day, April 7th, Donato Giannotti wrote to Pietro Vettori, his go-between in Florence, saying, 'Tell Alamanno de' Medici as regards his affair, that here I have to deal with an old man who is suspicious, and he there with a young one who is too timid, and therefore the enterprise is difficult' (Giannotti, P.V., p. 128). See postscript, Plate 14. The truth of this observation is borne out by the fact that Lionardo had so far lost his nerve that he was proposing to escape on a pilgrimage to Loreto.*

2. *[Sic.] Loreto, a city in the Marches, was a famous place of pilgrimage because of the Santa Casa, or Holy House of the Virgin, which was alleged to have been miraculously transported from Nazareth to Loreto in the thirteenth century.*

¶ To Lionardo di Buonarroto Simoni in Florence

304

Lionardo — I have received, together with a letter of yours, a copy of the contract for the Company you have formed in the Arte della Lana. There was no need to send it, as it doesn't mean anything to me. I assume that you have considered it carefully and that it is all right. Please God it may be so.

As to the matter of Santa Caterina, about which you write me, do what you think, provided you make things clear, so that there may be no cause for dispute. As to the Tornabuoni house, it is true that it is outside our Quarter;[1] everything depends however on its price and on its being a sound proposition. So let me know about it.

Buonarroti Archives Mil. cxcvii From Rome April 14th 1548

14. *Facsimile of a Letter from Donato Giannotti to Piero Vettori* British Museum, London

I think that's all. Would you send me the entry of my birth,[2] which you sent me once before, exactly as it is given in our father's book, because I've lost it.

On the 14th day of April 1548.

MICHELANGELO BUONARROTI IN ROME

1. *The Quarter of Santa Croce.*

2. *See Appendix 35.*

¶ To Lionardo di Buonarroto Simoni in Florence

305

Buonarroti Archives Mil. cxcviii From Rome April 28th 1548

Lionardo — I have renounced my right as heir to Giovansimone, the deed for which will be enclosed with this.[1]

As regards the house in the Via de' Servi and the other one, I give you permission to do whatever you think best and to please yourself, provided you get a sound proposition and take something imposing, and don't be particular as to the money.

Commend me to Messer Giovan Francesco and tell him that as he has offered to get that receipt I asked of him made out by Bernardo Bini in the form of a deed, I should be very grateful; he will be doing me a great favour. You are to pay for the deed,[2] which will be a small amount, and to send it to me. Thank him and commend me to him.

MICHELANGELO BUONARROTI IN ROME

1. *According to an earlier letter, No. 301, Michelangelo thought he would be excluded from his right to the inheritance, owing, we may suppose, to his non-residence in Florence. But this turned out not to be the case.*

2. *Perhaps a further reference to the public quittance. See No. 268, n. 1.*

¶ To Lionardo di Buonarroto Simoni in Florence

306

Buonarroti Archives Mil. cxcix From Rome May 2nd 1548

Lionardo — I got the barrel of pears, which numbered eighty-six. I sent thirty-three of them to the Pope; he thought them excellent and was very grateful for them. As to the barrel of cheese, the Customs say that the carrier is a scamp, and that he never brought it into the Customs, so that when I find out that he's in Rome, I'll see that he gets his deserts – not on account of the cheese, but in order to teach him to show a little respect for people.

I've been very ill recently through not being able to urinate, as a result of which I'm extremely weak. However, I'm better now. I'm writing to you about this so that some chatterbox may not write and tell you a thousand lies to alarm you.

Tell the priest not to address me any more as 'Michelangelo sculptor', because here I'm only known as Michelangelo Buonarroti, and that if a Florentine citizen wants to have an altar-piece painted, he must find a painter – and that I was never a painter or a sculptor like those who set up shop for that purpose. I always refrained from doing so out of respect for my father and brothers; although I have served three Popes, it has been under compulsion. I think that's all.

From my letter of the last day of last month you will have learnt my opinion as regards the lady. Don't say anything to the priest about these few lines I've written about him, because I wish to indicate that I haven't had his letter.[1]

MICHELANGELO BUONARROTI IN ROME

---

1. *Presumably to make it appear that letters incorrectly addressed were not promptly delivered, there being lesser men who might be addressed 'Michelangelo, sculptor' – as indeed there were.*

307

Buonarroti Archives Mil. cc From Rome May 12th 1548

¶ TO LIONARDO DI BUONARROTO SIMONI IN FLORENCE

Lionardo — I've written to you several times telling you to do as you think about the house and the lands at Santa Caterina and about everything else. As to buying, I advise you to assure yourselves on every point, so that there are no grounds for litigation. I would remind you that the lands I bought at Santa Caterina I bought free of encumbrances and thus I have held them until to-day, so that you might not have to lease them at so much a year, like those you want to buy. Therefore, make a clear line of demarcation between the one and the other. I think that's all.

Thank Messer Giovan Francesco, because he has done me a great favour, although it's not a matter of any great importance.

Take the greatest care of every little item among the documents in the box I sent you, because they're very valuable. On the twelfth day of May 1548.

MICHELANGELO BUONARROTI IN ROME

¶ To Lionardo di Buonarroto Simoni in Florence

308

*Buonarroti
Archives
Mil. cci
From Rome
June 1548*

Lionardo — I've received a pack-load of *trebbiano* for which I'm grateful. Never-theless, I tell you not to send me anything else unless I send and ask you for it, be-cause I'll send you the money for what I want. As regards the shop I should be glad if you would let me know how you're succeeding. That's all I have to say. Commend me to Guicciardino and to Francesca and to Messer Giovan Francesco.

MICHELANGELO IN ROME

¶ To Lionardo di Buonarroto Simoni in Florence

309

*British
Museum
Mil. cxl
From Rome
(July) 1548*

Lionardo — I've received the ravioli, that is, six *coppie*; I imagine it was excellent in Florence, but it was completely ruined when it arrived here. I think it got wet. Therefore such soft things as this ought not to be sent. It suffices, in short, that I've re-ceived it; that's all there is to say about it.

I am very pleased that things are going well, as you write me, both with the pro-perties and with the shop. One must thank God for it, and try to do one's best. I think that's all.

MICHELANGELO IN ROME

¶ To Lionardo di Buonarroto Simoni in Florence

310

*Buonarroti
Archives
Mil. ccii
From Rome
July 28th
1548*

Lionardo — You write me that you enquired whether you could buy the house belonging to the Buondelmonte and on what terms. I reply that I like the house, but the method of buying it seems to me nothing but making a loan of the money. I should therefore dismiss the agent who made you the proposition, because to buy a house and not to know whether one has it to live in or not seems to me madness. I think that's all. Commend me to Guicciardino and to Francesca.

MICHELANGELO IN ROME

311

*Buonarroti
Archives
Mil. cciii
From Rome
August 10th
1548*

¶ TO LIONARDO DI BUONARROTO SIMONI IN FLORENCE

Lionardo — You write me that you have an offer of a farm at one thousand three hundred florins outside the Prato gate. If it is a good proposition I think you should certainly take it, provided that you get a sound title, so that there are no grounds for dispute. You must be careful that it's not in a place that can be flooded by the Arno. If a large sum – that is to say three or four thousand *scudi* – could be invested in a property ten or fifteen miles distant from Florence, I would take it, if I could have the income from it for myself; because, having lost the ferry, I am in need of providing myself with an income that cannot be taken away from me, and I would more gladly secure it in Florence than elsewhere. I'm writing you about this because, if you should hear of something good round about the price, you could let me know – but don't go talking about it.

I think that's all. Greet everyone on my behalf and commend me to Messer Giovan Francesco. On the tenth day of August 1548.

MICHELANGELO IN ROME

312

*Buonarroti
Archives
Mil. ccv
From Rome
September 15th
1548*

¶ TO LIONARDO DI BUONARROTO SIMONI IN FLORENCE

Lionardo — As I have no need to write to you this time, this is merely to act as a cover to a letter to Giuliano Bugiardini in reply to one of his. So give it to him, and if you don't know him, get Messer Giovan Francesco to point him out.

I've been a little depressed owing to being unable to urinate; however, I'm all right now. Let me know how things are going as regards the shop and if anyone comes from here and says anything to you on my behalf, don't believe him unless you have letters about it from me. On the fifteenth day of September 1548.

MICHELANGELO BUONARROTI IN ROME

313

*Buonarroti
Archives
Mil. ccvi
From Rome
October 20th
1548*

¶ TO LIONARDO DI BUONARROTO SIMONI IN FLORENCE

Lionardo — I learn from your letter of the properties that are for sale in the region of San Miniato al Tedesco. I do declare that there is no region in the country round Florence that for a number of reasons would please me less. Nevertheless, we ought to find out what they are like, because they and their titles might be such that we ought to take them. So find out about them, but as discreetly as you can. I think that's all for the present. I have little time for writing.

MICHELANGELO IN ROME

¶ To Lionardo di Buonarroto Simoni in Florence

314

*Buonarroti
Archives
Mil. ccvii
From Rome
December 29th
1548*

Lionardo — I've recently been approached again, as regards your proposed marriage, about two girls, concerning whom I believe I myself wrote to you last year. One is a daughter of Alamanno de' Medici[1] and the other the daughter of Cherubino Fortini.[2] In the case of the Medici girl I think there is very little money and also that she may be too old. Of the other one I can say even less; so that I am unable to advise you as to the one rather than the other, because I have little information. But since there is no one else left of us but you, I think you should marry. But we are living in times when for a number of reasons one should keep one's eyes wide open. So think it over, and when you have a fancy one way or another, let me know.

You wrote to me about a month ago concerning a certain property. I had, as I wrote you several times, a desire to secure an income in Florence, in order to be able to live here without having to work, because I'm an old man and unable to do so any more; but for a month now I've lost the desire.[3] I'll consider some other means of livelihood. I hope God will help me. I think that's all. On the twenty-ninth day of December 1548.

MICHELANGELO IN ROME

1. *Apparently he had not given up hope, but his efforts proved unsuccessful. He eventually married his daughter, Caterina, to Giovanbattista Botti (Litta, II, tav. vi).*

2. *Cherubino Fortini had held office as one of the Cinque Sindaci in 1527 and after the siege of Florence had been banished for three years (Varchi, pp. 112 and 453).*

3. *He had been granted the revenues of the office of Civil Notary to the Romagna, as from the new year, on October 2nd (Schiavo, Vita, p. 271).*

¶ To the Overseers of the Fabric of St. Peter's

315

*Vatican
Archives
Mil. cdxci
From Rome
(1548/9)*

You are aware that I told Balduccio[1] that he was not to send his lime unless it was good. Now, having sent it when it was poor, without the expectation of having to take it back, it may be thought that he was in league with the man who took delivery of it. This is playing into the hands of those whom I have dismissed from the fabric on like account. Whoever takes delivery of materials necessary to the fabric, but of inferior quality, which I have forbidden, does nothing but treat as friends those whom I have treated as enemies. This, I think, would be a new confederacy.

Promises, gratuities and presents corrupt justice. I therefore pray you, with that authority I have from the Pope, henceforward not to take delivery of anything that is not suitable, even if it comes from Heaven, so that I may not appear to be what I am not – partial.

YOUR MICHELANGELO

1. *Jacopo Balducci, one of the contractors responsible for the delivery of travertine, which Michelangelo used extensively in the building. His name appears in the list of suppliers given in an account book of the fabric for 1548–9 (Frey, 1916, p. 23).*

316

Buonarroti Archives Mil. ccviii From Rome January 18th 1549

¶ TO LIONARDO DI BUONARROTO SIMONI IN FLORENCE

Lionardo — I think you said that the house about which you wrote me was, according to what you tell me, one of those which Gagliano used to own in the Via del Cocomero, to the right going towards San Marco, near the corner of the Piazza di San Niccolò. If it's that one, I have no information about it whatsoever. So try to have a look at it and if it's suitable and the locality pleases you, take it; and above all, it behoves you to be careful about the title and to ensure that it is an imposing house.

As regards your taking a wife, I've heard that the two of whom I wrote you are married. We must suppose it was not to be, and must commend ourselves to God, and have faith that He will reveal someone suitable.

I am an old man, as you know, and as each hour might be my last, and as I have a certain amount of capital here, although it is not a vast amount, I should not like it to be wasted, because I earned it with much exertion. I've been considering whether it would be safe if I deposited it in Florence at Santa Maria Nuova, until we have come to a decision, and again I should be able to use it if I needed it, as in the case of illness or other necessity, and it could not be taken from me. Talk it over with Gismondo and let me know your opinion.

Since writing I've discussed the house, which is among those belonging to Gagliano, with a friend of mine who highly approves of it. If it's the one about which you wrote me, I think you should certainly take it, and don't be particular within a hundred *scudi*, provided the title is sound, and let me know how much money is needed and to whom I must pay it here, so that it may be made payable to you. I think that's all.

MICHELANGELO BUONARROTI IN ROME

On the eighteenth day of January 1549.

Tell Messer Giovan Francesco that I've been about very little for a month now, because I haven't been feeling too well; but that I'll go and see Bettino, who has more dealings at the Court than I have, and I'll see that together we do the best we can for him. My connections in Rome are very few and I do not know who might be able to serve him, and if I ask anything of these people, they ask a thousand things of me in return. So I'm obliged to have few connections. However, I'll do what I can. Commend me to him.

¶ TO LIONARDO DI BUONARROTO SIMONI IN FLORENCE

Buonarroti Archives Mil. ccix From Rome January 25th 1549

317

Lionardo — The cheese you've sent me – I've had the letter – but I haven't yet had the cheese. I believe the muleteer who brought it has sold it to someone else, because I sent to the Customs for it several times. The said muleteer has invented a thousand tales and talked so much that he must have made off with it – so I make no doubt he's a rogue. So don't send me anything more; because it's more nuisance than use.

As to the house about which you informed me, if it's one of those belonging to Gagliano, as I said in my reply to your letter, I think you should take it, as I wrote you, because I've had a very good account of it.

As regards your taking a wife, I had information this morning about several marriageable girls. I believe it was a broker[1] who wrote, although he didn't give his name. I'm sending you the said list enclosed with this, so that if you haven't had the information, you may acquire it. And I'll tell you my opinion next time I write, as I haven't time now. Don't let anyone know that I've sent you the said list.

MICHELANGELO BUONARROTI IN ROME

1. *Marriage negotiations were 'always conducted by a middleman, a relative or a marriage-broker', and generally involved prolonged bargaining, particularly about the dowery (Origo, pp. 188 et seq.)*

¶ TO LIONARDO DI BUONARROTO SIMONI IN FLORENCE

Buonarroti Archives Mil. ccx From Rome February 1st 1549

318

Lionardo — In my last letter I sent you a list of marriageable girls which was sent to me from Florence, I think by some broker. He must be a man of little sense, because as I have been resident in Rome for sixteen, or rather seventeen years, he should have realized how little information I could have about Florentine families.

I therefore impress upon you that if you want to take a wife you should not delay on my account, because I cannot advise you as to the best choice, but I do tell you not to go after money, but solely after a nice disposition and good repute.

I believe there may be many families in Florence who are noble though poor, with

97

whom it would be a charity to ally oneself, even if there were no dowery – since there would be no arrogance either! You need someone who would stay beside you, who would do your bidding and who would not want to live in a showy way or to go to parties and weddings every day; because where there is open house it is easy to become a wanton, and particularly for anyone without relatives.[1] But that is no reason for people to say that you apparently wish to ennoble yourself, because it is well known that we are old Florentine citizens and as noble as any other family. So commend yourself to God and pray Him to reveal to you what you need. And when you find someone you think suitable I should be very grateful if you would let me know before an alliance is arranged.[2]

As regards the house about which you write me, I replied that I had had a good account of it and that you should not be particular within a hundred *scudi*.

You also informed me about a farm at Monte Spertoli. I replied that I had lost the desire for it, not because the property is as it is, but for another reason. I now want you to let me know should you find some good property of which I could enjoy the income; because if it were a sound proposition, I'd take it. And as to the house, if you take it, let me know how much money I should send. And do what must be done quickly, because time is short.[3]

As to what I wrote about Santa Maria Nuova, I am advised against it, so think no more about it.

On the first day of February 1549.

[Unsigned]

1. *As Lionardo was motherless and Gismondo was unmarried, there would be no older women in the house to provide a sobering influence.*

2. *In a letter dated April 20th 1545, Luigi del Riccio had wisely advised Lionardo to do nothing without telling Michelangelo, because 'you would make a great mistake and do yourself a great deal of harm' (Steinmann, p. 52).*

3. *He was at this time suffering from symptoms of the stone. His condition became more acute later.*

319

¶ To Lionardo di Buonarroto Simoni in Florence

British Museum Mil. ccxi From Rome February 9th 1549

Lionardo — I've sent Urbino to the Customs several times for the cheese which you sent me. The men at the Customs say that the carrier either sold it at the inn, or left it in Florence, because here they don't put less than five barrels of cheese in bond and all these the Customs consign direct to their owners. It may be that the said carrier himself is an out-and-out glutton, because he did everything he could to avoid Urbino while he was in Rome. But if he returns here, will you let me have news.

As to the house, you informed me that you were not satisfied with the title. I assure you it is better not to buy at all than to buy a liability. As to Santa Maria Nuova, I have had the information and there's no need to think any more about it.

As to your taking a wife, I sent you the note I received. The letter was brought to the house I know not by whom. And when you have a fancy for one lady rather than another, I should be glad if you would let me know about it before you do anything. I think that's all, anyway I've no time now.

On the ninth day of February 1549.

MICHELANGELO BUONARROTI IN ROME

¶ To Lionardo di Buonarroto Simoni in Florence

320

*British
Museum
Mil. ccxii
From Rome
February 16th
1549*

Lionardo — Enclosed with this there will be a letter for Francesca, who, according to what Michele writes me, is very unhappy. I've done my best to comfort her; so take it to her and commend me to her.

As to the house and the farm, I've nothing further to add. And although I wrote that matters should be dealt with quickly, because time is short, there is no need to deal with them so quickly that the agent makes mistakes. One should only do what can be done properly. I haven't time to write more now.

On the sixteenth day of February 1549.

MICHELANGELO IN ROME

¶ To Lionardo di Buonarroto Simoni in Florence

321

*British
Museum
Mil. ccxiii
From Rome
February 21st
1549*

Lionardo — I've written to you several times about your taking a wife, telling you not to believe anyone who speaks to you about it on my behalf, unless you see letters from me. This I again repeat, because for more than a year now Bartolomeo Bettini has been trying to induce me to give you one of his nieces in marriage.[1] I've always made excuses. Now he is making another determined attempt through a friend of mine. I've replied that I know that you're inclined towards someone you like, and that you've practically made your intentions known and that I don't want to unsettle you. I'm informing you of this, so that you may know how to reply, because I believe that the proposal will be warmly recommended to you in Florence. Don't permit your-self to swallow the bait, just because the offers they are making are such that you would never be in want. Bartolomeo is a man of honour, able and obliging, but he is not our equal and your sister has married into the Guicciardini family. I don't think I need say more to you, because I know that you realize that honour is of more worth than possessions. That's all I have to say to you.

Commend me to Guicciardino and to Francesca and tell her on my behalf not to fret, because she has many companions in tribulation, particularly to-day because the better one is the more one suffers.[2] On the 21st day of February 1549.

MICHELANGELO BUONARROTI IN ROME

1. *Bartolomeo Bettini had been trying to arrange this alliance since 1545 (Steinmann, p. 52).*

2. *Cf. the line from Michelangelo's sonnet on Dante, 'C' a' più perfetti abonda di più guai' (Guasti, p. 155).*

322

¶ TO LIONARDO DI BUONARROTO SIMONI IN FLORENCE

British Museum Mil. cciv From Rome March (2nd) 1549

Lionardo — As I was unable to read your last letter or to make it out, I threw it in the fire. I am therefore unable to reply to you about anything. I have written and told you several times that every time I get a letter from you I'm thrown into a fever before I manage to read it. I therefore forbid you to write to me again from now on, and if you have anything to communicate to me, get hold of someone who knows how to write, because I've other things to occupy me without having to struggle over your letters.[1]

Messer Giovan Francesco writes me that you would like to come to Rome for a few days. I'm astonished that you can get away, having formed a partnership, as you wrote me. So take care not to waste the money I sent you. Similarly, Gismondo ought also to take care of it, since those who haven't earned it don't appreciate it. One knows this from experience, because the majority of those born into wealth waste it and come to ruin. So wake up and try to realize what a miserable life of toil I lead, old as I am.

Recently a Florentine citizen came to me and suggested one of the Ginori[2] daughters, who has been suggested to you in Florence and whom, he tells me, you like. I don't believe this is true, but again I am unable to advise you about it, as I have no information. But it would not please me at all that you should take as a wife someone whose father, if he could afford to give her a suitable dowery, would not give her to you. I should like anyone wishing to give you his daughter to wife, to think of doing so for yourself and not for your possessions. It seems to me that in seeking a wife it is for you to take the initiative, and not for others to make proposals when no dowery can be offered. So

A uolere imparare regolarmente questa
Eccellente virtu de lo Scriuere,
Qual si uoglia Sorte di
lettere, è necessa-
rio
primieramente sapere tenere ben la penna
in mano,
Senza, la quale auuertenza, è impossibi-
le peruenre alla uera perfettione de lo
Scriuere.
& però auuertirte che la penna si
deue tenere con le due prime
dita appoggiandole so-
pra 'l terzo,
Perche tenendola altrimenti, Il tratto no
uerria sicuro, ma
tremolante,

B

15. *A page from 'Libro nuovo d'imparare a scrivere'*   G. B. Palatino
British Museum, London

it is only soundness of mind and body and nobility of birth and upbringing that you need to consider, besides seeing what her parents are like, which is very important.

That's all I have to say. Commend me to Messer Giovan Francesco.

MICHELANGELO BUONARROTI IN ROME

1. *In his own interest Lionardo would have been well advised to study Palatino's manual. Plate 15.*

2. *As Lionardo Ginori had had to flee his creditors during the reign of Alessandro de' Medici, he had evidently died without being able to provide doweries for his daughters (Ginori, p. 216).*

323

*British
Museum
Mil. ccxiv
From Rome
March 15th
1549*

¶ TO LIONARDO DI BUONARROTO SIMONI IN FLORENCE

Lionardo — There's no need to add anything further to what I told you in my last letter.

As regards my malady – being unable to urinate – I have been very ill with it since then, groaning day and night, unable to sleep or to get any rest whatever. As far as they can make out, the doctors say I'm suffering from the stone. They're still not certain. However, they continue to treat me for the said malady and are very hopeful. Nevertheless, as I'm an old man suffering from such a cruel malady, they're not making me any promises. I'm advised to go and take the baths at Viterbo, but one cannot go until the beginning of May.[1] In the meantime I'll manage as best I can and perhaps it will turn out, mercifully, that the malady will prove not to be the stone, or that a cure will be found. I am therefore in need of God's help. So tell Francesca to pray for me and tell her that if she knew the state I have been in, she would see that she is not without companions in affliction. In other respects I am almost as I was at thirty years of age. This malady has come upon me through the hardships I have suffered and through taking too little care of myself.[2] But there it is. Perhaps with God's help it will turn out better than I expect, and if otherwise I'll let you know, because I want to put my spiritual and temporal affairs in order, and for this it will be necessary for you to come here. When I think the time has come, I'll let you know. But without letters from me make no move, whatever anyone else says. If it is the stone, the doctors tell me that it is at an early stage and that it is a small one. They're therefore very hopeful, as I've said.

If you know of any noble family in a state of real need, which I think may well be the case, let me know about it, because I'll send you up to fifty *scudi*, so that you may make a donation for the good of my soul. This will in no way diminish what I have arranged to leave you, so see to it without fail.

On the 15th day of March 1549.

MICHELANGELO BUONARROTI IN ROME

1. *The baths at Viterbo are still open from May to October.*

2. *Cf. in his letter of December 19th 1500, his father had warned him that when he grew older he would regret having taken too little care of himself in his youth (Frey, Briefe, p. 1).*

¶ To Lionardo di Buonarroto Simoni in Florence

324

British Museum Mil. ccxv From Rome March 23rd 1549

Lionardo — In my last letter I wrote and told you about my being ill with the stone, which is something cruel, as those who have had it know. Since then, having been given a certain kind of water to drink, it has caused me to discharge so much thick white matter in the urine, together with some fragments of the stone, that I am much better and they hope that in a short time I shall be free of it – thanks to God and to some good soul. As to what ensues you shall be informed. There is no need to repeat what I wrote you about almsgiving. I know that you'll see into it diligently.

This illness has caused me to think more about putting my affairs, both temporal and spiritual, in better order than I would have done, and I've sketched out a will that I think suitable, which I'll copy out next time, if I can, and you can give me your opinion. But I should have to make sure the letters were sent by a safe route. I think that's all for the present.

On the 23rd day of March 1549.

MICHELANGELO BUONARROTI IN ROME

¶ To Lionardo di Buonarroto Simoni in Florence

325

British Museum Mil. ccxvi From Rome March 29th 1549

Lionardo — I've sent Bartolomeo Bettini fifty gold *scudi* in gold by Urbino this morning, the twenty-ninth day of March 1549, in order that you may spend the money as I wrote and told you to. You've sent me information about a member of the Cerretani family,[1] who has to place his daughter in a monastery; I know nothing whatsoever about them. Take care to give where there is a need, and not out of friendship or kinship, but for the love of God. Arrange to get a receipt for it and don't say where it comes from. Bettino's draft for the said money will be enclosed with this. Go and get it and acknowledge it.

I have other things to write and tell you, as I wrote you, but writing is a trouble to me, because I don't feel well. However, compared with the state I have been in, I think

I've recovered; and as I've begun to discharge some fragments of the stone, I'm very hopeful.

MICHELANGELO BUONARROTI IN ROME

1. *In Lionardo's Ricordi which he kept between 1540 and 1565, the entry of this donation of 50 ducats, made on behalf of the daughter of Niccolò di Giovanni Cerretani, who entered the monastery of Santa Verdiana in Florence, may still be seen (Segnato A, carte 92, verso) (Milanesi, p. 244). The Cerretani, who came from Cerreto, are described by Mecatti (p. 44) as 'antichissimi e Nobilissimi in Firenze'.*

326

¶ TO LIONARDO DI BUONARROTO SIMONI IN FLORENCE

British Museum Mil. ccxvii From Rome April 5th 1549

Lionardo — Last week I sent Bettino fifty gold ducats in gold by Urbino to be made payable to you in Florence. I assume you will have received them and will use them, as I wrote you, on behalf either of one of the Cerretani or of someone else whom you find has need of them, and will let me know what you have done.

As regards putting my affairs in order, concerning which I wrote you, I only wished to say that being old and ill, I thought it advisable to make a will. And the will is as follows – that is to say, I intend to leave what I possess to you and to Gismondo on this basis, that Gismondo my brother shall have as much for his use as you, my nephew, for yours, and neither of you may make a decision about my estate without the consent of the other; and if you think it advisable to have this formulated by a notary, I will ratify it at any time.

As regards my malady, I'm very much better. We are now certain that I'm suffering from the stone, but it is a small one and thanks to God and to the virtues of the water I'm drinking, it's being dissolved little by little, so that I'm hopeful of being free of it. But as I'm an old man, and for many other reasons, I should be glad if the money I have here could be kept in Florence, so that it might be available if I needed it, and would afterwards pass to you. This would be a matter of about four thousand *scudi*. I should like to have as few encumbrances here as possible, especially now that I have to go to the baths. See Gismondo about it and give it a little thought, and give me your advice, because it matters no less to you than to me.

As regards your taking a wife, a friend of mine has been to see me this morning and asked me to let you know about one of Lionardo Ginori's[1] daughters, whose mother was a Soderini. I'm letting you know about her, as I was asked, but I am unable to say anything further to you about it, because I have no information. So think it over carefully and have no scruples about anything, and when you've come to a decision, answer me, so that I can answer my friend either yes or no.

On the fifth day of April 1549.

MICHELANGELO BUONARROTI IN ROME

I should much have preferred it if, before you get married, you had bought a larger and more imposing house than the one where you are living, and I would have sent you the money.

What I'm writing to you about the Ginori girl I'm writing only because I've been asked to do so, and not to the end that you should choose one rather than another. However, do as you feel inclined and, as I've written you on other occasions, have no scruples whatever. For me it suffices that I should know about it before you act. So make enquiries, think it over and don't delay in a matter like this once you've made up your mind.

1. *Lionardo di Bartolomeo Ginori (1502–1548), who belonged to the Ottimati party and had favoured the policy of Niccolò Capponi during the siege, married the beautiful Caterina di Tommaso Soderini, for whom Duke Alessandro de' Medici conceived an illicit passion. Though innocent of all intrigue herself, she was the ostensible decoy on the night of his murder in January 1537 (Ginori, pp. 214 et seq.).*

¶ TO LIONARDO DI BUONARROTO SIMONI IN FLORENCE

327

British Museum Mil. ccxviii From Rome April 13th 1549

Lionardo — I've got the receipt for fifty *scudi* from the Monastery. I'm pleased that you have allocated the money so well, and there's no need to say more about it.

In my last letter I wrote you that I had been asked to let you know about one of Lionardo Ginori's daughters, and this I did. I'm awaiting your reply about this, in order to be able to reply to my friend. Although I gave you this information, don't act on it unless it pleases you, and pay no attention to my having written. Consider it carefully, and if it's not to your satisfaction, tell me without hesitation, so that I can release my friend from his engagement to us.

I wrote you that I should be glad, as you are aware, to keep certain moneys in Florence, in order to live here with fewer anxieties, particularly as I am an old man. Therefore, if it can be done so that I may be sure of it, I would do so willingly, but I do not want to fall out of the frying-pan into the fire. I believe the only sure method is to find a means of investing it in property, that is to say either in lands or houses. You must both consider it, because it is in your own interest.

As regards the house near the Proconsolo, about which you wrote me, the locality doesn't please me as much as the one in the Via Cocomero which, had it been obtainable with a good title, could not in my opinion have been bettered.

As to my malady, I'm very hopeful about it, because I'm still improving, thank God, but I still think I shall have to go to the baths – so the doctors tell me.

I had a letter from Bugiardino, enclosed with yours. Another time don't enclose anyone else's with your letters. I have my reasons for saying this. Bugiardino is a good fellow – but simple[1] – and that suffices. If you are asked to enclose letters with yours, say that you have no occasion to write to me.

On the 13th day of April 1549.

MICHELANGELO BUONARROTI IN ROME

---

1.   *A true observation. cf. Vasari, VI, pp. 201 et seq.*

328

*Sta. Maria
Nuova
Archives
Mil. cdlxi
From Rome
April 19th
1549*

¶ [TO THE MAGNIFICENT MESSER BENVENUTO ULIVIERI AND PARTNERS IN ROME]

Magnificent Messer Benvenuto and partners of Rome — Please will you pay Bartolomeo Bettini and Company twenty-two gold *scudi* in gold each month, beginning the first payment from the month of January last. Prompt settlement will be appreciated, because I draw it month by month from the said Bettini – being the twenty-two gold *scudi* in gold remitted from my office of Civil Notary at Romagna.[1] May it please your lordships to continue the payment until further notice.

On the nineteenth day of April 1549.

I, MICHELANGELO BUONARROTI, by my own hand

---

1.   *The revenues of this office were granted him by Pope Paul III from the beginning of 1549, in lieu of those lost to him in 1547, when the Po ferry at Piacenza ceased to be in the gift of the Pope. See Appendix 33.*

¶ To Lionardo di Buonarroto Simoni in Florence

329

*British
Museum
Mil. ccxix
From Rome
April 25th
1549*

Lionardo — I couldn't write to you on Saturday, because I got your letter too late, and to-day, the 25th day of April 1549, I received another of yours of the twentieth of the said month to the same effect.

As regards the Chianti farm, my reply is that I would rather buy than hold the money. And if the said farm is a good proposition I think it should be taken without fail, particularly as it has a sound title, as you write me. But I should certainly look at it first, and if it is to your liking, take it without fail and don't be particular within fifty *scudi*. And this I commission you to do – if it's to your liking, take it without fail and don't be particular about the money. Keep me informed and I'll immediately have paid to you there whatever it amounts to. And if some other property were for sale for as much again, with a like title, I instruct you to look into it and I'll send the money for that also, because it's better than to keep it idle – or else in a house, if one is to be found.

As regards my malady, I'm hopeful and very much better – to many people's amazement, because I was given up for dead, and so I thought myself. I've had a good doctor,[1] but I believe more in prayers than in medicines. That's all. Next time I'll write to you about other things.

[Unsigned]

1. *Realdo Colombo da Cremona (c. 1520–1559). A professor first at the University of Padua and afterwards at Pisa, he was summoned to Rome by Paul III in 1549. He specialized in the study of anatomy, on which he published a treatise. He was a great friend of Michelangelo's (Condivi, lx).*

¶ To Lionardo di Buonarroto Simoni in Florence

330

*British
Museum
Mil. ccxx
From Rome
May 2nd 1549*

Lionardo — What I wrote you previously I here reaffirm – that is to say, that you should go and look at the Chianti farm, about which you wrote me. And if it's to your liking, take it without fail and don't be particular within fifty *scudi*. This I commissioned you to do with a free hand – that is, to take it without fail, if it is a good proposition, and not to be particular as to the money. Let me know, because I'll immediately send you whatever it amounts to.

As regards your taking a wife, I wrote to you about one of Lionardo Ginori's daughters, as I was asked to do by a friend of mine here. You replied, reminding me of what I wrote you about this last year.[1] I wrote you of this because I'm apprehensive about the airs and graces which this sort of family looks for and because there is no need for you to bow down to a wife. Nevertheless, if the girl is to your liking, you need pay no attention to what I write, because I know nothing whatsoever about the citizens of Florence. Therefore, if such a relationship is to your liking, don't bother about what I write you, and if is not to your liking, do nothing about it, since it is you who have to content yourself with a wife. And if you are content with her, I too shall be content. Reply without reserve, because I am not under any obligation to my friend here that I should consider him more than you.

As to the cruel malady I've had, I'm so well – having been given up for dead – that I think I've recovered.

I think that's all. Reply when you've come to a decision, and never dance to anyone's tune if it doesn't entirely content you.

MICHELANGELO BUONARROTI IN ROME

1. *See No. 322. According to Florentine dating, 'March 2nd' would be 'last year'.*

331

British Museum Mil. ccxxi From Rome May 11th 1549

¶ To Lionardo di Buonarroto Simoni in Florence

Lionardo — From your last letter I have all the information about the Chianti farm. Therefore, as it is a good proposition, endeavour to acquire it without fail and don't be particular as to the money.

You write me again about the one at Monte Spertoli and about a shop that is for sale in Porta Rossa; my answer is that if you find the title is sound take a shop as well as the farm, if it is a good proposition, and I commission you to spend with a free hand up to four thousand gold *scudi* in gold and to have no scruples, except about the titles. This will be better than keeping the money in banks because, rightly or wrongly, I place no reliance on them.

As to your taking a wife, I've released my friend from his engagement to us and told him to try his luck elsewhere, as I've had no answer from you to the contrary concerning the girl mentioned to me by a friend of mine, about whom I wrote you. I think that's all. As I've said above, buy with a free hand where the titles are sound and as soon as you can, and keep me informed.

On the eleventh day of May 1549.

MICHELANGELO BUONARROTI IN ROME

¶ To Lionardo di Buonarroto Simoni in Florence

332

*British
Museum
Mil. ccxxii
From Rome
May 25th
1549*

Lionardo — I learn from your last letter that the Chianti[1] properties are yours. I think you say for two thousand, three hundred florins, at seven *lire* each. If they're good properties, as you write, you've done well not to be particular as to the money. I've taken five hundred gold *scudi* in gold to Bartolomeo Bettini to be made payable to you in Florence, as a first instalment. Next Saturday I'll send you five hundred more through the Altoviti. And when Urbino, who went to Urbino several days ago, returns here, which will be within eight or ten days, I'll send you the rest. The gold *scudi* in gold I'm sending you are worth eleven julians here.

As to the properties at Monte Spertoli, if it is a good proposition and is for sale by the Public Trustee,[2] endeavour to acquire these also and don't be particular as to the money. I think that's all. Go and fetch the said money and acknowledge it. The draft of exchange will be enclosed with this.

On the twenty-fifth day of May 1549.

[Unsigned]

1. *This property lay in the parishes of San Giorgio and San Lorenzo in the 'Podestaria' di Rada. Michelangelo bought it from the Uffiziali de' Pupilli, the custodians of the heritage of Pierantonio di Giovan Francesco de' Nobili, who died on September 28th 1548. The contract was executed by the Florentine notary, Ser Piero dell' Orafo, on June 18th 1549 (Milanesi, p. 251).*

2. *The Uffiziali de' Pupilli were officials, equivalent to the Public Trustee in England, who were responsible for minors and for the administration of their estates.*

¶ To Lionardo di Buonarroto Simoni in Florence

333

*British
Museum
Mil. ccxxiii
From Rome
June 1st
1549*

Lionardo — This morning, the first of June 1549, I've taken one thousand gold *scudi* in gold to the Altoviti and I've taken five hundred to Bartolomeo Bettini, so that they may make them payable to you in Florence, in respect of the payment for the Chianti farm. The drafts of exchange, both from the Altoviti and from Bettino, will be enclosed in this. Go and fetch the money and write and tell me what the balance is, so that it may be paid promptly in view of the harvest, as you wrote me.

As to the Monte Spertoli farm, my instructions are that you should see whether it is a good proposition and should not be particular as to the money, but on that account I do not mean that you are to pay double what it's worth in order to get it, as I believe you did in the case of the Chianti – but not to be particular within fifty *scudi*.

As to my malady, I'm much better, which was not expected. I think that's all. Tell me what's needed.

MICHELANGELO BUONARROTI IN ROME

334

*British
Museum
Mil. ccxxiv
From Rome
June 8th
1549*

¶ To Lionardo di Buonarroto Simoni in Florence

Lionardo — As regards the Monte Spertoli farm, if you have to pay four hundred *scudi* more for it than it's worth, it seems to me to be a dishonest deal. I suspect that you seemed too keen and could be made to jump at it. I don't believe there's anyone who'll buy it for so many *scudi* more than it's worth. Within fifty or a hundred *scudi* there's no need to be particular. However, I leave it to you; if you think it advisable to take it, take it, because whatever you do will be satisfactory.

I haven't been able to see to the power of attorney. But I have such difficulty in making out your letters that I'm thrown into a fever every time I have to read one. I'll see to it next week – if I can make out what you want.

I've had the *trebbiano*, but the small parcel, about which you write me, hasn't arrived yet.

As to my malady, I'm very much better than I have been. Morning and evening for about two months I've been drinking the water from a spring about forty miles from Rome,[1] which breaks up the stone. It has done this for mine and has caused me to discharge a large part of it in the urine. I have had to lay in a supply at home and cannot drink or cook with anything else, and must lead a life to which I am not accustomed.

[Unsigned]

1. *The medicinal waters of Viterbo.*

335

*British
Museum
Mil. ccxxv
From Rome
June (22nd)
1549*

¶ To Lionardo di Buonarroto Simoni in Florence

Lionardo — I received the roll of *rascia*,[1] which I think excellent, but it would have been better had you given it to some poor person for the love of God.

As regards the contract, about which you write me, I assure you that the Public Trustee's office is frequently unscrupulous. So you must keep your eyes open and it would be as well to have the contract translated, so that everyone can understand it. Bettino, through whom I had the money made payable to you in Florence, thought you would soon be getting it, but I believe it is still here, so that the year's harvest, about which you wrote me, will be lost.

As to the Monte Spertoli farm, you've written me enough about it. Four hundred *scudi* more than it's worth would be the price of another farm. So I think one should go slowly. The power of attorney you asked for will be enclosed with this.

MICHELANGELO BUONARROTI IN ROME

---

1. *'Rascia', a fine woollen and silk cloth made especially for men's clothing. It was the most expensive woollen cloth manufactured in Florence during the sixteenth century.*

¶ TO LIONARDO DI BUONARROTO SIMONI IN FLORENCE

336

*British
Museum
Mil. ccxxvi
From Rome
July (6th)
1549*

Lionardo — I think the lands, about which you wrote me, which are at Chianti, near near *[sic] [those]* you've bought, should certainly be acquired for two hundred and fifty *scudi*, if the title is sound; because for me it suffices, in view of what you wrote concerning the copy of the contract and the other accounts that things should be honestly transacted and should be in order. I'm not bothered about anything else. Let me know what is needed. I've no time to write about anything else.

MICHELANGELO IN ROME

¶ TO LIONARDO DI BUONARROTO SIMONI IN FLORENCE

337

*British
Museum
Mil. ccxxvii
From Rome
July 19th
1549*

Lionardo — In your last letter I had an account of all the expenses incurred over the Chianti property, which was unnecessary, because if the money was well spent, as you write me, everything is all right. As to the lands bordering the said property, about which you wrote me, I replied that you should acquire them if there is a sound title. As to Monte Spertoli, there is, then, nothing further. It would be well to take it, if it were for sale, if the title is guaranteed by the Public Trustee, as you wrote me.

I've recently had a letter from that woman, the master weaver's wife, who says she wanted to give you to wife a girl whose father is a Capponi and whose mother is a Niccolini,[1] who is in the monastery of the Candeli. She has written me a long rigmarole, together with a sermon urging me to live a good life and to give alms. She says

111

she has been urging you to live like a Christian, and has probably told you she was inspired by God to give you the said girl. I maintain that she would do much better to attend to her spinning and weaving than to go round professing so much sanctity. It seems to me she is trying to be another Sister Domenica,[2] so don't trust her. But as regards your taking a wife, which seems to me necessary, I cannot advise you in favour of one girl rather than another, because I've no information about the citizens, as you may imagine and as I've written you on other occasions. So you must think it over yourself and make careful enquiries, and pray to God to be with you. And when you find a girl to your liking, I should be grateful if you would let me know of it before you act. I think that's all.

On the 19th day of July 1549.

MICHELANGELO IN ROME

1. *Niccolò Capponi (1481–1539) married Lisabetta di Simone Niccolini as his fourth wife in 1533. Despite the tactless but well-meant exhortations of the master weaver's wife, their daughter Margherita died unmarried, but without having taken the veil, among the nuns in the convent of Santa Maria dei Candeli at about thirty-three years of age in 1567 (Litta, X, tav. vii).*

2. *Sister Domenica is mentioned by Busini in his Letters to Varchi. She was a worthy woman who believed herself to be a prophetess. During the siege of Florence she was held in repute by men of the highest standing (Milanesi, p. 256).*

338 ¶ TO LIONARDO DI BUONARROTO SIMONI IN FLORENCE

*British
Museum
Mil. ccxxviii
From Rome
August (9th)
1549*

Lionardo — You write me in your last letter that the Monte Spertoli farm is unsuitable. There's no need to think further of it.

As regards the house, since you haven't found one to buy, you tell me that our own house, where you're living, could be adapted for an outlay of sixty *scudi*. You have my permission to do it, if you think it advisable, so that this may not delay your taking a wife. But as the house is in a bad position, owing to the river, I don't think it is worth spending a lot on it, if you have to buy another. However, do as much as you find necessary. I think that's all – I've no time for writing.

On the . . . day of August 1549.

MICHELANGELO IN ROME

¶ To Lionardo di Buonarroto Simoni in Florence

339

*British
Museum
Mil. ccxxix
From Rome
August (23rd)
1549*

Lionardo — A fortnight ago to-day I replied to you regarding the house in the Via Ghibellina[1] that you should adapt it as you thought advisable, until such time as you find another. This I repeat. That's all I'm writing you now, because I haven't time.

MICHELANGELO IN ROME

1. *As far as can be ascertained from the correspondence, Lionardo never acquired another house.*

¶ To Lionardo di Buonarroto Simoni in Florence

340

*British
Museum
Mil. ccxxx
From Rome
September (7th)
1549*

Lionardo — This is a covering note for a letter to Francesca. Give it to her at once. I think that's all.

As to adapting the house, I wrote and told you to do as much as you think necessary. As to the Chianti lands next to the ones you bought, I wrote you that you might buy them at a reasonable price, if the title were sound, and this I repeat.

MICHELANGELO IN ROME

¶ To Lionardo di Buonarroto Simoni in Florence

341

*British
Museum
Mil. ccxxxi
From Rome
December 21st
1549*

Lionardo — In reply to your last letter, it is true that the death of the Pope[1] has been a great sorrow to me and a loss no less, because I received many benefits from His Holiness and hoped to receive still more. But it has pleased God that it should be thus and we must be resigned. He died a beautiful death and was conscious to the last. May God have mercy on his soul. I think that's all concerning this.

I believe things in Florence are going well, and as to the question of your taking a wife, I don't think there's any more to be said. I think you're thinking it over and have not yet found anyone suitable.

As regards myself, I'm putting up with my malady as best I can and in comparison with other old men I've no cause for complaint, thank God.

Here we are awaiting a new Pope from hour to hour.[2] It suffices that God knows the needs of Christendom. Commend me to the priest. I think that's all.

On the twenty-first day of December 1549.

MICHELANGELO IN ROME

1. *Paul III had died on November 10th.*

2. *Rome was disappointed in the hope of an early election of a new Pope. The Cardinals entered the conclave on November 29th 1549 and did not emerge until February 8th 1550, one of the longest conclaves on record.*

XIII

LETTERS
342 - 396

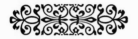

From Rome
1550 - 1555

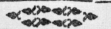

IVLIVS III· PONTIFEX· CCXXV·
ANNO DOMINI MDL·

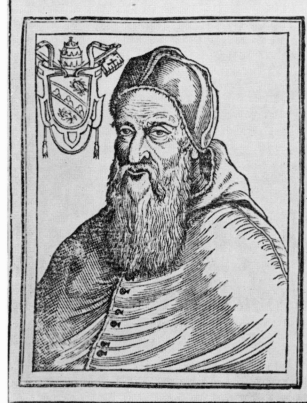 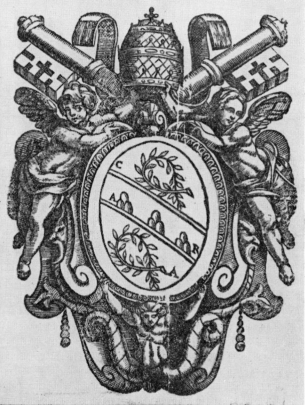

16. *Pope Julius III*   *Chacon, III, 741, 742*

XIII. From Rome : 1550-1555

342

Vatican
Archives
Frey, 1910
From Rome
January 1550

¶ [To Monsignore Cristoforo Spiriti da Cesena]

Monsignore[1] — I commend me to Your Lordship and beg you to give me your help and advice, as you have kindly done countless times, although I do not merit it.

The point is this. Since Paul's death the overseers of the fabric of St. Peter's have remained at the said fabric to guard it and to defend the muniments and other things against the soldiery,[2] and have done so at the risk of their lives and without any salary for about three months.[3] But being necessitous and unable to continue this any longer, they have given me to understand that, unless I am able to assist their case, they will be obliged to abandon the said fabric, owing to which the loss of several thousands of *scudi* might ensue. I have no means of paying them their usual salary, nor do I wish such a scandal to ensue. I therefore beg Your Lordship, for the love of St. Peter, to advise me what to do and to pardon my too great presumption.[4]

YOUR LORDSHIP'S SERVANT MICHELANGELO

1. *Cristoforo Spiriti da Viterbo (d. 1556) had been appointed Bishop of Cesena in 1510 and had held the see until 1545. An apostolic referendary, he was appointed titular Patriarch of Jerusalem on February 28th 1550 (Steinmann, Rep. f. Kunst., xxix, p. 312). According to Condivi, 'Michelangelo often conversed familiarly with him, as one whose open and liberal nature much pleased him' (Condivi, LXIII).*

2. *On the death of a Pope, when the normal authority was suspended, it was customary to augment the guard in the city, though the soldiers were apparently held to be as much of a menace as a protection. During the prolonged conclave, prior to the election of Julius III, Rome remained, however, comparatively quiet and the guard was twice reduced.*

3. *Following the death of Paul III on November 10th 1549 the Cardinals entered the conclave on November 29th, but did not emerge until February 8th 1550. 'Cut off from the outside world', the conclave was thus prolonged owing to the division between the Imperialist and French parties, one of which 'awaited the Holy Ghost from Flanders and the other from France'. By February 5th, when eighty superfluous conclavists left and many Cardinals had been taken ill, owing to the polluted atmosphere, a compromise had to be reached and both parties were disappointed (Pastor XIII, p. 28 et seq.).*

4. *The text of this letter was published by Karl Frey in Jahrbuch der k. p. Kunstsammlungen, xxxi, 1910, Beiheft, p. 94. It is endorsed in another hand '1550 on the . . . . day of January from Michelangelo Buonarroti to Mons. da Cesena'.*

343

*Buonarroti
Archives
Mil. cdlxvi
From Rome
February
(16th)
1550*

¶ To Messer Giovan Francesco Fattucci, priest of Santa Maria del Fiore, dearest friend, in Florence

Messer Giovan Francesco, dear friend — Although it is now several months since we have written to each other, our long and close friendship has not, on that account, been forgotten, nor is it that I do not desire your well-being, as I have always done, nor that I do not care for you with all my heart and even more so owing to the innumerable kindnesses I have received from you.

As regards old age, the state in which we both alike find ourselves, I should be glad to know how you, for your part, are faring, because I, for mine, am not well content. I beg you, therefore, to send me a line.

You are aware that we have a new Pope and who he is;[1] the whole of Rome is rejoiced about it, thank God, and nothing but the greatest good is expected of him, particularly for the poor, owing to his liberality.[2]

As regards my own affairs, I should be grateful, and you would be doing me the greatest kindness, if you would let me know, truthfully and without scruple, how Lionardo's affairs are going, because he is young and I am anxious about him, and more so because he is alone and without guidance.

I think that's all, except that Messer Tommaso de' Cavalieri has recently asked me to thank Varchi on his behalf for a certain admirable small book of his that has been published,[3] in which he says he speaks of him in the most honourable terms[4] and of me no less. He [Cavalieri] has given me a sonnet I wrote for him at that time, begging me to send it to him as a justification; the which I am sending you with this. If you like it, give it to him; if not, consign it to the fire, reflecting that I contend with death and that my mind is on other things. However, one sometimes has to do things like this. Please thank the said Messer Benedetto for the honour he does me in his sonnets,[5] and offer him my services, poor though they are.

Your Michelangelo in Rome

---

1. *Cardinal Giovanni Maria Ciocchi del Monte (1487–1555), who took the name of Julius III, had been elected on February 8th 1550. For his prediction of his own elevation, see Vasari VII, p. 692.*

2. *'The Romans rejoiced when the new Pope at once abolished the flour tax, introduced by Paul III, and distributed gifts and benefits on all sides with a generous hand' (Pastor, XIII, p. 52).*

3. *'Due Lezione di Messer Benedetto Varchi'. It was published on January 12th 1550 (O.S. 1549).*

4. *For the passage referred to see Guasti, p. cviii.*

5. *Varchi wrote one sonnet in praise of Michelangelo, namely 'Ben vi devea bastar chiaro Scultore', and one in praise of Cavalieri, 'Quel ben, che dentro informa, e fuor reluce' in which Michelangelo is mentioned (Varchi, Son. p. 92).*

¶ To Lionardo di Buonarroto Simoni in Florence

*Buonarroti
Archives
Mil. ccxxxii
From Rome
February 16th
1550*

344

Lionardo — As regards the Chianti lands about which you write me I cannot reply, unless I know how you are placed for money.

Some time ago you wrote me that, not having found another house to buy, you wished to convert the house in the Via Ghibellina. Since then I do not know what you have done or spent, nor how much you have left.

If you look through my letters you will find that many months ago I wrote and told you that, as I doubted whether the Pope would need me owing to my age, I wanted to provide an income in Florence rather than elsewhere, so that I might not have to beg in my old age, particularly as I have made others rich through my stupendous labours. So let me know how things stand and I'll reply to you. I have little capital here and if I were to spend that little in Florence I could die of hunger here. So let me know, as I've said, how things are going and I too will consider my position and will reply to you. I think that's all.

On the sixteenth day of February 1550.

MICHELANGELO IN ROME

¶ To Lionardo di Buonarroto Simoni in Florence

*Buonarroti
Archives
Mil. ccxxxiii
From Rome
March 1st
1550*

345

Lionardo — I did not write and tell you to render me accounts in such detail, but said that I could not reply to you about the Chianti lands unless you informed me how you were off for money, because with the capital that remains to me here I wished to provide an income for myself. It now seems to me, according to what you tell me, that enough money is left to enable you to buy the said lands. So see to it and if you find that there is a sound title, certainly take them, if you think it is a good and suitable proposition and I'll take thought here for my own affairs.

The truth is that if you had found the means of providing me with an income of a hundred *scudi* a year in Florence, I would have accepted the provision and still would, if you were able, or thought it possible, to supply my need. But I do not think there is anything to be had, as you wrote.

On the first day of March 1550.

MICHELANGELO IN ROME

346

*British
Museum
Mil. clvii
From Rome
June 21st
1550*

¶ To Lionardo di Buonarroto Simoni in Florence

Lionardo — I wrote you last Saturday that I would rather have had two flasks of *trebbiano* than the eight shirts you sent me. I now inform you that I have received a pack-load of *trebbiano*, that is 44 flasks, of which I have sent six to the Pope and the rest to friends, so that I have disposed of nearly all of them, because I can't drink.[1] But although I write you in this way, it is not because I want you to send me one thing rather than another. For me it is enough that you should be a man of honour and that you should do yourself and us credit.

MICHELANGELO IN ROME

1. *Owing to his recent attack of the stone he was restricted to drinking only the medicinal waters of Viterbo. Cf. Nos. 323, 334.*

347

*Buonarroti
Archives
Mil. cdlxvii
From Rome
August 1st
1550*

¶ [To Messer Giovan Francesco Fattucci in Florence]

Messer Giovan Francesco, dear friend — As I have occasion to write to the painter Giorgio[1] in Florence, I'm taking the liberty of putting you to a little trouble, that is to say, assuming that he is a friend of yours, would you give him the letter that will be enclosed with this.

Not having anything else to write about and in order not to write to you too briefly, I'm sending you one or two of the verses I used to write for the Marchesa di Pescara, who was devoted to me and I no less to her. Death deprived me of a very great friend. I think that's all. I go on as usual, bearing with patience the failings of old age. I expect you do the same.

On the first day of August 1550.

[Unsigned]

1. *Giorgio Vasari (1511–1574) the architect, painter and art historian. For his friendship with Michelangelo see Appendix 39.*

348

*Casa Vasari
Mil. cdlxviii
From Rome
August 1st
1550*

¶ To Messer Giorgio Vasari, painter and special friend, in Florence

Messer Giorgio, dear friend — I did not write to tell you that the Pope had changed his mind about the San Pietro in Montorio foundation,[1] knowing that you are kept informed by your agent here. I must now tell you what has happened, which is this. Yesterday morning, having gone to the said Montorio, the Pope sent for me. I did not get there in time, but met him on the bridge[2] as he was returning. I had a long

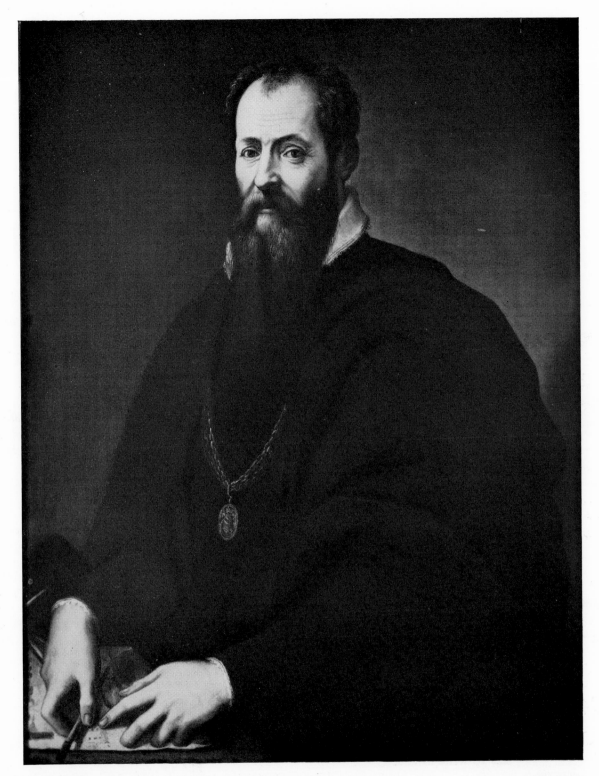

17. *Giorgio Vasari*

Self portrait
Galleria Uffizi, Florence

discussion with him about the tombs[3] that have been entrusted to you and he ended by saying that he had decided that he did not want to erect the said tombs on that hill, but in the Church of the Florentines,[4] and he asked me my opinion and proposals. I encouraged him considerably in this, thinking that this might be a means of getting the said church completed.

As regards the last three letters I have received from you – my pen is incapable of replying to such high praises. But I should be grateful to be in some sort that which you make me out to be, if for no other reason than that you would have a servant worth at least something. But seeing that you revive the dead,[5] I am not surprised that you should prolong the life of the living or rather the half-living, long since hastening to the grave. In short, I am wholly yours, such as I am.

On the 1st day of August 1550.[6]

YOUR MICHELANGELO BUONARROTI IN ROME

1. *The Pope, Julius III, intended to build a chapel at San Pietro in Montorio to house the tombs referred to below.*

2. *The Ponte Sisto.*

3. *The tombs referred to were (i) that of Cardinal Antonio del Monte, uncle of Julius III, (ii) that of Fabbiano del Monte, his grandfather. The designs were by Vasari. The work was allocated to Bartolomeo Ammanati under Michelangelo's supervision. They were eventually erected in San Pietro in Montorio and not in the Church of the Florentines after all. See Vasari, VII, p. 226.*

4. *For the history of San Giovanni de' Fiorentini see Vasari, VII, pp. 261 et seq.*

5. *Vasari painted a number of historical scenes, containing portraits of the dead.*

6. *Milanesi's text of Michelangelo's letters to Vasari is not based on the originals, but on eighteenth century copies, in the hand of Cavaliere Bustelli, which had formerly been copied by Michelangelo the Younger from the originals then in the possession of Vasari's nephew, Giorgio Vasari the Younger (Milanesi, p. 529). Vasari's 'Carteggio', which had been thought to be lost was discovered in 1908 in the Rasponi Spinelli Archives by Giovanni Poggi, the Director of the Museo Nazionale, Florence (Schlosser, p. 340), and is now housed in the Casa Vasari, in Arezzo. Milanesi's text has been collated with the text of the originals, as published by Karl Frey, and emended where necessary.*

349

¶ TO LIONARDO DI BUONARROTO SIMONI IN FLORENCE

*Buonarroti
Archives
Mil. ccxxxiv
From Rome
August 7th
1550*

Lionardo — Since the receipt of the *trebbiano* and the shirts I have had no occasion to write to you.

Now, as it would be to my advantage to have the two briefs[1] of Pope Paul, in which His Holiness grants me a salary for life, if I remain in his service in Rome – the which briefs I sent to Florence with the other documents in the box you received – I know you'll recognize them as they have leaden seals on them *[sic]*. So you can wrap them in a piece of waxed cloth and put them in a little box, well corded; and if you find that you can send them to me by someone to be trusted, so that they do not go astray, send them to me, consigning them as you think best, so that I may be sure of getting them. I wish to show them to the Pope so that he may see that according to them I am His Holiness's creditor, I believe, for more than two thousand *scudi*; not indeed that it will be of much avail to me to do this, but it would give me satisfaction. I think the courier could bring it, because it is a small parcel.

As to the matter of your taking a wife, you say nothing more about it. Everyone tells me that I ought to present you with a wife, as if I had a thousand of them in my pocket. I am in no position to make suggestions, because I have no information about our fellow citizens. You ought to marry and I should be very glad if you would, but I cannot help, as I've written you several times.

I think that's all. Commend me to the priest and to our friends. On the 7th day of August 1550.

MICHELANGELO BUONARROTI IN ROME

1. See Appendix 40.

¶ To Lionardo di Buonarroto Simoni in Florence

350

*Buonarroti
Archives
Mil. ccxxxv
From Rome
August 16th
1550*

Lionardo — You told me in your last letter that Cepperello[1] wants to sell the farm adjoining ours at Settignano and that that woman who has it has it for life. If she is really entitled to keep it during her lifetime and if the said Cepperello must sell it now, he should ask a price in proportion to the said woman's expectation of life, if possession is only to be had after her death. I don't think it is something we should undertake, because many things could happen that might be risky if we were not in possession. We must therefore wait until she dies, and if Cepperello comes to see me about it I'll tell him what I think; I certainly have no intention of going to see him.

You wrote me that you understand about the two briefs. If you have an opportunity of sending them to me by someone trustworthy so that I may get them, do so; if not, let them be.

As regards your taking a wife, you write that you want to come here to discuss it with me by word of mouth first. I, as regards my household arrangements, am very badly off and at great expense, as you'll see; by which I do not mean that you should not come, but I think it would be better to wait until the middle of September and if, in the meantime, you could find me a maidservant who is clean and respectable – which is difficult, because they are all pigs and prostitutes – let me know. I pay ten julians a month; I live poorly, but I pay well.

Recently I have been approached about a daughter of Alto Altoviti's[2] for you; she has neither father nor mother and is in the monastery of San Martino. I don't know her and don't know what to say to you about this.

On the 16th day of August 1550.

MICHELANGELO BUONARROTI IN ROME

1. *Giannozzo di Gherardo da Cepperello. Cf. No. 421.*

2. *Probably Altovito di Alamanno Altoviti, 1479–1548 (Passerini, Altoviti, tav. v).*

351

*Buonarroti
Archives
Mil. ccxxxvi
From Rome
August 22nd
1550*

¶ TO LIONARDO DI BUONARROTO SIMONI IN FLORENCE

Lionardo — I've received the briefs and paid the three julians as you wrote me.

As to Cepperello's farm, I replied to you saying that to pay now and not to get possession now did not seem to me a good thing to do. I've heard nothing more since.

In my last letter I wrote to you with reference to a maidservant. I now think I'm provided with one, so don't look elsewhere.

As to your taking a wife, you wrote me that you wanted to talk it over with me first. I replied that you could come when you like after the middle of September; although you could do without coming, because I can write and tell you as much as I know about our fellow citizens as I can tell you here by word of mouth – that I know nothing about them, because I have no truck with any of them, nor with anyone else. I think that's all.

Greet Francesca on my behalf and tell her that I'll reply to her letter when I can, and tell her to try and keep well.

On the 22nd of August 1550.

MICHELANGELO IN ROME

352

*Buonarroti
Archives
Mil. ccxxxvii
From Rome
August 31st
1550*

¶ TO LIONARDO DI BUONARROTO SIMONI IN FLORENCE

Lionardo — As regards Cepperello's farm, you write me that someone might buy it whom we shouldn't like. I care little about that, because I know that in Florence one can give as good as one gets. But as it seems all right to you, take it if you find it to be a good proposition. But I don't know where you'll find the money, as I'm not prepared to send you any more, because from the capital I have left I want to provide an income for myself here.

I wrote you that the briefs had come, according to which we see that I am owed more than two thousand gold *scudi*. I don't know what will ensue. I have no hope of it whatsoever.

As to the maidservant, I wrote and told you that I'm provided with one. Let me know what they are asking for the aforesaid farm.

On the last day of August 1550.

MICHELANGELO IN ROME

¶ To Lionardo di Buonarroto Simoni in Florence

353

Buonarroti Archives Mil. ccxxxviii From Rome September 6th 1550

Lionardo — You wrote me about Cepperello's farm that someone might buy it whom we shouldn't like and in my last letter I replied that you could buy it, but that I was not prepared to send you any more money. I've heard nothing else from you since.

About your coming here – as far as coming here to see me goes, I now know what kind of visits these are. Unless you have to come for something else, you needn't come on that account. But if you like to come for the reason you gave me, come as soon as you can before the rains start again in Florence. I think that's all.

On the sixth day of September 1550.

MICHELANGELO IN ROME

¶ To Lionardo di Buonarroto Simoni in Florence

354

Buonarroti Archives Mil. ccxxxix From Rome October 4th 1550

Lionardo — In your last letter you inform me that you are ready to come to Rome, and that before you leave you will await a letter from me and then leave. I think that's all I have to tell you.

As soon as you receive this, leave when you like. I think you'll know how to find the house in Rome; it is opposite Santa Maria del Loreto near to the Macello de' Corvi.[1]

On the 4th day of October 1550.

MICHELANGELO BUONARROTI IN ROME

1. *See the detail from Bufalini's plan of Rome, Plate 18.*

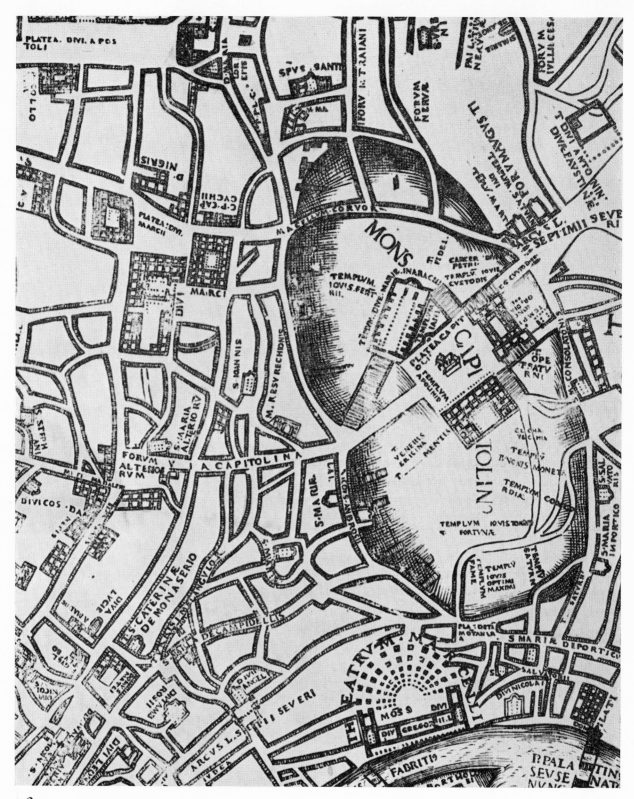

18. *The Capitoline Hill and the Macel de' Corvi*

Leonardo Bufalini

¶ To Messer Giorgio Vasari, painter and special friend, in Florence

355

*Casa Vasari
Mil. cdlxx
From Rome
October 13th
1550*

Messer Giorgio, my dear signor — As soon as Bartolomeo[1] arrived here I went at once to speak to the Pope. When I saw that he wished to proceed with the foundation for the tombs at Montorio I supplied a builder from St. Peter's. Tantecose[2] heard of this and wanted to send one of his own choosing. Not wishing to contend with one who sets the winds in motion, I withdrew; because, being a slight man I had no wish to be blown into some thicket. All that matters is that I don't think there's any need to consider the Church of the Florentines further. I think that's all.

On the 13th day of October 1550.

[Unsigned]

1. *Bartolomeo Ammanati (1511–1592). He was subsequently employed by Duke Cosimo and was responsible, together with Benvenuto Cellini, Angelo Bronzino and Giorgio Vasari, for the preparation of Michelangelo's obsequies in Florence (Vasari, VII, p. 287).*

2. *Tantecose or 'Busybody', i.e. Piergiovanni Aliotti. See No. 226, n. 1.*

¶ To Lionardo di Buonarroto Simoni in Florence

356

*Buonarroti
Archives
Mil. ccxl
November 14th
1550*

Lionardo — I got your letter from Aqualagnia telling me all you've been doing; and to-day, the 14th day of November, I've got the one saying you've arrived in Florence in good weather, for all of which may God be thanked.

About the ravioli – I got it, but all stuck together and spoilt. I think it was too fresh when it was boxed, or perhaps it got wet on the way. Otherwise it was excellent. I've nothing else to write to you about at present.

MICHELANGELO IN ROME

¶ To Lionardo di Buonarroto Simoni in Florence

357

*British
Museum
Mil. ccxli
From Rome
December 20th
1550*

Lionardo — I got the *marzolini*, that is to say, twelve cheeses. They are excellent. I shall give some of them to friends and keep the rest for the household, but as I've written and told you on other occasions – do not send me anything else unless I ask for it, particularly not things that cost you money.

About your taking a wife – which is necessary – I've nothing to say to you, except that you should not be particular as to the dowery, because possessions are of less value

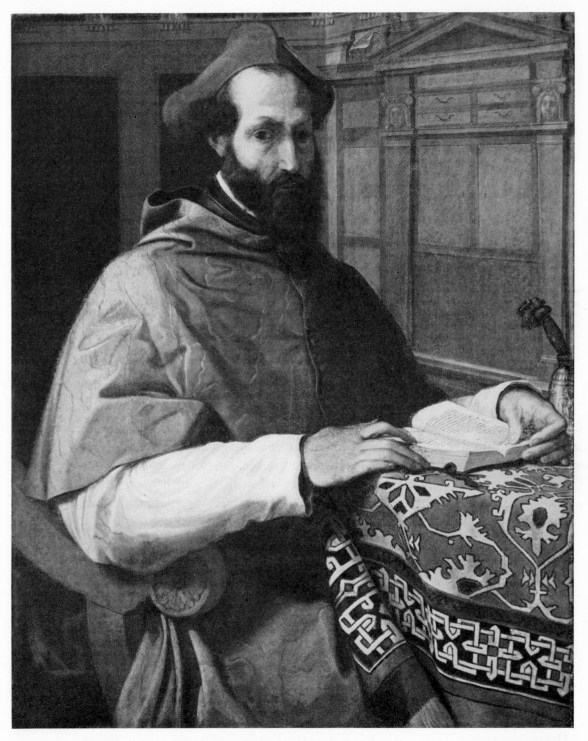

19. *Cardinal Marcello Cervini (afterwards Marcellus II)*

Jacopo da Pontormo
Galleria Borghese, Rome

than people. All you need have an eye to is birth, good health and, above all, a nice disposition. As regards beauty, not being, after all, the most handsome youth in Florence yourself, you need not bother overmuch,[1] provided she is neither deformed nor ill-favoured. I think that's all on this point.

I had a letter yesterday from Messer Giovan Francesco asking me whether I had anything of the Marchesa di Pescara's.[2] Would you tell him that I'll have a look and will answer him this coming Saturday, although I don't think I have anything; because when I was away ill, many things were stolen from me.

I should be glad if you would let me know if you were to hear of any citizen of noble birth in dire need, particularly someone who has daughters in the family, because I would do them a kindness for the welfare of my soul.

On the 20th day of December 1550.

MICHELANGELO BUONARROTI IN ROME

1. *Those who think this sentiment capable of a Neo-Platonic interpretation are, of course, entitled to the benefit of their erudition. Cf. Clements, p. 9.*

2. *That is to say, poems by Vittoria Colonna.*

¶ [TO THE MOST REVEREND MONSIGNORE, CARDINAL . . . . .]

358

Vatican Archives Mil. cdxc From Rome (December 1550)

Most Reverend Monsignore[1] — When a plan has diverse parts[2] all those that are of the same character and dimension must be decorated in the same way and in the same manner; and their counterparts likewise. But when a plan changes its form entirely[3] it is not only permissible, but necessary to vary the ornament also and *[that of]* their counterparts likewise. The central features are always as independent as one chooses – just as the nose, being in the middle of the face, is related neither to one eye nor to the other, though one hand is certainly related to the other and one eye to the other, owing to their being at the sides and having counterparts.

It is therefore indisputable that the limbs of architecture are derived from the limbs of man. No-one who has not been or is not a good master of the human figure, particularly of anatomy, can comprehend this.

MICHELANGELO BUONARROTI

1. *For the possible identification of the Cardinal addressed and for the date of the letter see Appendix 42.*

2. *The whole argument of this letter is based upon the principles of Vitruvius, notably those discussed in the Third Book of 'De Architectura', his treatise on architecture.*

3. *Michelangelo is apparently discussing the changes made in his own model of St. Peter's, which had superseded that of his predecessor, Antonio da Sangallo. In Sangallo's model (Letarouilly, pl. 34) the Tuscan order is used in the main elevation, the Ionic in the lower arcades of the drum and the Corinthian in the upper arcade. In Michelangelo's model the Corinthian order is used throughout.*

359   ¶ To Lionardo di Buonarroto Simoni in Florence

Buonarroti Archives Mil. ccxlii From Rome February 28th 1551

Lionardo — From your last letter about taking a wife I learn that as yet you've found no-one. I'm sorry, because it is surely necessary for you to marry, and as I've written you on other occasions, I do not think, having what you have and will have, that you need be particular about the dowery, but only about a nice disposition, a sound constitution and noble birth. If you were to marry someone well brought up, in good health and well born, but penniless, you should consider that you do so as a charity. If you were to do this you would not be subject to the airs and graces of women, and there would be more peace at home. As to your appearing to desire to ennoble yourself, as you wrote me before, it is a groundless charge, because it is well known that we are ancient Florentine citizens. So think over what I'm telling you, because neither by position nor by appearance are you worthy of the most beautiful woman in Florence. Commend yourself *[to God]* so that you may not make a mistake.

As to the alms which I wrote and told you to donate in Florence, you replied asking me to let you know how much I wanted to give, as if I had the means to give some hundreds of *scudi*. When you were here last time you brought me a piece of cloth, which I think I understood had cost you from twenty to twenty-five *scudi*, and this amount and this amount *[sic]* I then thought of donating in Florence for the souls of all of us. Afterwards, because of the great dearth here[1] it was converted into bread, yet even so unless some other assistance is forthcoming I make no doubt that we shall all die of hunger.

I think that's all. Commend me to the priest and when I can I'll reply to the request he has made of me.

On the last day of February 1551.

Michelangelo in Rome

1. *There was a great scarcity of provisions in Rome at this time, partly owing to the failure of the crops and partly owing to the vast influx of pilgrims during the Jubilee Year of 1550. In anticipation of the shortage the Pope had already taken steps to secure the necessary importation of corn from Spain and Provence (Pastor, XIII, p. 60 et seq.).*

¶ To Lionardo di Buonarroto Simoni in Florence

360

*British
Museum
Mil. ccxliii
From Rome
March 7th
1551*

Lionardo — I've had the pears, that is to say ninety-seven *bronche*,[1] for so they are called. I think that's all about this.

As to the matter of your taking a wife, I wrote and told you my opinion last Saturday, that is to say that you should not consider the dowery, but only whether she is of noble blood, of a sound constitution and well brought up. I don't know what else to say to you in particular, because I know no more about Florence than someone who has never been there. One of the Alessandri daughters was mentioned to me recently, but I learnt nothing in particular. If I hear anything I'll let you know next time.

About a month ago Messer Giovan Francesco asked me for something by the Marchesa di Pescara, if I had anything. I have a little book on parchment which she gave me about ten years ago, in which there are a hundred and three sonnets, apart from those on paper which she afterwards sent me from Viterbo, which number forty, which I had bound in the same little book, and at that time I lent them to many people, so they are all in print. I have besides many letters which she wrote me from Orvieto and from Viterbo. That's all I have of the Marchesa's. So show this to the said priest and let me know what he says to you.

As regards the money about which I wrote to you, which was to be given in charity in Florence, I must convert it into bread, as I think I wrote you last Saturday, because of the dearth there is here, which is such that, unless some other assistance is forthcoming, I make no doubt that we shall all die of hunger.[2]

On the 7th day of March 1551.

MICHELANGELO IN ROME

1. *A variety of yellow pear.*

2. *See Appendix 43, pt. III.*

¶ To Lionardo di Buonarroto Simoni in Florence

361

*Buonarroti
Archives
Mil. ccxliv
From Rome
May 8th
1551*

Lionardo — As regards your taking a wife, you are now writing and telling me the same thing that you told me when you were here, and I then made enquiries and learnt nothing but good.

I therefore tell you that the girl pleases me very well on the father's side and on the mother's. The other things, that is to say as to her age and constitution, you can find out better there, so if you are inclined to enter into discussions about it, as you write me, I leave it to you and may God grant that we decide for the best.

As regards the book of the Marchesa's sonnets, I'm not sending it, as I'll have it copied first and then I'll send it. I think that's all.

On the 8th day of May 1551.

MICHELANGELO IN ROME

362

Buonarroti Archives Mil. ccxlv From Rome May 22nd 1551

¶ TO LIONARDO DI BUONARROTO SIMONI IN FLORENCE

Lionardo — I replied to you last time that I've made some enquiries about the Nasi girl and that I've heard nothing but good. Afterwards I was again approached about a daughter of Filippo Girolami's,[1] whose mother is a sister of Bindo Altoviti's. I've no information as to what she's like; however I did not wish to fail to let you know about it. This Nasi daughter, according to the information I've had about her, if it's true – and I write you accordingly – would please me, so when you've looked into it there I should be glad if you'd let me know what ensues and also let me know what you learn about the other one, the Girolami daughter.

On the 22nd day of May 1551.

MICHELANGELO IN ROME

1. *Filippo di Francesco Girolami married Clarenza di Antonio Altoviti in 1519 (Passerini, Altoviti, tav. iv).*

363

Buonarroti Archives Mil. ccxlvi From Rome, June 28th 1551

¶ TO LIONARDO DI BUONARROTO SIMONI IN FLORENCE

Lionardo — eight days ago to-day I received a pack-load of *trebbiano*, that is to say, forty 4 flasks; I've presented some of it to several friends and it's said to be the best that has reached Rome this year. My thanks to you, which is all I have to say as to this.

As to the Nasi girl, you write me that you have not yet had a reply from Andrea Quaratesi; I don't think you should place much reliance on him in a matter like this; time passes with this waiting about and does not return. It seems to me that if you were to find a girl of noble birth, who is well brought up, of a nice disposition, but very poor – which would be very conducive to a quiet life – that you should marry her without a dowery for the love of God. I believe someone like this could be found in Florence, which would please me very much, because you would not be committed to airs and graces and you would be the means of bringing good fortune to others, as others have been to you, for you find yourself rich without knowing how. I do not want to expatiate further nor to describe to you the state of misery in which I found our family when I began to help them, because a book would not suffice – and never have I found anything but ingratitude. So give God recognition for the position in which you find yourself and do not go trailing after airs and graces.

On the 28th day of June 1551.

MICHELANGELO IN ROME

¶ To Messer Giorgio Vasari, friend and excellent painter

364

Casa Vasari
Mil. cdlxix
From Rome
August 22nd
1551

Messer Giorgio, dear friend — I received a letter of yours some time ago; I did not reply at once so that I might not appear mercenary. I now assure you that if, of the many praises which you bestow upon me in the said letter, I merited one only, it would seem to me to be in having given you at least something when I gave you myself body and soul, and in having discharged some minute part of that for which I am indebted to you; in respect of which I recognize hourly for how much more you are my creditor than I can pay. And being an old man I can never hope to settle my account in this world, but only in the next. I therefore beg you to have patience.

About your work.[1] I have seen Bartolomeo and it seems to me that it is going as well as it possibly can. He is working faithfully and putting his heart into it, and is a clever young man, as you know, and so much a man of honour that he might be called Bartolomeo the angel.[2]

On the 22nd day of August 1551.

YOUR MICHELANGELO BUONARROTI IN ROME

---

1. *i.e. the tombs in San Pietro in Montorio.*

2. *Michelangelo had agreed to Vasari's employing Ammanati on the tombs in preference to Raffaello da Montelupo, although he had conceived a dislike for him personally. Many years previously Ammanati had purloined some of Michelangelo's drawings from Antonio Mini. Vasari had placated Michelangelo by saying that in Ammanati's place he would have taken, not some of the drawings, but the lot, in order to learn all he could about art (Vasari, VII, p. 227). The above remark was therefore made in order to please and to reassure Vasari.*

133

365

*Buonarroti
Archives
Mil. ccxlvii
From Rome
October 17th
1551*

¶ To Lionardo di Buonarroto Simoni in Florence

Lionardo — From your last letter I learn that you have made enquiries about that Girolami daughter and have heard nothing but good. Therefore, if the other things to be desired in cases like this are as they should be, I don't think the dowery should stand in the way of the alliance. Therefore think it over well; because the alliance seems to me to be sufficiently distinguished and it would please me if the other things are satisfactory, as I've said; that is to say, if she is well brought up and has a good reputation and good manners, which is desirable. This you can proceed to enquire into carefully, but give credence to few. I think that's all. I'm very desirous that some descendant should survive you. If anyone were to approach you about someone on my behalf, I would remind you not to place any reliance on it unless you see letters from me.

On the . . . . day of October 1551.

MICHELANGELO BUONARROTI IN ROME

366

*Buonarroti
Archives
Mil. ccxlviii
From Rome
December 19th
1551*

¶ To Lionardo di Buonarroto Simoni in Florence

Lionardo — I learn from your last letter about the short sight, which seems to me no small defect; so my reply to you is that I have made no promises here, and if you have not yet made any there either, I don't think we need involve ourselves, if you're sure, because as you write me it is hereditary.

I now tell you again what I've told you before; that you should look for someone with a sound constitution and should marry rather for the love of God than because of the dowery, provided that she is nice and of noble birth. And don't bother yourself about her being poor, because it makes for a more peaceful life, and I will give you a suitable dowery myself. I think that's all as to this.

I find myself to be an old man with a little capital, which I do not want to spend here; so if you were to find a good house or property in Florence, that would be a sound investment for an expenditure of one thousand five hundred *scudi*, I should be in favour of taking it. So make enquiries in order that the money may not be wasted, if I were to die here, which might happen at any time.

On the 19th day of December 1551.

MICHELANGELO BUONARROTI IN ROME

¶ To Lionardo di Buonarroto Simoni in Florence

367

*British
Museum
Mil. ccxlix
From Rome
December 19th
1551*

Lionardo — As to the matter about which you write me, if you are sure about it, I don't think we need involve ourselves, as you have made no promises there, nor I here. But as I've written you on other occasions, you should look for someone with a sound constitution and should marry her rather for the love of God than for anything else, provided she is nice and of noble birth. And don't bother yourself about her being poor, because it makes for a more peaceful life. I've no time to expatiate further, but I've written more fully by a *scarpellino* called Fantasia, who is leaving here tomorrow morning. Seek him out and get him to give you the letter.

On the 19th of December.

MICHELANGELO IN ROME

¶ To Lionardo di Buonarroto Simoni in Florence

368

*Buonarroti
Archives
Mil. ccl
From Rome
February 20th
1552*

Lionardo — When I was talking here recently to that girl's uncle, he told me that he was very surprised that she had been turned down and that he supposed that some niggard had interposed in order to get possession of her property, or to inherit it. I thought I'd better let you know about what was said.

Now, as I write, a letter of yours has been brought to me, from which I learn of a daughter[1] of Carlo di Giovanni Strozzi's. I knew Giovanni Strozzi[2] when I was a child; he was a man of honour. That's all I can tell you about it. I also knew Carlo[3] and I believe it might be a good match.

As regards the properties which you tell me about, those near Florence are not to my liking; I think towards Chianti would be more suitable. So if you were to find a sound investment there, I should be in favour of making it, and do not be particular within two hundred *scudi*.

As regards your taking a wife, I've no means of learning of anyone here, because I have no truck with any of the Florentines, much less with anyone else.

I am an old man, as I wrote you in my last letter, and in order to dispel the vain hope of anyone, should any exist, I'm thinking of making a Will and leaving what I have in Florence to Gismondo my brother and to you, my nephew, neither of whom may make a decision of any kind without the consent of the other. And if you remain without legitimate issue, San Martino[4] will inherit everything – that is to say, the income will be given for the love of God to those ashamed to beg, that is to say, to poor fellow-citizens, or otherwise as may be best, as you advise me.

On the twentieth day of February one thousand five hundred and fifty-two.[5]

MICHELANGELO BUONARROTI IN ROME

1. *Francesca, daughter of Carlo Strozzi and Margareta di Lutozzo Nasi. She married Pierfrancesco di Tommaso Ginori in 1553 (Litta, IV, tav. viii).*

2. *Giovanni di Carlo Strozzi, who married Francesca d'Angelo Manetti (ibid.).*

3. *Carlo Strozzi, who had been active in the cause of Florentine liberty and died in exile. His son Giovanni (1517–1570) wrote the famous quatrain 'Sopra la Notte del Buonarroto' (Guasti, p. 3).*

4. *The Congregation of San Martino, was instituted in 1441 to help the 'poveri vergognosi' (Staley, pp. 550 et seq.).*

5. *The letter is endorsed in an unknown hand, 'Deliver safely, because it is from Messer Michelangelo Buonarroti'.*

369 ¶ To Lionardo di Buonarroto Simoni in Florence

*Buonarroti
Archives
Mil. ccli
From Rome
April 1st
1552*

Lionardo — As regards your taking a wife, I hear from a friend of mine that the report about the defect which caused you to withdraw from that match isn't true – that is to say about the short sight – but that it was told you by a friend of yours in order that he might give you a girl related to himself; and because she is not yet of marriageable age he has done everything possible to postpone your decision, in order to marry her to you. Therefore, if that report about the sight is not true and if there is no other defect, it seems to be a match to be considered.

So take care not to be led by the nose by people much inferior to her. That's all I have to say to you as to this. I would remind you that time passes, and I do not want to be importuned all my life by strangers; but I hope the Will may assist.

On the first day of April 1552.

MICHELANGELO IN ROME

370 ¶ To Lionardo di Buonarroto Simoni in Florence

*Buonarroti
Archives
Mil. cclii
From Rome
April 23rd
1552*

Lionardo — I wrote and told you about the information I had received from Florence, that is to say, among other things, that the statement you heard about that defect of vision wasn't true. Now you tell me in reply that you are certain it is not, and that if I wish it, you will marry her. But if the position is as you write, I tell you there is no need to say any more about it, but that you should certainly take a wife, and should not be particular as to the dowery, provided she is a fellow citizen and of a nice disposition. And don't dilly-dally with the parents, because perhaps it may not please them that you should marry her. Try to find someone who wouldn't be ashamed, if need be, to wash the dishes and to do other things about the house, so that you do not waste money on airs and graces.

I hear that there is great poverty in Florence, especially among the nobility. Therefore, if you are not looking for a dowery, I think it may be possible to find someone suitable. As I wrote you before, look upon it as the performance of an act of charity.

On the 23rd day of April 1552.

MICHELANGELO IN ROME

¶ To Lionardo di Buonarroto Simoni in Florence

371

*Buonarroti
Archives
Mil. ccliii
From Rome
June 24th
1552*

Lionardo — I've had the *trebbiano*, that is to say forty-four flasks, for which I thank you. It seems to me very good, but I am unable to enjoy much of it, because even when I have given a few flasks of it to friends, what I have left turns sour in a few days. Therefore, another year, if I am here, it will be sufficient to send ten flasks – if there is a way of doing so – with someone else's pack-load.

Bishop de' Minerbetti[1] was here recently and when I met him with Messer Giorgio, the painter,[2] he asked me about you and about your taking a wife. We discussed it and he told me that he had a nice girl to present to you and also that she doesn't have to be married out of charity. I did not enquire further, because he seemed to me to be rushing ahead.

Now you write me that I have no idea who among her relatives talked to you in Florence and encouraged you to take a wife, and told you that I greatly desired it. This you know for yourself from the letters I have written you on several occasions, and this I repeat, to the end that our race may not end here – not that the world would come to an end on that account; albeit every animal strives to preserve its species. I therefore desire you to take a wife, if you can find someone suitable, that is to say, someone with a sound constitution and well brought up and related to people of good repute; and if the other things that must be sought in matters like this are all right, do not consider the dowery.

If, however, you do not feel physically capable of marriage, it is better to contrive to keep alive oneself than to commit suicide in order to beget others. This I'm saying to you finally, because I see the affair is being long drawn out, and I should not like you to do something at my instance that is contrary to your own inclination, because it would never succeed and I should never be content.

As to my finding you someone suitable here, you may imagine that I am not in the way of things of this kind, because I have no truck with anyone, and particularly not with the Florentines, but I should be very glad when you have anything on hand, if you would let me know before the affair is finalized. I have nothing else to say to you. Pray God He may give us someone nice. On the 24th day of June 1552.

MICHELANGELO BUONARROTI IN ROME

1. *Bernadetto de' Minerbetti (1507–1574) a canon of Santa Maria del Fiore and Bishop of Arezzo.*

2. *Giorgio Vasari.*

372

British Museum Mil. ccliv From Rome October 22nd 1552

¶ TO LIONARDO DI BUONARROTO SIMONI IN FLORENCE

Lionardo — I was extremely glad to learn from your letter that the girl satisfies you. But take care, as you are not sure which of the two you saw together is being proposed, that you may not be presented with the one in place of the other, as once happened to a friend of mine. So keep your eyes open and don't be in a hurry.

As regards the dowery, I'll secure it and will do as you'll tell me; but here I've been told that there is no dowery at all. So proceed cautiously, because one can never turn back, and I should be extremely upset if, owing either to the dowery or to anything else, you weren't satisfied with it. The alliance, as I wrote you, pleases me well enough and as the other things that are desirable in a matter like this are not wanting, I don't think you should be particular if the dowery is not what you might desire. I've told you to keep your eyes open, because you're being pressed as I do not think you should be, and they being from every point of view who they are, one must pray and have prayers said to the end that what is for the best may ensue, because things like this are only done once.

MICHELANGELO IN ROME

373

Buonarroti Archives Mil. cclv From Rome October 28th 1552

¶ TO LIONARDO DI BUONARROTO SIMONI IN FLORENCE

Lionardo — The reply to Michele Guicciardini about your taking a wife will be enclosed with this. I'm writing to tell him that I'm prepared to secure the dowery on my own property as and where you think suitable, and I'm asking him to take a little trouble in this matter. So take him the letter and he will make clear to you what I'm thinking of doing about the security – or otherwise, as you think best. My advice to you is not to buy a pig in a poke, but to have a good look with your own eyes, because she might be crippled or unhealthy, so that you would never be content. So use all the diligence you can and commend yourself to God. I think that's all, and writing is very irksome to me.

On the 28th day of October 1552.[1]

MICHELANGELO BUONARROTI IN ROME

---

1. *The letter is endorsed '1552. From Rome, on the 28th day of October; on the 22nd of the said month'. October 28th was a Friday, but from what he says in his next letter, he more probably wrote on Saturday 29th and misdated it the 28th in error. For an explanation of the endorsement see the Dating and Sequence of the Letters, No. 372.*

¶ TO LIONARDO DI BUONARROTO SIMONI IN FLORENCE

374

*Buonarroti
Archives
Mil. cclvi
From Rome
November 5th
1552*

Lionardo — I've had a letter of yours with one of Michele's, to which I do not think I have any answer to make other than that which I wrote you a week ago to-day, which I assume you will have had. I repeat the same thing in this. That is to say, that not being there, I have no information about the Florentine families; but that I have such faith in Guicciardino that I do not believe he would advocate anyone who was unsuitable; and that you should take a look at her with your own eyes. As to the dowery, I wrote you that I would secure it on my own property wherever you thought suitable, and that you should send me the contract that I might ratify what you have done. I assume you have had the letters. That's all I have to say to you about this.

I should be glad if, when you were to find a house to buy at a thousand or up to two thousand *scudi*, you would let me know about it. Make enquiries about it and have careful enquiries made. I've no time to say more to you about it now.

On the fifth day of November 1552.

MICHELANGELO BUONARROTI IN ROME

¶ TO LIONARDO DI BUONARROTO SIMONI IN FLORENCE

375

*Buonarroti
Archives
Mil. cclvii
From Rome
November (19th)
1552*

Lionardo — It seems to me that things which begin badly cannot end well. I am informed by your last letter that they have failed in the promise voluntarily made to you about that girl. Although I have written to you several times telling you not to be particular about the money, I assure you I see no reason why they should fail in the promises made to you, and since the slight is of no small consequence, it seems to me better not to discuss it further, unless you find so many other things in its favour that you are prepared to overlook a small one. As I do not understand the details in this matter, I do not know what to say to you about it. Commend yourself to God and believe that what ensues is for the best; nor do I think one should fail to prepare to avail oneself of His grace.

In my last letter I wrote and told you to look out for an imposing house in a good position, because if I should happen to return to Florence I should want to have somewhere to live, and also as I am an old man I want to find a lodgment for the little capital I have here and to live here as unencumbered as I can. I think that's all. I'm not replying to Guicciardino, because I haven't yet been able to read his letter. I do not know where you two learnt to write. Make my apologies and commend me to him and to Francesca.

[Unsigned]

376

¶ To Lionardo di Buonarroto Simoni in Florence

*Buonarroti
Archives
Mil. cclviii
From Rome
December 17th
1552*

Lionardo — You write me of two matrimonial proposals that have been put before you. They please me much better than the first one, but as I have no-one to advise me in such a matter, I cannot write to you in detail about anything. You must look into it yourself and pray God that He may grant you the better one. It seems to me that you should pay attention to a nice disposition and a sound constitution rather than to anything else. That's all I can say to you about this.

As to the house about which I wrote to you, I repeat that if you were to find one in a good position, that is imposing and has a sound title, that I should not be particular as to the money up to the amount I mentioned to you.

On the 17th day of December 1552.

Michelangelo in Rome

377

¶ To Lionardo di Buonarroto Simoni in Florence

*British
Museum
Mil. cclix
(February 8th)
1553*

Lionardo — You've already written to me about a daughter of Donato Ridolfi's,[1] whose mother is a member of the Benino family, and now in your reply to Urbino you again remind me of it. I cannot advise you for or against it, because, as I've written and told you before, I have no information about any of the families in Florence and here I have no truck with any of the Florentines. But as you have discussed it with Guicciardino and as he is a relative and good and conscientious, I well believe the match may be suitable. I therefore tell you to beg him, on my behalf, to put himself to a little trouble in this matter, for the love of God, whether over this daughter of Ridolfi's or over someone else, so long as someone suitable is found. I should be most obliged to him for this and let Francesca pray about it, too, and commend me to them. I have written and told you before not to be particular about the dowery, but only about noble birth, a sound constitution and a nice disposition. And when you meet with these things you need have no scruples about anything else, because as you yourself are a man of means you will not want for anything.

Urbino[2] wrote and told you what was said about you here, which made me angry. So have no truck with the fellows at Settignano, because you will only be abused.

MICHELANGELO BUONARROTI IN ROME

1. *Cassandra (d. 1593) di Donato di Vincenzio Ridolfi (1489–1546). Donato had been elected senator on December 17th 1546, but died twelve days later (Manni, pp. 49, 85).*

2. *Urbino had evidently learnt to write by this time, though Luigi del Riccio had signed the Contract of May 16th 1542 for him, 'he not knowing how to write' (Milanesi, p. 711).*

¶ TO LIONARDO DI BUONARROTO SIMONI IN FLORENCE

Lionardo — I gather from your last letter that you have renewed negotiations for the Ridolfi daughter. It must be four months or more since I replied to you about the two girls about whom you wrote me, saying that I was agreeable. Afterwards you wrote me nothing further about them; so much so that I don't understand you and I don't know what you have in mind. This affair has gone on so long that I've grown weary of it, so that I no longer know what to say to you. If you have a good account of this Ridolfi daughter and are pleased about it, marry her and what I've written to you on other occasions about the security I reaffirm. And if it does not please you to take a wife – either this girl or anyone else – I leave the decision to you. I've attended to the affairs of all of you for sixty years; now I'm old and must think of my own. So decide about it as you think best, because whatever you do must be on your own account, not on mine, for I haven't long in this world.

When I received your letter, I also had one from Guicciardino which, as it is to the same effect, I have no occasion to answer separately. Commend me to him and to Francesca. I think that's all. On the 25th day of March 1553.

MICHELANGELO IN ROME

378

Buonarroti Archives Mil. cclx From Rome March 25th 1553

379

*Buonarroti
Archives
Mil. cclxi
From Rome
April 22nd
1553*

¶ To Lionardo di Buonarroto Simoni in Florence

Lionardo — I gather that the renewed negotiations for Donato Ridolfi's daughter have been successful, for which we must thank God; praying that by His grace it may be brought to fruition.

As regards the security for the dowery, I've had the power of attorney registered in your name, which I'm sending you with this, so that you may secure the dowery, which you write me is one thousand five hundred ducats, at seven lire each, on my property wherever you think best. I've spoken to Messer Lorenzo Ridolfi[1] and said all the correct things, better than I thought I could. I think that's all for the present. Write to me later and tell me how the affair proceeds, and I'll think about sending some gift as is customary.

On the 22nd day of April 1553.

MICHELANGELO BUONARROTI IN ROME

1. *Lorenzo Ridolfi (1503–1576), sometime Apostolic Secretary. He was the younger brother of Cardinal Niccolò Ridolfi (Mecatti, p. 208).*

380

*Buonarroti
Archives
Mil. cclxii
From Rome
April 30th
1553*

¶ To Lionardo di Buonarroto Simoni in Florence

Lionardo — As soon as I had your letter about the alliance that has been arranged I sent you the power of attorney, so that you might secure the dowery on my property, that is to say one thousand five hundred ducats at seven lire each.[1] I assume that you have had it and that it's in order. The notary who drew it up is well qualified, because he is notary to the Florentine Consulate and to the Camera.

From your last letter I understand that both sides are satisfied with the alliance, for which we must thank God. And when Urbino returns from Urbino, which will be within a fortnight, I'll discharge my obligation.

On the last day of April 1553.

MICHELANGELO IN ROME

1. *The acknowledgment of the receipt of the dowery of 1,500 ducats was made out on May 16th 1553 by an instrument drawn up by Ser Ottaviano da Ronta, a Florentine notary (Milanesi, p. 292).*

¶ To Lionardo di Buonarroto Simoni in Florence

381

British Museum Mil. cclxiii From Rome May 20th 1553

Lionardo — I gather from your last letter that you have taken your bride home and that you are very satisfied; that you greet me on her behalf, and that you have not yet given security for the dowery. I have derived the greatest pleasure from your satisfaction and I think we should continually give God thanks to the utmost of our power.

As to giving security for the dowery, if you haven't done so, don't secure it and keep your eyes open, because these money affairs always give rise to disagreements. I don't understand these things, but it seems to me that it would have been desirable to arrange everything before you brought your bride home.

As regards your greeting me on her behalf, thank her and make her those offers on my behalf which you will know how to do by word of mouth better than I by writing. I want it to be evident, however, that she is the wife of a nephew of mine, but I have not yet been able to give any indication of this, because Urbino hasn't been here. He has now been back for two days, so I'm thinking of giving some token of the relationship. I'm told that a fine necklace of valuable pearls would be appropriate. I've set a goldsmith, a friend of Urbino's, to look for it and hope to find one, but don't say anything to her about it yet, and if you think I should do anything else, let me know. I think that's all. Look after yourself, be prudent and use your judgment, because the number of widows is always much greater than the number of widowers.

On the twentieth day of May 1553.

MICHELANGELO BUONARROTI IN ROME

¶ To Lionardo di Buonarroto Simoni in Florence

382

Buonarroti Archives Mil. cclxiv From Rome June 21st 1553

Lionardo — I've received the pack-load of *trebbiano*, which you sent me, that is to say forty-four flasks; it is very good, but it's too much, because I no longer have anyone to give it to, as I used to have. So if I'm alive next year I don't want you to send me any more.

I've obtained two rings for Cassandra, a diamond and a ruby. I don't know whom to send them by. Urbino tells me that a certain Lattanzio da San Gimignano,[1] a friend of yours, is leaving here after San Giovanni.[2] I've thought of giving them to him to bring to you, or you can send someone who is to be trusted, so that they may not be exchanged or go astray. Let me know as soon as you can what you think I should do. When you get them I should be glad if you'd have them valued to see whether I've been cheated, because I know nothing about these things.

On the 21st day of June 1553.

MICHELANGELO BUONARROTI IN ROME

1. *According to Milanesi, perhaps Lattanzio Cortesi (p. 294).*
2. *The feast of St. John the Baptist, June 24th.*

383

*Buonarroti
Archives
Mil. cclxv
From Rome
July 22nd
1553*

¶ To Lionardo di Buonarroto Simoni in Florence

Lionardo — I'm sending you the rings by the courier, that is to say, one diamond and one ruby, and I'm sending them in a little box corded, as you wrote me. Give the carrier three julians for bringing them, and I've promised him three julians if he brings me the receipt, so make it out for him. I should be glad if you'd have the said rings examined and let me know what they're worth. I think that's all.

On the 22nd day of July 1553.[1]

MICHELANGELO BUONARROTI IN ROME

1. *The letter is endorsed in Michelangelo's hand 'Give the courier three julians for the carriage'.*

384

*British
Museum
Mil. cclxvi
From Rome
August 5th
1553*

¶ To Lionardo di Buonarroto Simoni in Florence

Lionardo — I've had the shirts, that is to say eight shirts; They're really beautiful, particularly the quality of the linen. I'm very grateful for them. But all the same I don't like taking them from you, because I don't lack for anything. Thank Cassandra on my behalf and offer her anything I can get in Rome or elsewhere, because I won't fail her.

I've had the receipt for the two rings and the estimate of their value. I'm grateful, because I'm assured that I wasn't cheated. Although the gift I've sent is a small one, we'll supplement it some other time with something else for which she may have a fancy, of which you must advise me. I think that's all as to this. Look after yourself and rest content.

On the 5th day of August 1553.

MICHELANGELO BUONARROTI IN ROME

¶ To Lionardo di Buonarroto Simoni in Florence

385

*British
Museum
Mil. cclxvii
From Rome
October 24th
1553*

Lionardo — I learn from your letter that Cassandra is pregnant. I'm very pleased about it, because I hope that at least some heir may remain after us, whether a girl or a boy, whichever it may be; for everything one must thank God.

Cepperello recently returned here from Florence and has told Urbino that he wants to talk to me. I think it's about that farm of his which is adjacent to ours. Let me know whether he has said anything to your people there, because if it is to be had, it would be very suitable.

I think that's all. Greet Messer Giovan Francesco on my behalf and let me know how *[he is]*.

On the 24th day of October 1553.

MICHELANGELO BUONARROTI IN ROME

¶ To Lionardo di Buonarroto Simoni in Florence

386

*British
Museum
Mil. cclxviii
From Rome
(March)
1554*

Lionardo — I had a letter of yours last week in which you write me of your continued happiness with Cassandra. We must thank *[God]* for it and all the more so because this is something sufficiently rare. Thank her and commend me to her and if anything here would please her, let me know of it.

As regards the name of the child you are awaiting, I think you should name it after your father, and if it's a girl, after our mother – that is to say Buonarroto or Francesca. Nevertheless, I leave it to you. I think that's all. See that you look after yourself.

MICHELANGELO BUONARROTI IN ROME

¶ To Lionardo di Buonarroto Simoni in Florence

387

*British
Museum
Mil. cclxix
From Rome
(April) 1554*

Lionardo — I gather from your letter that Cassandra is about to give birth and that you would like to know my view as to the child's name. For a girl, if it be a girl, you tell me you have made up your mind, because of her amiable behaviour.[1] For a boy, if it be a boy, I don't know what to say. I should be glad if the name Buonarroto were kept in the family, as it has now survived in our family for three hundred years.

That's all I have to say. Writing bothers me. Take care of yourself.

MICHELANGELO BUONARROTI IN ROME

1. *i.e. out of compliment to Cassandra, as she was proving to be so good a wife.*

388

*Buonarroti
Archives
Mil. cclxx
From Rome
April 21st
1554*

¶ To Lionardo di Buonarroto Simoni in Florence

Lionardo — I learn from your letter that Cassandra has given birth to a fine son and that she is well, and that you have named him Buonarroto.[1] All this has afforded me the greatest delight. God be thanked for it, and may He make him a good man, so that he may do honour to the family and uphold it. Thank Cassandra on my behalf and commend me to her.

I think that's all. I write briefly, because I've no time. On the twenty-first day of April 1554.

Michelangelo in Rome

1. *Buonarroto (1554–1628) was born on April 14th. The family descended through him in a direct line until 1858, when it became extinct with the death of Cosimo Buonarroti (Volume I, Appendix 1).*

389

*Casa Vasari
Mil. cdlxxii
From Rome
April 1554*

¶ To Giorgio Vasari

Messer Giorgio, dear friend — Your letter has afforded me the greatest pleasure, seeing that you still remember the poor old man, and still more so for having attended the triumph of which you write me and for having witnessed the beginnings of another Buonarroto. I thank you whole-heartedly for this account. But such pomp displeases me all the same. One ought not to laugh when the whole world weeps;[1] on which account it seems to me that Lionardo hasn't much judgment, and particularly not in making such a feast for the new-born with the rejoicing that should be reserved for the death of someone who has lived a good life. I think that's all.

I thank you above all for the love you bear me, unworthy of it though I am. On I know not what day of April 1554.

Your Michelangelo Buonarroti in Rome

1. *The full import of this remark is obscure. Cf. Giannotti, p. 68.*

390

*Casa Vasari
Mil. cdlxxiii
From Rome
September 19th
1554*

¶ To Messer Giorgio most excellent painter in Florence

Messer Giorgio, dear friend — You will say rightly that I am old and foolish in wishing to write sonnets, but because many people say that I am in my second childhood[1] I've tried to fulfil my part.[2]

From your letter[3] I realize the love you bear me and you may be sure that I should be glad to lay my feeble bones beside my father's, as you beg me. But if I were to leave here now, it would be the utter ruin of the fabric of St. Peter's, a great disgrace and a greater sin.

But when the structure has completely taken shape, so that it cannot be altered, I hope to do as you suggest, unless of course it be a sin to keep a few sharks waiting who anticipate my early departure.[4]

On the 19th day of September 1554.

YOUR MICHELANGELO BUONARROTI IN ROME

1. *This rumour was first put about by Pirro Ligorio (1510–1583), the architect who succeeded Michelangelo at St. Peter's (Vasari, VII, p. 245 and Gotti, I, p. 323).*

2. *This letter accompanied the now famous sonnet 'Giunto è già 'l corso della vita mia' (Guasti, p. 230).*

3. *Vasari had written to him on August 20th begging him to return to Florence (Vasari, VIII, p. 318).*

4. *He refers to all those who were opposing him in the work at St. Peter's. See Appendixes 39 and 44.*

¶ TO LIONARDO DI BUONARROTO SIMONI IN FLORENCE

391

Buonarroti Archives Mil. cclxxi From Rome December 8th 1554

Lionardo — I've received the cheeses which you sent me, that is to say, twelve *marzolini*; they are excellent and most delicious. I gave some of them to friends and kept the rest for the household. I think that's all about this.

As to my state of health, in view of my age I don't think I'm worse off than others of the same age. As to all of you I assume you are well and Cassandra likewise. Commend me to her and tell her I pray God that she may have another fine son. I think that's all.

MICHELANGELO BUONARROTI IN ROME

¶ TO LIONARDO DI BUONARROTO SIMONI IN FLORENCE

392

Buonarroti Archives Mil. cclxxii From Rome January 26th 1555

Lionardo — I've sent to Florence one hundred gold *scudi* in gold, and these I've paid here, or rather sent by Urbino, my assistant, to Messer Bartolomeo Bussotti[1] in Rome, so that they may be made payable to you there at your pleasure. So go and see Messer Simone Rinuccini[2] with the draft that will be enclosed with this and he'll pay you the money. And with the said money I want you to buy nineteen *palmi*[3] of dark violet *rascia*,[4] the finest to be found, to make a dress for Urbino's wife;[5] the rest I would like you to spend on charity where there is most need, particularly for girls.

I wrote you that I had received the *marzolini*. I think that's all. Let me know what happens about the said *scudi* and send the *rascia* as soon as you can. On the 26th day of January 1555.

MICHELANGELO BUONARROTI IN ROME

1. Bartolomeo Bussotti, a Florentine banker in Rome, who later became treasurer-general to Pius V (Pecchiai, p. 133 and Vasari, VII, p. 31).

2. The Rinuccini were the corresponding bankers in Florence with the Bussotti in Rome, the principal papal bankers at this period.

3. The 'palmo' was equivalent to $\frac{1}{8}$ or $\frac{1}{9}$ of a 'canna', and therefore measured about $\frac{1}{3}$ of a 'braccio', i.e. about $7\frac{1}{2}$ inches.

4. 'Rascia' is now the term for a coarse serge, but in the sixteenth century it was the name of the finest of all the woollen cloths manufactured in Florence. It was exported to England, where it was known as rash (Edler, p. 420).

5. Cornelia Colonelli da Castel Durante. Urbino had married her in 1551 and returned with her to Rome on September 25th of that year (Milanesi, p. 606).

---

393 ¶ TO LIONARDO DI BUONARROTO SIMONI IN FLORENCE

Buonarroti Archives Mil. cclxxiii From Rome February 9th 1555

Lionardo — I learn from your letter that you have received the hundred *scudi* that I sent you and that you have understood from mine what you are to do with them, that is to say you are to send me nineteen *palmi* of dark violet *rascia*, and to use the rest of them for charity, where and how you think best, and to let me know about it.

As regards the baby you are awaiting, you write me that you are thinking of naming him Michelangelo. I assure you that if this pleases you, it also pleases me, but if it's a girl I don't know what to say. Please yourselves, particularly Cassandra. Will you commend me to her. I think that's all. As to the charity about which I wrote you, don't make an ado about it. On the 9th day of February 1555.

MICHELANGELO BUONARROTI IN ROME

¶ To Lionardo di Buonarroto Simoni in Florence

394

Buonarroti
Archives
Mil. cclxxiv
From Rome
March 2nd
1555

Lionardo — I've received the *rascia*; it is really excellent. To buy it here would have cost much more and it would not have been as fine. Urbino thanks you wholeheartedly.

As regards that member of the Bardi family,[1] I'm pleased with what you've done. Follow it up without making an ado about it. It is said here that there is great dearth and poverty in Florence.[2] This therefore is the time for a man to do what he can for the welfare of his soul. I think that's all. Follow it up and let me know about it. I think that's all *[sic]*. On the 2nd day of March 1555.

MICHELANGELO BUONARROTI IN ROME

1. *This refers apparently to the almsgiving. In the fourteenth century the Bardi had been among the richest and most influential citizens in Florence (Tiribilli-Giuliani, I, no. 20) and as bankers 'perhaps the most famous of all' (Staley, p. 181), but in common with the Peruzzi and other leading banking houses had fallen on evil days prior to the rise of the Medici bank.*

2. *As a result of the war between Florence and Siena. Siena fell to the besiegers a few weeks later. See Appendix 43, pt. II.*

¶ To Lionardo di Buonarroto Simoni in Florence

395

Buonarroti
Archives
Mil. cclxxv
From Rome
March 1555

Lionardo — In your last letter I had the news of the death of Michelangelo. It has been as great a grief to me as it had been a joy – indeed much more so.[1] We must bear it patiently in the belief that it is better than if he had died in old age. Do your best to keep alive yourself, because without men to look after it our property would be so much wasted labour.

Cepperello has told Urbino that he is coming to Florence and that the woman who had a life interest in the farm, who was mentioned before, is dead. I think he will come to terms with you. If he likes to offer it to you at a reasonable price with good security, take it and let me know, and I'll send you the money.

MICHELANGELO BUONARROTI IN ROME

1. *This elliptical form of expression is characteristic.*

396   ❡ To Lionardo di Buonarroto Simoni in Florence

*Buonarroti
Archives
Mil. cclxxvi
From Rome
March 30th
1555*

Lionardo — Messer Francesco Bandini[1] has asked me whether I wish to sell the land I have near Santa Caterina, because he has a friend who would like to buy it. I've told him that everything I have there is yours; whatever you do with it will be satisfactory, and this I reaffirm. Therefore agree together, you and Gismondo, and see which will be the more to your advantage – the money or to keep the land; and reply to me decisively so that I can reply to the said Messer Francesco. I think that's all as to this.

A labourer[2] working here on the fabric of St. Peter's has here given me two gold *scudi* to send to his mother; therefore read the draft that will be enclosed with this and give them to the person named, because I have no means of sending them otherwise.

On the 30th day of March 1555.

Michelangelo Buonarroti in Rome

1. *Francesco Bandini was another of the many Florentine bankers in Rome and was one of the Deputies of the church of San Giovanni de' Fiorentini. He became an intimate friend of Michelangelo's and to some extent took the place of Luigi del Riccio (Gotti, I, p. 318 et seq.).*

2. *Masino da Macia.*

XIV

LETTERS
397 - 449

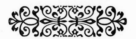

From Rome
1555 - 1559

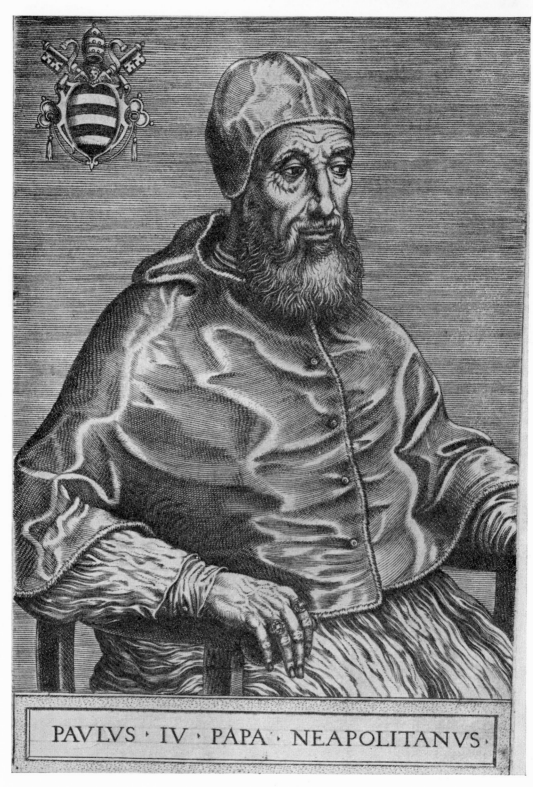

PAVLVS · IV · PAPA · NEAPOLITANVS ·

20. *Pope Paul IV*

XIV. From Rome: 1555-1559

¶ To Lionardo di Buonarroto Simoni in Florence

397

*Buonarroti
Archives
Mil. cclxxvii
From Rome
May 10th
1555*

Lionardo — I wrote you about a month ago, asking you to give two gold *scudi* to the mother of Masino da Macia, who is working here as a labourer, which he here gave me to send to her. I've had no reply. I should be glad if you would let me know whether you had the letter and whether you gave them to her – whether yes or no. I think that's all this time.

A letter for Messer Giorgio, the painter, will be enclosed with this. I would be glad if you would give it into his own hand, because it is a matter of some importance to me.[1] On the tenth day of May 1555.

MICHELANGELO BUONARROTI IN ROME

1. *On the death of Julius III and the accession of Marcellus II (Cardinal Cervini), who was ill disposed towards him, Michelangelo had decided to leave Rome and had written to Vasari to this effect. But with the death of the new Pope on May 1st, three weeks after his election, Michelangelo had decided to remain. The letter, enclosed for Vasari, No. 398, explains the position. Both these letters were written prior to the conclave which resulted in the elevation on May 23rd of Cardinal Gianpietro Caraffa, who took the name Paul IV out of compliment to the Farnese Pope Paul III.*

¶ To Messer Giorgio, most excellent painter, in Florence

398

*Casa Vasari
Mil. cdlxxv
From Rome
May 11th
1555*

I was forced to undertake the work on the fabric of St. Peter's[1] and for about eight years I have served not only for nothing, but at great cost and trouble to myself. But now that the work is advanced, that there is money to spend on it, and that I am almost ready to vault the dome, it would be the ruin of the said fabric if I were to depart; it would disgrace me utterly throughout Christendom and would lay a grievous sin upon my soul.

Therefore, my dear Messer Giorgio, I beg you to thank the Duke on my behalf for the splendid offers of which you write me,[2] and to beg His Lordship to allow me to continue here with his kind permission until I can leave with a good reputation, with honour and without sin.

On the eleventh day of May 1555.

YOUR MICHELANGELO BUONARROTI IN ROME

1. *See Appendix 44.*
2. *See Appendix 39.*

399

¶ [TO MESSER GIORGIO VASARI]

Casa Vasari Guasti lxvi From Rome (May 11th 1555)

Messer Giorgio — I'm sending you two sonnets[1] and although they're simple I do so that you may see whither my thoughts are tending, and when you have reached eighty-one years,[2] as I have, you will believe me. Please give them to Messer Giovan Francesco Fattucci, who has asked me for them.

YOUR MICHELANGELO BUONARROTI IN ROME

1. *This note is written under the sonnet 'Le favole del mondo m'hanno tolto'. The second sonnet, 'Non e più bassa o vil cosa terrena' (Guasti, pp. 232, 234) is written overleaf. For the arguments in favour of dating the letter May 11th 1555 see Dating and Sequence of the Letters.*

2. *Michelangelo was in his eighty-first year. As by Florentine dating he was born in 1474, he probably thought of himself as being eighty-one in 1555, Roman dating notwithstanding.*

400

¶ TO LIONARDO DI BUONARROTO SIMONI IN FLORENCE

Buonarroti Archives Mil. cclxxviii From Rome May 25th 1555

Lionardo — As regards the Santa Caterina lands, I wrote you that you should reach agreement with Gismondo and that you should come to that decision about it that would be most to your advantage. Now you write me that you think it best to sell it, which could not please me more. So sell it without waiting for anything else, and arrange between yourselves about the money.

Have you given the money to Masino's mother? That's all I have to say. Take care of yourself and may God help you. On the 25th day 1555 of May *[sic]*.

MICHELANGELO IN ROME

¶ To Lionardo di Buonarroto Simoni in Florence

401

*Buonarroti
Archives
Mil. cclxxix
From Rome
June 22nd
1555*

Lionardo — I'm sending a letter enclosed with this for you to give to Messer Giorgio Vasari. Commend me to him.

As to the Santa Caterina lands, I wrote you that I was very pleased that you should sell them, and that when you sold them you could use the money as you think best, as if it were your own. Therefore when you've agreed with the purchaser, let me know and I'll send you a power of attorney. I think that's all. Try to keep well and enjoy life.

On the 22nd day of June 1555.

MICHELANGELO BUONARROTI IN ROME

¶ To my dear Messer Giorgio Vasari in Florence

402

*Casa Vasari
Mil. cdlxxvi
From Rome
June 22nd
1555*

Messer Giorgio, dear friend — One evening recently a very discreet and worthy young man came to my house to see me, that is to say, Messer Lionardo,[1] Chamberlain to the Duke, who with great consideration and affection made the same offers on behalf of His Lordship as you made in your last letter. I made him the same reply I made to you, that is to say, I asked him to do his best to thank the Duke on my behalf and to beg His Lordship that I might, with his permission, continue to work here on the fabric of St. Peter's until it had reached a stage at which it could not be altered into another form, because if I were to leave earlier it would be the cause of great ruin, of great disgrace and of great sin. And this I beg you, for the love of God and of St. Peter, to beg of the Duke and to commend me to His Lordship.

My dear Messer Giorgio, I know that you realize from my writing that I am at the eleventh hour and that I conceive of no thought in which Death is not engraved. God grant that I may keep him waiting for another year or so.

On the 22nd day of June 1555.

YOUR MICHELANGELO BUONARROTI IN ROME

---

1. *Lionardo Marinozzi da Ancona, a Chamberlain to Cosimo I and his 'Obedientia' envoy to Paul IV, following his recent elevation. See Appendix 43, pt. III.*

403

*Buonarroti
Archives
Mil. cclxxx
From Rome
July 5th
1555*

¶ To Lionardo di Buonarroto Simoni in Florence

Lionardo — You write me in your last letter that you have come to an agreement with the *Spedalingo* di Bonifazio[1] about my lands near Santa Caterina, that is to say to sell them to him for three hundred and twenty *scudi*; and you ask me to send you the power of attorney. I'll send it to you this coming week without fail. I haven't been able to do so before, because of the cruellest pain I've had in one foot, which has prevented me from going out and has been a nuisance to me in a number of ways. They say it's a kind of gout; it's the last straw in my old age. However, I'm much better now and, as I've said, this coming week I'll send it to you without fail. Stand firm by the agreement, because I'm very pleased about it. I think that's all.

On the fifth day of July 1555.

MICHELANGELO BUONARROTI IN ROME

1. *The Hospital of Bonifazio Lupi stood in the Via San Gallo and adjacent to the land Michelangelo was selling in the same street (Vasari, VII, p. 395).*

404

*Buonarroti
Archives
Mil. cclxxxi
From Rome
July 13th
1555*

¶ To Lionardo di Buonarroto Simoni in Florence

Lionardo — I'm sending you the power of attorney so that you can sell the lands called Santa Caterina to the *Spedalingo* or to anyone else you think suitable, and as to the money, you can do with it whatever you and Gismondo think best. As to the lands that belonged to Niccolò della Buca, they would please me, as you wrote me, if there is a sound title.

A letter for Gismondo will be enclosed with this. Encourage him on my behalf to be patient and tell him that I too have my share of troubles and that he shall not want for anything. On the 13th day of July 1555.

MICHELANGELO BUONARROTI IN ROME

405

*Casa Vasari
Mil. cclxxxii
From Rome
September 28th
1555*

¶ To Lionardo di Buonarroto Simoni in Florence

Lionardo — I learn from your last letter that the Duke[1] has been to see the models of the façade of San Lorenzo and that His Lordship asked to have them. I instruct you to send them to His Lordship at once wherever he wants to have them sent, without writing to me again; and you must do the same with anything else of ours, if we have anything that would please him.

The reply to Messer Giorgio's letter will be enclosed with this and as regards the staircase of the Library, I'm giving him, as if in a dream, the little information I can recall about it. I'm sending you his letter open, so that you may read it; give it to him in the same way, open.[2]

I'm pleased that you and Cassandra and the little one are well, but I'm very worried and grieved about Gismondo. But I myself am not without infirmities either and beset with many worries and troubles, and the more so as I've had Urbino ill in bed for three months now and he's still in bed, which has been a great anxiety and trouble to me. [*One must*] thank God for everything.[3] Encourage him on my behalf and help him when you can. On the 28th day of September 1555.

MICHELANGELO BUONARROTI IN ROME

1. *Cosimo I de' Medici.*

2. *Surely a supreme courtesy.*

3. *Cf. Vol. I, No. 27, for the expression of a similar sentiment in face of adversity.*

¶ TO MESSER GIORGIO VASARI, MOST RARE OF PAINTERS, IN FLORENCE

406

*Published
Source
Mil. cdlxxxv
From Rome
September 28th
1555*

Messer Giorgio, dear friend — As regards the staircase for the Library, of which I have heard so much, believe me, if I were able to remember what I proposed to do with it no entreaties would have been necessary.

I recall a certain staircase, as it were in a dream, but I do not think it is exactly what I thought of then, because it is a clumsy affair, as I recall it. However, I will here describe it.

Thus, if you take a number of oval boxes, each a *palmo*[1] in depth, but not of the same length and breadth; first place the largest upon the paved floor, as far distant from the door in the wall as you require, according to whether the staircase is to be shallow or steep; upon this place another, which should be smaller in each direction and should project over the first one below as evenly as is required by the foot as it ascends, diminishing and narrowing them one after the other continuously as they ascend towards the door. The aforesaid section of the oval staircase should have, as it were, two wings, one on one side and one on the other, the steps of which should correspond to the others, but should be straight, not oval; these being for the servants and the middle for the master; from the middle upwards of the said staircase the ends of the said wings are towards the wall; from the middle downwards to the paved floor they, together with the whole staircase, are separated from the wall by about three *palmi*,[2] so that the entrance to the vestibule is entirely unencumbered and is free on all sides. I'm writing

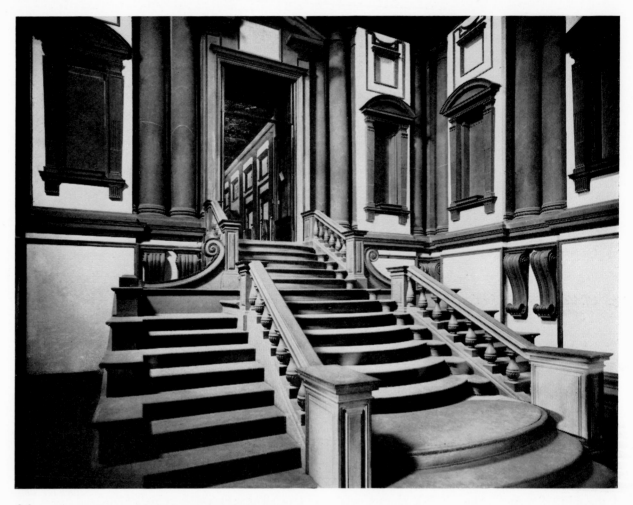

21. *The Staircase of the Laurentian Library*   *San Lorenzo, Florence*

nonsense, but I know very well that you and Messer Bartolomeo will make something of it.

As to the model of which you write me, do you not know that there was no need to write to me about it at all, but only to send it to the Duke, wherever he wanted it? And not only the model, but if God wills that any good thing of mine should be found there, I should not hesitate to send it to His Lordship. I beg you to thank His Lordship for his splendid offers. I know very well that I don't deserve them, but at least I can make capital out of them.

Rome. September 28th 1555.[3]

YOUR MICHELANGELO IN ROME

1. About 7½ inches.

2. The staircase, as finally constructed, is in fact separated from the side walls by about three 'braccia', and a measurement of only three 'palmi', which is only some 22½ inches, would in fact have been insufficient to allow for the effect Michelangelo apparently had in mind. See also Draft 11.

3. The autograph was not included among those discovered by Giovanni Poggi in the Rasponi Spinelli Archives. Milanesi's text, which differs slightly from that given by Vasari (VII, p. 237), is based on a sixteenth-century copy, then in the possession of Cavaliere Giuseppe Palagi. For a further discussion of the text see Appendix 39.

¶ TO LIONARDO DI BUONARROTO SIMONI IN FLORENCE   *407*

Lionardo — In your last letter I had the news of the death of Gismondo,[1] my brother, but not without great sorrow. We must be resigned; and since he died fully conscious and with all the sacraments ordained by the Church, we must thank God for it.

Buonarroti Archives Mil. cclxxxiii From Rome November 30th 1555

Here I'm beset by many anxieties. Urbino is still in bed and in a very poor condition. I do not know what will ensue.[2] I'm as upset about it as if he were my own son, because he has served me faithfully for twenty-five years and as I'm an old man I haven't time to train anyone else to suit me. I'm therefore very grieved. So if you have some devout soul there, I beg you to get him to pray to God for his recovery.

On the thirtieth day of November 1555.

MICHELANGELO BUONARROTI IN ROME

1. Gismondo had died on November 13th.

2. Urbino had made his will on November 24th. A copy exists in the Buonarroti Archives and is published by Gotti, (II, p. 137 et seq.). He expressed a wish to be buried in 'the church of the Minerva'.

408

*Buonarroti
Archives
Mil. clxxxiv
From Rome
December 4th
1555*

¶ To Lionardo di Buonarroto Simoni in Florence

Lionardo — As regards the property left by Gismondo, of which you write me, I tell you that everything is to be yours. See that the terms of his Will are carried out and have prayers said for his soul, as there is nothing else one can do for him.

I must tell you that last night, the third day of December at 9 o'clock, Francesco, called Urbino, passed from this life to my intense grief, leaving me so stricken and troubled that it would have been more easeful to die with him, because of the love I bore him, which he merited no less;[1] for he was a fine man, full of loyalty and devotion; so that owing to his death I now seem to be lifeless myself and can find no peace.

I should therefore be glad to see you, but I do not know when you can leave Florence on account of your wife. Let me know if you could come here within a month or six weeks; always, be it understood, with the Duke's permission. I've said that your coming should be with the Duke's permission to be on the safe side, but I don't think it's necessary. Manage it as you think fit and reply to me. Write and tell me whether you can come and I'll write and tell you when you must leave, because I want it to be after the departure of Urbino's wife.

Michelangelo Buonarroti in Rome

1. *Urbino could not have wished for a nobler epitaph.*

409

*Buonarroti
Archives
Mil. cclxxxv
From Rome
January 11th
1556*

¶ To Lionardo di Buonarroto Simoni in Florence

Lionardo — Last week[1] I wrote and told you of Urbino's death and that I was left in a state of great confusion and was very unhappy[2] and that I would be glad if you could come here. I'm writing you again to say that when you can arrange your affairs, without loss or risk for a month, you should get ready to come. If it were against your interests, or if some loss or some danger on the roads were involved, or anything else, wait until you think the time has come, and when you think it has, come, because I am an old man and should be glad to talk to you before I die. I think that's all. If anything were written you to the contrary, pay no attention, except to my letter. On the eleventh day of January 1556.[3]

Michelangelo Buonarroti in Rome

1. *He had in fact written over a month earlier.*

2. *The phrasing of the letter as a whole is indicative of his state of mind.*

3. *In the autograph he altered 1556 to 1559, but 1556 is manifestly the correct date.*

¶ To Messer Giorgio Vasari, dear friend, in Florence

410

Casa Vasari
Mil. cdlxxvii
From Rome
February 23rd
1556

My dear Messer Giorgio, — I am hardly able to write, but at least I'll make some attempt to answer your letter.

You know that Urbino is dead; through whom God has granted me his greatest favour, but to my grievous loss and infinite sorrow. The favour lay in this – that while living he kept me alive, and in dying he taught me to die, not with regret, but with a desire for death.

I have had him twenty-six years and found him entirely loyal and devoted; and now that I had made him rich and that I had expected him to be a support and stay to me in my old age, he has vanished from me, and nothing is left to me but the hope of seeing him again in Paradise. And of this God has given me a sign in the happy death he died; for he was far less grieved at dying than at leaving me here in this treacherous world with so many burdens; though the greater part of me has gone with him, and nothing but unending wretchedness remains to me.

I commend me to you and beg you, if it is not a trouble, to make my apologies to Messer Benvenuto[1] for not replying to his letter, because in thoughts such as these I am so overwhelmed with emotion that I cannot write. Commend me to him and to you do I commend myself.

On the 23rd day of February 1556.

Your Michelangelo Buonarroti in Rome

1. *Benvenuto Cellini (1500–1571), the goldsmith and sculptor.*

¶ To Lionardo di Buonarroto Simoni in Florence

411

Buonarroti
Archives
Mil. cclxxxvi
From Rome
March 7th
1556

Lionardo — I learn from your letter of your safe arrival, which gave me great pleasure, especially as Cassandra and the others are well. Here I remain in the same state in which you left me, and as to regaining my due,[1] nothing has yet resulted but prevarications. I'll wait as long as I can to see what happens.

As to spending some two thousand *scudi* in Florence, either on a house or on a country property, which I told you to do when you were here, I remain of the same mind. So when you find something suitable let me know of it.

Urbino's wife has sent to ask me for seven *braccia* of black cloth, which must be light and of a good quality, and says that she will send the money for it immediately. I should therefore be glad if you would send it to me. Pay for it and make the donation we agreed upon, less the amount it will cost, and as I have occasion to send you money, I will remit the amount in the total of the hundred. I think that's all. Thank Cassandra and commend me to her.

On the 7th day of March 1556.

MICHELANGELO BUONARROTI IN ROME

1. *i.e. the restoration of the revenues from the office of Civil Notary of the Romagna, of which he had been deprived on the elevation of Paul IV. See Appendix 33.*

412

¶ TO LIONARDO DI BUONARROTO SIMONI IN FLORENCE

*Buonarroti
Archives
Mil. cclxxxvii
From Rome
April 11th
1556*

Lionardo — A fine rascal you hit upon to entrust with that cloth. I've been awaiting it here for a month and have kept others waiting, to my great displeasure. Please will you find out what that rascal of a muleteer has done with it, and if it's found send it to me as quickly as you can. If it is not found, and if there are good grounds, have this rascal of a muleteer punished, make him pay for it, and send me another seven *braccia*. As if I hadn't burdens enough! I've had and I have so many vexations and troubles that they cannot be numbered.

I'll reply to Francesca's letter another time, because I don't feel like writing now. Commend me to her and to Michele and to all the others. On the eleventh day of April 1556.

MICHELANGELO BUONARROTI IN ROME

413

¶ TO LIONARDO DI BUONARROTO SIMONI IN FLORENCE

*Buonarroti
Archives
Mil. cclxxxviii
From Rome
April 25th
1556*

Lionardo — I've had the cloth, thank God, and when I find a muleteer to be trusted I'll send it to Cornelia.

I never replied to you as to the house for sale, about which you wrote me, because I've had other things to think about. I now tell you that the locality is not to my liking, because it seems to me too narrow and depressing. I should like one in a more airy and open situation, and don't be particular as to the cost – and if not a house, a country property, because here I should like to reduce the little capital I have in Rome as much as I can, because I'm very much weakened since Urbino died, and every hour might be my last, and God knows what would happen to my affairs then. Therefore think over what I'm writing you, because it is very much in your interest.

I could wish, and would be glad, if you would give me a little information as to how you managed the matter of the almsgiving and how one could do it again, if one were able. I think that's all. Commend me to Cassandra and do your best to live as long as you can, so that our possessions may not be left without anyone to enjoy them.

On the 25th day of April 1556.

MICHELANGELO BUONARROTI IN ROME

¶ To Lionardo di Buonarroto Simoni in Florence

*Buonarroti
Archives
Mil. cclxxxix
From Rome
May 8th
1556*

414

Lionardo — I've had a number of receipts with your letter; I did not want to see them and was very put out, because it appears that you think I don't trust you. I wanted to know how you distributed the money and where, in order to learn what persons are existing in a state of poverty; it would have been enough to have given me a little information by letter.

You write me that Cassandra is not feeling well; I'm concerned and very sorry about it. So do not go in want of anything, and if I can do anything, let me know, and commend me to her.

As to the house about which you wrote me, the locality isn't to my liking. It is better to stay as you are than not to be content with it. I wrote you that I wished to find a lodgment for the little capital I have, on account of what may happen,[1] as I am an old man and not in good health. I have not wished, after all, to accept a stipend for more reasons than I care to say.

On the 8th day of May 1556.

MICHELANGELO BUONARROTI IN ROME

1. *Rome was in a state of perturbation owing to the war with Spain (Appendix 43, pt. III).*

¶ To Messer Giorgio Vasari, dearest friend, in Florence

*Casa Vasari
Mil. cdlxxviii
From Rome
May 28th
1556*

415

Messer Giorgio — Only the day before yesterday did I speak to Messer Salustio[1] and not before, because he hasn't been in Rome. I think he is disposed to do your pleasure in every way, but he thinks it better to await his opportunity. He says that as the Pope wishes to place your picture[2] elsewhere and as His Holiness does nothing of this kind without consulting him, it will devolve upon him to put it where it seems best to him. Then will be the time to express your thanks to him and I have hopes that he will be of assistance to you, for such is his desire.

On the 28th day of May 1556.

YOUR MICHELANGELO IN ROME

1. *Giovanni Salustio di Baldassare Peruzzi (d. 1573), architect to the Pope (Vasari, VII, p. 241).*

2. *The picture commissioned from Vasari by Pope Julius III for a chapel in the Vatican. It was never paid for and was ultimately returned, by order of Pius IV, to Vasari, who hung it in the Pieve di Santa Maria at Arezzo (Vasari, VII, pp. 36, 693).*

416

*Buonarroti
Archives
Mil. ccxc
From Rome
May 31st
1556*

¶ TO LIONARDO DI BUONARROTO SIMONI IN FLORENCE

Lionardo — I haven't replied to your other letters because I wasn't able to. I now say, as regards Cepperello's farm, that if a reasonable price is agreed you may certainly take it, and in addition to Cepperello's farm I also authorize you to spend two thousand *scudi* as you think fit, because, as far as the house goes, if I do not find anything suitable – that is to say in a situation that is open and spacious – I would sooner that you acquired a country property.

I've had a letter from Francesca in which she begs me to make a donation of ten *scudi* to her confessor for a penniless young girl whom he is placing in the monastery of Santa Lucia. I want to do so for Francesca's sake, because I know that if it were not a deserving charity she would not ask it of me. But I don't know how to make the money payable there. So, if he has a friend here whom he can trust, to whom I could give it, I should like the said confessor to let me know of it.

I'm very pleased indeed that Cassandra is well, as you write me. Commend me to her and take care of yourself.

On the last day of May 1556.

MICHELANGELO BUONARROTI IN ROME

417

*British
Museum
Mil. ccxci
From Rome
(June) 1556*

¶ TO LIONARDO DI BUONARROTO SIMONI IN FLORENCE

Lionardo — I got the cask of white and red chick-peas, of peas and of apples. If I haven't written to you before, it hasn't seemed to me to matter, as writing is very irksome and fatiguing to me. I think that's all. Look after yourself.

I am old and in poor health; if anything serious befalls me I'll let you know, if I have time.

If you see Messer Giorgio,[1] tell him that as to that affair of his, I cannot help him, that I would do so willingly and that I have talked it over with Messer Salustio who replied to me that he has taken great pains over it and that he doesn't see a way out. In my view he'd better approach Messer Piergiovanni.[2]

MICHELANGELO BUONARROTI IN ROME

1. *Giorgio Vasari.*

2. *Piergiovanni Aleotti, i.e. 'Tantecose'.*

¶ TO LIONARDO DI BUONARROTO SIMONI IN FLORENCE

418

Lionardo — I'm sending you *[ten]* gold *[scudi]* in gold, the amount which I have paid here to Messer Francesco Bandini to make payable to you there; the draft will be enclosed with this. Take the money to Francesca so that she may pay it on behalf of that young girl of whom she wrote me.

As to Cepperello, you must take thought, because he is quite sure that you want to buy that farm and might contrive to cheat you of at least a hundred *scudi*. So do the best you can. In my other letters I wrote and told you how much you might spend on what you thought suitable.

That's that's *[sic]* all.

On the twenty 7th day of June 1556.

MICHELANGELO IN ROME

Buonarroti
Archives
Mil. ccxcii
From Rome
June 27th
1556

¶ TO LIONARDO DI BUONARROTO SIMONI IN FLORENCE

419

Lionardo — I did not acknowledge the *trebbiano*, as I was pressed when I received it – that is to say, thirty-six flasks. It's the best you've ever sent me, for which I thank you, but I'm sorry you put yourself to this expense, particularly as I've no longer anyone to give it to, since all my friends are dead.

As to Cepperello's farm, you showed you were too keen to have it – just the opposite of what I told you to do when you were here. It suffices that the lusty widow was willing to give a fortune for it – stupid ruses to make me rush after it. However, be it as it may, do the best you can; take it and let me know when and where I must pay the

Buonarroti
Archives
Mil. ccxciii
From Rome
July 4th
1556

money, and with as little ado as you can. I think that's all. I'm pleased you're all well. May God be thanked.

On the 4th day of July 1556.

MICHELANGELO BUONARROTI IN ROME

420

Buonarroti Archives Mil. ccxciv From Rome July 25th 1556

¶ TO LIONARDO DI BUONARROTO SIMONI IN FLORENCE

Lionardo — I learn from your last letter about the agreement you've reached with Cepperello and about the price. I now tell you that although it may be overpriced by a hundred *scudi*, you've done well. But before I have the money paid in Florence, I should like you to enquire into the title carefully and not to rush at it as you have done up till now, and to let me know exactly how much money I must arrange to have paid to you there, that is to say how many *scudi* I must have paid to you there, either in gold or in silver. The gold *scudi* is worth eleven julians here and the silver ten.[1] If I have to delay a few days in having the money paid to you, I cannot help it, because there are other things to think about – more than you would believe – and I've no-one to serve me in matters like this. Bastiano[2] is very ill and I'm afraid he will die.

Stand firm by the bargain with Cepperello. I think that's all. I assume you are all well and Cassandra likewise. Commend me to her and let us pray God to help us, because there is great need.[3] On the twenty-fifth day of July 1556.

MICHELANGELO BUONARROTI IN ROME

1. *See Vol. I, Appendix 3.*

2. *Sebastiano Malenotti, an overseer employed at St. Peter's. He was living in Michelangelo's house at this time and had been one of the witnesses to Urbino's Will (Gotti, II, p. 139).*

3. *Fears of a Spanish attack upon Rome were rife, see Appendix 43, pt. III.*

421

Buonarroti Archives Mil. ccxcv From Rome August 1st 1556

¶ TO LIONARDO DI BUONARROTO SIMONI IN FLORENCE

Lionardo — Owing to your impetuosity I'm worse off by at least fifty gold *scudi*, but it grieves me much more that you should set more store by a piece of land than by what I say. You know what I told you – that you should indicate that I didn't want it, and that we should be begged to buy it. But as soon as you reached Florence you were off to the brokers in a state of great anxiety. Now, since it's done, look after yourself and enjoy it.

Yesterday I had a letter of yours sent in a great hurry, in which you write me that they're ready to draw up the contract[1] and that in all it amounts to six hundred and fifty gold *scudi* in gold and that I should pay the said *scudi* to Messer Francesco Bandini to be made payable in Florence to the Capponi. This I'll do, but I cannot do so before next week, because as Bastiano is better, he'll begin going out and will go to the bank and pay the money down, because I've no-one else to serve me.

On the first day of August 1556.

MICHELANGELO BUONARROTI IN ROME

1. *The instrument by which Michelangelo bought the farm called Scopeto, in the parish of Santa Maria da Settignano, from Messer Giannozzo di Gherardo da Cepperello was drawn up by Ser Niccolò Parenti on July 28th 1556 (Milanesi, p. 326).*

¶ TO LIONARDO DI BUONARROTO SIMONI IN FLORENCE

422

Buonarroti Archives Mil. ccxcvi From Rome August 8th 1556

Lionardo — Bastiano is beginning to go out and on Monday or Tuesday he'll go to the Bandini and pay down the money, so that it will be paid to you there in the way you wrote me. As regards the purchase, you have managed it in your way, not in mine, and I'm worse off by at least fifty *scudi*. It is very true that self-love leads all men astray. Remember your father and how he died, while I, thank God, am still alive. I think that's all.

On the 8th day of August 1556.

MICHELANGELO BUONARROTI IN ROME

¶ TO LIONARDO DI BUONARROTO SIMONI IN FLORENCE

423

Buonarroti Archives Mil. ccxcvii From Rome August 15th 1556

Lionardo — Yesterday morning I took six hundred and fifty gold *scudi* in gold to the Bandini bank and the letter[1] will be enclosed with this. Go and pay them as you agreed.

You write me about the money I told you you might spend as you like. You know very well it was not meant for Cepperello's farm, which is an old affair already under discussion more than twenty years ago, and in our own minds we had already bought it. But you wanted to approach the matter and to manage it according to your own bent. The thing is done. Take care of yourself and make little ado about it, particularly at Settignano, because it is the last straw that you and your wife should be gossiped about here and in Florence by people from Settignano.[2] I'm not writing to you without anything to go upon, because your way of thinking is very different from mine. I think that's all. On the 15th day of August 1556.

The letter for the said *scudi* will be will be *[sic]* enclosed with this.

MICHELANGELO BUONARROTI IN ROME

1. *i.e. the letter of exchange.*

2. *Cf. No. 377.*

424

Buonarroti Archives Mil. ccxcviii From Rome September 1556

¶ TO LIONARDO DI BUONARROTO SIMONI IN FLORENCE

Lionardo — As regards fulfilling the vow, about which you write me, I tell you it doesn't seem to me to be the time to go hither and yon. This is my opinion at the moment. As to giving the infant you are awaiting the name Michelangelo, this would please me – or any other, provided it were a family name. Giovansimone would also be all right. Do as you like, because I shall be content with it. I think that's all.

On the . . . . day of September 1556.

MICHELANGELO BUONARROTI IN ROME

425

British Museum Mil. ccxcix From Rome October 31st 1556

¶ TO LIONARDO BUONARROTI SIMONI, DEAREST NEPHEW, IN FLORENCE
ENTRUSTED TO THE CORTESI FOR IMMEDIATE DELIVERY IN FLORENCE

Lionardo, dearest nephew[1] — Some days ago I received a letter of yours, to which I have not been able to reply before, as I have not had an opportunity. I will now make up for everything, in order that you may not be alarmed and so that you may understand.

Finding over a month ago that the work on the fabric of St. Peter's was slackening, I made ready to go to Loreto in order to make my devotions.[2] Then finding at Spoleto that I was a little tired, I stayed to rest for a while, with the result that I was unable to carry out my intention, because someone was sent expressly to say that I must return to Rome. For which reason, in order not to disobey, I set out for Rome, where, thank God, I find myself and where things are as God wills with respect to the misfortunes here. So I will not enlarge further, except to say that here there are good hopes of peace, the which may God grant. Fare you well, praying God to help us. From Rome on the last day of October 1556.

Yours, as a father,

[signed] MICHELANGELO BUONARROTI IN ROME

1. *From the embellishments in the opening address and the concluding salutation, as well as from its general style, it is obvious that this letter, which was only signed by Michelangelo, was written by someone else on his behalf, probably by Sebastiano Malenotti, who had accompanied him to Spoleto. Michelangelo had been away from Rome for five weeks. He returned on October 31st, having left on September 25th (Milanesi, p. 608).*

2. *This was not his only reason for leaving Rome. An attack upon the city was anticipated and four days after he left, the Spaniards, under the Duke of Alba, crossed the frontier into the Papal States (Appendix 43, pt. III).*

¶ TO MESSER GIORGIO VASARI IN FLORENCE

426

Casa Vasari
Mil. cdlxxix
From Rome
December 18th
1556

Messer Giorgio — I've received Messer Cosimo's book[1] which you sent me; a letter of thanks to his lordship will be enclosed with this. Please would you give it to him and commend me to him.

Recently, at great inconvenience and expense, I have had the great pleasure of a visit to the hermits in the mountains of Spoleto, so that less than half of me has returned to Rome, because peace is not really to be found save in the woods. That's all I have to tell you. I'm pleased that you're well and cheerful. And to you do I commend me.

On the 18th day of December.

YOUR MICHELANGELO BUONARROTI IN ROME

1. *Cosimo di Matteo Bartoli (1503–c.1573) Provost of San Lorenzo and a member of the Florentine Academy. The work in question was 'Difesa della lingua fiorentina e di Dante, con le regole di far bella e numerosa la prosa', by Carlo Lenzoni, which, having been completed after his death by Pierfrancesco Giambullari (1495–1555) passed on the death of the latter into the hands of Bartoli, who had it printed in Florence in 1556. In accordance with Lenzoni's wishes Bartoli dedicated it to Michelangelo.*

427

*Buonarroti
Archives
Mil. ccc
From Rome
December 19th
1556*

¶ To Lionardo di Buonarroto Simoni in Florence

Lionardo — I wrote you about my return to Rome. Afterwards I had a letter of yours from which I learnt that Cassandra had given birth to a baby girl who died a few days later, which has caused me much regret. But I'm not surprised about it, because it is not the lot of our family to multiply in Florence. So pray God that the one you have may live, and see that you keep alive yourself, so that everything may not have to be left to the Hospital.[1] I think that's all. Commend me to Cassandra and to God, because I am in great need of this. A letter for Messer Giorgio, the painter, will be enclosed with this; give it to him as soon as you can. On the 19th day of December 1556.

MICHELANGELO BUONARROTI IN ROME

1. *The Congregation of San Martino. Cf. No. 368.*

428

*Buonarroti
Archives
Mil. cccviii
From Rome
January 16th
1557*

¶ To Lionardo di Buonarroto Simoni in Florence

Lionardo — You write me in your last letter that if I need either maidservants or anyone else to look after me, I should let you know, and that you'll send me whatever I need. I assure you that at present I don't need anyone else, because I have two good lads who serve me well enough.

That's all I have to tell you. For an old man I'm pretty well and not discouraged. Look after yourself and let us pray God to help us. On the sixteenth day of December 1557.[1]

[*Unsigned*]

1. *The letter is endorsed in Lionardo's hand, employing the old style dating, '1556 from Rome, received on 22nd day of January from the said 16th'. As Michelangelo was often uncertain about the date at this period, we must suppose from the endorsement that he wrote December instead of January.*

429

*Buonarroti
Archives
Mil. ccci
From Rome
February 6th
1557*

¶ To his dearest Lionardo Buonarroti, dearest nephew, in Florence

Dearest Lionardo — I have received your letter and seen what you say about His Excellency,[1] therefore would you give the enclosed to Messer Lionardo[2] and make my apologies, because I do not wish to fail in my promise to His Excellency, and when I see that the time has come, I will not fail. But I cannot do so at once, because I need to put my affairs in order here. Therefore I'm not saying anything else to you now, as

I only had the letters at 6 o'clock on Saturday. May you fare well and may God keep you.[3]

From Rome, the 6th day of February 1557.

[signed] Michelangelo

1. *Cosimo I, Duke of Florence.*

2. *Lionardo Marinozzi da Ancona. See No. 402.*

3. *Once again the phraseology alone would indicate that the letter was not written by Michelangelo himself.*

¶ To Lionardo di Buonarroto Simoni in Florence

430

Buonarroti Archives Mil. cccii From Rome February 13th 1557

When he came to see me here in Rome about two years ago Messer Lionardo, the agent of the Duke of Florence, told me that His Lordship would be greatly pleased if I were to return to Florence and he made me many offers on his behalf. I replied to him that I begged His Lordship to concede me enough time to enable me to leave the fabric of St. Peter's at such a stage that it could not be changed in accordance with some other design which I have not authorized.[1] I have since continued with the said fabric, not having heard anything to the contrary, but it is not yet at the said stage; furthermore, I am obliged to make a large model in wood,[2] including the cupola and the lantern, in order to leave it completed as it is to be, finished in every detail. This I have been begged to do by the whole of Rome, and particularly by the Most Reverend Cardinal di Carpi;[3] so that I think it will be necessary for me to stay here for at least a year in order to do this. For the love of Christ and of St. Peter I beg the Duke to concede me this length of time, so that I may return to Florence without this goad,[4] in the knowledge that I should not be obliged to return to Rome any more. As regards the fabric being closed down[5] there is no truth in this, because, as may be seen, there are still sixty men working here, counting *scarpellini*, bricklayers and labourers, and doing so with the expectation of continuing.

I would like you to read this letter to the Duke and to beg His Lordship on my behalf to grant me the necessary grace mentioned above, which I need before I can return to Florence, for if the form of the said fabric were changed, as envy is seeking to do, I might as well have done nothing up till now.

[Unsigned]

1. *This is in fact what ultimately happened.*

2. *The model of the cupola was not completed until 1561; in an altered form it is still preserved in the Basilica.*

3. *Cardinal Ridolfo Pio di Carpi (1499–1564), archpriest of the Basilica, a diplomat, and a very eminent and cultured man. He was at this time a Deputy of the fabric.*

4. *i.e. to return to Rome to complete the work on the model.*

5. *Rumours that the work on St. Peter's was to be discontinued were due, no doubt, to the continued threat of a Spanish invasion. This, together with the heavy expenses which the war entailed, would account for the relatively small body of workmen employed at the Basilica. For the political situation see Appendix 43.*

431

*Vatican
Codex
Mil. cdlxxx
From Rome
April 28th
1557*

¶ [To Mona Cornelia di Guido Colonello, widow of Francesco d'Amadore, at Castel Durante]

I perceived that you were offended with me, but I did not know the reason. Now, from your last letter, I think I know why. When you sent me the cheeses you wrote me that you wished to send several other things, but that the handkerchiefs were not yet finished. And I, in order that you might not incur expenses on my behalf, wrote to you saying that you shouldn't send me anything more and should do me the very great pleasure of asking something of me, knowing – nay rather, being certain, as you ought to be – of the love I still have for Urbino, although he is dead, and for his family.

As regards my coming to Castel Durante to see the little ones, or your sending Michelangelo[1] here, I must tell you how I am placed. It would not be possible to send Michelangelo here, because I have no women[2] in the house and no-one to look after things and the little one is still too young and something might befall which I should very much regret.

Then, about a month ago the Duke of Florence very kindly brought great pressure to bear upon me and offered me great inducements to return to Florence. I have asked him for such time as will allow me to arrange my affairs here and to leave the fabric of St. Peter's at a satisfactory stage, so that I expect to be here until the end of the summer.

Having arranged my affairs, and yours as regards the Public Funds,[3] I shall leave for Florence this winter for good, since I am an old man and time will not remain for me to return to Rome any more. I'll pass through Castel Durante *[on my way]* and if you are willing to entrust Michelangelo to me, I'll cherish him in Florence with more affection than the children of my nephew, Lionardo, teaching him what I know his father wished him to learn. I received your last letter yesterday, the twenty-seventh day of March.[4]

Michelangelo Buonarroti in Rome

1. *Urbino's elder son and Michelangelo's godson.*

2. *Normally Michelangelo had two or three women in the house, but, perhaps owing to the troubled*

times (Appendix 43, pt. III), he had sent them back to Castel Durante where they came from, since only 'the two Antonii' are mentioned in the extant list of wage payments for 1557 (B.M., Add. MSS., 23.209, f. 29 and verso). At this time the place of Urbino, who had managed Michelangelo's day-to-day domestic affairs, had not yet been taken by Pierluigi Gaeta.

3. *In accordance with the terms of Urbino's Will (Gotti, II, p. 137 et seq.) Michelangelo had invested the specified six hundred and sixty scudi in the Monte on behalf of Urbino's heirs. The first payment from this investment was received on May 4th 1556 (Milanesi, p. 607).*

4. *March is a slip for April. See Dating and Sequence of Letters. Milanesi's text is based on a published source. The original is in the Vatican Codex (Symonds, II, p. 302).*

¶ To Lionardo di Buonarroto Simoni in Florence

432

*Buonarroti
Archives
Mil. ccciii
From Rome
May 4th
1557*

Lionardo — I'm sending to you in Florence through Messer Francesco Bandini fifty gold *scudi* in gold, in order that you may send me eight *braccia* of black *rascia*, the lightest and best to be had there, and two *braccia* of sarcenet. Urbino's wife has sent asking me for these things; so send them to me as soon as you can and let me know what the expenses amount to. Spend the balance of the fifty *scudi* I'm sending you on charity where you think there's most need. I think that's all as to this.

I'm old, as you know, and I've many bodily disabilities which make me feel that death is not far off, so that I should be glad if you would come here this September, if I'm alive, in order to settle my affairs and ours. Have prayers said to God for me – if I don't get there first, be it understood.

The letter for the money will be enclosed with this, and one for Messer Giorgio Vasari. Give it to him as soon as you can and commend me to him and let me know about everything. On other occasions I've written and told you not to believe anyone who talks about me, unless you see letters from me.

In order to cause me to return to Florence, perhaps in order to redress the dishonour of his departure from here, he – I speak of Bastiano da San Gimignano[1] – has told many lies there, perhaps to some purpose. On the 4th day of May 1557.[2]

Michelangelo Buonarroti in Rome

1. *Sebastiano Malenotti, formerly an overseer at the fabric of St. Peter's, who had been dismissed because of the serious mistake he had made over the building of the vault of the chapel of the King of France. Cf. Nos. 433, 437, 439.*

2. *The letter is endorsed in another hand 'D. Capponi, please deliver safely'.*

433

*State Archives
Florence
Mil. cdlxxxi
From Rome
May 1557*

¶ To the Illustrious Lord Cosimo, Duke of Florence

Lord Duke — About three months ago, or a little less, I made known to Your Lordship that I could not yet leave the fabric of St. Peter's without causing great damage to the fabric and bringing the greatest disgrace upon myself, and that I needed not less than another year, supposing the necessary conditions for this were available, if I wished to leave it at the stage I should desire; and that I thought Your Lordship would consent to grant me this space of time.

I now have another letter from Your Lordship urging me to return earlier than I anticipated, which has caused me no little consternation, because I am in a state of greater anxiety and difficulty over the affairs of the said fabric than I have ever been. This is because, owing to my being old and unable to go there often enough, a mistake has arisen over the vault of the chapel of the King of France, which is unusual and cunningly contrived, and I shall have to take down a great part of what has been done.[1] As to which this chapel is and of how much importance to the rest of the fabric, Bastiano da San Gimignano can bear witness, because he was the overseer here. I do not think the correction to the said chapel will be finished until the end of the summer; then there will be nothing more for me to do except to leave the model of the whole work here as I am begged to do by everyone, particularly by Carpi, and then to return to Florence with my mind upon my repose with death, to which I seek to accustom myself day and night, that he may not treat me worse than other old men.

Now to return to the subject, I beg Your Lordship to concede the required time of another year[2] on account of the fabric, as I thought you would concede it when I last wrote.

The least of Your Lordship's servants

Michelangelo Buonarroti in Rome

1. *See Nos. 437, 439.*

2. *As usual Michelangelo greatly underestimated the time needed.*

434

*Casa Vasari
Mil. cdlxxxii
From Rome
May (22nd)
1557*

¶ To Messer Giorgio Vasari, dearest friend

Messer Giorgio, dear friend — I call God to witness that ten years ago I was put in charge of the fabric of St. Peter's by Pope Pagolo,[1] under duress and against my will. And if the work on the said fabric had continued until to-day in the way in which it was then being conducted, I should now be at the stage on the said fabric which I desired to reach in order to be able to return to Florence. But through lack of money[2]

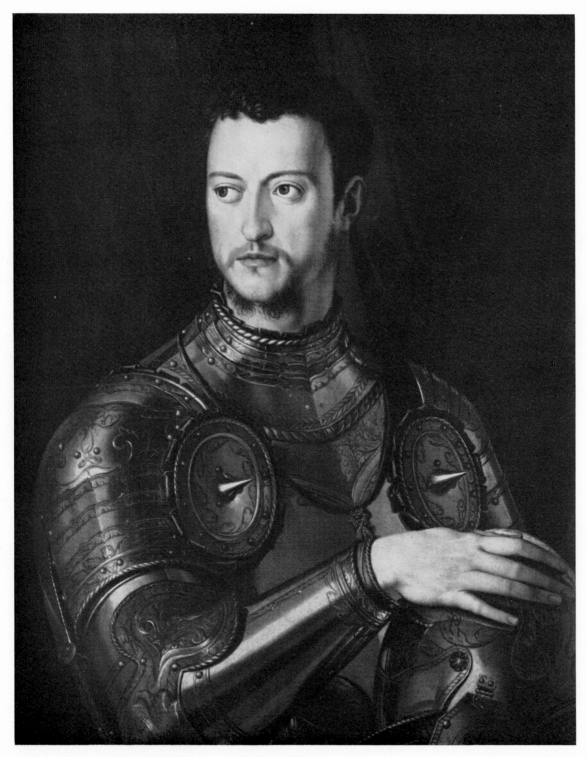

22. *Cosimo I, Duke of Florence*

Angelo Bronzino
Palazzo Vecchio, Florence

the work has been retarded and is being retarded, when it has reached the most toilsome and difficult part, so that if I were to abandon it now, it would result in nothing but the uttermost disgrace and the loss of the whole reward for the pains I have endured for the love of God during the said ten years.

I have delivered you this discourse as a reply to your letter and because I have a letter from the Duke[3] which has caused me much amazement, in that His Lordship should deign to write to me with such amiability. I thank God and His Excellency with all my heart. I'm straying from the point, because I've lost my memory and my judgment and writing is a great effort to me, as it's not my function.

This finally is the position – so that you may understand what would ensue if I were to abandon the above-mentioned fabric and to leave here. Firstly, it would gratify sundry thieves and robbers, and would be the cause of its ruin and perhaps even of its closing down for ever. Secondly, I have certain obligations here, a house and other things worth some thousands of *scudi* in all, and if I were to leave here without permission I don't know what might happen. Thirdly, I'm physically enfeebled like all old men, by kidney trouble, the stone and the colic, and Messer Eraldo[4] can bear witness to this, because I owe my life to him. I haven't therefore the courage to return to Florence in order to come back here, and if I were to return for good, it would take some time to arrange matters here so that there would be no need to give them further thought. The fact is that I left Florence so long ago that when I arrived here Pope Clement, who died two days afterwards, was still alive.

Messer Giorgio, I commend me to you and beg you to commend me to the Duke and to make my *[apologies]*, because I now have no courage except the courage to die, and what I have written about my circumstances here is abundantly true.

The reply I made to the Duke I made because I was told I must reply, although I lacked the courage to write to His Lordship, particularly so hastily; but if I had felt able to ride, I should at once have come to Florence and back, without anyone here being any the wiser.[5]

[Unsigned]

1. *Pope Paul III.*

2. *In the copy used by Milanesi the word 'danari' was wrongly transcribed as 'lavori'. This and one or two other corrections have been made in accordance with the autograph (Frey, Lit., I, p. 477).*

3. *Both Vasari and Duke Cosimo had written to Michelangelo on May 8th offering him every possible inducement to return to Florence (Vasari, VIII, p. 323).*

4. *Realdo Colombo, the physician who had attended him since his first attack of the stone in 1549. Colombo himself died in 1559, leaving Michelangelo bereft of even this consolation in his old age (Giornale Storico, III, p. 72).*

5. *It seems so likely that Michelangelo could have gone to Florence and back without anyone's knowledge!*

¶ To Lionardo di Buonarroto Simoni in Florence

435

*Buonarroti
Archives
Mil. ccciv
From Rome
June 16th
1557*

Lionardo — I've received the rash and the sarcenet; when I find someone to take it, I'll send it and she'll[1] send me the money immediately. As to the balance of the money, will you let me know when you've spent it, as I wrote you.

As regards my physical state, I'm ill, that is to say with all the ills to which old men are prone – with the stone, so that I cannot urinate, with the colic, with the back-ache, so that often I am unable to walk upstairs – and worse still, I'm full of worries, because if I leave the conveniences I have here for my ills, I should not survive three days; and yet I should not like to lose the Duke's favour on this account; neither do I wish to fail the fabric of St. Peter's here, nor do I wish to fail myself. I pray God to help and guide me. But if I become ill, that is to say with a dangerous fever, I'll send for you at once. But don't think of it and don't arrange to come unless you get letters from me telling you to come.

Commend me to Messer Giorgio, as he can, if he will, be of service to me, because I know that the Duke is well disposed towards him.

On the sixteenth day of June 1557.

MICHELANGELO BUONARROTI IN ROME

1. *Cornelia, Urbino's widow.*

¶ [To Lionardo di Buonarroto Simoni in Florence]

436

*Casa Vasari
Mil. cccv
From Rome
July 1st
1557*

Lionardo — I would rather die than be in disfavour with the Duke. In all my affairs I have always endeavoured to be true to my word, and if I have delayed in coming to Florence as I promised, I always had this proviso in mind, that I should not leave here until I had brought the fabric of St. Peter's to a stage at which my design could not be spoilt or altered nor an occasion given to thieves and robbers to return there to thieve and to rob as they are wont, and as they are waiting to do.[1] I have always been, and am, thus diligent, because many people believe, as I do myself, that I was put there by God.

But I have not yet reached the said stage of the said fabric owing to a lack of money and men. Because I am an old man and have no-one to leave in my place, I have not wished to abandon it, and also because I serve for the love of God, in Whom is all my hope.

In order that the Duke may understand the reason for my delay, I am explaining the mistake in the enclosed letter, by means of a small sketch, in order that Messer Giorgio may notify the Duke.

On the first day of July 1557.

MICHELANGELO BUONARROTI IN ROME

1. *See Appendix 44 in regard to these and similar references.*

---

437   ¶ TO MESSER GIORGIO VASARI IN FLORENCE

Casa Vasari
Mil. cdlxxxiii
From Rome
July 1st
1557

The clerk of works[1] took the centering marked in red to be the construction of the whole vault. Afterwards, when they began to approach the half *tondo*, which is in the middle of the said vault, it came short, owing to the mistake made over the said centering, as may be seen here in the drawing, because it was supported by one centering only, where there should have been a number, which are here marked in black on the drawing. Owing to this mistake, the vault has gone so far ahead that a number of the blocks will have to be taken down; for there is no brickwork in the said vault, but only travertine, and the diameter of the *tondi*, without the frame which surrounds them, is twenty-two *[palmi]*.

As the model, such as I make for everything, was exact, this mistake *[ought never to have been made]* but it happened through my not being able to go there often enough, owing to old age, and whereas I believed that the said vault would now be finished, it will not be finished until the end of this winter, and if one could die of shame and grief I should not be alive. I beg you to explain to the Duke why I am not now in Florence; although I am detained by other things more than I can say.[2]

YOUR MICHELANGELO IN ROME

1. *Sebastiano Malenotti who had made the mistake over the vault of the chapel of the King of France. See No. 433.*

2. *Milanesi's text was based on a copy of the original letter, which differs from the autograph in one or two minor details, which have been incorporated in the translation. The note is written beneath the drawings to which he refers. See Plate 23.*

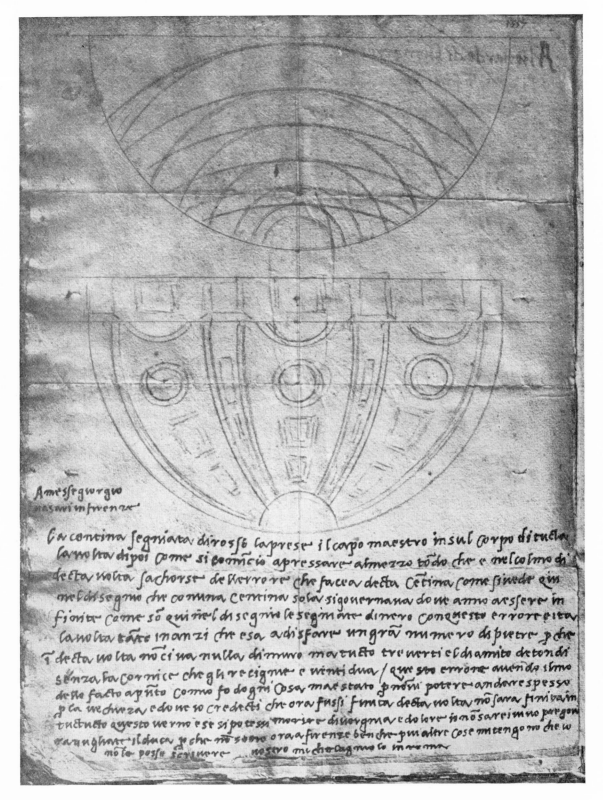

438

*Casa Vasari
Mil. cccvi
From Rome
August 17th
1557*

¶ [TO LIONARDO DI BUONARROTO SIMONI IN FLORENCE]

Lionardo — In your last letter, as in others, you urge me to return to Florence, but I tell you that those who are neither within sight nor hearing of me do not know what my life here is like. So there's no need to tell me differently. I'm doing my best in the circumstances in which I find myself.

As regards the exceeding courtesy, consideration and kindness of the Duke, I'm so overcome that I do not know what to say. I need Messer Giorgio Vasari to help me, because he knows how needful it is and in what terms to thank someone who values my life more than I do myself, and particularly someone without a peer.

I think that's all. Writing is very irksome to me as I am old and full of confusion. On the 17th day of August 1557.

MICHELANGELO BUONARROTI IN ROME

Tear off half this sheet and give it to Messer Giorgio, because it's for him. I have had to write like this, as I have no more paper in the house.

439

*Casa Vasari
Mil. cdlxxxiv
From Rome
August 17th
1557*

¶ [MESSER GIORGIO]

Messer Giorgio — In order that the difficulty over the vault, of which I sent you a drawing, may be better understood, I'm sending you the plan[1] of it which I did not send then – that is to say the plan of the said vault, in order that you may see how it springs from the ground.

It has been imperative to divide it into three vaults, corresponding to the windows below, which are divided by pilasters which rise, as you see, in the form of a pyramid to the half *tondo* at the top of the vault, as do the beds and the sides of the vaults. Similarly, it was necessary to support them with numbers of centerings, which change so much from so many sides and from point to point that one cannot keep to a set rule. And the *tondi* and coffers which go in the middle of their beds have to diminish and to increase on so many sides and to pass through so many points that it is difficult to find the correct method. Nevertheless, having the model, such as I make for everything, so great a mistake ought never to have been made as to try to support all three of these sections with a single centering; whence, with shame and loss, the necessity has arisen of taking it down and also of spoiling a great number of the blocks. The vaulting, the ornaments and the interstices are all of travertine, which is unusual in Rome.

I thank the Duke for his kindness with all my heart, and may God grant that I may

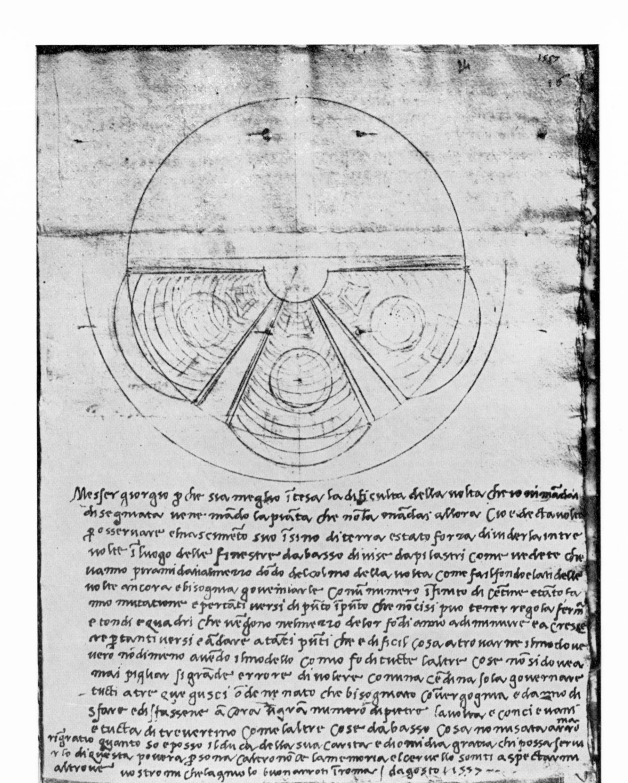

24. *Facsimile of Letter No. 439*   *Casa Vasari, Arezzo*

be able to serve him with this poor body, for there is nothing else. My brain and my memory have gone to await me elsewhere.

YOUR MICHELANGELO BUONARROTI IN ROME

August 1557

1. *See Plate 24.*

440

British Museum Mil. cccvii From Rome (September 25th) 1557

¶ TO LIONARDO DI BUONARROTO SIMONI IN FLORENCE

Lionardo — I learn from your last letter of the terrible destruction of bridges, monasteries and houses and of the loss of life that the flooding[1] has caused in Florence, but that, in comparison with others, you have escaped pretty well. I had already heard about it and I expect you, too, will have heard from here of similar destruction and loss of life from the flooding of the Tiber,[2] but being on high ground we have escaped pretty well in comparison with others. I pray God He may preserve us from worse, such as I apprehend on account of our sins.

My affairs here are not going too well, I mean as regards the fabric of St. Peter's, because to arrange things properly is not enough, since the overseers, either through ignorance or malice, always do the opposite and the bitterness of my infirmities is borne in upon me.[3] As for the rest, you can imagine it, I being as old as I am. I think that's all.

MICHELANGELO BUONARROTI

---

1. *The Arno overflowed its banks on September 13th 1557. The Ponte Santa Trinità, which was subsequently rebuilt by Bartolomeo Ammanati, was destroyed.*

2. *The Tiber broke its banks at midnight on September 15th. Among others the Ponte Santa Maria, for the strengthening of which Nanni di Baccio Bigio had been made responsible (Vasari, VII, p. 234 et seq.), was completely destroyed. The bridge which replaced it has been known as the Ponte Rotto ever since. The height of the flood-waters, which was recorded on the façade of Santa Maria sopra Minerva, reached 18.95 metres on this occasion (Lanciani, p. 94).*

3. *The original autograph contains a correction, which was misinterpreted by Milanesi's copyist. The word transcribed as 'errore' should read 'essere' (B.M., Add. MSS., 23.142, f. 86).*

¶ To Lionardo di Buonarroto Simoni in Florence

441

British Museum Mil. cccix From Rome June 25th 1558

Lionardo — I've had the *trebbiano*, but not without shame and consternation, because I gave some of it away without tasting it, believing it to be good. Afterwards I was disgusted with it. However good it was, you shouldn't have sent it, because these are not the times for such things. Take care of yourself and don't worry about me. When I need anything I'll let you know. I haven't replied to several of your letters, because writing is very fatiguing and irksome to me and because my mind is on other things. As they were not important, I passed them over and this I'll do in future.

MICHELANGELO BUONARROTI IN ROME

¶ To Lionardo di Buonarroto Simoni in Florence

442

Buonarroti Archives Mil. cccx From Rome July 2nd 1558

Lionardo — I wrote you about the receipt of the *trebbiano* and how, believing it to be like the rest you've often sent me, I gave a few flasks away without tasting it first, which has caused me shame and consternation. If you found that it was good in Florence, the muleteer must have committed some rascality on the way. So don't send me anything more, unless I ask you for it, because everything puts me to trouble. Make the most of life and manage as best you can, and don't worry about affairs here. And when I need one thing rather than another I'll let you know.

On the 2nd day of July.

MICHELANGELO BUONARROTI IN ROME

¶ To Lionardo di Buonarroto Simoni in Florence

443

Buonarroti Archives Mil. cccxi From Rome July 16th 1558

Lionardo — I had a letter of yours last week from which I learn that you are well and the little one also. May God grant her a long and good life, and for everything may He be thanked.

As regards the *trebbiano* about which you write me. There was no need to apologize for it, but another time I would be grateful if you would give in charity the money you would spend on sending it to me, because I believe there are people in need and according to what is said here there is great dearth in Florence. It looks as if it is going to be the same here. I think that's all. Contrive to keep alive and well and commend me to Cassandra.

MICHELANGELO BUONARROTI IN ROME

444

Buonarroti Archives Mil. cccxii From Rome December 2nd 1558

¶ To Lionardo di Buonarroto Simoni in Florence

Lionardo — I have learnt of the death of the baby girl; this does not surprise me, because in our family there was never more than one at a time.[1]

I wrote and told you before to buy a house in Florence, if it were imposing and well situated. I'm of the same mind, because I invested about nine hundred *scudi* here in the Funds from which I would withdraw it willingly and with the house I have here *[sic]*, and would buy there. So let me know if you were to find anything suitable up to two thousand *scudi*.

I think that's all. I'm an old man and here I am bearing great burdens, which is hardly recognized, and I do so for the love of God, in Whom is all my hope and in nothing else.

On the 2nd day of December 1558.

Michelangelo Buonarroti

1. *Cf. No. 461.*

445

Buonarroti Archives Mil. cccxiii From Rome December 16th 1558

¶ To Lionardo di Buonarroto Simoni in Florence

Lionardo — Bartolomeo Ammanati, clerk of works at the *Opera* of Santa Maria del Fiore, writes to ask my advice, on behalf of the Duke, about a certain staircase which is to be built in the Library at San Lorenzo. I've made, rather roughly, a little sketch of sorts for it in clay, as I think it might be done. And I thought of packing it up here in a box and giving it to whomsoever he writes and tells me to give it to, to send to him. So speak to him and let him know of this as soon as you can.

In my last letter I wrote you about a house, because if I am able to free myself from my obligations here, I should like to know that I have a nest just for myself and my crowd in Florence, and in order to do this I'm thinking of using some of the money I have here; and the sooner I can do so with free leave from Florence and from here, the sooner I shall, because, as I wrote you, my lot here is a hard one.

On the sixteenth day of December 1558.

Michelangelo Buonarroti in Rome

¶ To Lionardo di Buonarroto Simoni in Florence

446

*British
Museum
Mil. cccxvii
From Rome
January 7th
1559*

Lionardo — I've received fifteen *marzolini* cheeses and fourteen pounds of sausages delivered by Simon del Bernia.[1] I was glad of the sausages and likewise of the *marzolini*, because there is a scarcity of things like this. But I do not want you to incur further expense for things like this because I take the smallest share of it here.

I wrote to you about *[buying]* a house in order that what I have here might be transferred to Florence before my death. I do not know what will ensue, because I've many encumbrances here.

Would you tell Ammanato that on Saturday I'll send him the small model of the staircase for the Library by the hand either of his relative or of the courier, whichever may be the quicker and better.

Since he wrote I agreed with his relative, that is to say with his wife's[2] father, that he would send it by a muleteer, either yesterday or to-day, which is Saturday, because it might be damaged by the courier, but up till tonight the said relative is not to be found. I sent to his house; he is not in Rome. When he returns I'll give it to him, as I've been directed.

MICHELANGELO IN ROME

Let Ammanato know of this and commend me to him.

1. *A muleteer.*

2. *Laura di Giovanni Antonio Battifero da Urbino (1523–1589). She enjoyed a considerable reputation as a poet in her own lifetime.*

¶ To Lionardo di Buonarroto Simoni in Florence

447

*Buonarroti
Archives
Mil. cccxviii
From Rome
January 14th
1559*

Lionardo — Yesterday morning the muleteer, who is taking Ammanato the small model I promised him, left for Florence. The said muleteer is called Marco da Lucca. That Battifero, to whom I was directed to give it in order that he might send it on, had never been in Rome up to the time I sent it. When the said Marco comes to see you with the corded box containing the model, have it taken to the said Ammanato, so that he may give him something, because he only received one julian here. Commend me to him. On the 14th day of January 1559.[1]

MICHELANGELO BUONARROTI IN ROME

1. *See Dating and Sequence of Letters.*

448

*Buonarroti
Archives
Mil. cdlxxxvi
From Rome
(January 14th)
1559*

¶ [TO MESSER BARTOLOMEO AMMANATI IN FLORENCE]

Messer Bartolomeo — I wrote you that I had made a little clay model of the Library staircase; I'm now sending it to you in a box, and as it's a small affair, I have not been able to do more than give you an idea, remembering that what I formerly proposed was free-standing and only abutted on to the door of the Library. I've contrived to maintain the same method; I do not want the side stairs to have balusters at the ends, like the main flight, but a seat between every two steps, as indicated by the embellishments. There is no need for me to tell you anything about bases, fillets for these plinths and other ornaments, because you are resourceful, and being on the spot will see what is needed much better than I can.

As to the height and length, take up as little space as you can by narrowing the extremity as you think fit. It is my opinion that if the said staircase were made in wood – that is to say in a fine walnut – it would be better than in stone, and more in keeping with the desks, the ceiling and the door.

I think that's all. I'm all yours, old, blind, deaf and inept in hands and in body.[1]

YOUR MICHELANGELO BUONARROTI IN ROME

1. *The whereabouts of the original autograph, if it is extant, is unknown. Milanesi's text is based on a copy in the Bustelli Collection which was acquired for the Casa Buonarroti in 1861. See also Draft 11.*

449

*Buonarroti
Archives
Mil. cccxiv
From Rome
July 15th
1559*

¶ TO LIONARDO DI BUONARROTO SIMONI IN FLORENCE

Lionardo — I've received the shirts and the other things mentioned in the letter. Thank Cassandra on my behalf, as you will know how to do.

I've had two letters begging me very warmly to return to Florence. I don't think you know that about four months ago, through the Cardinal di Carpi,[1] who is one of the Deputies of the fabric of St. Peter's, I had permission from the Duke of Florence to continue with the fabric of St. Peter's in Rome. I derived great pleasure from this for which I returned thanks to God. Now I do not know whether what you write me so warmly, as I've said, is from your desire that I should return, or whether there is some other reason. So make it a little clearer, because everything is a worry and trouble to me.

It is incumbent upon me to tell you that the Florentines wish to build a fine edifice here, that is to say, a church of their own,[2] and all with one accord have tried and are trying to prevail upon me to consider it. I have replied that I am here at the instance of the Duke for the work on Saint *[Peter's]* and that without his permission they are not likely to get anything from me.

On the fifteenth day of June[3] 1559.

MICHELANGELO BUONARROTI IN ROME

Writing is extremely irksome to me – my hand, my sight and my memory.[4]

1. *Cardinal Ridolfo Pio di Carpi had written to the Duke on May 28th 1558, expressing the Pope's desire that Michelangelo might be allowed to remain quietly in Rome to finish the model of St. Peter's on which he was engaged. To this request the Duke acceded (Gotti, I, p. 316).*

2. *San Giovanni de' Fiorentini, for which, on the foundations laid by Jacopo Sansovino, Michelangelo eventually produced four ground plans. Of these the Deputies chose the most compact, but the most elaborate. The present church was completed in 1588 by Giacomo della Porta to a design of his own (Schiavo, figs. 125–129).*

3. *Corrected in Lionardo's hand to 'July'.*

4. *The truth of this remark is proved by the mistake made in the month and by his impression that the Cardinal had written to the Duke not a year, but only a few months previously.*

XV

LETTERS
450 – 480

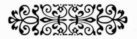

From Rome
1559 - 1563

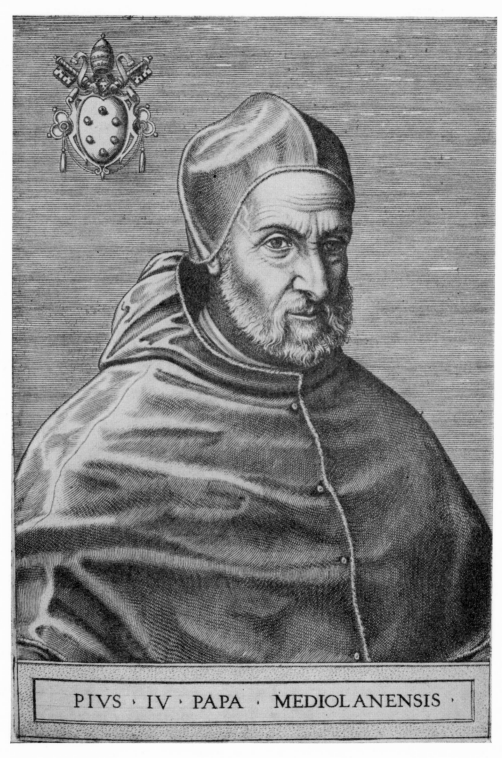

PIVS · IV · PAPA · MEDIOLANENSIS ·

25. *Pope Pius IV*

XV. From Rome: 1559-1563

¶ [To the Most Illustrious Lord Duke of Florence]

450

*State Archives
Florence
Mil. cdlxxxvii
From Rome
November 1st
1559*

Most Illustrious Lord Duke of Florence — The Florentines have often before had a great desire to build a church to San Giovanni here in Rome. Now, in Your Lordship's time, being in expectation of better facilities,[1] they are resolved upon it and have appointed five men[2] to take charge of it, who have asked me, nay begged me several times, for a design for the said building. Knowing that Pope Leo began the said church, I replied that I did not want to turn my attention to it without the permission and commission of the Duke of Florence.

Now, as it afterwards transpires, I have received a most kind and gracious letter from Your Most Illustrious Lordship, which enjoins me by express command to turn my attention to the above-mentioned Church of the Florentines, from which the great pleasure You have in it is manifest.

I have already done several designs suited to the site for this building, which the above-mentioned Deputies have shown me. They, being men of great judgment and discretion, have selected one of them, which I frankly think is the most imposing. This will be copied and drawn out more clearly than I am able to do myself, because of old age, and will be sent to Your Most Illustrious Lordship.[3] What ensues will be as Your Lordship deems best.

I regret in this instance that I am so old and so ill-attuned to life that I can promise little of myself to the said fabric; albeit from my own house I will endeavour to do what is asked of me on behalf of Your Lordship, and may God grant me not to fail You in any way.

On the first day of November 1559.

Your Excellency's servant

MICHELANGELO BUONARROTI IN ROME

1. *This letter was written during the conclave that had opened on September 5th following the death of Paul IV on August 18th 1559. At this period Cosimo I was using all the influence in his power to secure the election of Cardinal Gian Angelo de' Medici of Milan 'in whom he hoped to find an accommodating tool' (Pastor, XV, pp. 12 et seq. and Booth, p. 199). The Florentines in Rome evidently thought this an excellent opportunity to enlist Michelangelo's services under the patronage of the Duke, whose candidate, Pius IV (1559–1565), was finally elected on December 25th.*

2. *Of these five Deputies Vasari lists three, namely, Francesco Bandini, Uberto Ubaldini and Tommaso de' Bardi (Vasari, VII, p. 261).*

3. *Having received the drawing, the Duke acknowledged Michelangelo's letter on December 22nd and in the most flattering and honourable terms (Gaye, III, p. 22).*

451

*Buonarroti
Archives
Mil. cccxvi
From Rome
December 16th
1559*

¶ To Lionardo di Buonarroto Simoni in Florence

Lionardo — I've received the twelve *marzolini* cheeses which you sent me; they're delicious. I shared them with a few friends. I thank you for them and am pleased to learn that everyone is well.

As for me, I am old and have many disabilities such as old age brings. I should therefore be glad, for a number of reasons, if you would come here in the spring, when I write, but not before. I think that's all. On the sixteenth day of December 1559.

MICHELANGELO BUONARROTI IN ROME

452

*British
Museum
Mil. cccxv
From Rome
(December
23rd 1559)*

¶ To Lionardo di Buonarroto Simoni in Florence

Lionardo — I've had all the things mentioned in the letter, for which I thank you, and have shared them with friends.

The other matter about which you write me will soon be properly arranged and I'll send you everything in order.

MICHELANGELO IN ROME

453

*Buonarroti
Archives
Mil. cdxcii
From Rome
January 10th
1560*

¶ To the Magnificent Messer Pier Filippo Vandini at Castel Durante

Magnificent Messer Pier Filippo[1] — In answer to your letter of the tenth of this month,[2] I must tell you that I too have taken the opinion of the lawyers, to the effect that, as it is true that the house was allocated to Cornelia not as a dowery provision but as a security for 500 florins, she is not obliged to take over the house again, but can have the money if she wishes. But because it is my belief that Cornelia wants to remain in the house, to have the 500 florins and to get hold of the more valuable lands there belonging to these poor little wards – she not being, in my opinion, a good mother in this respect – I think that we, in order to discharge our obligation, must arrange matters in such a way that the estate of the wards may not be impaired. It might therefore perhaps be as well to see whether the house could be sold for 500 florins, and if possible for 800, which I understand it is worth, or, in effect, for the highest price possible, seeing that if one has to transfer real estate, it would be much better for the wards that the house rather than the lands should be transferred or the money in the Funds withdrawn, which is steadily increasing all the time, particularly as the wards could have a suitable house at an annual rent of three or four *scudi*, and would not wish more profitable possessions to be transferred.

Perhaps Cornelia, when she understands that you wish to sell the house, will change her mind and will decide to take the house, not being able to realize the ends she has in view. This is my opinion, always deferring to your judgment and friendship, as you are on the spot and can judge and can advise much better than I can myself. I should also be glad if, before any other concessions are made, you would be kind enough to come to Rome, as you have courteously offered to do, so that we could talk it over together, because the better we understand each other the better we shall decide and the better shall we be able to arrange the affairs of these poor little orphans.

I beg you then, with all my heart, as soon as it is convenient to you to let us have this talk. I commend me to you and to the wards with all my heart.

From Rome on the . . . . .

[Unsigned]

1. *Pier Filippo Vandini and Rosso de' Rossi, both of Castel Durante, were, together with Michelangelo, Urbino's executors and the guardians of his widow, Cornelia, and her two sons. There was a long correspondence between 1557 and 1561 (Frey, Briefe, pp. 351 et seq.) about the management of the estate, in connection with which numerous difficulties and disputes arose, particularly after Cornelia's marriage to Giulio Brunelli in April 1559. Of Michelangelo's letters this is the only one extant. From its style it would appear to have been drafted for him, perhaps by the lawyer.*

2. *On the evidence of Vandini's letter of March 1st 1560 (Frey, Briefe, p. 374) we know that Michelangelo's letter was dated January 10th. The reference to Vandini's letter of that date is therefore a mistake, as Michelangelo's letter was an answer to Vandini's letter of December 27th (Frey, Briefe, p. 372).*

¶ To the Most Illustrious and Most Excellent Lord Duke of Florence and Siena and my Most Honoured Patron

454

State Archives Florence Mil. cdlxxxviii From Rome March 5th 1560

My Most Honoured and Illustrious Lord — The Deputies of the fabric of the Church of the Florentines have decided to send Tiberio Calcagni[1] to Your Most Illustrious Excellency. This decision is very pleasing to me, because from the designs which he is bringing, You will the better understand what would need to be done here than from my plan which You saw. And if these were to Your satisfaction, with Your Excellency's aid, a beginning could be made on the foundations and the holy enterprise could be put in hand.

As Your Excellency has commanded me to give my attention to this fabric, it has seemed to me my duty to tell You in these few lines that to the best of my ability I will not fail, although owing to my age and indisposition I cannot do as I would wish and as it would be my duty to do in the service of Your Excellency and of the Nation. To You with all my heart do I offer my services and commend me and I pray God to hold You in felicity.[2]

From Rome on the V of March 1560.

[Signed] Your Excellency's servant

MICHELANGELO BUONARROTI

1. *Tiberio Calcagni (1532–1565), a young Florentine sculptor who studied architecture and worked with Michelangelo during his last years. He it was who redrew the plan mentioned in No. 450. He is described by Vasari as being of 'gentle manners and discreet behaviour' (Vasari, VII, p. 262).*

2. *This letter was drafted and written by someone else and only signed by Michelangelo.*

455

*Buonarroti
Archives
Mil. cccxix
From Rome
March (10th)
1560*

¶ TO LIONARDO DI BUONARROTO SIMONI IN FLORENCE

Lionardo — I've had the red and white chick-peas, the peas and the kidney beans. I am very grateful for them, though I am ill-able to keep Lent, being old as I am. I wrote you some months ago that I should be glad if you would come here and this I re-affirm; that is to say I will expect you at the end of this coming May. If you do not feel like coming or are unable to, let me know.

MICHELANGELO IN ROME

456

*Buonarroti
Archives
Mil. cccxx
From Rome
March (17th)
1560*

¶ TO LIONARDO DI BUONARROTO SIMONI IN FLORENCE

Lionardo — I did not reply to your last letter on Saturday, because I did not have time. I now tell you that I was delighted that you've had a daughter, because as we alone remain it will surely be a good thing to make some good alliance. You must therefore be careful about it, although I shan't be here when that time comes. I wrote about your coming to Rome. I'll let you know when, as I've written you before. Bear in mind that the greatest vexation I have in Rome is having to answer letters.

MICHELANGELO BUONARROTI IN ROME

¶ To Lionardo di Buonarroto Simoni in Florence

457

*Buonarroti
Archives
Mil. cccxxi
From Rome
April 11th
1560*

Lionardo — You write me that you wish to go to Loreto this spring and will pass through Rome. It seems to me that it would be better to go to Loreto first and to pass through Rome on your return. You could stay here for a few days. So write and tell me the day you will be leaving and arrange to be in good company, because it never does any harm. I think that's all. I think you should go before the hot weather.

On the eleventh day of April fifteen hundred and sixty.

Michelangelo Buonarroti in Rome

¶ To the Most Illustrious Duke of Florence

458

*State Archives
Florence
Mil. cdlxxxix
From Rome
April 25th
1560*

Most Illustrious Lord Duke — I have seen the designs of the rooms painted by Messer Giorgio[1] and the model of the Great Hall,[2] together with Messer Bartolomeo's design for the fountain that is to go in the same place.

As regards the picture, it appears to me a thing wonderful to behold, as is everything that is and will be executed under Your Excellency's patronage. As regards the model of the Hall, it seems to me to be rather low as it is; since so much is being spent on it, I think it should be raised by at least 12 *braccia*.[3] As regards the alteration to the Palace, from the designs I have seen it seems to me it could not be better incorporated. As to Messer Bartolomeo's fountain, which is to go in the said Hall, it seems to me a beautiful idea and should succeed admirably; for which reason I pray God He may grant You long life, that You may accomplish these and other things.

As regards the Church of the Florentines here, it grieves me that, being so old and near to death, I am unable to satisfy Your desire in everything. However, while I live I will do what I can. And to You do I commend me. From Rome on the 25th day of April 1560.[4]

Servant of Your Most Illustrious Excellency

Michelangelo Buonarroti

1. *For the alterations to the Palazzo Vecchio undertaken at this time see Vasari, VII, p. 696 et seq.*

2. *The so-called Hall of the Five Hundred.*

3. *It was finally raised by thirteen braccia (Vasari, VII, p. 700).*

4. As in his other letters to the Duke, Michelangelo uses the formal mode of address which cannot be rendered in English. Save for the signature, the letter is in the hand of an unknown writer, who probably added the flourishes. Milanesi suggests that the hand may be that of Daniele Ricciarelli da Volterra (c. 1509–1566), the painter, who was closely associated with Michelangelo at this period. After Michelangelo's death he rented the house in the Macel de' Corvi from Lionardo (Gasparoni, p. 158 et seq.).

459

Buonarroti Archives Mil. cccxxii From Rome May 18th 1560

¶ To Lionardo di Buonarroto Simoni in Florence

Lionardo — From your last letter I learn of your return from Loreto. I was expecting you in Rome on your way back; but I see that you did not get my letter before you left Florence. Now as it turns out, since we are once more at a distance, I think, for several reasons, that it would be better to delay your coming until September and then I will expect you. I think that's all for the present. I go on bearing with old age as best as I can, with all the ills and the impediments it brings with it. I commend me to Him, in Whom is my help.

On the . . . . .[1] day of May.

Michelangelo Buonarroti in Rome

1. *The missing date, as in other letters, is supplied from the endorsement.*

460

Buonarroti Archives Mil. cccxxiii From Rome June 1st 1560

¶ To Lionardo di Buonarroto Simoni in Florence

Lionardo — Since you did not come here on your return from Loreto, as you did not get my letter before you left Florence, it is better to leave it until after the summer, and to come this September. That's all I have to write you at present.

Michelangelo in Rome

¶ To Lionardo di Buonarroto Simoni in Florence

461

*Buonarroti
Archives
Mil. cccxxiv
From Rome
July 27th
1560*

Lionardo — I had a letter of yours a few days ago with the news of the death of your daughter, Lessandra. I was very sorry about it, but I should have been surprised if she had survived, because in our family there is never more than one at a time.[1] We must resign ourselves and take all the more care of the one that remains to us. I think that's all. When the hot weather is over I should like you to come here if you can, as I've written you before, and when you think it's convenient, let me know first.

On the 27th day of July.

MICHELANGELO IN ROME

1. *Presumably a general reflection on the unfruitfulness of the Buonarroti. Cf. No. 444.*

¶ To the Most Illustrious and Most Reverend Lord and Most Worshipful Patron, The Lord Cardinal di Carpi

462

*Buonarroti
Archives
Mil. cdxciii
From Rome
September 13th
1560*

Most Illustrious and Most Reverend Lord and Most Worshipful Patron — Messer Francesco Bandini told me yesterday that Your Most Illustrious and Most Reverend Lordship had told him that the fabric of St. Peter's could not be going worse than it is. This has truly grieved me very much, both because You have not been told the truth, and because I, too, as I must, desire more than all other men that it should go well. But, if I am not mistaken, I can affirm with truth that, as far as the work that is being done at present is concerned, it could not be proceeding better. But since I may perhaps be easily deceived by self-interest and old age and, contrary to my intention, may in consequence, be cause of damage and loss to the aforesaid fabric, I intend, as soon as I can, to ask His Holiness Our Lord for my release. Nay rather, in order to save time, I would entreat Your Most Illustrious and Most Reverend Lordship, as I do, to be pleased to relieve me of this burden, which, as You know, by the commands of the Popes, I have now borne voluntarily and without reward for 17 years.[1] The progress that has been made through my efforts in the above-mentioned fabric during this time is manifest. Returning to the issue, I earnestly beg You to grant me my release, than which for once You could not do me a more singular favour, and with all reverence I humbly kiss the hand of Your Most Illustrious and Most Reverend Lordship.

From my house in Rome on the 13th day of September in 1560.[2]

Your Most Illustrious and Most Reverend Lordship's humble servant

[Unsigned]

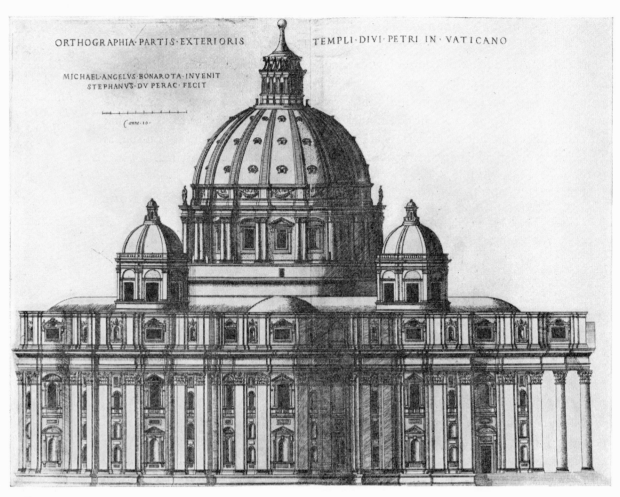

26. *Michelangelo's Project for St. Peter's*

Engraved by Stephan Dupérac
British Museum, London

1. *Apparently a prophetic reckoning. He was never relieved of his office and served for seventeen years in all. After his death his project for the Basilica (Plate 26) was substantially altered for the worse.*

2. *Milanesi's text is from a contemporary copy. The flourishes are clearly not by Michelangelo.*

¶ To Lionardo di Buonarroto Simoni in Florence

463

Lionardo — I wrote you several months ago that I should be glad if you would come here. Now I learn from your letter that it seems to you better to wait until October [sic]. I assure you that 4 months more or less makes no difference. It will therefore be better to delay until the spring, which would be a better time both to come and to return. I think that's all. When it's convenient I'll let you know. On the . . . . day of October 1560.

MICHELANGELO IN ROME

Buonarroti Archives Mil. cccxxv From Rome October (26th) 1560

¶ To Lionardo di Buonarroto Simoni in Florence

464

Lionardo — I had twelve *marzolini* cheeses from you a few days ago; which were excellent and most delicious and for which I thank you. I have not acknowledged them before, because I wasn't able to and because writing, being old as I am, writing [sic] is very irksome to me. I think that's all. As to your coming here now, it's not convenient, because I'm so placed that it would increase my burdens and vexations. When it's convenient I'll let you know.

On the twelfth day of January 15sixty-one.

MICHELANGELO BUONARROTI IN ROME

Buonarroti Archives Mil. cccxxvi From Rome January 12th 1561

¶ To Lionardo di Buonarroto Simoni in Florence

465

Lionardo — I'm expecting you here at Easter. I have not thought it convenient before this. So if it is convenient to you, don't fail.

On the 8th[1] day of February 15sixty-one.

MICHELANGELO IN ROME

Buonarroti Archives Mil. cccxxvii From Rome February 18th 1561

1. *From Lionardo's endorsement it would appear that the letter should have been dated the 18th instead of the 8th, as it was received on February 23rd.*

466

Buonarroti
Archives
Mil. cccxxviii
From Rome
March 22nd
1561

❡ To Lionardo Buonarroti in Florence

Lionardo — I'm expecting you after the festival or when it suits you, because it is not a matter of any importance. Arrange to come in good company, but don't bring anyone with you whom I should have to put up here, because here I have women in the house[1] and few furnishings. You will be able to return to Florence within two or three days, because I'll explain to you in a few words what I have in mind.

On the twenty-second of March one thousand five hundred and sixty-one.

MICHELANGELO BUONARROTI IN ROME

1. Cf. No. 431.

467

Buonarroti
Archives
Mil. cccxxix
From Rome
June 22nd
1561

❡ To Lionardo di Buonarroto Simoni in Florence

Lionardo — I've received to-day, the twenty-second of June, forty-two flasks of *trebbiano* for which I thank you. It is very good. I'll share it with friends. The name of the muleteer is Domenico da Feggine. Thank you for the two caps.[1] I should be glad if you would let me know how Francesca is.

MICHELANGELO IN ROME

1. *Two black sarcenet caps were in his wardrobe, according to the inventory of his effects taken after his death (Gotti, II, p. 149).*

468

British
Museum
Mil. cccxxx
From Rome
July 18th
1561

❡ To Lionardo di Buonarroto Simoni in Florence

Lionardo — I wrote to you acknowledging the *trebbiano* and saying at the end that I should be glad to learn how Francesca is, but I have had no answer.

And now, because I am an old man, as you know, I should like to do something in Florence for the welfare of my soul, that is to say, to give alms, since there is nothing else one can do that I know of. For this purpose I wish to have a certain number of *scudi* made payable in Florence, so that you can go and pay, or rather give in charity where there is most need. The said *scudi* will amount to about three hundred. I have asked Bandino, who is the one who will make them payable for me there, about it, and he replied that within four months he would take them himself.[1] I do not want to delay

Lionardo io ti scrissi lari ciè che desiderei bisogno e ultimamente
comio auero chiaro ditenere come sta la Francesca
e noro no auuto risposta ... ssuna e ora ... io so nechio come
sai uorrei fare costà qualche bene p lanima mia e le
limosine che altro bene no me posso fare m sso se p que
sto uorrei far pagare i firèze una certa quatità di
di scudi che tu ghadassi pagando ouero dando p limosina
doue e maggior bisognio e detti scudi saranno circa
ore cèto scudi o mo ui chiesto il badino cioè che meglio
facci pagare costà ma ui sposto che i fra quatro mesi
gli portera no uoglio i dugiar tato po se ai qua qualche
ami fiorètino a chi io possa dargnieue sicuramète
che togli diapagi costà dame ne auiso e tato faro
e auiserami della ri ceuuta

a di dicio tto di luglio
mille cinque cèto sessantino

Michelagnolo buonarroti
i Roma

as long as that. So if you have some Florentine friend to whom I could safely give them to give to you there, let me know and I'll do this. Advise me of the receipt.

On the eighteenth day of July one thousand fifteen hundred and sixty one.

MICHELANGELO BUONARROTI IN ROME

1. *Why this money could not be remitted in the ordinary way by a bill of exchange remains a mystery.*

469

Buonarroti
Archives
Mil. cccxxxi
From Rome
September 20th
1561

¶ TO LIONARDO DI BUONARROTO SIMONI IN FLORENCE

Lionardo — I would like you to search among the papers of Lodovico, our father, to see whether there is a copy of a contract *in forma Camera*, drawn up in respect of certain figures which I promised to execute for Pope Pius the Second[1] after his death. But because the said work has been suspended, owing to certain differences, for about fifty years now and because I am an old man, I should like to settle up the said matter, so that after me it may not unfairly be a cause of annoyance to you. I think I recall that the notary who drew up the said contract in the Bishop's palace was called Ser Donato Ciampelli. I'm told that all his papers were deposited with Ser Lorenzo Violi. So that if the copy is not found in the house, it could be enquired for from the son[2] of the said Ser Lorenzo and if he has it and the said contract *in forma Camera* is found, don't be particular as to the expense in getting a copy of it.

On the twentieth day of September 1561.

I, MICHELANGELO BUONARROTI

1. *Not Pius II but Pius III (Francesco Piccolomini) who succeeded Alexander VI in 1503. His ponti-ficate lasted only four weeks. The contract of 1501 was ratified by the heirs in 1504 (Milanesi, pp. 615, 616).*

2. *Vincenzio Violi. Michelangelo had received this information in a letter of May 1st from Paolo Panciatichi da Pistoia (Frey, Briefe, p. 382).*

470

Buonarroti
Archives
Mil. cdxciv
From Rome
(November
1561)

¶ [TO THE LORD DEPUTIES OF THE FABRIC OF ST. PETER'S]

Lord Deputies — As I am an old man and as I see that Cesare[1] is so occupied in dis-charging his own office at the fabric that the men often remain without any super-vision, I have thought it necessary to appoint Pierluigi[2] as his colleague, whom I know to be an honest and capable person suited to work at the fabric. Also, because he is accustomed to the work and lives in my house, he can explain to me in the evening what is to be done the next day.

Will Your Lordships authorize the payment of his salary, beginning the first of this month, at the same rate as that paid to Cesare; otherwise I'll pay him out of my own pocket; because, knowing the needs and requirements of the fabric I am determined that he shall be there.

And to Your Lordships do I commend me.[3]

[*Unsigned*]

1. *Cesare Bettini da Castel Durante, one of the overseers of the building work at St. Peter's. He was stabbed to death on August 8th 1563 (Appendix 44 and Daelli, 25).*

2. *Pierluigi Gaeta, who replaced Urbino in Michelangelo's service.*

3. *This copy is written in an unknown hand on the back of a letter from Vasari, dated November 4th 1561.*

¶ To Lionardo di Buonarroto Simoni in Florence   *471*

Lionardo — I've had two of your letters and one from Antonio Maria Piccolomini[1] and a contract. I can't tell you any more, because the Archbishop of Siena has kindly undertaken to arrange this affair and as he is a man of honour and resourceful I believe it will be successfully concluded. I'll let you know what ensues. That's all.

From Rome, on the last day of November.

I, Michelangelo Buonarroti

*Buonarroti
Archives
Mil. cccxxxii
From Rome
November 30th
1561*

1. *The matter was not in fact concluded until after Michelangelo's death. On April 21st 1564 Lionardo repaid the one hundred scudi to the heirs of Pius III, which had been advanced to Michelangelo in respect of the fifteen statues commissioned in 1501 for the Piccolomini chapel in Siena (Tolnay, I, p. 230 and Milanesi, p. 615. Cf. Vol. I, No. 60).*

¶ To Lionardo di Buonarroto Simoni in Florence   *472*

Lionardo — Some years ago I sent you a box of very important documents,[1] so that they might not come to harm, owing to certain risks there were here. It now happens that it would be to my honour and advantage to show them to the Pope.[2] So I should now like you to send them back to me as soon as you can by someone to be trusted; and consign them in any way you like, provided that they are delivered here.

From Rome on the twelfth day of January fifteen hundred and sixty-two.[3]

Michelangelo Buonarroti

*Buonarroti
Archives
Mil. cccxxxiii
From Rome
January 12th
1562*

1. *See No. 298.*

2. *Pius IV. These negotiations concerned the restoration of the income derived from the office of Civil Notary at Rimini, of which he had been deprived on the accession of Paul IV (Vasari, VII, p. 257 and Appendix 33).*

3. *The letter is endorsed by Lionardo, who received it on the 15th, as being written on the 15th, which was clearly a slip for the 12th. It was sent through D[onato] Capponi and is also endorsed in another hand 'Kindly have it delivered'.*

473

Buonarroti Archives Mil. cccxxiv From Rome January 31st 1562

¶ To Lionardo di Buonarroto Simoni in Florence

Lionardo — I've had the box of documents. In it I've found several things relating to the matter, which I want to be able to produce, as I wrote you. I want to have copies made of those I need and then I'll put them back with the others and send them to you. On the last day of January fifteen hundred and sixty-two. From Rome.

I, Michelangelo Buonarroti

474

Buonarroti Archives Mil. cccxxv From Rome February 14th 1562

¶ To Lionardo di Buonarroto Simoni in Florence

Lionardo — I haven't yet sent you back the documents which you sent me, because I haven't been able to do anything about the matter as I wished, owing to the Carnival and to my feeling indisposed. I've had the most cruel pains with the colic; I'm all right now. When I have dealt with the said documents, the copy will do for me and I'll send everything back to you with those I had before. Look after them, because it's useful to keep them at home.

On the fourteenth day of February one thousand five hundred and sixty-two.

I, Michelangelo Buonarroti in Rome

¶ To Lionardo di Buonarroto Simoni in Florence

475

Lionardo — I've had a barrel and three small bags of pulse, red and white chick-peas and green peas, for which I thank you. I think that's all. I've been a trifle unwell with the colic, but it's passed and I'm well enough now.

On the twentieth day of February one thousand five hundred and sixty-two.

I, Michelangelo

Buonarroti Archives Mil. cccxxxvi From Rome February 20th 1562

¶ [To Lionardo di Buonarroto Simoni in Florence]

476

Dearest Nephew[1] — This is to inform you that I have received the *trebbiano*, amounting to 43 flasks, which has been, as usual, very welcome to me. Don't be surprised if I don't write to you myself, because I'm an old man, as you know, and I cannot endure the fatigue of writing. I'm well and hoping the same of all of you. Pray to God for me. If Cassandra has a son, give him the name of Buonarroto; if it is a daughter, give her the name Francesca. I've no more to write. May the Lord God guard you from harm and me together with you. From Rome on the 27th day of June 1562.

[*signed*] Michelangelo Buonarroti

Buonarroti Archives Mil. cccxxxvii From Rome June 27th 1562

1. *Phrased by the amanuensis.*

¶ To Lionardo di Buonarroto Simoni in Florence

477

Lionardo — I've received the cloth through Simon del Bernia, the muleteer. Thank you. As to your coming to Rome, it would do nothing but add vexations to my worries for the time being. I think that's all. On the last day of January of sixty 3.

Michelangelo in Rome

Buonarroti Archives Mil. cccxxxviii From Rome January 31st 1563

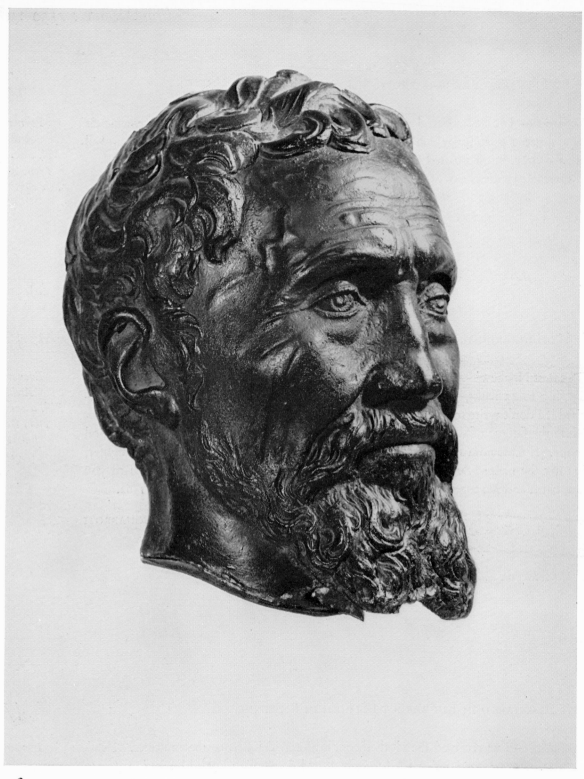

28. Michelangelo

Attributed to Daniele Ricciarelli da Volterra
Ashmolean Museum, Oxford

¶ To Lionardo di Buonarroto Simoni in Florence

478

*Buonarroti
Archives
Mil. cccxxxix
From Rome
June 25th
1563*

On the 25th day of June 1563

Lionardo — I've received the *trebbiano* and other letters of yours and of Francesca's. I haven't replied before, because I can't use my hand to write; I said the same to his lordship, the Duke's ambassador.[1] Thank you for the letter from Messer Giorgio; make my apologies to Messer Giorgio, because I'm an old man. To you do I commend me.

I, Michelangelo Buonarroti

1. *Averardo d'Antonio Serristori (1497–1569). He had been the Duke's ambassador in Rome since the time of Paul III (Mecatti, p. 213). The date of his death is incorrectly given as 1566 by Mecatti. See Serristori, p. xx.*

¶ To Lionardo di Buonarroto Simoni in Florence

479

*Buonarroti
Archives
Mil. cccxl
From Rome
August 21st
1563*

Lionardo — I see from your letter that you are lending credence to certain envious rascals who, being unable either to manage me or to rob me, write you a pack of lies. They are a lot of sharks and you are such a fool as to lend credence to them about my affairs, as if I were an infant. Spurn them as envious, scandalmongering, low-living rascals.

As regards allowing myself to be looked after, about which you write me, and about the other thing – I tell you, as to being looked after, I could not be better off; neither could I be more faithfully treated and looked after in every way. As regards my being robbed, which I believe you mean, I assure you I don't need to worry about the people I have in the house, whom I can rely upon. Therefore look after yourself and don't worry about my affairs, because I know how to look after myself, if I need to, and I am not an infant.[1] Farewell.

From Rome on the 21st day of August 1563.[2]

Michelangelo

1. *The head attributed to Daniele Ricciarelli (Plate 28) shows Michelangelo as he appeared at the end of his life. The problem presented by the various existing heads and busts, which has been fully discussed by Paul Garnault, is a vexed one and has never been finally resolved.*

2. *This letter is endorsed in another hand 'To Jacopo Buonsigniori, please deliver'.*

480

*Buonarroti
Archives
Mil. cccxli
From Rome
December 28th
1563*

¶ To Lionardo di Buonarroto Simoni in Florence

Lionardo — I had your last letter with twelve most excellent and delicious *marzolini* cheeses, for which I thank you. I'm delighted at your well-being; the same is true of me. Having received several letters of yours recently and not having replied, I have omitted to do so, because I can't use my hand to write; therefore from now on I'll get others to write and I'll sign. I think that's all. From Rome on the 28th Day of December 1563.

I, Michelangelo Buonarroti

DRAFTS
7 - 11

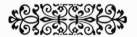

From Rome
1540 - 1555

Drafts 7-11. From Rome : 1540-1555

¶ To Messer Salvestro da Montaguto in Rome

Draft 7

Biblioteca
Nazionale
Florence
Mil. cdlii
From Rome
(February)
1545

Magnificent Messer Salvestro da Montaguto and Partners of Rome *per l'adrieto e per loro*[1] Antonio Covoni and Partners — Of the payment for the three marble figures done, or rather finished by Raffaello da Montelupo, sculptor, there remains on deposit with you a hundred and seventy *scudi* in silver, that is, at ten julians each. And the said Raffaello, having finished the figures as stated and set them up at San Piero in Vincola in the Tomb of Pope Julius, will you be pleased to pay him, at his convenience, as his last payment, the above-mentioned one hundred and seventy *scudi*; because he has done all that was required of him respecting the said three figures – that is, Our Lady with the Child in her arms, a Prophet and a Sibyl, all over life size.[2]

YOUR MICHELANGELO BUONARROTI IN ROME

1. *The meaning of this phrase remains obscure.*
2. *Draft of No. 248.*

¶ To Giovan Simone di Lodovico Buonarroti in Florence

Draft 8

Buonarroti
Archives
Mil. cxxxiii
From Rome
(1540/47)

Giovan Simone — I have had several letters from Ser Giovan Francesco about your illness which greatly distresses me; and still more so as I am not there to be able to help you, as I have always endeavoured to do. However, I'll do what I can and will endeavour to see that you do not want for anything.

With this letter I'm now sending you ten *scudi*, and again I promise you that while I am here I will not let you want for anything I can send you in future. So cheer up and try to get well and do not think of anything else. Because when you are in want, I shall be too; since, as I see it, goods endure longer than men. I think that's all. Commend yourself to God, because He can help you better than I can, and get someone to write and tell me what you need when the occasion arises.[1]

MICHELANGELO IN ROME

1. *Though this is not a draft, but the letter itself, it has been placed among the drafts because it is undatable. See The Dating and Sequence of the Letters.*

Draft 9   ¶ To Giovan Francesco, priest in Santa Maria in Florence

*Biblioteca
Nazionale
Florence
Mil. cdlxiv
From Rome
(March) 1547*

Messer Giovan Francesco — As it is some time since I've written to you and in order to prove to you by this that I'm still alive, and in order to learn from a letter of yours the same of you, I'm writing these few lines. I commend me to you and beg you to see that the enclosed letter reaches Messer Benedetto Varchi, the light and splendour of the Florentine Academy.[1] Give it to him and thank him on my behalf better than I am doing or can do. I think that's all. Write to me about something.

Overwhelmed with grief as I am,[2] I have been at home lately and among some of my things I found a great number of these things,[3] which I used to send you, of which I'm sending you four – I may perhaps have sent them before.[4]

YOUR MICHELANGELO BUONARROTI IN ROME

1. *Cf. Volume I, Draft 4, n. 3.*

2. *Vittoria Colonna had died in February and Luigi del Riccio four months previously.*

3. *i.e. his sonnets and madrigals.*

4. *Draft of No. 281.*

Draft 10   ¶ [To Benvenuto Cellini]

*Published
Source
Mil. cdlxxi
From Rome
(1550)*

My Benvenuto — I've recognized you for many years as the greatest goldsmith of whom we have ever heard, and now I shall recognize you equally as a sculptor. I must tell you that Messer Bindo Altoviti took me to see a portrait head of his in bronze[1] and he told me that it was by your hand. It pleased me very much, but I only regret that it had been placed in a bad light, because if it had been given its proper light, it would be seen to be the beautiful work it is.[2]

1. *This bust is now in the Gardner Museum, Boston, U.S.A. It was executed in 1550.*

2. *This letter, which Benvenuto Cellini quotes in his autobiography as being part of a letter which he received from Michelangelo, is known only in this version. Venturi thinks that it may be spurious (X, pt. 2, p. 471). For the probable date of the letter see The Dating and Sequence of the Letters.*

¶ [To Messer Giorgio Vasari in Florence]

Draft
11

*Vatican Codex
Frey ccxxiii (b)
From Rome
September 26th
1555*

. . . The middle oval section I intend for the master, the side sections for the servants going to see the library. The returns of the said wings from half-way up to the landing of the staircase are attached to the wall. From the middle down to the paved floor the said staircase is detached from the wall by about four *palmi*, so that the entrance of the vestibule is not encroached upon and allows free passage. I seem to have dreamt something like this and rely on you to serve your Lord Duke and *[on]* Messer Bartolomeo to find a means of doing the said staircase other than mine.

On the first day of January 1554.

On the 26th day of September 1555.[1]

---

1. *'1555' is added in an unknown hand. See The Dating and Sequence of the Letters. For other versions of the letter about the design of the staircase of the Laurentian Library, see Nos. 406, 448. This draft is published by Karl Frey in his edition of Vasari's 'Carteggio' (Lit. I, p. 420).*

The Dating and Sequence of
the Letters

The Dating and Sequence of the Letters

The problem of assigning correct or approximate dates to misdated, partially dated or un-dated letters has already been discussed in the first volume. In this second volume the same method has been adopted where Milanesi's dating has proved to be unacceptable.

Two additional letters *(Nos. 342 and 399)* and one Draft *(Draft 11)*, which were apparently unknown to Milanesi, have here been included.

Sequence of Letters the dates of which have been emended

Any date or any part of a date that is in doubt has been shown in brackets.

200	Assumed	. . . . *(1537)* . . . . —	. . . . —
	Milanesi	. . . . *(1540)* . . . . —	. . . . —

This letter cannot be accurately dated, but a date earlier than 1540 is to be pre-ferred for two reasons: *(i)* Michelangelo was remitting ducats, not *scudi (see Appendix 3)*. *(ii)* His reference to his nephew, Lionardo, who was born in 1519, suggests some-one younger than twenty-one. But while it has been placed here for convenience, it may well belong to a somewhat earlier date.

201	Assumed	. . . . *(1538/9)* . . . *(Winter)*	. . . . —
	Milanesi	. . . . *(1545)* . . . . —	. . . . —
202	Assumed	. . . . *(1539)* . . . . *(Spring)*	. . . . —
	Milanesi	. . . . *(1545)* . . . . —	. . . . —

For the arguments in favour of redating these letters see Appendix 26.

203	Assumed	. . . . 1540 . . . . *July*	. . . . *(10th/17th)*
	Milanesi	. . . . *(1540)* . . . . *(July)*	. . . . —

The seven hundred and fifty *scudi* to redeem the farm at Pazzolatica were sent on Saturday, August 7th *(No. 204)*. In this letter of his to Lionardo *(No. 203)* Michelangelo says he will be sending money in two or three weeks time, so that it must have been written either on Saturday (the day of the week on which he usually wrote letters), July 10th or on Saturday, July 17th. The letter is endorsed 'Assumption' (August 15th) presumably the day on which the money was received.

205	Ascertained	1540	September	. . . . 25th
	Milanesi	(1540)	—	. . . . —
206	Ascertained	1540	November	. . . . 13th
	Milanesi	(1540)	(November)	. . . . —
207	Corrected	1540	December	. . . . 18th
	Milanesi	(1541)	—	. . . . —

The full dating of these letters is derived from the endorsements.

208	Assumed	(1541)	(March)	. . . . —
	Milanesi	(1545)	(January)	. . . . —

From the formality of its style this letter must belong to the early years of Michelangelo's correspondence with Luigi del Riccio. It cannot be as late as 1545. A few months before he completed *The Last Judgment* Michelangelo fell from the scaffolding and injured his leg. He was attended on this occasion by the Florentine physician, Bartolomeo Rontini, mentioned in the letter. Reference is made to Rontini's care of Michelangelo in Niccolò Martelli's letter to Rontini of April 10th 1541 *(Martelli, 10v)*.

210	Corrected	1541	August	. . . . 20th
	Milanesi	1541	August	. . . . 25th

Lionardo's endorsement '1541. From Rome 25th August' is presumably the date of reception. Saturday, August 20th, may therefore be accepted as the date on which the letter was written.

214	Corrected	. . . .	1542	. . . .	May	. . . .	—
	Milanesi	. . . .	*(1542)*	. . . .	*(July)*	. . . .	—

The contract referred to in this letter is dated May 16th *(Milanesi, p. 710)*. It was cancelled however in favour of another dated June 1st. The letter therefore belongs not to July but to the second half of May.

215	Assumed	. . . .	*(1542)*	. . . .	*(May)*	. . . .	—
	Milanesi	. . . .	*(1542)*	. . . .	—	. . . .	—
216	Assumed	. . . .	*(1542)*	. . . .	*(May/June)*	. . . .	—
	Milanesi	. . . .	*(1542)*	. . . .	—	. . . .	—
217	Assumed	. . . .	*(1542)*	. . . .	*(May/June)*	. . . .	—
	Milanesi	. . . .	*(1542)*	. . . .	—	. . . .	—

For the tentative dating of these letters to May/June 1542 see Appendix 29.

220	Assumed	. . . .	1542	. . . .	*(July/August)*	. . . .	—
	Milanesi	. . . .	*(1542)*	. . . .	—	. . . .	—

The documents mentioned in this note were those connected with the contract for the Tomb of Julius II *(Appendix 28)*.

222	Ascertained	. . . .	1542	. . . .	August	. . . .	30th
	Milanesi	. . . .	*(1542)*	. . . .	—	. . . .	—

Luigi del Riccio had sent Michelangelo a note on August 29th asking him to dinner on the same evening *(Frey, Dicht., p. 530)*. Michelangelo was unable to attend for the reasons given in this note of apology which he wrote the next day.

223	Assumed	. . . .	*(1542)*	. . . .	*(August/September)*	.	—
	Milanesi	. . . .	*(1542)*	. . . .	—	. . . .	—

There seems no reason to dispute Frey's conjectural assignment of this note to August/September 1542 *(Frey, Dicht., p. 530)*.

224   *Assumed*   ....   *1542*   ....   *(September)*   ....   —

       Milanesi   ....   *(1542)* ....   —   ....   —

The last contract for the Tomb of Julius II was drawn up on August 20th 1542. In this note Michelangelo refers to the non-arrival of the expected ratification. But he does so without alarm. We may therefore suppose that the note was written some time in September.

228   *Corrected*   ....   *1542*   ....   *November*   ....   —

       Milanesi   ....   *(1542)* ....   *(October)*   ....   —

According to the Duke of Urbino's letter to his envoy Girolamo Tiranno, his emissary, Girolamo Genga, left Urbino for Rome shortly after November 11th *(Vasari, VII, Prosp. Chron., p. 388)*.

229   *Corrected*   ....   *1542*   ....   *November*   ....   —

       Milanesi   ....   *(1542)* ....   *(October)*   ....   —

This letter, which follows No. 228, also belongs to November and not to October.

232   *Ascertained* ....   *1543*   ....   *April*   ....   *(28th)*

       Milanesi   ....   *(1543)* ....   *(March)*   ....   —

This letter follows the dated letter of April 14th *(No. 231)* and cannot therefore have been written in March.

233   *Assumed*   ....   *1543*   ....   *(May)*   ....   *(12th)*

       Milanesi   ....   *(1543)* ....   *(April)*   ....   —

This letter follows that of April 28th *(No. 232)*. It is the last letter dealing with the subject of the missing contract and from a calculation of the time taken to exchange the relevant letters between Florence and Rome would appear to have been written on Saturday, May 12th.

234	Corrected	. . . .	1544	. . . .	February	. . . .	—
	Milanesi	. . . .	*(1545)*	. . . .	*(January)*	. . . .	*(26th)*

In dating this letter, like the following one, to 1545, Milanesi was evidently under the impression that 1544 was an *ab Incarnatione* reckoning of the year, which it was not. Donato Giannotti's sonnet, *Messer Luigi mio, di noi che sia, (Frey, Dicht., p. 269),* was written in honour of Cecchino de' Bracci, who died on January 8th 1544. Giannotti's note to Messer Luigi del Riccio asking him to show the sonnet to Michelangelo is dated January 30th 1544. This note of Michelangelo's in reply must therefore be assigned to February 1544.

235	Assumed	. . . .	1544	. . . .	*(February)*	. . . .	—
	Milanesi	. . . .	*(1545)*	. . . .	—	. . . .	—

As this note accompanied the epigram No. 8 *(Guasti, p. 7)* in the series of forty-eight which Michelangelo wrote for Luigi del Riccio, it has been assigned to the early part of 1544.

239	Assumed	. . . .	*(1544)*	. . . .	*(July/August)*	. . . .	—
	Milanesi	. . . .	*(1545)*	. . . .	—	. . . .	—

This note, accompanying epigram No. 28 in the Magliabechiano Codex *(Guasti, p. 13)* probably belongs to the weeks immediately following Michelangelo's return to his own house after his illness in the summer of 1544, when he had been nursed by Luigi del Riccio in the Strozzi Palace. Steinmann assigns it to July/August 1544 *(p. 39).* The mention of melons suggests the early part of August at the latest, as melons were to be had in Rome from July onwards *(Cartwright, II, p. 221)* and would have been a delicacy earlier rather than later in the season.

240	Assumed	. . . .	*(1544)*	. . . .	*(August)*	. . . .	—
	Milanesi	. . . .	*(1543)*	. . . .	—	. . . .	—

There are no means of dating this note precisely, but for two reasons 1544 seems more likely than 1543. *(i)* At this period *(i.e.* in 1544) Michelangelo was in the habit of acknowledging his indebtedness to Luigi del Riccio for gifts and services of one kind or another in a few lines of verse which he referred to as *berlingozzi* or trifles *(Guasti, p. 19).* *(ii)* Though the Bishop, Federico Cesi, might have sent Michelangelo a gift (apparently a delicacy which he proposed to share with del Riccio) at any time, some period not long after his recovery from the illness which had alarmed the whole of Rome, would seem not unlikely.

244	Assumed	. . . .	(1545)	. . . .	(January)	. . . .	—
	Milanesi	. . . .	(1546)	. . . .	—	. . . .	—

For the arguments in favour of dating this letter January 1545 see Appendix 27, pt. III.

245	Assumed	. . . .	1545	. . . .	January	. . . .	(10th)
	Milanesi	. . . .	(1545)	. . . .	(January)	. . . .	—

The letter is endorsed '1544 *[N.S. 1545]* from Rome received on the 16th day of January'. Saturday, January 10th was therefore almost certainly the date of writing.

246	Assumed	. . . .	1545	. . . .	(January)	. . . .	—
	Milanesi	. . . .	(1545)	. . . .	—	. . . .	—

The fire to which this letter refers, which damaged the roof of the Sistine Chapel (not the Pauline, as stated by Milanesi) broke out on the night of December 31st 1544. This letter therefore presumably belongs to January 1545.

249	Assumed	. . . .	(1545)	. . . .	(February)	. . . .	—
	Milanesi	. . . .	1545	. . . .	—	. . . .	—

For the argument in favour of dating this letter February 1545 see Appendix 27, pt. II.

250	Assumed	. . . .	(1545)	. . . .	(February)	. . . .	(14th)
	Milanesi	. . . .	(1545)	. . . .	—	. . . .	—

The date of this letter cannot be determined with certainty. Frey *(Dicht., p. 445)* advances arguments in favour of assigning it to 1546, when Ash Wednesday fell on March 10th. But in view of the fact that Luigi del Riccio left Rome for Venice a few days later, his cousin Francesco del Riccio's letter which refers to his departure being dated March 13th *(Steinmann, p. 61)*, it seems highly improbable that Michelangelo would have attempted to postpone the proposed outing. As Ash Wednesday fell on February 18th in 1545 and as Luigi was apparently in the habit of seeing Michelangelo on Sundays *(Steinmann, op. cit., p. 55)* the most probable date for this communication is Saturday, February 14th.

251	Ascertained	. . . .	1545	. . . .	February	. . . .	*(14th)*
	Milanesi	. . . .	1545	. . . .	February	. . . .	*(15th)*

Lionardo's endorsement gives February 20th as the date of receipt. Allowing the usual five days Milanesi dated the letter February 15th. As Michelangelo normally wrote letters on Saturday, February 14th (see above) is probably the correct date.

253	Ascertained	. . . .	1545	. . . .	April	. . . .	*(4th)*
	Milanesi	. . . .	*(1545)*	. . . .	*(April)*	. . . .	*(5th)*

The same argument as that advanced for No. 251 holds good.

256	Ascertained	. . . .	1545	. . . .	July	. . . .	4th
	Milanesi	. . . .	*(1545)*	. . . .	July	. . . .	—

From Luigi del Riccio's letters to Lionardo *(Steinmann, p. 53)* we know that the *trebbiano* arrived on Friday, June 26th. Michelangelo appears to have acknowledged its receipt on Saturday, June 27th. This letter refers to the previous letter and may accordingly be assigned to the following Saturday, July 4th.

257	Assumed	. . . .	*(1545)*	. . . .	*(Summer)*	. . . .	—
	Milanesi	. . . .	*(1545)*	. . . .	—	. . . .	—
258	Assumed	. . . .	*(1545)*	. . . .	*(Autumn)*	. . . .	—
	Milanesi	. . . .	*(1545)*	. . . .	—	. . . .	—

Neither of these letters can be dated precisely. On the assumption that both are connected with Luigi del Riccio's visit to Lyons some time between July and December 1545 they have been assigned to this period. The first *(No. 257)* appears to deal with the appointment of someone to look after Michelangelo's affairs during del Riccio's absence. The second is almost equally enigmatic and may have been addressed to del Riccio while he was in Lyons, where Roberto Strozzi and Giuliano de' Medici were resident. As to the dates – there is a lacuna in del Riccio's correspondence with Lionardo between July 11th 1545 and January 9th 1546 *(Steinmann, p. 57)* while Donato Giannotti (who is mentioned in No. 257) can be presumed to have been absent from Rome between July 14th and the end of October 1545 with his patron, Cardinal Ridolfi, who was at Bagnaia during this period *(Giannotti, Lettere, p. 22)*. For a different conclusion as to the date, see *Frey, Dicht., p. 362.*

259	*Assumed*	. . . .	1545	. . . .	*(November)*	. . . .	—
	Milanesi	. . . .	*(1545)*	. . . .	*(December)*	. . . .	—

If this letter had been sent to Lyons and returned to Rome by December 22nd it must have been written in November since the time allowed for the couriers from Florence to Venice and back was about three weeks *(Staley, p. 188)*, so that an even longer period must be allowed between Lyons and Rome.

263	*Assumed*	. . . .	1546	. . . .	*February*	. . . .	*(13th)*
	Milanesi	. . . .	*(1546)*	. . . .	*(February)*	. . . .	*(15th)*

This letter is endorsed with the date of reception only, February 20th. As it is extremely unlikely that Michelangelo wrote on the Monday, it has been here dated Saturday, February 13th.

273	*Corrected*	. . . .	1546	. . . .	*December*	. . . .	31st
	Milanesi	. . . .	*(1545)*	. . . .	*(December)*	. . . .	31st

The 1545 date accepted by Milanesi is an *ab Incarnatione* dating and therefore requires the adjustment to 1546. In any case this letter is related to No. 275.

274	*Assumed*	. . . .	*(1547)*	. . . .	*(January)*	. . . .	—
	Milanesi	. . . .	*(1555)*	. . . .	—	. . . .	—

For the dating of this letter see Appendix 36.

278 Ascertained . . . . *1547* . . . . March *26th*

   Milanesi . . . . *(1547)* . . . . *(March)* . . . . —

   The date has been completed from the endorsement.

279 Corrected . . . . *1547* . . . . *(March)* . . . . —

&

280 *Milanesi* . . . . *(1549)* . . . . — . . . . —

   For the redating of these letters see Appendix 37.

281 Corrected . . . . *1547* . . . . *(March)* . . . . —

   Milanesi . . . . *(1549)* . . . . — . . . . —

   This letter is related to Nos. 279 and 280.

282 Corrected . . . . *1547* . . . . April *29th*

   Milanesi . . . . *(1546)* . . . . April *29th*

   The year is corrected from the endorsement. In any case the contents of the letter relate to 1547 and not to 1546.

283 Assumed . . . . *(1547)* . . . . *(May)* . . . . *(14th)*

   Milanesi . . . . *(1547)* . . . . — . . . . —

   The endorsement, in so far as Lionardo's almost indecipherable hand may be deciphered, appears to read 'Received on the 21st'. Having regard to the contents and date of No. 284, the letter must therefore be assigned to Saturday, May 14th.

284 Ascertained . . . . *1547* . . . . June *18th*

   Milanesi . . . . *(1547)* . . . . — . . . . —

285 Ascertained . . . . *1547* . . . . July *30th*

   Milanesi . . . . *(1547)* . . . . *(July)* . . . . —

   The dates have been completed from the endorsements.

287	Corrected	....	1547	....	September	....	3rd
	Milanesi	....	(1547)	....	(August)	....	—
289	Ascertained	....	1547	....	October	....	1st
	Milanesi	....	(1547)	....	—	....	—
290	Ascertained	....	1547	....	October	....	15th
	Milanesi	....	(1547)	....	—	....	—
291	Corrected	....	1547	....	October	....	22nd
	Milanesi	....	(1548)	....	(March)	....	—
292	Ascertained	....	1547	....	November	....	5th
	Milanesi	....	(1547)	....	—	....	—
293	Ascertained	....	1547	....	November	....	12th
	Milanesi	....	(1547)	....	—	....	—
294	Ascertained	....	1547	....	November	....	19th
	Milanesi	....	(1547)	....	—	....	—
295	Corrected	....	1547	....	December	....	3rd
	Milanesi	....	(1546)	....	(December)	....	—
300	Ascertained	....	1548	....	January	....	28th
	Milanesi	....	(1548)	....	(January)	....	—
301	Ascertained	....	1548	....	February	....	4th
	Milanesi	....	(1548)	....	(February)	....	—

All these dates have been completed and where necessary corrected from the endorsements.

| 302 | Ascertained | .... | 1548 | .... | February | .... | 18th |
| | Milanesi | .... | (1548) | .... | (February) | .... | 23rd |

A close examination of this almost indecipherable endorsement reveals February

18th to have been the date of writing and February 24th (or possibly 23rd) as the date of the receipt. Milanesi's copyist evidently took the figure which he read as 23 to be the date of writing. As the 18th was a Saturday, the 18th may be accepted as correct.

309	Assumed	....	1548	....	*(July)*	....	—
	Milanesi	....	*(1541)*	....	—	....	—

This letter, which is not endorsed, cannot belong to 1541, as the shop to which it refers was not bought until April 1548 *(No. 304)*. In his letter of June 1548 *(No. 308)* Michelangelo had enquired about the shop and having received a reply, he here proceeds to comment on it. The letter may therefore very well be assigned to July.

315	Assumed	....	*(1548/1549)*	.	—	....	—
	Milanesi	....	*(1560)*	....	—	....	—

The date of this letter is a matter of conjecture, but an earlier rather than a later date during the time that Michelangelo was responsible for the work at St. Peter's is to be preferred for the following reasons: *(i)* From the building accounts *(Frey, Jahrbuch, 1916, p. 23)* we know that Jacopo Balducci, the contractor mentioned in the letter, was employed in 1548/9. *(ii)* The terms of the letter suggest the beginning of Michelangelo's stewardship and a time prior to the brief of October 1549 which granted him absolute powers. The handwriting suggests an earlier rather than a later date.

322	Assumed	....	1549	....	*(March)*	....	*(2nd)*
	Milanesi	....	*(1549)*	....	*(August)*	....	—

The reference to the 'Ginori daughters' dates this letter to the spring of 1549. The letter was received on March 8th and would therefore have been written on the previous Saturday.

335	Assumed	....	1549	....	June	....	*(22nd)*
	Milanesi	....	*(1549)*	....	*(June)*	....	*(15th)*
336	Assumed	....	1549	....	July	....	*(6th)*
	Milanesi	....	*(1549)*	....	*(July)*	....	*(12th)*

338	Assumed	. . . .	1549	. . . .	August	. . . .	(9th)
	Milanesi	. . . .	(1549)	. . . .	(August)	. . . .	(3rd)
339	Assumed	. . . .	1549	. . . .	August	. . . .	(23rd)
	Milanesi	. . . .	(1549)	. . . .	(August)	. . . .	(18th)
340	Assumed	. . . .	1549	. . . .	September	. . . .	(7th)
	Milanesi	. . . .	(1549)	. . . .	(August)	. . . .	25th

These endorsements are very difficult to decipher, but the amended dates appear to be correct – Lionardo's handwriting notwithstanding.

| 343 | Corrected | . . . . | 1550 | . . . . | February | . . . . | (15th/16th) |
| | Milanesi | . . . . | (1549) | . . . . | (October) | . . . . | — |

How Milanesi came to date this letter October 1549 is a question impossible to answer, seeing that the new Pope, Julius III, was not elected until February 8th 1550. The following Sunday (*Cf. No. 344*) would therefore seem a likely date for it.

| 346 | Corrected | . . . . | 1550 | . . . . | June | . . . . | 21st |
| | Milanesi | . . . . | (1545) | . . . . | — | . . . . | — |

The correct date is supplied from the endorsement, but in any case it can only be after Michelangelo's dangerous attack of the stone in 1549 that he can have been prohibited from drinking wine.

| 358 | Assumed | . . . . | (1550) | . . . . | (December) | . . . . | — |
| | Milanesi | . . . . | (1560) | . . . . | — | . . . . | — |

For the assumed date of this letter see Appendix 42.

| 372 | Ascertained | . . . . | 1552 | . . . . | October | . . . . | 22nd |
| | Milanesi | . . . . | (1552) | . . . . | (October) | . . . . | — |

From the endorsement this letter would appear to have been received on November 7th or 9th (these figures being indistinguishable in Lionardo's hand), while No. 373, which was written on October 28th is endorsed '1552 from Rome on the 28th day of October from the 22nd of the said month', which makes no sense at all. It is therefore obvious that Lionardo endorsed both letters after the arrival of the second and confused the two. No. 372, which was written on October 22nd should have been endorsed 'received on October 28th' and No. 373, which was written on October 28th, should have been endorsed with the November date.

375	*Assumed*	. . . .	*1552*	. . . .	*November*	. . . .	*(19th)*
	Milanesi	. . . .	*(1552)*	. . . .	*(November)*	. . . .	*(21st)*

As it is extremely unlikely that Michelangelo wrote on a Monday (November 21st) this letter has been dated Saturday, November 19th.

399	*Assumed*	. . . .	*(1555)*	. . . .	*(May)*	. . . .	*(11th)*
	Guasti	. . . .	—	. . . .	—	. . . .	—

This note is written under the sonnet *Le favole del mondo m' hanno tolto*, the other sonnet referred to, *Non è più bassa o vil cosa terrena*, being written overleaf *(Guasti, pp. 232, 234)*. The original autograph, which was discovered in the Rasponi Spinelli Archives, in 1908 and is now in the Casa Vasari, Arezzo, was not known to Guasti when he published the *Rime* in 1863. The text used by him was a copy in the Anonimo collection. On the ground that there is in the Casa Buonarroti a copy in Lionardo's hand of the two sonnets, together with the letter to Vasari of May 11th 1555 *(No. 398)* which Michelangelo had enclosed in a letter to Lionardo of May 10th *(No. 397)* Frey assumed that this note to Vasari was also enclosed and must therefore be dated May 11th 1555, so that under one cover the post of Saturday May 11th, addressed to Lionardo, comprised two letters, two sonnets and one note *(Frey, Dicht., p. 488 and Lit., I, p. 408)*. As there is nothing to contradict this argument, Frey's conjectural dating may be accepted.

406	*Corrected*	. . . .	*1555*	. . . .	*September*	. . . .	*28th*
	Milanesi	. . . .	*1558*	. . . .	*September*	. . . .	*28th*

If the autograph of this letter is extant it has not been traced. Milanesi's text is based on a misdated version published by Bottari *(I, p. 4)*. The accepted date is that given by Vasari in his published text of the letter *(Vasari, VII, p. 237)*. A partial draft of it is preserved in the Vatican Codex *(Draft 11)*.

428	Corrected	. . . .	1557	. . . .	January	. . . .	16th
	Milanesi	. . . .	1557	. . . .	December	. . . .	16th

This letter is endorsed in Lionardo's hand '1556 *(O.S.)* from Rome, received on the 22nd day of January from the 16th day of the said *[month]*'. As Michelangelo was very uncertain about dates at this period, we may be confident, in view of the endorsement, that he wrote 'December' when he should have written 'January'.

431	Corrected	. . . .	1557	. . . .	April	. . . .	28th
	Milanesi	. . . .	(1557)	. . . .	March	. . . .	28th

Cornelia Colonelli, Urbino's widow, had written to Michelangelo on April 25th. He received the letter on April 27th and replied on the following day. To this letter Cornelia replied on May 10th. As there can be no doubt about this sequence of letters, Michelangelo's date of March 28th must be a slip for April 28th *(Frey, Briefe, p. 353)*.

434	Ascertained	. . . .	1557	. . . .	May	. . . .	(22nd)
	Milanesi	. . . .	(1557)	. . . .	(May)	. . . .	—

This letter is a reply to Vasari's of May 8th, on receipt of which Vasari sent it to the Duke to read on May 30th. Saturday, May 22nd, would therefore appear to be the date of Michelangelo's letter. Cf. *Frey, Lit., I, p. 477 et seq.*

437	Corrected	. . . .	1557	. . . .	July	. . . .	1st
	Milanesi	. . . .	(1557)	. . . .	(August)	. . . .	17th

This letter to Vasari was enclosed in Michelangelo's letter to Lionardo of July 1st *(No. 436)*.

440	Assumed	. . . .	1557	. . . .	(September)	. . . .	(25th)
	Milanesi	. . . .	1557	. . . .	(September)	. . . .	—

From the terms of the letter Milanesi assumed that it was written shortly after the flooding in Florence and in Rome, which occurred on September 13th and 15th respectively. The letter is not endorsed, but Saturday, September 25th, would seem a not unlikely date for it.

446	Corrected	....	1559	....	January	....	7th
	Milanesi	....	1560	....	January	....	7th
447	Corrected	....	1559	....	January	....	14th
	Milanesi	....	1560	....	January	....	14th

On December 16th 1558 *(No. 445)* Michelangelo wrote to Lionardo saying that he had made a rough model of the staircase for the Laurentian Library and asked him to find out from Bartolomeo Ammanati by whom he should send it. In this letter of January 7th of the following year he wrote saying he was about to send it, and on January 14th that he has sent it. No. 446 is not endorsed, but No. 447 is endorsed '1559 on the 23rd day of January from the said 14th day'. Milanesi therefore automatically made what he assumed to be the necessary adjustment as between the Old Style dating and the New, supposing, not unnaturally, that both Michelangelo and Lionardo were using the Florentine system, whereas Michelangelo was in fact using the Roman system, as he generally did, and by some aberration the Roman dating was copied by Lionardo. In view of the sequence of the letters *(Nos. 445–448)* no other conclusion is possible. A whole year could not have elapsed between the making of the model and its despatch.

452	Assumed	....	(1559)	....	(December)	....	(23rd)
	Milanesi	....	(1559)	....	(December)	....	—

Milanesi's assumption that this undated note, which is not endorsed, belongs to December is almost certainly correct, in which case Saturday 23rd can likewise be assumed to be correct.

463	Assumed	....	1560	....	October	....	(26th)
	Milanesi	....	(1560)	....	(October)	....	(27th)

October 26th fell on a Saturday, the more probable date of writing.

Drafts, fragments and undatable letters

Draft   Undatable   . . . .   *(1540/47)* . .   —   . . . .   —

  8   *Milanesi*   . . . .   *(1547)* . . . .   —   . . . .   —

This letter is undatable. On the grounds that Giovansimone died in January 1548 Milanesi tentatively assigned it to 1547. For several reasons this assumption seems untenable. *(i)* Giovansimone was frequently ill and there seems to be no reason to relate this indisposition to his last illness. *(ii)* There is no mention of Giovansimone in Michelangelo's letters to Lionardo at this time. *(iii)* The news of the illness referred to had been conveyed to Michelangelo by Fattucci and not by Lionardo. *(iv)* The general terms of the letter suggest an earlier date than 1547. It cannot, however, be much earlier than 1540, as *scudi* and not *ducati* are mentioned *(Appendix 3)*. As the letter may well have been written at any time from about 1540 onwards and belongs to no sequence, it seemed better to exclude it from the main series.

Draft   Corrected   . . . .   *1547*   . . . .   *(March)*   . . . .   —

  9   *Milanesi*   . . . .   *(1549)*   . . . .   *(October)*   . . . .   —

This is a draft of No. 281 and is related to Nos. 279 and 280 *(Appendix 37)*.

Draft   Assumed   . . . .   *(1550)* . . . .   —   . . . .   —

 10   *Milanesi*   . . . .   *(1552)* . . . .   —   . . . .   —

This fragment is part of a letter purporting to have been written to Benvenuto Cellini by Michelangelo. The letter itself has not survived and Cellini, who published it in his autobiography, may or may not be truthful in saying that he received such a letter. In view of its style the letter would appear to be a recollected version, suitably embellished by Cellini, of one which he had in fact received.

Its date is problematical, because there is a lacuna in the autobiography for the years 1550–1552. For some reason best known to himself, Cellini wished to conceal details of a visit to Rome in 1550, since the passage referring to it is cancelled in the original MS. *(Ferrero, p. 497)*. But from the references to the casting of the *Perseus* (1549) and to the execution of the bust of Bindo Altoviti, which was completed at about the same time and had been sent to Rome prior to Cellini's visit 'during the first years of Pope Giulio del Monte' (Julius III), and from the fact that he says he showed Duke Cosimo Michelangelo's letter before he left, 1550 rather than 1552 would seem a likely date for it.

Draft

11   *Assumed*   . . . .   *(1555)* . . . .   *September* *26th*

  This draft, of which the original is in the Vatican Codex and was published by Frey *(Lit., I, p. 420 et seq.)*, is related to No. 406. It bears two dates, of which both are probably correct, unless the first, namely January 1st 1554 is an *ab Incarnatione* date, which seems unlikely. The probable explanation is that Michelangelo jotted this note down on January 1st 1554/55, since we know that the question of the staircase had been under discussion for some time. Then in September 1555, when he finally wrote to Vasari about it, he added the date September 26th, when he looked out the note he had previously made. The year 1555 has, according to Frey, been added in another hand, probably, we may suppose, when the connection with the letter to Vasari of September 28th 1555 was perceived.

APPENDIXES
26 - 44

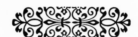

Appendix 26

Michelangelo and Vittoria Colonna

As it is nowhere stated when, or by whom, Michelangelo was introduced to Vittoria Colonna, the widowed Marchesa di Pescara (1490–1547), the date of their meeting can only be established by a process of elimination – that is to say, by the elimination of those periods, which were both frequent and prolonged, when the Marchesa is known to have been absent from Rome.

Michelangelo himself settled there permanently, as we know, in September 1534, which provides us, we may suppose, with a *terminus post quem*. It was not until the spring of 1536, however, that the Marchesa took up her residence for any length of time in Rome. Following the death of her husband, Ferrante Francesco d'Avalos di Pescara, who died in November 1525 from the wounds he had received at the battle of Pavia, she had lived for the most part either in the island of Ischia, where she had been brought up, or on one or other of the Colonna estates. But some time in the early part of 1536, certainly before the end of March, she arrived in Rome, and except perhaps for a few weeks during the height of the summer, remained there for the greater part of the year. It would therefore seem highly probable that it was in 1536 that Michelangelo was first presented to her. Opinions differ, however, and two other dates have been suggested, namely, 1532 or 1533 and 1538.

On the absurd assumption that Michelangelo's letters of 1533 addressed to Tommaso de' Cavalieri were only ostensibly so addressed and were really intended for Vittoria Colonna, both Gotti and Milanesi advanced the theory that they met during one of Michelangelo's periodic visits to Rome, either in 1532 or 1533. Apart from the fact that there is no evidence that the Marchesa was in Rome during these years, the greater part of which she spent in Ischia, one would have thought that the inherent improbability of such a proceeding, which would be wholly out of character, would have been sufficient to discredit it, even if Cavalieri's letters written in reply to Michelangelo's were not extant to disprove it. Yet neither the absurdity of the assumption, on which the earlier date has been put forward, nor the availability of the relevant correspondence, has deterred Armando Schiavo, a more recent biographer, from perpetuating this extraordinary farrago of nonsense.

Though less patently ridiculous, 1538, the other date proposed for their meeting, is hardly more feasible, owing to the Marchesa's peregrinations.

After a visit of approximately eight months, she left Rome some time between November 8th and December 15th 1536. Thence she went first to Arpino, and then to Ferrara, where she remained from June until February of the following year. From Ferrara, after visiting Bologna, she went on to Pisa, attracted thither by the preaching of the Capuchin, Bernardino

Ochino (1487–1564), to whose influence she had succumbed. Later, during the season of the baths, she left for Lucca, which was already a centre of religious controversy, and there she remained during the greater part of 1538, as we learn from her letter of September 25th to Pietro Aretino, to whom she wrote, saying that she continued to content herself in Lucca, being unable to proceed, as she had hoped, to the Holy Land, but added that the Pope now wished her to return to Rome. This command she obeyed at the beginning of October, as she is known to have been present at the church of San Silvestro di Monte Cavallo on Sunday, October 13th, when she attended a discourse on the Epistles of St. Paul, given by the noted Dominican preacher, Frate Ambrosio Politi. Of this we are informed by the Portuguese miniature painter, Francisco d'Ollanda, who was present at the meeting which took place in the sacristy afterwards between Lattanzio Tolomei, the Sienese envoy, Vittoria Colonna and Michelangelo himself. Now from the account he has left us, in his so-called Portuguese Dialogues, it is evident beyond all doubt that by this time the Marchesa not only knew Michelangelo very well indeed, but knew exactly how to manage him, and did so, as Ollanda observed, 'with an art I could not describe'. The Marchesa and Michelangelo must therefore have known each other for some time, which establishes 1536 as the date from which their friendship took its rise, since, owing to the Marchesa's movements, as shown above, no other year seems feasible.

Of the many letters which passed between them, only two of his and five of hers have survived, and all are, regrettably, undated *(Frey, Dicht., pp. 533, 534)*.

Although Milanesi has given an assumed date of 1545 to both Michelangelo's letters, there is no authority for this, and Alfredo Reumont, Ferrero and Müller have included them with the correspondence of 1539/40. A slightly earlier date might, however, be preferred, and the first *(No. 201)* has accordingly been assigned to the turn of the year 1538/9; the second *(No. 202)* to the first months of 1539. But no unassailable case can be made out for dating them either earlier or later within the presumed period.

On her return from Lucca in October 1538 Vittoria Colonna again took up her residence with the Sisters of San Silvestro in Capite, as Francisco d'Ollanda records at the end of his first dialogue, where he says, 'Messer Lattanzio left with Michelangelo, and I and Diogo Zapata, a Spaniard, went with the Marchesa from the monastery of San Silvestro at Monte Cavallo to the other monastery, where the head of St. John the Baptist is preserved and where the Marchesa resides.'

After an absence of two years, and on her return from a journey that might almost be described as a religious pilgrimage, the Marchesa may well have been anxious to present Michelangelo with gifts of the kind indicated in his letter, that is to say, with gifts of a devotional character. 'What the gifts referred to in his letter were', writes M. F. Jerrold in her life of Vittoria Colonna *(p. 131)*, 'we have no certain means of knowing, but it seems likely, from the way in which they are mentioned, that they were pictures.' At first the notion of giving paintings to a painter may seem to lack verisimilitude, but if this letter and the sonnet *Per esser manco almen, signiora, indegnio (Guasti, p. 169)* he sent with it, which echoes the letter, are to be related, in accordance with Jerrold's suggestion, to the two sonnets of hers addressed to him – *Perchè la mente vostra, ornata e cinta* and *Quanto intender qui puote umano ingegno (Colonna, pp. 365, 366)*, there can be no doubt that both refer to an image of Christ, one of which appears to have been a painting, perhaps a small altar-piece, and the other a crucifix. Various lesser items may also have been included in the gift, which, judging from what Michelangelo says about being in paradise, because he would then be in their house, not they in his, may reasonably be thought to have been the simple furnishings of a private oratory. This interpretation of the letter and of the sonnets would be entirely consonant, not only with the religious attitude of the circle in which Vittoria Colonna moved, but also with the spiritual relationship in which she and Michelangelo stood to each other.

Ever since the founding of the Oratory of Divine Love, during the pontificate of Leo X, there had been a strong movement among the more thoughtful churchmen to make their faith less a matter of profession than of practice, and with the increasing influence of the *spirituali*, a group which originally centred in the teaching of the Spanish mystic, Juan de Valdés, in Naples, a new spirit of devotion had been abroad. So that not only churchmen, such as Gaspero Contarini, Gian Matteo Giberti, Reginald Pole and others, but also laymen, such as Pietro Carnesecchi, Marcantonio Flaminio and Alvise Priuli, with all of whom Vittoria Colonna was closely associated, were wholly intent upon the practice of the Christian life, believing, not perfunctorily but sincerely with Thomas à Kempis, that it is 'our chief pursuit to meditate upon the life of Jesus Christ' and to 'imitate His life and manners'.

There is, accordingly, nothing surprising in the Marchesa's wish to present Michelangelo with gifts designed to aid his devotions, especially as it is demonstrable from certain poems which he addressed to her, how dependent he felt himself to be upon her spiritual guidance, as, for example, when he wrote:

> *Porgo la carta bianca*
> *A' vostri sacri inchiostri*
> *Ch' amor mi sganni, e pietà 'l ver ne scriva:*
> > (Guasti, p. 30)

It is significant, moreover, that the three works he executed for her, of which we have any notice, were all religious subjects. 'Michelangelo designed for her', writes Vasari, 'a marvellous Pietà with two little angels, and a Christ on the Cross, expiring, a divine thing, as well as Christ and the Woman of Samaria.' From what Condivi says about the type of the Christ in the Pietà, which he contrasts with the Christ of the early Pietà – the *Madonna della Febbre*, in Rome – and the last *Deposition*, in Florence *(Condivi, LIV)* a sculptured work is suggested, but from what the Marchesa herself says in her letter referring to it, one must suppose a painting. A painting is likewise suggested in her letter of July 20th *[1542]* from Viterbo, when she wrote: 'I would rather wait with a well-prepared mind for some substantial occasion of serving you, praying that Lord of Whom you spoke to me with such a fervent and humble heart, on my departure from Rome, that I may find you on my return with His image so renewed and alive by true faith in your soul, as you have so well painted it in my Woman of Samaria' *(Jerrold, p. 134)*.

Curiously enough, of the five extant letters which the Marchesa wrote to Michelangelo, four refer to one or other of the three works he executed for her. It is therefore the more disappointing that the circumstances which occasioned the letter of mild rebuke *(No. 202)* which he wrote her about the *Crucifixion* should not be known to us.

One may suppose, however, that in return for the gifts she gave him, he later offered her the drawing of *Christ on the Cross*, mentioned by both Vasari and Condivi, to which she referred in the following short and delightfully informal note:

My most cordial Signor Michelangelo – I beg you to let me have the Christ on the Cross for a short time, although it is not finished, because I want to show it to the gentlemen in the Cardinal of Mantua's suite. And if you are not working to-day, could you come and talk to me at a time convenient to you?

Yours to command,
The Marchesa di Pescara
(Ferrero & Müller, p. 207)

If Michelangelo complied with her request, he probably left the almost completed drawing with her for some time and she, not knowing quite how she stood in the matter, finally left it with Tommaso de' Cavalieri, who, as an unneeded go-between, indicated that Michelangelo was engaged on something else for her, thereby spoiling the surprise he had had in store for her, to which he refers in the letter. As the references to the three works he executed for her are all relatively obscure, it is impossible to be categorical, but from the second letter she wrote to him about the *Crucifixion,* which is rather curiously phrased, the completed work would appear to have been a painting, based on the original design, and that it was for this reason that he had not retrieved the drawing. But whatever the final explanation, it seems certain from the tentative wording of her letter of acknowledgment that for some reason or other Michelangelo had failed to make his intention clear.

Whether or not the drawing of *Christ on the Cross* in the British Museum *(Wilde, Pl. ciii)*, of which there are several copies, is the original is a matter of dispute. Dr. Wilde, while frankly admitting that 'Thode is the only critic of this century to speak in its favour', all other writers on Michelangelo believing it to be a copy, accepts it without reservation on the ground that 'it is completely finished in the manner of the Cavalieri sheets, a comparison with which vindicates its authenticity' *(p. 107)*. It is arguable, however, that in comparison with some of the so-called presentation drawings it is not completely finished, the skull in the foreground and the half-figures flanking the Cross being little more than sketched in. But whatever the state of advancement of the drawing which the Marchesa wished to show to the gentlemen in the suite of Ercole Gonzaga, Cardinal of Mantua (1505–1563), it seems reasonably certain that the sequence of letters in regard to it was as follows. The first would appear to be the Marchesa's, in which she asks for the loan of the unfinished drawing; the second, Michelangelo's, in which he gently blames her for using Tommaso de' Cavalieri as a go-between; the third the Marchesa's, in which she acknowledges 'The Crucifixion which has certainly crucified in my mind all other pictures that I have ever seen' *(Jerrold, p. 128)*. The use of the word *pittura* is significant, as is the phrase *più finita*, which she used to describe it, neither of which would seem to be entirely applicable to the British Museum drawing of *Christ on the Cross (Ferrero & Müller, p. 208)*.

At a time when the doctrine of justification had yet to be formulated, the choice of this image was particularly appropriate; since for those most sensibly aware of the religious controversies of the period and most deeply concerned to penetrate to the heart of the matter, the image of 'Christ, and Him crucified' was the supreme image of contemplation, for only, it was felt, through 'The Book of the Cross' could the ultimate 'benefits of His Passion' be assured. In this connection it is interesting to remark, moreover, that forty thousand copies of the second edition of *Del Beneficio di Gesù Christo Crocifisso* were sold in Venice alone. This work by the Augustinian, Benedetto da Mantova, which embodied the teaching of Valdés, was particularly esteemed by the *spirituali*, the group which gathered round Cardinal Pole, when, as Governor of the 'Patrimonium Petri', he held office at Viterbo.

In view of the intensity of the contemporary desire to focus attention upon the crucified Christ –

> . . . .*quell' Amor divino*
> *Ch' aperse, a prender noi, in croce le braccia . . .*
>
> *(Guasti, p. 230)*

the following extract from a letter addressed by Pietro Bertano, Bishop of Fano, to Ercole Gonzaga, Cardinal of Mantua, written in Trent on May 12th 1546, is not inapposite –

> My lord Pole, having heard that your lordship desired a painting of Christ by Michelangelo, charged me secretly to find out if such were the case, because he happens to have one from that painter's own hand, which he would willingly send you, but it is in the shape of a Pietà, although the whole figure is seen. He says it would be no deprivation for him, because he can get another from the Marchesa di Pescara. Will your lordship write to me about it? . . .
>
> *(Haile, p. 323)*

All things considered, it seems a rather rash assumption on Pole's part that he could so easily get another from the Marchesa di Pescara, unless the Marchesa, who, as we know, possessed a drawing of the same subject, had expressed the desire to give him hers, since, as she confessed to Cardinal Morone, she 'was never under such obligations to anyone as to Pole' *(Jerrold, p. 277)*. It can hardly imply that it would be easy for her to persuade Michelangelo to do another!

The Marchesa's residence in Rome since October 1538 was brought to an abrupt end in March 1541, owing to the outbreak of the Salt War between the Pope and her brother, Ascanio Colonna, who, because it affected his interests, had refused to comply with the papal decree imposed in February 1540, whereby the price of salt had been augmented and the citizens and provinces obliged to receive it from Rome. The Marchesa used every means in her power to persuade her brother to submit, but having failed she withdrew to the monastery of San Paolo at Orvieto, not because she herself was no longer *persona grata* with the Pope, but because she desired a life of greater retirement and tranquillity than was then possible in Rome. She remained at Orvieto until August when she returned to Rome by which time the Pope had triumphed; Ascanio himself was an exile in Naples, and all the Colonna estates were forfeit.

In her life of Vittoria Colonna, Mrs. Henry Roscoe makes the curious statement that the Marchesa was present at Ratisbon during the Diet which was in session there from April 5th to May 22nd 1541, and quotes as her authority the letter which Cardinal Pole, who was in Rome, wrote to Cardinal Contarini, the Papal Legate at Ratisbon, on April 2nd of that year. Apart from the fact that on the face of it such a visit would appear extremely unlikely, several letters addressed to the Marchesa, and others concerning her movements during the relevant period, when she was, in fact, at Orvieto, preclude such a possibility. According to Roscoe *(p. 257)*, Pole wrote to Contarini, saying:

> I rejoice greatly that the most reverend Lady Vittoria, with all her companions, having overcome the difficulties and dangers of the journey, arrived at Ratisbon as at a haven. . . .

There is, however, no mention of the Lady Vittoria in the original, which opens as follows:

> *Incolumen Reverendissimam D.V. cum suis comitibus omnibus, superatis itineris & molestiis & difficultatibus, Ratisbonam, tanquam in portus venisse . . . . . . valde gratulor . . .*
>
> *(Pole, III, p. 17)*

Though hardly excusable, the slip is not unamusing. Having once taken *Reverendissima D[ominatio] V[estra]* to mean *Reverendissima D[onna] V[ittoria]*, Roscoe inevitably went on, in an otherwise adequate translation, to make nonsense of the entire text. Well, therefore, might one have wondered why this is the only mention of Vittoria Colonna's visit to Ratisbon in 1541.

After a brief sojourn, the Marchesa once again left Rome, for Viterbo, where, in October 1541, she took up her residence with the sisters of Santa Caterina. Her choice of Viterbo was largely determined by the presence there of Cardinal Pole, who became her spiritual adviser, while she, for her part, stood to him in the relation of a second mother, after the execution of his own mother, the Countess of Salisbury, in May 1541. For the following three years she remained at Viterbo, though, as Condivi tells us, 'she often returned to Rome . . . for no other reason than to see Michelangelo'.

In the summer of 1543 she was taken seriously ill, to the great consternation of her friends, but she remained in Viterbo for some time afterwards and did not return to Rome until the late summer of 1544. Instead of taking up her abode in the monastery of San Silvestro, as she had formerly done, she moved to the Benedictine monastery of Sant' Anna de' Funari, where she remained, except for a visit to Viterbo in April 1545 (according to one of her letters to

Cardinal Pole), until the last days of her life, when she was removed to the Cesarini Palace, the home of her kinswoman, Cecilia Colonna and her husband, Giuliano Cesarini. Here, on February 15th 1547, she made her Will and expressed her wish to be buried simply, according to the style and custom of the monastery of Sant' Anna, in which she had lived. She died ten days later, on February 25th, in the fifty-seventh year of her age.

To Michelangelo, who was entirely devoted to her, it must have seemed unthinkable that she should have predeceased him; for, as Condivi tells us, in 'recalling this, her death, he often remained dazed, as one bereft of sense'. 'I remember to have heard him say', he writes, 'that nothing grieved him so much as that when he went to see her after she had passed away . . . he did not kiss her on the brow or on the cheek; as he did kiss her hand' *(Condivi, lxiii)*.

Appendix 27

Michelangelo and Luigi del Riccio

Part I

Although Michelangelo had always stood in need of having someone to *governare* for him, that is to say, of someone to manage his affairs, to act for him, and to look after his interests generally, it was not until after he settled permanently in Rome, towards the end of 1534, that he acquired the support and assistance he needed.

Unfortunately, there is a gap in the family correspondence from the time of his arrival until 1540, so that we do not know at exactly what date Bartolomeo Angiolini, who had long been devoted to him, became his man of business, but that he was acting in this capacity from 1537 onwards is certain from one of Fattucci's letters to Michelangelo, dated August 2nd of that year, in which he expressed his pleasure at Angiolini's diligence *(Frey, Dicht., p. 528)*. Michelangelo's last reference to him during his lifetime occurs in his letter of December 18th 1540 to Lionardo *(No. 207)*, since Angiolini died, perhaps suddenly, on December 28th of the same year. Some three months later, as far as can be ascertained, Luigi del Riccio figures for the first time in the correspondence *(No. 208)*. That del Riccio succeeded Angiolini finds confirmation in Michelangelo's comment to Lionardo that he had found no-one after Angiolini's death who managed his affairs better or more devotedly than Luigi del Riccio *(No. 291)*.

For obvious reasons, Frey believed that Luigi, the son of Giovanbattista del Riccio and Eleanora di Cristofano Bracci, a Florentine from the Santo Spirito Quarter, had been resident in Rome at least from 1534 onwards, but there is nothing to confirm this, for although he moved in the society of the *fuorusciti*, he was not himself an exile, since he remained on excellent terms with the Medici Duke, Cosimo I.

It is more than probable that Michelangelo and Luigi del Riccio, who was Roberto Strozzi's agent and the managing director of the Strozzi-Ulivieri bank in Rome, had been acquainted for some time before del Riccio took over the management of his affairs, but the beginning of the intimate and rather moving friendship which grew up between them dates from about 1541.

Like almost everyone whom Michelangelo had ever known, del Riccio's one desire was to serve him. 'How much I desire to serve you', he wrote on August 29th 1542, 'is known to everyone acquainted with me' *(Steinmann, p. 34)*, a statement that is borne out by the character of the correspondence that passed between them, extending as it did to matters far beyond the scope of an ordinary business association. For, in addition to many other courtesies and acts of kindness and consideration, del Riccio continually sought to give him pleasure by sending him gifts of one kind or another – usually delicacies such as caviar, trout, melons and wine, gifts which Michelangelo often acknowledged in verses, which he sometimes referred to as *polizzini* or 'drafts', and sometimes as *berlingozzi*, 'tartlets' or, as we might say, 'trifles'. And, as if not satisfied with this, del Riccio, who kept up an intermittent correspondence with Michelangelo's nephew, Lionardo, between September 1544 and February 1546, used also to encourage him to do the same, telling him not to be deterred if his uncle tried to discourage him from sending gifts, because, as Messer Luigi put it, 'it gratifies him and he sees that you think of him'. Again, when Lionardo's projected marriage was under discussion he strongly advised him not to do anything without Michelangelo's consent, because 'you would be making a great mistake, and would do yourself a great deal of harm'. Likewise, after Lionardo returned to Florence, having failed to see his uncle when he was ill in the summer of 1544 (Michelangelo being persuaded that he had come only to attend his obsequies and to secure the inheritance), del Riccio did his best to smooth matters over, saying, 'Since you left I have always written to you when I had occasion, and have not failed to commend you to your Messer Michelangelo, who certainly loves you as a son' *(Steinmann, p. 51)*. But despite del Riccio's kindly intervention and Lionardo's well-intentioned efforts, he seldom succeeded in pleasing his illustrious uncle – partly, perhaps, because he never 'learnt to write'.

In his *Dialoghi*, Donato Giannotti has preserved for us an obviously authentic picture of the wholly delightful relationship which existed between the three Florentines – Michelangelo, Messer Luigi, and Messer Donato himself. From the interchanges between them it is quite clear that, while the fourth speaker, Messer Antonio Petrio, knew Michelangelo well, the other two knew him intimately, particularly Messer Luigi, who treats him throughout with that degree of intimacy in which the affectionate respect he felt for him is in no way belied by an amused and gentle mocking at his foibles.

It was, however, in the way in which del Riccio received him into his house and took care of him on the two occasions when he was ill that the profoundness of his regard was finally shown. The first occasion was in July 1544; the second at the turn of the year 1545/46. There is no doubt that Michelangelo was seriously ill on both occasions and del Riccio probably found it imperative to have him moved into his own apartment in the Strozzi Palace, partly because no member of the household at the Macel de' Corvi was competent either to see that the doctor's orders were obeyed or to deal with the endless succession of callers, who came on behalf of 'all the prelates, the chief gentlemen of Rome, the Pope himself and the Farnese', who 'sent daily to enquire after the state of his health' *(Gaye, II, p. 296)*. It is therefore not surprising that Michelangelo afterwards felt that he owed his life to del Riccio and, presumably, we may add, to the good offices of del Riccio's wife. And that he was sensible of this *immensa cortesia* to the point of being overwhelmed, we know from the poems he subsequently addressed to his affectionate host.

As he was twice received into the del Riccio household, it cannot be said with certainty on which occasion the graceful exchange of verses between del Riccio and himself took place

(Guasti, p. 28), though the first may be confidently presumed. But on whichever occasion it was, del Riccio certainly surpassed himself, notwithstanding the fact that he had once remarked in a letter to Michelangelo that 'there is as much difference between my verses and yours as there is between Urbino and you' *(Steinmann, p. 36)*. From the poem *Perchè è troppo molesta*, to which del Riccio made so elegant a reply, we see beyond all doubt how deeply affected Michelangelo was by the extent of his indebtedness, and when we consider from his previous correspondence, as witness that concerning Festa and Arcadelt *(Nos. 194 and 217)*, how anxious he had always been to make a suitable presentation in acknowledgment of any kindness he received, we may well regard it as unthinkable that he should not have made some commensurate return to del Riccio in recognition of an unprecedented service, seeing that over a mere business transaction he had written, 'I presume too much on your kindness – God grant I may be able to repay you' *(No. 218)*. This being so, what presentation did he make to Luigi del Riccio comparable to the two *Captives* (originally intended for the Tomb of Julius II) which he later presented to Roberto Strozzi, who can have been regarded only indirectly as his host? Indeed, what was there equivalent to such a gift that he could have presented to his Messer Luigi, to whom he referred after his death as having been *molto mio amico*? Perhaps, however, the following questions might be more pertinent.

Did Michelangelo, in fact, present the *Captives* to Roberto Strozzi in the first instance? And is it not much more likely that he originally presented them to Luigi del Riccio, and that it was only after del Riccio's death in the autumn of 1546 that he offered them to Roberto Strozzi, partly because he had, in a sense, been a guest in his house; partly because the figures were already in the Strozzi Palace; and partly because he would not have wanted, and would have found it too painful, to take them back? Surely this is the explanation of how the Strozzi came to receive a gift so munificent and so out of all proportion to any claim they can be conceived to have had as to seem invidious? There are, moreover, three considerations which lend colour to this view. Firstly, in addition to having been Michelangelo's personal host, del Riccio, who had seen him through the troubles connected with the last contract for the Tomb of Julius, may reasonably be thought to have been a more probable recipient of these figures, to which the della Rovere family had no claim, once the Tomb was completed. Secondly, in a letter to Lionardo *(No. 291)* Michelangelo was at pains to emphasize that he considered himself to have been a guest in del Riccio's apartment, rather than in the Strozzi Palace itself. Thirdly, it is only on this assumption that the concluding sentence of the one bitter letter he ever wrote to del Riccio makes any sense at all *(No. 244)*.

Part II

The occasion of this letter was a difference of opinion over a print – not a print by Ennea Vico of *The Last Judgment*, as Milanesi and Symonds thought possible, nor of the printing of Michelangelo's poems, as Ludwig von Scheffler thought certain – but of an engraved portrait of Michelangelo himself. Milanesi's alternative suggestion that the print in question might have been by Giulio Bonasone, would therefore be plausible, if he was referring to a version of the line engraving of Michelangelo, published by Bonasone in 1545. The remote chance that the print in dispute may have been by some other hand cannot, however, be entirely ruled out.

But proceeding on the hypothesis that Bonasone was, in fact, the engraver in question, we may note that among his engravings of Michelangelo listed by Passerini *(p. 313)* there is one with the title *Michel Angelus Buonarrotus, Patricius Florentinus, Sculptor, Pictor, Architectus Unicus*, which is certainly significant in connection with the postscript to Michelangelo's letter. Moreover, there are two engravings, to one of which Michelangelo might reasonably and understandably have taken exception *(Steinmann, Portrait, pl. 37)*. Both were published in 1545, when Michelangelo was in his seventy-first year. The second, which may be accepted as an excellent likeness *(Plate 7, Vol. II)*, was reissued in 1546 with an amended title. The original drawing, probably commissioned at the instance of his friends, may therefore have been executed towards the end of 1544, when the master had recovered from the illness which had alarmed the whole of Rome in the summer of that year.

On this assumption and on the basis of Michelangelo's letter it is easy to reconstruct the occasion of the quarrel. Luigi del Riccio, acting in the unenviable role of a go-between, had shown Michelangelo a proof of the engraving, which he rejected, because he thought it made him look like a drunkard; but del Riccio, perhaps at the request of the engraver, unwisely submitted it a second time. Thereupon Michelangelo, who felt this to be an insult, became enraged and took it into his head that not only the engraver, but del Riccio himself, which could hardly be credited, was trying to make money out of him. That del Riccio can have had no such intention is beside the point, though it is difficult to imagine by what unwonted error of judgment he had sought to override Michelangelo in a personal matter of this kind.

Supposing this deduction to be correct, we still have two other problems to solve with reference to Michelangelo's 'wild' letter, as his biographers have been pleased to call it. One is the implication of the sentence with which it concludes; the other the approximate date of the letter itself.

With regard to the first problem, the crux of the matter lies in the meaning of the word *cose*, which can generally be translated either as 'things' or as 'affairs'. But to translate the sentence *Se fate di me mille pezzi, io ne farò altretanti, non di voi, ma delle cose vostre*, with Symonds, 'If you hack me into a thousand pieces, I will do the same, not indeed to yourself, but to what belongs to you', or, with Heath Wilson, 'If you make of me a thousand pieces, I will do as much not of you, but of your affairs', makes no sense at all, unless we can identify the *cose* referred to. We must therefore suppose that Michelangelo was not only referring to something specific, but to something that was at once in his possession and in his power to destroy. Now the *cose* in question can be none other than the *Captives*, which Michelangelo may well have promised to del Riccio, but had not yet actually given him. And that in this context *cose* might easily mean the *Captives* is proved almost conclusively by Condivi, who, in speaking of Michelangelo's generosity, wrote as follows: 'He has given away many of his things –

sue cose – which, if he had wished to sell them, would have brought him endless money, as for example the two statues that he gave to Messer Roberto Strozzi' *(Condivi, LXVII)*.

To put this construction upon the threat with which Michelangelo ended his letter does not involve any supposition that he was intending to be vindictive (a supposition that would be wholly out of keeping with all that we know of his character) for, terrible though this threat was, it was the measure not so much of the extent to which he had been enraged, as of the extent to which he had patently been hurt. The full implication of what he said is therefore, virtually this – 'If you persist in doing what I have asked you nor to do, our friendship will be at an end, and as I should then feel able neither to give the figures to you, nor to keep them myself, I should have no alternative but to smash them to pieces.'

The final problem to resolve is when this quarrel took place. On the whole, the consensus of opinion has been in favour of assigning it to 1546, shortly after Michelangelo's recovery from the second illness. But this is scarcely possible. According to del Riccio's letter to Lionardo, dated January 30th 1546 *(Steinmann, p. 57)*, it was only by the end of the month that Michelangelo has recovered sufficiently to be able to go out every day; and throughout February del Riccio was in correspondence with Lionardo about the purchase of a property Michelangelo had in view. His last letter is dated February 27th, and a fortnight later he left for Venice, as we know from a communication addressed to Lionardo by Francesco del Riccio, Luigi's cousin, on March 13th *(Steinmann, p. 61)*. It is therefore highly unlikely that he was concerned at this time with anything but the business affairs connected with his imminent departure. How long he was away, and when he returned to Rome we do not know, but we do know that he was there in August, by which time he may already have been ill, as he died, to Michelangelo's intense grief and consternation, a month or so later, probably in the October of that year.

Under these circumstances it would be more reasonable to suppose that the disagreement arose at a time not too long after Michelangelo's first illness, that is to say, some time between August 1544 and the following August, since del Riccio left for Lyons some time after July in 1545. Within that period certain times may be excluded, either by reason of Michelangelo's correspondence with del Riccio, or by reason of del Riccio's correspondence with Lionardo. Of the possible times remaining, which are relatively few, much the most feasible would appear to be some date between December 1544 and January 1545.

Such a date would coincide perfectly with the publication of the Bonasone engravings, besides which Michelangelo would then have been in a position to offer the *Captives* as a gift, the Tomb of Julius being virtually complete, since the final payment for the figures in the upper zone was authorized in January 1545 *(Nos. 247, 248)*. There is, however, a further argument which may be adduced in support of this theory; namely, the terms of Michelangelo's letter to del Riccio concerning the payment for the moving of his own figures into San Pietro in Vincoli *(No. 249)*. This letter, though undated, clearly belongs to January/February 1545. In it Michelangelo begins by asking del Riccio to treat him less formally, surely a rather strange request, considering that they had known each other intimately for several years – unless, of course, something had occurred to upset their normal relationship.

Supposing this to be the case, we may take it that the misunderstanding had been cleared up, but that del Riccio, perhaps from some feeling of embarrassment after what had happened, had tended to treat him with more reserve than he had done before, but that Michelangelo had said nothing, hoping that this sense of constraint would pass. Then, one morning he had gone into del Riccio's office, as he was in the habit of doing; had found him with Altoviti's son, and had been received with a formality he could no longer brook. The next day, having thought it over, he accordingly wrote a letter, half in earnest and half in jest, that was perfectly calculated to meet the situation – ostensibly blaming himself for behaving like a 'presumptuous buffalo', while in reality begging for a return to the old friendly relationship. It is, indeed, only in the light of the quarrel that this second letter has any meaning.

Although Michelangelo's biographers have never pretended to understand the implications of his letter of protest about the engraving, they have not for a moment been deterred from condemning him for what they have chosen to regard as a typical outburst of 'petulant rage'. Whereas, had they even remotely appreciated the circumstances in which it was written, they might have been less ready to imagine that he wrote without provocation and was therefore wholly to blame for what occurred. The incident, like all incidents which arise from misunderstandings, was obviously unfortunate, but one has only to consider the eloquence of the sonnet, with which the letter was closely, if not immediately, followed up, to realize the nature of Michelangelo's real feeling for his friend Luigi.

> *Nel dolce d'una immensa cortesia,*
> *Dell' onor, della vita alcuna offesa*
> *S' asconde e cela spesso; e tanto pesa,*
> *Che fa men cara la salute mia.*
> *Chi gli omer' altru' 'mpenna, e po' tra via*
> *A lungo andar la reta occulta ha tesa;*
> *L' ardente carità, d' amore accesa,*
> *La più l' ammorza ov' arder più desia.*
> *Pero, Luigi mio, tenete chiara*
> *La prima grazia, ond' io la vita porto,*
> *Che non si turbi per tempesta o vento.*
> *L' isdegnio ogni mercè vincere impara;*
> *E, s' i' son ben del vero amico accorto,*
> *Mille piacer non vaglion un tormento.*
>
> *(Guasti, p. 161)*

Here, while not withdrawing the accusation that del Riccio had tricked him (an accusation in which he still believed, since, when Michelangelo wrote the sonnet, del Riccio had had, presumably, no time to deny it), he makes a moving appeal for the preservation of the old affection to which he owed his life, averring that the shock of the hurt he had sustained was in proportion to the warmth of the feeling he had cherished. The last line, *Mille piacer non vaglion un tormento*, is not original; it is a line from Petrarch's sonnet *I' mi vivea di mia sorte contento*, and had therefore an epigrammatic significance, with which del Riccio would certainly have been familiar, as it was a common practice at this period to conclude poems with quotations from Petrarch.

The strength of Michelangelo's attachment to Luigi del Riccio, no less than the extent to which he was dependent upon him, is finally confirmed by the grief with which he was overwhelmed, when del Riccio died in his prime in the autumn of 1546. In his letter of November 13th to Pier Luigi Farnese, Duke of Parma and Piacenza, the Treasurer-General, Bernardino della Croce, Bishop of Casale, referred to this, saying, 'Now that Luigi del Riccio is dead, who used to manage his affairs, he is so stunned that he can do nothing but give himself up to despair' *(Steinmann, p. 28)*, a state of mind which, incidentally, belies the notion that the quarrel took place in 1546 and brought their friendship to an end.

But if Michelangelo was distraught, so, apparently, was the Pope, as we learn from another letter, also addressed to the Duke, by his agent Fabio Cappalati a few days later. 'If ever he *[the Pope]* had need of him, he has need of him now,' he wrote, 'in particular for the building of St. Peter's and of his Palace here, since Sangallo is dead; and if ever it was difficult to conciliate him, and to induce him to do anything, it is now that that Messer Luigi is dead, who used to manage him and was the means of inducing him to comply with the wishes of His Beatitude' *(ibid., p. 28)*.

Thus, from everyone's point of view, del Riccio's death was a calamity. And thus, in the words of Steinmann, 'the noble figure of Luigi del Riccio recedes into the shadows; a true gentleman in every respect; a Florentine, destined to end his days, like Michelangelo himself, in Rome; but the fidelity, the affection and the self-abnegation with which he served his great compatriot have rendered him immortal and endeared his image to posterity for ever'.

The Tomb of Pope Julius II : 1505-1545

Part II 1532-1545

*The history of the earlier negotiations and Contracts for the Tomb of Julius II is given in
Volume I, Appendix 11*

1532-1542. The Fourth and Last Contract with the Heirs of Julius II

THE Third Contract for the Tomb of Pope Julius II, which had been agreed on April 29th 1532, expired in 1535, but once more little progress had been made with the work, which was scarcely more advanced than before; since Clement VII, not satisfied with employing Michelangelo on the Medici Tombs, and long before the work at the New Sacristy was completed, had desired him to come to Rome to paint the fresco of *The Last Judgment* in the Sistine Chapel. Michelangelo did not arrive in Rome, however, until September 23rd 1534, two days before the death of Clement. As the fresco was still only projected, he hoped at last to be relieved of all papal commissions and left free to fulfil his obligations to the Duke of Urbino – a hope perhaps more vain than any he had ever cherished. For thirty years, it seems, Alessandro Farnese, who became Pope as Paul III, had desired to obtain Michelangelo's services, and having succeeded to the Papacy, was not to be denied, however much Michelangelo might plead his engagement to the Duke. Michelangelo was therefore obliged to proceed with *The Last Judgment* and by a papal brief, dated September 1st 1535, was nominated supreme architect, painter and sculptor to the Vatican and enrolled as a member of the Pope's household. A year later Paul III issued a *motu proprio* exempting him from the legal penalties for which he was liable owing to his non-fulfilment of the terms of the 1532 contract *(Steinmann, Sixt., II, p. 748)*.

Nevertheless, Michelangelo rightly felt that he remained under a moral obligation to the Duke to complete the Tomb, and in September 1539 the young Duke, Guidobaldo, who had succeeded his father in October 1538, and was amicably disposed towards Michelangelo, wrote expressing his willingness to 'let him have a breather' over the Tomb, while he was engaged in the Sistine, at the same time affirming his faith in Michelangelo's integrity and in his willingness to finish the Tomb when he was able to do so.

Paul III had, however, little or no consideration for the claims of others, and three weeks after the completion of *The Last Judgment* in October 1541, he informed the Duke, through Cardinal Ascanio Parisani *(Gaye, II, p. 290)*, that he required Michelangelo to undertake the painting of his new chapel, the Cappella Paolina, and that, in consequence, the completion of the Tomb would have to be entrusted to other masters, working on Michelangelo's designs and under his supervision. Accordingly, of the six statues which Michelangelo had undertaken to deliver finished by his own hand, three were allocated to Raffaello da Montelupo by a contract drawn up on February 27th 1542 *(Milanesi, p. 709)*. These were apparently the *Virgin*, the *Sibyl* and the *Prophet*, and in May he entered into an agreement with Giovanni de' Marchesi and Francesco d'Amadore da Urbino (his own assistant, Urbino), for the finishing of the frame *(Milanesi, p. 710, and No. 214)*. Then in July he presented a petition to the Pope *(No. 219)* asking to be entirely relieved of the charge of the Tomb, and to be allowed to allocate the finishing of the two statues, the *Active* and the *Contemplative Life*, which he proposed to substitute for the two *Captives*, which were unsuitable for the revised design, to Raffaello da Montelupo. Only the *Moses* he proposed to deliver finished by his own hand.

The Duke signified his willingness to make certain concessions and on August 20th 1542 a new contract – the fourth and last – was drawn up on the lines proposed by Michelangelo in his petition to the Pope *(Milanesi, p. 715)*. According to the terms of this agreement, Michelangelo agreed to deposit 1,400 *scudi* to pay for the completion of the work, and was at last confirmed in his possession of the house in the Macello de' Corvi, the possession of which had so long been in dispute. It is interesting to observe that the words *non mutata la substanzia delle cose predette* were significantly added, presumably at Michelangelo's request, in order to safeguard him against subsequent alterations, such as had been made to the Contract of 1532 *(No. 227)*.

The Duke's agent, Girolamo Tiranno, promised ratification of the contract within fifteen days. But the terms whereby only the *Moses* would be finished by Michelangelo's hand were unacceptable to the Duke, who refused to ratify, and wrote to the Bishop of Sinigaglia, Marco Vigerio, who had been party to the negotiations, to that effect on October 24th, and to Tiranno on November 11th *(Vasari, Prosp. Cron., pp. 387, 388)*. It must therefore have been at this juncture that Michelangelo sought and obtained leave to complete the *Leah* and the *Rachel* (i.e. the *Active* and the *Contemplative Life*) himself *(No. 248)*. The ratification presumably arrived shortly after this, but on precisely what date we do not know. The time allowed to Raffaello da Montelupo for the completion of the work assigned to him was approximately twenty months; that is to say, the figures were due for delivery in March 1544.

1542-1545. *The Completion of the Tomb*

In point of fact, the Tomb was not completed until the beginning of 1545, the final payments for the work being authorized in February of that year *(No. 247)*. But notwithstanding its completion, and as if to emphasize the irony of the whole affair, the so-called Tomb is not and has never been other than a cenotaph, as Julius II is still buried beside his uncle, Sixtus IV, in the Cappella del Santo Sacramento in St. Peter's, to which, on the demolition of the former Sistine or Giulia Chapel, both bodies were removed by order of Pope Paul III *(Tolnay, IV, p. 119)*.

Thus, after forty long years of anxiety, bitterness, tears and frustration, the Tragedy of the Tomb was brought to a close, the terms of the final contract being at last fulfilled, whereby *si ponga silenzio perpetuo a questo negocio di sepultura per conto di detto messer Michelagnolo*.

But while the negotiations over the Tomb might be legally at an end, this did not suffice to console Michelangelo for the tragic failure of a project which he had conceived on a scale so magnificent that it would be 'the mirror of all Italy'. A sense of bitterness and a feeling of guilt certainly remained with him, as is shown by the letter which Annibale Caro, secretary to Cardinal Alessandro Farnese, wrote to Antonio Gallo, secretary to the Duke of Urbino, on August 20th 1553 on the occasion of the publication of Condivi's *Life of Michelangelo*, in which the Tomb and the difficulties which Michelangelo had encountered were discussed.

In this letter the writer begged his correspondent to seek to effect a reconciliation between the Duke and Michelangelo, because, as he says, 'I assure you he is so upset at being in disgrace with the Duke that this alone might be the cause of bringing him to the grave before his time' *(Caro, II, p. 50)*. This view as to Michelangelo's attitude is further borne out by Condivi's observation, 'But what grieved Michelangelo most was that, instead of thanks, all he got was odium and disgrace in return for the effort he had made contending with two Popes for the love of the della Rovere' *(Condivi, lii)*.

Appendix 29

An Interpretation of Letter No. 215

IN this note to Luigi del Riccio Michelangelo began by saying, 'I sent this to Florence some time ago'. The unspecified 'this' is undoubtedly, and has always been assumed to be, a madrigal or sonnet, which we may suppose he had sent to Ser Giovan Francesco Fattucci, to whom he was in the habit of sending copies of his poems from time to time. This we know from one of Fattucci's letters to Michelangelo, written in 1537 and published in part by Frey *(Dicht., p. 528)*, in which Fattucci begged for a sight of some of Michelangelo's sonnets, saying that he had not seen anything for about a year.

To hazard a guess as to which particular madrigal or sonnet is here referred to would be rash, were it not for Frey's brilliant conjecture as to the probable meaning of the somewhat enigmatic postscript to the letter, in which Michelangelo said, 'If you like it, have it copied out properly and give it to those chords which hold men captive without distinction.' This Frey believes to be an oblique way of saying, 'have it copied out properly and give it to Arcadelt to set to music'. In this case, Frey goes on to say, the madrigal in question must have been one of the two set by the great Flemish composer, who was at that time a member of the Sistine Choir. That is to say, it must be either *Deh! dimmi, amor, se l'alma di costei (Guasti, p. 48)* or *Io dico che fra noi potenti dei, (ibid., p. 107)* the settings for both of which are extant. The suggestion is certainly a plausible one, and there is much internal evidence, which Frey has not been at pains to elaborate, which may be adduced in support of it.

From a careful perusal of the letter it would appear that the subject under discussion was something that in some way concerned all three Florentines – Michelangelo, Donato Giannotti and Luigi del Riccio. Thus, proceeding on the assumption that the word *corde* is here correctly translated as 'chords' or 'strings', it seems not unlikely, from the particular way in which Giannotti's name is introduced, that he had suggested that one of Michelangelo's poems should be set to music by Arcadelt; that Michelangelo had been asked to produce something suitable; and that del Riccio had undertaken to approach the composer. And that Michelangelo felt himself to be in some way especially indebted to his Messer Luigi on this occasion is shown by the unusual conclusion to the letter – 'Yours always and with infinite obligation' – a sense of obligation which we may understand, when we learn, from a subsequent letter *(No. 217)* that del Riccio did, in fact, commission the musical setting which gave Michelangelo so much pleasure.

Parallel to this somewhat cryptic (and perhaps rather bashful) injunction, 'If you like it . . . give it to those chords which hold men captive without distinction' – *quelle corde che legan gli uomini senza discrezione* – is another in the body of the letter, which is structurally similar, namely, 'If you like it, you may devote it to that flame *[or passion]* which consumes me' – *al fuoco . . . che m'arde* – which is even more difficult to interpret, and one for which, moreover, Frey has, inconsiderately, proposed no solution.

Left to our own resources, we may observe, on reflection, that both passages are distinctly Dantesque in character, which, in view of Michelangelo's known devotion to Dante, the exiled Florentine *par excellence*, is not surprising. Thus, just as 'those chords which hold men captive without distinction' may be said to echo those 'sacred chords' – *sante corde* – which held Dante and Beatrice captive in the fifth heaven; so 'the flame *[or passion]* . . . that consumes me – *il fuoco che m'arde* – may be said to echo 'the flame by which I am ever consumed' – *il fuoco ond' io sempre ardo* – the terms in which the poet describes his burning passion for Beatrice.

To what burning passion, we may then ask, does Michelangelo refer in this context? To this enquiry the answer is provided by the two madrigals in question, whichever of the two it was. Without a doubt, it is to his burning passion for Florence, the subject of both poems. So that, when he says to Luigi del Riccio, 'You may devote it to . . . the flame which consumes me', it is an equivocal way of saying 'You may devote it to Florence as personified by the Florentine exiles – the *fuorusciti*.'

In support of this argument, it may be noted that the fate of Florence was a subject with which Michelangelo was constantly preoccupied, as we know from various sources, among which Giannotti's *Dialoghi* may be cited as being of particular interest. In the opening passages Michelangelo is gently chided by del Riccio for his habit of reverting to the ills by which, with the loss of republican liberty, Florence had been beset. Again, in the same work special mention is made of his madrigal beginning,

Deh! dimmi, amor, se l'alma di costei

which is only one of several devoted to the subject of Florence and the *fuorusciti*. It is, moreover, in keeping with Michelangelo's unconceit, where his own achievements were concerned, that in writing to del Riccio he should have alluded to the matter obliquely.

Having carried our speculations thus far, we are tempted to carry them a little further and to ask ourselves whether Arcadelt's setting may not have been commissioned for some special occasion, than which none would have been more appropriate than the celebration of the pre-eminently Florentine festival, the Feast of St. John the Baptist, which is kept on June 24th and must always have been observed with particular devotion by the *fuorusciti*. On this assumption the three letters relating to Arcadelt *(Nos. 215, 216, 217)* have been tentatively assigned to the late spring or early summer of 1542, rather than to a period later in the year, as preferred by Frey. The precise dates on which they were written remain, however, problematical, since all that we know for certain is that both poems were included in Arcadelt's first book of madrigals, *Il Primo Libro de' Madrigali d'Arcadelt*, which was published in 1543.

Appendix 30

Cecchino de' Bracci

FRANCESCO DE' BRACCI, who was familiarly known as Cecchino, was the son of Zanobi di Giovanbattista de' Bracci and his wife, Contessa de' Castellani. He was born on April 23rd 1528, and was therefore six years of age when his parents, who were bitterly opposed to the hated Medici régime, left Florence to take refuge in Rome, there to make common cause with other Florentine exiles – the *fuorusciti*.

The Bracci were related to the del Riccio family, Cecchino's grandfather and Luigi's mother having been brother and sister, the children of Cristofano de' Bracci, who was elected a prior in 1472. Although Cecchino, who belonged to a younger generation, is generally referred to as Luigi's nephew, he was, strictly speaking, his first cousin once removed. The relation in which Cecchino stood to Luigi, who was childless, would seem, however, to have been rather that of an adopted son. They were constantly together, and after the boy's death del Riccio was responsible for all the arrangements. That Luigi had formally adopted his young cousin would, nevertheless, remain merely an assumption, were it not for an entry in his hand in the *Codex Riccardiano (Polidori, II, p. 385)*. It is in the form of a Latin epitaph and reads *Aloisius del Riccio orbatus affini et alumno dolcissimo desperatus futurae laetitiae pos[uit]*. Such adoptions were, after all, a common practice at this period, the childless Vittoria Colonna, for example, having likewise adopted a son; moreover, the fact that Luigi and Cecchino were so related explains various references which might otherwise be inexplicable. Why, but for this, should Cecchino, at the age of fourteen, have been one of the witnesses to the contract between Michelangelo on the one hand, and Giovanni de' Marchesi and Urbino on the other? *(Milanesi, p. 711)*.

As far as may be judged from the surviving references to him, hyperbole notwithstanding, Cecchino, who was one of several brothers, appears to have been a youth of singular beauty and extraordinary grace. It is therefore not in the least surprising that he should have been idolized by del Riccio and made much of by Michelangelo and Giannotti, and that these men, being childless and in exile, should have lavished their affection and set their hopes for the future upon this boy, who became in some sort a symbol of their patriotic ideals – *Fede tra noi del sommo ben divino* – as Giannotti wrote in one of the sonnets dedicated to del Riccio after Cecchino's death. So that, just as 'in Michelangelo the *fuorusciti* adored a relic of the beloved Republic', so in Cecchino they worshipped the image of its hoped-for restoration. Michelangelo's phrase *nostro idolo* and del Riccio's phrase, *idol mio*, thus epitomized the attitude of the Florentine circle towards him. At first sight, this may seem a trifle excessive, but there can be little doubt that he was an unusually attractive character, if we consider the appealing lines in one of del Riccio's sonnets, written after his death, which have a clear ring of truth,

> *Vedi i mie grani affanni e la mie doglia*
> *Deh, per quella bonta, per quella voglia*
> *Che havesti di piacermi et per quel zelo*
> *Di vero amor' fra noi* . . . .
>
> *(Frey, Dicht., p. 268)*

What caused Cecchino's death at the age of sixteen, on January 8th 1544, and how long he was ill, is, regrettably, not recorded. But four days later del Riccio wrote to Giannotti, who was then in Vicenza, in the following heart-broken terms:

Oymè, messer Donato mio, our Cecchino is dead. I would recall to you the love and reverence he bore us and his rare and excellent qualities, which had increased immeasurably since you left, so much so, that Heaven, which continually increased them, has taken him from us. All Rome weeps for him. Messer Michelangelo is doing me the design for a simple marble tomb, and you, would you deign to write the epitaph and to send it to me with a consoling letter – if it arrives in time, for he has reft my soul from me. Alas! Alas! Living, each hour I die a thousand deaths. O God, how Fortune changes her mood.
From Rome, on the 12th day of January 1544, style of the Nativity.
Your forlorn Luigi del Riccio

'All Rome weeps for him' – and many indeed were the verses written in his honour, as they had been in honour of Celso Mellini, a youth who, as Steinmann reminds us, had perished tragically in 1519. Giannotti addressed three sonnets to Luigi del Riccio in commemoration of Cecchino's 'goodness', 'grace', and 'beauty', and at the head of one, written by Michelangelo, are the words, 'From Michelangelo Buonarroti to Luigi del Riccio, on the portrait he did of Francesco Bracci'. Besides this drawing, to which Michelangelo refers in one of his letters *(No. 239)*, he also sent del Riccio a series of epigrams and epitaphs. For some reason or other, he originally promised to send him fifteen, but it became a habit with him to send one every time del Riccio sent a delicacy of any kind *(Guasti, p. 10)*. Thus, we find attached to one of the verses the words, 'When you don't want any more, don't send me anything else.' On another occasion he wrote, 'For the turtle-dove; Urbino will do one for the fish, because he has gobbled it up.' Again, 'This is rubbish; the fount is dry; you must wait till it rains, but you're in too much of a hurry.' Clearly, as time went on, he tried to cheer Luigi up and was still sending him quatrains as late in the year as November 9th, since on one of them he added a note, 'Till we meet the day after tomorrow, the Feast of St. Martin, unless it rains.' Another day he signed himself 'Michelangelo in the Macel de' Corvi', but, instead of writing the word *Corvi*, he drew a raven *(Guasti, p. 19)*. He wrote forty-eight epigrams and epitaphs, in all, but the one used on the tomb in the church of Santa Maria in Aracoeli – a tomb executed by Urbino, ostensibly to Michelangelo's design – is an inscription of the simplest kind –

Francesco Braccio Florentino nobili adolescenti immatura morte praerepto anno agenti XVI die VIII Januarii MDXLIIII. As we know, Luigi himself died two years later in fulfilment, it might almost seem, of the concluding lines of one of Giannotti's three sonnets addressed to him,

> *Che vogliam far più in questa afflitta valle?*
> *Deh, presto andiamo a ritrovarla in cielo.*
>
> *(Dicht., p. 269)*

The Identification of the Cardinal addressed in Letter No. 227

THERE has always been considerable speculation as to the identity of the recipient of Michelangelo's letter *(No. 227)*, written, presumably in the late autumn of 1542, which was discovered by Sebastiano Ciampi and first published in 1834.

Hitherto opinion as to the recipient has been divided between (i) Alessandro Rufini, steward to Pope Paul III, (ii) Marco Vigerio, Bishop of Sinigaglia, (iii) Cardinal Ascanio Parisani, Bishop of Rimini, and (iv) Messer Pier Giovanni Aliotti, Master of the Robes to Pope Paul.

The claims of the first, Rufini, are clearly inadmissible. In making this suggestion, Ciampi did so on the analogy that it was to the Pope's steward, Messer Agostino, that Michelangelo had entrusted his letter to Julius II, when he fled from Rome in 1506. The situation is, however, in no way analogous, since Michelangelo did not address the steward, but merely gave him the letter to deliver. Also, quite apart from the fact that Michelangelo would not be discussing his intimate affairs with a steward, the letter of 1542 is obviously addressed to some high-placed dignatory in the immediate entourage of the Pope. It may be added that Ciampi, perhaps understandably, adduces no arguments in support of this somewhat naïve suggestion.

As to the second, Marco Vigerio, Bishop of Sinigaglia, his name has been put forward because he acted as an intermediary between the Duke of Urbino and the Pope in the correspondence of 1542 about the completion of the Julius Tomb. This might indeed be regarded as a plausible suggestion, were it not that the Bishop was resident in Ancona, whereas the person addressed by Michelangelo was certainly a member of the Papal Court in Rome.

On the face of it, the most likely name advanced, and the one that has generally found favour, would appear to be that of Cardinal Ascanio Parisani, not only because he had long been a prominent member of the *Famiglia Palatina*, but also because it was he who, on November 23rd 1541, first wrote to the Duke, announcing the Pope's intention of employing Michelangelo to paint the frescoes in his new chapel, the Cappella Paolina, recently completed by Antonio da Sangallo, and asking the Duke's indulgence in the matter of the completion of the Tomb. After this, however, Parisani's name disappears from the correspondence, for the sufficient reason that he was appointed Legate to Umbria and Perugia in 1542.

The name of Messer Pier Giovanni Aliotti, though it was again advocated as recently as 1949 in a publication on the frescoes of the Pauline Chapel, may be dismissed even more summarily than the others, inasmuch as he is specifically mentioned by Michelangelo in the body of the letter. Nobody thinks!

We are therefore thrown back upon Milanesi's thoughtful conjecture that 'this letter may perhaps have been written to one of the many prelates at the Court of Paul III'.

Given this decisive lead, it is incumbent upon us first of all to examine the letter itself, in order to see whether it affords any internal evidence as to the probable identity of the recipient and, if such be the case, then to proceed to seek out any confirmatory evidence that may be available.

Now, it is obvious from the opening lines of the letter that the prelate in question was someone in a sufficiently high position to be able to send a message to Michelangelo telling him to paint, and sufficiently conversant with his affairs to be able to tell him not to worry. (Pier Giovanni Aliotti's habit of urging him to paint, as seen in No. 226 was a different matter, this being a direct communication between members of the papal household and not an indirect communication from a superior authority.) Then, at the close of the letter proper, and again in the middle of the postscript and at the end of it, Michelangelo urges the prelate addressed to explain matters to the Pope and, if the opportunity occurs, to show him the letter, in order that he may fully understand Michelangelo's point of view. The assumption that the dignitary to whom he was writing is not only likely to have such an opportunity, but was also in a position to influence the Pope, if he chose, is also implicit in the letter. Moreover, that he wrote at such length presupposes a conviction on Michelangelo's part that he was writing to someone who was both able and willing to understand his argument and to support his case.

In attempting to identify the prelate in question, we may assume him to be someone of the rank of Cardinal, and among the Cardinals resident in Rome at the time, someone intimately associated with the Pope, on the one hand, and fully conversant with Michelangelo's professional affairs, on the other.

At a first glance, the name of the Pope's eldest grandson, Cardinal Alessandro Farnese, would appear to be the most obvious, particularly as Paul III (whose children were all born before he entered the priesthood) was, as he himself confessed on his deathbed, notoriously given to nepotism. The fact that Michelangelo was on good terms with the Pope's family is further borne out by Condivi, who remarks on the regard Michelangelo always cherished for the House of Farnese.

From what is known of Cardinal Alessandro's character, tastes and interests, this would not seem at all improbable. Unlike his father, Pier Luigi, afterwards Duke of Parma, he was renowned for his probity, and he so excited the admiration of Charles V that the Emperor once said of him, 'If the Sacred College were composed of men such as Alessandro Farnese, it would be the most illustrious assembly in the world.' Since the Cardinal was, moreover, a typical man of the Renaissance, a lavish patron of learning, of the arts and perhaps more especially of letters, Michelangelo would not have been wrong in expecting to meet with a sympathetic hearing of his case.

Nevertheless, without some documentary evidence of a more or less direct kind, these facts would not in themselves be sufficient to warrant us in assuming Cardinal Farnese to have been the recipient of the letter; notwithstanding the fact that such was his admiration for Michelangelo's work that a few years after the completion of *The Last Judgment*, he had a copy, one-tenth the size of the original, made for the Farnese Palace by the Mantuan painter, Marcello Venusti. It was, furthermore, the Cardinal who purchased Tommaso de' Cavalieri's collection of drawings after his death in 1587.

One of the earliest of the Cardinal's letters relating to Michelangelo's affairs, though this is only incidental, is that dated September 19th 1538, addressed to the Legate della Gallia Cispadana, Cardinal Giovan Maria Ciocchi, respecting the rival ferry across the Po, which had been started at Piacenza to the detriment of Michelangelo, to whom the revenues had been allocated *(Appendix 33)*. The more important letters not only belong to the relevant years, but also touch upon the relevant subjects. The first, addressed to the Bishop of Sinigaglia, is dated October 12th 1541, and refers to the frescoes which the Pope desired Michelangelo to paint for the Pauline Chapel, which would prevent him completing the Julius Tomb. In the following year, 1542, when the Duke of Urbino failed to ratify the agreement negotiated on August 21st 1542 between his ambassador, Girolamo Tiranno, and Michelangelo, it was Cardinal Farnese who again wrote to the Bishop of Sinigaglia, as witness the Duke's letter to his ambassador, dated November 11th, in which he says that 'Monsignor di Sinigaglia recently sent his secretary with a letter from the Most Reverend Farnese', in which the Cardinal urged the sending of the ratification, which the Duke was not prepared to do, saying that instead he had ordered Girolamo Genga *(No. 228, n. 1)* to Rome to investigate matters *(Vasari, Pros. Cron., p. 388)*.

Now, this letter to which the Duke refers is all-important in connection with the present enquiry. It was discovered in the Archives of Parma by Amadeo Ronchini *(II, p. 29)* and published in 1864. It reads as follows:

The Cardinal Farnese to Monsignor Marco Vigerio,
Bishop of Sinigaglia

Rev. Mons.^{or}, come fratello,

For several days now I have been expecting our *Mons^{or} Rev^{mo}* di Carpi; on the occasion of whose arrival I wished to write to your lordship and to answer the two letters I received from you. But seeing that he has not appeared, for which I must therefore blame the evils of the present time, I will not delay longer to inform your lordship that the resistance put up by the Lord Duke of Urbino, in declining to ratify that contract, which was legally drawn up by his ambassador in the presence of Our Lord, while in the meantime His Excellency expresses no intention other than that which appears up to now to have been intended, cannot be otherwise than a cause of dissatisfaction to His Holiness, who is beyond measure desirous of having Michelangelo free and liberated from all embarrassments, in order that he may be able to devote himself to the work of this new chapel. However, His Excellency will appreciate the circumstances and will of his bounty, as I believe and anticipate, do everything to find a means of satisfying His Beatitude, particularly as Michelangelo for his part has paid down the money, and has placed the work in the hands of capable masters, who will complete it, which is what His Excellency chiefly desires. But of this I shall perhaps have to write to your lordship another time, when it is more convenient. For the present I will confine myself to this.

From Rome on the 6th day of November 1542.

From this correspondence it is clear beyond all reasonable doubt that it was to Cardinal Alessandro Farnese, who was personally concerned in the negotiations over the Tomb, that Michelangelo addressed himself in the letter under discussion, which, from the date of the Cardinal's letter to the Bishop, would appear to have been written either at the very end of October or the beginning of November 1542. Apart from its obvious importance, as providing documentary evidence as to the identity of the hitherto 'unknown' prelate, the Cardinal's letter is valuable for two other reasons. In the first place, it shows how he responded to Michelangelo's appeal and what steps he took to ameliorate the position. In the second, it shows that Michelangelo's confidence was not misplaced, when he laid his case freely and frankly before a man who was as considerate as he was fair, and whose letters, generally, reveal him to have been as likeable as he was eminent.

Appendix 32

The Fortification of the Borgo

WHEN Cardinal Alessandro Farnese became Pope as Paul III in October 1534 one of the first matters to claim his attention was the urgent need of putting Rome into a state of defence, owing to the proneness of the city to attack from the infidel Turk on the one hand and from the Holy Roman Emperor on the other. Already, in the August of that year, the fleet of Soliman II, under the formidable Khair-ed-Din Barbarossa, had appeared at the mouth of the Tiber, while the possibility of a recurrence of the appalling disaster which had overtaken the city seven years before rendered the construction of adequate defences imperative. Of the two the Emperor, Charles V, was in fact, the greater potential danger by far, if one may judge by the amiable words with which he dismissed the Papal Legate, Cardinal Alessandro Farnese, the Pope's grandson, who at the beginning of 1544 delivered to the Emperor a letter from the Pope exhorting peace. Alleging that 'the Vicar of Christ . . . is ready to join forces with the King of France or rather, should we say, with the Turk', Charles concluded by saying 'He may well look to it that we do not deal the same measure to him that we dealt to Clement VII' *(Pastor, XII, p. 188).*

The defensive works already begun at Ancona and Civitavecchia were therefore carried forward without delay, while the most eminent military architects and engineers in Italy were summoned to Rome to prepare plans for the fortifications. After prolonged deliberations under the chairmanship of Pier Luigi, Duke of Castro, the Pope's eldest son, and after what would appear, under the circumstances, to have been an inordinate delay, work was finally begun in the autumn of 1537, the direction of the operation being entrusted to the Pope's architect, Antonio da Sangallo.

It was originally intended to build an enceinte, incorporating no less than eighteen bastions, according to Sangallo's design, on the lines of the old Servian and Aurelian walls. But when by 1542 only two bastions had been completed the experts came to the conclusion that the scheme was beyond realization, being altogether too extensive, too costly and, by reason of the grain tax imposed to meet the expenses, too unpopular an undertaking to be carried out. They were therefore obliged to fall back upon the expedient of fortifying the Borgo only, that is to say, the area on the right bank of the Tiber, between Monte Mario on the north and the Janiculum on the south.

This decision was taken in November 1542, and in December the renowned general and military architect, Alessandro Vitelli, who had been partly responsible for the building of the great citadel at the Faenza gate in Florence, was summoned to Rome to preside. Associated with him, among others, were Giovan Francesco Montemellino of Perugia, a military engineer and later Captain of the Guard at the Castel Sant' Angelo, Jacopo Fusti da Urbino, nicknamed Castriotto, who afterwards carried out a great part of the work, Jacopo Melighini of Ferrara, an architect who had been in the Pope's service since 1537, and Prospero Mochi, who enjoyed the title of Commissary General of the Fortifications and who, in the absence of Pier Luigi, especially after he received the Duchy of Parma, kept the Duke fully informed as to the progress of the work. A fresh start was made on April 18th 1543, and Sangallo remained in supreme charge of the operations.

As if all this were not enough, Michelangelo, whose reputation as a military architect, which was founded on his organization of the defences of San Miniato during the siege of Florence, had been enhanced by his completion of the fortress of Civitavecchia in 1535, was also called in, and required to take part in the formal discussions at which the Pope himself was frequently present.

As always in matters of expertise, opinions were divided and disagreements often arose, as was evidently the case at the meeting on February 25th 1544, referred to by Michelangelo in his letter to the Constable of Castel Sant' Angelo *(No. 236)*. Precisely on what points Michelangelo disagreed with Montemellino on this occasion we do not know, though it might be conjectured that he favoured Castriotto's view that the line of the fortifications should be carried along the ridge of the hills, and was opposed to Montemellino, who had always advocated shortening, rather than extending, the line of defence, and continued, at a considerably later date, to urge the erection of fortifications at the foot of the Vatican Hill. Notwithstanding this disagreement, Michelangelo expressed his willingness to serve under Montemellino in the supervision of the works, if he were to replace Sangallo, under whom he implied that he would decline to serve, though whether this indicates that the famous altercation with Sangallo had already taken place cannot be determined. The date generally assigned to the dispute is October 1545, though on what authority is not established, since an earlier date seems more probable. Gotti assumes that the argument took place on February 25th 1544, but Schiavo *(Vita, p. 254)* supposes that on that date only Montemellino's model was under discussion, and that Sangallo was not involved.

The episode in question, which took place in the presence of the Pope when the fortifications were being discussed, is related by Vasari, who says that when his opinion was asked, Michelangelo, being opposed to the advice of Sangallo and the others, said so frankly, whereupon 'Sangallo retorted that sculpture and painting were his arts, not fortification, to which Michelangelo replied that he knew very little of sculpture and painting, but that as he had thought a great deal about fortification, of which he had had experience, he thought he knew more about it than Antonio or any other member of his family'. In the presence of the company he then proceeded to point out many of the errors they had committed. And, as Vasari goes on to say, 'the dispute waxed so hot that the Pope was obliged to impose silence upon both of them'. Before long, it is said, Michelangelo brought designs for the entire fortification of the Borgo, which prepared the way for all that was done afterwards.

It would appear, however, that it was only after the death of his distinguished rival that Michelangelo played any active part in the work of fortification, since Sangallo remained in charge until his death, which took place on August 3rd 1546. The progress made by that time was not startling, however, since, despite the Pope's anxiety to hasten the work, relatively little advance had been made, for at his death Sangallo left only three bastions completed, though it should be added that considerable progress had been made with the imposing *ornamental* gateway of Santo Spirito.

It was not Michelangelo, however, but Melighini, who was nominally appointed director of the fortifications at Sangallo's death, though only on the express understanding that he was to defer 'in all questions to the opinion of Michelangelo', who, although by right subordinate to Melighini, now became *de facto* the leading architect under whose direction the Belvedere bastion was completed between 1547 and 1548. On its completion, Michelangelo passed the direction to Castriotto, and subsequently to Francesco Laparelli, under whom the work was finally finished, during the pontificate of Paul IV.

The history of the fortifications of the Borgo is summed up by Alberto Guglielmotti as follows: 'The enceinte of the Borgo, first designed by Sangallo, afterwards modified by Michelangelo, then begun by Castriotto, was finally brought to completion by Laparelli and the others . . . taking as a basis the bulwarks of Santo Spirito, and as a guide that of the Belvedere. Three kilometres of ramparted enceinte, ten majestic bulwarks, five main gates, four detached bastions and two outworks, ten years' work' *(Schiavo, p. 160)*.

Appendix 33

The Po Ferry above Piacenza

WHEN Michelangelo was appointed supreme architect, painter and sculptor to the Vatican, and became a member of the Pope's household, he was granted a salary of 1,200 *scudi* a year. Of this sum 600 *scudi* were to be raised from the revenues of the Po ferry – *il Porto del Po* – above Piacenza, which was at that time a possession of the Holy See. These revenues were granted to him for life, but the grant proved to be a troublesome source of income. For although the bimonthly payments were made more or less regularly during his twelve years' tenure, they never amounted to more than 550 *scudi* annually, and his right to possession was repeatedly challenged.

The brief conceding these revenues was dated September 1st 1535, but it was some time before Michelangelo actually gained possession. According to the entry in the *Ricordi (Milanesi, p. 604)*, he acknowledged receipt of a payment in respect of October and November 1536, made to him by his agent, Agostino da Lodi, who had received it from Francesco Durante da Piacenza, to whom Michelangelo had leased the ferry, on January 2nd 1537. The letter addressed to Michelangelo by his agent, and quoted in part by Gotti *(I, p. 263)*, in which the said agent, Agostino, says that he has taken possession of the ferry in Michelangelo's name, should therefore, presumably, be dated September 30th 1536 and not, as cited by Gotti, September 30th 1537, more especially as the payment from the previous October and November, received in January 1537, would be consistent with such a supposition. It was not until May 4th 1538, however, when by order of the Cardinal Camerlengo, Guido Ascanio Sforza, the brief was entered in the *Libri della Camera Apostolica*, that the concession officially became his.

Scarcely had this formal acknowledgment of his claim been made, when the news of the establishment of a rival ferry, operating to Michelangelo's detriment, reached Rome. But although the Pope sent orders requiring the rival enterprise to cease operations immediately, these orders had no effect, and the Signora Beatrice Trivulzio, who was responsible for the innovation, continued to operate the rival service. Whereupon, on September 19th 1538, Cardinal Alessandro Farnese addressed a peremptory letter to the Legate della Gallia Cispadana, Cardinal Giovan Maria Ciocchi del Monte (afterwards Julius III), giving express orders in the name of the Pope for the immediate destruction – *subito, subito, et de facto* – of the new ferry, orders which were this time obeyed.

The following year, in 1539, Michelangelo's interests were again assailed, this time by the Municipality of Piacenza, which made an attempt to obtain the revenues of the ferry for itself; but despite the alternative source of income which the authorities were willing to provide in lieu thereof, the Pope refused to entertain any such proposal, the reason given being that 'he did not wish Michelangelo to be distracted from the work he wished him to undertake'. The Pope having thus intervened for the second time, Michelangelo was left in peace until Pier Luigi Farnese became Duke of Parma and Piacenza in August 1545. Thereupon, his agents at once possessed themselves of the ferry, and would have remained in possession, regardless of Michelangelo, had not the Pope successfully intervened for the third time.

The usual bimonthly payments were, however, suspended, and Michelangelo received nothing between August 1545 and February 1546. It was during this time that he wrote to Luigi del Riccio, who was in Lyons, saying he could not remain in Rome without an income *(No. 259)*, while the need of providing himself with an alternative source of revenue is reiterated in his letters to Lionardo, to whom, however, del Riccio wrote on January 30th 1546, saying 'The Lord Duke of Parma and Piacenza has restored the Po ferry to Messer Michelangelo, which is a very good thing.' But Michelangelo had evidently had enough of incomes 'based upon water', since in his letter to Lionardo of February 13th, del Riccio wrote as follows: 'The Duke has restored the ferry to him, as I told you; now he seems to be disinclined to keep it, because he says he is very old and no longer able to endure fatigue or to work, and for this reason does not want the rewards. We'll have to wait and see what he'll do, because you know what he is – one cannot anticipate.' *(Steinmann, p. 58)*.

Although regular bimonthly payments were then resumed, a new and more formidable claim to the Po revenues was put forward in April of the same year, this time by Baldassare and Niccolò Pusterli, who, with the support of Maria d'Aragona, the Marchesa del Vasto, now laid claim to them by right of inheritance. With this claim the new Duke, Pier Luigi, was disposed to sympathize, a disposition which is a little difficult to understand, in view of his professed affection for Michelangelo. The claim being allowed, the matter was placed in the hands of a member of the Council of Justice, and Michelangelo was summoned to give answer before the Tribunal.

As may be imagined, this new and unlooked for calamity caused him the utmost consternation, but the Pope, whose one anxiety was not to disturb his peace of mind, again refused to countenance a change in the ownership of the ferry, notwithstanding Pier Luigi's offer to provide Michelangelo with another source of income. When writing from Rome to express the Pope's satisfaction on learning that Michelangelo would not be molested further, the Duke's ambassador, Fabio Cappalati, added, 'it is fitting that this should be so, having regard to Michelangelo's personal distinction'.

The matter was not yet at an end, however, as the Pusterli persisted in pressing their claim, and it was only after renewed correspondence that the dispute was eventually settled in Michelangelo's favour. In a letter to the Duke, dated November 17th 1546, Cappalati began by saying that the Pope had had a long discussion with him about Michelangelo's affairs, and had gone on to explain his cogent reasons for wishing at all costs to placate him. 'Our Lord spoke at length,' he wrote, 'saying that if ever he had need of him *[i.e. of Michelangelo]* he had need of him now, in particular for the building of St. Peter's and of his Palace here, since Sangallo is dead; and if ever it was difficult to conciliate him and to induce him to do anything, it is so now, that that Messer Luigi *[del Riccio]* is dead, who used to manage him and was the means of inducing him to comply with the wishes of His Beatitude', adding that Michelangelo, having heard from Piacenza that the case instituted by the Pusterli about the ferry was again being proceeded with, was thoroughly upset. Having reiterated the urgency of the need of preventing further litigation, and having emphasized the Pope's contention that the Po ferry was in the gift of the Holy See, the ambassador then went on to say that His Holiness had informed Michelangelo of the instructions he had given him, and that he could rest assured that no further action would be taken against him *(Ronchini, II, p. 33)*.

On November 25th, the Duke wrote substantiating the Pope's assurances and Michelangelo's right to the revenues of the ferry appeared to be finally settled, but this was not the case. Within less than a year he was to be deprived of them altogether. On September 10th 1547, with the connivance of Charles V, Pier Luigi was overthrown by Ferrante Gonzaga, Viceroy of Milan, and as a result Parma and Piacenza passed into the possession of the Emperor. Four years later, in 1551, Charles acknowledged the Pusterli claim to the disputed revenues and confirmed them in their possession.

To compensate him for the loss of this troublesome, though regular, source of income, on October 1st 1548 the Pope granted Michelangelo an office as Civil Notary in the Chancellery of Rimini *(Schiavo, Vita, p. 271)*, an office which he retained until May 23rd 1555, when, on the day of his election as Pope Paul IV, Cardinal Caraffa took it from him *(Milanesi, p. 609)*. Strictly speaking, it was not Paul IV himself, but his cup-bearer, who took it from him, proposing to pay him a hundred *scudi* a month in exchange. But Michelangelo, who always refused to mention this to the Pope, who knew nothing about it, declined to accept the money when it was sent round to his house *(Vasari, VII, p. 240)*. The matter was later reopened under Pius IV, as we know from Michelangelo's letter to his nephew in January 1562 *(No. 472)*, but nothing seems to have come of it.

Lionardo Buonarroti and his Uncle's illness in 1546

SOME time in December 1545, probably towards the end of the month, Michelangelo was taken seriously ill for the second time in eighteen months. We do not know the predisposing cause of his illness, but the onset of fever may well have been precipitated, partly by anxiety over his financial position, the Po ferry payments having been suspended since the August of that year *(Appendix 33)*, and partly by the cumulative effect of Pietro Aretino's abusive letter about *The Last Judgment*. This letter, with its 'cruel insinuations' of every kind, in which, as Symonds wrote, Aretino 'used every means he could devise to wound and irritate a sensitive nature', must have reached him at about this time, having been written in Venice in November 1545. *[For the emendation of the date given in the letter, namely MDLXV, instead of MDXLV, which may certainly be accepted as correct, see Gaye, II, p. 335.]*

On the occasion of this second illness, as on the first, Luigi del Riccio, who had been ill himself, and had only recently returned from Lyons, received him into his own apartments in the Strozzi Palace, and took care of him. The letter to Lionardo *(No. 260)*, which Michelangelo began and del Riccio finished on Saturday, January 9th, 1546, was therefore written from the Strozzi Palace, as is made clear by del Riccio's covering letter to Lionardo, which reads as follows:

My honoured Messer Lionardo,

Above is a copy of the receipt you must give Piero Capponi for the 600 *scudi* remitted to you by your Messer Michelangelo, who has certainly been very ill and has deigned to come here to me, as he did last time, where he is already so much better that one might say he has recovered. So be reassured about him. He confessed and took communion and made his will, which I wrote down. Being so much better that he is out of danger, he did not afterwards have it legalized by a notary. Be reassured that whenever need arises I will not fail you or your family in doing as you would do yourselves. Now turn your attention to a way in which to invest these 3,000 *scudi*, which he has assigned to you, as you will see by his letter. With other moneys he intends to provide himself with an independent income, which will afterwards come to you. So be reassured. As I think that's all, I remain at your command. God prosper you.

In Rome on the 9th day of January 1546. Style of the Nativity.

Your Luigi del Riccio

(Steinmann, p. 57)

This, like his other letters, bears witness to del Riccio's charming consideration for everyone concerned. To make quite sure that Lionardo did not make a mistake in the wording of the quittance, he enclosed a copy, just as on other occasions, when a particularly tactful letter was needed, he had sent Lionardo drafts of the kind of letter he should address to his uncle.

The news of Michelangelo's illness had, however, already reached Florence, and three days later, on January 12th, Lionardo, riding post, left for Rome, which he reached, according to his own *ricordo*, on January 15th *(Milanesi, p. 605)*, but according to his letter to Giovansimone, on the 14th. The letter in question was published by Frey *(Dicht., p. 532)* and runs thus:

> Jesus. On the XVI day of January 1545 [*Style of the Incarnation*] Lionardo Buonarroti to Giovansimone Buonarroti, being honoured in the place of a father – greetings.
>
> On Thursday I arrived well and cheerful in Rome, and sent at once to find out about Michelangelo and learnt that he was in Luigi del Riccio's house and that he was free of fever and about in his room, for which I was very grateful. Later, this morning, he returned to his own house and is in good spirits and within a day or two will be able to go about, God willing. I don't think there's anything else to tell you for the moment. I shall be in Florence by the end of the month and will explain everything by word of mouth. Christ protect you. There is no need to write to me or to reply, because I shall be leaving, etc.

As Michelangelo wrote to his nephew, whom he supposed to be in Florence, on the same day *(No. 261)*, it is clear that Lionardo had not by this time made his presence in Rome known either to his uncle or to Luigi del Riccio.

Meanwhile, rumours that Michelangelo was dead were spreading in Florence, though it seems strange that as late as Friday, January 22nd, Michele Guicciardini should have written to Giovansimone in the following terms *(Gotti, I, p. 299)*:

> Since I wrote to you, I had news from Niccolò Buondelmonte that Michelangelo was dead, that Lionardo hadn't arrived in time, that he was dead on his arrival and that later they would get confirmation. I will leave you to imagine Francesca's terrible grief at the news. The same evening I had a letter from Bartolomeo Ratti, who works in the shop belonging to Francesco and Averardo Ratti, that according to the last letters from Rome they are informed that the doctors have saved him. God grant this may be so.

Four days later, on Tuesday, January 26th, Lionardo was back in Florence, with the reassuring news of Michelangelo's recovery; perhaps without having attempted to see his uncle, after the reception he had been given in the July of 1544 *(No. 238)*; certainly without having succeeded. This is made clear from del Riccio's letter of January 30th, in which he said that he had told Michelangelo about his departure, and about the farm which was for sale adjoining Lionardo's property. Further reference is made to this farm in del Riccio's letter of

February 6th, in which he said that Michelangelo was awaiting details of the farm 'about which you spoke to me'. It is therefore evident that although Lionardo failed to see his uncle, he had had at least one interview with Luigi del Riccio.

The question then arises – Why did Michelangelo refuse to see him? The answer to this question is given in his letter of February 6th *(No. 262)*, which is the same as that given on the previous occasion, namely that Lionardo had hastened to Rome, not for his uncle's sake, but for the sake of the inheritance. The letter of February 6th is undeniably harsh. Was it justifiably so? And was Michelangelo right in his conjectures? To both questions the answer is in the affirmative. The reason that Lionardo went to Rome *con tanta furia* was undoubtedly, first and foremost, to find out how things stood in relation to Michelangelo's possessions, in the event of his death, and to be at hand to lay claim to anything that he had not otherwise bequeathed. This information is supplied by the letter of introduction from Ottaviano de' Medici in Florence to Lorenzo Ridolfi, brother of Cardinal Niccolò Ridolfi, in Rome, which he had been careful to obtain before his departure on January 12th *(Steinmann, p. 48)*. The terms are unmistakable; in case the illness proved fatal, Lionardo wished 'to be in Rome to see that there were no concealments of his property' and to find out from del Riccio, with whom Ridolfi was asked to use his influence, how things stood in the matter of his affairs. In other words, Lionardo went to Rome for one reason and for one reason only, as Michelangelo was well aware; namely to assert his claims to the inheritance. For the love Lionardo affected to have for his uncle, Michelangelo had therefore one phrase, and one phrase only – cupboard love – for which, characteristically, he had no use whatsoever.

Appendix 35

The Record of Michelangelo's Birth

AMONG the documents in the Buonarroti Archives is a contemporary copy of the record of Michelangelo's birth made by his father, Lodovico, in his *Ricordanza*. The extract (*Milanesi, p. 223*) is as follows:

I record that to-day, this 6th day of March 1474 *[N.S. 1475]* a son was born to me. I named him Michelangelo. He was born on Monday morning 4 or 5 hours before day-break while I was Podestà at Caprese. He was born at Caprese and these named below were his godfathers. He was baptized on the 8th day of the said month in the church of Santo Giovanni at Caprese. These are his godfathers –
Don Daniello di Ser Bonaguida da Firenze, Rector of Santo Giovanni di Caprese.
Don Andrea di.... da Poppi, Rector of the Badia di Diariano *[Larniano?]*
Giovanni di Nanni da Caprese
Jacopo di Francesco da Casurio
Marco di Giorgio da Caprese
Giovanni di Biaggio da Caprese
Andrea di Biaggio da Caprese
Francesco di Jacopo del Anduino da Caprese
Ser Bartolomeo di Santi del Lanse, notary.

The Identification of the Prelate addressed in Letter No. 274

'THERE can be no doubt', wrote Milanesi in his footnote to the undated letter which Michelangelo addressed to a certain 'Messer Bartolomeo', 'that the Messer Bartolomeo in question was Bartolomeo Ammanati.' This assumption, which five minutes' thought shows to be wrong, has, nevertheless, been generally, though not invariably accepted, but for no better reason, one must suppose, than that 'thought is difficult', as A. E. Housman once remarked, 'and five minutes is a long time'. The date Milanesi proposed for the letter, namely 1555, is, if anything, more palpably incorrect and has, accordingly, from time to time been questioned. Not, however, by Venturi, who unaccountably accepted both conjectures, though neither he nor Milanesi paused to tell us why Bartolomeo Ammanati, Michelangelo's junior by thirty-six years, a sculptor who had nothing whatever to do with the building of St. Peter's and who in 1555 was in Florence, while the Pope was of course in Rome, should have been thought to be in a better position than Michelangelo to influence the Pope, and that, more especially, over matters which in 1555 had long been settled.

From its contents it is quite clear that this letter must have been written shortly after Michelangelo had been forced by command of Paul III to continue the building of St. Peter's in succession to Antonio da Sangallo, who died in the summer of 1546. Michelangelo's appointment took effect from January 1st 1547. Now we learn from Vasari that it was after his appointment that he made an official inspection of Sangallo's ornate and costly model of the Basilica, while, from the internal evidence of the letter itself, it is clear that it was written after Michelangelo had examined the model and at a time when he was himself personally involved. The first weeks of 1547 would, therefore, seem the most probable date for it, since we have no means of dating it more precisely.

The identity of the recipient would be more difficult to establish were it not for a letter in the Buonarroti Archives, the text of which has been quoted by Gotti in full *(I, p. 309 et seq.)*. This letter was addressed to Michelangelo on May 14th 1547 by a friend of his in Florence, Giovan Francesco Ughi, in which the writer informed him of the rumours that were being spread in Florence by the painter, Jacopo del Conte, a partisan of Nanni di Baccio Bigio's, who fancied himself as a rival to Michelangelo at St. Peter's. In this letter Ughi gives a detailed account of the way in which Michelangelo's abilities as an architect were being impugned in regard to his work both at the Farnese Palace and at St. Peter's. On receipt of this highly defamatory letter Michelangelo immediately sent it round to a certain Messer Bartolomeo Ferratini, one of the Deputies of the fabric of St. Peter's, probably at this time the Prefect, since he was manifestly influential. At the head of the letter Michelangelo added this note:

> Messer Bartolomeo – Kindly read this letter and consider who these two sharks are, who have thus lied about what I have done at the Farnese Palace. They lie in the same way over the information they give to the Deputies of the fabric of St. Peter's. This is what I get in return for the kindnesses I have done them. But one can expect nothing else from such vicious, low-born churls.

Bartolomeo Ferratini was, as we know from his epitaph in the Cathedral Church at Emilia, a canon of St. Peter's and Prefect of the fabric. He had been bishop, first of Sora and afterwards of Chiusi *(Gams, pp. 925, 754)* and had held various important offices during the pontificates of Julius II and Clement VII *(Ughelli, III, 649).* This being so, there can be no doubt whatever that the Messer Bartolomeo addressed in the note appended to Ughi's letter and the Messer Bartolomeo addressed in the letter about Sangallo's model were in fact one and the same, since no-one would have been in a better position to present Michelangelo's proposals to the Pope and to support them if he were so disposed, than the Prefect of the Deputies of the fabric.

> *This conclusion was also reached by Carl Frey (Die*
> *Briefe des M.B., pp. 199, 324) and has since been*
> *accepted by James Ackerman (Catalogue, p. 88).*

Appendix 37

Michelangelo and the Proceedings of the Accademia Fiorentina

OR a variety of reasons, some of which may not be immediately obvious, Michelangelo's letter to Luca Martini *(No. 279)*, no less than the one which he addressed to Benedetto Varchi at the same time *(No. 280)*, is at once both interesting and important. Both were occasioned by the proceedings of the Accademia Fiorentina and relate, the one to the second, and the other to the first of two discourses delivered by Varchi before a public audience and 'The magnificent and most worthy Consul and most noble and learned Academicians' on the second and third Sundays in Lent in 1547.

The Accademia Fiorentina, or as it was originally called the Accademia degli Umidi, had been founded in November 1540 with the object of fostering the study of Italian literature, Dante and Petrarch in particular, and of preserving and perfecting the Tuscan tongue in its *purità e sincerità*. The Academy, which enjoyed the patronage of the Duke, Cosimo I, who had sanctioned the change to the new name three months after the foundation of the society, included among its members the most eminent men in Florence, churchmen and laymen alike, of whom the following may be mentioned – Giovanni Mazzuoli, with whom the idea had originated; Niccolò Martelli, the poet; Benedetto Varchi, the scholar and historian; Cosimo Bartoli, the provost of San Giovanni; Luca Martini, a civil engineer and man of letters; Bartolomeo Rontini, the physician, and Giovanbattista da Ricasoli, Bishop of Cortona, one of the Duke's most trusted envoys. Although he was no longer resident in Florence, Michelangelo was elected a member and is proudly referred to by Varchi in the introduction to his first discourse, which was given on March 6th 1547, as *nobilissimo cittadino ed accademico nostro (Guasti, p. lxxxvii)*.

Taking as his subject what he described as Michelangelo's *altissimo Sonnetto*, namely the one beginning,

> *Non ha l'ottimo artista alcun concetto,*
> *Ch' un marmo solo in sè non circonscriva*

> *(Guasti, pp. lxxxv, 173),*

he proceeded to a long, learned and detailed exposition of the poem, to a study of comparative material, showing to what extent Michelangelo had been influenced by Dante and Petrarch, in whose works he was steeped, and, in true academic fashion, to an analysis of his vocabulary according to its classical or Tuscan bias, the comparative virtues of Latin and the vernacular being a common topic of interest at this period. Assuming, on the authority of the opening lines of the sonnet, that Michelangelo held sculpture to be the noblest of all the arts, Varchi next proposed, *piacendo a Dio ed al Consolo nostro*, to deliver a second lecture on the following Sunday, March 13th, in order to consider the relative merits of painting and sculpture – a subject frequently debated at this time, as witness, for example, Vasari's letter of February 1547 to Varchi *(Due Lez., p. 121)*, in which he said that, following a similar discussion in Rome, he himself had already consulted Michelangelo on the point. Prior to the lecture Varchi had elicited the opinions of a number of artists living in Florence and intended, as he said in the course of this second lecture, to defer to Michelangelo himself, whom he considered to be perfect in both arts.

From a letter which Varchi sent to his fellow Academician, Luca Martini, on Monday, March 14th, following the delivery of the second lecture, we find that he did not himself approach Michelangelo on the subject, but left it to Martini, who proposed, with Varchi's consent, to send copies of both discourses to Rome, Varchi himself being anxious only to acknowledge his own ignorance and presumption in face of the man whom he reverenced as much as he admired him. The letter to Martini, which has not survived, is known to us from its inclusion with the printed text of the two lectures *(p. 55)* which was published by Lorenzo Torrentino under the title *Due Lezioni di Benedetto Varchi* in 1549. Although the date of publication, as printed, is 1549, it happens to be an *ab Incarnatione* dating, as is evident from the publisher's preface, addressed to Bartolomeo Bettini, which is dated January 12th 1549. The date of the first edition should therefore properly be given as 1550.

Somewhat mistakenly, one may feel, Milanesi did not consult the *Due Lezioni*, to which he alludes in a footnote to the Italian text of Michelangelo's letter to Varchi. Had he done so, he must instantly have recognized firstly, that the date of the publication of the first edition of the work was in fact 1550 and not 1549; secondly, that in acknowledging Varchi's *libretto*, Michelangelo was acknowledging the receipt not of the published volume, but of the work in manuscript, presented in book form; and would accordingly have realized that the date of the letter to Martini and of that to Varchi likewise, is not, as he supposed, 1549, but, without a doubt, March/April 1547.

It is a pity that Luca Martini's covering letter has not been preserved, particularly as he appears to have been an attractive personality, if one may judge from Vasari's account of him as a patron of the arts *(VI, pp. 125 et seq.)* and from Niccolò Martelli's assurances of the esteem in which he was held by his many friends *(p. 17)*, as well as from the tone of another letter to Michelangelo, written many years later in May 1560 *(Frey, Briefe, p. 378)*, in which he signed himself 'your most affectionate servant'. Besides being active in humanistic and artistic circles, as is shown by his extant correspondence with the leading men of his day, he was also *persona grata* with the Duke, for whom he performed services of a more practical nature, as for instance when he was appointed *ministro e provveditore* at Pisa for the purpose of draining the marshes, with the plans for which he is shown in his portrait by Bronzino.

From Michelangelo's reception of Martini's letter and of the commentary it is obvious that he was both flattered and delighted by the honour done him, notwithstanding the note of sadness at the end, which, on reflection, is not difficult to interpret. Although his immediate reaction to the letter and to the *si bello e dotto commento* was one of intense pride and pleasure, the sense of grief and desolation into which he had been plunged by the death of Vittoria Colonna some three weeks before was, after a moment's pause, perhaps intensified by the realization that neither she nor Luigi del Riccio, who had died in the previous October, were any longer at hand to share his pleasure in this unexpected recognition of his poetic achievement. Happily, however, Donato Giannotti was in Rome at the time, and Michelangelo had evidently lost no time in communicating the gratifying news to an almost equally sympathetic ear, while Giannotti, for his part, must have been thankful for what was probably the first respite since the Marchesa's death on February 25th.

The letter to Varchi from whom, as already stated, he had received no direct communication, is rather different in tone and betrays, unwittingly, a certain impatience with the amount of time and thought spent upon the resolution of problems which, in face of the anomalies of destiny and of the unresolved mysteries of life and death with which he was overtaken, must necessarily, and despite his gratitude, have seemed to him not only purely academic, but altogether trivial and unreal. And that this is unquestionably what he felt is further borne out by his letter and perhaps even more poignantly by the draft *(Draft No. 9)* of the letter *(No. 281)* which he wrote to his old friend Fattucci, enclosing his reply to Varchi, which, together with letters from other artists on the same subject, was published three years later in the *Due Lezioni di Benedetto Varchi*.

Appendix 38

The Fuorusciti and the Decree of 1547

IN the absence of an autograph date or of any internal evidence as to the approximate period at which they were written, Michelangelo's letters to his nephew can only be dated from the endorsements in Lionardo's hand – always supposing, of course, that these can be deciphered, intermittent onsets of 'fever' notwithstanding. Unfortunately for Milanesi, his copyist in London sometimes failed to supply him with these essential details, so that as far as the letters in the British Museum are concerned he was bound from time to time to be at a loss and cannot therefore be blamed for his misdating of No. 291, which is a case in point. But in associating the *bando* or proclamation, to which the letter refers, with the so-called *Polverina* – a law against lese-majesty and misprision of treason, promulgated on March 11th 1548 by Jacopo Polverini, *Auditore Fiscale* to Cosimo I, Milanesi can be blamed for his failure to observe that this is an *ab Incarnatione* dating and therefore requires adjustment in order to conform to modern usage. In other words, both the law and – on Milanesi's conjecture that it is to the *Polverina* that Michelangelo refers – the letter likewise should have been assigned, not to March 1548, but to March 1549. A not dissimilar error in regard to the dating of this legislation seems, incidentally, to have been made by the contemporary historian, Giovambattista Adriani, who refers it to the beginning instead of to the end of the Florentine year *(Adriani, III, p. 7)*.

It is not, however, the *Polverina* to which Michelangelo's letter relates, but to the *bando* of '*27 Novembre 1547 ab Incarnat.*' *(Cantini, Leg., I, p. 363)*, since his letter is endorsed by Lionardo – as clearly as makes no matter – *1547 da Roma. Ricevuta 29 ottobre di ottobre 22.* Nor, indeed, do the terms of the letter itself admit of any doubt of this being so, besides which, no other *bando* was promulgated during this period, to which Michelangelo might be referring. But in view of the fact that the letter was written not after, but before the promulgation of the decree, we must suppose that rumour, as always in Florence, was rife and that Lionardo hastened to pass on the information to his uncle. The correctness of this supposition that the *bando* was, in fact, the main topic of the day is further borne out by Luca Martini's observation in his letter of October 8th to Benedetto Varchi, in which he said that there was no news in Florence, except that the *bando* against the *fuorusciti* had been printed *(Martini, p. 267)*. But in order to appreciate the implications of the letter some mention must be made of the historical events which preceded the promulgation of the said *bando*.

Ever since the fall of the Florentine Republic and the inception of the ducal rule in 1532, Tuscan loyalties had been divided and as between those who accepted and those who rejected the new order of things there was a great gulf fixed. Apart from those who were banished, the malcontents were divided into two categories; those who, though opposed to the new régime, deemed it more politic to submit, and those who, finding it impossible to remain, went into voluntary exile and were ultimately declared rebels.

Although the opposition of the rebels, or *fuorusciti* as they were called, declared itself from the outset, it was not until after Alessandro, the first Duke, had been murdered by Lorenzino de' Medici, and Cosimo, Lorenzino's second cousin, had seized power and established himself as absolute ruler in Florence in Alessandro's stead, that the full force of their hostility became evident. Under the leadership of Filippo Strozzi, whose son Piero held the military command of the considerable force that had been assembled, an ill-advised and precipitate attempt was made to overthrow the newly constituted tyrant, which resulted in the complete defeat of the rebels. Most of those who fell into the hands of the Florentine commander, Alessandro Vitelli, were conducted to Florence, thrown into the Bargello and put to death, with the exception of Filippo Strozzi, whom Cosimo dared not execute. Instead, he was imprisoned in the citadel at the Faenza gate, where he died by his own hand in September 1538.

But while the *fuorusciti* could do little to assist their own cause after the defeat at Montemurlo, they remained a formidable centre of intrigue and could and did do everything in their power to comfort the Duke's enemies, as witness their implication, for example, in the attempted rising of Burlamarcchi in 1546, for as Adriani remarks, they 'were men of great daring, ready to face any danger', if by so doing they saw an opportunity of furthering the cause of Florentine liberty, to which they remained consistently devoted.

Such being the situation, it was inevitable that stern measures should be taken in Florence to prohibit and, as far as possible, to prevent all communications with the *fuorusciti* and legislation was promulgated to that effect in 1537 and again in 1539, severe penalties being imposed for the infringement of the regulations, while in 1540 further measures were concerted in order to put a stop to the 'emigration of citizens', numbers of whom were leaving Tuscany to seek service elsewhere. The *bando* of November 1547 confirmed the provisions of the foregoing years. In it all dealings with the rebels of any kind whatsoever, either within or beyond the confines of the State, were expressly forbidden on pain, not only of the imposition of heavy fines, but of punishment being visited upon their next of kin in the case of those who themselves escaped the penalties of the law.

It is therefore understandable that for the sake of his relatives in Florence Michelangelo should have been at pains to avoid all appearance of implication with the *fuorusciti*, and that he should have been careful to stress the fact that he did not consider himself to have been the guest of the Strozzi when he was ill in Rome in 1544 and again 1545/6, but of Luigi del Riccio, who, like Michelangelo himself, was not a *fuoruscito*. But while it is true that at the period in question Michelangelo was probably unaware as to exactly who were *fuorusciti* and who were not, he had long been on more or less intimate terms with known *fuorusciti*, men like Cardinal Ridolfi, Donato Giannotti, Bindo Altoviti and others – with whom he certainly remained on the same terms – since there is no doubt where his own sympathies lay, he being, as Giannotti emphasizes in his *Dialoghi*, an incorrigible old Republican at heart. Later, however, he became reconciled, owing to the Duke's exceeding amiability towards him.

Appendix 39

Michelangelo and Giorgio Vasari

MILANESI'S text of Michelangelo's letters to Giorgio Vasari was based, as we know, on copies in the hand of Cavaliere Bustelli, the Portuguese consul at Civitavecchia, whose collection had been acquired for the Casa Buonarroti in 1861 *(Giornale, V, p. 338)*. The originals, once in the possession of Vasari's nephew, Giorgio Vasari the Younger, had been copied by Michelangelo the Younger, but all trace of them was subsequently lost until 1908, when, together with many other letters addressed to Vasari, Signor Giovanni Poggi, Director of the Museo Nazionale in Florence, discovered them, in the private archives of Conte Rasponi Spinelli, a descendant of one of Vasari's executors *(Schlosser, p. 340)*. This invaluable collection is now housed in the Casa Vasari at Arezzo.

Of the fifteen letters from Michelangelo to Vasari published by Milanesi, fourteen are still extant, but of Vasari's letters to Michelangelo only five have been preserved. A further insight into the relationship of the two men is afforded, however, by numerous references to Michelangelo which occur in Vasari's letters to other correspondents, in which he speaks of him in affectionate terms, sometimes as *il mio gran' Michelagnolo*, and sometimes as *il mio rarissimo vecchio*.

Although their correspondence did not begin until 1550, they had known each other for a long time. When about twelve years of age Vasari had studied design, albeit briefly, under Michelangelo who, when he was summoned to Rome by Clement VII to discuss the plans for the Laurentian Library, placed the boy in Andrea del Sarto's charge *(Vasari, VII, p. 7 et seq.)*. Nearly twenty years later, when Vasari found himself in Rome, where he habitually stayed in the house of Bindo Altoviti, he resolved to make the most of his opportunities. 'In those days I courted Michelangelo assiduously and consulted him about all my affairs', he wrote, adding (as one might anticipate) 'and he was good enough to show me great friendship' *(ibid., VII, p. 672)*.

Although Vasari did not remain permanently in Rome, he returned there from time to time and in 1550 under rather unusual circumstances. When leaving Florence on his way to the conclave of 1549/50, Cardinal Giovanni Maria del Monte had said to him, 'I am going to Rome and shall assuredly be made Pope. . . . When you hear the news set out for Rome at once, without waiting for a summons' *(ibid., VII, p. 692)*. This Vasari accordingly proceeded to do, 'being glad of such employment,' as he said, 'which brought me near to Michelangelo' *(ibid., VII, p. 226)*.

The first work on which the new Pope, Julius III, employed him was on the building of a chapel in San Pietro in Montorio, to contain the tombs of his uncle, Cardinal Antonio del

280

Monte, and of his grandfather, Messer Fabiano Ciocchi. At one stage, as we know from Michelangelo's letter to Vasari of August 1st, 1550 *(No. 348)*, the Pope considered the church of San Giovanni dei Fiorentini as an alternative site for the tombs, but this proposal was afterwards abandoned.

Among various other projects Julius III also commissioned him to prepare designs for his *vigna*, the villa Julia, but despite the auspicious beginnings of their association the Pope, who was for ever changing his mind, did not, as a patron, commend himself to Vasari who, finding himself constantly at the Pope's beck and call and unable to do himself justice in any commission he undertook, decided to return to Florence and to enter the service of the Duke who had signified his desire to employ him. But it was not until the spring of 1554 that he was at last able to leave for Florence, which he did with many regrets at having wasted so much time in the service of 'asses clothed in silk'. It is therefore after this date that his main correspondence with Michelangelo begins.

On his return to Tuscany Vasari found that his property at Arezzo had been extensively damaged by the French soldiery marauding over the territory, who were there in support of the Sienese cause *(Appendix 43)*. These misfortunes he contrived to bear, however, as he told Michelangelo, in his letter of August 20th 1554 'with that long-suffering which I learnt from you when I was in Rome'. After expressing his affectionate respect and saying that having heard from Sebastiano Malenotti, Michelangelo's deputy at St. Peter's and the bearer of this letter to him, of the cruel usage to which he was being subjected at the Basilica, he went on to beg him to return to Florence, there to enjoy the peace that would be his under the rule of a prince who recognized and appreciated his genius. To this letter Michelangelo replied on September 19th, giving his reasons for being unable to comply with Vasari's suggestion *(No. 390)*.

The opposition which Michelangelo encountered in his work at St. Peter's was in no way diminished when, on the death of Julius III, Cardinal Marcello Cervini, who supported the rival faction, became Pope as Marcellus II in April 1555. As Michelangelo had, so to speak, crossed swords with him only a few years earlier *(Appendixes 42 and 44)* he prudently considered the possibility of leaving Rome, reluctant though he would have been to abandon the work at the Basilica. As soon as this was known in Florence every inducement to return to Florence was offered him on behalf of the Duke, in reply to whose flattering offers Michelangelo wrote to Vasari on May 11th 1555 *(No. 398)*, declining the invitation and advancing in support of his refusal appreciably the same arguments that he had used to Vasari before, since by this time circumstances had again changed with the death of Marcellus on May 1st. On a renewal of the Duke's offers through his chamberlain, Lionardo Marinozzi, when he was in Rome on the embassy of obedience to the new Pope, Paul IV, Michelangelo wrote once more, on June 22nd *(No. 402)*, explaining his inability to leave the work on the fabric at the stage it had then reached.

On May 8th 1557 the same offers were once again renewed, this time not only by Vasari on behalf of the Duke, but by the Duke himself in the following letter, the terms of which do him credit as a prince:

Magnifico nostro carissimo – Since the nature of the times and the reports of your friends give us some hope that you are not altogether disinclined to visit Florence to see your native land and your kindred once again after so many years – which would give us the pleasure we have always so much desired – we have thought it fitting hereby to exhort and entreat you to do so, as we do exhort and entreat you with all our heart, assuring you that to us it would be most gratifying to see you. And let no suspicion that we intend to burden you with any labour or vexation deter you, since we know the respect due to your age and to your singular genius. But come freely in the expectation of being able to pass such time as suits you, living here entirely as you choose and to your own satisfaction, because to us it will suffice to see you here – and for the rest our pleasure will be in proportion to your recreation and repose, nor shall we ever think to do aught but to your honour and advantage. May the Lord our God preserve you.

From Florence viii May MDLVII.

Vostro el duca di Firenze

(Cosimo, I, p. 196).

To this gratifying and persuasive communication Michelangelo replied in a letter *(No. 433)* which, from what he says in another to Vasari written at about the same time *(No. 434)*, he judged to be inadequate, but being old and easily moved by kindness, he wrote as he did and before he had had time to adjust himself to so amiable a gesture on the part of the Duke or to reflect upon the terms of his reply. It is therefore understandable that he should have enlarged upon his difficulties at the Basilica, the subject uppermost in his mind, being, as he was, much upset by the mistake made in the vaulting of the chapel of the King of France, of which this is the first mention and of which fuller explanations were forthcoming later in his two letters to Vasari in the summer of the same year *(Nos. 437, 439)*.

Although these two letters are the last of those surviving addressed by Michelangelo to his old friend, they remained closely in touch. Vasari always saw as much of him as possible when he was in Rome and continued as before to consult him about his affairs, and notably about the projects for the Duke at the Palazzo Vecchio, in which connection it may not be uninteresting to anticipate the circumstances in which Michelangelo wrote to the Duke about the alterations and decorations in question *(No. 458)*.

On the death of Paul IV in August 1559 Cosimo was determined to use every means in his power to secure the election of his chosen candidate, Cardinal Gian Angelo de' Medici of Milan, and had written to his agent in Rome, Gian Francesco Lottini, who had failed to satisfy him on the two previous occasions, saying 'if for the third time with your caprices over yonder you bring about the election of another such, all the waters in the Arno will not wash you' *(Booth, p. 199)*. Luckily for Lottini, the Cardinal of Cosimo's choice was elected on December 25th 1559 and in token of his gratitude for the support he had received, the new Pope, Pius IV, immediately raised the Duke's second son, Giovanni, to the purple. The prince, accompanied by Vasari, accordingly left for Rome in March 1560. In addition to acting as an escort to the young Cardinal, Vasari had also been commissioned to consult Michelangelo about the work being undertaken at the Palazzo. About this he apparently had some qualms, perhaps owing to the amount of advice needed, and on reaching Siena he wrote to the Duke on March 5th in these terms:

> My Most Illustrious and Most Excellent Lord – I am on my way to Rome with your son, the Most Reverend and Most Illustrious Cardinal de' Medici. And as I wrote You how necessary it is for me to get Michelangelo's opinion regarding those matters with which I have to deal, I had hoped that You would send me a note containing a message for Buonarroto, in order that he may give ear to me and advise me about all those things which I have to discuss with him on Your Illustrious Excellency's account. For although I know that he would do so willingly in the ordinary way, he will be obliged to do so much more diligently if You ask him . . . *(Vasari, VIII, p. 349).*

Although the Duke apparently wrote as requested, Vasari need not have entertained a moment's doubt about Michelangelo's readiness to do what was asked of him, such was the pleasure of his *rarissimo vecchio* at seeing him. On his arrival Vasari at once went to see Michelangelo and on April 9th he wrote to the Duke to inform him of what had taken place. His letter opens with these words –

> My Most Illustrious and Most Excellent Lord – I arrived in Rome and as soon as the Most Reverend and Most Illustrious Medici had made his entry and received the hat from Our Lord *[the Pope]* I immediately went to see *il mio gran Michelagnolo*. He did not know of my coming and with the tenderness of a father unexpectedly finding a long lost son he threw his arms round my neck and kissed me a thousand times, weeping with pleasure, so glad was he to see me and I him . . . *(ibid., VIII, p. 330).*

After this they discussed all manner of things – St. Peter's and the model of the cupola and lantern, which filled Vasari with amazement; the rebuilding of the Ponte S. Trinità, which had been destroyed in the flooding of the Arno in 1557 and was subsequently replaced by Ammanati's beautiful and brilliantly contrived structure and, by no means least, Vasari's work at the Palazzo Vecchio, which Michelangelo approved and on which he commented in his letter to the Duke of April 25th 1560 *(No. 458).*

In November of the same year Duke Cosimo and his Duchess, Eleanora of Toledo, made a state visit to Rome, where they were received with all the pomp and circumstance due to their rank. On this occasion Michelangelo was received by the Duke with every mark of affection and respect, and prior to the visit of Don Francesco, the Duke's eldest son, in the autumn of 1561, Vasari sent Michelangelo word to this effect:

> Our Prince is coming to Rome and last night, prior to his departure, he commissioned me to write to you, since he, knowing how much the Duke, his father, loves and honours

you, and wishing to do no less himself, is most insistent upon his desire to see you. Therefore when you go to St. Peter's – he will be staying at the Palace – I should be grateful if you would go to see him. . . . .

Michelangelo took a liking to the young prince, who always addressed him standing with his hat in his hand, and, in a letter no longer extant, wrote and told Vasari that he was grieved that he was old and ailing, as he would have liked to execute something for the youth, for whom he had tried to buy a valuable antique *(ibid., VII, p. 260)*.

Vasari's last surviving letter to Michelangelo is dated March 17th 1563 *(ibid., VIII, p. 366)*. In it he informs him, among other things, of the foundation of the new *Accademia del Disegno*, of which the leading members, elected from the main body of artists by secret ballot, were to be known as Academicians. The Duke, as patron, was to rank as the first Academician, and then, as Vasari proceeded, 'next to him, by reason of the debt owed by all art to you, they wished to elect you as the head, patron and master of them all, as excelling in these three professions more than anyone whom the city and perhaps the world has ever known. And this they have done unanimously and to everyone's complete satisfaction.' The letter concluded with a long and importunate plea on behalf of the Duke for Michelangelo's guidance as to how the New Sacristy at San Lorenzo should be completed, as all the Academicians were only waiting to do him honour, if he would but give them *un poco di splendore del animo suo*. But it was already too late; and the only thing they could now do in acknowledgment of his perfection in the three arts, painting, sculpture and architecture, was to change his own device of three rings, interlaced, into three crowns of laurel, interlaced, with this legend: He assumes a crown of triple honours – *Tergeminis tollit honoribus*.

Two Briefs of Pope Paul III

Aᴄᴄᴏʀᴅɪɴɢ to Milanesi the two briefs of Paul III which Michelangelo asked his nephew, Lionardo, to send to him in August 1550 *(No. 349)* were *(i)* the brief of September 1st 1535, by which he had been appointed supreme architect, sculptor and painter to the Vatican and granted the privileges and prerogatives of a *familiaris* to the Pope; *(ii)* the brief of December 18th 1537 (September 18th, according to Gotti *(I, p. 263)*, who refers to it in a different connection) relating to Michelangelo's inability to fulfil his obligations to the Duke of Urbino in the matter of completing the long-commissioned Tomb of Julius II, owing to his commitments to the Pope when painting *The Last Judgment*.

Milanesi's conjecture as to which were the briefs in question is obviously as correct in the first instance as it is incorrect in the second, since the one was as irrelevant as the other was relevant to the matter under discussion, namely the grounds on which Michelangelo might be deemed to be a creditor of the Pope in respect of some two thousand *scudi*.

By the brief of 1535 Michelangelo had been granted a salary of twelve hundred *scudi* a year for life, as long as he remained in the Pope's service and of this amount, as already shown *(Appendix 33)*, six hundred *scudi* were to be secured on the revenues of the Po ferry at Piacenza, in regard to which a second brief, substantially the same as the first, but dealing specifically with the matter of his salary, was also addressed to him. Both briefs concluded with the words *Datum Roma apud S. Marcum, primus septembris, 1535, anno primo (Gotti, II, pp. 123, 124)*.

There can therefore be no doubt at all that it was to these two briefs, and not to the brief of 1537, that Michelangelo was referring in his letter of August 7th 1550.

A further point of interest arising out of this letter is that concerning the sum of approximately two thousand *scudi*, for which Michelangelo believed himself to be a creditor of the Pope. The deficit on his salary was due, of course, to the amount by which the revenues of the Po ferry, and of the Romagna office which replaced it, had fallen short of the amount estimated, namely six hundred *scudi* a year. On the basis of the existing records of the payments received, his computation is found on examination to be correct and is made up as follows:

(i) The revenues of the Po ferry were granted to Michelangelo in September 1535, but no payment was received until a year later.

The deficit therefore amounted to . . . . 600 *scudi*

(ii) Over a period of ten years the annual income from this source fell short of the estimated six hundred by approximately fifty *scudi* a year.

The deficit therefore amounted to . . . . . . 500 *scudi*

(iii) The revenues of the Po ferry were lost to him in 1547 (the last recorded bimonthly payment was for February and March) and the income from the office of Civil Notary to the Romagna, by which it was replaced, was not granted to him until October 1548, so that the loss was in excess of the income for one year.

The deficit therefore amounted to . . . . . . 600 *scudi*
+

(iv) The office of Civil Notary to the Romagna was worth approximately half the value of the Po ferry.

The deficit therefore amounted to . . . . . . 300 *scudi*
±

Total 2,000 *scudi*
deficit ±

Appendix 41

The Dowery System in sixteenth-century Florence

'A WOMAN who seeks a greater station than her own,' wrote Fra Giovanni Dominici in his *Regolo del governo di cura familiare*, 'or a husband who will only take her for her money, may be said to add a further servitude to a natural yoke.' Despite this sage counsel, the preoccupation of the Florentines in their marriage negotiations was primarily with money and with birth. In urging his nephew, Lionardo, to dispense with a dowery and to look only for nobility of blood, excellence of character and soundness of health in the ladies offered for his consideration, Michelangelo was to some extent running counter to the general feeling of his period. Indeed, so essential was the provision of a dowery, that a girl without one could rarely obtain a husband, and the fact that one of those suggested to Lionardo as a possible bride died unmarried in a monastery without having taken the veil *(No. 337, n. 1)* may well be attributed to her penniless state, since without endowment she could hardly even have become a nun in a house of suitable standing.

Michelangelo, though himself a bachelor, was, perforce, involved on various occasions throughout his life in transactions concerned with such endowments.

The first occasion was the lawsuit brought by Mona Cassandra, the widow of his father's elder brother, Francesco, for the return of her dowery, following the death of her husband in June 1508 *(Nos. 45 et seq.)*. The money given with a bride upon her marriage became the temporary property of her husband, and if she predeceased him it apparently passed, automatically and absolutely, to him or to his legitimate issue, even if they were not the children of his marriage with her. This had been the case with the dowery of Michelangelo's stepmother, Lucrezia Ubaldini da Gagliano *(No. 153, n. 1)*. If, however, the husband predeceased his wife, her dowery was repaid to her by her husband's relatives. The estate of Michelangelo's uncle had consisted largely of unpaid debts, which there were insufficient assets to meet, and in the hope of escaping their legal obligation towards the widow and the rest of Francesco's creditors, Lodovico and his sons, including Michelangelo, had all formally renounced their, in fact, non-existent inheritance under Francesco's Will. The subterfuge proved unavailing, however, for Mona Cassandra apparently succeeded in her lawsuit, if we may judge from the remarks made by Michelangelo to his father in his letter of September 15th 1509 *(No. 50)*.

The experience gained from this legal reverse doubtless accounted for the extreme promptitude with which, on September 16th 1528, only eleven weeks after the death of their brother Buonarroto, Michelangelo and Gismondo repaid her dowery to the widowed Bartolomea della Casa, in the presence of ten witnesses, including her mother and two notaries, one of whom, acting on behalf of the Buonarroti family, drew up an appropriate deed. The sum involved was five hundred and twenty-two ducats, counted out to the widow in coins of different denominations, part gold and part silver, drawn from a small store found in Buonarroto's house *(Milanesi, p. 600)*.

The dowery of Buonarroto's daughter, Francesca, who married Michele Guicciardini in 1537, was paid by Michelangelo himself, though its size is nowhere stated. That Michelangelo was personally responsible for it is shown by his references to the matter in letters written to Giovansimone and to Lionardo between July and November 1540 *(Nos. 204, 206)*, from which it appears that the dowery had originally consisted, in part at least, of Michelangelo's own farm property at Pazzolatica. In the summer of 1540 Guicciardini decided that he would prefer capital to land, and Michelangelo therefore agreed to redeem the farm from him for the sum of seven hundred ducats.

This transaction emphasizes certain peculiarities about the system at this period. Doweries may, indeed, be regarded as having had the dual character of both marriage settlements on the bride and of loans to the bridegroom, and the bride's family seem to have retained some degree of direct interest in and responsibility for the dowery. Thus, Michele Guicciardini had presumably no prescriptive right to demand, after three years of marriage, that the farm bestowed upon Francesca as a marriage portion should be commuted for a capital payment, nor could he himself exchange or alienate it without permission.

It is in certain of the letters to Lionardo di Buonarroto concerning his proposed marriage that the loan aspect of the dowery fully emerges *(Nos. 372–380)*, since it is clear that the bride's family had the right to demand that the dowery they provided should be secured upon landed estates of equivalent value. In other words, houses, farms and lands were in fact mortgaged to the bride's family, who could foreclose upon them, if the dowery were not returned in the event of the husband predeceasing his wife. The deeds covering such a provision were, of course, drawn up by notaries, but even so it appears that differences of interpretation might arise, if we may judge from the references to Cornelia Colonelli's claim for possession of a house, on the death of her husband. This claim was regarded by Michelangelo and the other executors of Urbino's Will as being detrimental to the interests of the children, who were the principal heirs, and they seem to have been in a position to dispute the legality of Cornelia's claim *(No. 453)*.

Curiously enough, the practice of demanding security was waived when Lionardo finally found in Cassandra Ridolfi a wife to his liking, although her dowery amounted to the not inconsiderable sum of one thousand five hundred *scudi*, and in the preceeding negotiations Michelangelo had given his nephew leave to secure it upon whatever properties he thought fit. The marriage having taken place, however, without any reference to security for the marriage portion, Michelangelo's astute business sense asserted itself, and he counselled his nephew not to raise the question, lest it should involve them both in endless disputes regarding the value of the security proposed *(No. 381)*. Since no further allusion to the subject is made in subsequent letters, it may be presumed that the Ridolfi family were willing to dispense with the formality, in view of the fact that it was well known that Lionardo was sole heir to his uncle's substantial fortune and that there would therefore be little difficulty about repayment, should Cassandra's husband die before her.

Cassandra was well endowed; but such had not been the case with many of the ladies of noble birth who had been suggested to Lionardo, and Michelangelo had consistently urged his nephew to pay no heed to their lack of portion, but to marry, if need be, as an act of charity, and had even gone so far as to offer to provide a dowery for his nephew's bride himself *(No. 366)*.

This generous attitude with regard to the marriage of a member of his own family throws an interesting light on Michelangelo's charitable activities for the love of God and the welfare of his own soul. It will be seen how constantly, in sending to Florence money to be bestowed in alms *(Nos. 287, 335 etc.)*, he expressed the wish that it might be expended on making some provision for the penniless daughters of noble families, to enable them either to marry or to enter monasteries. The sums involved in these charitable benefactions were comparatively small, but it is probable that it was Michelangelo's intention that the donations should be made to families whose daughters were still small children. In that case, the fathers or guardians of the girls concerned would presumably have invested the small capital sum in the Public Funds, there to accrue at a generous rate of compound interest until the girls were of marriageable age. Such means of providing doweries was an inherent part of the *Monte* system and serves, as does so much of the evidence in Michelangelo's own letters, to underline the concern of the Florentines with the financial provisions required for the marriage of their daughters.

M.E.E.

Appendix 42

The Recipient of Letter No. 358: A Possible Identification

No letter in the whole range of Michelangelo's correspondence presents greater difficulties than this. It is undated; the name of the Cardinal to whom it was addressed is wanting, and the precise architectural problem with which it is concerned remains a matter of conjecture.

In his footnote to the published text of the signed draft or copy of the letter Milanesi proposed Cardinal Ridolfo Pio da Carpi, Archpriest of St. Peter's and a Deputy of the fabric, as a possible recipient and 1560 as a possible date. Both suggestions are plausible. The Cardinal was at this time closely associated with the work at the Basilica and it was to him that Michelangelo addressed his letter of resignation on September 13th 1560. It would therefore be easy to accept Carpi as the probable Cardinal, if it were equally easy to accept 1560 as the probable date. But it is not. Milanesi himself had certain misgivings on the point and frankly acknowledged that an earlier date might well be preferred.

In the absence of any proof to the contrary, both Milanesi's conjectures have hitherto been tacitly accepted, but when Schiavo says that the letter was addressed to Cardinal Ridolfo Pio da Carpi, 'who had considered superfluous the re-making of some decorations left to Michelangelo by other artists who worked previously on the fabric *(p. 96)*, he is presumably only improvising and is not adducing new evidence in support of Milanesi's suggestions.

The first question to be considered, however, is the subject-matter of the letter itself, which is devoted to a consideration of certain aspects of the architectural principles of Vitruvius, upon whom all the architects of the period based themselves. The theory on which Michelangelo's argument is developed is that advanced by Vitruvius, where he says that 'the planning of temples depends upon symmetry . . . . for without symmetry and proportion no temple can have a regular plan; that is to say it must have an exact proportion worked out after the fashion of a finely-shaped human body' *(Vitruvius, Bk. III, p. 159 et seq.)*.

No mention is made of Vitruvius, manifestly because Michelangelo was in no doubt that his correspondent would recognize the reference and appreciate its implications. But with regard to the nature of the practical problem with which they were engaged we have little to go upon beyond a conviction that it was St. Peter's that was under discussion, and that it was the changes made in his own plan of the Basilica that Michelangelo was defending. In his final project *(Letarouilly, pl. 34)* Antonio Sangallo used the Tuscan Order (i.e. the Roman version of the Doric) in the main elevation; the Ionic in the lower and the Corinthian in the upper arcades of the drum; whereas Michelangelo used the Corinthian order throughout. Furthermore, the analogy of the nose is indicative, since in such a context it could only typify the dome, the exterior decorations of which would appear to have been called in question, as differing from those being used in other parts of the building. Michelangelo's contention that a central architectural feature having, like the nose, no counterpart, is 'as independent as one chooses', seems obvious enough, but it is possible that in an age in which a rigorous observance of classical modes was required, the comparative freedom of the handling of the proposed decorations of the attic and perhaps, more particularly, the imaginative use of the figures rayed round the dome above the drum, a feature not repeated elsewhere, may have alarmed the purists, who were ever on the watch to fault Michelangelo, whose creative genius presented a challenge to which, for all their pedantry, they were unequal. But in this connection it may be remarked as a matter of moment, that when the dome was finally completed by Giacomo della Porta in 1590 these figures, together with the socles on which they were raised and the *speroni* of which they formed the terminals, were omitted, to the detriment of the fabric in the estimation of some of the experts who were consulted in 1742, when evidence of the spreading of the dome, the proportion of which had been altered by della Porta, who had built a structure both higher and heavier than Michelangelo had intended, began to appear. Since in their opinion this original device, which can be seen to admirable advantage in Gotti's reproduction of the drawing of the cupola, albeit as partly altered by della Porta *(Gotti, II, p. 136 et seq.)* and to less effect in Dupérac's engraving of the whole project *(Pl. 26)* was intended to provide not only an ornament but a buttress to the outward thrust of the dome *(Poleni, III, 245, para. 289)*.

The point next to be determined is that as to whether Michelangelo was dealing with the model of the whole Basilica, in respect of which he received the brief of October 1549, which no longer exists, or the detailed model of the cupola, which was begun in 1558 and completed in 1561, which is still preserved. All things considered, there is so little likelihood that it was on the basis of the second and not of the first that the objections were raised that the possibility may be virtually ruled out. By 1560/61 it would have been too late to cavil over architectural details and in any case by this time Michelangelo's unique prerogatives at the Basilica were too well, and had been too long established to permit of the work being subjected to criticisms of this particular kind, however much his ability to supervise the work in progress might, owing to his age and infirmities, be questioned by those who sought to calumniate him. It must be emphasized, moreover, that it was at the express wish, notably, of the Cardinal da Carpi that the definitive – or what was intended to be the definitive – model of the cupola was initially undertaken.

If we therefore reject 1560/61, as being too late a date for the letter, we are immediately faced with the problem of proposing an alternative, than which none would seem more likely than 1550/51, since in view of the authoritative and uncompromising tone of the letter it is almost certain that it must have been written some time after October 1549, when absolute powers in respect of the Basilica were conferred upon him by Paul III and some time before January 1552, when those powers were confirmed by Julius III. For though carping criticisms of one kind or another were probably always rife, the likelihood of objections being afterwards raised such as those which prompted the Vitruvian letter, if it may be so called, seems extremely remote.

Both from Vasari *(VII, p. 232)* and from Bonanni *(p. 63)*, who published an extract from the *Acta sub Julio* we learn that from the beginning of the new pontificate a concerted effort had been made by Michelangelo's would-be rivals at the Basilica, especially by the Sangallo faction, to discredit him in the eyes of the Pope from whom they hoped, by their much importuning, to obtain a revocation of Michelangelo's appointment. According to Vasari, matters were brought to a head towards the end of 1550 and as a result an enquiry was held, in the presence of the Pope, early in the new year.

At this meeting the Deputies of the Basilica, headed by Cardinals Cervini and Salviati, who had been won over to the views of those who, looking with 'livid eyes' on the proceedings at the Basilica, alleged many things against him, now came forward with the accusation, which was only one among others, that Michelangelo was 'constructing a temple in the image of the sun's rays', which we may interpret with some certainty as meaning that they were opposed to Michelangelo's decision to revert to Bramante's original plan of building the Basilica in the form, not of a Latin, but of a Greek cross, dominated by a central dome. This being the case, one can well imagine that they would be even more strongly opposed to the use of any form of decoration, such as the motifs we have discussed, which, in their estimation, might serve to emphasize 'the image of the sun's rays', more especially if it might be conceived to violate the sacrosanct canons of Vitruvius.

This, however, is merely an hypothesis, but it is sufficiently well based to be worth pursuing. If, then, the Vitruvian letter may be related to this controversy and dated accordingly (and there are more grounds for thinking that it may than that it may not be so related) it cannot have been addressed to Cardinal Pio da Carpi, who was not, at this time, concerned with the affairs of the Basilica, as in 1551 he was appointed to the governorship of the Patrimony, which required his residence at Viterbo *(Bussi, p. 391)*. Happily, the problem of proposing an alternative Cardinal presents no difficulty at all. For just as it may be said, with a fair presumption of truth, that if the letter belongs to 1560/61 then the Cardinal to whom it was addressed was Cardinal Ridolfo Pio da Carpi, so it may be said, with an equal presumption of truth, that if it belongs to 1550/51, then the Cardinal in question was Cardinal Marcello Cervini, the future Pope.

Cardinal Cervini, who was, as we know, a Deputy of the fabric at the relevant time and had been appointed Prefect of the Vatican Library by Paul III in 1548, an appointment which had been confirmed by Julius III by a brief of February 24th 1550, was a man of extraordinary erudition and versed in a number of subjects, among which architecture was not the least, for, as his biographer, Pietro Pollidori, informs us *(p. 17)*, he was able to discourse learnedly on the subject with Sangallo and with Michelangelo himself. He was, in addition, together with his intimate friend and fellow Cardinal, Bernardino Maffei, a member of the Academy of Vitruvius, which had been founded by Claudio Tolmei in 1542, probably as an extension of the Academy of Virtù, which he had founded twelve years previously under the patronage of Cardinal Ippolito de' Medici *(Maylender, V, p. 478 et seq. and Bottari, II, p. 1)*.

There is moreover a further argument which may be advanced in support of this hypothesis and that is the abrupt tone of the letter, which is very similar to the sharpness of the retort which Michelangelo made to Cervini in reply to another criticism raised at the enquiry of 1551 *(Appendix 44, pt. III)* which certainly suggests that there was no love lost between himself and the Cardinal, despite Condivi's assertion (which in 1553 may perhaps have been merely politic) that Michelangelo entertained for him both affection and esteem. If we may judge from his bigoted expression, the Cardinal would certainly not appear to be a man likely to commend himself to Michelangelo and still less so when he attempted to dictate to him in architectural matters of which, for all his learning, he had no practical experience. There is, besides, very little doubt that Cervini was the Deputy who professed to understand Vitruvius, mentioned by Vasari, of whom when someone remarked that he had at the Basilica a man of great gifts, Michelangelo retorted: 'that is true; but of poor judgment'. It is extremely significant, moreover, that on Cervini's elevation to the Papacy Michelangelo seriously thought of leaving Rome *(Vasari, VII, p. 238)*. Indeed, it would be difficult to adduce more conclusive evidence in support of the argument that although Michelangelo had originally been on friendly terms with Cardinal Cervini, these good relations had afterwards declined, most probably as a result of these acrimonious interchanges.

If then, proceeding on this hypothesis, we may assume Cervini to have been the recipient of the Vitruvian letter, the *post* and *ante quem* is shortly after the beginning of November 1550, when the Cardinal returned to Rome from Gubbio, where he had been recuperating after a severe illness, and before the end of May 1551, when he returned to Gubbio, where he held the bishopric, though he was never formally installed *(B.M. Add. MSS. 10.274, ff. 17, 26)*. Within this period a date prior to the 1551 enquiry, when the Pope afforded Michelangelo such singular proof of his favour and approbation, would seem the most tenable and the letter has, in accordance with this assumption, been tentatively assigned to December 1550.

Finally, the holograph itself remains to be considered. Though by no means an infallible guide as to the time at which any given letter was written, the handwriting affords at least some slight indication as to the approximate period. Although Michelangelo's highly characteristic and singularly beautiful italic hand shows remarkably little variation over the years, the variations, such as they are, being due less to his age than to his health and to his state of mind when writing, there is obviously a difference between the steadiness of the hand, seen in a letter of 1542 *(Pl. 5)* and the unsteadiness of the hand seen in a letter of 1561 *(Pl. 27)*. Yet even so, it is rather in the erasures and corrections to the text than in the actual calligraphy that the evidence of his advancing age becomes most evident. Thus on mature reflection the unfaltering and uncorrected draft under review, which is preserved in the Vatican Archives, appears to be nearer in date to the letters of 1550 than to those of 1560, a time at which Michelangelo complained that he found letter writing the greatest of the many burdens he had to bear. The opening lines of the two unfinished sonnets which are written on the verso, namely *Di più cose s'attristan gli occhi miei* and *Non più per altro da me stesso togli (Guasti, pp. 261, 268)*, provide, disappointingly, no additional information or confirmatory evidence one way or the other. The sentiments expressed in them are typical of much of his poetry composed both before and after 1550, though perhaps hardly as late as 1560. But as regards the autograph it may be remarked, for what it is worth, that neither sonnet has been either amended or corrected.

Despite this exhaustive examination of the data available to us, the case in favour of one date rather than the other has not been conclusively proved, and in all probability never will be. It can be said, however, with some degree of assurance, that on the whole the balance of evidence is in favour of 1550/51 rather than of 1560/61, in which case the recipient of the letter was Cardinal Marcello Cervini, and not Cardinal Ridolfo Pio da Carpi, as has hitherto been supposed.

Mo S.re X quado una piata a diuerse parte
tucte quelle che sono an modo di qualita
e quatita anno aessere adorne i nu me
desimo modo e duna medesima maniera
e simyl meti i lor riscotri / ma quado la
piata muta de tucto forma e no solamete
lecito ma necessario mutare di tucta a
coraghadormeti e similmete i lor risco
trise mezzi sempre son liberi come no
ghono si come il naso che e nel mezzo del
uiso nome obrigato ne alluno ne a laltro
ochio ma luna mana che ne obrigata ae
sere come laltra e luno ochio come la
ltro prispecto de gh illati e de riscotri
e p e cosa certa che sembra del sar chitettura
di pe duno dalle mebra delluomo chi no ne
stato o no ne buo maestro di figure e me
simo chi notomia no sem puo i tenderi

Appendix 43

The Political Scene in Europe from the Accession of Paul III (1534) to the Death of Pius IV (1565)

Part I

WHEN, in October 1534, as Pope Paul III – the greatest pontiff of the Renaissance – Cardinal Alessandro Farnese received the tiara, in succession to Clement VII, the political scene in Europe was not appreciably different, apart from the addition of the religious controversies of the Reformation and of the Counter-Reformation, from what it had been since the beginning of the century. The names of the players had changed; but the main outlines of the plot remained the same. The enmity existing between the Holy Roman Emperor, in the person of Charles V of Spain, and the Most Christian King of France, in the person of Francis I, persisted as before; the great aim of the one, as of the other, being to gain Papal support for the furtherance of his claims upon Italy, in which each sought to be supreme. But in this endeavour both were to be disappointed.

From the beginning of his pontificate Paul III was determined, as a matter of principle, to preserve the neutrality of the Church and to exert his influence in the interests of peace. But despite his efforts, which were unremitting, and notwithstanding a conference between himself and the two princes at Nice in 1538 and between himself and the Emperor at Lucca in 1541, war could not be averted and hostilities broke out in the summer of 1542. To the scandal of Christendom, Francis entered into an alliance with the Sultan, but the appearance of the Turkish fleet, under its commander Khair-ed-din Barbarossa, at the mouth of the Tiber in June of the following year constituted rather an act of defiance than any serious menace to the Papal States. It was sufficient, however, to alarm the City and to hasten plans for her defence against the infidel. Following a further conference with the Emperor at Busseto in 1543 the Pope therefore decided to despatch his eldest grandson, Cardinal Alessandro Farnese, on an embassy exhorting peace, first to the French King and then to the Emperor. Although the Cardinal failed in his mission, terms were subsequently arranged without Papal intervention, and the Peace of Crespy was signed in September 1544.

One of the more serious results of the war had been the inevitable suspension of the Council of Trent, which had originally been convoked to meet in November 1542. Once the war was over, however, the way became clear for its resumption, but for a number of reasons the formal opening was delayed until December 1545. Despite both its importance and its fascination, the history of the Council, in which Monsignor d'Inghilterra, Cardinal Reginald Pole, played so prominent a part, cannot be discussed here. It is enough to say that during the eighteen years of its intermittent deliberations (the last session being held in December 1563) it was continually hindered in its proceedings by political objections raised for one reason or another by the reigning sovereigns, who were prepared to support the Council to the extent to which it served their own ends. Charles V, for instance, though himself a devout Catholic, frequently intervened in the interest of his Protestant subjects, even after the virtual overthrow of the Schmalkaldic League, so that it was almost in defiance of his wishes that the Decree of Justification was eventually promulgated. Indeed, it was Charles's desire for toleration that exacerbated the strained relations between himself and the Pope, who under great provocation conducted himself with commendable forbearance, though on one occasion he found himself impelled to remind the Emperor that 'though he might well consider himself to be the eldest son of the Church, he *[the Pope]*, however unworthy, was the Church itself'.

Their relations were strained still further by the disputes over the Duchy of Parma and Piacenza with which the Pope's son, Pierluigi Farnese, had been invested in 1545, an investiture which the Emperor had, from the first, refused to recognize. When, therefore, his generalissimo, Ferrante Gonzaga, whom he appointed to the viceroyalty of Milan in April 1546, proposed to overthrow the Duke in furtherance of his policy of Spanish aggrandizement in the peninsula and to seize the Duchy, Charles was not disposed to discourage him, more particularly as Pierluigi had not been slow to invoke French support in face of the Emperor's hostile attitude. But while agreeing to Gonzaga's proposal to seize the Duchy, he specifically forbade the murder of the Duke himself. But Gonzaga was not to be restrained. On the night of September 10th 1547, Pierluigi was surprised in the citadel of Piacenza and brutally, though not undeservedly, put to death in defiance of the Emperor's orders, and Piacenza (though not Parma which was retained by the Farnese during seven generations) passed into Imperial possession.

The news of his son's murder, and of what may well have appeared as the Emperor's perfidy, came as a terrible blow to the aging Pope, who nevertheless retained his self-possession with exemplary fortitude. But when, added to the news of this disaster, fears, albeit unfounded, of another Spanish attack upon the City became rife, the Pope was finally forced to abandon his policy of neutrality and to enter into negotiations for a French alliance. The terms proposed were not, however, acceptable to him, as they involved ceding Parma to Pierluigi's third son, Orazio, recently betrothed to Diane de France, the illegitimate daughter of Henry II of France. The Pope replied with counter proposals to the effect that both Parma and Piacenza should be restored to the Church and that Ottaviano, Orazio's elder brother, husband of Margaret, the illegitimate daughter of Charles V, should be compensated with Camerino. But these terms were not to be entertained by Ottaviano, who in an attempt to regain possession of Parma (which had been occupied in the Pope's name) appealed to Ferrante Gonzaga, who agreed to support him, if he consented to hold the Duchy as an imperial fief. These terms, which he set forth in a letter addressed to his grandfather, Ottaviano threatened to accept, if the Pope refused to surrender the city. The letter reached Rome on November 5th and its contents were communicated to the Pope by Cardinal Farnese who read him the letter in the Quirinal Palace on the same evening. The shock of his grandson's defection might in itself have been sufficient to overset the Pope, who was in declining health, but when he perceived that the Cardinal's sympathies lay with his brother, his fury knew no bounds. Unable to sustain the shock, the old man was thrown into a fever, to which he succumbed five days later, on the morning of November 10th 1549. 'No man', wrote Matteo Dandolo, the Venetian ambassador, 'was ever more worthy to be called magnanimous,' and, as Pastor continues, 'nepotism, his besetting fault, he acknowledged himself and in his last hours, he repeated the words of the Psalm, "My sin is ever before me", "If they had not had the mastery over me, then should I have been without great offence" ' *(Pastor, XII, p. 453).*

Part II

On November 29th the Cardinals entered the conclave; but owing largely to the conflicting interests of the Spanish and French parties and to the right of veto possessed at that time by the two sovereigns, it proved to be one of the most prolonged in the history of the Church. Eventually, however, on the morning of February 8th 1550 Cardinal Gianmaria Ciocchi del Monte (who, as Vasari relates, had foretold his own elevation on his way to the conclave) was formally elected, and out of compliment to the della Rovere Pope, took the name Julius III.

As usual, much was expected of the new Pope, who had a considerable reputation for liberality, though it was not on this account that his financial resources were soon exhausted, but rather owing to his lack of political wisdom in allowing himself to become embroiled in the ensuing war over Parma. Ottaviano Farnese being determined, with the assistance of the French, to assert his rights, invaded the States of the Church in the summer of 1551 but was repulsed by the Papal troops. Although these were joined by the Imperial troops under Ferrante Gonzaga, the Pope found himself more involved than he had intended and in receipt of less support from the Emperor than he had anticipated and had been led to expect. He was in any case temperamentally unsuited to an enterprise of this kind and was soon forced to agree to an armistice with France, but not before the costs of the undertaking had risen out of all proportion to what, if anything, had been gained. Terms were arranged in April 1552, but the war between France (in alliance with the Electors of Mayence and Saxony) and the Emperor continued, all efforts on the part of the Pope to end it having proved unavailing.

A much more serious disturbance, as far as Italy was concerned, occurred a few months later. At this time Siena was nominally under the domination of Spain. But in July 1552 the inhabitants having risen in rebellion to the rallying cry of 'France, Victory and Freedom' and having forced the Spanish garrison to retire, placed themselves under French protection. Thus once again both powers became engaged in defending what they were pleased to regard as their respective rights in Italy. To add to the turmoil, the Duke of Florence, who supported the Emperor, and the *fuorusciti* who supported the Sienese and the French, also became involved. Incidentally, it was at this juncture that Bindo Altoviti and his son, Giovanbattista, were declared rebels, since, although hitherto the Duke had found it convenient to do so, owing to the wealth and influence of the Altoviti, he could now no longer remain oblivious of their participation in *fuorusciti* activities.

For a short period after the initial uprising Siena was left in peace to enjoy her newly acquired freedom, but the struggle was soon renewed, Cosimo, Duke of Florence and Piero di Filippo Strozzi being the protagonists. The campaign was carried on throughout the Sienese territory and the whole countryside between Siena and Florence became a frequently fought-over battlefield. But in August 1554 Piero Strozzi suffered a crushing defeat on the field of Marciano and the investment of the city followed. For eight months Siena sustained all the terrors and deprivations of a siege prolonged throughout the winter, but when everything that could be eaten had been consumed and only 6,000 out of 40,000 inhabitants remained alive, she was forced to open her gates to the besiegers. The remnant of the garrison marched out with the honours of war in April 1555. In spite of the barbarity with which the war had been carried on, Siena submitted to a better fate at the hands of Cosimo than might have been expected. Many of her ancient institutions were preserved and thereafter the Sienese appeared to have had little cause for discontent. Cosimo received formal investiture of the territory as a Spanish fief in 1557.

Julius III, who had spared no effort in trying to bring the unhappy war to an end, did not survive to see the issue of the struggle. He died on March 23rd 1555 after a protracted period of declining health. His successor, Cardinal Marcello Cervini, who retained his own name as Marcellus II, had like himself played a prominent part at the Council of Trent, but unlike the easy-going, pleasure-loving Julius, was an uncompromising churchman, a man stern and unbending, who scarcely knew what it was to smile. Happily for Rome, his pontificate lasted only three weeks, but quite long enough for the Romans to have become exceedingly despondent, as invariably with a pontiff bent upon reform. 'Everything was sad, gloomy and disheartening', according to an entry in the diary of Angelo Massarelli, secretary to the Tridentine Council, since all in Rome recognized that they had nothing to hope from him. Indeed such was the prospect, that 'many members of the Curia feared the Pope's reform measures so much that they sold the offices they had bought at a high price for a mere trifle' *(Pastor, XIV, p. 47)*.

Part III

Marcellus II was succeeded on May 23rd 1555 by the formidable Caraffa Pope, Gianpietro, one of the founders of the Theatines, who assumed the name of Paul IV. From the Roman point of view this election can hardly have been regarded as much improvement on the last, since he was a reformer, zealous to the point of fanaticism, as witness his pitiless persecution of heresy and his 'burning' ardour for the Inquisition, for the reintroduction of which, under Paul III, he had been largely responsible.

But more inimical to the peace and well-being of Italy than his zeal for reform, was the rabid anti-Spanish policy of the new Pope. As a Catholic and as a Neapolitan he was determined from the very beginning of his pontificate to liberate Italy from foreign interference in general and from Spanish domination in particular. As could have been foretold and as it transpired, no policy could have been more disastrous. Neither the Pope himself nor the States of the Church were in any way equipped to challenge the power of Spain. In addition, the situation was worsened by the intrigues of the Sforza and of the Colonna, both Imperialist in sympathy, and by the duplicity of the Cardinal nephew, Carlo Caraffa, to whom everything was entrusted and who, together with his brothers, was prepared to employ any means, however unscrupulous and corrupt, to further his own interests, a fact of which the Pope long remained entirely unaware.

Being anxious to pursue his plans against Spain, the Pope lost no time in entering into negotiations for French support, but failed of his objective as, notwithstanding the signature of a draft for such an alliance on October 14th 1555, a Franco-Spanish armistice was arranged shortly afterwards which shattered his hopes. But he was not to be so easily frustrated and in May 1556 Cardinal Caraffa was sent on a legation to France with the same end in view. Meanwhile fears of a Spanish attack upon Rome were rising and when a spy was intercepted in the following July and a letter from Garcilasso della Vega, the Spanish envoy, addressed to the Duke of Alba, Viceroy of Naples, inciting such an attack, was discovered on him, Rome was thoroughly alarmed. The fortifications of the Borgo were extended and the City was put into a state of defence, but at so enormous a cost (estimated by the Venetian envoy, Bernardo Navagero to be some eighty thousand *scudi* a month) that new taxes had to be imposed to meet the extraordinary expense. Thus on his return from France on September 7th 1556 with promises of help from the French king, Cardinal Caraffa 'found the Eternal City in a state of indescribable confusion'. The horrors of the sack of 1527 were still a living memory too awful to contemplate, and 'had the gates not been closed', as Pastor goes on to say, 'most of the inhabitants would have fled'. On August 27th the Duke of Alba had sent an ultimatum to the Pope, but no decisive answer was forthcoming and on September 25th he crossed the frontier into the Papal States. On November 18th Ostia fell to the invaders and Rome was cut off from the sea. Alba, who was not in fact anxious to follow up his advantage then offered an armistice, which was later extended from November 28th to January 9th 1557, while an embassy was sent to Philip II, who had succeeded to the Spanish throne on the abdication of his father Charles V, in 1556. In the meantime the Caraffa nephews were in secret negotiation with both France and Spain and were trying to determine what course would best be to their personal advantage. French reinforcements had already arrived and news that the French army was on the move now intensified the conflict, as the Spaniards lost no time in advancing against them in the Low Countries, and to such purpose that on August 10th the French were heavily defeated at the battle of St. Quentin and the Spaniards had nothing further to hinder their advance. Alba at once approached the gates of Rome, his army awfully equipped with scaling ladders. The worst was anticipated; but nothing happened. The City was lit up and, from the beating of drums and the shouts of command that could be heard within, appeared to be in readiness to meet the attack, and Alba withdrew. But while this might be the ostensible reason for his withdrawal, the real reason probably lay in the fact that he never intended to do otherwise. He may well have wished to frighten the Pope for his temerity, but he clearly had no wish to incur the guilt of another sack or to suffer the execrations of Christendom for the perpetration of such a crime. Negotiations were opened, and on April 14th 1557 a treaty was signed. A consistory was arranged for September 15th, but the night before the Tiber burst its banks and the greater part of Rome was flooded. The waters subsided, however, almost as quickly as they had risen and four days later the Duke of Alba entered Rome in state to make his submission of obedience to the Pope, as a loyal son of the Church.

During the remaining years of his reign Paul IV was free to devote himself to the real work of his life, the work of Catholic reform, a task in which he showed himself to be as impartial as he was energetic. But if he was relentless in his correction of the abuses by which ecclesiastical offices were held in order to augment the revenues of the holders, he was no less relentless in his stern denunciation of his own kindred when he at length discovered the crimes of which they had been guilty. But in stripping the Caraffa of their offices and sending them ignominiously into exile he did not conceal from himself or from the Curia his recognition of the sin of nepotism of which he himself, in spite of all his professions, had been guilty.

But in the eyes of the people nothing could make amends and when on August 18th 1559 Paul IV breathed his last, the name of the hated Caraffa was shown to be anathema. The fury of the Roman populace was released and was scarcely to be satiated, so much so that it was found necessary to bury the body temporarily, in an obscure grave, and to mount a guard over it, lest it should be dragged from its resting place and cast, like the dead Pope's effigy, into the Tiber.

The man who was finally elected in his stead, on December 25th 1559, Cardinal Gian Angelo de' Medici of Milan, who took the name of Pius IV, because 'he wished to be what the name signified', was a man of very different type and temperament. And in Pastor's words 'great was the jubilation of the city when the new Pope announced that he would secure peace, justice and an ample supply of provisions to the Eternal City' – promises which in a large measure he was able to fulfil.

Of these needs the most immediate was to secure the necessary supplies, a need which, for different reasons, had been only intermittently met ever since the jubilee year of Julius III's accession, when pilgrims from all parts of Christendom had rendered the prevailing shortage consequent upon a poor harvest even more acute *(Cf. Nos. 359, 443)*. The Pope likewise took steps to reform the administration in the interests of efficiency and justice, but it was, above all, in preserving peace in Italy that his success as a potentate lay. Fortunately, France, under the regency of Catherine de' Medici, was preoccupied with her own religious difficulties and dissensions, nor was a Medici in any case likely to provoke trouble in Italy. Relations between the Holy See and Spain, on the other hand, were far from being all that might have been wished, but they were not strained to breaking point for whatever their personal animosities may have been, neither Pius nor Philip was in any position, financial or otherwise, to make war. The Turk, in addition, continued to constitute a menace to the peace of Christendom, which neither could afford to disregard.

The Pope was thus enabled to accomplish the most important task of his pontificate – the reopening of the Council of Trent, which was reconvened on January 18th 1562 and concluded on December 3rd 1563. Though it had failed in certain of its objectives, notably that of securing religious unity in Europe, it nevertheless succeeded in performing work of immense value to the Church – not only in the way of Catholic reform and of the correction of abuses, but more importantly in the rigorous definition of the doctrines of the Church. Immediately on the successful termination of its labours, which was a cause of immense satisfaction and rejoicing to him, the Pope proceeded, in spite of some opposition from the Curia, to confirm and publish its decrees and canons in full and to make the Tridentine profession obligatory. The Bull of Confirmation was finally published in November 1564.

The Pope, who had been guided and supported throughout by his nephew, Cardinal Carlo Borromeo, only survived this triumph of the Counter-Reformation for a brief period. A year later he was taken ill; and as if in premonition of his death, the candle nearest the Papal throne twice went out, for no accountable reason, at a mass at which he was not present on December 2nd. He died with great composure a week afterwards, on the evening of December 9th 1565.

It was against this historical background that Michelangelo lived out the remaining years of his life in Rome from 1534 to 1564; it was by these tumultuous events that he was hampered and hindered in the work imposed upon him by successive Popes; it was in this religious atmosphere, the atmosphere of the Counter-Reformation, that he toiled and struggled and endured.

Appendix 44

The Rebuilding of the Basilica of St. Peter

Part I

THE history of the rebuilding of St. Peter's is a complex one. The corner stone was laid by Julius II on Sunday, April 18th 1506: the dome was completed in 1590 under Sixtus V and the lantern in 1592 under Gregory XIV. The cross was raised in 1593 and on November 18th of the same year the Basilica was dedicated by Clement VIII. But it was not until 1607, when Paul V commissioned the nave and narthex, which were completed in 1614, that the last remains of the old Basilica, which had been founded in the fourth century by the Emperor Constantine during the pontificate of Sylvester I, were finally swept away.

The decision to build *una nuova e più amplia tribuna*, which had been taken with the advice of Leon Battista Alberti by Nicholas V, had been reached half a century before the laying of the foundation stone, but Bernardo Rossellini, the architect appointed, had scarcely begun work on the choir when the Pope died, and little further progress was made.

The real incentive to continue was provided by Michelangelo, whose design for the Tomb of Julius II was conceived on so stupendous a scale that the Pope, stimulated by the project, decided upon nothing less than the entire rebuilding of the Basilica in order to accommodate it and forthwith invited Giuliano da Sangallo and Donato Bramante to prepare designs. Of these the Pope preferred Bramante's, which 'took the form of a Greek Cross, with a hexastyle portico and an immense cupola resembling the dome of the Pantheon' *(Letarouilly, p. 3)*. The work was begun with tremendous energy and no less than two thousand five hundred workmen were employed in pulling down (with almost indecent haste) those parts of the old Basilica which interfered with the work on the new *fabbrica*, and in raising the four great central piers to support the dome. These, according to Vasari, Bramante 'vaulted with the utmost rapidity and great art', but, as with so much of Bramante's work, they were insecurely built and had subsequently to be strongly reinforced. They remain, however, as Bramante's contribution to the building, the form of which they largely conditioned. Bramante also completed the choir which Rossellini had begun half a century before, but in order to equalize the arms of the cross, this had eventually to be demolished and was pulled down in 1585 *(Ackerman, Cat., p. 84)*. At Bramante's death, a year after that of his patron Julius II in 1513, some 70,653 ducats had been expended on the building *(Turco, p. 24)*.

Under Leo X three architects were appointed: Giuliano da Sangallo, who retired shortly afterwards, Fra Giocondo, whose tenure of office appears to have been almost equally brief, and Raphael, to whom, according to Serlio, a design in the form of a Latin cross may be attributed, but little further was undertaken. On Raphael's death in 1520, Baldassare Peruzzi da Siena, who was next appointed, reverted to the form of a Greek cross, but he appears to have been so preoccupied with other commissions and to have suffered so many vicissitudes, that the work on the Basilica, which had in any case been interrupted by the sack of Rome and all that had ensued, remained virtually suspended until the death of Clement VII in 1534.

His successor, Paul III, resolved to proceed with the enterprise and vigorous measures were at once concerted to enable him to do so. To finance it the Confraternity of St. Peter, of which the Pope himself and the cardinals were members, was founded; appeals were made to all the princes of Christendom; graces and indulgences were offered to all who supported the undertaking and the privileges granted to the Commissioners of the fabric, a body which had been constituted by Clement in 1533, were confirmed. In addition, the riparian rights of the river Anio, from Ponte Lucano to its junction with the Tiber, were later bestowed upon the fabric for the easier transport of materials and especially of travertine *(Pastor, XII, pp. 635 et seq.)*. Antonio da Sangallo, who had been employed at the Basilica ever since the retirement of his uncle, Giuliano, many years before, and was already in the service of the Farnese, was promoted to the office of chief architect, while, until his death in 1537, Baldassare Peruzzi acted as his coadjutor.

Sangallo's conception of what the Church of the Prince of the Apostles should be was very different, however, from Bramante's. In place of the original clear, coherent and compact plan of his predecessor *(Plan 1)* he devised an edifice on a larger, more extended and altogether more grandiose scale. But what he gained in complexity he lost in effect, with his confusion of orders, his endless ranges of columns, 'his arches upon arches, his cornices upon cornices', his bewildering array of parapets, pinnacles and panels, and the use of almost every device known to the classical repertory. But it did not require the scale model built by his assistant, Antonio Labacco, over a period of seven years and at a cost of more than four thousand *scudi*, to demonstrate his want of architectural judgment, since the faults inherent in the design were manifest from the ground plan *(Plan 2)*, which, being an awkward compromise between the Greek cross and the Latin, lost the coherence of the first without gaining the majesty of the second.

Little advance seems to have been made during the early years of Sangallo's stewardship, but once the new project had been approved in 1540, the work on the fabric went ahead reasonably fast – as far as may be judged from the account books and from contemporary drawings (the main source of our information) – so that when Sangallo died on August 3rd 1546, a good deal, some of it regrettable, had been accomplished.

On his demise, the appointment was first of all offered to Giulio Romano, but being in poor health and unwilling to leave Mantua, he declined the position, perhaps propitiously, as he too died shortly afterwards, on November 1st of the same year.

Now, more than ever before, had the Pope need of Michelangelo's services *(cf. Appendix 27, Pt. III)*. But when His Holiness sent for him, he refused to undertake so heavy a burden in his old age and pleaded that architecture was not his art. Paul III was not, however, to be

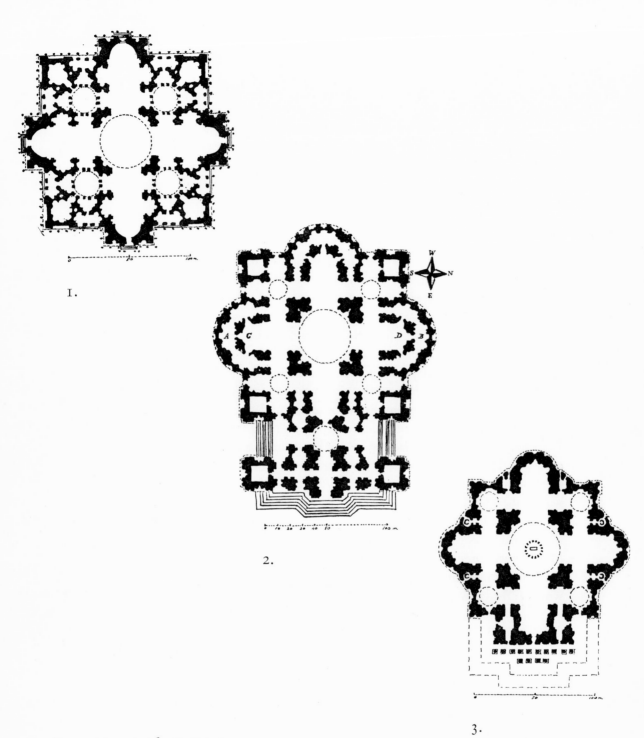

1.   *Bramante's project for St. Peter's.*

2.   *Sangallo's project for St. Peter's.*

3.   *Michelangelo's project for St. Peter's.*

gainsaid, and just as in 1505 Michelangelo had been forced to leave the unfinished Cartoon of *The Battle of Cascina* in obedience to the orders of Julius II, so now, with the second Pauline fresco still unfinished, he found himself, at the age of seventy-one and after over forty years' compulsory service to a succession of pontiffs, constrained once again to bow to the will of the Pope, who refused to listen either to his protests or his prayers, but finally commanded him to accept the charge imposed upon him.

Part II

When Michelangelo took over the direction of the work at St. Peter's much of the old Basilica was still standing, as the beginnings that had been made on the west end (the liturgical east, St. Peter's being incorrectly orientated) had not necessitated further demolition. The progress that had been made on the work of rebuilding during the forty years that had elapsed since the laying of the foundation stone in 1506 had not been spectacular.

Proceeding from Bramante's four great piers and their connecting arches at the crossing, which formed the fixed point of departure for all future developments, Sangallo had concentrated his building operations mainly on the eastern and southern arms of the cross, leaving the choir to the west, begun by Rossellini and completed by Bramante, as he found it, and the northern arm of the cross untouched except for part of the foundations. Thus, beside building the pendentives which defined the base of the drum, Sangallo had completed the eastern hemicycle and raised the vault towards the entrance. He had also raised the vault of the south transept and had begun, but had not completed the terminal hemicycle which formed the inner wall of the ambulatory, while the outer hemicycle (subsequently demolished by Michelangelo) he had carried to door level at the time of his death *(Ackerman, Cat. pp. 85 et seq.)*. This then, in the main, was the stage that had been reached when, in obedience to the Pope's command, Michelangelo prepared, within fifteen days and at a cost of only twenty-five *scudi*, the rough clay model illustrating his own proposals for the completion of the Basilica, on the strength of which at the beginning of January 1547 he officially succeeded Sangallo at St. Peter's.

Until 1881 the *motu proprio* conferring upon Michelangelo the office of *soprastante alla fabbrica* had not been discovered, but in that year the document, which is in the form of a *minuta* and is dated January 2nd 1547, was included by Alessandro Gherardi, Director of the Florentine State Archives, in his Catalogue of the MSS. in the Buonarroti Archives in Florence *(Frey, Jahrbuch, 1916, p. 32)*. Unfortunately Milanesi mistakenly supposed the text of the brief of Paul III, published without a date by Bonanni in 1696 *(first ed. p. 77)* to be the *motu proprio* of 1547 *(Pros. Chron. p. 391)*, whereas it is, in fact, the brief of October 11th 1549, by which Paul III granted Michelangelo absolute authority over the building operations at the Basilica. The text of the first *motu proprio* has never been published; that of the second was first published in full by Steinmann and Pogatcher in 1906.

Shortly after having assumed office, which he did with so much reluctance, Michelangelo went to St. Peter's to inspect Sangallo's wooden model of the Basilica. There he was met by 'all the Sangallo faction, who, putting the best face on the matter, came forward and said how glad they were that the work had been given to him and that the model was a meadow that would always afford inexhaustible pasture', to which Michelangelo replied that they spoke truly, meaning, 'as he afterwards told a friend, that it would serve for sheep and oxen who know nothing of art' *(Vasari, VII, p. 218)*. As we have already seen *(Appendix 36)*, having inspected the model, Michelangelo wrote to the Prefect of the Deputies, Bartolomeo Ferratini *(No. 274)* criticizing the project and giving his reasons for wishing to revert, in principle, to Bramante's original design *(Plan 3)*. He proposed, in the first place, to do away with Sangallo's ambulatories, which would involve demolishing the half-erected hemicycle to the south, a proposal which he recognized from the outset would be highly prejudicial to his personal interests, but which he nevertheless felt bound to advocate on artistic grounds.

As may well be imagined, this move alone would have been sufficient to set 'the Sangallo faction' against him, even had it not been hostile from the beginning, since he made no secret of the fact that in his opinion 'Sangallo had made the building without sufficient light, that he had used too many ranges of columns on the exterior, one above the other, and that with his numerous projections and angles, his style had much more of the German than of the good antique or modern manner' *(Vasari, VII, p. 218)*. These views, publicly expressed, together with his announcement prior to his appointment that if he were put in charge he would employ none of those who had intrigued against him, naturally served to provoke his enemies still further, so that 'when they saw him change all the dispositions both inside and out . . . . they never gave him any peace and were always seeking fresh means of annoying him' *(ibid., VII, p. 219)*.

From the relevant account books for the building of St. Peter's *(Pollak, Jahrbuch, 1915, p. 21 et seq.)* we learn that from December 1546 until August 1548 payments were being made in respect of the new wooden model which Michelangelo caused to be built in his own house in the Macel de' Corvi, while the work on the fabric itself was going ahead without interruption. Orders for columns and for the carving of capitals were put in hand, construction of the walls of the northern arm, which was to terminate in the *Cappella del Imperatore,* just as the southern arm was to terminate in the *Cappella del Re di Francia,* was continued and, most importantly of all, preparations were made for the building of the cornice at the base of the drum *(Ackerman, Cat., p. 92)*, while from July 1548 onwards large quantities of travertine were being delivered.

It was not until October 11th 1549, however, that Michelangelo was granted absolute powers at the Basilica. What it was that lead to the issuing of the second brief we do not know. Possibly it was only at this time and, almost certainly, in the face of considerable opposition that Michelangelo's model of a smaller but grander building, was finally approved; possibly it was only on condition that he was given absolute authority and some measure of Papal protection against the persecution he was continually encountering, that Michelangelo consented to proceed with the work. But be this as it may, it is at least certain that never in the history of art can such powers as these have been granted to any architect:

The Motu Proprio of Paul III

Motu proprio etc., Forasmuch as our beloved son, Michael Angelo Buonarroti, a Florentine citizen, a member of our household, and our regular dining-companion, has remade and designed in a better shape, a model or plan of the fabric of the Basilica of the Prince of the Apostles in Rome, which had been produced by other skilled architects, and has done the same to the building itself or its plan without accepting the reward or fee which we have repeatedly offered to him, but has done so because of the unfeigned affection and single-minded devotion which he has for that church;

We ratify and confirm the matters aforementioned, desirous that they be respected and put into effect in perpetuity, since they contribute to the grace and beauty of that church, and because they will have been executed at our request and on our clear orders, as by these present we fully and unambiguously testify and affirm;

Of our sure knowledge and in the fulness of our Apostolic power, we hereby approve and confirm the aforementioned new design and alteration, and all and several demolitions and constructions of whatever kind are caused to be done in the said fabric by the same Michael Angelo or on his orders, and whatever else he may do there, even if these things shall have been caused to be done at considerable expense and with damage to and destruction of the fabric; and these conditions, together with the model or plan for or in respect of the said fabric, drawn up and submitted by the same Michael Angelo, are to be observed and carried out in perpetuity, so that they may not be changed, re-fashioned, or altered; and the same Michael Angelo, or the master craftsmen he commissions for that work, or their assistants, or their heirs and assigns, cannot be held responsible to give any estimate or account of the damages and expenses brought about and caused by reason of the matters aforesaid, either concerning the matters themselves, or concerning other matters managed by them, nor can they be required in any way to prove or verify those matters, or any one of them, nor can they be compelled or coerced thereto; and thus we declare and decree in all and several of the matters set out above and below, by whomsoever etc., borne etc., also incited etc.;

And, moreover, trusting in the good faith, experience and earnest care of Michael Angelo himself, but above all trusting in God, we appoint and commission him the prefect, overseer *[operarius]* and architect of the building and fabric of the aforementioned Basilica on behalf of ourselves and of the Apostolic See for as long as he shall live. And we grant him full, free and complete permission and authority to change, re-fashion, enlarge and contract the model and plan and the construction of the building as shall seem best to him; to choose and commission all and several helpers and prefects and other men needed to work in that said building, and to arrange their due and customary wages and fees; and to release, dismiss and withdraw at will those same men, and others chosen previously, and his deputies; and to provide others as it shall seem best to him to do; and to do and perform all and several other things which shall be necessary, or in any way appropriate for the aforesaid work, without seeking permission from the Deputies of that fabric who shall be in office at that time, or from anyone else whatsoever. Moreover, in order that Michael Angelo himself shall be able more freely to direct the work of the said building, we entirely and completely release and free him and his assistants and deputies from the power, jurisdiction and authority of the Deputies of the same fabric. This notwithstanding earlier constitutions of any kind in favour of the Deputies of the aforesaid Basilica, or of its Chapter, or of anyone else whomsoever; and notwithstanding Apostolic ordinances and statutes, even if they have been confirmed etc., by oath, or privileges, indulgences and letters Apostolic, whatever their contents are etc., even if they are inspired in a like way etc., have been granted etc., are to be granted etc., to whom even if of those etc., We completely revoke them and all other enactments to the contrary of any kind whatsoever, with appropriate clauses. (Let the petition be granted.)

And absolution from censures to take effect even when breaches of the rule occur, with modification of it. And that the fashion and shape of single models of the same fabric and of changes made to it, and the expenses incurred in this work, and the damages consequent upon it, may be taken as expressed and may be inserted and expressed most fully and word for word.

And that the attestation, confirmation, license, permission, faculty, decree, abrogation and other matters set out above (which have been partly recorded one by one) may be most fully developed. And that the signature of these present alone may suffice for universal recognition, any regulation to the contrary notwithstanding, or, if it appears that letters have been issued from above through our brief, even with the delegation of executors, who shall assist, etc., with power to cite etc., even through a public edict summarily concerning not having the agreed access, and of restraining etc., even under ecclesiastical pains and penalties and monetary fines; the complete suspension of such a constitution being extended for one or two days but not more than three, these matters may be provided for under our brief with a greater and more accurate description of names, surnames, and other conditions, which need to be set down about the foregoing together and severally.

(And let this be well-pleasing to us.)

Given at Rome in the church of St. Mark on the fifth day of the Ides of October and in the fifteenth year of our reign.

V. Boncompagnus

(Steinmann and Pogatcher, Repertorium, 1906, p. 400)

Part III

Less than a month after having given such singular proof of his confidence in Michelangelo as prefect, *operarius* and architect of St. Peter's, Paul III was dead. With the election of his successor, Julius III, Michelangelo was at first in some doubt as to whether the new pontiff would wish to retain his service owing to his age *(No. 344)*, but he was soon reassured, as Julius had for him a respect at least equal to that which Paul III had entertained for him. But Michelangelo's detractors, the Sangallo faction and those whom he had dismissed from the fabric, seeing in the advent of a new pontificate a fresh opportunity for conspiring against him, 'constantly attacked him with malicious tongue' in a ceaseless effort to induce the Pope to revoke the powers that had been conferred upon him.

At last, towards the end of 1550, matters had reached such a pitch that the Pope found it necessary to institute an enquiry into the position. A meeting was summoned in the new year, at which Julius himself presided and at which Michelangelo was granted permission to answer the disaffected Deputies who had, no doubt without much difficulty, been persuaded of the justness of the grievances of the opposing party. The grounds of their objections are effectively summarized in an extract from the *Acta sub Julio*, published by Bonanni *(p. 63)*, according to which it is said that 'they asserted that the noble Basilica, planned by Bramante and most beautifully embellished by Antonio . . . had been completely destroyed by Michael, and that the distinguished names of these men had perished together with the stones that had been removed, and that vast sums of gold had been expended to no purpose and that the labours of so many learned pontiffs had been rendered void and that the honour of the Prince of the Apostles had been diminished by the erection of a smaller Basilica, and finally, that everything had been thrown into confusion by the decisions of a single man, contrary to the feeling of the whole City'. All these things and worse than these his envious rivals preferred against him, alleging first and foremost that 'he was constructing a Temple in the image of the sun's rays'. This particular charge, the possible implications of which have already been discussed *(Appendix 42)*, is not mentioned by Vasari in his account of what took place on this momentous occasion. Instead, he deals with the second criticism raised by the Deputies, namely, that concerning the lighting of the Basilica from the side apses – the *Cappella del Re* on the south being, at that time, under construction – which they deemed to be insufficient. To this objection, which had been put forward by Cardinal Cervini, speaking on behalf of the Deputies, Michelangelo replied saying, 'Monsignor, above these windows, in the travertine vaults which are to be built, there will be three others.' 'You have never informed us of this,' objected the Cardinal, to whom Michelangelo retorted in the now famous words, 'I am not obliged and I certainly do not intend to tell either Your Eminence or anyone else what I should be about or what I propose to do. Your office is to provide the money and to see that it is not stolen and to leave the design of the building to me.' Then, turning to the Pope, he said, 'Holy Father, You see my reward; if the pains I endure profit not my soul, I am losing both time and labour.' At this the Pope, who loved him, placed his hands on his shoulders, saying, 'Doubt not that you are gaining good reward both for soul and body.' And, in the words of the *Acta*, 'he renewed the diploma of Paul III'.

But even this was insufficient to secure Michelangelo against the calumnies of envious tongues and before the year was out the trouble began again. This time the spleen of the Deputies (which is understandable) was expressed in a letter to the Pope couched in these words:

From the year 1540 when the rebuilding of St. Peter's was resumed with new vigour to the year 1547, when Michelangelo began to do and undo, to destroy and rebuild at his own will, we have spent 162,624 ducats. From 1547 to the present day, during which time we deputies of the Fabbrica have counted for absolutely nothing and have been kept by Michelangelo in absolute ignorance of his plans and doings – because such was the will of the late Pope Paul III and of the reigning Pope, the expense has reached the total of 136,881 ducats. As regards the progress and the designs and the prospects of the basilica, the deputies know nothing whatever, Michelangelo despising them worse than if they were outsiders. They must, however, make the following declaration to ease their conscience; they highly disapprove Michelangelo's methods, especially in demolishing and destroying the work of his predecessors. This mania for pulling to pieces what has already been erected at such enormous cost is criticized by everybody; however, if the Pope is pleased with it, we have nothing to say.

(Fea, p. 32: translated by Lanciani, p. 166)

By some unaccountable aberration, Ackerman places this letter in 1547 *(Cat., p. 90)*, to which year it could not possibly belong, as it was written during the pontificate of Julius III, besides which the moneys referred to in it date the letter to about the end of 1551. According to Fea *(p. 35)* between January 1st 1547 and May 8th 1551, 121,454 *scudi* were expended on the fabric. This gives an average expenditure of some 28,000 *scudi* annually, or 2,300 a month. The difference between 121,554 and the sum of 136,381 mentioned in the letter is nearly 15,000 *scudi*, which would bring the payments approximately to the end of the year, when the accounts were probably made up.

If the letter be correctly dated to the end of 1551 or the beginning of 1552, its repercussions, as far as the Deputies were concerned, could not be described as other than extremely unfortunate, as the only effect it had upon the Pope was to cause him 'to confirm Michelangelo in the Prefecture of the fabric by a new papal diploma, so that the uncommon integrity of his character should be made clear not in the City alone, but throughout the whole world' *(Bonanni, p. 63)*.

The new *motu proprio* was not substantially different from the previous one, except that the Pope, having reaffirmed his confidence in the master, proceeded, in addition, to appoint certain persons, two of them being Deputies, who were favourably disposed towards him, who were empowered to protect him and to safeguard his interests. The relevant paragraph reads as follows:

On that account, by these present, and with like knowledge and impulse, we entrust and delegate our revered brothers the Patriarch of Jerusalem *[Cristoforo Spiriti]* and the Bishop of Lipari *[Baldo Ferratini]*, and to our beloved son the Auditor of Curial Pleas of the Apostolic Camera *[unidentified]*, that they, or two, or one of them, through themselves or another or others, helping you in the aforesaid effective ways with the support of their protection, shall make these present letters and whatever is contained in them produce their full effect, and shall make you to be at peace to enjoy and reap the benefit of these letters and all and singular things which are contained in them, not allowing you to be disturbed, or hindered, or disquieted in any way contrary to the intention of these present.

The above-mentioned *motu proprio* is dated January 23rd 1552. On February 24th of the same year a *colazione* was provided for the workmen to celebrate the completion of the cornice at the base of the drum. This repast was similar to that which had been provided two years previously, on December 23rd 1550, for those who had been employed on the stone-work for the said cornice. The entry in the account book in respect of the first repast includes a variety of items:

From the 22nd day of December until the 23rd, the under-mentioned expenses were incurred by order of Messer Michel Angelo as a reward to those who had been employed on the stone-work for the first great cornice.

For 100 pounds of sausages bought from the butcher Nanno at 2½ *bol[ognini]* per pound	*[scudi]*	2 : 50
For 90 pounds of flank of pork bought from the aforesaid		1 : 45
For four pigs' livers from the aforesaid, 30 *bol*.		30
For bread bought from Cristofano, baker to *[Monsignor]* Cesis, amounting to		2 : 20
For two barrels of wine *di Campagna* bought from Messer Domenico della Porta, amounting to		2 : 10
For bringing the meat from the Paradiso *[the inn in the garden near S. Andrea della Valle, where Nanno the butcher was employed]* to St. Peter's		: 5½

311

For two and a half dozen caps bought from Messer Ambrosio Marliano to give
to all those who had served as above, at 33 julians a dozen, amounting to   8 : 25
For the cooking of the above-mentioned things, cooked by Trenchetto, the
inn-keeper, amounting to   : 60
On the aforesaid day, to Maestro Pierantonio da Cerone for the cost of the first
repast given to all the labourers and bricklayers for the cornice, including the
caps   *[scudi]*   17 : 45½

(Frey, Jahrbuch, 1916, p. 69 et seq.).

The entry for the second celebration is less detailed, but lists an item for the hire of plates and drinking vessels, including breakages.

Unhappily for Michelangelo, the completion of the lower cornice marked the end of the first phase of his building activity. Thereafter, having been temporarily brought to a standstill, the work of actual construction could only be continued at a much slower pace, owing partly to the depletion of the papal coffers and partly to the interruption of political events *(Appendix 43)*. But although Julius III did what he could to encourage donations to the fabric by the granting of privileges and indulgences to those who subscribed, the amount expended during the next four years amounted to only 62,911 *scudi (Fea, p. 35)*, which may have included, though this is by no means certain, the 50,000 *scudi* received in 1554 from the Sigismondo de' Conti inheritance *(Pastor, XIII, p. 336)*.

Part IV

Despite the unsettled state of affairs during the beginning of the pontificate of Paul IV, some progress was made on the building between 1555 and 1557, mainly on the drum and on the *Cappella del Re*, the entablature of which had been completed and the travertine vault partially constructed by April 1557, when the mistake made by the overseer, Bastiano Malenotti in the centering for the vault was discovered. This mistake, which led to Malenotti's dismissal and required the dismantling and rebuilding of the vault, which was not completed until May 1558 *(Frey, Jahrbuch, 1916, p. 75)*, caused Michelangelo immense chagrin, as may be seen from his letters to Vasari, to Lionardo and to the Duke *(Nos. 437, 439, 440, 433)*. In the meantime, the detailed model of the cupola had been initiated with a view to obtaining a record of Michelangelo's intentions as to its construction, and perhaps also as a means of preventing comparable mistakes in the future.

It is significant that in a letter of February 1557 to Lionardo *(No. 430)*, Michelangelo referred to a rumour that building operations at the Basilica were to be closed down altogether, but said that this rumour was unfounded, as there were still sixty workmen, including *scarpellini*, bricklayers and labourers, working on the site. This in itself is indicative of the slowness of the pace at which he was having to proceed, a state of affairs that had not improved five months later, when he again complained of the lack of men and of money by which his activities were being hampered *(No. 436)*.

Although between April 1555 and June 1561 there was a slight increase in the funds available, the sum expended during this period being 105,115 *scudi (Fea, p. 35)*, it was wholly inadequate for Michelangelo's requirements, so that when he died in February 1564 much less had been accomplished than was warranted by the creative, as opposed to the physical, effort of which he had been capable. What he accomplished was, nevertheless, of fundamental importance for the future, by reason not only of what he built, but of what he destroyed.

At Michelangelo's death Sangallo's outer hemicycles had been eliminated from the plan and the only one that had actually been begun (namely that on the south side) had been pulled down. For the rest, the completed hemicycle terminating the eastern arm of the Greek cross, which Sangallo had intended to lengthen by the addition of a nave extending beyond the hemicycle to the entrance, remained, like the west end, as it was, Michelangelo having been mainly engaged on the construction of the drum and of the great apses of the transepts, the *Cappella del Re* to the south and the *Cappella del Imperatore* to the north. By 1564 the former was virtually complete and the latter almost so, save for part of the vaulting. Besides strengthening Bramante's four great piers still further (the speed with which they were built having been, like much of Bramante's work, in inverse proportion to their stability) Michelangelo also began work on the corner chapels and on the *Cappella Gregoriana* on the north side. But most important of all, having completed the first great cornice, which Vasari described as being of marvellous grace and originality and impossible to better, he raised the whole of the drum to the level of the pilaster and buttress capitals and, on the eastern side, above this point, to the level of the imposts and entablature *(Ackerman, Cat., p. 95)*. In addition, by 1561, he had completed the scale model of the cupola, which was of such a size that, as Vasari relates, the columns, bases, capitals, doors and windows, cornices and projections, were perfect in every detail.

But the frustration consequent upon the shortage of money and men, with which Michelangelo was continually beset, was by no means all that he had to endure. Throughout the time during which he was in charge at the Basilica, he was constantly pursued by the jealousies and animosities of his rivals, who contrived to hurt and torment him at every opportunity. As we have already seen, Julius III did his best to protect him, but immediately on his death, the Sangallo faction, which was favoured by Marcellus II, began to molest him, as everyone supposed, no doubt, with impunity, so much so that Michelangelo considered the possibility of retiring to Florence. Haply, however, the Pope died, and Michelangelo remained in Rome to continue his labours, only to be subjected to the insults of Pirro Ligorio, the Neapolitan architect whom Paul IV had promoted on his accession. He desired to supplant Michelangelo and put it about that he was in his dotage and incapable of continuing, but the Pope was very far from being convinced of this, and confirmed his powers over the Basilica. Then in 1562, notwithstanding the fact that Pius IV, like his predecessor Paul IV, had given ample proof of his confidence in anything that Michelangelo proposed, Nanni di Baccio Bigio, who had made trouble from the outset *(Appendix 36)*, had the temerity to ask the Duke of Florence to use his influence to get him promoted to Michelangelo's post at St. Peter's. To this egregious piece of insolence he received the following reply:

To Maestro Nanni, architect. 19th April, 1562.
We are disposed, by reason of your abilities, to do you every service and favour, but in the matter which you desire we shall never do you such an office while Michelangelo is alive, because it would too much disparage his merits and the love we bear him; but we promise you that at an opportune moment we will not fail you.

(Gaye, III, p. 66)

But not to the end of his days was Michelangelo to enjoy the peace he had so long desired *(No. 76)*. In August of the following year Cesare Bettini da Castel Durante, *soprastante* at St. Peter's, was murdered by the Bishop of Forli's cook, who discovered him with his wife *(Daelli, p. 25)*. In his place Michelangelo wished to appoint his young assistant, Pierluigi Gaeta *(No. 470)* to act for him, at least temporarily; but Gaeta did not prove acceptable to the Deputies, who desired to appoint Nanni di Baccio Bigio to take over the supervision of the work at the fabric.

Various rumours were put about and certain allegations were made, to the effect that more harm than good was being done by Michelangelo's workmen at the Basilica, and in self-defence Michelangelo sent his protégé, Daniele Ricciarelli da Volterra, to the former Bishop of Lipari, Baldo Ferratini, one of the two Deputies whom Julius III had previously appointed to see that the privileges granted to Michelangelo were respected. But whether through disinclination or through inability, Ferratini effected nothing, and Nanni was eventually appointed. Thereupon, according to Vasari, Michelangelo at once went in search of the Pope, who was at the Campidoglio and loudly demanded admission; but this is not entirely accurate, as at the time, according to Tiberio Calcagni's letter to Lionardo Buonarroti, dated September 2nd, the Pope being at Tivoli, Michelangelo took counsel with the Pope's nephew, Gabrio Serbelloni, who promised him satisfaction on the Pope's return *(Daelli, 26, and Gotti, I, pp. 321 et seq.)*. At the audience that was granted him shortly afterwards Michelangelo offered his resignation, saying, 'Holy Father, the Deputies have appointed in my place someone whom I do not know, but if they and Your Holiness think me no longer capable, I will return to take my ease in Florence and to enjoy the favour of the Duke, as he has so much desired, and will there end my days in my own house. I therefore ask for my discharge.' But Pius, knowing that the complaints of the Deputies were unfounded, had no wish to dispense with his services and promised to investigate the matter. Having heard the Deputies, he accordingly sent Serbelloni to inspect the fabric, and on being informed that Nanni's accusations proceeded merely from malignity, he caused him to be ignominiously dismissed and, while confirming Michelangelo in his office, the Pope threatened condign punishment to all who disobeyed the master's orders. At the same time he appointed an independent architect, Francesco da Cortona, to deputize for Michelangelo who was no longer able to supervise the work himself.

Nanni's insolence, however, knew no bounds and on the very night of Michelangelo's death, under cover of Averardo Serristori's letter to the Duke announcing this event, he wrote reminding him of his promise and asking for his intervention with the Pope to obtain for him the office now left vacant, 'it having pleased God to terminate Michelangelo's days, to the greatest loss and sorrow of the whole world' *(Gaye, III, p. 129)*.

But the Duke had no intention of committing himself to so arrant a hypocrite without first obtaining certain assurances from Nanni himself. All we know of his reactions to the request made of him is revealed at the conclusion of his letter to his envoy, Serristori, dated March 5th 1564, where he writes, 'We will write to Our Lord *[the Pope]* regarding Maestro Nanni, the architect, only when he has promised to follow Michelangelo's model without any alteration whatsoever' *(Cosimo, I, p. 197)*.

Part V

In the *motu proprio* of Paul III it had been laid down that the plan *(Plan 3)* and model of the Basilica that had been remade and designed in a better shape by Michelangelo were to be 'respected and put into effect in perpetuity, since they contribute to the grace and beauty of that church'. These stipulations Pius IV, like Julius III and Paul IV, confirmed and it was on these conditions that Michelangelo's successors were appointed, but not until August 1564, when Pirro Ligorio (1510–1583) became chief architect, only to be dismissed the following year for daring to suggest alterations to Michelangelo's plan. He was succeeded in turn by his coadjutor, Vignola (1507–1573), and, in 1573/4 by Giacomo della Porta (c. 1537–1602). Up to that time relatively little more had been accomplished beyond the completion of work already initiated. Between 1580 and 1585 the western, or choir apse was replaced, but it was not until 1588 that any significant progress was made, when, under Sixtus V and with immense energy, the building of the cupola, to a revised design by Giacomo della Porta, was undertaken. It had been estimated that it would cost a million ducats to build and would take ten years to complete; whereas it was in fact erected at a cost of two hundred thousand ducats in only twenty-two months *(Turcio, p. 30)*, by eight hundred men working day and night. The mass to celebrate its completion was sung in May 1590 and the lantern, orb and cross were added three years later.

Only in 1607, however, during the pontificate of Paul V, when the last remains of the old Basilica with its atrium were finally demolished, was the decision reached to spoil Michelangelo's design, if not entirely, at least as far as was possible, by the addition of a long nave and an enormous narthex and façade. The former, by changing the plan once more from a Greek into a Latin cross, had the effect of spoiling the essential coherence of the whole design; the latter, by changing the exterior perspective, of losing the tremendous impact of the cupola when the building is viewed from the piazza. It is thus only when it is seen from the Vatican gardens that any conception of what Michelangelo had intended can now be gained. This commission, assigned to Carlo Maderno, was executed in seven years, but it was not until 1626 that the completely rebuilt Basilica was finally dedicated by Urban VIII.

It would perhaps have been too much to hope that, of all the plans prepared for St. Peter's, that of the greatest master, among the many who had worked at the Basilica, should have been realized. But if, despite his efforts, Michelangelo was not destined to leave the fabric at such a stage that it could not afterwards be altered or spoilt, it is to him that it owes the preservation of the essential elements of Bramante's design, to the exclusion of those features projected by Sangallo; it is to him that it owes the organic unity of the great crossing; it is to him that it owes the exterior grandeur of the west end; it is to him that it owes the austere simplicity of the drum and, subsequent modifications notwithstanding, it is, in all essential respects, to him, that it owes the greatest cupola in the world.

Bibliography

In the text, works are cited by the name of the author or editor, with an abbreviated title where necessary. In the bibliography Michelangelo's name is abbreviated to M. or M.B., irrespective of the spelling in the original title.

ACKERMAN, James S.
  The Architecture of M., 2 vols., London, 1961

ADRIANI, Giovanbattista
  Istoria de' suoi tempi, 6 vols., Prato, 1822

ADY, Cecilia M.
  The Bentivoglio of Bologna, London, 1937

ALBERTINI, Francesco degli
  Memoriale di molti statue et pitture della città di Firenze, 1510, ed. G. Milanesi, Florence, 1863
  Opusculum de mirabilibus . . . . urbis Romae, Rome, 1510

AMMIRATO, Scipione
  Istorie Fiorentine, 6 vols., Florence, 1846–1849

ANZILOTTI, A.
  La Constituzione interna della Stato Fiorentino sotto il Duca Cosimo I de' Medici, Florence, 1910

ARMENINI, Giovanbattista
  De' veri Precetti della Pittura, Ravenna, 1587

BARRACLOUGH, Geoffrey
  Public Notaries and The Papal Curia, Brit. S., Rome, 1934

BECCADELLI, Lodovico
  Tre Lettere inedite di L.B. a M.B. ed alcuni notizie, ed. A. Vital, Conegliano, 1901

BENRATH, Karl
  Bernardino Ochino of Siena, trans. H. Zimmern, London, 1876

BONANNI (BUONANNI), Filippo
  Numismata Summorum Pontificum Templi Vaticani ect., Rome, 1715 (first ed. 1696)

BOOTH, Cecily
  Cosimo I, Duke of Florence, Cambridge, 1921

BOTTARI, G.
  Raccolta di Lettere sulla Pittura, Scultura ed Architectura, 8 vols., cont. S. Ticozzi, Rome, 1822–1825

BRÉQUIGNY, M. de
  Notices et extraits des MSS. de la Bibliothéque du Roi (J. Burchard, Paris de Grassis, etc.) in La Bibliothèque Nationale, II, Paris, 1789

BUFALINI, Lionardo
  Le Piante maggiore di Roma, Vatican Library, Rome, 1911

BUSSI, Feliciano
  Istoria della Città di Viterbo, Rome, 1742

BORGHINI, Raffaello,
  Il Riposo, Florence, 1584

CAMBI, Giovanni
  Storia di Giovanni Cambi, 4 vols., Florence, 1785

CAMPORI, G.
  Memorie Biografiche degli Sculptori, Architecturi, Pittori di Carrara, Modena, 1873

CANTINI, Lorenzo
  Legislatione Toscana, 32 vols., Florence, 1800
  Saggi istorichi d'Antichita Toscana, 10 vols., Florence, 1796–1800

CAPPONI, Gino
  Storia della Repubblica di Firenze, 2 vols., Florence, 1875

CARDELLA, L.
  Memorie storiche de' Cardinali della S. Romana Chiesa, 9 vols., Rome, 1793

CARDEN, Robert W.
  M. – A Record of his life as told in his own letters and papers, London, 1913

CARO, Annibale
  Delle Lettere famigliare del Annibal Caro, 3 vols., Padua, 1748

CARTWRIGHT, Julia
  Baldassare Castiglione, 2 vols., London, 1907

CASIMIRO, P. F.
  Memorie storiche del' Chiesa e Convento di S. Maria in Araceli, Rome, 1736

CASTIGLIONE, Baldassare
  Lettere, ed. P. Serassi, 2 vols., Padua, 1769

CELLINI, Benvenuto
  Vita di B.C., ed. F. Tassi, 3 vols., Florence, 1829
  Vita di B.C., ed. G. Ferrero, Turin, 1959

CHACON, Alonso
  Vitae et Res Gestae Pontificum Romanorum, 4 vols., Rome, 1667

CHINALI, G.
  Caprese e M.B., Arezzo, 1904

CIANFOGNI, P. M. N.
  Memorie istoriche dell' Ambrosiana R. Basilica di S. Lorenzo di Firenze, cont. D. Moreni, Florence, 1804–1816

CIOMPI, Sebastiano
  Lettera di M.B., Florence, 1834

CLAUSSE, G.
  Les Sangallo, 3 vols., Paris, 1900–1902

COLONNA, Vittoria
  Carteggio di V.C., ed. E. Ferrero and G. Muller, Turin, 1889
  Lettere inedite, ed. C. Piccioni, Rome, 1875
  Le Rime di V.C., con la vita, ec., ed. P. E. Visconti, Rome, 1840

CONDIVI, Ascanio
  La Vita di M.B., Rome, 1553
  La Vita di M.B., ed. A. F. Gori, Florence, 1746

CORBINELLI, J.
  Histoire de la Maison de Gondi, 2 vols., Paris, 1705

Bibliography

Cosimo I de' Medici
Lettere, ed. Spini, Florence, 1940

Daelli, G.
Carte Michelangiolesche inedite, Milan, 1865

Dorez, Léon
La Cour de Paul III, 2 vols., Paris, 1952
Nouvelles Recherches sur M. et son entourage, in Bibliothèque de l'Ecole de Chartes, LXXVII–LXXVIII, Paris, 1916–1917

Dovizi da Bibbiena, Bernardo
La Calandria, Siena, 1521

Duppa, R.
Life of M.B., 3rd ed., London, 1816

Edler, Florence
Glossary of Medieval Terms of Business; Italian Series 1200–1600, Cambridge, Mass., 1934

Ellis, Havelock
L'Inversion Sexuelle, trans. A. van Gennep, Paris, 1934

Eubel, Conrad, and others
Hierarchia Cattolica Medii Aevi, 6 vols., Monastir, 1901

Fea, Carlo
Notizie intorno Raffaello . . . Bramante, Giuliano da Sangallo . . . M.B. . . . come architetti di Pietro, Rome, 1822

Fracastoro, Girolamo
Fracastor – Syphilis or the French Disease, ed. with trans. H. Wynne-Finch, London, 1935

Frediani, Carlo
Ragionamento storico su le diverse gite che fece a Carrara M.B., Massa, 1837

Frey, Carl (or Karl)
Die Briefe des M.B., Berlin, 1914
Denunzia dei Beni della famiglia Buonarroti, in Jahrbuch der Preussischen Kunstsammlungen, VI, Berlin, 1885
Die Dichtungen des M.B., Berlin 1897 *(Dicht)*
M.B. Quellen und Forschungen, Berlin, 1907 *(Quellen)*
Sammlung ausgewählter Briefe an. M.B., Berlin, 1899 *(Briefe)*
Articles in Jahrbuch der Preussischen Kunstsammlungen, Berlin, XVI, 1895, XVII, 1896, XXX, 1909 *(Studien),* XXXI, 1910, XXXVII, 1916 *(Jahrbuch)*

Frey, Carl and W. H. (eds.)
Der Literarische Nachlass Giorgio Vasaris, 2 vols., Munich, 1923–30 *(Lit)*

Gams, P. P. B.
Episcoporum Ecclesiae Catholicae, Ratisbon, 1873

Garnault, Paul
Les Portraits de M., Paris, 1913

Gasparoni, Benvenuto
La Casa di M. nel Macel de' Corvi, in Il Buonarroti, Rome, 1866

Gaye, G.
Carteggio inedito d'artisti dei secoli XIV, XV, XVI, 3 vols., Florence, 1839–40

Giannotti, Donato
Dialogi (Dialoghi) di D.G., ed. D. Redig de Campos, Florence, 1939
Lettere a Piero Vettori, ed. R. Ridolfi and C. Roth, Florence, 1932
Nove Lettere inedite, ed. J. del Budia, Florence, 1870
Opere Politiche e Litterarie di D.G., ed. F. L. Polidori, 2 vols., 1850

Ginori Conti, P.
La Basilica di S. Lorenzo di Firenze e la famiglia Ginori, Florence, 1940

Giornale Storico
Giornale Storico degli Archivi Toscani, 7 vols., Florence, 1857–1863

Gotti, Aurelio
Vita di M.B., 2 vols., Florence, 1876

Gould, Cecil (ed.)
National Gallery Catalogue – Sixteenth-Century Italian Schools, London, 1962

Grimm, Herman
The Life of M.B., trans. Bunnett, 2 vols., London, 1865

Gronau, Georg
Dokumente z. Entstehung. d. neu. Sakristie, etc., in Jahrbuch des Preussischen Kunstsammlungen, XXXII, Berlin, 1911

Guasti, Cesare
Due Motu propri di Paolo III, in Archivio Storico Italiano, Ser. IV, Tome xviii, Florence, 1886
Le Rime di M.B., Florence, 1863

Haile, Martin
Life of Reginald Pole, London, 1911

Hale, J. R.
England and the Italian Renaissance, London, 1954

Harford, J. S.
The Life of M.B., 2 vols., London, 1857

Holroyd, Charles
M.B., with translations of the life of the master by . . . Condivi and three Dialogues from the Portuguese . . . , London, 1911

Inghirami, F.
Storia della Toscana, 16 vols., Fiesole, 1841–1843

Jerrold, M. F.
Vittoria Colonna, London, 1906

Justi, G.
M. Neue Beiträge z. Erklärung seiner Werke, Berlin, 1900

Lanciani, R.
The Golden Days of the Renaissance in Rome, London, 1906

Landucci, Luca
Diario Fiorentino 1450–1516, continuato da un anonimo fino al 1542, ed. I. del Badia, Florence, 1883

Langéard, Pierre
L'Intersexualité dans l'Art, Montpelier, 1936

Lapini, Agostino
Diario Fiorentino, ed. G. O. Corazzini, Florence, 1900

LAWLEY, Alethea
Vittoria Colonna, London, 1889

LETAROUILLY, Paul
The Basilica of St. Peter, London, 1953

LIMBURGER, W.
Die Gebände von Florenz, Leipzig, 1910

LITTA, Pompeo
Famiglie Celebri Italiane, 10 vols., Milan and Turin, 1847–1899

MANNI, Giuseppe
Serie de' Senatori Fiorentini, Florence, 1722

MANSFIELD, M.
A Family of Decent Folk, 1200–1741. A Study in the Centuries' Growth of the Lanfredini, Florence, 1922

MARTELLI, Niccolò
Il Primo Libro delle Lettere di N.M., Florence, 1547

MARTINI, Luca
[Select letters] in *Lettere serie, erudite e famigliare di diversi Uomini Scienziate*, Venice, 1735

MARTINORI, E.
La Moneta, Rome, 1915

MARZI, Demetrio
La Cancellaria della Republica Fiorentina, Florence, 1910

MAYLENDER, Michele
Storia delle accademie d'Italia, 5 vols., Bologna, 1926–1930

MECATTI, G. M.
Storia Genealogica della nobilità e cittadinanza di Firenze, Naples, 1754

MIGNANTI, Filippo Maria
Istoria della Basilica Vaticana, 2 vols., Rome, 1867

MILANESI, Gaetano
Les Correspondants de M. – I. Sebastiano del Piombo with French trans. A. le Pileur, Paris, 1890 *(Corr)*
Le Lettere di M.B. edite e inedite, coi ricordi e contratti artistici, Florence, 1875

MONCALLERO, G. L.
Il Cardinale Bernardo Dovizi da Bibbiena, Rome, 1953
Epistolario di Bernardo Dovizi da Bibbiena, Florence, 1955

NARDI, Jacopo
Istoria della Città di Firenze, 2 vols., Florence, 1858

O'BRIEN, Grace
The Golden Age of Italian Music, London [1948]

O'DEA, W. T.
The Social History of Lighting, London, 1958

ORIGO, Iris
The Merchant of Prato, London, 1959

PAPINI, Giovanni
Vita di M. nella vita del suo tempo, Milan, 1951

PASSERINI, Luigi
Bibliografia di M.B. e gli Incisori delle sue Opere, Florence, 1875
Genealogia e Storia della Famiglia Altoviti, Florence, 1871
Genealogia ec. Ricasoli, Florence, 1861
Genealogia ec. Ruccellai, Florence, 1861
Storia degli Stabilimente di Beneficenza della Città di Firenze, Florence, 1853

PASTOR, Ludwig
History of the Popes, 40 vols., London, 1891–1953

PECCHIAI, Pio
Roma nel Cinquecento, Bologna, 1948

PETRARCA, Francesco
Rime, Trionfi e Poesie Latine, ed. F. Neri, Milan and Naples, 1951

PINO, Bernardino
Nuova Scelta di Lettere di diversi nobilissimi ingegni, etc., Venice, 1574

PODESTÀ, B.
Documenti inedite relativi a M.B., in Il Buonarroti, X, Rome, 1875
Intorno alle due Statue erette in Bologna a Giulio II, in Atti e Memorie della R. Deputazione . . . di Romagna, 1868

POGGI, G.
M.B. nel IV Centenario del Giudizio Universale, Florence, 1942

POLE, Reginald
Epistolarum R.P. S.R.E. Cardinalis et aliorum ad ipsum Collectio, ed. Quirini, 5 vols., Brescia, 1744–1757

POLENI, Giovanni
Memorie istoriche della gran' Cupola, Padua, 1748

POLIDORI, Petrus
De Vita Gestis et Moribus Marcelli II, Pont. Max., Rome, 1744

POLLAK, Oscar
Ausgewählter Akten z. Geschichte der Romischen Peterskirche, in Jahrbuch der Preussischen Kunstsammlungen, XXXVI, Berlin, 1915

PONNELLE, L. and BORDET, L.
St. Philip Neri and the Roman Society of his times, trans. R. F. Kerr, London, 1937

POPHAM, A. E. and WILDE, Johannes
The Italian Drawings of the XV and XVI Centuries in the Collection of H.M. the King at Windsor Castle, London, 1949

PUCCINELLI, Placido
Istoria dell' eroiche attioni di Ugo il grande Duca e le memorie di Pescia, Milan, 1664

RAYMOND, I. W. and LOPEZ, R. S.
Medieval Trade in the Mediterranean World, New York, 1955

RE, Niccolò del
La Curia Romana, Rome, 1952

REDIG DE CAMPOS, Diocletio
M.: Affreschi della Capella Paolina in Vaticano, Milan, 1949

REUMONT, Alfredo
Vittoria Colonna, Turin, 1892

RILLI, Jacopo
Notizie Letterarie ed Istoriche intorno agli Uomini Illustri dell' Accademia Fiorentina, Florence, 1700

Bibliography

ROLLAND, Romain
Vie de M., Paris, 1913

RONCHINI, Armando
M. e il porto del Po a Piacenza, in Atti e Memorie della
R. Deputazione di . . . Modenesi e Parmenesi, II, 1864

ROOVER, Raymond de
The Medici Bank, New York, 1948

ROSCOE, Mrs. Henry
Vittoria Colonna, London, 1868

ROSCOE, William
Life and Pontificate of Leo X, 6 vols., London, 1806

SALVINI, Salvo
*Catalogo Genealogico dei Canonici della Chiesa Metropolitana
in Firenze,* Florence, 1782 *(Cat)*
Fasti, Consolari del' Accademia Fiorentina, Florence, 1717

SANUTO, Marius
I Diarii 1496–1533, ed. Berchet, Barozzi, Stefani and Fulin,
58 vols., Venice, 1879–1903

SAPORI, A.
Il giusto prezzo, in Archivio Storico Italiano, Ser. VII, Vol.
xviii, Florence, 1932

SCHENK, W.
Reginald Pole, Cardinal of England, London, 1950

SCHIAVO, Armando
La Vita e le Opere architettoniche di M., Rome, 1953
(Vita)
M. Architetto, Rome, 1949

SCHLOSSER, Julius von
La Letteratura Artistica, trans. F. Rossi, 2nd. ed., Florence,
1956

SCHOLA SALTERNITANA
Regimen Sanitatis Salternitanum, with trans. Sir J. Harring-
ton, London, 1922

SEGNI, Bernardo
Storia Fiorentina, 3 vols., Milan, 1805

SERRISTORI, A.
*Legazione di A. Serristori – Ambasciatore di Cosimo I a Carlo
V e in Corte di Roma,* ed. L. Serristori, Florence, 1853

SHAW, W. A.
The History of Currency 1252–1894, London (1895)

STALEY, Edgcumbe
The Guilds of Florence, London, 1906

STEINMANN, E.
Die Sixtinische Kapelle, 2 vols., Munich, 1905   *(Sixt)*
M. e Luigi del Riccio, Florence, 1932
Portraitdarstellungen des M., Leipzig, 1913

STEINMANN, E. and POGATCHER, H.
Dokumente u. Forschungen z M., in Repertorium für Kunst-
wissenchaft, XXIX, 1906

STEINMANN, E. and WITTKOWER, R.
M. Bibliographie, 1510–1926, Leipzig, 1927

SYMONDS, John Addington
The Life of M.B., 2 vols., London, 1899

THODE, H.
M. und das Ende der Renaissance, 3 vols., Berlin, 1902–1912

TOLNAY, Charles de
Michelangelo, 5 vols., Princeton, 1938–1960
    I. *The Youth of M.*
    II. *The Sistine Ceiling*
    III. *The Medici Chapel*
    IV. *The Tomb of Julius II*
    V. *The Final Period*

TURCIO, Genesio
La Basilica di San Pietro, Florence, 1946

TUSIANI, Joseph
The Complete Poems of M., New York, 1960

TOLOMEI, Claudio
Delle Lettere di M. C.T., Naples, 1829

TIRIBILLI-GIULIANI, D.
Sommario storico delle famiglie celebri Toscane, 3 vols., Florence, 1855–1864

UGHELLI, Ferdinand
Italia Sacra, sive de episcopis Italie et insularum adjacentium,
10 vols., Venice, 1717–1722

VARCHI, Benedetto
*Due Lezioni di Mess. B.V., nella prima di quali si dichiara un
Sonetto di Mess. M.B.,* Florence, 1549/50
Sonetti, Florence, 1555
Storia Fiorentina, Florence, 1721

VASARI, Giorgio
Le Opere di G.V., ed. G. Milanesi, 9 vols., Florence, 1878–
1883
    I–VII. *Le vite de' piu eccellenti pittori, ec.*
    VIII. *Le Lettere di G.V. ec.*
    IX. *Index*
        *(The Life of M.B., with Prospetto Cronologico, is in-
        cluded in Vol. VII)*
Il Libro delle Ricordanze di G.V., ed. A. del Vita, Arezzo,
1927

VENTURI, Adolfo
Storia dell'Arte Italiana, 11 vols., Milan, 1901–39
    IX. *pts. i, ii 'La Pittura nel Cinquecento'*
    X. *pts. i, ii 'La Scultura'*

VITRUVIUS
De Architectura, ed. with trans. F. Granger, 2 vols., London,
1931

WILDE, Johannes
*Italian Drawings in the Department of Prints and Drawings in
the British Museum,* London, 1953

WILSON, C. Heath
Life and Works of M.B., London, 1876

WOLF, Rosina
Documenti inedite su M., Budapest, 1931

YOUNG, G. F.
The Medici, 2 vols., London, 1909

ZANONI, Enrico
Donato Giannotti, Rome, 1900

Concordance

The Roman numbers given to the Letters in *Le Lettere di Michelangelo Buonarroti, coi Ricordi e Contratti Artistici*, edited by Gaetano Milanesi and published in Florence in 1875, are given on the left of each column; the Arabic numerals on the right denote the numbers accorded to the same letters in the present edition.

The word 'Omitted', appearing in the right-hand column of figures, indicates that the letter published by Milanesi either duplicates another or is too fragmentary to be suitable for translation. The word 'Excluded' denotes that the letter in question has been rejected by the present Editor as not being by Michelangelo.

Letters No. 342 and 399 and Draft 11, included among the translations, were not published by Milanesi. The source in each case is given in the relevant footnotes.

i	2	xxii	50	xliii	153	lxiv	29
ii	3	xxiii	63	xliv	154	lxv	30
iii	6	xxiv	64	xlv	Draft 1	lxvi	31
iv	13	xxv	62	xlvi	Excluded	lxvii	32
v	46	xxvi	65	xlvii	4	lxviii	33
vi	47	xxvii	59	xlviii	9	lxix	34
vii	48	xxviii	67	xlix	10	lxx	35
viii	5	xxix	68	l	11	lxxi	36
ix	86	xxx	69	li	12	lxxii	37
x	45	xxxi	70	lii	14	lxxiii	38
xi	60	xxxii	87	liii	15	lxxiv	39
xii	74	xxxiii	75	liv	16	lxxv	40
xiii	72	xxxiv	76	lv	17	lxxvi	42
xiv	73	xxxv	78	lvi	18	lxxvii	7
xv	83	xxxvi	85	lvii	19	lxxviii	43
xvi	88	xxxvii	82	lviii	20	lxxix	44
xvii	89	xxxviii	71	lix	21	lxxx	51
xviii	90	xxxix	149	lx	25	lxxxi	52
xix	91	xl	112	lxi	26	lxxxii	55
xx	53	xli	117	lxii	27	lxxxiii	56
xxi	54	xlii	118	lxiii	28	lxxxiv	57

Concordance

Index of Correspondents

Index

The Index relates to the Introduction, the Letters and the Appendixes only. The folios shown in Roman numerals refer to the Introduction; the folios shown in Arabic numerals refer to the text and footnotes of the Letters, and, where preceded by an asterisk, to the Appendixes.

Erratum

p. 169, No. 426, n.1.   *For* Provost of San Lorenzo *read* Provost of San Giovanni